Nelson ESSENTIALS OF PEDIATRICS

EIGHTH EDITION

KAREN J. MARCDANTE, MD
Professor
Department of Pediatrics
Medical College of Wisconsin
Children's Hospital of Wisconsin
Milwaukee, Wisconsin

ROBERT M. KLIEGMAN, MD
Professor and Chair Emeritus
Department of Pediatrics
Medical College of Wisconsin
Children's Hospital of Wisconsin
Milwaukee, Wisconsin

ELSEVIER

ELSEVIER

1600 John F. Kennedy Blvd.
Ste 1800
Philadelphia, PA 19103-2899

NELSON ESSENTIALS OF PEDIATRICS, EIGHTH EDITION
INTERNATIONAL EDITION

ISBN: 978-0-323-51145-2
ISBN: 978-0-323-52735-4

Notices

Knowledge and best practice in this field are constantly changing. As new research and experience broaden our understanding, changes in research methods, professional practices, or medical treatment may become necessary.

Practitioners and researchers must always rely on their own experience and knowledge in evaluating and using any information, methods, compounds, or experiments described herein. In using such information or methods they should be mindful of their own safety and the safety of others, including parties for whom they have a professional responsibility.

With respect to any drug or pharmaceutical products identified, readers are advised to check the most current information provided (i) on procedures featured or (ii) by the manufacturer of each product to be administered, to verify the recommended dose or formula, the method and duration of administration, and contraindications. It is the responsibility of practitioners, relying on their own experience and knowledge of their patients, to make diagnoses, to determine dosages and the best treatment for each individual patient, and to take all appropriate safety precautions.

To the fullest extent of the law, neither the Publisher nor the authors, contributors, or editors, assume any liability for any injury and/or damage to persons or property as a matter of products liability, negligence or otherwise, or from any use or operation of any methods, products, instructions, or ideas contained in the material herein.

Previous editions copyrighted 2015, 2011, 2006, 2002, 1998, 1994, 1990.

Library of Congress Cataloging-in-Publication Data
Names: Marcdante, Karen J., editor. | Kliegman, Robert, editor.
Title: Nelson essentials of pediatrics / [edited by] Karen J. Marcdante, Robert M. Kliegman.
Other titles: Essentials of pediatrics
Description: Eighth edition. | Philadelphia, PA : Elsevier, [2019] | Includes bibliographical references and index.
Identifiers: LCCN 2017057316 | ISBN 9780323511452 (pbk. : alk. paper)
Subjects: | MESH: Pediatrics
Classification: LCC RJ45 | NLM WS 100 | DDC 618.92–dc23 LC record available at https://lccn.loc.gov/2017057316

Executive Content Strategist: James Merritt
Senior Content Development Specialist: Jennifer Shreiner
Publishing Services Manager: Patricia Tannian
Senior Project Manager: Amanda Mincher
Design Direction: Amy Buxton

Printed in Canada

Last digit is the print number: 9 8 7 6 5 4 3 2

This book is dedicated to our patients, who inspire us to learn more, and to our mentors and colleagues, the dedicated medical professionals whose curiosity and focus on providing excellent care spur the advancement of our medical practice.

CONTRIBUTORS

Lisa M. Allen, MD, FRCSC
Professor of Pediatric and Adolescent Gynecology
Department of Obstetrics and Gynecology
University of Toronto;
Head, Section of Pediatric and Gynecology
Hospital for Sick Children;
Head, Department of Gynecology
Mt. Sinai Hospital;
Site Chief, Department of Obstetrics and Gynecology
Women's College Hospital
Toronto, Ontario, Canada
Adolescent Medicine

Warren P. Bishop, MD
Professor of Pediatrics
University of Iowa Carver College of Medicine
University of Iowa Children's Hospital
Iowa City, Iowa
Digestive System

Kim Blake, MD, MRCP, FRCPC
Professor of Medicine
Department of General Pediatrics
IWK Health Centre;
Division of Medical Education
Dalhousie University
Halifax, Nova Scotia, Canada
Adolescent Medicine

Amanda Brandow, DO, MS
Associate Professor of Pediatrics
Section of Hematology and Oncology
Medical College of Wisconsin
Milwaukee, Wisconsin
Hematology

April O. Buchanan, MD
Associate Professor of Pediatrics
Assistant Dean for Academic Affairs
University of South Carolina School of Medicine Greenville;
Pediatric Hospitalist
Children's Hospital of the Greenville Health System
Greenville, South Carolina
Pediatric Nutrition and Nutritional Disorders

Gray M. Buchanan, PhD
Associate Professor of Family Medicine
Medical University of South Carolina
Charleston, South Carolina;
Director, Behavioral Medicine
Family Medicine Residency Program
Self Regional Healthcare
Greenwood, South Carolina
Psychiatric Disorders

Asriani M. Chiu, MD
Professor of Pediatrics (Allergy and Immunology) and Medicine
Director, Asthma and Allergy Clinic
Medical College of Wisconsin
Milwaukee, Wisconsin
Allergy

Yvonne E. Chiu, MD
Associate Professor of Dermatology and Pediatrics
Medical College of Wisconsin
Milwaukee, Wisconsin
Dermatology

Claudia S. Crowell, MD, MPH
Assistant Professor of Pediatric Infectious Diseases
University of Washington School of Medicine;
Program Director, Infectious Diseases QAPI
Seattle Children's Hospital
Seattle, Washington
Infectious Diseases

David Dimmock, MD
Medical Director
Rady Children's Institute for Genomic Medicine
San Diego, California
Metabolic Disorders

Alison H. Downes, MD
Assistant Professor of Clinical Pediatrics
Perelman School of Medicine at the University of Pennsylvania;
Division of Developmental and Behavioral Pediatrics
Children's Hospital of Philadelphia
Philadelphia, Pennsylvania
Psychosocial Issues

Dawn R. Ebach, MD
Clinical Professor of Pediatrics
University of Iowa Carver College of Medicine;
Division of Gastroenterology
University of Iowa Children's Hospital
Iowa City, Iowa
Digestive System

Kristine Fortin, MD, MPH
Assistant Professor of Clinical Pediatrics
Perelman School of Medicine at the University of Pennsylvania;
Safe Place: Center for Child Protection and Health
Children's Hospital of Philadelphia
Philadelphia, Pennsylvania
Psychosocial Issues

Ahmeneh Ghavam, MD
Pediatric Critical Care Fellow
Medical College of Wisconsin
Children's Hospital of Wisconsin
Milwaukee, Wisconsin
Profession of Pediatrics

Clarence W. Gowen Jr., MD
Professor and EVMS Foundation Chair
Department of Pediatrics
Eastern Virginia Medical School;
Senior Vice-President for Academic Affairs
Children's Hospital of (The) King's Daughters
Norfolk, Virginia
Fetal and Neonatal Medicine

Larry A. Greenbaum, MD, PhD
Marcus Professor of Pediatrics
Director, Division of Pediatric Nephrology
Emory University School of Medicine
Children's Healthcare of Atlanta
Atlanta, Georgia
Fluids and Electrolytes

Hilary M. Haftel, MD, MHPE
Professor of Pediatrics and Communicable Diseases, Internal Medicine, and Learning Health Sciences
Associate Chair and Director, Pediatric Education
Director, Pediatric Rheumatology
University of Michigan Medical School
Ann Arbor, Michigan
Rheumatic Diseases of Childhood

MaryKathleen Heneghan, MD
Attending Physician
Division of Pediatric Endocrinology
Advocate Children's Hospital
Park Ridge, Illinois
Endocrinology

Alana M. Karp, MD
Pediatric Nephrology Fellow
Emory University School of Medicine
Atlanta, Georgia
Fluids and Electrolytes

Mary Kim, MD
Department of Dermatology
Medical College of Wisconsin
Milwaukee, Wisconsin
Dermatology

Matthew P. Kronman, MD, MSCE
Associate Professor of Pediatric Infectious Diseases
University of Washington School of Medicine;
Associate Medical Director of Infection Prevention
Seattle Children's Hospital
Seattle, Washington
Infectious Diseases

K. Jane Lee, MD
Associate Professor of Pediatrics
Division of Special Needs
Medical College of Wisconsin
Milwaukee, Wisconsin
Acutely Ill or Injured Child

David A. Levine, MD, FAAP
Professor of Pediatrics
Chief, Division of Predoctoral Education
Morehouse School of Medicine
Atlanta, Georgia
Growth and Development

Paul A. Levy, MD
Assistant Professor of Pediatrics and Pathology
Albert Einstein College of Medicine
Children's Hospital at Montefiore
Bronx, New York
Human Genetics and Dysmorphology

John D. Mahan, MD
Professor of Pediatrics
The Ohio State University College of Medicine;
Director, Metabolic Bone Clinic
Medical Director, Transplant Program
Nationwide Children's Hospital
Columbus, Ohio
Nephrology and Urology

Karen J. Marcdante, MD
Professor
Department of Pediatrics
Medical College of Wisconsin
Children's Hospital of Wisconsin
Milwaukee, Wisconsin
Profession of Pediatrics

Robert W. Marion, MD
Professor of Pediatrics
Professor of Obstetrics and Gynecology and Women's Health
Albert Einstein College of Medicine;
Chief Emeritus, Divisions of Genetic Medicine and Developmental Medicine
Department of Pediatrics
Montefiore Medical Center
Bronx, New York
Human Genetics and Dysmorphology

Maria L. Marquez, MD
Professor of Pediatrics
MedStar Georgetown University Hospital;
Associate Dean, Reflection and Professional Development
Georgetown University School of Medicine;
Medical Director
Mary's Center Fort Totten
Washington, DC
Pediatric Nutrition and Nutritional Disorders

Susan G. Marshall, MD
Professor and Vice Chair for Education
Department of Pediatrics
University of Washington School of Medicine;
Director of Medical Education
Seattle Children's Hospital
Seattle, Washington
Respiratory System

Thomas W. McLean, MD
Professor of Pediatrics
Wake Forest Baptist Medical Center
Winston-Salem, North Carolina
Oncology

Thida Ong, MD
Assistant Professor of Pediatrics
University of Washington School of Medicine;
Associate Director, Cystic Fibrosis Center
Seattle Children's Hospital
Seattle, Washington
Respiratory System

Hiren P. Patel, MD
Clinical Associate Professor of Pediatrics
The Ohio State University College of Medicine;
Chief, Section of Nephrology
Medical Director, Kidney Transplant Program
Nationwide Children's Hospital
Columbus, Ohio
Nephrology and Urology

Caroline R. Paul, MD
Assistant Professor of Pediatrics
University of Wisconsin School of Medicine and Public Health
Madison, Wisconsin
Behavioral Disorders

Tara L. Petersen, MD
Assistant Professor of Pediatrics
Division of Pediatric Critical Care
Medical College of Wisconsin
Milwaukee, Wisconsin
Acutely Ill or Injured Child

Thomas B. Russell, MD
Assistant Professor of Pediatrics
Wake Forest Baptist Medical Center
Winston-Salem, North Carolina
Oncology

Jocelyn Huang Schiller, MD
Associate Professor of Pediatrics
University of Michigan Medical School
Ann Arbor, Michigan
Neurology

Daniel S. Schneider, MD
Associate Professor of Pediatrics
Division of Pediatric Cardiology
University of Virginia School of Medicine
Charlottesville, Virginia
Cardiovascular System

J. Paul Scott, MD
Professor of Pediatrics
Medical College of Wisconsin;
Medical Director, Wisconsin Sickle Cell Center
The Children's Research Institute of the Children's Hospital of Wisconsin
Milwaukee, Wisconsin
Hematology

Renée A. Shellhaas, MD
Associate Professor of Pediatrics
University of Michigan Medical School
Ann Arbor, Michigan
Neurology

Paola Palma Sisto, MD
Associate Professor of Pediatrics
Department of Pediatrics
Division of Endocrinology
Medical College of Wisconsin
Milwaukee, Wisconsin
Endocrinology

Amanda Striegl, MD, MS
Assistant Professor of Pediatrics
University of Washington School of Medicine;
Medical Director, Respiratory Care
Seattle Children's Hospital
Seattle, Washington
Respiratory System

J. Channing Tassone, MD
Associate Professor of Orthopedic Surgery
Medical College of Wisconsin;
Clinical Vice President, Surgical Services and Anesthesia
Section Chief, Pediatric Orthopedics
Children's Hospital of Wisconsin
Milwaukee, Wisconsin
Orthopedics

James W. Verbsky, MD, PhD
Associate Professor of Pediatrics and Microbiology/Immunology
Medical Director, Clinical Immunology Research Laboratory
Medical Director, Clinical and Translational Research
Medical College of Wisconsin
Children's Hospital of Wisconsin
Milwaukee, Wisconsin
Immunology

Kristen K. Volkman, MD
Assistant Professor of Pediatrics (Allergy and Immunology) and Medicine
Medical College of Wisconsin
Milwaukee, Wisconsin
Allergy

Surabhi B. Vora, MD, MPH
Assistant Professor of Pediatric Infectious Diseases
University of Washington School of Medicine
Seattle Children's Hospital
Seattle, Washington
Infectious Diseases

Colleen M. Wallace, MD
Assistant Professor of Pediatrics
Division of Hospitalist Medicine
Director, Pediatrics Clerkship
Director, Program for Humanities in Medicine
Washington University School of Medicine
St. Louis, Missouri
Behavioral Disorders

Kevin D. Walter, MD, FAAP
Associate Professor of Orthopedic Surgery and Pediatrics
Medical College of Wisconsin;
Program Director, Sports Medicine
Children's Hospital of Wisconsin
Milwaukee, Wisconsin
Orthopedics

PREFACE

It has been said that knowledge doubles every two years and computing power doubles every eighteen months. These dynamic changes will allow us to use technology in new ways as quickly as we can learn them. The interface of medicine and technology will help us provide better, safer care with each passing year as the amazing advancements of our scientist colleagues further delineate the pathophysiology and mechanisms of diseases. Our goal as the editors and authors of this textbook is not only to provide the classic, foundational knowledge we use every day, but to include recent advances in a readable, searchable, and concise text for medical learners as they move toward their careers as physicians and advanced practice providers.

We have once again provided updated information, including the advances that have occurred since the last edition. We believe this integration will help you investigate the common and classic pediatric disorders in a time-honored, logical format, helping you to both acquire knowledge and apply knowledge to your patients. The authors again include our colleagues who serve as clerkship directors so that medical students and advanced practice providers can gain the knowledge and skills necessary to succeed in caring for patients and in preparing for clerkship or in-service examinations.

We are honored to be part of the journey of the thousands of learners who rotate through pediatrics and of those who will become new providers of pediatric care in the years to come.

Karen J. Marcdante, MD
Robert M. Kliegman, MD

ACKNOWLEDGMENTS

The editors profusely thank James Merritt, Jennifer Shreiner, Amanda Mincher, and their team for their assistance and attention to detail. We also again thank our colleague, Carolyn Redman, whose prompting, organizing, and overseeing of the process helped us create this new edition. Finally we thank our spouses for their patient support throughout the process.

CONTENTS

SECTION 1
PROFESSION OF PEDIATRICS
Ahmeneh Ghavam and Karen J. Marcdante

1 Population and Culture 1
2 Professionalism 3
3 Ethics and Legal Issues 4
4 Palliative Care and End-of-Life Issues 6

SECTION 2
GROWTH AND DEVELOPMENT
David A. Levine

5 Normal Growth 11
6 Disorders of Growth 13
7 Normal Development 14
8 Disorders of Development 16
9 Evaluation of the Well Child 19
10 Evaluation of the Child With Special Needs 28

SECTION 3
BEHAVIORAL DISORDERS
Caroline R. Paul and Colleen M. Wallace

11 Crying and Colic 41
12 Temper Tantrums 43
13 Attention-Deficit/Hyperactivity Disorder 45
14 Control of Elimination 47
15 Normal Sleep and Pediatric Sleep Disorders 52

SECTION 4
PSYCHIATRIC DISORDERS
Gray M. Buchanan

16 Somatic Symptom and Related Disorders 59
17 Anxiety Disorders 61
18 Depressive Disorders and Bipolar Disorders 64
19 Obsessive-Compulsive Disorder 68
20 Autism Spectrum Disorder and Schizophrenia Spectrum Disorders 70

SECTION 5
PSYCHOSOCIAL ISSUES
Kristine Fortin and Alison H. Downes

21 Failure to Thrive 77
22 Child Abuse and Neglect 80
23 Homosexuality and Gender Identity 84
24 Family Structure and Function 87
25 Violence 91
26 Divorce, Separation, and Bereavement 93

SECTION 6
PEDIATRIC NUTRITION AND NUTRITIONAL DISORDERS
April O. Buchanan and Maria L. Marquez

27 Diet of the Normal Infant 99
28 Diet of the Normal Child and Adolescent 102
29 Obesity 104
30 Pediatric Undernutrition 109
31 Vitamin and Mineral Deficiencies 112

SECTION 7
FLUIDS AND ELECTROLYTES
Alana M. Karp and Larry A. Greenbaum

32 Maintenance Fluid Therapy 125
33 Dehydration and Replacement Therapy 126
34 Parenteral Nutrition 130
35 Sodium Disorders 131
36 Potassium Disorders 134
37 Acid-Base Disorders 138

SECTION 8
ACUTELY ILL OR INJURED CHILD
Tara L. Petersen and K. Jane Lee

38 Assessment and Resuscitation 145
39 Respiratory Failure 149
40 Shock 151
41 Injury Prevention 154
42 Major Trauma 155
43 Drowning 157
44 Burns 158
45 Poisoning 160
46 Sedation and Analgesia 165

SECTION 9
HUMAN GENETICS AND DYSMORPHOLOGY
Robert W. Marion and Paul A. Levy

47 Patterns of Inheritance 169
48 Genetic Assessment 177
49 Chromosomal Disorders 179
50 Approach to the Dysmorphic Child 183

SECTION 10
METABOLIC DISORDERS
David Dimmock

51 Metabolic Assessment 191
52 Carbohydrate Disorders 199
53 Amino Acid Disorders 201
54 Organic Acid Disorders 205
55 Disorders of Fat Metabolism 207
56 Lysosomal and Peroxisomal Disorders 208
57 Mitochondrial Disorders 213

SECTION 11
FETAL AND NEONATAL MEDICINE
Clarence W. Gowen Jr.

58 Assessment of the Mother, Fetus, and Newborn 217
59 Maternal Diseases Affecting the Newborn 235
60 Diseases of the Fetus 239
61 Respiratory Diseases of the Newborn 240
62 Anemia and Hyperbilirubinemia 247
63 Necrotizing Enterocolitis 254
64 Hypoxic-Ischemic Encephalopathy, Intracranial Hemorrhage, and Seizures 255
65 Sepsis and Meningitis 258
66 Congenital Infections 259

SECTION 12
ADOLESCENT MEDICINE
Kim Blake and Lisa M. Allen

67 Overview and Assessment of Adolescents 267
68 Well-Adolescent Care 273
69 Adolescent Gynecology 275
70 Eating Disorders 281
71 Substance Abuse 283

SECTION 13
IMMUNOLOGY
James W. Verbsky

72 Immunological Assessment 289
73 Lymphocyte Disorders 293
74 Neutrophil Disorders 300
75 Complement System 304
76 Hematopoietic Stem Cell Transplantation 306

SECTION 14
ALLERGY
Kristen K. Volkman and Asriani M. Chiu

77 Allergy Assessment 311
78 Asthma 313
79 Allergic Rhinitis 323
80 Atopic Dermatitis 325
81 Urticaria, Angioedema, and Anaphylaxis 328
82 Serum Sickness 332
83 Insect Allergies 333
84 Adverse Reactions to Foods 334
85 Adverse Reactions to Drugs 338

SECTION 15
RHEUMATIC DISEASES OF CHILDHOOD
Hilary M. Haftel

86 Rheumatic Assessment 343
87 Henoch-Schönlein Purpura 345
88 Kawasaki Disease 347
89 Juvenile Idiopathic Arthritis 349
90 Systemic Lupus Erythematosus 353
91 Juvenile Dermatomyositis 355
92 Musculoskeletal Pain Syndromes 356

SECTION 16
INFECTIOUS DISEASES
Matthew P. Kronman, Claudia S. Crowell, and Surabhi B. Vora

93 Infectious Disease Assessment 361
94 Immunization and Prophylaxis 363
95 Antiinfective Therapy 367
96 Fever Without a Focus 368
97 Infections Characterized by Fever and Rash 373
98 Cutaneous Infections 379
99 Lymphadenopathy 383
100 Meningitis 386
101 Encephalitis 389
102 Upper Respiratory Tract Infection 391
103 Pharyngitis 392
104 Sinusitis 394
105 Otitis Media 395
106 Otitis Externa 397
107 Croup (Laryngotracheobronchitis) 398
108 Pertussis 400
109 Bronchiolitis 401
110 Pneumonia 402
111 Infective Endocarditis 408
112 Acute Gastroenteritis 410
113 Viral Hepatitis 413
114 Urinary Tract Infection 416
115 Vulvovaginitis 417
116 Sexually Transmitted Infections 419
117 Osteomyelitis 425
118 Infectious Arthritis 428
119 Ocular Infections 430
120 Infection in the Immunocompromised Person 434
121 Infections Associated With Medical Devices 437
122 Zoonoses and Vector Borne Infections 439
123 Parasitic Diseases 447
124 Tuberculosis 452
125 Human Immunodeficiency Virus and Acquired Immunodeficiency Syndrome 457

SECTION 17
DIGESTIVE SYSTEM
Warren P. Bishop and Dawn R. Ebach

126 Digestive System Assessment 467
127 Oral Cavity 479
128 Esophagus and Stomach 480
129 Intestinal Tract 487
130 Liver Disease 494
131 Pancreatic Disease 501
132 Peritonitis 504

SECTION 18
RESPIRATORY SYSTEM
Amanda Striegl, Thida Ong, and Susan G. Marshall

133 Respiratory System Assessment 507
134 Control of Breathing 513
135 Upper Airway Obstruction 516

136 Lower Airway, Parenchymal, and Pulmonary Vascular Diseases 519
137 Cystic Fibrosis 526
138 Chest Wall and Pleura 529

SECTION **19**
CARDIOVASCULAR SYSTEM
Daniel S. Schneider

139 Cardiovascular System Assessment 535
140 Syncope 540
141 Chest Pain 541
142 Dysrhythmias 542
143 Acyanotic Congenital Heart Disease 545
144 Cyanotic Congenital Heart Disease 549
145 Heart Failure 553
146 Rheumatic Fever 556
147 Cardiomyopathies 556
148 Pericarditis 558

SECTION **20**
HEMATOLOGY
Amanda Brandow and J. Paul Scott

149 Hematology Assessment 563
150 Anemia 566
151 Hemostatic Disorders 580
152 Blood Component Therapy 589

SECTION **21**
ONCOLOGY
Thomas B. Russell and Thomas W. McLean

153 Oncology Assessment 595
154 Principles of Cancer Treatment 599
155 Leukemia 603
156 Lymphoma 605
157 Central Nervous System Tumors 607
158 Neuroblastoma 608
159 Wilms Tumor 610
160 Sarcomas 611

SECTION **22**
NEPHROLOGY AND UROLOGY
Hiren P. Patel and John D. Mahan

161 Nephrology and Urology Assessment 617
162 Nephrotic Syndrome and Proteinuria 620
163 Glomerulonephritis and Hematuria 622
164 Hemolytic Uremic Syndrome 624
165 Acute and Chronic Renal Failure 625
166 Hypertension 627
167 Vesicoureteral Reflux 628
168 Congenital and Developmental Abnormalities of the Urinary Tract 629
169 Other Urinary Tract and Genital Disorders 631

SECTION **23**
ENDOCRINOLOGY
Paola Palma Sisto and MaryKathleen Heneghan

170 Endocrinology Assessment 637
171 Diabetes Mellitus 639
172 Hypoglycemia 646
173 Short Stature 650
174 Disorders of Puberty 656
175 Thyroid Disease 663
176 Disorders of Parathyroid Bone and Mineral Endocrinology 669
177 Disorders of Sexual Development 670
178 Adrenal Gland Dysfunction 674

SECTION **24**
NEUROLOGY
Jocelyn Huang Schiller and Renée A. Shellhaas

179 Neurology Assessment 681
180 Headache and Migraine 685
181 Seizures 687
182 Weakness and Hypotonia 692
183 Ataxia and Movement Disorders 700
184 Altered Mental Status 703
185 Neurodegenerative Disorders 711
186 Neurocutaneous Disorders 714
187 Congenital Malformations of the Central Nervous System 716

SECTION **25**
DERMATOLOGY
Mary Kim and Yvonne E. Chiu

188 Dermatology Assessment 721
189 Acne 723
190 Atopic Dermatitis 724
191 Contact Dermatitis 727
192 Seborrheic Dermatitis 728
193 Pigmented Lesions 730
194 Vascular Anomalies 732
195 Erythema Multiforme, Stevens-Johnson Syndrome, and Toxic Epidermal Necrolysis 733
196 Cutaneous Infestations 735

SECTION **26**
ORTHOPEDICS
Kevin D. Walter and J. Channing Tassone

197 Orthopedics Assessment 739
198 Fractures 742
199 Hip 744
200 Lower Extremity and Knee 748
201 Foot 752
202 Spine 756
203 Upper Extremity 763
204 Benign Bone Tumors and Cystic Lesions 765

Index 769

PROFESSION OF PEDIATRICS

Ahmeneh Ghavam | Karen J. Marcdante

CHAPTER 1

Population and Culture

CARE OF CHILDREN IN SOCIETY

Health care professionals need to appreciate the interactions between medical conditions and social, economic, and environmental influences associated with the provision of pediatric care. New technologies and treatments improve morbidity, mortality, and the quality of life for children and their families, but the costs may exacerbate disparities in medical care. The challenge for pediatricians is to deliver care that is socially equitable; integrates psychosocial, cultural, and ethical issues into practice; and ensures that health care is available to all children.

CURRENT CHALLENGES

Challenges that affect children's health outcomes include access to health care; health disparities; supporting their social, cognitive, and emotional lives in the context of families and communities; and addressing environmental factors, especially poverty. Early experiences and environmental stresses interact with the genetic predisposition of every child and, ultimately, may lead to the development of diseases seen in adulthood. Pediatricians have the unique opportunity to address not only acute and chronic illnesses but also the aforementioned issues and toxic stressors to promote wellness and health maintenance in children.

Many scientific advances have an impact on the growing role of pediatricians. Newer genetic technologies allow the diagnosis of diseases at the molecular level, aid in the selection of medications and therapies, and may provide information on prognosis. Prenatal diagnosis and newborn screening improve the accuracy of early diagnosis and treatment, even when a cure is impossible. Functional magnetic resonance imaging allows a greater understanding of psychiatric and neurologic problems, such as dyslexia and attention-deficit/hyperactivity disorder.

Challenges persist as the incidence and prevalence of chronic illness increase over recent decades. Chronic illness is now the most common reason for hospital admissions among children (excluding trauma and newborn admissions). From middle school and beyond, mental illness is the main non–childbirth-related reason for hospitalization among children. Pediatricians must also address the increasing concern about environmental toxins and the prevalence of physical, emotional, and sexual abuse, and violence. World unrest and terrorism, such as the September 11 attack on New York's World Trade Center, have caused an increased level of anxiety and fear for many families and children.

To address these ongoing challenges, many pediatricians now practice as part of a health care team that includes psychiatrists, psychologists, nurses, and social workers. This **patient-centered medical home model** of care is designed to provide continuous and coordinated care to maximize health outcomes. Other models, such as school-based health clinical and retail medical facilities, may improve access but may not support continuity and coordination of care.

Childhood antecedents of adult health conditions, such as alcoholism, depression, obesity, hypertension, and hyperlipidemias, are increasingly recognized. Infants who are relatively underweight at birth due to maternal malnutrition are at higher risk of developing certain health conditions later in life, including diabetes, heart disease, hypertension, metabolic syndrome, and obesity. Improved neonatal care results in greater survival of preterm, low birthweight, or very low birthweight newborns, increasing the number of children with chronic medical conditions and developmental delays with their lifelong implications.

LANDSCAPE OF HEALTH CARE FOR CHILDREN IN THE UNITED STATES

Complex health, economic, and psychosocial challenges greatly influence the well-being and health outcomes of children. National reports from the Centers for Disease Control and Prevention (CDC) (e.g., http://www.cdc.gov/nchs/data/hus/hus15.pdf) provide information about many of these issues. Some of the key issues include the following:

- **Health insurance coverage.** Medicaid and the State Children's Health Insurance Program provide coverage to health care access to more than 45 million children in 2013.The slow drop in uninsured children nationally over the past decade leaves 5.5% of U.S. children lacking insurance in 2014. Despite public sector insurance, the rate of unvaccinated children remains unchanged over the past 5 years.
- **Prenatal and perinatal care.** Ten to 25% of women do not receive prenatal care during the first trimester. In addition, a significant percentage of women continue to smoke, use illicit drugs, and consume alcohol during pregnancy.
- **Preterm births.** The incidence of preterm births (<37 weeks) peaked in 2006 and has been slowly declining (9.6% in 2014). However, the rates of low birthweight infants (≤2,500 g [8% of all births]) and very low birthweight infants (≤1,500 g [1.4% of all births]) are essentially unchanged since 2006.

- **Birthrate in adolescents.** The national birthrate among adolescents has been steadily dropping since 1990, reaching its lowest rate (24.2 per 1000) for 15- to 19-year-old adolescents in 2014.
- **Adolescent abortions.** In 2010 the percent of adolescent pregnancies that ended in abortion was 30%. The rate of abortions among adolescents has been dropping since its peak in 1988 and is now at its lowest rate since abortion was legalized in 1973.
- **Infant mortality.** Internationally, infant mortality decreased from 63 deaths per 1000 live births in 1990 to 32 deaths per 1000 live births in 2015. In the United States, overall infant mortality rate decreased to a record low 5.96 per 1000 live births in 2013. A persistent disparity remains among ethnic groups. The infant mortality rate (in deaths per 1000 live births) is 4.96 for non-Hispanic white infant mortality, 5.27 for Hispanic infants, and 11.61 black infants. U.S. geographic variability persists with highest mortality rates in the South.
- **Initiation and maintenance of breast-feeding.** Seventy-nine percent of newborn infants start to breast-feed after birth. Breast-feeding rates vary by ethnicity (higher rates in non-Hispanic whites and Hispanic mothers) and education (highest in women with a bachelor's degree or higher). Only 49% of women continue breast-feeding for 6 months, with about 27% continuing at 12 months.
- **Cause of death in U.S. children.** The overall causes of death in all children (1-24 years of age) in the United States in 2014, in order of frequency, were accidents (unintentional injuries), suicide, assaults (homicide), malignant neoplasms, and congenital malformations (Table 1.1). There was a slight improvement in the rate of death from all causes.
- **Hospital admissions for children and adolescents.** In 2014, 7.2% of children were admitted to a hospital at least once. Respiratory illnesses are the predominant cause of hospitalization for children 1-9 years of age, while mental illness is the most common cause of admission for adolescents.

TABLE 1.1 Causes of Death by Age in the United States, 2014

AGE GROUP (YEAR)	CAUSES OF DEATH IN ORDER OF FREQUENCY
1-4	Unintentional injuries (accidents) Congenital anomalies Homicide Malignant neoplasms Diseases of the heart
5-14	Unintentional injuries (accidents) Malignant neoplasms Suicide Congenital anomalies Homicide Diseases of the heart
15-24	Unintentional injuries (accidents) Suicide Homicide Malignant neoplasms Diseases of the heart

From National Center for Health Statistics (US). Health, United States, 2015: with special feature on racial and ethnic health disparities. http://www.cdc.gov/nchs/data/hus/hus15.pdf.

- **Significant adolescent health challenges: substance use and abuse.** There is considerable substance use and abuse among U.S. adolescents, although the overall trend in use is declining. Current estimates are that between 36% and 50% of high school students currently drink alcohol. Overall illicit drug use by adolescents is slowly declining (23.6% 12th graders reporting drug use in 2015). The teen smoking rate is also declining (13% in 2002; 5.5% in 2015). However, in 2014 more teens reported using electronic nicotine delivery systems (ENDS) than any other tobacco product. ENDS, commonly referred to as e-cigarettes, pose significant health risks to both users and nonusers.
- **Children in foster care.** In 2013 just over 400,000 children were in the foster care system. Children in foster care often have significant developmental, behavioral, and emotional problems that require access to quality health and mental health care services. Although adoptions account for nearly 20% of children exiting foster care annually, 25-50% of children leaving the welfare system experience homelessness and/or joblessness and will not graduate from high school.

OTHER HEALTH ISSUES THAT AFFECT CHILDREN IN THE UNITED STATES

- **Obesity.** Obesity is the second leading cause of death in the United States (estimated 300,000 deaths annually). Childhood obesity has more than doubled in children and quadrupled in adolescents over the past 30 years. The prevalence of obese children 6-19 years of age in 2012 was estimated at 39%.
- **Sedentary lifestyle.** Currently, only 1 in 3 children are physically active every day. As technology continues to advance, children spend more time in front of a screen (television, video games, computer, etc.), with some spending more than 7.5 hours per day.
- **Motor vehicle accidents and injuries.** In 2014, 602 children 12 years of age or younger died in motor vehicle crashes, and more than 121,350 were injured. Preliminary data suggest a slight increase in 2015. The impact of mobile device use and increased speed limits is being considered. Carseat and seatbelt use can reduce the risk of serious injury and death by half for infants and children. On average, more than 12,000 children ages 0-19 years die each year of unintentional injury in the United States. Other causes of childhood injury included drowning, suffocation, burns, child abuse, and poisonings.
- **Child maltreatment.** In 2014 there were an estimated 702,000 reported cases of maltreatment with 1,580 deaths as a result of abuse and neglect. The majority of children (75%) were neglected; 17% suffered physical abuse, and nearly 8.3% were victims of sexual abuse.
- **Toxic stress in childhood leading to adult health challenges.** The growing understanding of the interrelationship between biologic and developmental stresses, environmental exposure, and the genetic potential of patients is helping us recognize the adverse impact of toxic stressors on health and well-being. Screening for and acting upon factors that promote or hinder early development provides the best opportunity for long-term health. The field of epigenetics is demonstrating that exposure to environmental stress impacts genetic expression and can result in long-term effects on development, health, and behaviors.

- **Military deployment and children.** Current armed conflicts and political unrest have affected millions of adults and their children. There are an estimated 1.3 million active duty and National Guard/Reserve servicemen and servicewomen, parents to more than a million children. An estimated 30% of troops returning from armed conflicts have a mental health condition (alcoholism, depression, and post-traumatic stress disorder) or report having experienced a traumatic brain injury. Their children are affected by these morbidities, as well as by the psychologic impact of deployment. Child maltreatment is more prevalent in families of U.S.-enlisted soldiers during combat deployment than in nondeployed soldiers.

HEALTH DISPARITIES IN HEALTH CARE FOR CHILDREN

Health disparities are the differences that remain after taking into account patients' needs, preferences, and the availability of health care. Social conditions, social inequity, discrimination, social stress, language barriers, and poverty are antecedents to and associated causes of health disparities. Disparities in infant mortality relate to poor access to prenatal care and the lack of access and appropriate health services for women, such as preventive services, family planning, and appropriate nutrition and health care.

- Infant mortality increases as the mother's level of education decreases.
- Children from poor families are less likely to be immunized at 4 years of age and less likely to receive dental care.
- Children with Medicaid/public coverage are less likely to be in excellent health than children with private health insurance.
- Rates of hospital admission are higher for people who live in low-income areas.
- Children of ethnic minorities and those from poor families are less likely to have physician office or hospital outpatient visits and more likely to have hospital emergency department visits.

CHANGING MORBIDITY: SOCIAL/EMOTIONAL ASPECTS OF PEDIATRIC PRACTICE

- **Changing morbidity** reflects the relationship among environmental, social, emotional, and developmental issues; child health status; and outcome. These observations are based on significant interactions of **biopsychosocial** influences on health and illness, such as school problems, learning disabilities, and attention problems; child and adolescent mood and anxiety disorders; adolescent suicide and homicide; firearms in the home; school violence; effects of media violence, obesity, and sexual activity; and substance use and abuse by adolescents.
- It is estimated that 1 in 5 children, ages 13-18 years, has a mental health condition. Fifty percent of all lifetime cases of mental illness begin by age 14 years. The average delay between onset of symptoms and intervention is 8-10 years. Suicide is the second leading cause of death for children ages 10-24 years, making early recognition of mental illness paramount. Children from poor families are twice as likely to have psychosocial problems as children from higher-income families. Nationwide, there is a lack of adequate mental health services for children.

Important influences on children's health, in addition to poverty, include homelessness, single-parent families, parental divorce, domestic violence, both parents working, and inadequate child care. Related pediatric challenges include improving the quality of health care, social justice, equality in health care access, and improving the public health system. For adolescents, there are special concerns about sexuality, sexual orientation, pregnancy, substance use and abuse, violence, depression, and suicide.

CULTURE

The growing diversity of the United States requires that health care workers make an attempt to understand the impact of health, illness, and treatment on the patient and family from their perspective. Facilitating a discussion of parental thoughts and feelings about illness and its causes requires open-ended questions, such as: "What *worries* you the most about your child's illness?" and "What do you *think* has caused your child's illness?" One must address concepts and beliefs about how patients/families interact with health professionals, as well as their spiritual and religious approach to health and health care from a cultural perspective; this allows all to incorporate differences in perspectives, values, or beliefs into the care plan. Significant conflicts may arise because religious or cultural practices may lead to the possibility of child abuse and neglect. In this circumstance, the suspected child abuse and neglect is required, by law, to be reported to the appropriate social service authorities (see Chapter 22).

Complementary and alternative medicine (CAM) practices constitute a part of the broad cultural perspective. Therapeutic modalities for CAM include biochemical, lifestyle, biomechanical, and bioenergetic treatments, as well as homeopathy. It is estimated that 20-40% of healthy children and more than 60% of children with chronic illness use CAM. Only 30-60% of these children and families tell their physicians about their use of CAM. Screening for CAM use can aid the pediatrician's counseling and minimize unintentional adverse interactions.

CHAPTER 2

Professionalism

CONCEPT OF PROFESSIONALISM

Society provides a profession with economic, political, and social rewards. Professions have specialized knowledge and the potential to maintain a monopoly on power and control, remaining relatively autonomous. A profession exists as long as it fulfills its responsibilities for the social good.

Today the activities of medical professionals are subject to explicit public rules of accountability. Governmental and other authorities at city, state, and federal levels grant limited autonomy to professional organizations and their membership thorough regulations, licensing requirement, and standards of service (e.g., Medicare, Medicaid, and the Food and Drug Administration). The Department of Health and Human Services regulates physician behavior in conducting research with the goal of protecting human subjects. The National Practitioner Data Bank, created in 1986, contains information about physicians and other health care practitioners who have been disciplined by a state licensing board, professional society, hospital, or health plan or named in medical malpractice judgments or settlements. Hospitals are required to review information in this data bank every 2 years as part of clinician recredentialing. There are accrediting agencies for medical schools, such as the Liaison Committee on Medical Education (LCME), and postgraduate training, such as the Accreditation Council for Graduate Medical Education (ACGME).

The public trust of physicians is based on the physician's commitment to altruism, which is a cornerstone of the Hippocratic Oath, an important rite of passage and part of medical school commencement ceremonies. The core of professionalism is embedded in the daily healing work of the physician and encompasses the patient-physician relationship. Professionalism includes an appreciation for the cultural and religious/spiritual health beliefs of the patient, incorporating the ethical and moral values of the profession and the moral values of the patient. Unfortunately, the inappropriate actions of a few practicing physicians, physician investigators, and physicians in positions of power have created a societal demand to punish those involved and lead to the erosion of respect for the medical profession.

PROFESSIONALISM FOR PEDIATRICIANS

The American Board of Pediatrics (ABP) adopted professional standards in 2000, and the American Academy of Pediatrics (AAP) updated the policy statement and technical report on Professionalism in 2007, as follows:

- **Honesty/integrity** is the consistent regard for the highest standards of behavior and the refusal to violate one's personal and professional codes. Maintaining integrity requires awareness of situations that may result in conflict of interest or that may result in personal gain at the expense of the best interest of the patient.
- **Reliability/responsibility** includes accountability to one's patients, their families, to society, and the medical community to ensure that all needs are addressed. There also must be a willingness to accept responsibility for errors.
- **Respect for others** requires the pediatrician to treat all persons with respect and regard for their individual worth and dignity; be aware of emotional, personal, family, and cultural influences on a patient's well-being, rights, and choices of medical care; and respect appropriate patient confidentiality.
- **Compassion/empathy** requires the pediatrician to listen attentively, respond humanely to the concerns of patients and family members, and provide appropriate empathy for and relief of pain, discomfort, and anxiety as part of daily practice.
- **Self-improvement** is the pursuit of and commitment to providing the highest quality of health care through lifelong learning and education. The pediatrician must seek to learn from errors and aspire to excellence through self-evaluation and acceptance of the critiques of others.
- **Self-awareness/knowledge of limits** includes recognition of the need for guidance and supervision when faced with new or complex responsibilities, the impact of his or her behavior on others, and appropriate professional boundaries.
- **Communication/collaboration** is crucial to providing the best care for patients. Pediatricians must work cooperatively and communicate effectively with patients and their families and with all health care providers involved in the care of their patients.
- **Altruism/advocacy** refers to unselfish regard for and devotion to the welfare of others. It is a key element of professionalism. Self-interest or the interests of other parties should not interfere with the care of one's patients and their families.

CHAPTER 3

Ethics and Legal Issues

ETHICS IN HEALTH CARE

The ethics of health care and medical decision-making relies on **values**. Sometimes, ethical decision making in medical care is a matter of choosing the least harmful option among many adverse alternatives. In the day-to-day practice of medicine, although all clinical encounters may have an ethical component, major ethical challenges are infrequent.

The legal system defines the minimal standards of behavior required of physicians and the rest of society through the legislative, regulatory, and judicial systems. Laws support the principle of **confidentiality** for teenagers who are competent to decide about medical issues. Using the concept of **limited confidentiality**, parents, teenagers, and the pediatrician may all agree to openly discuss serious health challenges, such as suicidal ideation and pregnancy. This reinforces the long-term goal of supporting the autonomy and identity of the teenager while encouraging appropriate conversations with parents.

Ethical problems derive from **value differences** among patients, families, and clinicians regarding choices and options in the provision of health care. Resolving these value differences involves several important ethical principles. **Autonomy**, which is based on the principle of **respect for persons**, means that competent adult patients can make choices about health care that they perceive to be in their best interests after being appropriately informed about their particular health condition and the risks and benefits of alternative diagnostic tests and treatments. **Paternalism** challenges the principle of autonomy and involves the clinician deciding what is best for the patient based on how much information is provided. Paternalism under certain circumstances (e.g., when a patient has a life-threatening medical condition or a significant psychiatric disorder and is threatening self or others) may be more appropriate than autonomy.

Other important ethical principles are those of **beneficence** (doing good), **nonmaleficence** (doing no harm or as little harm as possible), and **justice** (the values involved in the equality of the distribution of goods, services, benefits, and burdens to the individual, family, or society).

ETHICAL PRINCIPLES RELATED TO INFANTS, CHILDREN, AND ADOLESCENTS

Infants and young children do not have the capacity for making medical decisions. Paternalism by parents and pediatricians in these circumstances is appropriate. Adolescents (<18 years of age), if competent, have the legal right to make medical decisions for themselves. Children 8-9 years old can understand how the body works and the meaning of certain procedures; by age 14-15, young adolescents may be considered autonomous through the process of being designated a mature or emancipated minor or by having certain medical conditions. Obtaining the

assent of a child is the process by which the pediatrician involves the child in the decision-making process with information appropriate to their capacity to understand.

The principle of shared medical decision-making is appropriate, but the process may be limited because of issues of confidentiality. A parent's concern about the side effects of immunization raises a conflict between the need to protect and support the health of the individual and of the public.

LEGAL ISSUES

All competent patients of an age defined legally by each state (usually ≥18 years of age) are considered autonomous regarding their health decisions. To have the capacity to decide, patients must meet the following requirements:

- Understand the nature of the medical interventions and procedures, understand the risks and benefits of these interventions, and be able to communicate their decision.
- Reason, deliberate, and weigh the risks and benefits using their understanding about the implications of the decision on their own welfare.
- Apply a set of personal values to the decision-making process and show an awareness of the possible conflicts or differences in values as applied to the decisions to be made.

These requirements must be placed within the context of medical care and applied to each case with its unique characteristics. Most young children are not able to meet these requirements and need others, usually the parent, to serve as the legal surrogate decision maker. However, when child abuse and neglect are present, a further legal process may determine the best interests of the child.

It is important to become familiar with state law as it, not federal law, determines when an adolescent can consent to medical care and when parents may access confidential adolescent medical information. The Health Insurance Portability and Accountability Act (HIPAA), which became effective in 2003, requires a minimal standard of confidentiality protection. The law confers less confidentiality protection to minors than to adults. It is the pediatrician's responsibility to inform minors of their confidentiality rights and help them exercise these rights under the HIPAA regulations.

Under special circumstances, nonautonomous adolescents are granted the legal right to consent under state law when they are considered mature or emancipated minors or because of certain public health considerations, as follows:

- **Mature minors.** Some states have legally recognized that many adolescents can meet the cognitive criteria and emotional maturity for competence and may decide independently. The Supreme Court has decided that pregnant, mature minors have the constitutional right to make decisions about abortion without parental consent. Although many state legislatures require parental notification, pregnant adolescents wishing to have an abortion do not have to seek parental consent. The state must provide a judicial procedure to facilitate this decision making for adolescents.
- **Emancipated minors.** Children who are legally emancipated from parental control may seek medical treatment without parental consent. The definition varies from state to state but generally includes children who have graduated from high school, are members of the armed forces, married, pregnant, runaways, are parents, live apart from their parents, and are financially independent or declared emancipated by a court.
- **Interests of the state (public health).** State legislatures have concluded that minors with certain medical conditions, such as sexually transmitted infections and other contagious diseases, pregnancy (including prevention with the use of birth control), certain mental illnesses, and drug and alcohol abuse, may seek treatment for these conditions autonomously. States have an interest in limiting the spread of disease that may endanger the public health and in eliminating barriers to access for the treatment of certain conditions.

ETHICAL ISSUES IN PRACTICE

Clinicians should engage children and adolescents based on their developmental capacity in discussions about medical plans so that the child has a good understanding of the nature of the treatments and alternatives, the side effects, and expected outcomes. There should be an assessment of the patient's understanding of the clinical situation, how the patient is responding, and the factors that may influence the patient's decisions. Pediatricians should always listen to and appreciate patients' requests for confidentiality and their hopes and wishes. The ultimate goal is to help nourish children's capacity to become as autonomous as is appropriate to their developmental stage.

Confidentiality

Confidentiality is crucial to the provision of medical care and is an important part of the basis for a trusting patient-family-physician relationship. Confidentiality means that information about a patient should not be shared without consent. If confidentiality is broken, patients may experience great harm and may not seek needed medical care. See Chapter 67 for a discussion of confidentiality in the care of adolescents.

Ethical Issues in Genetic Testing and Screening in Children

The goal of **screening** is to identify diseases when there is no clinically identifiable risk factor for disease. Screening should take place only when there is a treatment available or when a diagnosis would benefit the child. **Testing** usually is performed when there is some clinically identifiable risk factor. Genetic testing and screening present special problems because test results have important implications. Some genetic screening (sickle cell anemia or cystic fibrosis) may reveal a carrier state, which may lead to choices about reproduction or create financial, psychosocial, and interpersonal problems (e.g., guilt, shame, social stigma, and discrimination in insurance and jobs). Collaboration with, or referral to, a clinical geneticist is appropriate in helping the family with the complex issues of genetic counseling when a genetic disorder is detected or anticipated.

Newborn screening should not be used as a surrogate for parental testing. Examples of diseases that can be diagnosed by genetic screening, even though the manifestations of the disease process do not appear until later in life, are polycystic kidney disease; Huntington disease; certain cancers, such as breast cancer in some ethnic populations; and hemochromatosis. For their own purposes, parents may pressure the pediatrician to order genetic tests when the child is still young. Testing for these disorders should be delayed until the child has the capacity for informed consent or assent and is competent to make decisions, unless there is a direct benefit to the child at the time of testing.

Religious Issues and Ethics

The pediatrician is required to act in the best interests of the child, even when religious tenets may interfere with the health and well-being of the child. When an infant or child whose parents have a religious prohibition against a blood transfusion needs a transfusion to save his or her life, the courts always intervene to allow a transfusion. In contrast, parents with strong religious beliefs under some state laws may refuse immunizations for their children. States may use the principle of **distributive justice** to require immunization of all during outbreaks or epidemics, including individuals who object on religious grounds.

Children as Human Subjects in Research

The goal of research is to develop new and generalized knowledge. Parents may give informed permission for children to participate in research under certain conditions. Children cannot give consent but may assent or dissent to research protocols. Special federal regulations have been developed to protect child and adolescent participants in human investigation. These regulations provide additional safeguards beyond those for adult participants while still providing the opportunity for children to benefit from the scientific advances of research.

Many parents with seriously ill children hope that the research protocol will have a direct benefit for their particular child. The greatest challenge for researchers is to be clear with parents that research is not treatment. This fact should be addressed as sensitively and compassionately as possible.

CHAPTER 4

Palliative Care and End-of-Life Issues

The death of a child is one of life's most difficult experiences. The **palliative care** approach is defined as patient- and family-centered care that optimizes quality of life by anticipating, preventing, and treating suffering. This approach should be instituted when medical diagnosis, intervention, and treatment cannot reasonably be expected to affect the imminence of death. Central to this approach is the willingness of clinicians to look beyond the traditional medical goals of curing disease and preserving life and towards enhancing the life of the child with assistance from family members and close friends. High-quality palliative care is an expected standard at the end of life.

Palliative care in pediatrics is not simply end-of-life care. Children needing palliative care have been described as having conditions that fall into four basic groups based on the goal of treatment. These include conditions of the following scenarios:

- A cure is possible, but failure is not uncommon (e.g., cancer with a poor prognosis).
- Long-term treatment is provided with a goal of maintaining quality of life (e.g., cystic fibrosis).
- Treatment that is exclusively palliative after the diagnosis of a progressive condition is made (e.g., trisomy 13 syndrome).
- Treatments are available for severe, non-progressive disability in patients who are vulnerable to health complications (e.g., severe spastic quadriparesis with difficulty in controlling symptoms).

These conditions present different timelines and different models of medical intervention while sharing the need to attend to concrete elements affecting the quality of a child's death and mediated by medical, psychosocial, cultural, and spiritual concerns.

Families without time to prepare for the tragedy of an unexpected death require considerable support. Palliative care can make important contributions to the end-of-life and bereavement issues that families face in these circumstances. This may become complicated in circumstances where the cause of the death must be fully explored. The need to investigate the possibility of child abuse or neglect subjects the family to intense scrutiny and may create guilt and anger directed at the medical team.

PALLIATIVE AND END-OF-LIFE CARE

Palliative treatment is directed toward the relief of symptoms as well as assistance with anticipated adaptations that may cause distress and diminish the quality of life of the dying child. Elements of palliative care include pain management; expertise with feeding and nutritional issues at the end of life; and management of symptoms, such as minimizing nausea and vomiting, bowel obstruction, labored breathing, and fatigue. Psychologic elements of palliative care have a profound importance and include sensitivity to bereavement, a developmental perspective of a child's understanding of death, clarification of the goals of care, and ethical issues. Palliative care is delivered through a multidisciplinary approach, giving a broad range of expertise to patients and families as well as providing a supportive network for the caregivers. Caregivers involved may be pediatricians, nurses, mental health professionals, social workers, and pastors.

A model of integrated palliative care rests on the following principles:

- **Respect for the dignity of patients and families.** The clinician should respect and listen to patient and family goals, preferences, and choices. School-age children can articulate preferences about how they wish to be treated. Adolescents can engage in decision-making (see Section 12). **Advanced care** (advance directives) should be instituted with the child and parents, allowing discussions about what they would like as treatment options as the end of life nears. Differences of opinion between the family and the pediatrician should be addressed by identifying the multiple perspectives, reflecting on possible conflicts, and altruistically coming to agreements that validate the patient and family perspectives yet reflect sound practice. **Hospital ethics committees** and consultation services are important resources for the pediatrician and family members.
- **Access to comprehensive and compassionate palliative care.** The clinician should address the physical symptoms, comfort, and functional capacity, with special attention to pain and other symptoms associated with the dying process, and respond empathically to the psychologic distress and

human suffering, providing treatment options. Respite should be available at any time during the illness to allow the family caregivers to rest and renew.

- **Use of interdisciplinary resources.** Because of the complexity of care, no one clinician can provide all of the needed services. The team members may include primary and subspecialty physicians, nurses in the hospital/facility or for home visits, the pain management team, psychologists, social workers, pastoral ministers, schoolteachers, friends of the family, and peers of the child. The child and family should be in a position to decide who should know what during all phases of the illness process.
- **Acknowledgment and support provisions for caregivers.** The primary caregivers of the child, family, and friends need opportunities to address their own emotional concerns. Team meetings to address thoughts and feelings of team members are crucial. Institutional support may include time to attend funerals, counseling for the staff, opportunities for families to return to the hospital, and scheduled ceremonies to commemorate the death of the child.
- **Commitment to quality improvement of palliative care through research and education.** Hospitals should develop support systems and staff to monitor the quality of care continually, assess the need for appropriate resources, and evaluate the responses of the patient and family members to the treatment program.

Hospice care is a treatment program for the end of life that provides the range of palliative care services by an interdisciplinary team including specialists in the bereavement and end-of-life process. In 2010, legislation was passed allowing children covered under Medicaid or the Children's Health Insurance Program (CHIP) to receive access simultaneously to hospice care and curative care.

BEREAVEMENT

Bereavement refers to the process of psychologic and spiritual accommodation to death on the part of the child and the child's family. **Grief** has been defined as the emotional response caused by a loss which may include pain, distress, and physical and emotional suffering. It is a normal adaptive human response to death. Assessing the coping resources and vulnerabilities of the affected family before death occurs is central to the palliative care approach.

Parental grief is recognized as being more intense and sustained than other types of grief. Most parents work through their grief. Complicated grief, a pathologic manifestation of continued and disabling grief, is rare. Parents who share their problems with others during the child's illness, who have access to psychologic support during the last month of their child's life, and who have had closure sessions with the attending staff are more likely to resolve their grief. In the era of technology, some parents may find solace in connecting with other parents with similar experiences in an online forum.

A particularly difficult issue for parents is whether to talk with their child about the child's imminent death. Although evidence suggests that sharing accurate and truthful information with a dying child is beneficial, each individual case presents its own complexities, based on the child's age, cognitive development, disease, timeline of disease, and parental psychologic state. Parents are more likely to regret not talking with their child about death than having done so.

COGNITIVE ISSUES IN CHILDREN AND ADOLESCENTS: UNDERSTANDING DEATH AND DYING

The pediatrician should communicate with children about what is happening to them while respecting the cultural and personal preferences of the family. A developmental understanding of children's concepts of health and illness helps frame the discussion and can help parents understand how their child is grappling with the situation. Piaget's theories of cognitive development, which help illustrate children's concepts of death and disease, are categorized as sensorimotor, preoperational, concrete operations, and formal operations.

For children up to 2 years of age (sensorimotor), death is seen as a separation without a specific concept of death. The associated behaviors in grieving children of this age usually include protesting and difficulty of attachment to other adults. The degree of difficulty depends on the availability of other nurturing people with whom the child has a good previous attachment.

Children from 3-5 years of age (preoperational; sometimes called *the magic years*) have trouble grasping the meaning of the illness and the permanence of the death. Their language skills at this age make understanding their moods and behavior difficult. Because of a developing sense of guilt, death may be viewed as punishment. If a child previously wished a younger sibling dead, the death may be seen psychologically as being caused by the child's wishful thinking. They can feel overwhelmed when confronted with the strong emotional reactions of their parents.

In children ages 6-11 years of age (late preoperational to concrete operational), the finality of death gradually comes to be understood. Magical thinking gives way to a need for detailed information to gain a sense of control. Older children in this range have a strong need to control their emotions by compartmentalizing and intellectualizing.

In adolescents (≥12 years of age) (formal operations), death is a reality and is seen as universal and irreversible. Adolescents handle death issues at the abstract or philosophical level and can be realistic. They may also avoid emotional expression and information, instead relying on anger or disdain. Adolescents can discuss withholding treatments. Their wishes, hopes, and fears should be attended to and respected.

CULTURAL, RELIGIOUS, AND SPIRITUAL CONCERNS ABOUT PALLIATIVE CARE AND END-OF-LIFE DECISIONS

Understanding the family's religious/spiritual or cultural beliefs and values about death and dying can help the pediatrician work with the family to integrate these beliefs, values, and practices into the palliative care plan. Cultures vary regarding the roles family members have, the site of treatment for dying people, and the preparation of the body. Some ethnic groups expect the clinical team to speak with the oldest family member or to only the head of the family outside of the patient's presence, while others involve the entire extended family in decision-making. For some families, dying at home can bring the family bad luck; others believe that the patient's spirit will become lost if the death occurs in the hospital. In some traditions, the health care team cleans and prepares the body, whereas in others, family members prefer to complete this ritual. Religious/

spiritual or cultural practices may include prayer, anointing, laying on of the hands, an exorcism ceremony to undo a curse, amulets, and other religious objects placed on the child or at the bedside. Families differ in the idea of organ donation and the acceptance of autopsy. Decisions, rituals, and withholding of palliative or lifesaving procedures that could harm the child or are not in the best interests of the child should be addressed. Quality palliative care attends to this complexity and helps parents and families through the death of a child while honoring the familial, cultural, and spiritual values.

ETHICAL ISSUES IN END-OF-LIFE DECISION-MAKING

Before speaking with a child about death, the caregiver should assess the child's age, experience, and level of development; the child's understanding and involvement in end-of-life decision-making; the parents' emotional acceptance of death; their coping strategies; and their philosophical, spiritual, and cultural views of death. These may change over time. The use of open-ended questions to repeatedly assess these areas contributes to the end-of-life process. The care of a dying child can create **ethical dilemmas** involving **autonomy, beneficence** (doing good), **nonmaleficence** (doing no harm), truth telling, confidentiality, or the physician's duty. It is extremely difficult for parents to know when the burdens of continued medical care are no longer appropriate for their child and may, at times, rely on the medical team for guidance. The beliefs and values of what constitutes quality of life, when life ceases to be worth living, and religious/spiritual, cultural, and philosophical beliefs may differ between families and health care workers. The most important ethical principle is what is in the **best interest** of the child as determined through the process of **shared decision-making**, **informed permission/consent** from the parents, and **assent** from the child. Sensitive and meaningful communication with the family, in their own terms, is essential. The physician, patient, and family must **negotiate** the goals of continued medical treatment while recognizing the burdens and benefits of the medical intervention plan. There is no ethical or legal difference between withholding treatment and withdrawing treatment, although many parents and physicians see the latter as more challenging. Family members and the patient should agree about what are appropriate **do not resuscitate** (also called **DNR**) orders. Foregoing some measures does not preclude other measures being implemented based on the needs and wishes of the patient and family. When there are serious differences among parents, children, and physicians on these matters, the physician may consult with the **hospital ethics committee** or, as a last resort, turn to the legal system by filing a report about potential abuse or neglect.

ORGAN DONATION IN PEDIATRICS

The gap between supply and demand of transplantable organs in children is widening as more patients need a transplant without a concomitant increase in the organ donor pool. Organ donation can occur one of two ways: after fulfilling criteria for neurologic (brain) death or through a process of donation after circulatory death (DCD). DCD has only recently gained acceptance in pediatrics. Organ procurement, donation, and transplantation are strictly regulated by governmental agencies to ensure proper and fair allocation of donated organs for transplantation. It is important that pediatric medical specialists and pediatricians be well acquainted with the strategies and methods of organ donation to help acquaint both the donor family and the recipient family with the process and address expectations. Areas of concern within pediatric organ donation include availability of and access to donor organs; oversight and control of the process; pediatric medical and surgical consultation and continued care throughout the transplantation process; ethical, social, financial, and follow-up; insurance-coverage; and public awareness of the need for organ donors. Organ donation and organ transplantation can provide significant life-extending benefits to a child who has a failing organ and is awaiting transplant, while at the same time place a high emotional impact on the donor family after the loss of a child.

Suggested Readings

American Academy of Pediatrics, Committee on Bioethics, Fallat ME, Glover J. Professionalism in pediatrics: statement of principles. *Pediatrics*. 2007;120(4):895–897.

American Academy of Pediatrics, Committee on Hospital Care, Section on Surgery and Section on Critical Care. Policy statement—pediatric organ donation and transplantation. *Pediatrics*. 2010;125(4):822–828.

Bloom B, Jones LI, Freeman G. Summary health statistics for U.S. children: National Health Interview Survey, 2012. National Center for Health Statistics. *Vital Health Stat*. 2013;10(258):1–72.

National Center for Health Statistics. *Health, United States, 2015: With Special Feature on Racial and Ethnic Health Disparities*. Hyattsville, MD: National Center for Health Statistics (US); 2016.

National Consensus Project for Quality Palliative Care. *Clinical Practice Guidelines for Quality Palliative Care*. Pittsburgh: National Consensus Project for Quality Palliative Care; 2013.

PEARLS FOR PRACTITIONERS

CHAPTER 1

Population and Culture

- Pediatricians must continue to address major issues impacting children's health outcomes including access to care, health disparities, and environmental factors including toxic stressors such as poverty and violence.
- The significant increase in the number of children with a chronic medical condition (e.g., asthma, obesity, attention-deficit/hyperactivity disorder) affects both inpatient and outpatient care.
- Addressing the following as a part of routine health care allows pediatricians to impact health care outcomes:
  - Toxic stressors (e.g., maternal stress, poverty, exposure to violence)

- The use of electronic nicotine delivery systems or e-cigarettes
- The sedentary lifestyle as children spend an increased amount of time in front of a screen (TV, videogames, computers, cell phones)
- Early recognition of mental illness (It is estimated that 1 in 5 adolescents has a mental health condition.)
- Use of complementary and alternative medicine (to minimize unintended interactions)

CHAPTER 2

Professionalism

- The activities of medical professionals are subject to explicit public rules of accountability developed by governmental and other authorities.
- The public trust of physicians is based on the physician's commitment to altruism.
- The policy statement on professionalism released by The American Board of Pediatrics emphasizes: honesty/integrity, reliability/responsibility, respect for others, compassion/empathy, self-improvement, self-awareness/knowledge of limits, communication/collaboration, and altruism/advocacy.

CHAPTER 3

Ethics and Legal Issues

- Key ethical principles in the care of pediatric patients include autonomy (addressing when minor patients can make their own medical decisions), informed consent by parents and assent by the child, and confidentiality.

CHAPTER 4

Palliative Care and End-of-Life Issues

- Children needing palliative care generally fall into four basic categories: (1) when a cure is possible but unlikely; (2) long-term treatment with a goal of maintaining quality of life (e.g., cystic fibrosis); (3) treatment that is exclusively palliative after the diagnosis of a progressive condition is made (e.g., trisomy 13); and (4) when treatments are available for severe, non-progressive disabilities.
- Organ donation can occur after fulfilling criteria for neurologic death or through donation after circulatory death.

GROWTH AND DEVELOPMENT

David A. Levine

CHAPTER 5

Normal Growth

HEALTH MAINTENANCE VISIT

The frequent office visits for health maintenance in the first 2 years of life are more than *physicals*. Although a somatic history and physical examination are important parts of each visit, many other issues are discussed, including nutrition, behavior, development, safety, and **anticipatory guidance**.

Disorders of growth and development are often associated with chronic or severe illness or may be the only symptom of parental neglect or abuse. Although normal growth and development does not eliminate a serious or chronic illness, in general, it supports a judgment that a child is healthy except for acute, often benign, illnesses that do not affect growth and development.

The processes of growth and development are intertwined. However, it is convenient to refer to **growth** as the increase in size and **development** as an increase in function of processes related to body and mind. Being familiar with normal patterns of growth and development allows those practitioners who care for children to recognize and manage abnormal variations.

The genetic makeup and the physical, emotional, and social environment of the individual determine how a child grows and develops throughout childhood. One goal of pediatrics is to help each child achieve his or her individual potential through periodically monitoring and screening for the normal progression or abnormalities of growth and development. The American Academy of Pediatrics recommends routine office visits in the first week of life (depending on timing of nursery discharge); at 2 weeks; at 1, 2, 4, 6, 9, 12, 15, and 18 months; at 2, 2½, and 3 years; and then annually through adolescence/young adulthood (see Fig. 9.1; the *Bright Futures'* "Recommendations for Preventive Pediatric Health Care" found at https://www.aap.org/en-us/documents/periodicity_schedule.pdf).

Deviations in growth patterns may be nonspecific or may be important indicators of serious and chronic medical disorders. An accurate measurement of length/height, weight, and head circumference should be obtained at every health supervision visit and compared with statistical norms on growth charts. Table 5.1 summarizes several convenient benchmarks to evaluate normal growth. Serial measurements are much more useful than single measurements to detect deviations from a particular growth pattern even if the value remains within statistically defined normal limits (percentiles). Following the trend helps define whether growth is within acceptable limits or warrants further evaluation.

Growth is assessed by plotting accurate measurements on growth charts and comparing each set of measurements with previous measurements obtained at health visits. Please see examples in Figs. 5.1-5.4. Complete charts can be found at www.cdc.gov/growthcharts. The body mass index is defined as body weight in kilograms divided by height in meters squared; it is used to classify adiposity and is recommended as a screening tool for children and adolescents to identify those overweight or at risk for being overweight (see Chapter 29).

Normal growth patterns have spurts and plateaus, so some shifting on percentile graphs can be expected. Large shifts in percentiles warrant attention, as do large discrepancies in height, weight, and head circumference percentiles. When caloric intake is inadequate, the weight percentile falls first, then the height, and the head circumference is last. Caloric intake may be poor as a result of inadequate feeding or because the child is not receiving adequate attention and stimulation (*nonorganic* failure to thrive [see Chapter 21]).

Caloric intake also may be inadequate because of increased caloric needs. Children with chronic illnesses, such as heart failure or cystic fibrosis, may require a significantly higher caloric intake to sustain growth. An increasing weight percentile in

TABLE 5.1 Rules of Thumb for Growth
WEIGHT
Weight loss in first few days: 5-10% of birthweight
Return to birthweight: 7-10 days of age
Double birthweight: 4-5 months
Triple birthweight: 1 year
Daily weight gain:
20-30 g for first 3-4 months
15-20 g for rest of the first year
HEIGHT
Average length: 20 in. at birth, 30 in. at 1 year
At age 4 years, the average child is double birth length or 40 in.
HEAD CIRCUMFERENCE (HC)
Average HC: 35 cm at birth (13.5 in.)
HC increases: 1 cm per month for first year (2 cm per month for first 3 months, then slower)

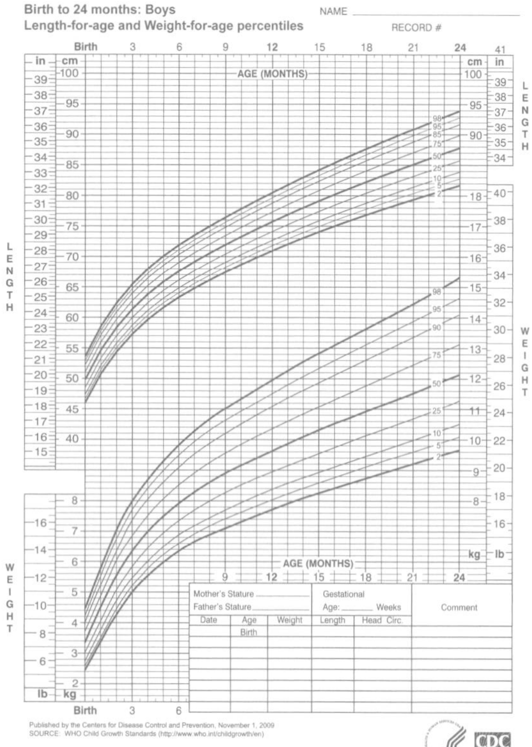

FIGURE 5.1 Length-by-age and weight-by-age percentiles for boys, birth to 2 years of age. Developed by the National Center for Health Statistics in collaboration with the National Center for Chronic Disease Prevention and Health Promotion. (From Centers for Disease Control and Prevention. *WHO Child Growth Standards.* Atlanta, GA; 2009. Available at http://www.cdc.gov/growthcharts/who_charts.htm.)

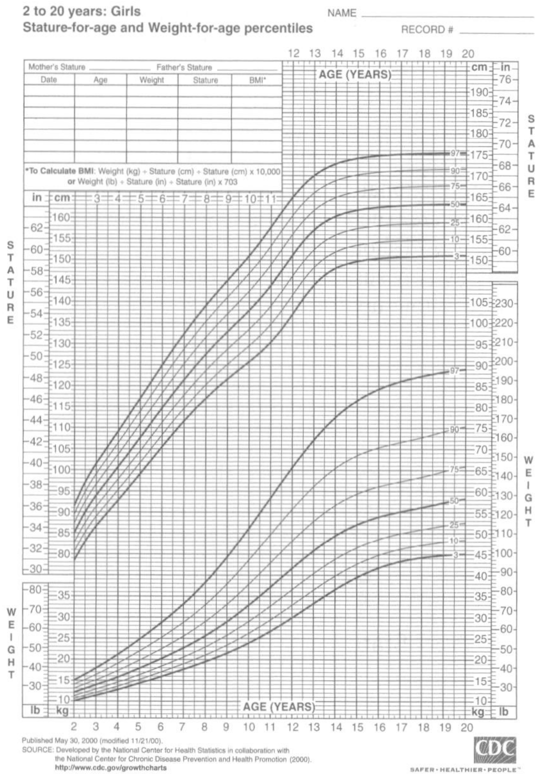

FIGURE 5.3 Stature-for-age and weight-for-age percentiles for girls, 2-20 years of age. Developed by the National Center for Health Statistics in collaboration with the National Center for Chronic Disease Prevention and Health Promotion. (From Centers for Disease Control and Prevention. Atlanta, GA; 2001. Available at http://www.cdc.gov/growthcharts.)

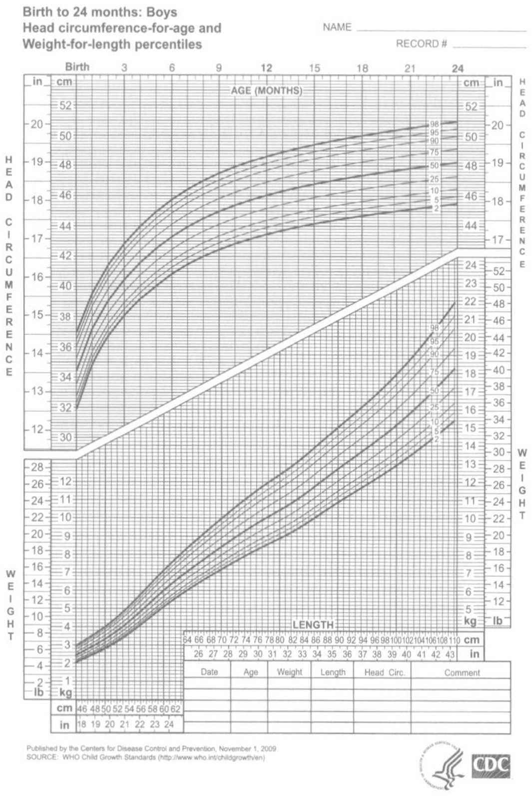

FIGURE 5.2 Head circumference and weight-by-length percentiles for boys, birth to 2 years of age. Developed by the National Center for Health Statistics in collaboration with the National Center for Chronic Disease Prevention and Health Promotion. (From Centers for Disease Control and Prevention. *WHO Child Growth Standards.* Atlanta, GA; 2009. Available at http://www.cdc.gov/growthcharts/who_charts.htm.)

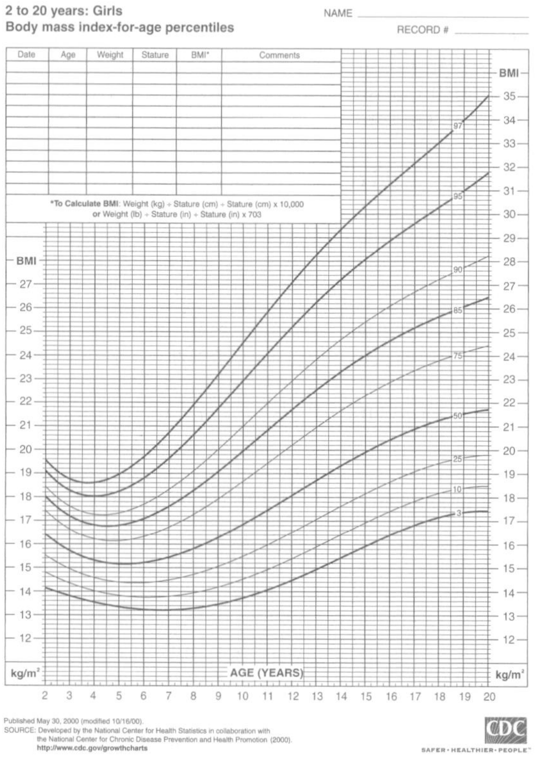

FIGURE 5.4 Body mass index–for-age percentiles for girls, 2-20 years of age. Developed by the National Center for Health Statistics in collaboration with the National Center for Chronic Disease Prevention and Health Promotion. (From Centers for Disease Control and Prevention. Atlanta, GA; 2001. Available at http://www.cdc.gov/growthcharts.)

the face of a falling height percentile suggests hypothyroidism. Head circumference may be disproportionately large when there is familial megalocephaly, hydrocephalus, or merely *catch-up* growth in a neurologically normal premature infant. A child is considered microcephalic if the head circumference is less than the third percentile, even if length and weight measurements also are proportionately low. Serial measurements of head circumference are crucial during infancy, a period of rapid brain development, and should be plotted regularly until the child is 2 years of age. Any suspicion of abnormal growth warrants at least a close follow-up, further evaluation, or both.

CHAPTER 6

Disorders of Growth

Decision-Making Algorithm
Available @ StudentConsult.com

Short Stature

The most common reasons for deviant measurements are technical (i.e., faulty equipment and human errors). Repeating a deviant measurement is the first step. Separate growth charts are available and should be used for very low birthweight infants (weight <1,500 g) and for those with Turner syndrome, Down syndrome, achondroplasia, and various other dysmorphology syndromes.

Variability in body proportions occurs from fetal to adult life. Newborns' heads are significantly larger in proportion to the rest of their body. This difference gradually disappears. Certain growth disturbances result in characteristic changes in the proportional sizes of the trunk, extremities, and head. Patterns requiring further assessment are summarized in Table 6.1.

TABLE 6.1 Specific Growth Patterns Requiring Further Evaluation

PATTERN	REPRESENTATIVE DIAGNOSES TO CONSIDER	FURTHER EVALUATION
Weight, length, head circumference all <5th percentile	Familial short stature Constitutional short stature Intrauterine insult Genetic abnormality	Midparental heights Evaluation of pubertal development Examination of prenatal records Chromosome analysis
Discrepant percentiles (e.g., weight 5th, length 5th, head circumference 50th, or other discrepancies)	Normal variant (familial or constitutional) Endocrine growth failure Caloric insufficiency	Midparental heights Thyroid hormone Growth factors, growth hormone testing Evaluation of pubertal development
Declining percentiles	*Catch-down growth* Caloric insufficiency Endocrine growth failure	Complete history and physical examination Dietary and social history Growth factors, growth hormone testing

Evaluating a child over time, coupled with a careful history and physical examination, helps determine whether the growth pattern is normal or abnormal. Parental heights may be useful when deciding whether to proceed with a further evaluation. Children, in general, follow their parents' growth pattern, although there are many exceptions.

For a girl, midparental height is calculated as follows:

$$\frac{\text{Paternal height (inches)} + \text{Maternal height (inches)}}{2} - 2.5$$

For a boy, midparental height is calculated as follows:

$$\frac{\textit{Paternal height (inches)} + \textit{Maternal height (inches)}}{2} + 2.5$$

Actual growth depends on too many variables to make an accurate prediction from midparental height determination for every child. The growth pattern of a child with low weight, length, and head circumference is commonly associated with **familial short stature** (see Chapter 173). These children are genetically normal but are smaller than most children. A child who, by age, is preadolescent or adolescent and who starts puberty later than others may have the normal variant called **constitutional short stature** (see Chapter 173); careful examination for abnormalities of pubertal development should be done. An evaluation for primary amenorrhea should be considered for any female adolescent who has not reached menarche by 15 years or has not done so within 3 years of thelarche (beginning of breast development). Lack of breast development by age 13 years also should be evaluated (see Chapter 174).

Starting out in high growth percentiles, many children assume a lower percentile between 6 and 18 months of age until they match their genetic programming; then they grow along new, lower percentiles. They usually do not decrease more than two major percentiles and have normal developmental, behavioral, and physical examinations. These children with *catch-down growth* should be followed closely, but no further evaluation is warranted.

Infants born small for gestational age, or prematurely, ingest more breast milk or formula and, unless there are complications that require extra calories, usually exhibit *catch-up growth* in the first 6 months. These infants should be fed on demand and provided as much as they want unless they are vomiting (not just spitting up [see Chapter 128]). Some may benefit from a higher caloric content formula. Many psychosocial risk factors that may have led to being born small or early may contribute to nonorganic failure to thrive (see Chapter 21). Conversely infants who recover from being low birthweight or premature have an increased risk of developing childhood obesity.

Growth of the nervous system is most rapid in the first 2 years, correlating with increasing physical, emotional, behavioral, and cognitive development. There is again rapid change during adolescence. Osseous maturation (bone age) is determined from radiographs on the basis of the number and size of calcified epiphyseal centers; the size, shape, density, and sharpness of outline of the ends of bones; and the distance separating the epiphyseal center from the zone of provisional calcification.

CHAPTER 7

Normal Development

PHYSICAL DEVELOPMENT

Parallel to the changes in the developing brain (i.e., cognition, language, behavior) are changes in the physical development of the body.

NEWBORN PERIOD

Observation of any asymmetric movement or altered muscle tone and function may indicate a significant central nervous system abnormality or a nerve palsy resulting from the delivery and requires further evaluation. Primitive neonatal reflexes are unique in the newborn period and can further elucidate or eliminate concerns over asymmetric function. The most important reflexes to assess during the newborn period are as follows:

The **Moro reflex** is elicited by allowing the infant's head to gently move back suddenly (from a few inches off of the mattress onto the examiner's hand), resulting in a startle, then abduction and upward movement of the arms followed by adduction and flexion. The legs respond with flexion.

The **rooting reflex** is elicited by touching the corner of the infant's mouth, resulting in lowering of the lower lip on the same side with tongue movement toward the stimulus. The face also turns toward the stimulus.

The **sucking reflex** occurs with almost any object placed in the newborn's mouth. The infant responds with vigorous sucking. The sucking reflex is replaced later by voluntary sucking.

The **asymmetric tonic neck reflex** is elicited by placing the infant supine and turning the head to the side. This placement results in ipsilateral extension of the arm and the leg into a "fencing" position. The contralateral side flexes as well.

A delay in the expected disappearance of the reflexes may also warrant an evaluation of the central nervous system.

See Sections 11 and 26 for additional information on the newborn period.

LATER INFANCY

With the development of gross motor skills, the infant is first able to control his or her posture, then proximal musculature, and, last, distal musculature. As the infant progresses through these stages, the parents may notice orthopedic deformities (see Chapters 202 and 203). The infant also may have deformities that are related to intrauterine positioning. Physical examination should indicate whether the deformity is fixed or can be moved passively into the proper position. When a joint held in an abnormal fashion can be moved passively into the proper position, there is a high likelihood of resolving with the progression of gross motor development. Fixed deformities warrant immediate pediatric orthopedic consultation (see Section 26).

Evaluation of vision and ocular movements is important to prevent the serious outcome of strabismus. The cover test and light reflex should be performed at early health maintenance visits; interventions after age 2 decrease the chance of preserving binocular vision or normal visual acuity (see Chapter 179).

SCHOOL AGE/PREADOLESCENT

Older school-age children who begin to participate in competitive sports should have a comprehensive sports history and physical examination, including a careful evaluation of the cardiovascular system. The American Academy of Pediatrics 4th edition sports preparticipation form is excellent for documenting cardiovascular and other risks. The patient and parent should complete the history form and be interviewed to assess cardiovascular risk. Any history of heart disease or a murmur must be referred for evaluation by a pediatric cardiologist. A child with a history of dyspnea or chest pain on exertion, irregular heart rate (i.e., skipped beats, palpitations), or syncope should also be referred to a pediatric cardiologist. A family history of a primary (immediate family) or secondary (immediate family's immediate family) atherosclerotic disease (myocardial infarction or cerebrovascular disease) before 50 years of age or sudden unexplained death at any age also requires additional assessment.

Children interested in contact sports should be assessed for special vulnerabilities. Similarly, vision should be assessed as a crucial part of the evaluation before participation in sports.

ADOLESCENCE

Adolescents need annual comprehensive health assessments to ensure progression through puberty without major problems (see Chapters 67 and 68). Sexual maturity is an important issue in adolescents, and all adolescents should be assessed to monitor progression through sexual maturity rating stages (see Chapter 67). Other issues in physical development include scoliosis, obesity, and common orthopedic growth issues (e.g., Osgood Schlatter; see Chapters 29 and 203). Most scoliosis is mild and requires only observation for resolution. Obesity may first manifest during childhood and is a growing public health for many adolescents.

DEVELOPMENTAL MILESTONES

The use of milestones to assess development focuses on discrete behaviors that the clinician can observe or accept as present by parental report. This approach is based on comparing the patient's behavior with that of many normal children whose behaviors evolve in a uniform sequence within specific age ranges (see Chapter 8). The development of the neuromuscular system, similar to that of other organ systems, is determined first by genetic endowment and then is molded by environmental influences.

Although a sequence of specific, easily measured behaviors can adequately represent some areas of development (**gross motor, fine motor**, and **language**), other areas, particularly social and emotional development, are not as easy to assess. Easily measured developmental milestones are well established through age 6 years only. Other types of assessment (e.g., intelligence tests, school performance, and personality profiles) that expand the developmental milestone approach are available for older children.

PSYCHOSOCIAL ASSESSMENT

Bonding and Attachment in Infancy

The terms *bonding* and *attachment* describe the affective relationships between parents and infants. **Bonding** occurs shortly after birth and reflects the feelings of the parents toward the newborn (unidirectional). **Attachment** involves reciprocal feelings between parent and infant and develops gradually over the first year.

Attachment of infants outside of the newborn period is crucial for optimal development. Infants who receive extra attention, such as parents responding immediately to any crying or fussiness in the first 4 months, show less crying and fussiness at the end of the first year. **Stranger anxiety** develops between 9 and 18 months of age, when infants normally become insecure about separation from the primary caregiver. The infant's new motor skills and attraction to novelty may lead to headlong plunges into new adventures that result in fright or pain followed by frantic efforts to find and cling to the primary caregiver. The result is dramatic swings from stubborn independence to clinging dependence that can be frustrating and confusing to parents. With secure attachment, this period of ambivalence may be shorter and less tumultuous.

Developing Autonomy in Early Childhood

Toddlers build on attachment and begin developing autonomy that allows separation from parents. In times of stress, toddlers often cling to their parents, but in their usual activities they may be actively separated. Ages 2-3 years are a time of major accomplishments in fine motor skills, social skills, cognitive skills, and language skills. The dependency of infancy yields to developing independence and the "I can do it myself" age. Limit setting is essential to a balance of the child's emerging independence.

Early Childhood Education

There is a growing body of evidence that notes that children who are in high quality early learning environments are more prepared to succeed in school. Every dollar invested in early childhood education may save taxpayers up to 13 dollars in future costs. These children commit fewer crimes and are better prepared to enter the workforce after school. Early Head Start (less than 3 years); Head Start (3-4 years), and prekindergarten programs (4-5 years) all demonstrate better educational attainment, although the earlier the start, the better the results.

School Readiness

Readiness for preschool depends on the development of autonomy and the ability of the parent and the child to separate for hours at a time. Preschool experiences help children develop socialization skills; improve language; increase skill building in areas such as colors, numbers, and letters; and increase problem solving (puzzles).

Readiness for school (kindergarten) requires emotional maturity, peer group and individual social skills, cognitive abilities, and fine and gross motor skills (Table 7.1). Other issues include chronological age and gender. Children tend to do better in kindergarten if their fifth birthday is at least 4-6 months before the beginning of school. Girls usually are ready earlier than boys.

TABLE 7.1 Evaluating School Readiness

PHYSICIAN OBSERVATIONS (BEHAVIORS OBSERVED IN THE OFFICE)
Ease of separation of the child from the parent
Speech development and articulation
Understanding of and ability to follow complex directions
Specific pre-academic skills
Knowledge of colors
Counts to 10
Knows age, first and last names, address, and phone number
Ability to copy shapes
Motor skills
Stand on one foot, skip, and catch a bounced ball
Dresses and undresses without assistance
PARENT OBSERVATIONS (QUESTIONS ANSWERED BY HISTORY)
Does the child play well with other children?
Does the child separate well, such as a child playing in the backyard alone with occasional monitoring by the parent?
Does the child show interest in books, letters, and numbers?
Can the child sustain attention to quiet activities?
How frequent are toilet-training *accidents*?

If the child is in less than the average developmental range, he or she should not be forced into early kindergarten. Holding a child back for reasons of developmental delay, in the false hope that the child will catch up, can also lead to difficulties. The child should enroll on schedule, and educational planning should be initiated to address any deficiencies.

Physicians should be able to identify children at risk for school difficulties, such as those who have developmental delays or physical disabilities. These children may require specialized school services in an individualized education plan (IEP).

Adolescence

Some define adolescence as 10-25 years of age, but adolescence is perhaps better characterized by the developmental stages (*early, middle,* and *late* adolescence) that all teens must negotiate to develop into healthy, functional adults. Different behavioral and developmental issues characterize each stage. The age at which each issue manifests and the importance of these issues vary widely among individuals, as do the rates of cognitive, psychosexual, psychosocial, and physical development.

During **early adolescence**, attention is focused on the present and on the peer group. Concerns are primarily related to the body's physical changes and normality. Strivings for independence are ambivalent. These young adolescents are difficult to interview because they often respond with short, clipped conversation and may have little insight. They are just becoming accustomed to abstract thinking.

Middle adolescence can be a difficult time for adolescents and the adults who have contact with them. Cognitive processes are more sophisticated. Through abstract thinking, middle adolescents can experiment with ideas, consider things as they might be, develop insight, and reflect on their own feelings and the feelings of others. As they mature, these adolescents focus on issues of identity not limited solely to the physical aspects of their body. They explore their parents' and culture's values, sometimes by expressing the contrary side of the dominant value. Many middle adolescents explore these values in their minds only; others do so by challenging their parents' authority. Many engage in high-risk behaviors, including unprotected sexual intercourse, substance abuse, or dangerous driving. The strivings of middle adolescents for independence, limit testing, and need for autonomy often distress their families, teachers, or other authority figures. These adolescents are at higher risk for morbidity and mortality from accidents, homicide, or suicide.

Late adolescence usually is marked by formal operational thinking, including thoughts about the future (e.g., educational, vocational, and sexual). Late adolescents are usually more committed to their sexual partners than are middle adolescents. Unresolved separation anxiety from previous developmental stages may emerge, at this time, as the young person begins to move physically away from the family of origin to college or vocational school, a job, or military service.

MODIFYING PSYCHOSOCIAL BEHAVIORS

Child behavior is determined by heredity and by the environment. Behavioral theory postulates that behavior is primarily a product of external environmental determinants and that manipulation of the environmental antecedents and consequences of behavior can be used to modify maladaptive behavior and to increase desirable behavior (operant conditioning). The four major methods of operant conditioning are positive reinforcement, negative reinforcement, extinction, and punishment. Many common behavioral problems of children can be ameliorated by these methods.

Positive reinforcement increases the frequency of a behavior by following the behavior with a favorable event (e.g., praising a child for excellent school performance). **Negative reinforcement** usually decreases the frequency of a behavior by removal, cessation, or avoidance of an unpleasant event. Conversely, sometimes this reinforcement may occur unintentionally, increasing the frequency of an undesirable behavior. For example, a toddler may purposely try to stick a pencil in a light socket to obtain attention, whether it be positive or negative. **Extinction** occurs when there is a decrease in the frequency of a previously reinforced behavior because the reinforcement is withheld. Extinction is the principle behind the common advice to ignore behavior such as crying at bedtime or temper tantrums, which parents may unwittingly reinforce through attention and comforting. **Punishment** decreases the frequency of a behavior through unpleasant consequences.

Positive reinforcement is more effective than punishment. Punishment is more effective when combined with positive reinforcement. A toddler who draws on the wall with a crayon may be punished, but he or she learns much quicker when positive reinforcement is given for the proper use of the crayon—on paper, not the wall. Interrupting and modifying behaviors are discussed in detail in Section 3.

TEMPERAMENT

Significant individual differences exist within the normal development of temperament (behavioral style). Temperament must be appreciated because, if an expected pattern of behavior is too narrowly defined, normal behavior may be inappropriately labeled as abnormal or pathologic. Three common constellations of temperamental characteristics are as follows:

1. The **easy child** (about 40% of children) is characterized by regularity of biological functions (consistent, predictable times for eating, sleeping, and elimination), a positive approach to new stimuli, high adaptability to change, mild or moderate intensity in responses, and a positive mood.
2. The **difficult child** (about 10%) is characterized by irregularity of biological functions, negative withdrawal from new stimuli, poor adaptability, intense responses, and a negative mood.
3. The **slow to warm up child** (about 15%) is characterized by a low activity level, withdrawal from new stimuli, slow adaptability, mild intensity in responses, and a somewhat negative mood.

The remaining 35% of children have more mixed temperaments. The individual temperament of a child has important implications for parenting and for the advice a pediatrician may give in anticipatory guidance or behavioral problem counseling.

Although temperament may be hardwired *(nature)* in each child to some degree, the environment *(nurture)* in which the child grows has a strong effect on the child's adjustment. Social and cultural factors can have marked effects on the child through differences in parenting style, educational approaches, and behavioral expectations.

CHAPTER 8
Disorders of Development

DEVELOPMENTAL SURVEILLANCE AND SCREENING

Developmental and behavioral problems are more common than any category of problems in pediatrics, except acute infections and trauma. In 2008, 15% of children ages 3-7 had a developmental disability and others had behavioral disabilities. As many as 25% of children have serious psychosocial problems. Parents often neglect to mention these problems because they think the physician is uninterested or cannot help. It is necessary to monitor development and screen for the presence of these problems at health supervision visits, particularly in the years before preschool or early childhood learning center enrollment.

Development surveillance, done at every office visit, is an informal process comparing skill levels to lists of milestones. If suspicion of developmental or behavioral issues recurs, further evaluation is warranted (Table 8.1). Surveillance does not have a standard, and screening tests are necessary.

Developmental screening involves the use of standardized screening tests to identify children who require further diagnostic assessment. The American Academy of Pediatrics recommends the use of validated standardized screening tools at three of the health maintenance visits: 9 months, 18 months, and 30 months. Clinics and offices that serve a higher risk patient population (children living in poverty) often perform a screening test at *every* health maintenance visit. A child who fails to pass a developmental screening test requires more comprehensive evaluation but does not necessarily have a delay; definitive testing must confirm. Developmental evaluations for children with suspected delays and intervention services for children with diagnosed disabilities are available free to families. A combination of U.S. state and federal funds provides these services.

TABLE 8.1 Developmental Milestones

AGE	GROSS MOTOR	FINE MOTOR–ADAPTIVE	PERSONAL-SOCIAL	LANGUAGE	OTHER COGNITIVE
2 wk	Moves head side to side	—	Regards face	Alerts to bell	—
2 mo	Lifts shoulder while prone	Tracks past midline	Smiles responsively	Cooing Searches for sound with eyes	—
4 mo	Lifts up on hands Rolls front to back If pulled to sit from supine, no head lag	Reaches for object Raking grasp	Looks at hand Begins to work toward toy	Laughs and squeals	—
6 mo	Sits alone	Transfers object hand to hand	Feeds self Holds bottle	Babbles	—
9 mo	Pulls to stand Gets into sitting position	Starting to pincer grasp Bangs two blocks together	Waves bye-bye Plays pat-a-cake	Says *Dada* and *Mama*, but nonspecific Two-syllable sounds	
12 mo	Walks Stoops and stands	Puts block in cup	Drinks from a cup Imitates others	Says *Mama* and *Dada*, specific Says one to two other words	—
15 mo	Walks backward	Scribbles Stacks two blocks	Uses spoon and fork Helps in housework	Says three to six words Follows commands	—
18 mo	Runs	Stacks four blocks Kicks a ball	Removes garment "Feeds" doll	Says at least six words	—
2 yr	Walks up and down stairs Throws overhand	Stacks six blocks Copies line	Washes and dries hands Brushes teeth Puts on clothes	Puts two words together Points to pictures Knows body parts	Understands concept of *today*
3 yr	Walks steps alternating feet Broad jump	Stacks eight blocks Wiggles thumb	Uses spoon well, spilling little Puts on T-shirt	Names pictures Speech understandable to stranger 75% Says three-word sentences	Understands concepts of *tomorrow* and *yesterday*
4 yr	Balances well on each foot Hops on one foot	Copies **O**, maybe **+** Draws person with three parts	Brushes teeth without help Dresses without help	Names colors Understands adjectives	—
5 yr	Skips Heel-to-toe walks	Copies □	—	Counts Understands opposites	—
6 yr	Balances on each foot 6 sec	Copies Δ Draws person with six parts	—	Defines words	Begins to understand *right* and *left*

Mo, Month; *sec*, second; *wk*, week; *yr*, year.

Screening tests can be categorized as general screening tests that cover all behavioral domains or as targeted screens that focus on one area of development. Some may be administered in the office by professionals, while others may be completed at home (or in a waiting room) by parents. Good developmental/behavioral screening instruments have a sensitivity of 70-80% in detecting suspected problems and a specificity of 70-80% in detecting normal development. Although 30% of children screened may be *over-referred* for definitive developmental testing, this group also includes children whose skills are below average and who may benefit from testing that may help address relative developmental deficits. The 20-30% of children who have disabilities that are not detected by the single administration of a screening instrument are likely to be identified on repeat screening at subsequent health maintenance visits.

The Denver Developmental Screening Test II was the first test used by general pediatricians, but it is now out of date and the company has closed. The test required observation of objective behavior and was difficult to administer consistently.

Today's most used developmental screening tools include **Ages and Stages Questionnaires** (developmental milestone driven) and **Parents' Evaluation of Developmental Status (PEDS)**. The latter is a simple, 10-item questionnaire that parents complete at office visits based on concerns with function and progression of development. Parent-reported screens have good validity compared to office-based screening measures. Many offices combine PEDS with developmental surveillance to track milestone attainment.

Autism screening is mandated for all children at 18-24 months of age. Although there are several tools, many pediatricians use the **Modified Checklist for Autism in Toddlers—Revised (M-CHAT-R)**. M-CHAT-R is an office-based questionnaire that asks parents about typical behaviors, some of which are more predictive than others for autism or other pervasive developmental disorders. If the child demonstrates more than two predictive or three total behaviors, further assessment with an interview algorithm is indicated to distinguish normal variant behaviors from those children needing a referral for definitive testing. The test is freely distributed on the internet and is available at https://www.m-chat.org (see Chapter 20).

Language screening correlates best with cognitive development in the early years. Table 8.2 provides some rules of thumb for language development that focus on speech production (expressive language). Although expressive language is the most obvious language element, the most dramatic changes in language development in the first years involve recognition and understanding (receptive language).

Whenever there is a speech and/or language delay, a **hearing deficit** must be considered. The implementation of universal newborn hearing screening detects many, if not most, of these children in the newborn period, and appropriate early intervention services may be provided. Conditions that present a high risk of an associated hearing deficit are listed in Table 8.3. Dysfluency *(stuttering)* is common in a 3- and 4-year-old child. Unless the dysfluency is severe, is accompanied by tics or unusual posturing, or occurs after 4 years of age, parents should be counseled that it is normal and transient and to accept it calmly and patiently.

After the child's sixth birthday and until adolescence, developmental assessment is initially done by inquiring about school performance (academic achievement and behavior). Inquiring about concerns raised by teachers or other adults who care for the child (after-school program counselor, coach, religious leader) is prudent. Formal developmental testing of these older children is beyond the scope of the primary care pediatrician. Nonetheless, the health care provider should be the coordinator of the testing and evaluation performed by other specialists (e.g., psychologists, psychiatrists, developmental pediatricians, and educational professionals).

TABLE 8.2 Rules of Thumb for Speech Screening

AGE (YR)	SPEECH PRODUCTION	ARTICULATION (AMOUNT OF SPEECH UNDERSTOOD BY A STRANGER)	FOLLOWING COMMANDS
1	One to three words	—	One-step commands
2	Two- to three-word phrases	One half	Two-step commands
3	Routine use of sentences	Three fourths	—
4	Routine use of sentence sequences; conversational give-and-take	Almost all	—
5	Complex sentences; extensive use of modifiers, pronouns, and prepositions	Almost all	—

TABLE 8.3 Conditions Considered High Risk for Associated Hearing Deficit

Congenital hearing loss in first cousin or closer relative
Bilirubin level of ≥20 mg/dL
Congenital rubella or other nonbacterial intrauterine infection
Defects in the ear, nose, or throat
Birthweight of ≤1,500 g
Multiple apneic episodes
Exchange transfusion
Meningitis
Five-minute Apgar score of ≤5
Persistent fetal circulation (primary pulmonary hypertension)
Treatment with ototoxic drugs (e.g., aminoglycosides and loop diuretics)

OTHER ISSUES IN ASSESSING DEVELOPMENT AND BEHAVIOR

Ignorance of environmental influences on child behavior may result in ineffective or inappropriate management (or both). Table 8.4 lists some contextual factors that should be considered in the etiology of a child's behavioral or developmental problem.

Building rapport with the parents and the child is a prerequisite for obtaining the often sensitive information that is essential for understanding a behavioral or developmental issue. Rapport usually can be established quickly if the parents sense that the clinician respects them and is genuinely interested in listening to their concerns. The clinician develops rapport with the child by engaging the child in developmentally appropriate conversation or play, perhaps providing toys while interviewing the parents, and being sensitive to the fears the child may have. Too often, the child is ignored until it is

TABLE 8.4 Context of Behavioral Problems

CHILD FACTORS
Health (past and current)
Developmental status
Temperament (e.g., difficult, slow to warm up)
Coping mechanisms
PARENTAL FACTORS
Misinterpretations of stage-related behaviors
Mismatch of parental expectations and characteristics of child
Mismatch of personality style between parent and child
Parental characteristics (e.g., depression, lack of interest, rejection, overprotective, coping)
ENVIRONMENTAL FACTORS
Stress (e.g., marital discord, unemployment, personal loss)
Support (e.g., emotional, material, informational, child care)
Poverty—including poor housing, poorer education facilities, lack of access to healthy foods (food deserts), unsafe environments, toxic stress, poor access to primary care
Racism

time for the physical examination. Similar to their parents, children feel more comfortable if they are greeted by name and involved in pleasant interactions before they are asked sensitive questions or threatened with examinations. Young children can be engaged in conversation on the parent's lap, which provides security and places the child at the eye level of the examiner.

With adolescents, emphasis should be placed on building a physician-patient relationship that is distinct from the relationship with the parents. The parents should not be excluded; however, the adolescent should have the opportunity to express concerns to and ask questions of the physician in confidence. Two intertwined issues must be taken into consideration—consent and confidentiality. Although laws vary from state to state, in general, adolescents who are able to give informed consent (i.e., mature minors) may consent to visits and care related to high-risk behaviors (i.e., substance abuse; sexual health, including prevention, detection, and treatment of sexually transmitted infections; and pregnancy). Most states support the physician who wishes the visit to be confidential. Physicians should become familiar with the governing law in the state where they practice (see https://www.guttmacher.org). Providing confidentiality is crucial, allowing for optimal care (especially for obtaining a history of risk behaviors). When assessing development and behavior, confidentiality can be achieved by meeting with the adolescent alone for at least part of each visit. However, parents must be informed when the clinician has significant and immediate concerns about the health and safety of the child. Often, the clinician can convince the adolescent to inform the parents directly about a problem or can reach an agreement with the adolescent about how the parents will be informed by the physician (see Chapter 67).

EVALUATING DEVELOPMENTAL AND BEHAVIORAL ISSUES

Responses to open-ended questions often provide clues to underlying, unstated problems and identify the appropriate direction for further, more directed questions. Histories about developmental and behavioral problems are often vague and confusing; to reconcile apparent contradictions, the interviewer frequently must request clarification, more detail, or mere repetition. By summarizing an understanding of the information at frequent intervals and by recapitulating at the close of the visit, the interviewer and patient and family can ensure that they understand each other.

If the clinician's impression of the child differs markedly from the parent's description, there may be a crucial parental concern or issue that has not yet been expressed, either because it may be difficult to talk about (e.g., marital problems), because it is unconscious, or because the parent overlooks its relevance to the child's behavior. Alternatively, the physician's observations may be atypical, even with multiple visits. The observations of teachers, relatives, and other regular caregivers may be crucial in sorting out this possibility. The parent also may have a distorted image of the child, rooted in parental psychopathology. A sensitive, supportive, and noncritical approach to the parent is crucial to appropriate intervention. More information about referral and intervention for behavioral and developmental issues is covered in Chapter 10.

CHAPTER 9

Evaluation of the Well Child

Health maintenance or supervision visits should consist of a comprehensive assessment of the child's health and of the parent's/guardian's role in providing an environment for optimal growth, development, and health. The American Academy of Pediatrics' (AAP) Bright Futures information standardizes each of the health maintenance visits and provides resources for working with the children and families of different ages (see https://brightfutures.aap.org). Elements of each visit include evaluation and management of parental concerns; inquiry about any interval illness since the last physical, growth, development, and nutrition; anticipatory guidance (including safety information and counseling); physical examination; screening tests; and immunizations (Table 9.1). The Bright Futures Recommendations for Preventive Pediatric Health Care, found at https://www.aap.org/en-us/Documents/periodicity_schedule.pdf, summarizes requirements and indicates the ages that specific prevention measures should be undertaken, including risk screening and performance items for specific measurements. Bright Futures is now the enforced standard for the Medicaid and the Children's Health Insurance Program, along with many insurers. Health maintenance and immunizations now are covered without copays for insured patients as part of the Patient Protection and Affordable Care Act.

TABLE 9.1 Topics for Health Supervision Visits
FOCUS ON THE CHILD
Concerns (parent's or child's)
Past problem follow-up
Immunization and screening test update
Routine care (e.g., eating, sleeping, elimination, and health habits)
Developmental progress
Behavioral style and problems
FOCUS ON THE CHILD'S ENVIRONMENT
Family
Caregiving schedule for caregiver who lives at home
Parent-child and sibling-child interactions
Extended family role
Family stresses (e.g., work, move, finances, illness, death, marital, and other interpersonal relationships)
Family supports (relatives, friends, groups)
Community
Caregivers outside of the family
Peer interaction
School and work
Recreational activities
Physical Environment
Appropriate stimulation
Safety

SCREENING TESTS

Children usually are quite healthy and only the following screening tests are recommended: newborn metabolic screening with hemoglobin electrophoresis, hearing and vision evaluation, anemia and lead screening, and tuberculosis testing. Children born to families with dyslipidemias or early heart disease should also be screened for lipid disorders; in addition, all children should have a routine cholesterol test between ages 9 and 11. (Items marked by a *star* in the Bright Futures Recommendations should be performed if a risk factor is found.) Sexually experienced adolescents should be screened for sexually transmissible infections and have an HIV test at least once between 16 and 18. When an infant, child, or adolescent begins with a new physician, the pediatrician should perform any missing screening tests and immunizations.

Newborn Screening

Metabolic Screening

Every state in the United States mandates newborn metabolic screening. Each state determines its own priorities and procedures, but the following diseases are usually included in metabolic screening: phenylketonuria, galactosemia, congenital hypothyroidism, maple sugar urine disease, and organic aciduria (see Section 10). Many states now screen for cystic fibrosis (CF) by testing for immunoreactive trypsinogen. If that test is positive, then a DNA analysis for the most common cystic fibrosis mutations is performed. This is not a perfect test due to the myriad mutations that lead to CF. Clinical suspicion warrants evaluation even if there were no CF mutations noted on the DNA analysis.

Hemoglobin Electrophoresis

Children with hemoglobinopathies are at higher risk for infection and complications from anemia, which early detection may prevent or ameliorate. Infants with sickle cell disease are begun on oral penicillin prophylaxis to prevent sepsis, which is the major cause of mortality in these infants (see Chapter 150).

Critical Congenital Heart Disease Screening

New for the fourth edition of Bright Futures is newborn screening for critical congenital heart disease (CCHD). Newborns with cyanotic congenital heart disease may be missed if the ductus arteriosus is still open; when the ductus closes, these children become profoundly cyanotic, leading to complications and even death. The AAP now mandates screening with pulse oximetry of the right hand and foot. The baby passes screening if the oxygen saturation is 95% or greater in the right hand and foot and the difference is three percentage points or less between the right hand and foot. The screen is immediately failed if the oxygen saturation is less than 90% in the right hand and foot. Equivocal tests are repeated, or echocardiography and pediatric cardiology consultation are warranted (see Chapters 143 and 144).

Hearing Evaluation

Because speech and language are central to a child's cognitive development, the hearing screening is performed before discharge from the newborn nursery. An infant's hearing is tested by placing headphones over the infant's ears and electrodes on the head. Standard sounds are played, and the transmission of the impulse to the brain is documented. If abnormal, a further evaluation using evoked response technology of sound transmission is indicated.

Hearing and Vision Screening of Older Children

Infants and Toddlers

Inferences about hearing are drawn from asking parents about responses to sound and speech and by examining speech and language development closely. Inferences about vision may be made by examining gross motor milestones (children with vision problems may have a delay) and by physical examination of the eye. Parental concerns about vision should be sought until the child is 3 years of age and about hearing until the child is 4 years of age. If there are concerns, definitive testing should be arranged. Hearing can be screened by auditory evoked responses, as mentioned for newborns. For toddlers and older children who cannot cooperate with formal audiologic testing with headphones, behavioral audiology may be used. Sounds of a specific frequency or intensity are provided in a standard environment within a soundproof room, and responses are assessed by a trained audiologist. Vision may be assessed by referral to a pediatric ophthalmologist and by visual evoked responses.

Children 3 Years of Age and Older

At various ages, hearing and vision should be screened objectively using standard techniques as specified in the Bright Futures Recommendations. Asking the family and child about any concerns or consequences of poor hearing or vision accomplishes subjective evaluation. At 3 years of age, children are screened for vision for the first time if they are developmentally able to be tested. Many children at this age do not have the interactive language or interpersonal skills to perform a vision screen; these children should be re-examined at a 3-6-month interval to ensure that their vision is normal. Because most of these children do not yet identify letters, using a Snellen eye chart with standard shapes is recommended. When a child is able to identify letters, the more accurate letter-based chart should be used. Audiologic testing of sounds with headphones should be begun on the fourth birthday (although Head Start requires that pediatricians attempt the hearing screening at 3 years of age). Any suspected audiologic problem should be evaluated by a careful history and physical examination with referral for comprehensive testing. Children who have a documented vision problem, failed screening, or parental concern should be referred, preferably to a pediatric ophthalmologist.

Anemia Screening

Children are screened for anemia at ages when there is a higher incidence of iron deficiency anemia. Infants are screened at birth and again at 4 months if there is a documented risk, such as low birthweight or prematurity. All infants are screened at 12 months of age because this is when a high incidence of iron deficiency is noted. Children are assessed at other visits for risks or concerns related to anemia (denoted by a *star* in the Bright Futures Recommendations at http://brightfutures.aap.org/clinical_practice.html). Any abnormalities detected should be evaluated for etiology. Anemic infants do not perform as well on standard developmental testing. When iron deficiency is strongly suspected, a therapeutic trial of iron may be used (see Chapter 150).

Lead Screening

Lead intoxication may cause developmental and behavioral abnormalities that are not reversible, even if the hematologic and other metabolic complications are treated. Although the Centers for Disease Control and Prevention (CDC) recommends environmental investigation at blood lead levels of 20 µg/dL on a single visit or persistent 15 µg/dL over a 3-month period, levels of 5-10 µg/dL may cause learning problems. Risk factors for lead intoxication include living in older homes with cracked or peeling lead-based paint, industrial exposure, use of foreign remedies (e.g., a diarrhea remedy from Central or South America), and use of pottery with lead paint glaze. Because of the significant association of lead intoxication with poverty, the CDC recommends routine blood lead screening at 12 and 24 months. In addition, standardized screening questions for risk of lead intoxication should be asked for all children between 6 months and 6 years of age (Table 9.2). Any positive or suspect response is an indication for obtaining a blood lead level. Capillary blood sampling may produce false-positive results; thus, in most situations, a venous blood sample should be obtained or a mechanism implemented to get children tested with a venous sample if they had an elevated capillary level. County health departments, community organizations, and private companies provide lead inspection and detection services to determine the source of the lead. Standard decontamination techniques should be used to remove the lead while avoiding aerosolizing the toxic metal that a child might breathe or creating dust that a child might ingest (see Chapters 149 and 150).

Tuberculosis Testing

The prevalence of tuberculosis is increasing largely as a result of the adult HIV epidemic. Children often present with serious and multisystem disease (miliary tuberculosis). All children should be assessed for risk of tuberculosis at health maintenance visits at 1 month, 6 months, 12 months, and then annually. The high-risk groups, as defined by the CDC, are listed in Table 9.3. In general, the standardized purified protein derivative intradermal test is used with evaluation by a health care provider 48-72 hours after injection. The size of induration, not the color of any mark, denotes a positive test. For most patients, 10 mm of induration is a positive test. For HIV-positive patients, those with recent tuberculosis contacts, patients with evidence of old healed tuberculosis on chest film, or immunosuppressed patients, 5 mm is a positive test (see Chapter 124). The CDC has also approved the QuantiFERON-TB Gold Test, which has the advantage of needing one office visit only.

Cholesterol

Children and adolescents who have a family history of cardiovascular disease or have at least one parent with a high blood cholesterol level are at increased risk of having high blood cholesterol levels as adults and increased risk of coronary heart disease. The AAP recommends dyslipidemia screening in the context of regular health care for at-risk populations (Table 9.4) by obtaining a fasting lipid profile. The recommended screening levels are the same for all children 2-18 years. Total cholesterol of less than 170 mg/dL is normal, 170-199 mg/dL is borderline, and greater than 200 mg/dL is elevated. In addition, in 2011, the AAP endorsed the National Heart, Lung, and Blood Institute of the National Institutes of Health recommendation to test all children between ages 9 and 11.

Sexually Transmitted Infection Testing

Annual office visits are recommended for adolescents. A full adolescent psychosocial history should be obtained in

TABLE 9.2 Lead Poisoning Risk Assessment Questions to Be Asked Between 6 Months and 6 Years
Does the child spend any time in a building built before 1960 (e.g., home, school, barn) that has cracked or peeling paint?
Is there a brother, sister, housemate, playmate, or community member being followed or treated (or even rumored to be) for lead poisoning?
Does the child live with an adult whose job or hobby involves exposure to lead (e.g., lead smelting and automotive radiator repair)?
Does the child live near an active lead smelter, battery recycling plant, or other industry likely to release lead?
Does the family use home remedies or pottery from another country?

TABLE 9.3 Groups at High Risk for Tuberculosis
Close contact with persons known to have tuberculosis (TB), positive TB test, or suspected to have TB
Foreign-born persons from areas with high TB rates (Asia, Africa, Latin America, Eastern Europe, Russia)
Health care workers
High-risk racial or ethnic minorities or other populations at higher risk (Asian, Pacific Islander, Hispanic, African American, Native American, groups living in poverty [e.g., Medicaid recipients], migrant farm workers, homeless persons, substance abusers)
Infants, children, and adolescents exposed to adults in high-risk categories

TABLE 9.4 Cholesterol Risk Screening Recommendations
Risk screening at ages 2, 4, 6, 8, 10, and annually in adolescence: 1. Children and adolescents who have a family history of high cholesterol or heart disease
2. Children whose family history is unknown
3. Children who have other personal risk factors: obesity, high blood pressure, or diabetes
Universal screening at ages 9-11 and ages 18-20

confidential fashion (see Section 12). Part of this evaluation is a comprehensive sexual history that often requires creative questioning. Not all adolescents identify oral sex as sex, and some adolescents misinterpret the term *sexually active* to mean that one has many sexual partners or is very vigorous during intercourse. The questions, "Are you having sex?" and "Have you ever had sex?" should be asked. In the Bright Futures Guidelines, any child or adolescent who has had any form of sexual intercourse should have at least an annual evaluation (more often if there is a history of high-risk sex) for sexually transmitted diseases by physical examination (genital warts, genital herpes, and pediculosis) and laboratory testing (chlamydia, gonorrhea, syphilis, and HIV) (see Chapter 116). Young women should be assessed for human papillomavirus and precancerous lesions by Papanicolaou smear at 21 years of age.

Depression Screening

All adolescents, starting at age 11, should have annual depression screening with a validated tool. The Patient Health Questionnaires (PHQ) are commonly used. Both the short PHQ2 and its slightly longer PHQ9 are available on the Bright Futures website in the Tool and Resource Kit at https://brightfutures.aap.org/materials-and-tools/tool-and-resource-kit/Pages/default.aspx.

IMMUNIZATIONS

Immunization records should be checked at each office visit regardless of the reason. Appropriate vaccinations should be administered (see Chapter 94).

DENTAL CARE

Many families in the United States, particularly poor families and ethnic minorities, underuse dental health care. Pediatricians may identify gross abnormalities, such as large caries, gingival inflammation, or significant malocclusion. All children should have a dental examination by a dentist at least annually and a dental cleaning by a dentist or hygienist every 6 months. Dental health care visits should include instruction about preventive care practiced at home (brushing and flossing). Other prophylactic methods shown to be effective at preventing caries are concentrated fluoride topical treatments (dental varnish) and acrylic sealants on the molars. A new change for the Bright Futures 4th Edition is the recommendation for Pediatricians to apply dental fluoride varnish to infants and children every 3-6 months between 9 months and 5 years. Pediatric dentists recommend beginning visits at age 1 year to educate families and to screen for milk bottle caries. Fluoridation of water or fluoride supplements in communities that do not have fluoridation are important in the prevention of cavities (see Chapter 127).

NUTRITIONAL ASSESSMENT

Plotting a child's growth on the standard charts is a vital component of the nutritional assessment. A dietary history should be obtained because the content of the diet may suggest a risk of nutritional deficiency (see Chapters 27 and 28).

ANTICIPATORY GUIDANCE

Anticipatory guidance is information conveyed to parents verbally, in written materials, or even directing parents to certain Internet websites to assist them in facilitating optimal growth and development for their children. Anticipatory guidance that is age relevant is another part of the Bright Futures Guidelines. The Bright Futures Tool and Resource Kit includes the topics and one-page handouts for families (and for older children) about the highest yield issues for the specific age. Table 9.5 summarizes representative issues that might be discussed. It is important to review briefly the safety topics previously discussed at other visits for reinforcement. Age-appropriate discussions should occur at each visit.

Safety Issues

The most common cause of death for infants 1 month to 1 year of age is **motor vehicle crashes**. No newborn should be discharged from a nursery unless the parents have a functioning and properly installed car seat. Many automobile dealerships offer services to parents to ensure that safety seats are installed properly in their specific model. Most states have laws that mandate the use of safety seats until the child reaches 4 years of age or at least 40 pounds in weight. The following are age-appropriate recommendations for car safety:

1. Infants and toddlers should ride in a **rear-facing safety seat** until they are 2 years of age or until they reach the highest weight or height allowed by the safety seat manufacturer.
2. Toddlers and preschoolers over age 2 or who have outgrown the rear-facing car seat should use a **forward-facing car seat** with harness for as long as possible up to the highest weight or height recommended by the manufacturer.
3. School-age children, whose weight or height is above the forward-facing limit for their car seat, should use a **belt-positioning booster seat** until the vehicle seat belt fits properly, typically when they have reached 4 ft 9 in. in height and are between 8 and 12 years of age.
4. Older children should always use **lap and shoulder seat belts** for optimal protection. All children younger than 13 years should be restrained in the rear seats of vehicles for optimal protection. This is specifically to protect them from airbags, which may cause more injury than the crash in young children.

The ***Back to Sleep*** **initiative** has reduced the incidence of sudden infant death syndrome (SIDS). Before the initiative, infants routinely were placed prone to sleep. Since 1992, when the AAP recommended this program, the annual SIDS rate has decreased by more than 50%. Another initiative is aimed at day care providers, because 20% of SIDS deaths occur in day care settings.

Fostering Optimal Development

See Table 9.5 as well as the Bright Futures Recommendations (Fig. 9.1; also found at http://brightfutures.aap.org/clinical_practice.html) for presentation of age-appropriate activities that the pediatrician may advocate for families.

Discipline means to teach, not merely to punish. The ultimate goal is the child's self-control. Overbearing punishment to control a child's behavior interferes with the learning process and focuses on external control at the expense of the

TABLE 9.5 Anticipatory Guidance Topics Suggested by Age

AGES	INJURY PREVENTION	VIOLENCE PREVENTION	SLEEP POSITION	NUTRITIONAL COUNSELING	FOSTERING OPTIMAL DEVELOPMENT
Birth and/or 3-5 days	Crib safety Hot water heaters <120°F Car safety seats Smoke detectors	Assess bonding and attachment Identify family strife, lack of support, pathology Educate parents on nurturing	Back to sleep Crib safety	Exclusive breast-feeding encouraged Formula as a second-best option	Discuss parenting skills Refer for parenting education
2 weeks or 1 month	Falls	Reassess* Discuss sibling rivalry Assess if guns in the home	Back to sleep	Assess breast-feeding and offer encouragement, problem solving	Recognize and manage postpartum blues Child-care options
2 months	Burns/hot liquids	Reassess firearm safety	Back to sleep		Parent getting enough rest and managing returning to work
4 months	Infant walkers Choking/suffocation	Reassess	Back to sleep	Introduction of solid foods	Discuss central to peripheral motor development Praise good behavior
6 months	Burns/hot surfaces	Reassess		Assess status	Consistent limit-setting versus "spoiling" an infant Praise good behavior
9 months	Water safety Home safety review Ingestions/poisoning	Assess parents' ideas on discipline and "spoiling"		Avoiding juice Begin to encourage practice with cup drinking	Assisting infants to sleep through the night if not accomplished Praise good behavior
12 months	Firearm hazards Auto-pedestrian safety	Discuss time-out versus corporal punishment Avoiding media violence Review firearm safety		Introduction of whole cow's milk (and constipation with change discussed) Assess anemia, discuss iron-rich foods	Safe exploration Proper shoes Praise good behavior
15 months	Review and reassess topics	Encourage nonviolent punishments (time-out or natural consequences)		Discuss decline in eating with slower growth Assess food choices and variety	Fostering independence Reinforce good behavior Ignore annoying but not unsafe behaviors
18 months	Review and reassess topics	Limit punishment to high yield (not spilled milk!) Parents consistent in discipline		Discuss food choices, portions, "finicky" feeders	Preparation for toilet training Reinforce good behavior
2 years	Falls—play equipment	Assess and discuss any aggressive behaviors in the child		Assess body proportions and recommend low-fat milk Assess family cholesterol and atherosclerosis risk	Toilet training and resistance
3 years	Review and reassess topics	Review, especially avoiding media violence		Discuss optimal eating and the food pyramid Healthy snacks	Read to child Socializing with other children Head Start if possible
4 years	Booster seat versus seat belts			Healthy snacks	Read to child Head Start or pre-K options
5 years	Bicycle safety Water/pool safety	Developing consistent, clearly defined family rules and consequences Avoiding media violence		Assess for anemia Discuss iron-rich foods	Reinforcing school topics Read to child Library card Chores begun at home

Continued

TABLE 9.5 Anticipatory Guidance Topics Suggested by Age—cont'd

AGES	INJURY PREVENTION	VIOLENCE PREVENTION	SLEEP POSITION	NUTRITIONAL COUNSELING	FOSTERING OPTIMAL DEVELOPMENT
6 years	Fire safety	Reinforce consistent discipline Encourage nonviolent strategies Assess domestic violence Avoiding media violence		Assess content, offer specific suggestions	Reinforcing school topics After-school programs Responsibility given for chores (and enforced)
7-10 years	Sports safety Firearm hazard	Reinforcement Assess domestic violence Assess discipline techniques Avoiding media violence Walking away from fights (either victim or spectator)		Assess content, offer specific suggestions	Reviewing homework and reinforcing school topics After-school programs Introduce smoking and substance abuse prevention (concrete)
11-13 years	Review and reassess	Discuss strategies to avoid interpersonal conflicts Avoiding media violence Avoiding fights and walking away Discuss conflict resolution techniques		Junk food versus healthy eating	Reviewing homework and reinforcing school topics Smoking and substance abuse prevention (begin abstraction) Discuss and encourage abstinence; possibly discuss condoms and contraceptive options Avoiding violence Offer availability
14-16 years	Motor vehicle safety Avoiding riding with substance abuser	Establish new family rules related to curfews, school, and household responsibilities		Junk food versus healthy eating	Review school work Begin career discussions and college preparation (PSAT) Review substance abuse, sexuality, and violence regularly Discuss condoms, contraception options, including emergency contraception Discuss sexually transmitted diseases, HIV Providing "no questions asked" ride home from at-risk situations
17-21 years	Review and reassess	Establish new rules related to driving, dating, and substance abuse		Heart healthy diet for life	Continuation of above topics Off to college or employment New roles within the family

*Reassess *means to review the issues discussed at the prior health maintenance visit.*
PSAT, Preliminary scholastic aptitude test.

development of self-control. Parents who set too few reasonable limits may be frustrated by children who cannot control their own behavior. Discipline should teach a child exactly what is expected by supporting and reinforcing positive behaviors and responding appropriately to negative behaviors with proper limits. It is more important and effective to reinforce good behavior than to punish bad behavior.

Commonly used techniques to control undesirable behaviors in children include scolding, physical punishment, and threats. These techniques have potential adverse effects on children's sense of security and self-esteem. The effectiveness of scolding diminishes the more it is used. Scolding should not be allowed to expand from an expression of displeasure about a specific event to derogatory statements about the child. Scolding also may escalate to the level of psychological abuse. It is important to educate parents that they have a *good child who does bad things from time to time*, so parents do not think and tell the child that he or she is "bad."

Frequent mild physical punishment (corporal punishment) may become less effective over time and tempt the parent to escalate the physical punishment, increasing the risk of child abuse. Corporal punishment teaches a child that in certain situations it is proper to strike another person. Commonly, in households that use spanking, older children who have been raised with this technique are seen responding to younger sibling behavioral problems by hitting their siblings.

Threats by parents to leave or to give up the child are perhaps the most psychologically damaging ways to control a child's behavior. Children of any age may remain fearful and anxious about loss of the parent long after the threat is made; however, many children are able to see through empty threats. Threatening a mild loss of privileges (no video games for 1 week or grounding a teenager) may be appropriate, but the consequence must be enforced if there is a violation.

Parenting involves a dynamic balance between **setting limits** on the one hand and allowing and encouraging freedom of expression and exploration on the other. A child whose behavior is out of control improves when clear limits on their behavior are set and enforced. However, parents must agree on where the limit will be set and how it will be enforced. The limit and the consequence of breaking the limit must be clearly presented to the child. Enforcement of the limit should be consistent and firm. Too many limits are difficult to learn and may thwart the normal development of autonomy. The limit must be reasonable in terms of the child's age, temperament, and developmental level. To be effective, both parents (and other adults in the home) must enforce limits. Otherwise, children may effectively *split* the parents and seek to test the limits with the more indulgent parent. In all situations, to be effective, punishment must be brief and linked directly to a behavior. More effective behavioral change occurs when punishment also is linked to praise of the intended behavior.

Extinction is an effective and systematic way to eliminate a frequent, annoying, and relatively harmless behavior by ignoring it. First parents should note the frequency of the behavior to appreciate realistically the magnitude of the problem and to evaluate progress. Parents must determine what reinforces the child's behavior and what needs to be consistently eliminated. An appropriate behavior is identified to give the child a positive alternative that the parents can reinforce. Parents should be warned that the annoying behavior usually increases in frequency and intensity (and may last for weeks) before it decreases when the parent ignores it (removes the reinforcement). A child who has an attention-seeking temper tantrum should be ignored or placed in a secure environment. This action may anger the child more, and the behavior may get louder and angrier. Eventually with no audience for the tantrum, the tantrums decrease in intensity and frequency. In each specific instance, when the child's behavior has become appropriate, he or she should be praised, and extra attention should be given. This is an effective technique for early toddlers, before their capacity to understand and adhere to a time-out develops.

The **time-out** consists of a short period of isolation *immediately* after a problem behavior is observed. Time-out interrupts the behavior and immediately links it to an unpleasant consequence. This method requires considerable effort by the parents because the child does not wish to be isolated. A parent may need to hold the child physically in time-out. In this situation, the parent should become *part of the furniture* and should not respond to the child until the time-out period is over. When established, a simple isolation technique, such as making a child stand in the corner or sending a child to his or her room, may be effective. If such a technique is not helpful, a more systematic procedure may be needed. One effective protocol for the time-out procedure involves interrupting the child's play when the behavior occurs and having the child sit in a dull, isolated place for a brief period, measured by a portable kitchen timer (the clicking noises document that time is passing and the bell alarm at the end signals the end of the punishment). Time-out is simply punishment and is not a time for a young child to *think* about the behavior (these children do not possess the capacity for abstract thinking) or a time to de-escalate the behavior. The amount of time-out should be appropriate to the child's short attention span. One minute per year of a child's age is recommended. This inescapable and unpleasant consequence of the undesired behavior motivates the child to learn to avoid the behavior.

American Academy of Pediatrics
DEDICATED TO THE HEALTH OF ALL CHILDREN®

Recommendations for Preventive Pediatric Health Care

Bright Futures/American Academy of Pediatrics

Bright Futures. prevention and health promotion for infants, children, adolescents, and their families™

Each child and family is unique; therefore, these Recommendations for Preventive Pediatric Health Care are designed for the care of children who are receiving competent parenting, have no manifestations of any important health problems, and are growing and developing in a satisfactory fashion. Developmental, psychosocial, and chronic disease issues for children and adolescents may require frequent counseling and treatment visits separate from preventive care visits. Additional visits also may become necessary if circumstances suggest variations from normal.

These recommendations represent a consensus by the American Academy of Pediatrics (AAP) and Bright Futures. The AAP continues to emphasize the great importance of continuity of care in comprehensive health supervision and the need to avoid fragmentation of care.

Refer to the specific guidance by age as listed in the *Bright Futures Guidelines* (Hagan JF, Shaw JS, Duncan PM, eds. *Bright Futures: Guidelines for Health Supervision of Infants, Children, and Adolescents.* 4th ed. Elk Grove Village, IL: American Academy of Pediatrics; 2017).

The recommendations in this statement do not indicate an exclusive course of treatment or standard of medical care. Variations, taking into account individual circumstances, may be appropriate.

	INFANCY								EARLY CHILDHOOD							MIDDLE CHILDHOOD						ADOLESCENCE										
AGE[1]	**Prenatal**[2]	**Newborn**[3]	**3-5 d**[4]	**By 1 mo**	**2 mo**	**4 mo**	**6 mo**	**9 mo**	**12 mo**	**15 mo**	**18 mo**	**24 mo**	**30 mo**	**3 y**	**4 y**	**5 y**	**6 y**	**7 y**	**8 y**	**9 y**	**10 y**	**11 y**	**12 y**	**13 y**	**14 y**	**15 y**	**16 y**	**17 y**	**18 y**	**19 y**	**20 y**	**21 y**
HISTORY Initial/Interval	●	●	●	●	●	●	●	●	●	●	●	●	●	●	●	●	●	●	●	●	●	●	●	●	●	●	●	●	●	●	●	●
MEASUREMENTS																																
Length/Height and Weight		●	●	●	●	●	●	●	●	●	●	●	●	●	●	●	●	●	●	●	●	●	●	●	●	●	●	●	●	●	●	●
Head Circumference		●	●	●	●	●	●	●	●	●	●	●																				
Weight for Length		●	●	●	●	●	●	●	●	●	●																					
Body Mass Index[5]												●	●	●	●	●	●	●	●	●	●	●	●	●	●	●	●	●	●	●	●	●
Blood Pressure[6]		★	★	★	★	★	★	★	★	★	★	★	★	●	●	●	●	●	●	●	●	●	●	●	●	●	●	●	●	●	●	●
SENSORY SCREENING																																
Vision[7]		★	★	★	★	★	★	★	★	★	★	★	★	●	●	●	●	★	●	★	●	★	●	★	★	●	★	★	★	★	★	★
Hearing		●[8]	●[9] →	→	→	★	★	★	★	★	★	★	★	★	●	●	●	★	●	★	●	←	—	●[10]	→	←	●	→	←	—	●	→
DEVELOPMENTAL/BEHAVIORAL HEALTH																																
Developmental Screening[11]								●			●		●																			
Autism Spectrum Disorder Screening[12]											●	●																				
Developmental Surveillance		●	●	●	●	●	●		●	●		●		●	●	●	●	●	●	●	●	●	●	●	●	●	●	●	●	●	●	●
Psychosocial/Behavioral Assessment[13]		●	●	●	●	●	●	●	●	●	●	●	●	●	●	●	●	●	●	●	●	●	●	●	●	●	●	●	●	●	●	●
Tobacco, Alcohol, or Drug Use Assessment[14]																						★	★	★	★	★	★	★	★	★	★	★
Depression Screening[15]																							●	●	●	●	●	●	●	●	●	●
Maternal Depression Screening[16]				●	●	●	●																									
PHYSICAL EXAMINATION[17]		●	●	●	●	●	●	●	●	●	●	●	●	●	●	●	●	●	●	●	●	●	●	●	●	●	●	●	●	●	●	●
PROCEDURES[18]																																
Newborn Blood		●[19]	●[20] →	→	→																											
Newborn Bilirubin[21]		●																														
Critical Congenital Heart Defect[22]		●																														
Immunization[23]		●	●	●	●	●	●	●	●	●	●	●	●	●	●	●	●	●	●	●	●	●	●	●	●	●	●	●	●	●	●	●
Anemia[24]						★			●	★	★	★	★	★	★	★	★	★	★	★	★	★	★	★	★	★	★	★	★	★	★	★
Lead[25]							★	★	● or ★[26]		★	● or ★[26]		★	★	★	★															
Tuberculosis[27]				★			★		★			★		★	★	★	★	★	★	★	★	★	★	★	★	★	★	★	★	★	★	★
Dyslipidemia[28]												★			★		★		★	←	●	→	★	★	★	★	★	←	—	—	●	→
Sexually Transmitted Infections[29]																						★	★	★	★	★	★	★	★	★	★	★
HIV[30]																						★	★	★	★	←	—	●	→	★	★	★
Cervical Dysplasia[31]																																●
ORAL HEALTH[32]							●[33]	●[33]	★		★	★	★	★	★	★	★															
Fluoride Varnish[34]							←	—	—	—	●	—	—	—	—	→																
Fluoride Supplementation[35]							★	★	★		★	★	★	★	★	★	★	★	★	★	★	★	★	★	★	★	★					
ANTICIPATORY GUIDANCE	●	●	●	●	●	●	●	●	●	●	●	●	●	●	●	●	●	●	●	●	●	●	●	●	●	●	●	●	●	●	●	●

1. If a child comes under care for the first time at any point on the schedule, or if any items are not accomplished at the suggested age, the schedule should be brought up-to-date at the earliest possible time.
2. A prenatal visit is recommended for parents who are at high risk, for first-time parents, and for those who request a conference. The prenatal visit should include anticipatory guidance, pertinent medical history, and a discussion of benefits of breastfeeding and planned method of feeding, per "The Prenatal Visit" (http://pediatrics.aappublications.org/content/124/4/1227.full).
3. Newborns should have an evaluation after birth, and breastfeeding should be encouraged (and instruction and support should be offered).
4. Newborns should have an evaluation within 3 to 5 days of birth and within 48 to 72 hours after discharge from the hospital to include evaluation for feeding and jaundice. Breastfeeding newborns should receive formal breastfeeding evaluation, and their mothers should receive encouragement and instruction, as recommended in "Breastfeeding and the Use of Human Milk" (http://pediatrics.aappublications.org/content/129/3/e827.full). Newborns discharged less than 48 hours after delivery must be examined within 48 hours of discharge, per "Hospital Stay for Healthy Term Newborns" (http://pediatrics.aappublications.org/content/125/2/405.full).
5. Screen, per "Expert Committee Recommendations Regarding the Prevention, Assessment, and Treatment of Child and Adolescent Overweight and Obesity: Summary Report" (http://pediatrics.aappublications.org/content/120/Supplement_4/S164.full).
6. Blood pressure measurement in infants and children with specific risk conditions should be performed at visits before age 3 years.
7. A visual acuity screen is recommended at ages 4 and 5 years, as well as in cooperative 3-year-olds. Instrument-based screening may be used to assess risk at ages 12 and 24 months, in addition to the well visits at 3 through 5 years of age. See "Visual System Assessment in Infants, Children, and Young Adults by Pediatricians" (http://pediatrics.aappublications.org/content/137/1/e20153596) and "Procedures for the Evaluation of the Visual System by Pediatricians" (http://pediatrics.aappublications.org/content/137/1/e20153597).
8. Confirm initial screen was completed, verify results, and follow up, as appropriate. Newborns should be screened, per "Year 2007 Position Statement: Principles and Guidelines for Early Hearing Detection and Intervention Programs" (http://pediatrics.aappublications.org/content/120/4/898.full).
9. Verify results as soon as possible, and follow up, as appropriate.
10. Screen with audiometry including 6,000 and 8,000 Hz high frequencies once between 11 and 14 years, once between 15 and 17 years, and once between 18 and 21 years. See "The Sensitivity of Adolescent Hearing Screens Significantly Improves by Adding High Frequencies" (http://www.jahonline.org/article/S1054-139X(16)00048-3/fulltext).
11. See "Identifying Infants and Young Children With Developmental Disorders in the Medical Home: An Algorithm for Developmental Surveillance and Screening" (http://pediatrics.aappublications.org/content/118/1/405.full).
12. Screening should occur per "Identification and Evaluation of Children With Autism Spectrum Disorders" (http://pediatrics.aappublications.org/content/120/5/1183.full).
13. This assessment should be family centered and may include an assessment of child social-emotional health, caregiver depression, and social determinants of health. See "Promoting Optimal Development: Screening for Behavioral and Emotional Problems" (http://pediatrics.aappublications.org/content/135/2/384) and "Poverty and Child Health in the United States" (http://pediatrics.aappublications.org/content/137/4/e20160339).
14. A recommended assessment tool is available at http://www.ceasar-boston.org/CRAFFT/index.php.
15. Recommended screening using the Patient Health Questionnaire (PHQ)-2 or other tools available in the GLAD-PC toolkit and at http://www.aap.org/en-us/advocacy-and-policy/aap-health-initiatives/Mental-Health/Documents/MH_ScreeningChart.pdf.
16. Screening should occur per "Incorporating Recognition and Management of Perinatal and Postpartum Depression Into Pediatric Practice" (http://pediatrics.aappublications.org/content/126/5/1032).
17. At each visit, age-appropriate physical examination is essential, with infant totally unclothed and older children undressed and suitably draped. See "Use of Chaperones During the Physical Examination of the Pediatric Patient" (http://pediatrics.aappublications.org/content/127/5/991.full).
18. These may be modified, depending on entry point into schedule and individual need.

(continued)

KEY: ● = to be performed ★ = risk assessment to be performed with appropriate action to follow, if positive ←—●—→ = range during which a service may be provided

FIGURE 9.1 (From Bright Futures Guidelines for Health Supervision of Infants, Children, and Adolescents. 4th ed. Copyright 2017 by the American Academy of Pediatrics. Reproduced with permission. Available at https://www.aap.org/en-us/documents/periodicity_schedule.pdf.)

(continued)

19. Confirm initial screen was accomplished, verify results, and follow up, as appropriate. The Recommended Uniform Newborn Screening Panel (http://www.hrsa.gov/advisorycommittees/mchbadvisory/heritabledisorders/recommendedpanel/uniformscreeningpanel.pdf), as determined by The Secretary's Advisory Committee on Heritable Disorders in Newborns and Children, and state newborn screening laws/regulations (http://genes-r-us.uthscsa.edu/sites/genes-r-us/files/nbsdisorders.pdf) establish the criteria for and coverage of newborn screening procedures and programs.
20. Verify results as soon as possible, and follow up, as appropriate.
21. Confirm initial screening was accomplished, verify results, and follow up, as appropriate. See "Hyperbilirubinemia in the Newborn Infant ≥35 Weeks' Gestation: An Update With Clarifications" (http://pediatrics.aappublications.org/content/124/4/1193).
22. Screening for critical congenital heart disease using pulse oximetry should be performed in newborns, after 24 hours of age, before discharge from the hospital, per "Endorsement of Health and Human Services Recommendation for Pulse Oximetry Screening for Critical Congenital Heart Disease" (http://pediatrics.aappublications.org/content/129/1/190.full).
23. Schedules, per the AAP Committee on Infectious Diseases, are available at http://redbook.solutions.aap.org/SS/Immunization_Schedules.aspx. Every visit should be an opportunity to update and complete a child's immunizations.
24. See "Diagnosis and Prevention of Iron Deficiency and Iron-Deficiency Anemia in Infants and Young Children (0–3 Years of Age)" (http://pediatrics.aappublications.org/content/126/5/1040.full).
25. For children at risk of lead exposure, see "Low Level Lead Exposure Harms Children: A Renewed Call for Primary Prevention" (http://www.cdc.gov/nceh/lead/ACCLPP/Final_Document_030712.pdf).
26. Perform risk assessments or screenings as appropriate, based on universal screening requirements for patients with Medicaid or in high prevalence areas.
27. Tuberculosis testing per recommendations of the AAP Committee on Infectious Diseases, published in the current edition of the AAP *Red Book: Report of the Committee on Infectious Diseases*. Testing should be performed on recognition of high-risk factors.
28. See "Integrated Guidelines for Cardiovascular Health and Risk Reduction in Children and Adolescents" (http://www.nhlbi.nih.gov/guidelines/cvd_ped/index.htm).
29. Adolescents should be screened for sexually transmitted infections (STIs) per recommendations in the current edition of the AAP *Red Book: Report of the Committee on Infectious Diseases.*
30. Adolescents should be screened for HIV according to the USPSTF recommendations (http://www.uspreventiveservicestaskforce.org/uspstf/uspshivi.htm) once between the ages of 15 and 18, making every effort to preserve confidentiality of the adolescent. Those at increased risk of HIV infection, including those who are sexually active, participate in injection drug use, or are being tested for other STIs, should be tested for HIV and reassessed annually.
31. See USPSTF recommendations (http://www.uspreventiveservicestaskforce.org/uspstf/uspscerv.htm). Indications for pelvic examinations prior to age 21 are noted in "Gynecologic Examination for Adolescents in the Pediatric Office Setting" (http://pediatrics.aappublications.org/content/126/3/583.full).
32. Assess whether the child has a dental home. If no dental home is identified, perform a risk assessment (http://www2.aap.org/oralhealth/docs/RiskAssessmentTool.pdf) and refer to a dental home. Recommend brushing with fluoride toothpaste in the proper dosage for age. See "Maintaining and Improving the Oral Health of Young Children" (http://pediatrics.aappublications.org/content/134/6/1224).
33. Perform a risk assessment (http://www2.aap.org/oralhealth/docs/RiskAssessmentTool.pdf). See "Maintaining and Improving the Oral Health of Young Children" (http://pediatrics.aappublications.org/content/134/6/1224).
34. See USPSTF recommendations (http://www.uspreventiveservicestaskforce.org/uspstf/uspsdnch.htm). Once teeth are present, fluoride varnish may be applied to all children every 3–6 months in the primary care or dental office. Indications for fluoride use are noted in "Fluoride Use in Caries Prevention in the Primary Care Setting" (http://pediatrics.aappublications.org/content/134/3/626).
35. If primary water source is deficient in fluoride, consider oral fluoride supplementation. See "Fluoride Use in Caries Prevention in the Primary Care Setting" (http://pediatrics.aappublications.org/content/134/3/626).

Summary of Changes Made to the Bright Futures/AAP Recommendations for Preventive Pediatric Health Care
(Periodicity Schedule)

This schedule reflects changes approved in February 2017 and published in April 2017.
For updates, visit www.aap.org/periodicityschedule.
For further information, see the *Bright Futures Guidelines*, 4th Edition, *Evidence and Rationale chapter* (https://brightfutures.aap.org/Bright%20Futures%20Documents/BF4_Evidence_Rationale.pdf).

CHANGES MADE IN FEBRUARY 2017

HEARING

- Timing and follow-up of the screening recommendations for hearing during the infancy visits have been delineated. Adolescent risk assessment has changed to screening once during each time period.
- Footnote 8 has been updated to read as follows: "Confirm initial screen was completed, verify results, and follow up, as appropriate. Newborns should be screened, per 'Year 2007 Position Statement: Principles and Guidelines for Early Hearing Detection and Intervention Programs' (http://pediatrics.aappublications.org/content/120/4/898.full)."
- Footnote 9 has been added to read as follows: "Verify results as soon as possible, and follow up, as appropriate."
- Footnote 10 has been added to read as follows: "Screen with audiometry including 6,000 and 8,000 Hz high frequencies once between 11 and 14 years, once between 15 and 17 years, and once between 18 and 21 years. See 'The Sensitivity of Adolescent Hearing Screens Significantly Improves by Adding High Frequencies' (http://www.jahonline.org/article/S1054-139X(16)00048-3/fulltext)."

PSYCHOSOCIAL/BEHAVIORAL ASSESSMENT

- Footnote 13 has been added to read as follows: "This assessment should be family centered and may include an assessment of child social-emotional health, caregiver depression, and social determinants of health. See 'Promoting Optimal Development: Screening for Behavioral and Emotional Problems' (http://pediatrics.aappublications.org/content/135/2/384) and 'Poverty and Child Health in the United States' (http://pediatrics.aappublications.org/content/137/4/e20160339)."

TOBACCO, ALCOHOL, OR DRUG USE ASSESSMENT

- The header was updated to be consistent with recommendations.

DEPRESSION SCREENING

- Adolescent depression screening begins routinely at 12 years of age (to be consistent with recommendations of the US Preventive Services Task Force [USPSTF]).

MATERNAL DEPRESSION SCREENING

- Screening for maternal depression at 1-, 2-, 4-, and 6-month visits has been added.
- Footnote 16 was added to read as follows: "Screening should occur per 'Incorporating Recognition and Management of Perinatal and Postpartum Depression Into Pediatric Practice' (http://pediatrics.aappublications.org/content/126/5/1032)."

NEWBORN BLOOD

- Timing and follow-up of the newborn blood screening recommendations have been delineated.
- Footnote 19 has been updated to read as follows: "Confirm initial screen was accomplished, verify results, and follow up, as appropriate. The Recommended Uniform Newborn Screening Panel (http://www.hrsa.gov/advisorycommittees/mchbadvisory/heritabledisorders/recommendedpanel/uniformscreeningpanel.pdf), as determined by The Secretary's Advisory Committee on Heritable Disorders in Newborns and Children, and state newborn screening laws/regulations (http://genes-r-us.uthscsa.edu/sites/genes-r-us/files/nbsdisorders.pdf) establish the criteria for and coverage of newborn screening procedures and programs."
- Footnote 20 has been added to read as follows: "Verify results as soon as possible, and follow up, as appropriate."

NEWBORN BILIRUBIN

- Screening for bilirubin concentration at the newborn visit has been added.
- Footnote 21 has been added to read as follows: "Confirm initial screening was accomplished, verify results, and follow up, as appropriate. See 'Hyperbilirubinemia in the Newborn Infant ≥35 Weeks' Gestation: An Update With Clarifications' (http://pediatrics.aappublications.org/content/124/4/1193)."

DYSLIPIDEMIA

- Screening for dyslipidemia has been updated to occur once between 9 and 11 years of age, and once between 17 and 21 years of age (to be consistent with guidelines of the National Heart, Lung, and Blood Institute).

SEXUALLY TRANSMITTED INFECTIONS

- Footnote 29 has been updated to read as follows: "Adolescents should be screened for sexually transmitted infections (STIs) per recommendations in the current edition of the AAP *Red Book: Report of the Committee on Infectious Diseases.*"

HIV

- A subheading has been added for the HIV universal recommendation to avoid confusion with STIs selective screening recommendation.
- Screening for HIV has been updated to occur once between 15 and 18 years of age (to be consistent with recommendations of the USPSTF).
- Footnote 30 has been added to read as follows: "Adolescents should be screened for HIV according to the USPSTF recommendations (http://www.uspreventiveservicestaskforce.org/uspstf/uspshivi.htm) once between the ages of 15 and 18, making every effort to preserve confidentiality of the adolescent. Those at increased risk of HIV infection, including those who are sexually active, participate in injection drug use, or are being tested for other STIs, should be tested for HIV and reassessed annually."

ORAL HEALTH

- Assessing for a dental home has been updated to occur at the 12-month and 18-month through 6-year visits. A subheading has been added for fluoride supplementation, with a recommendation from the 6-month through 12-month and 18-month through 16-year visits.
- Footnote 32 has been updated to read as follows: "Assess whether the child has a dental home. If no dental home is identified, perform a risk assessment (http://www2.aap.org/oralhealth/docs/RiskAssessmentTool.pdf) and refer to a dental home. Recommend brushing with fluoride toothpaste in the proper dosage for age. See 'Maintaining and Improving the Oral Health of Young Children' (http://pediatrics.aappublications.org/content/134/6/1224)."
- Footnote 33 has been updated to read as follows: "Perform a risk assessment (http://www2.aap.org/oralhealth/docs/RiskAssessmentTool.pdf). See 'Maintaining and Improving the Oral Health of Young Children' (http://pediatrics.aappublications.org/content/134/6/1224)."
- Footnote 35 has been added to read as follows: "If primary water source is deficient in fluoride, consider oral fluoride supplementation. See 'Fluoride Use in Caries Prevention in the Primary Care Setting' (http://pediatrics.aappublications.org/content/134/3/626)."

FIGURE 9.1, cont'd

CHAPTER 10

Evaluation of the Child With Special Needs

Children with disabilities, severe chronic illnesses, congenital defects, and health-related educational and behavioral problems are **children with special health care needs (SHCN)**. Many of these children share a broad group of experiences and encounter similar problems, such as school difficulties and family stress. The term *children with special health care needs* defines these children noncategorically, without regard to specific diagnoses, in terms of increased service needs. Approximately 19% of children in the United States younger than 18 years of age have a physical, developmental, behavioral, or emotional condition requiring services of a type or amount beyond those generally required by most children.

The goal in managing a child with SHCN is to maximize the child's potential for productive adult functioning by treating the primary diagnosis and by helping the patient and family deal with the stresses and secondary impairments incurred because of the disease or disability. Whenever a chronic disease is diagnosed, family members typically grieve, show anger, denial, negotiation (in an attempt to forestall the inevitable), and depression. Because the child with SHCN is a constant reminder of the object of this grief, it may take family members a long time to accept the condition. A supportive physician can facilitate the process of acceptance by education and by allaying guilty feelings and fear. To minimize denial, it is helpful to confirm the family's observations about the child. The family may not be able to absorb any additional information initially, so written material and the option for further discussion at a later date should be offered.

The primary physician should provide a **medical home** to maintain close oversight of treatments and subspecialty services, provide preventive care, and facilitate interactions with school and community agencies. A major goal of *family-centered care* is for the family and child to feel in control. Although the medical management team usually directs treatment in the acute health care setting, the locus of control should shift to the family as the child moves into a more routine, home-based life. Treatment plans should allow the greatest degree of normalization of the child's life. As the child matures, self-management programs that provide health education, self-efficacy skills, and techniques such as symptom monitoring help promote good long-term health habits. These programs should be introduced at 6 or 7 years of age or when a child is at a developmental level to take on chores and benefit from being given responsibility. Self-management minimizes *learned helplessness* and the *vulnerable child syndrome*, both of which occur commonly in families with chronically ill or disabled children.

MULTIFACETED TEAM ASSESSMENT OF COMPLEX PROBLEMS

When developmental screening and surveillance suggest the presence of significant developmental lags, the physician should take responsibility for coordinating the further assessment of the child by the team of professionals and provide continuity of care. The physician should become aware of local facilities and programs for assessment and treatment. If the child is at high risk for delay (e.g., prematurity), a structured follow-up program to monitor the child's progress may already exist. Under federal law, all children are entitled to assessments if there is a suspected developmental delay or a risk factor for delay (e.g., prematurity, failure to thrive, and parental mental retardation [MR]). Special programs for children up to 3 years of age are developed by states to implement this policy. Developmental interventions are arranged in conjunction with third-party payers with local programs funding the cost only when there is no insurance coverage. After 3 years of age, development programs usually are administered by school districts. Federal laws mandate that special education programs be provided for all children with developmental disabilities from birth through 21 years of age.

Children with special needs may be enrolled in pre-K programs with a therapeutic core, including visits to the program by therapists, to work on challenges. Children who are of traditional school age (kindergarten through secondary school) should be evaluated by the school district and provided an **individualized educational plan (IEP)** to address any deficiencies. An IEP may feature individual tutoring time (resource time), placement in a special education program, placement in classes with children with severe behavioral problems, or other strategies to address deficiencies. As part of the comprehensive evaluation of developmental/behavioral issues, all children should receive a thorough medical assessment. A variety of other specialists may assist in the assessment and intervention, including subspecialist pediatricians (e.g., neurology, orthopedics, psychiatry, developmental/behavioral), therapists (e.g., occupational, physical, oral-motor), and others (e.g., psychologists, early childhood development specialists).

Medical Assessment

The physician's main goals in team assessment are to identify the cause of the developmental dysfunction, if possible (often a specific cause is not found), and identify and interpret other medical conditions that have a developmental impact. The comprehensive history (Table 10.1) and physical examination (Table 10.2) include a careful graphing of growth parameters and an accurate description of dysmorphic features. Many of the diagnoses are rare or unusual diseases or syndromes. Many of these diseases and syndromes are discussed further in Sections 9 and 24.

Motor Assessment

The comprehensive neurological examination is an excellent basis for evaluating motor function, but it should be supplemented by an adaptive functional evaluation (see Chapter 179). Observing the child at play aids assessment of function. Specialists in early childhood development and therapists (especially occupational and physical therapists who have experience with children) can provide excellent input into the evaluation of age-appropriate adaptive function.

Psychological Assessment

Psychological assessment includes the testing of cognitive ability (Table 10.3) and the evaluation of personality and emotional

TABLE 10.1 Information to Be Sought During the History Taking of a Child With Suspected Developmental Disabilities

ITEM	POSSIBLE SIGNIFICANCE
Parental concerns	Parents are quite accurate in identifying development problems in their children.
Current levels of developmental functioning	Should be used to monitor child's progress
Temperament	May interact with disability or may be confused with developmental delay
PRENATAL HISTORY	
Alcohol ingestion	Fetal alcohol syndrome; index of caregiving risk
Exposure to medication, illegal drug, or toxin	Development toxin (e.g., phenytoin); may be an index of caregiving risk
Radiation exposure	Damage to CNS
Nutrition	Inadequate fetal nutrition
Prenatal care	Index of social situation
Injuries, hyperthermia	Damage to CNS
Smoking	Possible CNS damage
HIV exposure	Congenital HIV infection
Maternal illness (so-called "**TORCH**" infections)	**T**oxoplasmosis, Syphilis (**O**ther in the mnemonic), **R**ubella, **C**ytomegalovirus, **H**erpes simplex virus infections
PERINATAL HISTORY	
Gestational age, birthweight	Biological risk from prematurity and small for gestational age
Labor and delivery	Hypoxia or index of abnormal prenatal development
APGAR scores	Hypoxia, cardiovascular impairment
Specific perinatal adverse events	Increased risk of CNS damage
NEONATAL HISTORY	
Illness—seizures, respiratory distress, hyperbilirubinemia, metabolic disorder	Increased risk of CNS damage
Malformations	May represent genetic syndrome or new mutation associated with developmental delay
FAMILY HISTORY	
Consanguinity	Autosomal recessive condition more likely
Mental functioning	Increased hereditary and environmental risks
Illnesses (e.g., metabolic diseases)	Hereditary illness associated with developmental delay
Family member died young or unexpectedly	May suggest inborn error of metabolism or storage disease
Family member requires special education	Hereditary causes of developmental delay
SOCIAL HISTORY	
Resources available (e.g., financial, social support)	Necessary to maximize child's potential
Educational level of parents	Family may need help to provide stimulation
Mental health problems	May exacerbate child's conditions
High-risk behaviors (e.g., illicit drugs, sex)	Increased risk for HIV infection; index of caregiving risk
Other stressors (e.g., marital discord)	May exacerbate child's conditions or compromise care
OTHER HISTORY	
Gender of child	Important for X-linked conditions
Developmental milestones	Index of developmental delay; regression may indicate progressive condition.
Head injury	Even moderate trauma may be associated with developmental delay or learning disabilities.
Serious infections (e.g., meningitis)	May be associated with developmental delay
Toxic exposure (e.g., lead)	May be associated with developmental delay
Physical growth	May indicate malnutrition; obesity, short stature, genetic syndrome
Recurrent otitis media	Associated with hearing loss and abnormal speech development
Visual and auditory functioning	Sensitive index of impaired vision and hearing
Nutrition	Malnutrition during infancy may lead to delayed development.
Chronic conditions such as renal disease	May be associated with delayed development or anemia

CNS, Central nervous system.
Modified and updated from Liptak G. Mental retardation and developmental disability. In: Kliegman RM, ed. Practical Strategies in Pediatric Diagnosis and Therapy. *Philadelphia: WB Saunders; 1996.*

well-being. The IQ and mental age scores, taken in isolation, are only partially descriptive of a person's functional abilities, which are a combination of cognitive, adaptive, and social skills. Tests of achievement are subject to variability based on culture, educational exposures, and experience and must be standardized for social factors. Projective and nonprojective tests are useful in understanding the child's emotional status. Although a child should not be labeled as having a problem solely on the basis of a standardized test, these tests provide important and reasonably objective data for evaluating a child's progress within a particular educational program.

Educational Assessment

Educational assessment involves the evaluation of areas of specific strengths and weaknesses in reading, spelling, written expression, and mathematical skills. Schools routinely screen children with grouped tests to aid in problem identification

TABLE 10.2 Information to Be Sought During the Physical Examination of a Child With Suspected Developmental Disabilities

ITEM	POSSIBLE SIGNIFICANCE
General appearance	May indicate significant delay in development or obvious syndrome
STATURE	
Short stature	Williams syndrome, malnutrition, Turner syndrome; many children with severe retardation have associated short stature.
Obesity	Prader-Willi syndrome
Large stature	Sotos syndrome
HEAD	
Macrocephaly	Alexander syndrome, Sotos syndrome, gangliosidosis, hydrocephalus, mucopolysaccharidosis, subdural effusion
Microcephaly	Virtually any condition that can retard brain growth (e.g., malnutrition, Angelman syndrome, de Lange syndrome, fetal alcohol effects)
FACE	
Coarse, triangular, round, or flat face; hypotelorism or hypertelorism, slanted or short palpebral fissure; unusual nose, maxilla, and mandible	Specific measurements may provide clues to inherited, metabolic, or other diseases such as fetal alcohol syndrome, cri du chat syndrome (5p-syndrome), or Williams syndrome.
EYES	
Prominent	Crouzon syndrome, Seckel syndrome, fragile X syndrome
Cataract	Galactosemia, Lowe syndrome, prenatal rubella, hypothyroidism
Cherry-red spot in macula	Gangliosidosis (GM_1), metachromatic leukodystrophy, mucolipidosis, Tay-Sachs disease, Niemann-Pick disease, Farber lipogranulomatosis, sialidosis III
Chorioretinitis	Congenital infection with cytomegalovirus, toxoplasmosis, or rubella
Corneal cloudiness	Mucopolysaccharidosis I and II, Lowe syndrome, congenital syphilis
EARS	
Pinnae, low set or malformed	Trisomies such as 18, Rubinstein-Taybi syndrome, Down syndrome, CHARGE association, cerebro-oculo-facio-skeletal syndrome, fetal phenytoin effects
Hearing	Loss of acuity in mucopolysaccharidosis; hyperacusis in many encephalopathies
HEART	
Structural anomaly or hypertrophy	CHARGE association, CATCH-22, velocardiofacial syndrome, glycogenosis II, fetal alcohol effects, mucopolysaccharidosis I; chromosomal anomalies such as Down syndrome; maternal phenylketonuria; chronic cyanosis may impair cognitive development.
LIVER	
Hepatomegaly	Fructose intolerance, galactosemia, glycogenosis types I to IV, mucopolysaccharidosis I and II, Niemann-Pick disease, Tay-Sachs disease, Zellweger syndrome, Gaucher disease, ceroid lipofuscinosis, gangliosidosis
GENITALIA	
Macro-orchidism (usually not noted until puberty)	Fragile X syndrome
Hypogenitalism	Prader-Willi syndrome, Klinefelter syndrome, CHARGE association
EXTREMITIES	
Hands, feet, dermatoglyphics, and creases	May indicate specific entity such as Rubinstein-Taybi syndrome or be associated with chromosomal anomaly
Joint contractures	Sign of muscle imbalance around joints (e.g., with meningomyelocele, cerebral palsy, arthrogryposis, muscular dystrophy; also occurs with cartilaginous problems such as mucopolysaccharidosis)
SKIN	
Café-au-lait spots	Neurofibromatosis, tuberous sclerosis, Bloom syndrome
Eczema	Phenylketonuria, histiocytosis
Hemangiomas and telangiectasia	Sturge-Weber syndrome, Bloom syndrome, ataxia-telangiectasia
Hypopigmented macules, streaks, adenoma sebaceum	Tuberous sclerosis, hypomelanosis of Ito
HAIR	
Hirsutism	de Lange syndrome, mucopolysaccharidosis, fetal phenytoin effects, cerebro-oculo-facio-skeletal syndrome, trisomy 18 syndrome
NEUROLOGICAL	
Asymmetry of strength and tone	Focal lesion, cerebral palsy
Hypotonia	Prader-Willi syndrome, Down syndrome, Angelman syndrome, gangliosidosis, early cerebral palsy
Hypertonia	Neurodegenerative conditions involving white matter, cerebral palsy, trisomy 18 syndrome
Ataxia	Ataxia-telangiectasia, metachromatic leukodystrophy, Angelman syndrome

CATCH-22, **C**ardiac defects, **a**bnormal face, **t**hymic hypoplasia, **c**left palate, **h**ypocalcemia, defects on chromosome **22**; *CHARGE,* **c**oloboma, **h**eart defects, **a**tresia choanae, **r**etarded growth, **g**enital anomalies, **e**ar anomalies (deafness).

Modified and updated from Liptak G. Mental retardation and developmental disability. In: Kliegman RM, Greenbaum LA, Lye PS, eds. Practical Strategies in Pediatric Diagnosis and Therapy. *2nd ed. Philadelphia: Saunders; 2004:540.*

TABLE 10.3 Tests of Cognition

TEST	AGE RANGE	SPECIAL FEATURES
INFANT SCALES		
Bayley Scales of Infant Development (3rd ed.)	1-42 mo	Mental, psychomotor scales, behavior record; weak intelligence predictor
Cattell Infant Intelligence Scale	2-30 mo	Used to extend Stanford-Binet downward
Gesell Developmental Observation-Revised (GDO-R)	Birth-3 yr	Used by many pediatricians
Ordinal Scales of Infant Psychological Development	Birth-24 mo	Six subscales; based on Piaget's stages; weak in predicting later intelligence
PRESCHOOL SCALES		
Stanford-Binet Intelligence Scale (4th ed.)	2 yr-adult	Four area scores, with subtests and composite IQ score
McCarthy Scales of Children's Abilities	2½-8½ yr	6-18 subtests; good at defining learning disabilities; strengths/weaknesses approach
Wechsler Primary and Preschool Test of Intelligence–Revised (WPPSI-R)	2½-7¼ yr	11 subtests; verbal, performance IQs; long administration time; good at defining learning disabilities
Merrill-Palmer Scale of Mental Tests	18 mo-4 yr	19 subtests cover language skills, motor skills, manual dexterity, and matching ability
Differential Abilities Scale—II (2nd ed.)	2½-18 yr	Special nonverbal composite; short administration time
SCHOOL-AGE SCALES		
Stanford-Binet Intelligence Scale (4th ed.)	2 yr-adult	Four area scores, with subtests and composite IQ score
Wechsler Intelligence Scale for Children (4th ed) (WISC IV)	6-16 yr	See comments on WPPSI-R
Leiter International Performance Scale, Revised	2-20 yr	Nonverbal measure of intelligence ideal for use with those who are cognitively delayed, non-English speaking, hearing impaired, speech impaired, or autistic
Wechsler Adult Intelligence Scale–Revised (WAIS-III)	16 yr-adult	See comments on WPPSI-R
Differential Abilities Scale—II (2nd ed.)	2½ yr-adult	Special nonverbal composite; short administration time
ADAPTIVE BEHAVIOR SCALES		
Vineland Adaptive Behavior Scale—II (2nd ed.)	Birth-90 yr	Interview/questionnaire; typical persons and blind, deaf, developmentally delayed, and retarded
American Association on Mental Retardation (AAMR) Adaptive Behavioral Scale	4-21 yr	Useful in mental retardation, other disabilities

and program evaluation. For the child with special needs, this screening ultimately should lead to individualized testing and the development of an IEP that would enable the child to progress comfortably in school. Diagnostic teaching, in which the child's response to various teaching techniques is assessed, also may be helpful.

Social Environment Assessment

Assessments of the environment in which the child is living, working, playing, and growing are important in understanding the child's development. A home visit by a social worker, community health nurse, and/or home-based intervention specialist can provide valuable information about the child's social milieu. Often, the home visitor can suggest additional adaptive equipment or renovations if there are challenges at home. If there is a suspicion of inadequate parenting, and, especially, if there is a suspicion of neglect or abuse (including emotional abuse), the child and family must be referred to the local child protection agency. Information about reporting hotlines and local child protection agencies usually is found inside the front cover of local telephone directories (see Chapter 22).

MANAGEMENT OF DEVELOPMENTAL PROBLEMS

Intervention in the Primary Care Setting

The clinician must decide whether a problem requires referral for further diagnostic work-up and management or whether management in the primary care setting is appropriate. Counseling roles required in caring for these children are listed in Table 10.4. When a child is young, much of the counseling interaction takes place between the parents and the clinician, and, as the child matures, direct counseling shifts increasingly toward the child.

The assessment process may be therapeutic in itself. By assuming the role of a nonjudgmental, supportive listener, the clinician creates a climate of trust, allowing the family to express difficult or painful thoughts and feelings. Expressing

TABLE 10.4 Primary Care Counseling Roles
Allow ventilation
Facilitate clarification
Support patient problem solving
Provide specific reassurance
Provide education
Provide specific parenting advice
Suggest environmental interventions
Provide follow-up
Facilitate appropriate referrals
Coordinate care and interpret reports after referrals

emotions may allow the parent or caregiver to move on to the work of understanding and resolving the problem.

Interview techniques may facilitate clarification of the problem for the family and for the clinician. The family's ideas about the causes of the problem and attempts at coping can provide a basis for developing strategies for problem management that are much more likely to be implemented successfully because they emanate, in part, from the family. The clinician shows respect by endorsing the parent's ideas when appropriate; this can increase self-esteem and sense of competency.

Educating parents about normal and aberrant development and behavior may prevent problems through early detection and anticipatory guidance and communicates the physician's interest in hearing parental concerns. Early detection allows intervention before the problem becomes entrenched and associated problems develop.

The severity of developmental and behavioral problems ranges from variations of normal to problematic responses to stressful situations to frank disorders. The clinician must try to establish the severity and scope of the patient's symptoms so that appropriate intervention can be planned.

Counseling Principles

For the child, behavioral change must be learned, not simply imposed. It is easiest to learn when the lesson is simple, clear, and consistent and presented in an atmosphere free of fear or intimidation. Parents often try to impose behavioral change in an emotionally charged atmosphere, most often at the time of a behavioral *violation*. Similarly, clinicians may try to *teach* parents with hastily presented advice when the parents are distracted by other concerns or not engaged in the suggested behavioral change.

Apart from management strategies directed specifically at the problem behavior, regular times for positive parent-child interaction should be instituted. Frequent, brief, affectionate physical contact over the day provides opportunities for positive reinforcement of desirable child behaviors and for building a sense of competence in the child and the parent.

Most parents feel guilty when their children have a developmental/behavioral problem. Guilt may be caused by the fear that the problem was caused by inadequate parenting or by previous angry responses to the child's behavior. If possible and appropriate, the clinician should find ways to alleviate guilt, which may be a serious impediment to problem solving.

Interdisciplinary Team Intervention

In many cases, a team of professionals is required to provide the breadth and quality of services needed to appropriately serve the child who has SHCN. The primary care physician should monitor the progress of the child and continually reassess that the requisite therapy is being accomplished.

Educational intervention for a young child begins as home-based infant stimulation, often with an early childhood specialist (e.g., nurse/therapist), providing direct stimulation for the child and training the family to provide the stimulation. As the child matures, a center-based early learning center program may be indicated. For the school-age child, special services may range from extra attention in the classroom to a self-contained special education classroom.

Psychological intervention may be directed to the parent or family or, with an older child, primarily child-directed. Examples of therapeutic approaches are guidance therapies, such as directive advice giving, counseling to create their own solutions to problems, psychotherapy, behavioral management techniques, psychopharmacologic methods (from a psychiatrist), and cognitive-behavioral therapy.

Motor intervention may be performed by a physical or occupational therapist. *Neurodevelopmental therapy* (NDT), the most commonly used method, is based on the concept that nervous system development is hierarchical and subject to some plasticity. The focus of NDT is on gait training and motor development, including daily living skills; perceptual abilities, such as eye-hand coordination; and spatial relationships. *Sensory integration therapy* is also used by occupational therapists to structure sensory experience from the tactile, proprioceptive, and vestibular systems to allow for adaptive motor responses.

Speech-language intervention by a speech and language therapist/pathologist (oral-motor therapist) is usually part of the overall educational program and is based on the tested language strengths and weaknesses of the child. Children needing this type of intervention may show difficulties in reading and other academic areas and develop social and behavioral problems because of their difficulties in being understood and in understanding others. **Hearing intervention**, performed by an audiologist (or an otolaryngologist), includes monitoring hearing acuity and providing amplification when necessary via hearing aids.

Social and environmental intervention generally includes nursing or social work involvement with the family. Frequently, the task of coordinating services falls to these specialists. Case managers may be in the private sector, from the child's insurance or Medicaid plan, or part of a child protection agency.

Medical intervention for a child with a developmental disability involves providing primary care as well as specific treatment of conditions associated with the disability. Although curative treatment often is not possible, functional impairment can be minimized through thoughtful medical management. Certain general medical problems are found more frequently in delayed and developmentally disabled people (Table 10.5), especially if the delay is part of a known syndrome. Some children may have a limited life expectancy. Supporting the family through palliative care, hospice, and bereavement is another important role of the primary care pediatrician.

TABLE 10.5 Recurring Medical Issues in Children With Developmental Disabilities

PROBLEM	ASK ABOUT OR CHECK
Motor	Range of motion examination; scoliosis check; assessment of mobility; interaction with orthopedist, physical medicine and rehabilitation, and physical therapist/occupational therapist as needed
Diet	Dietary history, feeding observation, growth parameter measurement and charting, supplementation as indicated by observations, oro-motor therapist as needed
Sensory impairments	Functional vision and hearing screening; interaction as needed with ophthalmologist, audiologist
Dermatologic	Examination of *all* skin areas for decubitus ulcers or infection
Dentistry	Examination of teeth and gums; confirmation of access to dental care (preferably with ability to use sedation)
Behavioral problems	Aggression, self-injury, pica; sleep problems; psychotropic drug levels and side effects
Seizures	Major motor, absence, other suspicious symptoms; monitoring of anticonvulsant levels and side effects
Infectious diseases	Ear infections, diarrhea, respiratory symptoms, aspiration pneumonia, immunizations (especially hepatitis B and influenza)
Gastrointestinal problems	Constipation, gastroesophageal reflux, gastrointestinal bleeding (stool for occult blood)
Sexuality	Sexuality education, preventing abuse, hygiene, contraception, menstrual suppression, genetic counseling
Other syndrome-specific problems	Ongoing evaluation of other "physical" problems as indicated by known mental retardation/developmental disability etiology
Advocacy for services and enhancing access to care	Educational program, family supports, financial supports, legislative advocacy to support programs

SELECTED CLINICAL PROBLEMS: THE SPECIAL NEEDS CHILD

Mental Retardation

MR is defined as significantly subnormal intellectual functioning for a child's developmental stage, existing concurrently with deficits in adaptive behaviors (self-care, home living, communication, and social interactions). MR is defined statistically as cognitive performance that is two standard deviations below the mean (roughly below the third percentile) of the general population as measured on standardized intelligence testing. The last known estimate of the prevalence of MR is that about 2% of the U.S. population is affected. Levels of MR from IQ scores derived from two typical tests are shown in Table 10.6. Caution must be exercised in interpretation because these categories do not reflect actual functional level of the tested individual.

TABLE 10.6 Levels of Mental Retardation

LEVEL OF RETARDATION	ICD-10 IQ SCORE	WISC-IV IQ SCORE	EDUCATIONAL LABEL
Mild	50-69	50-55 to 70	EMR
Moderate	35-49	35-40 to 50-55	TMR
Severe	20-34	20-25 to 35-50	
Profound	<20	<20 to 25	

EMR, Educable mentally retarded; *ICD-10*, International Classification of Diseases (WHO), ed 10; *TMR*, trainable mentally retarded; *WISC-IV*, Wechsler Intelligence Scale for children, ed 4.

The etiology of the central nervous system insult resulting in MR may involve genetic disorders, teratogenic influences, perinatal insults, acquired childhood disease, and environmental and social determinants of health (Table 10.7). Mild MR correlates with socioeconomic status, although profound MR does not. Although a single organic cause may be found, each individual's performance should be considered a function of the interaction of environmental influences with the individual's organic substrate. Behavioral difficulties resulting from MR itself and from the family's reaction to the child and the condition are common. More severe forms of MR can be traced to biological factors. The earlier the cognitive slowing is recognized, the more severe the deviation from normal is likely to be.

The first step in the diagnosis and management of a child with MR is to identify functional strengths and weaknesses for purposes of medical and rehabilitative therapies. A history and physical examination may suggest a diagnostic approach that, then, may be confirmed by laboratory testing and/or imaging. Frequently used laboratory tests include chromosomal analysis and magnetic resonance imaging of the brain. Almost one-third of individuals with MR do not have readily identifiable reasons for their disability.

Vision Impairment

Significant visual impairment is a problem in many children. **Partial vision** (defined as visual acuity between 20/70 and 20/200) occurs in 1 in 500 school-age children in the United States. **Legal blindness** is defined as distant visual acuity of 20/200 or worse and affects about 35,000 children in the United States. Such impairment can be a major barrier to optimal development.

The most common cause of **severe visual impairment** in children is retinopathy of prematurity (see Chapter 61). Congenital cataracts may lead to significant amblyopia. Cataracts also are associated with other ocular abnormalities and developmental disabilities. **Amblyopia** is a pathologic alteration of the visual system characterized by a reduction in visual acuity in one or both eyes with no clinically apparent organic abnormality that completely accounts for the visual loss. Amblyopia is due to a distortion of the normal clearly formed retinal image (from congenital cataracts or severe refractive errors); abnormal binocular interaction between the eyes, as one eye competitively inhibits the other (strabismus); or a combination of both mechanisms. Albinism, hydrocephalus, congenital cytomegalovirus infection, and birth asphyxia are other significant contributors to blindness in children.

TABLE 10.7 Differential Diagnosis of Mental Retardation*
EARLY ALTERATIONS OF EMBRYONIC DEVELOPMENT
Sporadic events affecting embryogenesis, usually a stable developmental challenge
Chromosomal changes (e.g., trisomy 21 syndrome)
Prenatal influences (e.g., substance abuse, teratogenic medications, intrauterine TORCH infections)†
UNKNOWN CAUSES
No definite issue is identified, or multiple elements present, none of which is diagnostic (may be multifactorial)
ENVIRONMENTAL AND SOCIAL PROBLEMS
Dynamic influences, commonly associated with other challenges
Deprivation (neglect)
Parental mental illness
Environmental intoxications (e.g., significant lead intoxication)*
PREGNANCY PROBLEMS AND PERINATAL MORBIDITY
Impingement on normal intrauterine development or delivery; neurological abnormalities frequent, challenges are stable or occasionally worsening
Fetal malnutrition and placental insufficiency
Perinatal complications (e.g., prematurity, birth asphyxia, birth trauma)
HEREDITARY DISORDERS
Preconceptual origin, variable expression in the individual infant, multiple somatic effects, frequently a progressive or degenerative course
Inborn errors of metabolism (e.g., Tay-Sachs disease, Hunter disease, phenylketonuria)
Single-gene abnormalities (e.g., neurofibromatosis or tuberous sclerosis)
Other chromosomal aberrations (e.g., fragile X syndrome, deletion mutations such as Prader-Willi syndrome)
Polygenic familial syndromes (pervasive developmental disorders)
ACQUIRED CHILDHOOD ILLNESS
Acute modification of developmental status, variable potential for functional recovery
Infections (all can ultimately lead to brain damage, but most significant are encephalitis and meningitis)
Cranial trauma (accidental and child abuse)
Accidents (e.g., near-drowning, electrocution)
Environmental intoxications (prototype is lead poisoning)

**Some health problems fit in several categories (e.g., lead intoxication may be involved in several areas).*
†This also may be considered as an acquired childhood disease.
TORCH, **T**oxoplasmosis, **o**ther (congenital syphilis), **r**ubella, **c**ytomegalovirus, and **h**erpes simplex virus.

Children with **mild to moderate visual impairment** usually have an uncorrected refractive error. The most common presentation is myopia or nearsightedness. Other causes are hyperopia (farsightedness) and astigmatism (alteration in the shape of the cornea leading to visual distortion). In children younger than 6 years, high refractive errors in one or both eyes also may cause amblyopia, aggravating visual impairment.

The diagnosis of severe visual impairment commonly is made when an infant is 4-8 months of age. Clinical suspicion is based on parental concerns aroused by unusual behavior, such as lack of smiling in response to appropriate stimuli, the presence of nystagmus, other wandering eye movements, or motor delays in beginning to reach for objects. Fixation and visual tracking behavior can be seen in most infants by 6 weeks of age. This behavior can be assessed by moving a brightly colored object (or the examiner's face) across the visual field of a quiet but alert infant at a distance of 1 ft. The eyes also should be examined for red reflexes and pupillary reactions to light. Optical alignment (binocular vision with both eyes consistently focusing on the same spot) should not be expected until the infant is beyond the newborn period. Persistent nystagmus is abnormal at any age. If ocular abnormalities are identified, referral to a pediatric ophthalmologist is indicated.

During the newborn period, vision may be assessed by physical examination and by **visual evoked response**. This test evaluates the conduction of electrical impulses from the optic nerve to the occipital cortex of the brain. The eye is stimulated by a bright flash of light or with an alternating checkerboard of black-and-white squares, and the resulting electrical response is recorded from electrodes strategically placed on the scalp, similar to an electroencephalogram.

There are many developmental implications of visual impairment. Perception of body image is abnormal, and imitative behavior, such as smiling, is delayed. Delays in mobility may occur in children who are visually impaired from birth, although their postural milestones (ability to sit) usually are achieved appropriately. Social bonding with the parents also is often affected.

Visually impaired children can be helped in various ways. Classroom settings may be augmented with resource-room assistance to present material in a nonvisual format. Fine motor activity development, listening skills, and Braille reading and writing are intrinsic to successful educational intervention for a child with severe visual impairment.

Hearing Impairment

Decision-Making Algorithm
Available @ StudentConsult.com
Hearing Loss

The clinical significance of hearing loss varies with its type (conductive vs. sensorineural), its frequency, and its severity as measured in the number of decibels heard or the number of decibels of hearing lost. The most common cause of mild to moderate hearing loss in children is a conduction abnormality caused by acquired middle ear disease (acute and chronic otitis media). This abnormality may have a significant effect on the development of speech and language development, particularly if there is chronic fluctuating middle ear fluid. If hearing impairment is more severe, sensorineural hearing loss is more common. Causes of sensorineural deafness include congenital infections (e.g., rubella and cytomegalovirus), meningitis, birth asphyxia, kernicterus, ototoxic drugs (especially aminoglycoside antibiotics), and tumors and their treatments. Genetic deafness may be either dominant or recessive in inheritance; this is the main cause of hearing impairment in schools for the deaf. In Down syndrome, there is a predisposition to conductive loss caused by middle-ear infection and sensorineural loss caused by cochlear disease. Any hearing loss may have a significant effect on the child's developing communication skills. These skills then affect all areas of the child's cognitive and skills development (Table 10.8).

It is sometimes quite difficult to accurately determine the presence of hearing in infants and young children. Inquiring about a newborn's or infant's response to sounds or even observing the response to sounds in the office is unreliable for identifying hearing-impaired children. Universal screening of newborns is required prior to nursery discharge and includes the following:

1. **Auditory brainstem response (ABR)** measures how the brain responds to sound. Clicks or tones are played through soft earphones into the infant's ears. Three electrodes placed on the infant's head measure the brain's response.
2. **Otoacoustic emissions** measure sound waves produced in the inner ear. A tiny probe is placed just inside the infant's ear canal. It measures the response (echo) when clicks or tones are played into the infant's ears.

TABLE 10.8 Neurodevelopmental-Behavioral Complications of Hearing Loss

SEVERITY OF HEARING LOSS	POSSIBLE ETIOLOGIC ORIGINS	COMPLICATIONS			TYPES OF THERAPY
		SPEECH-LANGUAGE	EDUCATIONAL	BEHAVIORAL	
Slight 15-25 dB (ASA)	Chronic otitis media/ middle ear effusions	Difficulty with hearing distant or faint speech	Possible auditory learning dysfunction	Usually none	May require favorable class setting, speech therapy, or auditory training
	Perforation of tympanic membrane		May reveal a slight verbal deficit		Possible value in hearing aid, surgery
	Sensorineural loss				Favorable class setting
	Tympanosclerosis				
Mild 25-40 dB (ASA)	Chronic otitis media/ middle ear effusions	Difficulty with conversational speech over 3-5 ft	May miss 50% of class discussions	Psychological problems	Special education resource help, surgery
	Perforation of tympanic membrane	May have limited vocabulary and speech disorders	Auditory learning dysfunction	May act inappropriately if directions are not heard well	Hearing aid, surgery
	Sensorineural loss			Acting out behavior	Favorable class setting
	Tympanosclerosis			Poor self-concept	Lip reading instruction
					Speech therapy
Moderate 40-65 dB (ASA)	Chronic otitis media/ middle ear effusions	Conversation must be loud to be understood.	Learning disability	Emotional and social problems	Special education resource or special class, surgery
	Middle ear anomaly	Defective speech	Difficulty with group learning or discussion	Behavioral reactions of childhood	Special help in speech-language development
	Sensorineural loss	Deficient language use and comprehension	Auditory processing dysfunction	Acting out	Hearing aid and lip reading
			Limited vocabulary	Poor self-concept	Speech therapy
Severe 65-95 dB (ASA)	Sensorineural loss	Loud voices may be heard 2 ft from ear.	Marked educational retardation	Emotional and social problems that are associated with handicap	Full-time special education for deaf children, cochlear implant
	Severe middle ear disease	Defective speech and language No spontaneous speech development if loss present before 1 yr	Marked learning disability, limited vocabulary	Poor self-concept	Full-time special education for deaf children, hearing aid, lip reading, speech therapy, surgery, cochlear implant
Profound ≥95 dB (ASA)	Sensorineural or mixed loss	Relies on vision rather than hearing Defective speech and language Speech and language will not develop spontaneously if loss present before 1 yr.	Marked learning disability because of lack of understanding of speech	Congenital and prelingually deaf may show severe emotional problems.	Full-time special education for deaf children, hearing aid, lip reading, speech therapy, surgery, cochlear implant

ASA, Acoustical Society of America.

Modified and updated from Gottlieb MI. Otitis media. In: Levine MD, Carey WB, Crocker AC, et al., eds. Developmental-Behavioral Pediatrics. *Philadelphia: WB Saunders; 1983.*

Both of these tests are quick (5-10 minutes), painless, and may be performed while the infant is sleeping or lying still. The tests are sensitive but not as specific as more definitive tests. Infants who do not pass these tests are referred for more comprehensive testing. Many of these infants have normal hearing on definitive testing. Infants who do not have normal hearing should be immediately evaluated or referred for etiologic diagnosis and early intervention.

For children not screened at birth (such as children of immigrant parents) or children with suspected acquired hearing loss, later testing may allow early appropriate intervention. Hearing can be screened by means of an office audiogram, but other techniques are needed (ABR, behavior audiology) for young, neurologically immature or impaired, and behaviorally difficult children. The typical audiologic assessment includes pure-tone audiometry over a variety of sound frequencies (pitches), especially over the range of frequencies in which most speech occurs. **Pneumatic otoscopic** examination and **tympanometry** are used to assess middle ear function and the tympanic membrane compliance for pathology in the middle ear, such as fluid, ossicular dysfunction, and eustachian tube dysfunction (see Chapter 9).

The treatment of conductive hearing loss (largely due to otitis media and middle ear effusions) is discussed in Chapter 105. Treatment of sensorineural hearing impairment may be medical or surgical. If amplification is indicated, hearing aids can be tuned preferentially to amplify the frequency ranges in which the patient has decreased acuity. Educational intervention typically includes speech-language therapy and teaching American Sign Language. Even with amplification, many hearing-impaired children show deficits in processing auditory information, requiring special educational services for helping to read and for other academic skills. **Cochlear implants** are surgically implantable devices that provide hearing sensation to individuals with severe to profound hearing loss. The implants are designed to substitute for the function of the middle ear, cochlear mechanical motion, and sensory cells, transforming sound energy into electrical energy that initiates impulses in the auditory nerve. Cochlear implants are indicated for children older than 12 months with profound bilateral sensorineural hearing loss who have limited benefit from hearing aids, have failed to progress in auditory skill development, and have no radiologic or medical contraindications. Implantation in children as young as possible gives them the most advantageous auditory environment for speech-language learning.

Speech-Language Impairment

Parents often bring the concern of speech delay to the physician's attention when they compare their young child with others of the same age (Table 10.9). The most common causes of the speech delay are MR, hearing impairment, social deprivation, autism, and oral-motor abnormalities. If a problem is suspected based on screening with tests such as Ages and Stages Questionnaires or the Parents' Evaluation of Developmental Status test (see Chapter 8) or other standard screening test (Early Language Milestone Scale), a referral to a specialized hearing and speech center is indicated. While awaiting the results of testing or initiation of speech-language therapy, parents should be advised to speak slowly and clearly to the child (and avoid *baby talk*). Parents and older siblings should read frequently to the speech-delayed child.

TABLE 10.9 Clues to When a Child With a Communication Disorder Needs Help

0-11 MONTHS
Before 6 months, the child does not startle, blink, or change immediate activity in response to sudden, loud sounds.
Before 6 months, the child does not attend to the human voice and is not soothed by mother's voice.
By 6 months, the child does not babble strings of consonant and vowel syllables or imitate gurgling or cooing sounds.
By 10 months, the child does not respond to his or her name.
At 10 months, the child's sound-making is limited to shrieks, grunts, or sustained vowel production.
12-23 MONTHS
At 12 months, the child's babbling or speech is limited to vowel sounds.
By 15 months, the child does not respond to "no," "bye-bye," or "bottle."
By 15 months, the child does not imitate sounds or words.
By 18 months, the child is not consistently using at least six words with appropriate meaning.
By 21 months, the child does not respond correctly to "Give me...," "Sit down," or "Come here" when spoken without gestural cues.
By 23 months, two-word phrases that are spoken as single units (e.g., "whatszit," "thankyou," "allgone") have not emerged.
24-36 MONTHS
By 24 months, at least 50% of the child's speech is not understood by familiar listeners.
By 24 months, the child does not point to body parts without gestural cues.
By 24 months, the child is not combining words into phrases (e.g., "go bye-bye," "go car," "want cookie").
By 30 months, the child does not show understanding of spatial concepts: on, in, under, front, and back.
By 30 months, the child is not using short sentences (e.g., "Daddy went bye-bye").
By 30 months, the child has not begun to ask questions (using *where, what, why*).
By 36 months, the child's speech is not understood by unfamiliar listeners.
ALL AGES
At any age, the child is consistently dysfluent with repetitions, hesitations; blocks or struggles to say words. Struggle may be accompanied by grimaces, eye blinks, or hand gestures.

Modified and updated from Weiss CE, Lillywhite HE. Communication Disorders: A Handbook for Prevention and Early Detection. *St Louis: Mosby; 1976.*

Speech disorders include **articulation, fluency,** and **resonance disorders.** Articulation disorders include difficulties producing sounds in syllables or saying words incorrectly to the point that other people cannot understand what is being said. Fluency disorders include problems such as **stuttering,** the condition in which the flow of speech is interrupted by abnormal stoppages, repetitions *(st-st-stuttering)*, or prolonged sounds and syllables *(ssssstuttering)*. Resonance or voice disorders include problems with the pitch, volume, or quality of a child's voice that distract listeners from what is being said.

Language disorders can be either receptive or expressive. Receptive disorders refer to difficulties understanding or processing language. Expressive disorders include difficulty putting words together, limited vocabulary, or inability to use language in a socially appropriate way.

Speech-language pathologists (also called speech or oral-motor therapists) assess the speech, language, cognitive communication, and swallowing skills of children; determine what types of communication problems exist; and identify the best way to treat these challenges. Speech-language pathologists skilled at working with infants and young children are also vital in training parents and infants in other oral-motor skills, such as how to feed an infant born with a cleft lip and palate.

Speech-language therapy involves having a speech-language specialist work with a child on a one-on-one basis, in a small group, or directly in a classroom to overcome a specific disorder using a variety of therapeutic strategies. Language intervention activities involve having a speech-language specialist interact with a child by playing and talking to him or her using pictures, books, objects, or ongoing events to stimulate language development. Articulation therapy involves having the therapist model correct sounds and syllables for a child, often during play activities.

Children enrolled in therapy early (<3 years of age) tend to have better outcomes than children who begin therapy later. Older children can make progress in therapy, but progress may occur more slowly because these children often have learned patterns that need to be modified or changed. Parental involvement is crucial to the success of a child's progress in speech-language therapy.

Cerebral Palsy

Decision-Making Algorithms
Available @ StudentConsult.com

Limp
In-Toeing, Out-Toeing, and Toe-Walking
Bowlegs and Knock-Knees
Hypotonia and Weakness

Cerebral palsy (CP) refers to a group of non-progressive, but often changing, motor impairment syndromes secondary to anomalies or lesions of the brain arising before or after birth. The prevalence of CP at age 8 in the United States is 1.5-4 per 1000; prevalence is much higher in premature and twin births. Prematurity and low birthweight infants (leading to perinatal asphyxia), congenital malformations, and kernicterus are causes of CP noted at birth. Ten percent of children with CP have acquired CP, developing at later ages. Meningitis and head injury (accidental and nonaccidental) are the most common causes of acquired CP (Table 10.10). Nearly 50% of children with CP have no identifiable risk factors. As genomic medicine advances, many of these causes of idiopathic CP may be identified.

Most children with CP, except in its mildest forms, are diagnosed in the first 18 months of life when they fail to attain motor milestones or show abnormalities such as asymmetric gross motor function, hypertonia, or hypotonia. CP can be characterized further by the affected parts of the body (Table 10.11) and descriptions of the predominant type of motor disorder (Table 10.12). Co-morbidities in these children often include epilepsy, learning difficulties, behavioral challenges, and sensory impairments. Many of these children have an isolated motor defect. Some affected children may be intellectually gifted.

TABLE 10.10 Risk Factors for Cerebral Palsy

PREGNANCY AND BIRTH
Low socioeconomic status
Prematurity
Low birthweight/fetal growth retardation (<1,500 g at birth)
Maternal seizures/seizure disorder
Maternal treatment with thyroid hormone, estrogen, or progesterone
Pregnancy complications
Polyhydramnios
Eclampsia
Third-trimester bleeding (including threatened abortion and placenta previa)
Multiple births
Abnormal fetal presentation
Maternal fever
Congenital malformations/syndromes
Newborn hypoxic-ischemic encephalopathy
Bilirubin (kernicterus)
ACQUIRED AFTER THE NEWBORN PERIOD
Meningitis
Head injury
Car crashes
Child abuse
Near-drowning
Stroke

TABLE 10.11 Descriptions of Cerebral Palsy by Site of Involvement

Hemiparesis (hemiplegia): predominantly unilateral impairment of the arm and leg on the same (e.g., right or left) side
Diplegia: motor impairment primarily of the legs (often with some limited involvement of the arms; some authors challenge this specific type as not being different from quadriplegia)
Quadriplegia: all four limbs (whole body) are functionally compromised.

Treatment depends on the pattern of dysfunction. Physical and occupational therapy can facilitate optimal positioning and movement patterns, increasing function of the affected parts. Spasticity management also may include oral medications (dantrolene, benzodiazepines, and baclofen), botulinum toxin injections, and implantation of intrathecal baclofen pumps. Management of seizures, spasticity, orthopedic impairments, and sensory impairments may help improve educational attainment. CP cannot be cured, but a host of interventions can

TABLE 10.12 Classification of Cerebral Palsy by Type of Motor Disorder

Spastic cerebral palsy: the most common form of cerebral palsy, it accounts for 70-80% of cases. It results from injury to the upper motor neurons of the pyramidal tract. It may occasionally be bilateral. It is characterized by at least two of the following: abnormal movement pattern, increased tone, or pathologic reflexes (e.g., Babinski response, hyperreflexia).
Dyskinetic cerebral palsy: occurs in 10-15% of cases. It is dominated by abnormal patterns of movement and involuntary, uncontrolled, recurring movements.
Ataxic cerebral palsy: accounts for <5% of cases. This form results from cerebellar injury and features abnormal posture or movement and loss of orderly muscle coordination or both.
Dystonic cerebral palsy: also uncommon. It is characterized by reduced activity and stiff movement (hypokinesia) and hypotonia.
Choreoathetotic cerebral palsy: rare now that excessive hyperbilirubinemia is aggressively prevented and treated. This form is dominated by increased and stormy movements (hyperkinesia) and hypotonia.
Mixed cerebral palsy: accounts for 10-15% of cases. This term is used when more than one type of motor pattern is present and when one pattern does not clearly dominate another. It typically is associated with more complications, including sensory deficits, seizures, and cognitive-perceptual impairments.

improve functional abilities, participation in society, and quality of life. Like all children, an assessment and reinforcement of strengths are important, especially for intellectually intact or gifted children who have simple motor deficits.

Suggested Readings

Brosco J, Mattingly M, Sanders L. Impact of specific medical interventions on reducing the prevalence of mental retardation. *Arch Pediatr Adolesc Med.* 2006;160:302–309.

Gardner HG; American Academy of Pediatrics Committee on Injury, Violence, and Poison Prevention. Office-based counseling for unintentional injury prevention. *Pediatrics.* 2007;119(1):202–206.

Hagan JF, Shaw JS, Duncan PM, eds. *Bright Futures: Guidelines for Health Supervision of Infants, Children, and Adolescents.* 4th ed. Elk Grove Village, IL: American Academy of Pediatrics; 2017.

Kliegman R, Behrman R, Jenson H, et al. *Nelson Textbook of Pediatrics.* 18th ed. Philadelphia: Elsevier; 2007.

McCrindle B, Kwiterovich P, McBride P, et al. Guidelines for lipid screening in children and adolescents: bringing evidence to the debate. *Pediatrics.* 2012;130(2):353–356.

PEARLS FOR PRACTITIONERS

CHAPTER 5

Normal Growth

- Standard growth charts are used; they are available free from the CDC
  - 0-2 years, use the WHO growth charts and measure weight, recumbent length, and head circumference and plot these as well as the weight for length
  - For >2 years, use the CDC growth charts and measure weight, standing height, and calculate BMI. All should be plotted.
- Rules of thumb
  - Double birthweight in 4-5 months
  - Double birth length by age 4 years.

CHAPTER 6

Disorders of Growth

- The pattern of decreased growth may assist in the evaluation.
  - Weight decreases first, then length, then head circumference: caloric inadequacy
    - May be organic (increased work of breathing with congestive heart failure)
    - Often is nonorganic (neglected child, material depression)
  - All growth parameters less than the fifth percentile
    - Normal variants: familial short stature, constitutional delay
    - Endocrine disorders (especially with pituitary dysfunction)
  - Declining percentiles but otherwise normal 6-18 months: “catch-down growth”

CHAPTER 7

Normal Development

- Selected age appropriate issues
  - Neonatal reflexes assist in evaluation of the newborn: moro, rooting, sucking, asymmetric tonic neck reflex
  - Contractures of the joints at birth should be followed if the joint can be moved to the proper position; fixed deformities require pediatric orthopedic evaluation
  - By no later than 1 year, examine for binocular vision with the light reflex and cover test
  - Older children and adolescents who participate in sports need a careful cardiovascular and orthopedic risk assessment
- Developmental milestones
  - Gross motor, fine motor, speech, and personal–social are the areas most used for comparison
  - Selected age appropriate issues

- Bonding and attachment in infancy are critical for optimal outcomes
- Developing autonomy in early childhood: child explores but needs quick access to the caregivers.
  - Stranger anxiety beginning at about 9 months: support the infant when they are exploring and when others are present
  - Terrible twos: reinforce the desired behavior and try extinguishing the undesired behavior (by not responding to the behavior)
  - Value of early childhood education: increases educational attainment and is preferably started before age 3.
- School readiness should be assessed, not just assumed, to have optimal educational outcome.
- Adolescent development divided into three phases
  - Early adolescent: "Am I normal?"
  - Middle adolescent: risk behaviors and exploration of parental and cultural values
  - Late adolescent: "been there, done that"; emerge from risk behaviors and planning for the future adult roles.

CHAPTER 8

Disorders of Development

- Developmental surveillance at every office visit; more careful attention at health maintenance visits
- Developmental screening using validated tool
  - Done at 9, 18, and 30 months at a minimum
  - Most common tools are Ages and Stages and Parents' Evaluation of Developmental Status
  - Abnormalities require definitive testing
- Autism screening using validated tool is done at 18 and 24 months
  - Most common is the M-CHAT-R
  - Abnormalities require definitive testing
- Language development is critical in early childhood
  - Highly correlates with cognitive development
  - Even with newborn hearing test, may need to re-test hearing at any age
  - Speech therapy is more effective the younger it is started
- After age 6, school performance is assessed; if there are performance issues (academic or behavioral), there should be elaborated testing; testing should be done by psychologists, psychiatrists, developmental pediatricians, or educational experts
- Context of Behavioral problems
  - Parental factors: mismatch in temperament of expectations between parent and child, depression, other health issues
  - Social determinants of health
    - Stress, lack of parental support, perceived prejudice, and racism
    - Poverty: housing with environmental exposures, poor access to quality education, poor access to healthy nutrition (food deserts), toxic stress
  - Adolescents are a special challenge; developing rapport and open communication is critical
  - Adolescents may usually consent for sexual health, mental health, and substance abuse services
    - As long as they are not homicidal, suicidal, or unable to give informed consent, adolescents should consent for above issues
    - Confidentiality is critical unless there is information that would seem to allow harm to come to the individual or others

CHAPTER 9

Evaluation of the Well Child

- Standardized by the American Academy of Pediatrics Bright Futures program; recommendations for Preventive Pediatric Health Care were updated in 2015
- Elements of the visits
  - Measurements: growth, blood pressure, sensory screening (vision and hearing)
  - Developmental/Behavioral Assessment
    - New in the 4th edition is mandated depression screening starting at age 11; PHQ2 and PHQ9 are available in Bright Futures resources
  - Physical examination
  - Procedures
    - Newborn screening, CCHD
    - Hemoglobin, lead, TB testing at certain ages or if risks are present
    - Lipid screening once at age 9-11, other ages if risk factors
    - STD/HIV risk assessment and screening between ages 16 and 18 (or if sexually active at earlier age)
    - Oral health: Dental referral starting at age 1 year; fluoride varnish every 3-6 months between ages 6 months to 6 years
  - Anticipatory guidance that is age and developmentally appropriate
    - Bright Futures has age-appropriate one-page handouts for each health maintenance visit by age in the Tool and Resource Kit
- Promoting optimal development
  - Discipline means to teach, not just to punish
  - Reinforcing positive behaviors and activities is the most effective
  - Time out technique is optimal for altering undesired behaviors; corporal punishment teaches children it is okay to hit
  - Setting limits that are agreed upon by all caregivers leads to optimal outcomes

CHAPTER 10

Evaluation of the Child With Special Needs

- Children with special health care needs share broad experiences in school difficulties and family stress; 19% of U.S. children have a special health care need

- Goal is to maximize potential by treating primary issue and helping the family and patient deal with the stresses and secondary impairments
- Optimal care
  - Primary care pediatrician in a medical home—provides big picture oversight, evaluates the concern and provides diagnosis, provides preventive care, and facilitates
    - Pediatric subspecialists
    - Pediatric therapists—OT, PT, speech
    - Social work or health navigator may assist by finding needed community services (e.g., medically fragile child care)
  - Developmental assessments under age 3 are mandated to happen with no charge to the family or insurance; over age 3, they are performed by school districts
  - Psychology, education, and social environment assessments
- Selected special health care needs
  - Mental retardation—myriad causes that should be investigated; children may often "outperform" their expected intelligence with excellent support
  - Vision impairment
    - Can be tested as early as newborn using visual evoked response
    - Diagnosed between 4 and 8 months; clues: the child does not respond to the parent's smile, has wandering eye movements, or has motor delays in reaching for objects
  - Hearing impairment
    - Newborns have their hearing tested but may need additional testing later if there is a clinical suspicion
    - Can be conductive or sensorineural, each has different available treatment
  - Speech disorders
    - Many causes: MR, hearing impairment, deprivation and poor use of language with caregivers, autism, oral-motor abnormalities
    - Immediate speech-language evaluation and hearing evaluation
    - Commence speech therapy as soon as a true deficit is found; outcomes are better the earlier speech therapy is started
    - Articulation, fluency, stuttering, and resonance disorders may be discovered and are amenable to speech-language therapy
  - Cerebral palsy: non-progressive motor impairment syndrome
    - Myriad causes: 50% no cause identified
      - Congenital: prematurity, low birthweight, congenital malformations, kernicterus in the past
      - Acquired: meningitis/encephalitis, head injury (crashes or child abuse)
    - May be associated with other deficits depending on the causes, but this is a motor deficiency definition; some children are even intellectually gifted
    - Team approach for optimal outcomes
      - Physicians provide antispasticity medications
      - Home health care and durable medical equipment
      - OT/PT/Speech therapy as needed
      - Social work/health navigator

BEHAVIORAL DISORDERS

Caroline R. Paul | Colleen M. Wallace

CHAPTER 11

Crying and Colic

Infant crying can be a sign of pain, distress, hunger, or fatigue and is interpreted by caregivers according to the context of the crying. The cry just after birth heralds the infant's health and vigor. The screams of the same infant, 6 weeks later, may be interpreted as a sign of illness, difficult temperament, or poor parenting. Crying is a manifestation of infant arousal influenced by the environment and interpreted through the lens of the family, social, and cultural context.

NORMAL DEVELOPMENT

Crying is best understood by the characteristics of timing, duration, frequency, intensity, and modifiability of the cry (Fig. 11.1). Most infants cry little during the first 2 weeks of life, gradually increasing to an average of 3 hours per day by 6 weeks and decreasing to an average of 1 hour per day by 12 weeks.

Cry **duration** differs by culture and infant care practices. For example, Kung San hunter–gatherer infants, who are continuously carried and fed four times per hour, cry 50% less than infants in the United States. Crying may also relate to health status and gestational age. Premature infants cry little before 40 weeks gestational age but tend to cry more than term infants at 6 weeks' corrected age. Crying behavior in former premature infants also may be influenced by ongoing medical conditions, such as bronchopulmonary dysplasia, visual impairments, and feeding disorders. The duration of crying is often modifiable by caregiving strategies.

Frequency of crying is less variable than duration of crying. At 6 weeks of age, the mean frequency of combined crying and fussing is 10 episodes in 24 hours. Diurnal variation in crying is the norm, with crying concentrated in the late afternoon and evening.

The **intensity** of infant crying varies, with descriptions ranging from fussing to screaming. An intense infant cry (pitch and loudness) is more likely to elicit concern or even alarm from parents and caregivers than an infant who frets more quietly. Pain cries of newborns are remarkably loud: 80 dB at a distance of 30.5 cm from the infant's mouth. Although pain cries have a higher frequency than hunger cries, when not attended to for a protracted period, hunger cries become acoustically similar to pain cries. Fortunately, most infant crying is of a lesser intensity, consistent with fussing.

COLIC

Colic often is diagnosed using **Wessel's rule of threes**—crying for more than 3 hours per day, at least 3 days per week, for more than 3 weeks. The limitations of this definition include the lack of specificity of the word *crying* (e.g., does this include fussing?) and the necessity to wait 3 weeks to make a diagnosis in an infant who has excessive crying. Colicky crying is often described as paroxysmal and may be characterized by facial grimacing, leg flexion, and passing flatus.

Etiology

Fewer than 5% of infants evaluated for excessive crying have an organic etiology, with no known association with feeding method or family history of food allergy or atopy. The etiology of colic is unknown and is likely multifactorial in etiology. Since it is a diagnosis of exclusion, evaluation of infants with excessive crying is necessary in order to rule out other serious diagnoses.

Epidemiology

Cumulative incidence rates of colic vary from 5% to 28% in different studies that vary by definition of colic and method

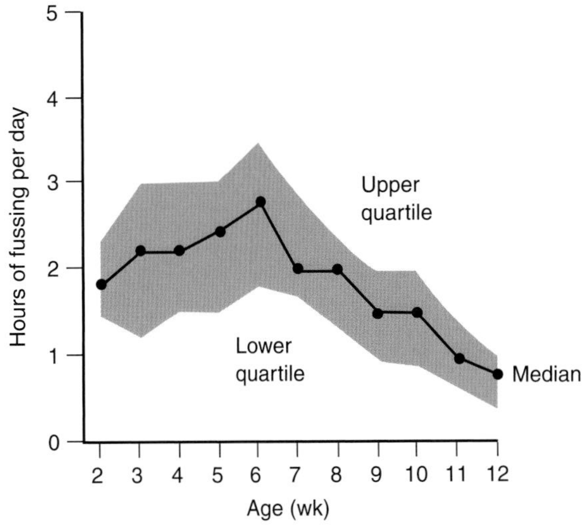

FIGURE 11.1 Distribution of total crying time among 80 infants studied from 2-12 weeks of age. Data derived from daily crying diaries recorded by mothers. (From Brazelton TB. Crying in infancy. *Pediatrics.* 1962;29:582.)

of data collection. There is no known association with gender or socioeconomic status. Concern about infant crying also varies by culture, and this may influence what is recorded as crying or fussing.

Clinical Manifestations

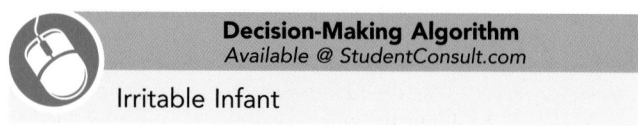

Decision-Making Algorithm
Available @ StudentConsult.com

Irritable Infant

The clinician who evaluates a crying infant must first rule out serious diseases and injuries that can mimic colic. The **history** should include a description of the crying (including onset, duration, frequency, diurnal pattern, intensity, periodicity, and relieving or exacerbating factors) as well as associated symptoms such as leg flexion, facial grimacing, vomiting, or back arching. A review of systems is helpful to identify or eliminate other serious conditions, and a birth history can help identify perinatal problems, which may increase the likelihood of neurologic causes of crying. A detailed feeding history can reveal feeding-related problems, including hunger, air swallowing (worsened by crying), gastroesophageal reflux, and food intolerance. Finally, questions concerning the family's ability to handle the stress of the infant's crying and their knowledge of infant soothing strategies assist the clinician in assessing risk for parental mental health comorbidities and developing an intervention plan suitable for the family.

The diagnosis of colic is made only when the **physical examination** reveals no organic cause for the infant's excessive crying. An infant who is not consolable is considered to be irritable and warrants further investigation for infant irritability. The examination begins with vital signs, weight, length, and head circumference, looking for effects of systemic illness on growth. A thorough inspection of the infant is important to identify possible sources of pain, including skin lesions, **corneal abrasions, hair tourniquets,** or signs of child abuse such as **bruising** or **fractures** (see Chapters 22 and 198). Other infant conditions that commonly cause pain include acute otitis media, urinary tract infections, oral ulcerations, and insect bites. A neurologic examination may reveal previously undiagnosed neurologic conditions, such as perinatal brain injuries. Observing the infant during a crying episode (or reviewing a recording of an episode) can be invaluable in assessing the infant's potential for calming and the parents' skills in soothing the infant.

Laboratory and imaging studies are warranted when the history or physical examination findings suggest an organic cause for excessive crying. An algorithm for the medical evaluation of an infant with excessive crying inconsistent with colic is presented in Fig. 11.2.

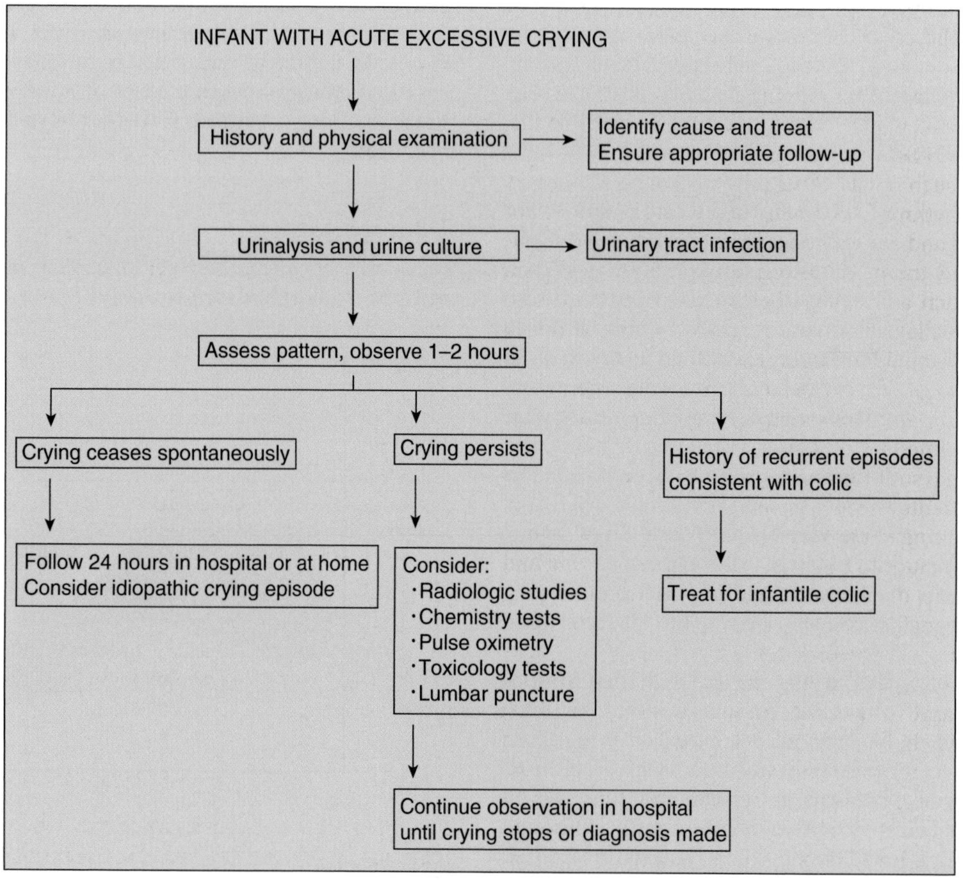

FIGURE 11.2 Algorithm for medical evaluation of infants with acute excessive crying. (From Barr RG, Hopkins B, Green JA, ed. Crying complaints in the emergency department. In: *Crying as a Sign, a Symptom, and a Signal*. London: MacKeith Press; 2000:99.)

Differential Diagnosis

The differential diagnosis for colic is broad and includes any condition that can cause pain or discomfort in the infant, including those above, as well as conditions associated with *nonpainful* distress, such as fatigue or sensory overload. Cow's milk protein intolerance, gastroesophageal reflux disease (GERD), maternal substance use including nicotine, and anomalous left coronary artery all have been reported as causes of persistent crying. In addition, situations associated with poor infant regulation, including fatigue, hunger, parental anxiety, and chaotic environmental conditions, may increase the risk of excessive crying. In most cases, the cause of crying in infants is unexplained. If the condition began before 3 weeks' corrected age, the crying has a diurnal pattern consistent with colic (afternoon and evening clustering), the infant is otherwise developing and thriving, and no organic cause is found, a diagnosis of colic may be made.

Anticipatory Guidance and Management

The management of colic begins with education and demystification. When the family and the physician are reassured that the infant is healthy, education about the normal pattern of infant crying is appropriate. Anticipatory guidance should also be provided regarding atypical crying that warrants further medical attention. Learning about the temporal pattern of colic can be reassuring; the mean crying duration begins to decrease at 6 weeks of age and decreases by half by 12 weeks of age. Colic frequently resolves by 3 months of age. Approximately 15% of infants with colic continue to have excessive crying after this age.

Helping families develop caregiving strategies for the infant's fussy period is useful. Techniques for calming infants include Dr. Harvey Karp's "5 Ss": swaddling, side or stomach holding, soothing noises (such as shushing, singing, or white noise), swinging or slow rhythmic movement (such as rocking, walking, or riding in a car), and sucking on a pacifier. Giving caregivers permission to allow the infant to rest or leave the infant alone in a safe place (such as a crib) when soothing strategies are not working may alleviate overstimulation in some infants; this also relieves families of guilt and allows them a wider range of responses to infant crying. It is important to encourage parents to seek help and support from others when they are becoming overwhelmed and to advise against harmful methods to soothe an infant (such as placing the infant on a vibrating clothes dryer). Parents should be specifically educated about the dangers of shaking babies.

Medications, including phenobarbital, diphenhydramine, alcohol, simethicone, dicyclomine, and lactase, have not been shown to be of benefit and may cause serious side effects; they are, therefore, not recommended. Some early studies have suggested that probiotics may be useful, but results have been conflicting, and further research is needed. Alternative treatments such as chamomile, fennel, vervain, licorice, and balm-mint teas have not been approved for use in infants and can cause serious side effects such as hyponatremia and anemia.

Some feeding measures may be helpful in alleviating the symptoms of colic. Educating parents regarding variable hunger cues, avoiding excessive caffeine and alcohol in nursing mothers, ensuring adequate yet not excessive bottle nipple flow, and cautioning against overfeeding may be helpful. In most circumstances, more specific **dietary changes** are not effective in reducing colic but should be considered in certain specific circumstances such as when there is concern for cow's milk protein allergy/intolerance or lactase deficiency.

Prognosis

The most serious complication of colic is child abuse from frustrated caretakers. It is important to reassure parents that there is no evidence that infants with colic have adverse long-term outcomes in health or temperament after the affected period. Similarly, infantile colic does not have untoward long-term effects on maternal mental health, as parental distress tends to resolve as colic subsides.

CHAPTER 12

Temper Tantrums

Temper tantrums are a very common childhood behavioral condition, which commonly cause concern for parents, prompting presentation to pediatric care providers and referrals to behavioral consultants.

Temper tantrums can be defined as episodes of extreme frustration and anger that manifest in an array of signs ranging from whining, screaming, stomping, hitting, head banging, and falling to more severe actions such as breath holding, vomiting, and aggression, including biting. Tantrums are seen most often when the young child experiences frustration, anger, or simple inability to cope with a situation. The behavior appears very disproportionate to the situation, and the child often appears to be "out of control."

ETIOLOGY

Temper tantrums are believed to be a normal human developmental stage. Child temperament may be a determinant of tantrum behavior.

EPIDEMIOLOGY

Temper tantrums are considered part of typical behavior in 1- to 4-year-old children. In U.S. studies, 50-80% of 2- to 3-year-old children have had regular tantrums, and 20% are reported to have daily tantrums. The behavior appears to peak late in the third year of life; however, approximately 20% of 4-year-olds are still having regular temper tantrums, and 10% of 4-year-old children have tantrums at least once a day. Explosive temper occurs in approximately 5% of school-aged children. Tantrums occur equally in boys and girls during the preschool period.

CLINICAL MANIFESTATIONS

It is important to recognize that there is not one set of behaviors that reliably differentiates typical and abnormal temper tantrums. However, some concerning elements that may signal abnormal tantrums are summarized and contrasted with typical tantrum characteristics in Table 12.1. Atypical tantrums (especially those

TABLE 12.1 Normal and Abnormal Tantrums

	NORMAL TEMPER TANTRUM	ABNORMAL TEMPER TANTRUM
Age	12 months up to age 4	Continuing past age 4
Behavior during tantrum	Crying, flailing arms or legs, falling to the floor, pushing, pulling, or biting	Injury to themselves or others during the tantrum
Duration	Up to 15 min	Lasting longer than 15 min
Frequency	Less than five times a day	More than five times a day
Mood	Should return to normal between tantrums	Persistent negative mood between tantrums

From Daniels E, Mandleco B, Luthy KE. Assessment, management, and prevention of childhood temper tantrums. J Amer Acad Nurse Pract. 2012;24(10):569–573 [Table 1].

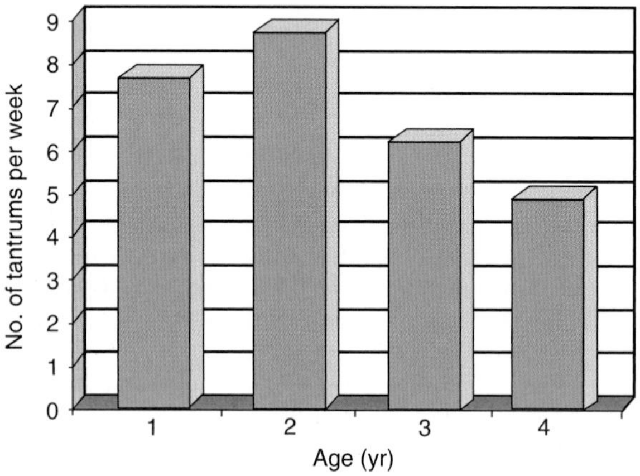

FIGURE 12.1 Mean tantrum frequency per week. Children 1-4 years of age who have tantrums typically have 4-9 tantrums per week.

involving violent, destructive, injurious, or aggressive displays) may be indicative of more serious behavioral, mood, or other medical problems. The frequency of tantrums typically decreases with age (Fig. 12.1), while the mean duration increases with age (Fig. 12.2). However, there is variability within the normal range, and about 5-7% of children between the age of 1 and 3 years have temper tantrums that last more than 15 minutes with a frequency of 3 times or more a week.

The **evaluation** of a child with tantrums starts with the intent to rule out other explanations for the behavior complaints. A comprehensive and detailed history including perinatal, developmental, family, and social history as well as review of systems is warranted to evaluate for other conditions and aid in the management of the temper tantrum episode. In particular, a social history that includes past and ongoing family stressors, including parental well-being, is important as these stressors can exacerbate or prolong what begins as a normal developmental phase. In general, parental mental hygiene is helpful for the management of temper tantrums. Atypical tantrum features or the coexistence of other behavioral problems and conditions,

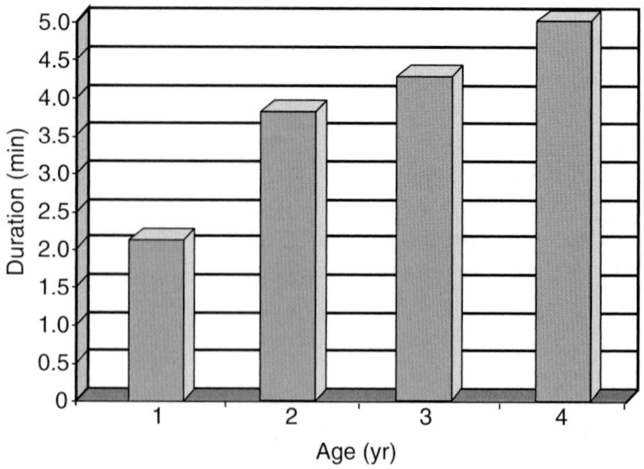

FIGURE 12.2 Mean duration of tantrums. The typical duration of a tantrum increases with the age of the child.

such as sleep disturbances, learning problems, attention-deficit/hyperactivity disorder (ADHD), autism spectrum disorder (ASD), and mood disorders, may suggest the possibility of a more serious mental health disorder.

A parental questionnaire of the tantrum episodes is valuable to both the evaluation and the management of temper tantrums. Helping the family identify the typical antecedents of the child's tantrums is essential to evaluation and intervention. For example, a child who has tantrums only when he or she misses a routine nap can be treated differently than a child who has frequent tantrums related to minor difficulties or disappointments. Careful attention to the child's daily routines may reveal problems associated with hunger, fatigue, inadequate physical activity, or overstimulation.

The physical examination focuses on discovering an underlying illness with symptoms that mimic temper tantrums or that can decrease the child's ability to self-regulate. A full exam is essential and includes vision and hearing and a developmental exam. Speech and language delay can frustrate a child and exacerbate tantrums. The examiner's general observation is very helpful. Behavioral observations reveal a child's ability to follow instructions, play with age-appropriate toys, and interact with parents and the clinician; observation of attention may be especially helpful in evaluating for ASD. Dysmorphic features may reveal a genetic syndrome, and a full skin exam may reveal neurocutaneous stigma as well as evidence of child abuse (see Chapter 22). Neurological exam includes the general disposition of the child, brief cognition assessment, and exploration for neurological deficits that could suggest brain tumors or other neurological conditions.

Laboratory studies screening for iron deficiency anemia, sleep disturbance such as restless sleep, and lead exposure are important. Other laboratory and imaging studies should be reserved for situations where the history and physical examination suggest a possible underlying etiology.

DIFFERENTIAL DIAGNOSIS

Most children who have temper tantrums have no underlying medical problem. The differential diagnosis for atypical tantrums includes hearing loss and language delay, which may contribute to the severity of temper tantrums. Children with brain injury and other brain disorders are at increased risk for prolonged temper tantrum behavior. These children include former premature infants and children with ASDs, traumatic brain injury, cognitive impairment, and Prader-Willi and Smith-Magenis syndromes. Children with rare conditions, such as congenital adrenal hyperplasia and precocious puberty, also may present with severe and persistent tantrums. Children with intellectual disability may exhibit tantrums when their developmental age is comparable to 3 to 4 years.

ANTICIPATORY GUIDANCE AND MANAGEMENT

Intervention begins with parental education about the nature of typical temper tantrums, stressing that tantrums are a normal developmental phase. It is very important to guide parents' expectations of their child's tantrums as related to normal development. Anticipatory guidance should occur at the 12-month well-child check, providing strategies for assisting children with emotional regulation, and emphasizing the importance of regular routines for sleeping, eating, and safe physical activity.

The clinician can help parents understand their role in helping the child by highlighting the importance of maintaining consistency regarding behavioral expectations and consequences, encouraging developmentally appropriate positive and negative reinforcements, and structure in a child's environment. Reviewing the child's daily routine is critical to understanding if the tantrums are communicating essential unmet needs. Parents should be educated on structuring the environment, avoiding age-inappropriate demands on the child, and addressing hunger, fatigue, loneliness, or hyperstimulation. Children who behave well all day at day care and exhibit temper tantrums at home in the evening may be signaling fatigue or need for parental attention. Identification of underlying stress is the cornerstone of treatment because many stressors can be eliminated.

In some cases, parents inadvertently reinforce tantrum behavior by complying with the child's demands. Parental ambivalence about acceptable toddler behavior also may lead to inconsistent expectations and restrictions. Helping parents clarify what behavior is allowed and what is off limits can avert the temptation to give in when the child screams loudly or publicly.

It is important for parents to model positive behavior and avoid tantrum-like behavior themselves (e.g., yelling) and to avoid physical punishment, which in turn can encourage physical aggression by the child. Other helpful strategies include offering children choices among acceptable alternatives, teaching alternate ways to communicate desires and frustrations (verbally, signing, etc.), and providing warnings prior to unpleasant transitions such as leaving a place the child enjoys.

Distraction is an effective means of short-circuiting impending tantrums. Physically removing the child from an environment that is associated with the child's difficulty is sometimes helpful. Further behavioral interventions are recommended only after engaging in strategies to help the child gain control by meeting basic needs, altering the environment, and anticipating meltdowns. Recommended behavioral strategies include behavior modification with positive and negative reinforcement or extinction. During the first week of any behavioral intervention, tantrum behavior may increase. While parents are working to extinguish or decrease the tantrums, it is important that they provide positive reinforcement for good behavior.

CHAPTER 13

Attention-Deficit/Hyperactivity Disorder

Attention-deficit/hyperactivity disorder (ADHD) is a chronic neurobehavioral disorder characterized by symptoms of inattention, hyperactivity, impulsivity, or a combination of these symptoms. It is typically diagnosed in childhood but frequently has long-term implications, including decreased likelihood of high school and postsecondary graduation as well as poor peer relations.

ETIOLOGY

ADHD is multifactorial in origin with genetic, neural, and environmental contributions. There are many studies that suggest variable degrees of genetic associations with ADHD, yet overall, clear and definitive associations are not well defined. Twin and family studies demonstrate high heritability (0.8) and greater risk of developing ADHD in first-degree relatives, especially those where ADHD persists into adolescence and adulthood. Candidate genes include those involving the dopaminergic and noradrenergic neurotransmitter systems. Neuroimaging studies (functional magnetic resonance imaging and positron emission tomography) have shown structural and functional differences, particularly of the frontal lobes, inferior parietal cortex, basal ganglia, corpus callus, and cerebellar vermis. Neuroimaging studies have demonstrated delay in cortical maturation and suggest that the pathophysiological features include large-scale neuronal networks including frontal to parietal cortical connections. Environmental links have been described with prenatal exposure to a variety of substances including nicotine, alcohol, prescription medications, and illicit substances. Environmental exposure to lead, organophosphate pesticides, or polychlorinated biphenyls has also been shown to be a risk factor. Additionally, damage to the central nervous system from trauma or infection can increase the risk of ADHD.

EPIDEMIOLOGY

U.S. prevalence rates for ADHD vary depending on criteria used and population studied, with approximately 11% of U.S. children diagnosed with ADHD today. The male to female ratio is 2-6:1, with greater male predominance for the hyperactive/impulsive and combined types. Girls often present with inattentive symptoms and are more likely to be underdiagnosed or to receive later diagnoses. Symptoms of ADHD, particularly impulsivity and inattention, frequently persist past childhood, with up to 80% of those affected having symptoms into adolescence, and 40% into adulthood.

Clinical Symptoms

Many of the symptoms of ADHD mimic typical findings of normal development; thus it is important to consider whether the child's symptoms are out of proportion to what would be expected for stage of development. Symptoms of inattention (e.g., failing to pay close attention to details, appearing to not listen when spoken to directly), hyperactivity (e.g., being fidgety or restless, leaving a seat when expected to remain seated), or impulsivity (e.g., blurting out answers before a question has been completed) may indicate a diagnosis of ADHD (Table 13.1).

Diagnosis and Evaluation

ADHD is diagnosed clinically by **history.** The reports of parents, teachers, and others, including teenage self-report, are core to its diagnosis. The history should rely on open-ended questions as much as possible to explore specific behaviors and their impact on academic performance, family and peer relationships, safety, self-esteem, and daily activities. However, ultimately, a diagnosis of ADHD requires that the symptoms be measured with validated rating scales to establish the diagnosis.

TABLE 13.1 Key Diagnostic Symptoms of Attention-Deficit/Hyperactivity Disorder

INATTENTIVE SYMPTOMS
• Does not give close attention to details or makes careless mistakes
• Has difficulty sustaining attention on tasks or play activities
• Does not seem to listen when directly spoken to
• Does not follow through on instructions and does not finish schoolwork, chores, or duties in the workplace
• Has trouble organizing tasks or activities
• Avoids, dislikes, or is reluctant to do tasks that need sustained mental effort
• Loses things needed for tasks or activities
• Easily distracted
• Forgetful in daily activities
HYPERACTIVITY OR IMPULSIVITY SYMPTOMS
• Fidgets with or taps hands or feet, or squirms in seat
• Leaves seat in situations when staying seated is expected
• Runs about or climbs when not appropriate (may present as feelings of restlessness in adolescents or adults)
• Unable to play or undertake leisure activities quietly
• "On the go," acting as if "driven by a motor"
• Talks excessively
• Blurts out answers before a question has been finished
• Has difficulty waiting his or her turn
• Interrupts or intrudes on others

From Thapar A, Cooper M. Attention deficit hyperactivity disorder. Lancet. 2016;387(10024):1240–1250.

Clinical guidelines emphasize the use of the *Diagnostic and Statistical Manual of Mental Health Disorders*, fifth edition, with specific criteria (available at http://www.cdc.gov/ncbddd/adhd/diagnosis.html) to diagnose ADHD. Symptoms must have been present prior to 12 years of age; evidence of significant impairment in social, academic, or work settings must occur; and other mental disorders must be excluded. Changes incorporated into the fifth edition include the age prior to which symptoms must occur (to identify the subset of older children (frequently female) who exhibit predominantly inattentive symptoms and who may not present with significant functional impairment early in childhood), the need for symptoms to occur in at least two settings, and the decrease in number of symptoms to five for adolescents 17 years of age or older.

A **physical examination** is essential to identify medical (e.g., neurologic, genetic) or developmental problems (e.g., cognitive impairment, language disorder, learning disability, autism spectrum disorder) that may underlie, coexist, or provide an alternative explanation for the child's behaviors. Observation of the child, the parents, and their interactions is part of the evaluation. Note that some children with ADHD will be able to maintain focus without hyperactivity in environments with low stimulation and little distraction (e.g., clinician's office).

Laboratory and imaging studies should be considered with the aim to exclude other conditions. Consider thyroid function studies, blood lead levels, genetic studies, anemia screening, and brain imaging studies if clearly indicated by medical history, environmental history, or physical examination.

DIFFERENTIAL DIAGNOSIS

The differential diagnosis can be challenging given that co-morbidities of ADHD overlap and intertwine with the differential diagnoses. The diagnostic process should evaluate for other conditions such as sleep disorders, seizure disorders, substance use, hyperthyroidism, lead intoxication, sensory processing issues, and vision or auditory deficits as possible causes for a child's hyperactivity and distractibility. Inattention and hyperactivity may be present as features of genetic disorders such as fragile X, 22q11.2 deletion syndrome, and neurofibromatosis 1. Psychological stress (e.g., bullying, abuse) and disruptive surroundings can also lead to symptoms of hyperactivity, impulsivity, and inattention *and* mimic indeed the symptoms of ADHD. Children who have symptoms of ADHD in only one setting may be having problems due to cognitive disability, level of emotional maturity, or feelings of inadequate well-being in that setting. Overall, it is prudent to investigate and ensure overall well-being including sleep and nutritional hygiene before embarking on an extensive evaluation of ADHD.

Co-morbidities

Co-morbidities are present in up to 60% of children with ADHD such as anxiety, learning disabilities, language disorders, tic disorders, mood disorders, coordination problems, oppositional defiant disorder, and other conduct disorder. Tourette syndrome and fragile X syndrome, in particular, are known conditions with associated ADHD. It is important to discern if the symptoms are due to the co-morbidities independently or as a co-morbidity with ADHD.

Treatment

Management begins with recognizing ADHD as a chronic condition and educating affected children and their parents about the diagnosis, treatment options, and prognosis. With appropriate management, including behavioral and academic interventions in conjunction with medication, up to 80% of children have significant response to treatment. Anticipatory guidance is important and includes providing proactive strategies to mediate adverse effects on learning, school functioning, social relationships, family life, and self-esteem.

Behavioral therapy is central to children of all ages with ADHD and must be the core of overall treatment. **Behavioral management** includes establishment of structure, routine, consistency in adult responses to behaviors, and appropriate behavioral goals. Children also benefit when parents and clinicians work with teachers to address the child's needs. Regular behavior report cards and other "check-in" aids may be helpful to the child in their respective environments such as for a classroom and the overall school day.

The pediatrician should advocate for **optimal educational settings** in the school. Children may qualify for individual education plans where school psychologists can establish organizational plans and charts for the individual child as part of a management plan. Social skills training or additional mental health interventions may assist some children with behavior change or preservation of self-esteem, particularly when they have coexisting developmental or mental health conditions also requiring treatment.

Stimulant medications (methylphenidate or amphetamine compounds) are the first-line agents for pharmacologic treatment of ADHD due to extensive evidence of efficacy and safety. Short-term studies have shown a significant clinical benefit of stimulant medications in reducing inattention, hyperactivity, and impulsivity. Stimulant medications are available in short-acting, intermediate-acting, and long-acting forms. Sustained and long-acting forms are often preferred, yet there are no definitive studies to establish the benefit of long-acting stimulants over short-acting stimulant medication. Preparations include liquid, chewables, tablets, capsules, and a transdermal patch, allowing the clinician to tailor the choice of medication to the child's needs. While stimulants have been shown to provide some benefit in short-term studies in preschool-aged children, behavioral management is still considered the standard of care for this age group.

Nonstimulant medications, including atomoxetine (norepinephrine-reuptake inhibitor), guanfacine, or clonidine (α-agonists), may be helpful in children that do not respond to stimulant medication, or for family preference, concerns about medication abuse or diversion, and contraindications to stimulant use.

Medications continue to be developed as researchers add to the knowledge of effectiveness and adverse side effects. Reputable resources such as the Centers for Disease Control and Prevention (CDC) and American Academy of Pediatrics (AAP) can provide up-to-date information on specific medications, dosing, contraindications, and other considerations to optimize management for these children.

Medication side effects are common, occurring in about one third of patients and severe enough to indicate changing or discontinuing the medication in 15% of patients. The most common side effects include appetite suppression and sleep disturbance with stimulant medications, gastrointestinal tract symptoms with atomoxetine, and sedation with α-agonists. Side effects must be assessed while children are undergoing treatment, including careful monitoring of the child's height and weight at regular follow-up appointments. In general, providers should titrate medication dosages and timing to minimize side effects and optimize treatment response. Screening for cardiac disease by history, family history, and physical exam, as well as monitoring the cardiac status of children on stimulant medication is prudent.

COMPLICATIONS

ADHD may be associated with academic underachievement, difficulties in interpersonal relationships, and poor self-esteem. These complications may have long-reaching effects including lower levels of educational and employment attainment. Adolescents with ADHD, particularly those who are untreated, are at increased risk for high-risk behaviors. Despite parental concerns of illicit drug use and addiction from stimulant medication, there is actually decreased risk of drug abuse in children and adolescents with ADHD who are appropriately medically managed.

ANTICIPATORY GUIDANCE

Child-rearing practices, including promoting calm environments and opportunities for age-appropriate activities that require increasing levels of focus, may be helpful in terms of behavioral modifications. Limiting time spent watching television and playing rapid-response video games also may be prudent as these activities may reinforce short attention span.

Early implementation of behavior management techniques may assist in curtailing problematic behaviors before they result in significant impairment and can help with the child's self-esteem and school performance concerns. Education of medical professionals and teachers about the signs and symptoms of ADHD and the most appropriate and timing behavioral and pharmaceutical interventions is helpful to the overall management of ADHD. Collaboration between health care providers, educational professionals, mental health clinicians, and families will enhance the early identification of, treatment, and provision of services to children with ADHD.

CHAPTER 14

Control of Elimination

NORMAL DEVELOPMENT OF ELIMINATION

Development of control of urination and defecation involves physical and cognitive maturation and is strongly influenced by cultural norms, socioeconomic status, and practices within the United States and throughout the world. In the first half of the 20th century, toilet mastery by 18 months of age was the norm in the United States. Brazelton's introduction of the *child-centered approach* and the invention of disposable diapers facilitated later toilet training. Social changes, including increased maternal work outside of the home and group child care, also have influenced the trend to later initiation of toilet training. Toilet training now usually begins after the second birthday and is achieved at about 3 years of age in middle-class white U.S. populations. Toilet training between 12 and 18 months of age continues to be accepted in lower-income families.

Prerequisites for achieving elimination in the toilet include the child's ability to recognize the urge for urination and defecation, to get to the toilet, to understand the sequence of tasks required, to avoid oppositional behavior, and to take pride in achievement. The entire process of toilet training can take 6 months and need not be hurried. Successful parent–child interaction around the goal of toilet mastery can set the stage for future active parental teaching and training (e.g., manners, kindness, rules and laws, and limit setting).

ENURESIS

Enuresis is urinary incontinence in a child who is adequately mature to have achieved continence. Enuresis is classified as diurnal (daytime) or nocturnal (nighttime). In the United States, daytime and nighttime dryness are expected by 4 and 6 years of age, respectively. Another useful classification of enuresis is **primary** (incontinence in a child who has never achieved dryness) and **secondary** (incontinence in a child who has been dry for at least 6 months).

Etiology

Enuresis is a symptom with multiple possible etiologic factors, including developmental difference, organic illness, or psychological distress. Primary enuresis often is associated with a family history of delayed acquisition of bladder control. A genetic etiology has been hypothesized, and familial groups with autosomal dominant phenotypic patterns for nocturnal enuresis have been identified. Although most children with enuresis do not have a psychiatric disorder, stressful life events can trigger loss of bladder control. Sleep physiology may play a role in the etiology of nocturnal enuresis, with a high arousal threshold commonly noted. In a subgroup of enuretic children, nocturnal polyuria relates to a lack of a nocturnal vasopressin peak. Another possible etiology is malfunction of the detrusor muscle with a tendency for involuntary contractions even when the bladder contains small amounts of urine. Reduced bladder capacity can be associated with enuresis and is commonly seen in children who have chronic constipation with a large dilated distal colon, which impinges on the bladder.

Epidemiology

Enuresis is the most common urologic condition in children. Nocturnal enuresis has a reported prevalence of 15% in 5-year-olds, 7% in 8-year-olds, and 1% in 15-year-olds. The spontaneous remission rate is reported to be 15% per year. The odds ratio of nocturnal enuresis in boys compared with girls is 1.4:1. The prevalence of daytime enuresis is lower than nocturnal enuresis but has a female predominance, 1.5:1 at 7 years of age. Of children with enuresis, 22% wet during the day only, 17% wet during the day and at night, and 61% wet at night only.

Clinical Manifestations

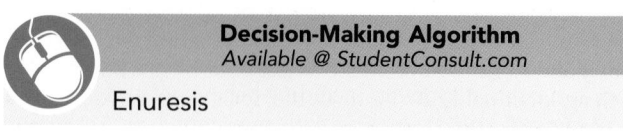

Decision-Making Algorithm
Available @ StudentConsult.com

Enuresis

The history focuses on elucidating the pattern of voiding including frequency, timing (diurnal/nocturnal), associated conditions or stressful events (e.g., bad dreams, consumption of caffeinated beverages, or exhausting days), and whether it is primary or secondary enuresis. A review of systems should include a developmental history and detailed information about the neurologic, urinary, and gastrointestinal systems (including patterns of defecation). A history of sleep patterns is important, including snoring, parasomnias, and timing of nighttime urination. A family history often reveals that one or both parents had enuresis as children. Although enuresis is rarely associated with child abuse, physical and sexual abuse history should be included as part of the psychosocial history. Many families have tried numerous interventions before seeking a physician's help. Identifying these interventions and how they were carried out aids the understanding of the child's condition and its role within the family.

The **physical examination** begins with observation of the child and the parent for clues about child developmental and parent-child interaction patterns. Special attention is paid to the abdominal, neurologic, and genital examination. A rectal examination is recommended if the child has constipation. Observation of voiding is recommended if a history of voiding problems, such as hesitancy or dribbling, is elicited. The lumbosacral spine should be examined for signs of spinal dysraphism or a tethered cord.

For most children with enuresis, the only laboratory test recommended is a clean catch urinalysis to look for chronic urinary tract infection (UTI), renal disease, and diabetes mellitus. Further testing, such as a urine culture, is based on the urinalysis. Children with complicated enuresis, including children with previous or current UTI, severe voiding dysfunction, or a neurologic finding, are evaluated with a renal sonogram and a voiding cystourethrogram. If vesicoureteral reflux, hydronephrosis, or posterior urethral valves are found, the child is referred to a urologist for further evaluation and treatment.

Differential Diagnosis

There is no commonly identified cause of enuresis and, in most cases, enuresis resolves by adolescence without treatment. Children with primary nocturnal enuresis are most likely to have a family history and are least likely to have an identified etiology. Children with secondary diurnal and nocturnal enuresis are more likely to have an organic etiology, such as UTI, diabetes mellitus, or diabetes insipidus, to explain their symptoms. Children with primary diurnal and nocturnal enuresis may have a neurodevelopmental condition or a problem with bladder function. Children with secondary nocturnal enuresis may have a psychosocial stressor or a sleep disturbance as a predisposing condition for enuresis.

Treatment

Treatment begins with treating any diagnosed underlying organic causes of enuresis. Elimination of underlying chronic constipation is often curative. For a child whose enuresis is not associated with an identifiable disorder, all therapies must be considered in terms of cost in time, money, disruption to the family, the treatment's known success rate, and the child's likelihood to recover from the condition without treatment. The most commonly used treatment options are **conditioning therapy** and **pharmacotherapy.** The clinician can also assist the family in making a plan to help the child cope with this problem until it is resolved. Many children have to live with enuresis for months to years before a cure is achieved; a few children have symptoms into adulthood. A plan for handling wet garments and linens in a nonhumiliating and hygienic manner preserves the child's self-esteem. The child should take as much responsibility as he or she is able, depending on age, development, and family culture.

The most widely used **conditioning therapy** for nocturnal enuresis is the **enuresis alarm.** Enuresis alarms have an initial success rate of 30-60% with a significant relapse rate. The alarm is worn on the wrist or clipped onto the pajama and has a probe that is placed in the underpants or pajamas in front of the urethra. The alarm sounds when the first drop of urine contacts the probe. The child is instructed to get up and finish voiding in the bathroom when the alarm sounds.

Pharmacotherapy for nighttime enuresis includes desmopressin acetate and, rarely, tricyclic antidepressants. **Desmopressin** decreases urine production and has proved to be safe in the treatment of enuresis. The oral medication is started at 0.2 mg per dose (one dose at bedtime) and on subsequent nights is increased to 0.4 mg and then to 0.6 mg if needed. This treatment must be considered symptomatic, not curative, and has a relapse rate of 90% when the medication is discontinued. **Imipramine,** now rarely used for enuresis, reduces the frequency of nighttime wetting, and the initial success rate is 50%. Imipramine is effective during treatment only, with a relapse rate of 90% on discontinuation of the medication. The most important contraindication is the risk of overdose (associated with fatal cardiac arrhythmia).

Complications

The psychological consequences can be severe. Families can minimize the impact on the child's self-esteem by avoiding punitive approaches and ensuring that the child is competent to handle issues of their own comfort, hygiene, and aesthetics.

Prevention

Appropriate anticipatory guidance to educate parents that bed-wetting is common in early childhood helps alleviate considerable anxiety.

FUNCTIONAL CONSTIPATION AND SOILING

Constipation is decreased frequency of bowel movements, usually associated with a hard stool consistency. The occurrence of pain at defecation frequently accompanies constipation. Although underlying gastrointestinal, endocrinologic, or neurologic disorders can cause constipation, *functional constipation* implies that there is no identifiable causative organic condition. **Encopresis** is the regular, voluntary, or involuntary passage of feces into a place other than the toilet after 4 years of age. Encopresis without constipation is uncommon and may be a symptom of oppositional defiant disorder or other psychiatric illness. *Soiling* is the involuntary passage of stool and often is associated with fecal impaction. The normal frequency of bowel movements declines between birth and 4 years of age, beginning with greater than four stools per day to approximately one per day.

Etiology

The etiology of functional constipation and soiling includes a low-fiber diet, slow gastrointestinal transit time for neurologic or genetic reasons, and chronic withholding of bowel movements, usually because of past painful defecation experiences. Approximately 95% of children referred to a subspecialist for encopresis have no other underlying pathologic condition.

Epidemiology

In U.S. studies, 16-37% of children experience constipation between 5 and 12 years of age. Constipation with overflow soiling occurs in 1-2% of preschool children and 4% of school-aged children. The incidence of constipation and soiling is equal in preschool girls and boys, whereas there is a male predominance during school age.

Clinical Manifestations

Decision-Making Algorithms
Available @ StudentConsult.com

Constipation
Irritable infant

The presenting complaint for constipation with soiling is typically a complaint of uncontrolled defecation. Parents may report that the child has diarrhea because of soiling of liquid stool. Soiling may be frequent or continuous. Children younger than 3 years of age often present with painful defecation, impaction, and withholding. The history should include a complete review of systems for gastrointestinal, endocrine, and neurologic disorders and a developmental and psychosocial history.

Stool impaction can be felt on abdominal examination in about 50% of patients at presentation. Firm packed stool in the rectum is highly predictive of fecal impaction. A rectal examination allows assessment of sphincter tone and size of the rectal vault. Evaluation of anal placement and existence of anal fissures also is helpful in considering etiology and severity. A neurologic examination, including lower extremity reflexes, anal wink, and cremasteric reflexes, may reveal underlying spinal cord abnormalities.

Abdominal x-ray is not required. It can be helpful to show to the family the degree of colonic distention and fecal impaction. In general, further studies, such as barium enema and rectal biopsy, are indicated only if an organic cause for the constipation is indicated by history or physical examination (see Chapter 129). Similarly, although endocrinologic conditions such as hypothyroidism can cause chronic constipation, laboratory studies are not indicated without history or physical examination suggesting such a disorder.

Differential Diagnosis

The differential diagnosis for functional constipation and soiling includes organic causes of constipation (e.g., neurogenic, anatomic, endocrinologic, gastrointestinal, and pharmacologic). A child with chronic constipation and soiling who had delayed passage of meconium and has an empty rectum and tight sphincter may have Hirschsprung disease (see Chapter 129). Chronic constipation may be a presenting sign of spinal cord abnormalities, such as a spinal cord tumor or a tethered cord. Physical examination findings of altered lower extremity reflexes, absent anal wink, or a sacral hairy tuft or sacral sinus may be a clue to these anomalies. Hypothyroidism can present with chronic constipation and typically is accompanied by poor linear growth and bradycardia. Anal stenosis may lead to chronic constipation. The use of opiates, phenothiazine, antidepressants, and anticholinergics also may lead to chronic constipation. Developmental problems, including mental retardation and autism, may be associated with chronic constipation.

Treatment

Treatment begins with education and demystification for the child and family about chronic constipation and soiling, emphasizing the chronic nature of this condition and the good prognosis with optimal management. Explaining the physiologic basis of constipation and soiling to the child and the family alleviates blame and enlists cooperation. Education may improve adherence to the long-term treatment plan (Table 14.1). One half to two thirds of children with functional constipation recover completely and no longer require medication. The younger the child is when diagnosis and treatment begin, the higher the success rate. Treatment involves a combination of behavioral training and laxative therapy. Successful treatment requires 6-24 months. The next step is adequate colonic cleanout or disimpaction. Cleanout methods include enemas alone or combinations of enema, suppository, and oral laxatives. High-dose oral mineral oil is a slower approach to cleanout. Choice of disimpaction method depends on the age of the child, family choice, and the clinician's experience with a particular method. Methods and side effects are summarized in Table 14.2. The child and family should be included in the process of choosing the cleanout method. Because enemas may be invasive and oral medication may be unpleasant, allowing points of choice and control for the child and praising all signs of cooperation are important.

Behavioral training is essential to the treatment of chronic constipation and soiling. The child and family are asked to monitor and document stool output. Routine toilet sitting is instituted for 5-10 minutes, three to four times per day. The child is asked to demonstrate proper toilet sitting position with the upper body flexed forward slightly and feet on the floor or foot support. The child should be praised for all components of cooperation with this program, and punishment and embarrassment should be avoided. As symptoms resolve, toilet sitting is decreased to twice daily and finally to once a day.

When disimpaction is achieved, the child begins the maintenance phase of treatment. This phase promotes regular stool production and prevents reimpaction. It involves attention to diet, medications to promote stool regularity, and behavioral training. Increasing dietary fiber and fluid are recommended. For children with chronic constipation, the recommended daily dose of fiber is calculated as 10 grams plus the child's age in years (e.g., a 10-year-old should take 20 g of fiber per day). At least 2 ounces of nondairy fluid intake per gram of fiber intake is recommended. Sorbitol-based juices, including prune, pear,

TABLE 14.1 Education About Chronic Constipation and Soiling
Constipation affects 16-37% of children.
One percent to 4% of children have functional constipation and soiling.
Functional constipation with/without soiling begins early in life due to a combination of factors:
Uncomfortable/painful stool passage
Withholding of stool to avoid discomfort
Diets higher in constipating foods and lower in fiber and fluid intake*
Use of medications that are constipating
Developmental features—increasing autonomy; perhaps toilet avoidance
Possible family genetic factors—slower colonic transit
When chronic impaction, physiologic changes at the rectum reduce a child's bowel control.
Dilated rectal vault results in reduced sensation to standard fecal volume.
Rehabilitation of rectal musculature and strength requires several months. Until then, dilated rectal musculature may be less able to expel stool effectively.
Paradoxical anal sphincter contraction may occur when the urge to defecate is felt; it can lead to incomplete emptying of stool at defecation attempt.
Many children do not recognize their soiling accidents owing to olfactory accommodation.
Low self-esteem or other behavioral concerns are common on presentation. Improve for most with education and management for the constipation and soiling.
Effective management of functional constipation requires a substantial commitment of the child/family, usually for 6–24 months.
Degree of child and family adherence is likely a predictor of the child's success.

**The common features of the transition to the toddler diet (decreased fluid intake, continued high dairy intake, and finicky eating patterns) make this a high-risk time during development for constipation problems.*

TABLE 14.2 Cleanout Disimpaction

MEDICATION	SIDE EFFECTS/COMMENTS
INFANTS	
Glycerin suppositories	No side effects
Enema—6 mL/kg up to 4.5 oz (135 mL)	If enemas are considered, administer first in physician's office.
CHILDREN	
Rapid Cleanout	
Enema—6 mL/kg up to 4.5 oz (135 mL) every 12–24 hr × 1–3	Invasive; risk of mechanical trauma Large impaction: mineral oil enema followed 1–3 hr later by normal saline or phosphate enema Small impaction: normal saline or phosphate enema
Mineral oil	Lubricates hard impaction; may not see return after administration
Normal saline	Abdominal cramping; may not be as effective as hypertonic phosphate
Hypertonic phosphate	Abdominal cramping; risk of hyperphosphatemia, hypokalemia, and hypocalcemia, especially with Hirschsprung or renal insufficiency or if retained. Some experts do not recommend phosphate enema for children <4 yr, others for children <2 yr.
Milk of molasses: 1:1 milk:molasses	For difficult to clear impaction
Combination: Enema, Suppository, Oral Laxative	
Day 1: Enema q12–24 hr	See enemas above
Day 2: Bisacodyl suppository (10 mg) q12–24 hr	Abdominal cramping, diarrhea, hypokalemia
Day 3: Bisacodyl tablet (5 mg) q12–24 hr	Abdominal cramping, diarrhea, hypokalemia
Repeat 3-day cycle if needed × 1–2	—
Oral/nasogastric tube: Polyethylene glycol electrolyte solution (GoLYTELY or NuLYTELY)—25 mL/kg/hr up to 1000 mL/hr × 4 hr/day	Nausea, cramping, vomiting, bloating, aspiration. Large volume. Usually requires nasogastric tube and hospitalization to administer
Slower Cleanout	
Oral high-dose mineral oil—15–30 mL per year of age per day up to 8 oz × 3–4 days	Aspiration—lipoid pneumonia. Give chilled.
X-Prep (senna): 15 mL q12 hr × 3	Abdominal cramping. May not see output until dose 2 or 3
Magnesium citrate: 1 oz/yr of age to maximum of 10 oz per day for 2–3 days	Hypermagnesemia
Maintenance medications—also may be used for cleanout	—

Limited data available for higher doses.

and apple juice, increase the water content of bowel movements. Lubricants or osmotic laxatives are used to promote regular soft bowel movements. Maintenance medications, including side effects, are listed in Table 14.3. Polyethylene glycol powder is well tolerated because the taste and texture are palatable. Some children may require the use of a lubricant in addition to an osmotic laxative; children with severe constipation may require a stimulant laxative. Treatment failure occurs in approximately one in five children secondary to problems with adherence or poor recognition of inadequate treatment resulting in reimpaction.

Complications

Chronic constipation and soiling interfere with social functioning and self-esteem. Discomfort and fear of accidents may distract children from their schoolwork and other important tasks. Children also may develop unusual eating habits in response to chronic constipation and their beliefs about this condition. Case reports of child abuse related to soiling have been published.

Prevention

The primary care physician can recommend adequate fiber intake in all children and encourage families to help their children institute regular toileting habits at an early age as preventive measures. Earlier diagnosis of chronic constipation can prevent much secondary disability and shorten the length of treatment required.

ACKNOWLEDGMENT

This chapter appeared in the previous edition and was written by Drs. Sheila Gahagan, Yi Hui Liu, and Scott J. Brown.

TABLE 14.3 Maintenance Medications*

MEDICATION	SIDE EFFECTS/COMMENTS
INFANTS	
Oral Medications/Other	
Juices containing sorbitol	Pear, prune, apple
Lactulose or sorbitol: 1–3 mL/kg/day ÷ doses bid	See below
Corn syrup (light or dark): 1–3 mL/kg/day ÷ doses bid *Per Rectum*	Not considered risk for *Clostridium botulinum* spores
Glycerin suppository	No side effects
CHILDREN	
Oral Medications	
Lubricant	Softens stool and eases passage
Mineral oil: 1–3 mL/kg day as one dose or ÷ bid	Aspiration—lipoid pneumonia Chill or give with juice Adherence problems Leakage: dose too high or impaction
Osmotics	Retain water in stool, aiding bulk and softness
Lactulose: 10 g/15 mL, 1–3 mL/kg/day ÷ doses bid	Synthetic disaccharide: abdominal cramping, flatus
Magnesium hydroxide (milk of magnesia): 400 mg/5 mL, 1–3 mL/kg/day ÷ bid 800 mg/5 mL, 0.5 mL/kg ÷ bid	Risk of hypermagnesemia, hypophosphatemia, secondary hypocalcemia with overdose or renal insufficiency
MiraLAX (polyethylene glycol powder): 17 g/240 mL water or juice stock, 1.0 g/kg/day ÷ doses bid (~15 mL/kg/day)	Titrate dose at 3-day intervals to achieve mushy stool consistency May make stock solutions to administer over 1–2 days Excellent adherence
Sorbitol: 1–3 mL/kg/day ÷ doses bid	Less costly than lactulose
Stimulants[†]	Improve effectiveness of colonic and rectal muscle contractions
Senna: syrup—8.8 g sennoside/5 mL	Idiosyncratic hepatitis, melanosis coli, hypertrophic osteoarthropathy, analgesic nephropathy, abdominal cramping
2–6 yr: 2.5–7.5 mL/day ÷ doses bid	—
6–12 yr: 5–15 mL/day ÷ doses bid (Tablets and granules available)	Improvement of melanosis coli after medication stopped
Bisacodyl: 5-mg tablets, 1–3 tablets/dose 1–2 × daily	Abdominal cramping, diarrhea, hypokalemia
Per Rectum	
Glycerin suppository	No side effects
Bisacodyl: 10-mg suppositories, 0.5–1 suppository, 1–2 × daily	Abdominal cramping, diarrhea, hypokalemia

**Single agent may suffice to achieve daily, comfortable stools.*
[†]Stimulants should be reserved for short-term use.

CHAPTER 15

Normal Sleep and Pediatric Sleep Disorders

Sleep is a universal phenomenon that is critical to child health, development, and daily functioning. Expectations and habits surrounding sleep vary greatly and must be interpreted in the context of each family and culture. Sleep is broadly categorized by polysomnographic patterns into rapid eye movement (REM) sleep and non-REM (NREM) sleep. REM sleep is characterized by an active, awake-like electroencephalography (EEG) pattern and muscle atonia. NREM sleep is further divided into three stages. Stage 1 (N1) is the lightest sleep stage and consists of low-amplitude, high-frequency EEG activity. Stage 2 (N2) is similar to Stage 1 although eye movements stop. Brain waves become slower with occasional bursts of rapid waves (called *sleep spindles* or *K complexes*). Stage 3 (N3), also known as *deep* or *slow-wave* sleep, is characterized by low-frequency, high-amplitude delta waves. REM and NREM sleep alternate in cycles throughout the night.

Sleep architecture changes from fetal life through infancy and childhood and parallels physical maturation and development. Newborns require the most sleep and have the most disrupted sleep patterns; newborn sleep cycles last approximately 60 minutes and gradually lengthen to 90 minutes in children and adults. Neonates typically begin their sleep cycle in REM sleep, whereas older children and adults begin sleep in NREM sleep. REM sleep comprises up to 50% of total sleep time in newborns and gradually decreases to 25-30% by adolescence.

Slow-wave sleep is not seen before 3-6 months of age. Starting at 6-12 months and continuing through adulthood, the amount of REM sleep shifts toward the last third of the night, while NREM sleep predominates during the first third of the night. Infants are capable of sleeping through the night without feeds at around 6 months of age; this age varies with many factors including gestational age, type of feeding (e.g., breast-fed infants tend to awaken more frequently than formula-fed infants), familial factors, and general cultural contexts.

The timing and duration of sleep also change with age. Sleep duration gradually decreases with age (0-12 years), while longest sleep period increases (0-2 years); number of night awakenings decrease in the first 2 years of life; number of daytime naps decreases (up to age 2). Sleep patterns also become more diurnal. Full-term infants sleep on average 16-18 hours per day in fragmented intervals throughout the day and night, and 1- to 3-year-old children sleep on average 10-16 hours. Naps begin to decrease from two naps to one starting around 15-18 months of age. The biological need for napping diminishes after age 2; significant consistent napping after age 2 has been associated with later sleep onset and reduced sleep quality and duration. However, 50% of 3-year-olds still nap. Napping in the older child and adolescent suggests insufficient sleep or a sleep disorder.

ADOLESCENT SLEEP

Adolescents also develop a physiologically based shift toward later sleep-onset and wake times relative to those in middle childhood. Most experts recommend that adolescents sleep at least 9 or 10 hours each night. However, only about 14-27% of adolescents worldwide achieve this amount of sleep. The average amount of adolescent sleep is 7.5 hours per day; up to 25% of adolescents achieve only 6 hours of sleep a night. Insufficient sleep in adolescents has been associated with morning tiredness, day sleepiness, and negative effects on cognitive function, moods, and motivation. Furthermore, sleep onset latency (the time it takes to fall sleep) in adolescents has been associated with fatigue, mood disorders, and anxiety. Early school start times have been associated with negative sleep adolescent profiles. Overall, adolescents should be advised to limit or reduce screen time exposure prior to overall bedtime to optimize sleep hygiene. Further studies on the use of electronic media on adolescent bedtime, sleep latency, and duration are warranted to understand the actual impact and neurophysiologic mechanisms of these associations. Similarly, the impact of substances (tobacco, caffeine, alcohol) has shown variable effects on adolescent sleep profiles.

SLEEP DISORDERS

Sleep problems are one of the most frequent complaints in pediatric practice. Numerous sleep disorders exist, including behavioral insomnias (bedtime refusal, delayed sleep onset, nighttime awakenings), parasomnias, and circadian rhythm disorders (Table 15.1). Obstructive sleep apnea (OSA) and sleep disorders associated with mental and physical illness should also be considered.

Epidemiology

Sleep problems occur in up to 50% of children at some point during childhood. The most common sequela of suboptimal sleep is daytime sleepiness. Other sequelae include irritability, behavioral problems, learning difficulties, and motor vehicle accidents in adolescents. Clear links between sleep disordered breathing and academic performance in the school-age child have been firmly established.

Behavioral sleep disorders are common and found across all age groups but are most prevalent from infancy through preschool age. Overall, behavioral insomnia of childhood has an estimated prevalence for 10-30%. Bedtime resistance occurs in 10-15% of toddlers, while 15-30% of preschool-aged children have difficulties achieving and/or maintaining sleep. Although generally benign, parasomnias such as sleepwalking (17% in children vs. 4% in adults) and sleep terrors (1-6%) occur commonly in young children. Sleepwalking peaks between 8 and 12 years of age, has a familial association, and is more common in males. Parasomnias typically resolve spontaneously by adolescence, and OSA is reported in 1-5% of children. Circadian rhythm disorders occur in 7-16% of adolescents.

Clinical Manifestations and Evaluation

Decision-Making Algorithms
Available @ StudentConsult.com

Seizures and other paroxysmal disorders
Sleep disturbances

Sleep disorders may manifest in a variety of ways and often go unrecognized. Some children present with daytime behavioral problems, including inattentiveness, hyperactivity, or irritability rather than overt sleepiness. Screening for sleep disorders is recommended as part of primary care practice. Clinicians should inquire about bedtime problems, excessive daytime sleepiness, and awakenings during the night, regularity and duration of sleep, and presence of snoring and sleep-disordered breathing.

The assessment of sleep complaints begins with a detailed history of sleep habits, including bedtime, sleep onset, and wake times. A detailed description of the sleep environment can result in a dynamic understanding of the challenges to and resources for achieving normal sleep. The recommended history includes the type of bed, who shares it, the ambient light, noise, temperature, and the bedtime routine. Household structure, routines, and cultural practices may be important and influence the timing and ease of sleep (e.g., parental work patterns, evening activities, number of household members). Dietary practices influence sleep, including timing of meals and caffeine intake. A detailed history assessing for symptoms of OSA (e.g., gasps, snorting noises, breathing pauses, etc.) should be obtained in all children who snore regularly. New-onset sleep disorders may be associated with a psychological trauma. When the history does not reveal the cause of the sleep disorder, a sleep diary can be helpful. Specifically for pre-adolescents and adolescents, a detailed history regarding bedtime routines, sleep onset time, wake times, electronic media, and light products in the room is valuable.

A complete **physical examination** is important to rule out medical causes of sleep disturbance such as conditions that cause pain, neurologic conditions that could be associated with seizure disorder, and other central nervous system disorders. Children with attention-deficit/hyperactivity disorder and fetal

TABLE **15.1** Sleep Disorders

	CAUSE	CLINICAL SYMPTOMS	DIAGNOSIS	TREATMENT	SPECIAL CONSIDERATIONS
ORGANIC					
Obstructive Sleep Apnea (OSA)	Adenotonsillar hypertrophy Overweight/obesity Allergic rhinitis Craniofacial abnormalities Neuromuscular diseases	Frequent snoring, unusual sleep positions, enlarged tonsils and adenoids, gasps/snorts, mouth breathing, episodes of apnea, labored breathing, daytime sleepiness, attention and/or learning and/or behavioral problems	PSG	Adenotonsillectomy Weight loss Noninvasive positive pressure support (CPAP/BiPAP)	Detailed history is often needed to detect early symptoms of OSA
Illness	Any chronically irritating disorder (e.g., AOM, Atopic Dermatitis, URI, GERD, Asthma) Triggers can be chronic or acute	Disrupted sleep, variant sleep patterns due to discomfort and pain	Hx & PE	Treat primary illness	Consider when an otherwise normal child presents with acute disruption in sleep Atypical sleep patterns may linger after resolution of instigating illness; behavioral interventions may be needed to restore to normal sleep patterns
Neurodevelopment and CNS disorders	Variable; may need to rule out seizures, OSA	Variable sleep disruptions	Hx & PE May need PSG, EEG, and imaging	Evaluate environment Sleep hygiene Depending on disorder, medications may be helpful	Consider use of sleep medicine or neurology specialist, especially when considering medication
Restless legs syndrome	Not fully defined but associated with genetics and iron deficiency	Unpleasant sensation in legs, urge to move legs often starting in the evening or during the night, difficulty falling asleep, lack of focus/hyperactivity, fatigue during the day	Hx, Family Hx, PSG, ferritin level	If ferritin is less than 50 µg, treat with iron replacement and recheck in 3 months. No other standard medications for children Consider referral to sleep medicine	Diagnosis can be a challenge
PARASOMNIAS					
Sleepwalking, sleep terrors	Stage N3 (deep) sleep instability Genetic predisposition	Awakening 1–3 hr after falling asleep with characteristic behaviors	Hx	Reassurance Protective environment	—
Confusional arousals	Irregular sleep patterns (e.g., night shift work); stress	Awakening in first 1/3 of night with confused thinking, slow speech	Hx, PSG	Sleep hygiene; treat other sleep disorders	—
BEHAVIORAL AND ENVIRONMENTAL					
Insomnia of childhood (Can have overlap of subtypes) • Sleep-onset association subtype • Limit setting subtype	10-30% prevalence Inability/unwillingness to fall asleep or return to sleep in absence of a specific conditions such as parental rocking Parental anxiety, unwillingness/inability to enforce bedtime rules and limits such as allowing child to sleep in parents' room	Frequent or prolonged night awakenings requiring intervention Bedtime resistance/refusal Excessive expression of "needs" by child	Hx	Prevention and education Put child to bed drowsy but awake; allow to fall asleep independently Minimize nocturnal parental response Modify parental behavior to improve limit setting (provide rewards/positive reinforcement, appropriate consequences)	Careful attention to detailed history and recognition of familial and cultural expectations is needed to negotiate an optimal sleep management plan with caregivers Recognize there are cultural norms for family sleep behavior

TABLE 15.1 Sleep Disorders—cont'd

	CAUSE	CLINICAL SYMPTOMS	DIAGNOSIS	TREATMENT	SPECIAL CONSIDERATIONS
Social disruptions	Family stressors	Night waking Refusal to sleep	Hx	Regularize routines Family counseling Family education regarding development and sleep needs of child	Respect family dynamics and refrain from blaming when providing guidance
Nighttime anxiety/ fears	Anxiety, stress, traumatic events, disruption in social surrounding such as change in house, bed type, although no specific trigger may be identified	Bedtime resistance Crying, clinging, seeking parental reassurance	Hx	Reassurance of safety Teach coping skills Nightlights, security objects Avoiding "drama" during the night awakening Avoid denial of fears; rather acknowledge and equip child with coping skills	Pay attention to any changes in child's environment and recognize normal development fears
CIRCADIAN RHYTHM DISORDERS					
Irregular sleep-wake pattern	No defined sleep schedule	Variable waking and sleeping	Hx	Regularize schedule	
Delayed sleep phase disorder	A shift in sleep-wake schedule with resetting of circadian rhythm Prevalence is 7-16% in adolescents due to longer circadian rhythm combined with increased social activity (delayed sleep onset)	Not sleepy at bedtime Sleep onset at a consistently late time Morning/daytime sleepiness	Hx	Depends on the trigger that is causing the discrepancy Good sleep hygiene Avoid bright light before bedtime Remove light-emitting devices in bedroom Melatonin	Detailed history and family education is helpful for optimal treatment response Sleep diary is helpful

AOM, Acute otitis media; *BiPAP*, bilevel positive airway pressure; *CNS*, central nervous system; *CPAP*, continuous positive airway pressure; *EEG*, electroencephalography; *GERD*, gastroesophageal reflux disease; *Hx*, history; *PE*, physical examination; *PSG*, polysomnography; *URI*, upper respiratory infection.

alcohol syndrome are at higher risk for sleep disorders than other children. Careful attention to the upper airway and pulmonary examination may reveal enlarged tonsils or adenoids or other signs of obstruction.

A **polysomnogram** is used to detect OSA, excessive limb movements, seizure disorder, and other sleep disorders. This consists of an all-night observation and recording performed in a sleep laboratory. Polysomnography is not indicated in children with primary insomnia (difficulty initiating or maintaining sleep), most circadian rhythm disorders, uncomplicated parasomnias, or behaviorally based sleep problems.

Differential Diagnosis

Behavioral insomnia of childhood is divided into two subtypes. *Sleep-onset association subtype* manifests as frequent or prolonged nighttime awakenings that occur in infants or young children. During periods of normal brief arousal with each sleep cycle, the child awakens under conditions different from those experienced as they fell asleep. Thus they are unable to return to sleep independently. *Limit-setting subtype* is most common in preschool-aged and older children and is characterized by bedtime resistance or refusal that stems from a caregiver's unwillingness or inability to enforce bedtime rules and expectations. Nighttime fears are also common causes of bedtime refusal.

Parasomnias include sleepwalking, sleep terrors, and confusional arousals. These occur during NREM sleep and are more likely during the first third of the night. They are most common in preschool children and are likely to resolve with time and developmental maturation. Sleepwalking is common and often benign but is sometimes associated with agitation or dangerous behaviors. Sleep terrors consist of an abrupt awakening with a loud scream or agitation that is unresponsive to caregivers' attempts to console. Sleep terrors are differentiated from nightmares, which occur later in the night and result from arousal in REM or dreaming sleep. Children typically remember their nightmares but have no recollection of sleep terrors. Confusional arousals are similar to sleep terrors but tend to be less dramatic and last longer.

Circadian rhythm disorders are most common during adolescence but can occur at any age. They consist of an exaggerated delayed sleep phase, leading to the inability to arouse in the mornings and failure to meet sleep requirements. Many adolescents attempt to recoup lost sleep on the weekends. The resulting sleep deprivation can lead to problems with cognition and emotional regulation.

OSA in childhood is not always obvious or easy to diagnose. OSA is commonly caused by tonsillar or adenoidal hypertrophy, and obesity is a risk factor. A history of snoring is typical, and some children may present with excessive daytime sleepiness. In toddlers OSA often is associated with poor growth, which improves when the obstruction is relieved by a tonsillectomy or adenoidectomy. Many children with OSA experience cognitive difficulties and school problems; hyperactivity is also more common in children with OSA than in age-matched controls.

Primary sleep disorders must be differentiated from sleep disorders associated with psychiatric and medical disorders. Psychoses, anxiety disorders, and substance abuse can present with disordered sleep. The clinician should also consider sleep-related epilepsy and developmental disorders.

Prevention and Treatment

Establishing a baseline of healthy sleep habits is essential to both prevention and treatment of sleep disorders at all ages. Recommendations include a consistent and appropriate bedtime and bedtime routine, as well as close attention to sleep hygiene (Table 15.2). A bedtime routine should last no more than 30 minutes and consist of three or four soothing activities that help calm the child and signal that it is time for sleep; activities may include bathing, brushing teeth, reading a story, or singing a song. Even older children and adolescents require a consistent pre-bed routine. A transitional object such as a blanket or stuffed animal can be used to promote positive sleep associations and encourage self-soothing. The bedtime should be set early enough to allow for sufficient nighttime sleep. Both bedtime and morning wake time should be consistent, including on weekends. Televisions and other electronic devices should be removed from the bedroom because they can lead to delayed sleep onset and maladaptive sleep associations.

Sleep-onset association disorder in infancy usually can be prevented by parental understanding of infant sleep physiology, developmentally appropriate expectations, and planning the infant sleep environment to coincide with family needs. It is important to recognize and respect cultural and other familial contexts when providing guidance. It is recommended that infants be put in bed drowsy, but still awake, after they have had a diaper change, food, and comfort. Some toleration of infant crying is required for the infant to achieve self-regulation of sleep. A safe sleep environment is essential. It is important for parents to understand that it is normal for their infant to wake frequently for the first 6 weeks before settling into a routine of waking every 3-4 hours for feeding. Infants typically do not sleep through the night before 6 months of age, and some do not sleep through the night before 12-18 months of age. Even though co-sleeping (infant sleeping with parent) is common and desired by many families for the purposes of convenience and closeness, it is contraindicated due to the increased risk of unexpected death.

Behavioral interventions comprise the mainstay of treatment for behavioral sleep disorders. In addition to meticulous attention to sleep hygiene and bedtime practices, difficulty falling asleep and bedtime resistance in young children are treated by specific behavioral strategies. *Systematic ignoring* consists of not responding to a child's demands for parental attention at bedtime. *Unmodified extinction* ("cry it out") involves putting the child to bed and then ignoring the child's demands until the next morning. *Graduated extinction* involves waiting successively longer periods of time before briefly checking on the child. Both methods are effective in decreasing bedtime resistance and enabling young children to fall asleep independently, but outcomes are dependent on several variables. Positive reinforcement strategies can also be used in preschool-aged and older children. These include rewards (e.g., stickers) for meeting a bedtime goal (e.g., staying in bed). Rewards should be provided immediately (first thing in the morning) to increase effectiveness and better link the reward with the positive behavior. Children with nighttime fears can benefit from behavioral therapy aimed at reinforcing feelings of safety.

Infrequent or nonintrusive parasomnias do not need treatment beyond education and reassurance. Ensuring a safe environment is essential. Sleep terrors are best managed by minimal intervention because conversation with the child is impossible during the episode and attempts at calming are unlikely to be successful. Anticipatory brief awakening of the child shortly before the typical occurrence of a parasomnia may be effective in aborting the event. Children with frequent or prolonged parasomnias may need a sleep study to evaluate for possible coexisting sleep disorders or nocturnal seizures. Medications that suppress slow-wave sleep may be indicated in severe cases.

Circadian rhythm disorders are best treated by ensuring sleep hygiene practices and gradual resetting of the biologic clock. Bedtime fading involves allowing the child to go to bed at the time he or she naturally feels tired and then gradually advancing the bedtime forward over the course of several weeks.

Rarely, children with insomnia are treated pharmacologically. Melatonin has soporific properties useful in treating delayed sleep phase syndrome. It has been used successfully in both children with normal development and those with developmental delays but should not be used unless after full evaluation and good medical surveillance. The α-agonist clonidine acts preferentially on presynaptic α_2 neurons to inhibit noradrenergic activity. Somnolence is a side effect of clonidine, which can be put to use in cases of refractory sleep difficulties; this is an *off-label* use in children. There are data on treating children as young as 4 years old with clonidine. Weaning off clonidine is recommended at the end of treatment. Optimally, clonidine should be considered only under specialty care such as sleep medicine or neurology.

TABLE 15.2 Prevention of Pediatric Behavioral Sleep Disorders
Consistent and appropriate bedtime and wake-up time
Consistent bedtime routine (~30 min) to cue sleep
Consistent ambient noise, light, temperature in bedroom
Adequate food, hydration, socialization, and physical activity during the day
No television, other electronics, electronic media, light emission products (e.g., chargers) in bedroom
Avoidance of naps (unless developmentally appropriate)
Caffeine avoidance
Child feels safe and protected
Child allowed to develop self-soothing strategies
Parents are comfortable setting limits/boundaries

Suggested Readings

Austerman J. ADHD and behavioral disorders: assessment, management, and an update from DSM-5. *Cleve Clin J Med.* 2015;82(11 suppl 1):S2–S7.

Bartel KA, Gradisar M, Williamson P. Protective and risk factors for adolescent sleep: a meta-analytic review. *Sleep Med Rev.* 2015;21:72–85.

Carter KA, Hathaway NE, Lettieri CF. Common sleep disorders in children. *Am Fam Physician.* 2014;89(5):368–377.

Feldman HM, Reiff MI. Clinical practice. Attention deficit-hyperactivity disorder in children and adolescents. *N Engl J Med.* 2014;370(9): 838–846.

Galland B, Meredith-Jones K, Gray A, et al. Criteria for nap identification in infants and young children using 24-h actigraphy and agreement with parental diary. *Sleep Med.* 2016;19:85–92.

Glazener CM, Evans JH, Peto RE. Alarm interventions for nocturnal enuresis in children. *Cochrane Database Syst Rev.* 2005;(2):CD002911.

National Sleep Foundation (NSF). Normal sleep. In: NSF, Kram JA, Kryger MH, et al, eds. *The Sleep Disorders.* NSF, 2017. Available at: http://sleepdisorders.sleepfoundation.org/chapter-1-normal-sleep/stages-of-human-sleep/.

Potegal M, Davidson RJ. Temper tantrums in young children: 1. Behavioral composition. 2. Tantrum duration and temporal organization. *J Dev Behav Pediatr.* 2003;24:140–154.

Subcommittee on Attention-Deficit/Hyperactivity Disorder; Steering Committee on Quality Improvement and Management, Wolraich M, Brown L, Brown RT, et al. ADHD: clinical practice guideline for the diagnosis, evaluation, and treatment of attention-deficit/hyperactivity disorder in children and adolescents. *Pediatrics.* 2011;128(5):1007–1022.

Thapar A, Cooper M. Attention deficit hyperactivity disorder. *Lancet.* 2016;387(10024):1240–1250.

Thorpe K, Staton S, Sawyer E, et al. Napping, development and health from 0 to 5 years: a systematic review. *Arch Dis Child.* 2015;100(7):615–622.

PEARLS FOR PRACTITIONERS

CHAPTER 11

Crying and Colic

- Colic is often diagnosed by using Wessel's Rule of Threes: crying for more than 3 hours per day, at least 3 days per week for more than 3 weeks.
- Colic is a diagnosis of exclusion; it is critical to evaluate for other conditions with a thorough history and physical exam.
- Management of colic includes parental education regarding natural, self-limited course of condition, parental coping mechanisms, and safe maneuvers to soothe baby such as the "5 Ss."
- Nonaccidental trauma can be a serious consequence of colic.

CHAPTER 12

Temper Tantrums

- Temper tantrums are commonplace in early childhood and are characterized by episodes of extreme frustration and anger, manifesting as a wide range of behaviors that appear disproportionate to the situation.
  - Evaluation should include a thorough history and physical examination to rule out for other etiologies such as development delay and hearing or visual deficits.
  - Atypical tantrums, particularly those that are destructive or injurious, may be indicative of a more serious underlying condition; consider sleep disturbances, attention-deficit/hyperactivity disorder (ADHD), mood disorders, or significant family stressors in these situations.
- Anticipatory guidance for parents should include tips for acute management of temper tantrums (e.g., staying calm, using distraction, cool-down techniques, not giving into the child's demands, and ignoring inappropriate behavior) as well as for prevention of future tantrums (e.g., setting clear limits, consistently enforcing limits, teaching communication skills, offering choices, role-modeling, and using positive and negative reinforcement).

CHAPTER 13

Attention-Deficit/Hyperactivity Disorder

- ADHD is multifactorial in origin with genetic, neural, and environmental contributions. It is characterized by symptoms of inattention, hyperactivity, and/or impulsivity that persist over a period of more than 6 months, are present prior to age 12, and lead to impairment in more than one setting.
- Diagnosis is by history including reports of the patient, parents, and teachers; diagnosis requires use of validated rating scales.
- Other diagnoses and co-morbidities should be considered, including learning disabilities, mood disorders, anxiety, and autism spectrum disorder.
- Behavior modification is the standard of care for management of ADHD in preschool-aged children.
- Management of ADHD for older children and adolescents should include behavioral management as well as parent training and classroom interventions.
  - Stimulant medications have been shown to be effective for the overall management of ADHD in these age groups. Side effects should be monitored carefully and doses titrated for optimal treatment response and diminished side effects.

CHAPTER 14

Control of Elimination

- Prerequisites for achieving elimination in the toilet include the child's ability to recognize the urge for urination and defecation, to get to the toilet, to understand the sequence of tasks required, to avoid oppositional behavior, and to take pride in achievement.
- Enuresis is classified as diurnal (daytime) or nocturnal (nighttime).
  - In the United States, daytime and nighttime dryness are expected by 4 and 6 years of age, respectively.

  - Nocturnal enuresis has a reported prevalence of 15% in 5-year-olds, 7% in 8-year-olds, and 1% in 15-year-olds.
- Enuresis can be classified as **primary** (incontinence in a child who has never achieved dryness) and **secondary** (incontinence in a child who has been dry for at least 6 months).
- The most commonly used treatment options are conditioning therapy and pharmacotherapy (usually desmopressin).
- **Encopresis** is the regular, voluntary, or involuntary passage of feces into a place other than the toilet after 4 years of age.
  - Encopresis without constipation is uncommon.
  - Approximately 95% of children referred to a subspecialist for encopresis have no other underlying pathologic condition.
- Treatment of constipation/encopresis involves a combination of behavioral training and laxative therapy. Successful treatment requires 6-24 months.

CHAPTER 15

Normal Sleep and Pediatric Sleep Disorders

- Sleep architecture changes from fetal life through infancy and childhood and parallels physical maturation and development.
- The timing and duration of sleep change with age.
- Establishing a baseline of healthy sleep habits is essential to both prevention and treatment of sleep disorders at all ages.
- Sleep disorders include behavioral insomnia of childhood, parasomnias, circadian rhythm disorders, and obstructive sleep apnea. Work-up should include a careful history, including a sleep diary, as well as a complete physical examination to rule out medical causes of sleep disturbance.
- Adolescents develop a physiologically based shift toward later sleep-onset and wake times relative to those in middle childhood. Insufficient sleep in adolescents is very common and has been associated with negative effects on cognitive function, moods, and motivation.

PSYCHIATRIC DISORDERS

Gray M. Buchanan

CHAPTER 16

Somatic Symptom and Related Disorders

Somatic symptom and related disorders (SSRDs) make up a new category in the Diagnostic and Statistical Manual of Mental Disorders (DSM)-5 which replaces the somatoform disorders from DSM-IV with the intent to eliminate diagnostic overlap across disorders. While DSM-IV emphasized medically unexplained symptoms, the current version allows for unexplained symptoms and those that may accompany diagnosed medical disorders. SSRDs involve physical symptoms (pain or loss of function), may occur in the context of a physical illness, and are identified by symptoms that go beyond the expected pathophysiology, affecting the child's school, home life, and peer relationships. SSRDs are often associated with psychosocial stress that persists beyond the acute stressor, leading to the belief by the child and family that the correct medical diagnosis has not yet been found.

The prevalence of SSRDs in children is not clearly known and represents only a minority of outpatient visits in the pediatric population. Adolescent girls tend to report nearly twice as many functional somatic symptoms as adolescent boys, whereas prior to puberty the ratio is equal. Affected children are more likely to have difficulty expressing emotional distress, come from families with a history of marital conflict, child maltreatment (including emotional, sexual, physical abuse), or history of physical illness. In early childhood, symptoms often include recurrent abdominal pain (RAP). Later, headaches, neurological symptoms, insomnia, and fatigue are more common.

Explainable medical conditions and an SSRD (e.g., seizures and pseudoseizures) can coexist in up to 50% of patients and present difficult diagnostic dilemmas. The list of systemic medical disorders that could present with unexplained physical symptoms includes chronic fatigue syndrome (CFS), multiple sclerosis, myasthenia gravis, endocrine disorders, chronic systemic infections, vocal cord dysfunction, periodic paralysis, acute intermittent porphyria, fibromyalgia, polymyositis, and other myopathies.

Depression is a common comorbid condition and frequently precedes the somatic symptoms. Anxiety and panic also commonly present with somatic complaints. Disorders included in the SSRD group include somatic symptom disorder (SSD), illness anxiety disorder, conversion disorder, factitious disorder, and psychological factors affecting other medical conditions. The diagnostic criteria for SSRDs are established for adults and need additional study in pediatric populations.

SSD typically involves one or more somatic symptoms that are distressing or result in significant disruption in daily life. The criteria used to diagnose this disorder are listed in Table 16.1. Individuals with SSD include the majority of those previously diagnosed with somatization disorder and hypochondriasis. Key symptoms of the disorder are excessive thoughts, feelings, or behaviors regarding the somatic complaint (e.g., excessive fatigue or pain). Prevalence estimates for SSD in children are unclear; however, between 5% and 7% of adults may be identified with SSD, with a greater proportion being female.

Illness Anxiety Disorder (Table 16.2) involves children who have a preoccupation with having or acquiring a serious illness. Typically, somatic symptoms are not present, and there is a high level of anxiety about health status. The child may be alarmed by illness in others, and they seldom respond to reassurance regarding their health. An elevated rate of medical utilization is common, and individuals may repeatedly seek reassurance from family, friends, and medical staff regarding their health. Approximately 25% of those previously diagnosed with hypochondriasis fall into this disorder and can be distinguished from those with SSD by their high anxiety and absence of somatic symptoms. Prevalence estimates in children are unknown due to the new DSM classification system; however, there appears to be similar prevalence rates in boys and girls.

Conversion disorder involves symptoms affecting voluntary motor or sensory function and is suggestive of a neurological illness in the absence of a disease process (Table 16.3). Adjustment difficulties, recent family stress, unresolved grief reactions, and family psychopathology occur at a high frequency in conversion symptoms. A physical condition and a conversion disorder (e.g., epileptic and nonepileptic seizures) may coexist in the same patient. There are multiple subtypes of conversion disorder based upon the symptoms present including difficulties with primarily motor, sensory, neurological, or mixed symptoms.

Presenting symptoms follow the psychological stressor by hours to weeks and may cause more distress for others than for the patient. This seeming lack of concern regarding potentially serious symptoms is referred to as *la belle indifference.* Symptoms are often self-limited but may be associated with chronic sequelae, such as contractures or iatrogenic injury.

Psychological factors affecting other medical conditions were minimally changed in the current version of the DSM and is marked by psychological or behavioral factors that adversely impact a medical condition by increasing the risk for suffering,

TABLE 16.1 Criteria for Diagnosis of Somatic Symptom Disorder

A. One or more somatic symptoms that are distressing or result in significant disruption of daily life.

B. Excessive thoughts, feelings, behaviors related to the somatic symptoms or associated health concerns as manifested by at least one of the following:

1. Disproportionate and persistent thoughts about the seriousness of one's symptoms.
2. Persistently high level of anxiety about health or symptoms.
3. Excessive time and energy devoted to these symptoms or health concerns.

C. Although any one somatic symptom may not be continuously present, the state of being symptomatic is persistent, more than 6 months.

Specify if:

With predominant pain (previously pain disorder): This specifier is for individuals whose somatic symptoms predominantly involve pain.

Persistent: A persistent course is characterized by severe symptoms, marked impairment, and long duration (more than 6 months).

Specify current severity:

Mild: Only one of the symptoms specified in Criterion B is fulfilled.

Moderate: Two or more of the symptoms specified in Criterion B are fulfilled.

Severe: Two or more of the symptoms specified in Criterion B are fulfilled, plus there are multiple somatic complaints (or one very severe somatic symptom).

TABLE 16.2 Criteria for Diagnosis of Illness Anxiety Disorder

A. Preoccupation with the idea that one has or will get a serious illness.

B. Somatic symptoms are not present or, if present, are only mild in intensity. If another medical condition is present or there is a high risk for developing a medical condition (e.g., strong family history is present), the preoccupation is clearly excessive or disproportionate.

C. There is a high level of anxiety about health, and the individual is easily alarmed about personal health status.

D. The individual performs excessive health-related behaviors (e.g., repeatedly checks his or her body for signs of illness) or exhibits maladaptive avoidance (e.g., avoids doctor appointments and hospitals).

E. Illness preoccupation has been present for at least 6 months, but the specific illness that is feared may change over that period of time.

F. The illness-related preoccupation is not better explained by another mental disorder, such as somatic symptom disorder, panic disorder, generalized anxiety disorder, body dysmorphic disorder, obsessive-compulsive disorder, or delusional disorder, somatic type.

Specify whether:

Care-seeking type: Medical care, including physician visits or undergoing tests and procedures, is frequently used.

Care-avoidant type: Medical care is rarely used.

TABLE 16.3 Diagnostic and Statistical Manual of Mental Disorders-5 Diagnostic Criteria for Conversion Disorder or Functional Neurological Symptom Disorder

A. One or more symptoms of altered voluntary motor or sensory function.

B. Clinical findings provide evidence of incompatibility between the symptom and recognized neurological or medical conditions.

C. The symptom or deficit is not better explained by another medical or mental disorder.

D. The symptom or deficit causes clinically significant distress or impairment in social, occupational, or other important areas of functioning or warrants medical evaluation.

Specify symptom type: weakness or paralysis, abnormal movements, swallowing symptoms, speech symptom, attacks/seizures, or anesthesia/sensory loss, special sensory symptom (visual, olfactory, or hearing), or mixed symptoms

Reprinted with permission from the Diagnostic and Statistical Manual of Mental Disorders. *5th ed. (Copyright 2013). American Psychiatric Association; 2013:318.*

TABLE 16.4 Diagnostic and Statistical Manual of Mental Disorders-5 Diagnostic Criteria for Psychological Factors Affecting Other Medical Conditions

A. A medical symptom or condition (other than a mental disorder) is present.

B. Psychological or behavioral factors adversely affect the medical condition in one of the following ways:

1. The factors have influenced the course of the medical condition as shown by a close temporal association between the psychological factors and the development or exacerbation of, or delayed recovery from, the medical condition.
2. The factors interfere with the treatment of the medical condition (e.g., poor adherence).
3. The factors constitute additional well-established health risks for the individual.
4. The factors influence the underlying pathophysiology, precipitating or exacerbating symptoms or necessitating medical attention.

C. The psychological and behavioral factors in Criterion B are not better explained by another mental disorder (e.g., panic disorder, major depressive disorder, post-traumatic stress disorder).

Reprinted with permission from the Diagnostic and Statistical Manual of Mental Disorders. *5th ed. (Copyright 2013). American Psychiatric Association; 2013:322.*

death, or disability (Table 16.4). The factors should interfere with the treatment of a medical condition (e.g., anxiety exacerbating asthma, poor medication adherence). This diagnosis is more common in young children and may require corroborative history from parents and the child's school. Prevalence is unclear. Some data suggest that this disorder is more prevalent than SSDs.

Factitious disorder is a condition in which physical or psychological symptoms are produced intentionally and often with the intent to assume a sick role (Table 16.5). This diagnosis is made either by direct observation or by eliminating other possible causes. This falsification of physical and psychological symptoms may also present as imposing illness

TABLE 16.5 Diagnostic and Statistical Manual of Mental Disorders-5 Diagnostic Criteria for Factitious Disorders
FACTITIOUS DISORDER IMPOSED ON SELF
A. Falsification of physical or psychological signs or symptoms, or induction of injury or disease, associated with identified deception.
B. The individual presents himself or herself to others as ill, impaired, or injured.
C. The deceptive behavior is evident even in the absence of obvious external rewards.
D. The behavior is not better explained by another mental disorder, such as delusional disorder or another psychotic disorder.
FACTITIOUS DISORDER IMPOSED ON ANOTHER (PREVIOUSLY FACTITIOUS DISORDER BY PROXY)
A. Falsification of physical or psychological signs or symptoms, or induction of injury or disease, in another, associated with identified deception.
B. The individual presents another individual (victim) to others as ill, impaired, or injured.
C. The deceptive behavior is evident even in the absence of obvious external rewards.
D. The behavior is not better explained by another mental disorder, such as delusional disorder or another psychotic disorder.
Note: The perpetrator, not the victim, receives this diagnosis.

Reprinted with permission from the Diagnostic and Statistical Manual of Mental Disorders. *5th ed. (Copyright 2013). American Psychiatric Association; 2013:324.*

or injury on another person (i.e., factitious disorder imposed on another [FDIA]; formerly Munchausen by proxy). Such a condition imposed on another commonly occurs following hospitalization of the child or another family member. Many patients demonstrate improvement when confronted with their behavior or acknowledge the factitious nature of their symptoms. Approximate answers (e.g., the patient provides 13 as the answer for 20 − 3) reported during a mental status examination are most commonly found in factitious disorders. The prevalence of factitious disorder in children is unknown. It is estimated that around 1% of individuals in hospital settings present with such a condition. FDIA is considered a type of child abuse and most commonly occurs in neonates and preschoolers.

Screening tools for SSRDs are currently being developed. Previous tools for somatoform disorders include the Children's Somatization Inventory (child and parent versions) and the Illness Attitude Scales and Soma Assessment Interview (parental interview questionnaires). The functional disability inventory assesses the severity of symptoms.

Treatment for SSRDs should employ an integrated medical and psychiatric approach. The goals are to identify concurrent psychiatric disorders, rule out concurrent physical disorders, improve overall functioning, and minimize unnecessary invasive tests and doctor shopping. This is most successful when mental health consultation is presented as part of a comprehensive evaluation, thereby minimizing stigma and distrust.

Antidepressant medications (e.g., fluoxetine, sertraline, citalopram, and clomipramine) may be of benefit in the treatment of some conditions such as unexplained headaches, fibromyalgia, body dysmorphic disorder, pain disorder, irritable bowel syndrome, and functional gastrointestinal disorders. Tricyclic antidepressants (e.g., clomipramine) should be avoided in youth with functional abdominal pain (FAP), because it has little proven efficacy in either pain management or mood disorders and is very dangerous in overdose. In CFS with comorbid depression and anxiety, a more activating antidepressant, such as bupropion, may be useful. Stimulants may also be helpful in CFS.

Therapies such as cognitive-behavioral methods, which reward health-promoting behaviors and discourage disability and illness behaviors, have been shown to help in the treatment of recurrent pain, CFS, fibromyalgia, and FAP. Additionally, self-management strategies such as self-monitoring, relaxation, hypnosis, and biofeedback provide some symptomatic relief and encourage more active coping strategies. Family therapy and family-based interventions may also be useful. Home schooling should be avoided. School attendance and performance should be emphasized as important indicators of appropriate functioning. In dealing with pain symptoms (e.g., headaches, stomachaches), parents should limit attention/reinforcement for pain behavior, strongly encourage normal routines/appropriate schedules (e.g., going to school), help the child identify stress at home and school, provide attention and special activities on days when the child does not have symptoms, and limit activities and interactions on sick days. Attempts to educate parents and personnel working with the child about limiting discussions about excessive discomfort or illness should occur. Caregivers and the child should also be taught methods of controlling their physiological and cognitive responses to discomfort via practicing relaxation techniques and mindfulness techniques.

Malingering is considered a V-code in the DSM-5 and involves the purposeful falsification or exaggeration of physical and/or psychological symptoms for external gain (e.g., money, avoidance of school, work, jail). The key feature of malingering is the seeking of an external reward. Symptoms may not lessen when the reward is attained. Unless the patient is directly observed or confesses to such falsification, malingering is difficult to prove.

CHAPTER 17
Anxiety Disorders

Anxiety disorders are characterized by uneasiness, excessive rumination, and apprehension about the future. The conditions tend to be chronic, recurring, and vary in intensity over time. They affect 5-10% of children and adolescents (Table 17.1) and have a lifetime prevalence of approximately 30%. Some common anxiety disorders are discussed in the following sections. Conditions such as obsessive-compulsive disorder (OCD) and post-traumatic stress disorder (PTSD) are no longer included in the DSM-5 section on anxiety but continue to share a close relationship with anxiety disorders.

Panic disorder is the presence of recurrent, unexpected panic attacks. A **panic attack** is a sudden unexpected onset of intense fear associated with a feeling of impending doom in the absence of real danger and may occur in the context of any anxiety disorder. The individual must experience four or more symptoms (e.g., sweating, palpitations, feeling of choking, chest

TABLE 17.1 Common Anxiety Disorders: Characteristics

FEATURE	PANIC DISORDER	GENERALIZED ANXIETY DISORDER	SEPARATION ANXIETY DISORDER	SPECIFIC PHOBIA
Epidemiology	Prevalence is 0.2-10%; Eight times more common and of early onset in family members of affected individuals than general population.	Prevalence is 2-4%. Sex ratio equal before puberty, but higher in female following puberty. Genetic factors play only a modest role in the etiology.	Prevalence is 3-4% of children and adolescents. The sex ratio is almost equal. Heritability of SAD is greater for girls than for boys.	Prevalence is 5% in children and approximately 16% in adolescence. Sex ratio is 2:1 females:males. Increased risk of specific phobias in first-degree relatives of patients with specific phobias.
Onset	Average age at onset is 20-24 years; <0.4% onset before 14 years of age.	The average age at onset is 10 years.	The average age at onset is 7 years.	Varies
Differential diagnosis	Anxiety disorder due to a general medical condition. Substance-related anxiety disorder due to caffeine or other stimulants.	Other anxiety disorders, OCD, PTSD, and depressive, bipolar, and psychotic disorders. Substance-related (caffeine and sedative-hypnotic withdrawal).	Other anxiety disorders and conduct, impulse-control, and disruptive behavior disorders.	Agoraphobia, panic disorder, OCD, and PTSD.
Co-morbidities	Separation anxiety disorder (common). Agoraphobia, substance use, major depression, OCD, and other anxiety disorders. Asthma patients have a high incidence of panic attacks.	Unipolar depression and other anxiety disorders.	GAD and specific phobia.	Depression and other anxiety disorders.
Prognosis	Frequently chronic with a relative high rate of suicide attempts and completions.	One study showed that 65% of children cease to have the diagnosis in 2 years.	Variable. The majority of children are not diagnosed with significant anxiety disorders as adults.	Social phobia in childhood may become associated with alcohol abuse in adolescence.

GAD, Generalized anxiety disorder; *OCD*, obsessive-compulsive disorder; *PTSD*, post-traumatic stress disorder; *SAD*, separation anxiety disorder.

pain, trembling/shaking, chills, paresthesias, fear of dying, fear of losing control, derealization, dizziness, nausea, or shortness of breath) during the attack. At least 1 month of persistent worrying about having another panic attack and/or a significant behavioral change following an attack (e.g., attempting to avoid another attack, avoidance of triggers such as exercise) is required to make the diagnosis.

Panic disorder often begins in adolescence or early adulthood. Symptom severity varies greatly. In children, the most commonly experienced symptoms include shortness of breath, palpitations, chest pain, a choking sensation, and a fear of losing control or going "crazy." Symptoms may be brief or may last for prolonged periods of time; however, they generally last less than 15 minutes. Patients may believe that they are experiencing an acute medical condition (e.g., a heart attack).

Agoraphobia is a disorder marked by anxiety or fear of situations where escape is difficult or would draw unwanted attention to the person. This is limited to situations involving two or more of five specific situations: fear/anxiety about the use of public transportation, being in open spaces, being in enclosed spaces, standing in line or being in a crowd, or being outside of the home alone. Agoraphobia is often persistent and can leave people homebound. While agoraphobia does commonly occur with panic disorder, a substantial number of individuals experience agoraphobia without panic symptoms. First onset of agoraphobia is rare in children but more commonly presents in adolescence. Females are approximately twice as likely to experience the disorder. Agoraphobia is a chronic condition. In children, being outside of the home alone and worries regarding becoming lost are common complaints.

Generalized anxiety disorder (GAD) is characterized by 6 or more months of persistent, excessive worry and anxiety about a variety of situations or activities. The worries should be multiple, not paroxysmal, not focused on a single theme and should cause significant impairment. The anxiety must be accompanied by at least one of the following symptoms: restlessness, fatigue, concentration difficulties, irritability, muscle tension, or sleep disturbance. Physiological signs of anxiety are often present, including shakiness, trembling, and myalgias. Gastrointestinal symptoms (nausea, vomiting, diarrhea) and autonomic symptoms (tachycardia, shortness of breath) also commonly coexist. In children and adolescents, the specific symptoms of autonomic arousal are less prominent. Symptoms are often related to school performance or sports. Patients also commonly present with concerns about punctuality and may be perfectionistic. Children with GAD are often exceedingly self-conscious, have low self-esteem, and have more sleep disturbance than patients with other kinds of anxiety disorder. Care must be taken to elicit internalizing symptoms of negative cognitions about the self (hopelessness, helplessness, worthlessness, suicidal ideation), as well as those concerning relationships (embarrassment, self-consciousness) and associated with anxieties. Inquiry about eating, weight, energy, and interests should also be performed to eliminate a mood disorder. GAD is slightly male predominant prior to puberty, but by adolescence, females outnumber males.

Unspecified anxiety disorder is a common condition in clinical practice. This diagnosis is used when there is impairing anxiety or phobic symptoms that do not meet full criteria for another anxiety disorder.

TABLE 17.2 Diagnostic and Statistical Manual of Mental Disorders-5 Diagnostic Criteria for Separation Anxiety Disorder

A. Developmentally inappropriate and excessive fear or anxiety concerning separation from those to whom the individual is attached, as evidenced by at least three of the following:

1. Recurrent, excessive distress when anticipating or experiencing separation from home or from major attachment figures.
2. Persistent and excessive worry about losing major attachment figures or about possible harm to them, such as illness, injury, disasters, or death.
3. Persistent and excessive worry about experiencing an untoward event (e.g., getting lost, being kidnapped, having an accident, becoming ill) that causes separation from a major attachment figure.
4. Persistent reluctance or refusal to go out, away from home, to school, to work, or elsewhere because of fear of separation.
5. Persistent and excessive fear of or reluctance about being alone or without major attachment figures at home or in other settings.
6. Persistent reluctance or refusal to sleep away from home or to go to sleep without being near a major attachment figure.
7. Repeated nightmares involving the theme of separation.
8. Repeated complaints of physical symptoms (e.g., headaches, stomachaches, nausea, vomiting) when separation from major attachment figures occurs or is anticipated.

B. The fear, anxiety, or avoidance is persistent, lasting at least 4 weeks in children and adolescents and typically 6 months or more in adults.

C. The disturbance causes clinically significant distress or impairment in social, academic, occupational, or other important areas of functioning.

D. The disturbance is not better explained by another mental disorder, such as refusing to leave home because of excessive resistance to change in autism spectrum disorder, delusions or hallucinations concerning separation in psychotic disorders, refusal to go outside without a trusted companion in agoraphobia, worries about ill health or other harm befalling significant others in generalized anxiety disorder, or concerns about having an illness in illness anxiety disorder.

Reprinted with permission from the Diagnostic and Statistical Manual of Mental Disorders. *5th ed. (Copyright 2013). American Psychiatric Association; 2013:190–191.*

Separation anxiety disorder (SAD) is marked by excessive distress or concern when separating from a major attachment figure (Table 17.2). Most commonly, children and adolescents express vague somatic symptoms (e.g., headaches, abdominal pain, fatigue) in an attempt to avoid going to school or leaving their home. Patients may have a valid or an irrational concern about a parent or have had an unpleasant experience in school, and the prospect of returning to school provokes extreme anxiety and escalating symptoms. Children may refuse to go to school or leave their home. Children with SAD may require constant attention and present with struggles with separation at bedtime. SAD is a strong (78%) risk factor for developing problems in adulthood, such as panic disorder, agoraphobia, and depression. SAD may be highly heritable with community samples estimating such genetic rates as high as 73%.

Selective mutism is present in up to 1% of children who consistently fail to speak in one or more social settings despite adequate receptive and expressive language skills. Symptoms are present for at least 1 month and interfere with educational or occupational achievement or social communication. Children with selective mutism will often speak at home in the presence of first-degree relatives but may refuse to speak to extended family or others in their environment. Between 25% and 50% of children with selective mutism exhibit some history of speech delay or speech disorder. Identification of selective mutism commonly occurs in kindergarten or first grade when there is an increased demand on speech and social interaction. Children of immigrants (who are non-English speaking) and a parental history of reticence and/or social anxiety are often found in children with selective mutism.

Specific phobias are marked, persistent fears of specific things/objects or situations that often lead to avoidance behaviors. The associated anxiety is almost always felt immediately when the person is confronted with the feared object or situation. The greater the proximity or the more difficult it is to escape, the higher the anxiety. Many patients have had actual fearful experiences with the object or situation (traumatic event). The response to the fear can range from limited symptoms of anxiety to full panic attacks. Children may not recognize that their fears are out of proportion to the circumstances, unlike adolescents and adults, and express their anxiety as crying, tantrums, freezing, or clinging. Many fears are normal in childhood; therefore only fears lasting greater than 6 months in duration should be considered diagnostically for children. Specific fears may be related to animals/insects, natural events (storms, flooding), blood-related events (injections, needles, medical procedures), situational events (elevator, airplane), or other circumstances/events (loud sounds, clowns).

Social anxiety disorder (formerly social phobia) is a common (~7% prevalence; girls predominate over boys) type of phobia characterized by a marked and persistent fear of social or performance situations in which embarrassment might occur (Table 17.3). In children, this apprehension must be present with peers and not just in the presence of adults. The vast majority of individuals with this disorder are identified prior to 15 years of age. Children appear to have a lower rate of negative cognitions (e.g., embarrassment, overconcern, self-consciousness) than adults. Left untreated or poorly treated, social anxiety disorder can become immobilizing and result in significant morbidity and functional impairments; however, approximately one third of individuals experience remission of symptoms within 1 year if untreated.

In the **management of anxiety disorders,** likely medical conditions should be carefully excluded including hyperthyroidism, medication side effects, substance abuse, or other medical conditions. Additionally, screening for co-morbid psychiatric disorders, such as mood disorders, eating disorders, tic disorders, and disruptive, impulse-control, and conduct disorders should occur. A collaborative history from multiple sources is important, as the child may be unable to effectively communicate symptoms. Screening with validated measures of anxiety can often be helpful.

Pharmacotherapy is the most common approach to helping those with anxiety. In general, for mild to moderate anxiety, evidence-based psychotherapies and psychoeducation should

TABLE 17.3 Diagnostic and Statistical Manual of Mental Disorders-V Diagnostic Criteria for Social Anxiety Disorder (Social Phobia)

A. Marked fear or anxiety about one or more social situations in which the individual is exposed to possible scrutiny by others. Examples include social interactions (e.g., having a conversation, meeting unfamiliar people), being observed (e.g., eating or drinking), and performing in front of others (e.g., giving a speech).

Note: In children, the anxiety must occur in peer settings and not just during interactions with adults.

B. The individual fears that he or she will act in a way or show anxiety symptoms that will be negatively evaluated (i.e., will be humiliating or embarrassing; will lead to rejection or offend others).

C. The social situations almost always provoke fear or anxiety.

Note: In children, the fear or anxiety may be expressed by crying, tantrums, freezing, clinging, shrinking, or failing to speak in social situations.

D. The social situations are avoided or endured with intense fear or anxiety.

E. The fear or anxiety is out of proportion to the actual threat posed by the social situation and to the sociocultural context.

F. The fear, anxiety, or avoidance is persistent, typically lasting for 6 months or more.

G. The fear, anxiety, or avoidance causes clinically significant distress or impairment in social, occupational, or other important areas of functioning.

H. The fear, anxiety, or avoidance is not attributable to the physiological effects of a substance (e.g., a drug of abuse, a medication) or another medical condition.

I. The fear, anxiety, or avoidance is not better explained by the symptoms of another mental disorder, such as panic disorder, body dysmorphic disorder, or autism spectrum disorder.

J. If another medical condition (e.g., Parkinson disease, obesity, disfigurement from burns or injury) is present, the anxiety or avoidance is clearly unrelated or is excessive.

Specify if:

Performance only: If the fear is restricted to speaking or performing in public.

Reprinted with permission from the Diagnostic and Statistical Manual of Mental Disorders. *5th ed. (Copyright 2013). American Psychiatric Association. 2013:202–203.*

be used first. Combined therapy usually has better efficacy than psychotherapy and psychopharmacology alone. Cognitive and behavioral therapy (e.g., systematic desensitization, exposure techniques, operant conditioning, modeling, and cognitive restructuring) can be beneficial in a variety of anxiety disorders. Children with anxiety disorders are often less tolerant of medication side effects. Supportive therapy may help them maintain treatment regimens and increase compliance rates.

Care coordination with a patient's school is often recommended and necessary. Reassurance that the patient does not have a life-threatening illness is important. Other psychosocial treatments that have demonstrated efficacy include stress management, supportive therapies, and biofeedback. Emphasis is placed on decreasing morbidity through proper treatment.

Selective serotonin reuptake inhibitors (SSRIs) are the medications of choice. The SSRIs approved for children by the U.S. Food and Drug Administration are fluoxetine, sertraline, and fluvoxamine. They can initially exacerbate anxiety or even panic symptoms, and tricyclic antidepressants have also shown efficacy. Benzodiazepines (alprazolam and clonazepam) include a risk of causing disinhibition in children. Alpha-2a-agonists (guanfacine and clonidine) may also be useful if autonomic symptoms are present. Anticonvulsant agents (gabapentin, topiramate, and oxcarbazepine) are used when other agents are ineffective, and β-Blockers help with performance anxiety.

Co-occurrence of the inattentive type of attention-deficit/hyperactivity disorder and an anxiety disorder is common. When using a stimulant, it is advisable to start at a low dose, increasing slowly to minimize the risk of increasing anxiety. Additionally, careful monitoring of sleep is important.

CHAPTER 18

Depressive Disorders and Bipolar Disorders

Depressive disorders and bipolar and related disorders comprise new categories in the DSM-5 and have been divided into separate sections in the newest edition. Several new diagnoses have been included in each chapter to aid with diagnostic clarity and assist in limiting overdiagnosis of some conditions, such as bipolar disorder in children.

Major depressive disorder (MDD) requires a minimum of 2 weeks of symptoms including either depressed mood or loss of interest or pleasure in nearly all activities. Four additional symptoms must also be present (Table 18.1). In children and adolescents, a new onset of irritability and/or restlessness may be present instead of depressed mood. Furthermore, many children/adolescents complain of pervasive boredom. A change in appetite (usually decreased but can be increased) with carbohydrate craving, with or without accompanying weight changes, and sleep disturbance along with somatic complaints (fatigue, vague aches and pains) may also be present. Furthermore, a key indicator in children may be declining performance in school. Psychotic symptoms, seen in severe cases of MDD, are generally mood-congruent (e.g., derogatory auditory hallucinations, guilt associated delusional thinking). Suicidal thoughts and attempts are common and should be evaluated. A prior history of suicidal thoughts/attempts and prominent feelings of hopelessness are risk factors that should be closely monitored.

Previously a bereavement exclusion existed in making a diagnosis of MDD. Current evidence suggests that although most people experience bereavement following a significant loss (e.g., loss of a loved one, financial ruin, etc.) without developing depression, many do, in fact, experience depressive symptoms related to depression. As such, evidence suggests that treatments for MDD and MDD with bereavement are often likely to help with the remittance of symptoms.

The prevalence of MDD in prepubertal children is approximately 2% with a 1 : 1 female-to-male ratio. In adolescence the prevalence is approximately 5% with a female-to-male ratio of 2 : 1 (similar to adults). If untreated, major depression can become chronic in 10% of patients.

TABLE 18.1 Diagnostic and Statistical Manual of Mental Disorders-5 Diagnostic Criteria for Major Depressive Disorder

A. Five (or more) of the following symptoms have been present during the same 2-week period and represent a change from previous functioning; at least one of the symptoms is either (1) depressed mood or (2) loss of interest or pleasure.

Note: Do not include symptoms that are clearly attributable to another medical condition.

1. Depressed most of the day, nearly every day, as indicated by either subjective report (e.g., feels sad, empty, hopeless) or observation made by others (e.g., appears tearful). Note: In children and adolescents, can be irritable mood.
2. Markedly diminished interest or pleasure in all, or almost all, activities most of the day, nearly every day (as indicated by either subjective account or observation).
3. Significant weight loss when not dieting or weight gain (e.g., a change of more than 5% of body weight in a month), or decrease or increase in appetite nearly every day. Note: In children, consider failure to make expected weight gain.
4. Insomnia or hypersomnia nearly every day.
5. Psychomotor agitation or retardation nearly every day (observable by others, not merely subjective feelings of restlessness or being slowed down).
6. Fatigue or loss of energy nearly every day.
7. Feelings of worthlessness or excessive or inappropriate guilt (which may be delusional) nearly every day (not merely self-reproach or guilt about being sick).
8. Diminished ability to think or concentrate, or indecisiveness, nearly every day (either by subjective account or as observed by others).
9. Recurrent thoughts of death (not just fear of dying), recurrent suicidal ideation without a specific plan, or a suicide attempt or a specific plan for committing suicide.

B. The symptoms cause clinically significant distress or impairment in social, occupational, or other important areas of functioning.

C. The episode is not attributable to the physiological effects of a substance or to another medical condition.

Reprinted with permission from the Diagnostic and Statistical Manual of Mental Disorders. *5th ed. (Copyright 2013). American Psychiatric Association; 2013:160–161.*

Genetic predisposition for MDD is present with twin studies showing 40-65% heritability. Additionally, family studies show a twofold to fourfold increased risk for depression in offspring of depressed parents. Other potential responsible factors for depression include dysregulation of central serotonergic and/or noradrenergic systems, hypothalamic-pituitary-adrenal axis dysfunction, and the influence of pubertal sex hormones. Stressful life events such as abuse and neglect have also been found to precipitate MDD, especially in young children.

Anxiety-related disorders (up to 80% prevalence), substance-related disorders (up to 30% prevalence), and conduct/disruptive disorders (up to 20% prevalence) frequently present as co-morbid with MDD. Onset of MDD in childhood is also more likely to be related to bipolar symptoms versus adult-onset bipolar disorder. This is especially true when a family history of bipolar disorder is present.

Differential diagnoses for MDD are diverse. It is always prudent to rule out mood disorder due to another medical condition or substance-related mood disorders before considering MDD. Dysphoria and concentration concerns related to untreated attention-deficit/hyperactivity disorder (ADHD) may also be mistakenly diagnosed as depression. Medically, conditions such as hypothyroidism, anemia, diabetes, and folate and B_{12} vitamin deficiencies need to be ruled out.

Persistent depressive disorder (formerly dysthymia and chronic MDD) (prevalence rate 0.5-2.0%) is a chronic form of depression characterized by a depressed or irritable mood (subjectively or described by others) present for at least 1 year. Two of the following symptoms are also required: changes in appetite, sleep difficulty, fatigue, low self-esteem, poor concentration or difficulty making decisions, and feelings of hopelessness. Approximately 70% of children and adolescents with persistent depressive disorder eventually develop major depression.

Disruptive mood dysregulation disorder (DMDD) has been added to DSM-5 and includes children ages 6-18 years who present with a chronic (12 or more months) pattern of severe irritability and behavioral dysregulation. The prevalence rate of DMDD is not known; however, estimates based upon the core feature of chronic irritability suggest a rate between 2% and 5%. DMDD typically first presents in school-age children and is more common among males. In distinguishing bipolar disorder in children from DMDD, particular attention should be given to the course of symptoms (with DMDD being chronic and persistent and bipolar disorder presenting with episodic mood changes). Co-morbidities with DMDD are relatively high, and conditions such as conduct, impulse-control, and disruptive behavior disorders should be assessed. Furthermore, children and adolescents with DMDD may also present with other mood concerns, anxiety, and/or autism spectrum disorder symptoms and diagnoses.

Premenstrual dysphoric disorder (PDD) was also added to DSM-5 and is marked by repeated irritability, anxiety, and mood lability that presents during the premenstrual cycle and remits near the onset of menses. Approximately 1.8-5.8% of adult women are thought to experience PDD with adolescent rates thought to be at a similar level. At least five physical (e.g., sleep disturbance, breast tenderness, joint/muscle pain, fatigue, appetite changes) and/or behavioral symptoms (e.g., affective lability, irritability, depressed mood, anxiety) must be present. Symptoms typically peak near the onset of menses. PDD differs from premenstrual syndrome in the number of symptoms present and in regard to the affective symptoms that are present. MDD is the most commonly presenting co-morbidity. However, other conditions such as anxiety disorders, allergies, migraine headaches, eating disorders, and substance abuse disorders may worsen during the premenstrual period.

Unspecified depressive disorder is a diagnosis used when patients have functionally impairing depressive symptoms that do not meet criteria for another condition.

Numerous **specifiers for depressive disorders** may also be identified. These include methods of noting additional struggles with anxious distress, mixed features (including elevated mood/hypomanic symptoms), melancholic features (loss of pleasure/lack of reactivity to pleasurable stimuli), psychotic features, and seasonal patterns (most common in northern or extreme southern latitudes, in which depressive symptoms occur in the late fall and early winter when the hours of daylight are shortening).

Treatment of depression involves psychopharmacological approaches and/or psychotherapy. Regardless of the treatment approach chosen, a thorough diagnostic interview and screening measures should be completed. There are a variety of screening tools such as Kovacs Children's Depression Inventory (CDI) that may be helpful. First-line pharmacological treatment involves selective serotonin reuptake inhibitors (SSRIs) that have demonstrated response rates of 50-70% despite high-placebo response rates. Fluoxetine is the only medication approved by the U.S. Food and Drug Administration (FDA) for treatment in youth 8 years and older. However, many other "off label" medications such as citalopram, escitalopram, paroxetine, and venlafaxine have positive clinical trial results as well. An antidepressant should be given an adequate trial (6 weeks at therapeutic doses) before switching or discontinuing unless there are serious side effects. For a first episode of depression in children and adolescents, treatment for 6-9 months after remission of symptoms is recommended. Patients with recurrent or persistent depression may need to take antidepressants for extended periods (years or even a lifetime). If a patient does not respond to adequate trials of two or more antidepressants, a child psychiatrist should be consulted. Following a thorough evaluation, the psychiatrist may use augmentation strategies that include other medications such as lithium, thyroid hormone, lamotrigine, or bupropion.

For acute depression, more frequent office visits are indicated, and the risks of medication (including suicidal and self-destructive behaviors) should always be discussed with caregivers and the patient. Higher frequency of monitoring should include regular telephone calls and/or collaborative care with a psychotherapist. Psychoeducation about the illness and a discussion about calling immediately if new symptoms occur should be held with the family. Notable side effects are thoughts of suicide, increased agitation, or restlessness. Other side effects include headache, dizziness, gastrointestinal symptoms, sleep cycle disturbance, sexual dysfunction, akathisia, serotonin syndrome, and risk of increased bruising (due to platelet inhibition).

In 2004, the FDA issued warnings regarding the potential for increased suicidal thoughts and/or behaviors when using an antidepressant. The data suggest that antidepressants pose a 4% risk, versus a 2% risk in placebo. An increase in suicides in children and adolescents since that year has many experts believing that it might be related to lowered prescription rates of antidepressants and resultant untreated depression. Substance use, concomitant conduct problems, and impulsivity increase the risk of suicide.

Psychotherapy appears to have good efficacy in mild to moderate depression. In moderate to severe depression, combined treatment with psychotherapy and medication has the greatest rate of response, although in severe cases, the efficacy was equivalent to medication alone. Cognitive-behavioral therapy (CBT) and interpersonal therapies have received the most empirical support. CBT involves a variety of behavioral techniques and skills-building to mitigate cognitive distortions and maladaptive processing. Interpersonal therapy focuses on collaborative decisions between the therapist and patient and is based on the exploration and recognition of precipitants of depression. Family therapy is often used as an adjunct to other treatments for depression. Light therapy has been shown to be beneficial for seasonal variants of MDD. Electroconvulsive therapy (ECT) is also used in refractory and life-threatening depression.

Suicide is a fatal complication of MDD and surpasses motor vehicle accidents as a cause of death in adolescents. It has high prevalence among high school students with 20% having contemplated suicide and 8% having attempted suicide each year. While the risk of suicide during an MDD episode is high, it can be paradoxically higher during start of treatment, as energy and motivation improve with cognitive recovery from depression.

Treatment is targeted toward decreasing morbidity and suicide. Along with treatments mentioned previously, modalities such as hospitalization, partial hospitalization, therapeutic after-school programs, or group therapies may be needed.

BIPOLAR AND RELATED DISORDERS

Bipolar I disorder (BD) consists of distinct periods of mania (elevated, expansive, or irritable moods and distractibility) and persistent goal-directed activity or energy (Table 18.2) that may alternate with periods of severe depression (Table 18.3).

To diagnose mania associated with BD, euphoria (elevated or expansive mood) with three additional symptoms or irritable mood with four additional symptoms are required. Children and adolescents with euphoric mood often present as bubbly, giggly, and "over-the-top" happy, to a degree that is socially unacceptable to others. Grandiosity in children is often dramatic, and they may believe they are superior to others in activities, sports, or academics even when it is obvious that it is not true. Racing thoughts and concentration difficulties are common in BD and speech can be loud and pressured. Periods of extreme rage may also present. Children with BD often present with rapid shifts in mood or lability over brief time frames (e.g., shifting between euphoria and dysphoria or irritability).

A decreased need for sleep without fatigue is a hallmark of mania. There are no other diagnoses where a child has a greatly decreased amount of total sleep (compared with age-appropriate norms) and is not fatigued. Sleep deprivation, substance abuse, and antidepressants may trigger mania. BD onset often begins with an episode of depression. Mania rarely occurs prior to adolescence. It is estimated that 33% of youth will develop BD within 5 years of a depressive episode and 20% of all patients with BD will experience their first manic episode during adolescence. *Hypomania* is used to describe a period of more than 4 but fewer than 7 days of manic symptoms. It also is used, less specifically, to describe less intense mania. The prevalence of psychosis in adolescents with BD (most often auditory hallucinations) is 16-60%. Although high, it is still less than its prevalence in adult BD.

Bipolar II disorder includes at least one current or past full major depressive episode and at least one period of current or past hypomania. **Unspecified bipolar and related disorder** is used to describe prominent symptoms of BD that do not meet full diagnostic criteria or when historical information is unclear or insufficient to make a specific diagnosis.

Cyclothymic disorder is a chronic (greater than 1 year) mood disorder characterized by several periods of hypomanic symptoms and depressive symptoms (which do not have to meet the full diagnostic criteria for hypomania or a depressive episode, respectively). The lifetime prevalence rate for cyclothymic disorder is around 1%. Childhood rates are not clearly established. The male to female ratio for the disorder is fairly equal, and in children, the mean age of onset is 6.5 years. ADHD has a strong co-morbidity with cyclothymic disorder

TABLE 18.2 Diagnostic and Statistical Manual of Mental Disorders-5 Diagnostic Criteria for a Manic Episode

A. A distinct period of abnormally and persistently elevated, expansive, or irritable mood and abnormally and persistently increased goal-directed activity or energy, lasting at least 1 wk and present most of the day, nearly every day (or any duration if hospitalization is necessary).

B. During the period of mood disturbance and increased energy or activity, three (or more) of the following symptoms (four if the mood is only irritable) are present to a significant degree and represent a noticeable change from usual behavior:

1. Inflated self-esteem or grandiosity.
2. Decreased need for sleep (e.g., feels rested after only 3 hours of sleep).
3. More talkative than usual or pressure to keep talking.
4. Flight of ideas or subjective experience that thoughts are racing.
5. Distractibility (i.e., attention too easily drawn to unimportant or irrelevant external stimuli), as reported or observed.
6. Increase in goal-directed activity (either socially, at work or school, or sexually) or psychomotor agitation (i.e., purposeless non-goal-directed activity).
7. Excessive involvement in activities that have a high potential for painful consequences (e.g., engaging in unrestrained buying sprees, sexual indiscretions, or foolish business investments).

C. The mood disturbance is sufficiently severe to cause marked impairment in social or occupational functioning or to necessitate hospitalization to prevent harm to self or others, or there are psychotic features.

D. The episode is not attributable to the physiological effects of a substance (e.g., a drug of abuse, a medication, other treatment) or to another medical condition.

Note: A full manic episode that emerges during antidepressant treatment (e.g., medication, electroconvulsive therapy) but persists at a fully syndromal level beyond the physiological effect of that treatment is sufficient evidence for a manic episode and, therefore, a bipolar I diagnosis.

Note: Criteria A-D constitute a manic episode. At least one lifetime manic episode is required for the diagnosis of bipolar I disorder.

Reprinted with permission from the Diagnostic and Statistical Manual of Mental Disorders. *5th ed. (Copyright 2013). American Psychiatric Association; 2013:124.*

in children. Other disorders, including sleep disorders and substance-related disorders, should be carefully assessed.

Numerous **specifiers for bipolar disorders** may also be identified. These include methods of noting additional struggles with anxious distress, mixed features (including elevated mood/hypomanic symptoms), melancholic features (loss of pleasure/lack of reactivity to pleasurable stimuli), psychotic features, seasonal patterns, and rapid cycling (four or more mood episodes during a 12-month period).

It is estimated that 1% of children and adolescents meet diagnostic criteria for BD. According to retrospective studies, 60% of BD onset occurs before 20 years of age, although it is often not until adulthood that BD is diagnosed. Although BD in adults tends to be gender neutral, it is estimated that prepubertal BD is almost four times more frequently diagnosed in boys.

TABLE 18.3 Diagnostic and Statistical Manual of Mental Disorders-5 Diagnostic Criteria for a Major Depressive Episode

A. Five (or more) of the following symptoms have been present during the same 2-week period and represent a change from previous functioning; at least one of the symptoms is either (1) depressed mood or (2) loss of interest or pleasure.

Note: Do not include symptoms that are clearly attributable to another medical condition.

1. Depressed mood most of the day, nearly every day, as indicated by either subjective report (e.g., feels sad, empty, or hopeless) or observation made by others (e.g., appears tearful). Note: In children and adolescents, can be irritable mood.
2. Markedly diminished interest or pleasure in all, or almost all, activities most of the day, nearly every day (as indicated by either subjective account or observation).
3. Significant weight loss when not dieting or weight gain (e.g., a change of more than 5% of body weight in a month), or decrease or increase in appetite nearly every day. Note: In children, consider failure to make expected weight gain.
4. Insomnia or hypersomnia nearly every day.
5. Psychomotor agitation or retardation nearly every day (observable by others; not merely subjective feelings of restlessness or being slowed down).
6. Fatigue or loss of energy nearly every day.
7. Feelings of worthlessness or excessive or inappropriate guilt (which may be delusional) nearly every day (not merely self-reproach or guilt about being sick).
8. Diminished ability to think or concentrate, or indecisiveness, early every day (either by subjective account or as observed by others).
9. Recurrent thoughts of death (not just fear of dying), recurrent suicidal ideation without a specific plan, or a suicide attempt or a specific plan for committing suicide.

B. The symptoms cause clinically significant distress or impairment in social, occupational, or other important areas of functioning.

C. The episode is not attributable to the physiological effects of a substance or another medical condition.

Reprinted with permission from the Diagnostic and Statistical Manual of Mental Disorders. *5th ed. (Copyright 2013). American Psychiatric Association; 2013:125.*

Familial etiology with a family history of mental illness, including MDD, BD, schizophrenia, or ADHD, is common in BD. A first-degree relative with BD leads to a 10-fold increase in a child's chance of developing BD. An earlier onset of BD in a parent increases the risk of early onset BD in offspring with a more chronic and debilitating course that may be less responsive to treatment. The differential diagnosis for BD includes ADHD, MDD, conduct disorder (CD), mood disorder due to a general medical condition, substance-related mood disorder, and schizophrenia.

Patients with BD often have concurrent conditions that warrant treatment. ADHD occurs in approximately 60-90% of children with BD. Anxiety disorders also commonly occur with BD and do not respond to antimanic agents. Substance abuse can precipitate and perpetuate mania and depression. The alteration between highs and lows related to some types of substance abuse often mimics BD. Patients with BD may also self-medicate in attempts to alleviate symptoms (with up to 50% of BD patients presenting with alcohol use disorder). It may be necessary to evaluate a patient in a substance-free state to make an accurate diagnosis of BD. Many patients with BD may meet criteria for CD due to aggression and impulsivity. In distinguishing BD from CD, patients with BD generally exhibit reactive aggression, whereas those with CD are more likely to preplan crimes.

No laboratory or imaging studies can diagnose BD. Physical examination, careful history, review of systems, and laboratory testing are done to rule out suspected medical etiologies, including neurological and substance-related disorders.

Treatment of BD initially includes targeting acute symptoms. If suicidal ideation and/or risk taking behaviors are present, hospitalization may be necessary. Treatment typically involves a variety of approaches depending upon the developmental level of the child/adolescent. Multiple FDA-approved medications including lithium, divalproex sodium, carbamazepine, olanzapine, risperidone, quetiapine, ziprasidone, and aripiprazole are available for adults with BD. Lithium is the oldest proven treatment for mania in adults and has been used in acute episodes and as a maintenance treatment in children and adolescents. Common side effects of lithium include hypothyroidism, polyuria, and acne. Anticonvulsants are also a first-line agent (preferable for mixed or rapid cycling cases) for adults. They have also been used effectively in youth, but are not FDA-approved in children for BD. Periodic monitoring of blood levels for select medications (lithium and divalproex sodium) can help ensure both treatment safety and the receipt of therapeutic amounts of the medication. Neuroleptics (e.g., risperidone, olanzapine, quetiapine, aripiprazole, and ziprasidone) have had positive results in youth with BD. The increased risk of tardive dyskinesia should be considered in using such agents. Benzodiazepines may also be helpful for alleviating insomnia and agitation during acute mania.

Treating co-morbid psychiatric disorders must be done carefully. Stimulants may be used to treat ADHD once the patient has been stabilized on a mood stabilizer. In contrast, antidepressants should be avoided; if the youth is depressed or has significant anxiety and is not responsive to other pharmacotherapy, cautious use of antidepressants may be necessary. Careful monitoring for manic reactivation, cycling, and suicidality is needed.

Cognitive and behavioral therapies are aimed at initially improving adherence to medication treatments and ameliorating anxiety and depressive symptoms. Psychoeducation and family therapy may also be needed to stabilize the patient's environment and improve prognosis. There should be ongoing safety assessment. Additionally, patients may display struggles with coping skills, impaired social/interpersonal relationships, and developmental deficits due to poor learning while symptomatic; therefore additional skills training and collaboration with the child's school regarding behavior management, special education needs, and an appropriate individualized education plan may also be needed.

When compared with depression, the rates of suicide and suicidal ideation are even higher in BD. Forty percent of children and 50% of adolescents with BD attempt suicide with approximately 10-15% completing attempts. High levels of irritability, impulsivity, and poor ability to consider consequences (e.g., substance abuse) increase the risk of completed suicide. Attempters are usually older, more likely to have mixed episodes and psychotic features, co-morbid substance use, panic disorder, nonsuicidal self-injurious behaviors, a family history of suicide attempts, history of hospitalizations, and history of physical or sexual abuse. Legal problems in adolescence is also a strong predictor of suicide attempts, with approximately one fourth of those attempting suicide having experienced legal concerns in the preceding 12 months. Ensuring safety should always be the first goal of treatment. Hospitalization, partial hospitalization, intensive outpatient treatment, and intensive in-home services are used as needed for stabilization and safety.

CHAPTER 19
Obsessive-Compulsive Disorder

Obsessive-compulsive disorder (OCD) is characterized by obsessions, compulsions, or both in the absence of another psychiatric disorder that better explains the symptoms (Table 19.1). Obsessions are recurring intrusive thoughts, images, or impulses. Compulsions are repetitive, nongratifying behaviors that a person feels driven to perform in order to reduce or prevent distress or anxiety. In children, rituals or compulsive symptoms may predominate over worries or obsessions, and the child may attempt to ignore or neutralize an obsessive thought by performing compulsions. Symptoms may or may not be recognized as being excessive or unreasonable. Some of the most common examples of obsessions in children are fears of contamination, fears of dirt/germs, repeated doubts, a need for orderliness or precision, and aggressive thoughts. Common compulsions include grooming rituals (e.g., handwashing, showering, teeth brushing), ordering, checking, requesting or demanding reassurance, praying, counting, repeating words silently, and touching rituals.

Prevalence of OCD in children and adolescents ranges from 1% to 4%, increasing with age. Boys typically have an earlier age of onset with approximately one quarter of boys being diagnosed prior to 10 years of age. It is most commonly diagnosed between the ages of 7 and 12 years. Symptoms typically have a gradual onset. Twin studies suggest that obsessive-compulsive symptoms are moderately heritable, with genetic factors accounting for 45-65% of variance.

Up to 50% of youth with OCD have at least one other psychiatric illness. Some of the most common psychiatric co-morbidities include mood and anxiety disorders (up to 75%), behavioral disorders (attention-deficit/hyperactivity disorder [ADHD] and oppositional defiant disorder) (up to 50%), tic disorders (20-30%), hoarding disorder, developmental disorders, body dysmorphic disorder, hypochondriasis, and obsessive-compulsive personality disorder (OCPD).

Streptococcal infection causing inflammation in the basal ganglia may account for 10% of childhood-onset OCD and is a part of a condition historically referred to as *pediatric autoimmune neuropsychiatric disorders associated with streptococcal* (PANDAS) infection. PANDAS is a subtype of *pediatric acute-onset neuropsychiatric syndrome* (PANS), which can, in part, be distinguished by an abrupt onset of moderate to severe OCD symptoms. Antistreptolysin O, antistreptococcal DNAase B titers, and a throat culture assist in diagnosing a group A beta-hemolytic streptococcal infection. Early antibiotic therapy may help treat these cases.

TABLE 19.1	Diagnostic and Statistical Manual of Mental Disorders-5 Criteria for Diagnosis of Obsessive-Compulsive Disorder

A. Presence of either obsessions or compulsions, or both.

Obsessions are defined by (1) and (2).

1. Recurrent and persistent thoughts, urges, or images that are experienced at some time during the disturbance as intrusive and unwanted, and that in most individuals cause marked anxiety or distress.
2. The individual attempts to ignore or suppress such thoughts, urges, or images or to neutralize them with some other thought or action (i.e., by performing a compulsion).

Compulsions are defined by (1) and (2).

1. Repetitive behaviors (e.g., handwashing, ordering, checking) or mental acts (e.g., praying, counting, repeating words silently) that the individual feels driven to perform in response to an obsession or according to rules that must be applied rigidly.
2. The behaviors or mental acts are aimed at preventing or reducing anxiety or distress or preventing some dreaded event or situation; however, these behaviors or mental acts are not connected in a realistic way with what they are designed to neutralize or prevent or are clearly excessive.

Note: Young children may not be able to articulate the aims of these behaviors or mental acts.

B. The obsessions or compulsions are time-consuming (taking >1 hour a day); or cause clinically significant distress or impairment in social, occupational, or other important areas of functioning.

C. The obsessive-compulsive symptoms are not attributable to the physiological effects of a substance (e.g., a drug of abuse, a medication) or a general medical condition.

D. The disturbance is not better explained by the symptoms of another mental disorder (e.g., excessive worries, as in generalized anxiety disorder; preoccupation with appearance, as in body dysmorphic disorder; difficulty discarding or parting with possessions, as in hoarding disorder; hair pulling, as in trichotillomania; skin picking, as in excoriation; stereotypies, as in stereotypical movement disorder; ritualized eating behavior, as in eating disorders; preoccupation with substances or gambling, as in substance-related and addictive disorders; preoccupation with having an illness, as in illness anxiety disorder; sexual urges or fantasies, as in paraphilic disorders; impulses, as in disruptive, impulse-control, and conduct disorders; guilty ruminations, as in major depressive disorder; thought insertion or delusional preoccupations, as in schizophrenia spectrum and other psychotic disorders; or repetitive patterns of behavior, as in autism spectrum disorder).

Specify if:

With good or fair insight: The individual recognizes that obsessive-compulsive disorder beliefs are definitely or probably not true or that they may or may not be true.

With poor insight: The individual thinks obsessive-compulsive disorder beliefs are probably true.

With absent insight/delusional beliefs: The individual is completely convinced that obsessive-compulsive disorder beliefs are true.

Specify if:

Tic related: The individual has a current or past history of a tic disorder.

Reprinted with permission from the Diagnostic and Statistical Manual of Mental Disorders. *5th ed. (Copyright 2013). American Psychiatric Association. 2013:237.*

OCD has been linked to a disruption in the brain's serotonin, glutamate, and dopamine systems. Overactivity in neural pathways involving orbital frontal cortex and the caudate nucleus has been implicated in OCD.

Physical examination may reveal rough, cracked skin as evidence of excessive handwashing. Other common complaints might include a persistent fear of illness, expressed concerns regarding the health of family members, and fear that something bad will happen to someone.

The Yale-Brown Obsessive-Compulsive Scale (Y-BOCS) is regarded as the gold standard measure of obsessive-compulsive symptom severity. Although somewhat lengthy, it can be helpful in the clinical setting. Additionally, there are numerous other diagnostic questionnaires available to assist in making an accurate diagnosis.

Cognitive-behavioral therapy (CBT) involving exposure and response prevention is considered the treatment of choice in mild to moderate cases. CBT provides durability of symptom relief and avoidance of potential pharmacotherapy-associated side effects. As with anxiety disorders, CBT is at least as good, if not better, than medications. The combination of medications and CBT has shown the best response. CBT typically involves gradually exposing the child to their fear/obsession paired with strategies that target preventing the child from performing the unwanted ritual/compulsion. Over time with repeated exposure and response prevention, the urge to repeat the compulsion(s) dissipates.

Selective serotonin reuptake inhibitors (SSRIs) are recommended for higher severity of symptoms and complications with co-morbidities or when cognitive or emotional ability are insufficient to demonstrate success in CBT. Additionally, if quality CBT is not available, treatment with medications alone while psychotherapy referral is pursued is a reasonable choice.

SSRI (e.g., paroxetine, fluoxetine, fluvoxamine, sertraline, citalopram, and escitalopram) treatment is generally thought to show a favorable risk-to-benefit ratio in OCD. Side effects such as activation, akathisia, disinhibition, impulsivity, and hyperactivity may be seen. Monitoring of height may be advisable due to possible growth suppression associated with the SSRIs.

Common protocols suggest three trials of an SSRI and, if unsuccessful, clomipramine can be tried next. Careful monitoring of potential anticholinergic side effects, lowering of blood pressure, and EKG monitoring is necessary. Combination therapy using an SSRI with an antipsychotic medication (risperidone or another atypical antipsychotic) may also be considered, especially with specific co-morbidities (e.g., tic disorders). Antipsychotics are also useful when the intrusive thoughts associated with OCD become nearly delusional in nature. Psychostimulants may be used with co-morbid ADHD, even though there is a risk that they may increase obsessional symptoms and tics. Children should be closely monitored for suicidal thoughts, as such ideation is not uncommon, increasing with symptom severity and depressive co-morbidities.

Most *responders* exhibit partial response only, and as many as one third of young people with OCD are refractory to treatment. Poor prognostic factors include co-morbid psychiatric illness and a poor initial treatment response.

Deep brain stimulation of the basal ganglia, through surgically implanted electrodes and surgical interventions (anterior capsulotomy, anterior cingulotomy, subcaudate tractotomy, and limbic leucotomy), are reserved for very severe cases or highly refractory cases.

The differential diagnosis for OCD includes MDD, other obsessive-compulsive and related disorders (e.g., hoarding, trichotillomania), psychotic disorders, tic disorders, other anxiety disorders, and OCPD. Although some children with OCD may have poor insight, they typically present with clear obsessions/compulsions that distinguish them from delusions. They lack hallucinations, which help to distinguish them from schizophrenia spectrum disorders. This may be at times difficult to discern. For instance, a delusional fixation on appearance in body dysmorphic disorder and impulsive hair pulling to relieve anxiety or tension in trichotillomania can be confused with OCD. OCPD is a character style involving preoccupation with orderliness, perfectionism, and control. It can be distinguished from OCD in that no true obsessions or compulsions are present in OCPD. However, if symptoms of both conditions are present, they can be co-morbid, although this is rare.

CHAPTER 20
Autism Spectrum Disorder and Schizophrenia Spectrum Disorders

The previous classification of four separate disorders, autism, Asperger syndrome, childhood disintegrative disorder, and pervasive developmental disorder not otherwise specified, have been combined in the DSM-5 under the category of autism spectrum disorder (ASD; Table 20.1). Specifiers of symptom severity in regard to core deficits in the domains of social communication impairments and restricted, repetitive patterns of behavior (RRPB) are also provided. A diagnosis of social (pragmatic) communication disorder (SCD) may be made in the absence of RRPBs.

Onset of ASD is in infancy and preschool years. Hallmarks of ASD include impaired communication and impaired social interaction as well as stereotypical behaviors, interests, and activities. Intellectual disability is common (~38% according to Centers for Disease Control and Prevention [CDC] estimates); although the majority of children demonstrate average to high intelligence scores, they often show uneven abilities.

ASD is seen in approximately 1% of the population with equal prevalence rates among all racial and ethnic groups. Boys appear to be diagnosed much more frequently than girls (4 : 1 ratio); however, girls with the disorder tend to be more severely affected regarding intellectual abilities and symptom severity.

ASD is characterized by lifelong marked impairment in social interaction and social communication in addition to RRPBs. Approximately 20% of parents report relatively normal development until 1-2 years of age, followed by a steady or sudden decline. In infants with ASD there is delayed or absent social smiling. The young child may spend hours in solitary play and be socially withdrawn with indifference to attempts at communication. Patients with autism often are not able to

TABLE 20.1 Diagnostic and Statistical Manual of Mental Disorders-5 Diagnostic Criteria for Autism Spectrum Disorder

A. Persistent deficits in social communication and social interaction across multiple contexts, as manifested by the following, currently or by history:
   1. Deficits in social-emotional reciprocity.
   2. Deficits in nonverbal communicative behaviors used for social interaction.
   3. Deficits in developing, maintaining, and understanding relationships.

B. Restricted, repetitive patterns of behavior, interests, or activities, as manifested by at least two of the following, currently or by history:
   1. Stereotyped or repetitive motor movements, use of objects, or speech.
   2. Insistence on sameness, inflexible adherence to routines, or ritualized patterns of verbal or nonverbal behavior.
   3. Highly restricted, fixated interests that are abnormal in intensity or focus.
   4. Hyper- or hyporeactivity to sensory input or unusual interest in sensory aspects of the environment.

C. Symptoms must be present in the early developmental period (but may not become fully manifest until social demands exceed limited capacities or may be masked by learned strategies in later life).

D. Symptoms cause clinically significant impairment in social, occupational, or other important areas of current functioning.

E. These disturbances are not better explained by intellectual disability (intellectual developmental disorder) or global developmental delay. Intellectual disability and spectrum disorder frequently co-occur; to make co-morbid diagnoses of autism spectrum disorder and intellectual disability, social communication should be below that expected for general developmental level.

Note: Individuals with a well-established Diagnostic and Statistical Manual of Mental Disorders-IV diagnosis of autistic disorder, Asperger disorder, or pervasive developmental disorder not otherwise specified should be given the diagnosis of autism spectrum disorder. Individuals who have marked deficits in social communication but whose symptoms do not otherwise meet criteria for autism spectrum disorder should be evaluated for social (pragmatic) communication disorder.

Specify if:

With or without accompanying intellectual impairment

With or without accompanying language impairment

Associated with a known medical or genetic condition or environmental factor

Associated with another neurodevelopmental, mental, or behavioral disorder

With catatonia (refer to the criteria for catatonia associated with another mental disorder)

Reprinted with permission from the Diagnostic and Statistical Manual of Mental Disorders. *5th ed. (Copyright 2013). American Psychiatric Association. 2013:50–51.*

understand nonverbal communication (e.g., eye contact, facial expressions) and do not interact with people as significantly different from objects. Communication and speech often are delayed and, when present, may be marked by echolalia (repetition of language of others), perseveration (prolonged repetition of words or behaviors of others), pronoun reversal, nonsense rhyming, and other abnormalities. Intense absorbing interests, ritualistic behavior, and compulsive routines are characteristic, and their disruption may invoke behavioral dysregulation. Self-injurious behaviors (head banging, biting), repetitive motor mannerisms (rocking, lining up objects, simple motor stereotypies), and hyperreactivity/hyporeactivity to their environment (diminished response to pain, adverse reactions to sounds/textures, or unusual visual inspection of objects) may be noted.

Although the full etiology of ASD is unknown, it is largely considered a genetic disorder. There is an increased risk of ASD in siblings compared to the general population. Twin studies have revealed high levels of concordance (36-95%) for identical twins. Family studies reveal prevalence rates of between 2% and 18% in siblings, and when absent, there may be increased risk for other language, learning, and social development problems.

It has been proposed that brain connectivity is adversely affected. Abnormalities in the limbic system, temporal, and frontal lobes have been suggested. Some postmortem studies reveal abnormalities in the brain microarchitecture, size, and neuronal packing. Functional magnetic resonance imaging (fMRI) studies show that hypoactivity of the fusiform gyrus of the amygdala, a location involved in face processing tasks and facial expression recognition involved in social and affective judgments, may be impacted in ASD.

There are no definitive laboratory studies for ASD, but they can help rule out other diagnoses. A hearing test (may account for the language deficits), chromosomal testing (to identify fragile X syndrome, tubular sclerosis, and genetic polymorphisms), congenital viral infections, and metabolic disorders (phenylketonuria) should be performed. Electroencephalography abnormalities may be seen in 20-25% of children with ASD, but they are not diagnostic.

The American Academy of Pediatrics (AAP) recommends screening for autism at 18 and 24 months of age. There are numerous screening measures that may be employed (e.g., Childhood Autism Rating Scale [CARS], Modified Checklist for Autism in Toddlers [M-CHAT], Gilliam Autism Rating Scale [GARS], and Screening Tool for Autism in Toddlers and Young Children [STAT]) to assist with appropriate referral for diagnostic evaluation. "Gold standard" psychological measures such as the Autism Diagnostic Observation Schedule (ADOS) and Autism Diagnostic Interview (ADI) are commonly recommended to confirm a diagnosis. Other measures of language, adaptive skills, and intelligence may also be administered if ASD is suspected. Psychological tests in children with ASD often show strengths in nonverbal tasks (e.g., puzzles) and marked deficiency in verbal cognitive abilities. Speech pathology consultation can be helpful in evaluating the communication difficulties.

Common psychiatric co-morbidities include intellectual disability, language/communication disorders, anxiety disorders, attention-deficit/hyperactivity disorder, developmental coordination disorder, and depressive disorders. Other medical complexities commonly seen in children with ASD include seizure disorder, sleep disorders, and gastrointestinal disorders (constipation, food selectivity). Intellectual abilities and language abilities are the strongest predictors of improved long-term prognosis. The earliest studies of autism suggested a relatively poor prognosis, with only a small number of individuals (1-2%) being able to function independently as adults. Recent research reveals major gains, but not a cure, with early diagnosis and treatment.

SCD involves difficulties with the social use of verbal and nonverbal communication. SCD involves struggles with using communication for social purposes (e.g., greeting others, sharing information, conversational rules, inferences, and pragmatic skills). SCD is marked by many of the same communication deficits seen in children with ASD with the absence of RRPBs. SCD is believed to be rare in children prior to 4 years of age; however, the prevalence rate is unclear because of its recent addition to the DSM-5. Typically, speech and language therapy and social skills training are employed to treat SCD.

Treatment of ASD is typically multimodal. At present, there are no pharmacological treatments for the core symptoms of ASDs. Antipsychotics (risperidone, olanzapine, quetiapine, aripiprazole, ziprasidone, paliperidone, haloperidol, thioridazine) are used for aggression, agitation, irritability, hyperactivity, and self-injurious behavior. Anticonvulsants have also been used for aggression. Naltrexone has been used to decrease self-injurious behavior, presumably by blocking endogenous opioids. Selective serotonin reuptake inhibitors are given for anxiety, perseveration, compulsions, depression, and social isolation. Stimulants are useful for hyperactivity and inattention; however, there are reports of significant worsening of irritability and aggression in some patients treated with stimulants. Alpha-2 agonists (guanfacine, clonidine) are used for hyperactivity, aggression, and sleep dysregulation, although melatonin is first-line medication for sleep dysregulation.

A variety of nonpharmacological interventions exist for ASD. Such interventions have largely fallen under the classification of behavioral training. Models have typically employed therapies individually tailored for children with ASD and their families/caregivers. Evidence suggests that useful therapies have included techniques from applied behavior analysis (ABA), discrete trial training (DTT), functional behavioral analysis (FBA), and structured teaching (TEACCH Model). Behavioral management training for parents has also demonstrated efficacy in helping with unwanted behaviors. Special education services should be individualized for the child. Occupational, speech, and physical therapy are often required. Referral for disability services and support is often warranted. Family support groups and individual supportive counseling for parents is useful. The prognosis for ASD is guarded and varies greatly from child to child. There are no known methods of primary prevention. Treatment and educational interventions are aimed at decreasing morbidity and maximizing function.

SCHIZOPHRENIA SPECTRUM AND OTHER PSYCHOTIC DISORDERS

Schizophrenia generally presents in adolescence or early adulthood. The same diagnostic criteria are applied as in adults but must be interpreted in terms of the developmental stage of the child (Table 20.2). Several significant changes to the diagnosis of schizophrenia were made within the DSM-5. The most significant changes involve requiring two or more of the core features of a psychotic disorder (delusion, hallucinations, disorganized speech, disorganized/catatonic behavior, negative symptoms) to be present, with at least one of the first three "positive symptoms" also being present. Additionally, subtypes of schizophrenia (e.g., paranoid, catatonic, undifferentiated)

TABLE 20.2 Diagnostic and Statistical Manual of Mental Disorders-5 Diagnostic Criteria for Brief Psychotic Disorder

A. Presence of one (or more) of the following symptoms. At least one of these must be (1), (2), or (3):
1. Delusions
2. Hallucinations
3. Disorganized speech (e.g., frequent derailment or incoherence)
4. Grossly disorganized or catatonic behavior
Note: Do not include a symptom if it is a culturally sanctioned response.
B. Duration of an episode of the disturbance is at least one day but less than 1 month, with eventual full return to premorbid level of functioning.
C. The disturbance is not better explained by major depressive or bipolar disorder with psychotic features or another psychotic disorder such as schizophrenia or catatonia, and is not attributable to the physiological effects of a substance (e.g., a drug of abuse, a medication) or another medical condition.
Specify if:
With marked stressor(s) (brief reactive psychosis): If symptoms occur in response to events that, singly or together, would be markedly stressful to almost anyone in similar circumstances in the individual's culture.
Without marked stressor(s): If the symptoms do not occur in response to events that, singly or together, would be would be markedly stressful to almost anyone in similar circumstances in the individual's culture.
With postpartum onset: If onset is during pregnancy or within 4 weeks postpartum.

Reprinted with permission from the Diagnostic and Statistical Manual of Mental Disorders. *5th ed. (Copyright 2013). American Psychiatric Association; 2013:94. All rights reserved.*

have been discarded, and severity ratings for the core symptoms have been included to reflect a more dimensional approach to the spectrum of schizophrenia.

Childhood-onset schizophrenia is a rare disorder (<1 in 10,000 children) and usually indicates a more severe form of schizophrenia. The frequency increases between 13 and 18 years of age, typically with the initial presentation of psychotic features. The incidence in boys is slightly greater than in girls, and the age of onset tends to be later for girls. The etiology of schizophrenia is not clearly known, but numerous studies have demonstrated a substantial genetic predisposition for the disorder. In addition, family studies consistently show a higher risk in monozygotic twins compared with dizygotic twins and siblings. First-degree relatives of patients with schizophrenia have a 10-fold higher risk.

The symptoms of schizophrenia typically fall into four broad categories:

- **Positive symptoms** include hallucinations and delusions. Hallucinations are auditory or visual misperceptions that occur without external stimuli. Delusions are fixed false beliefs and can be bizarre or non-bizarre depending on cultural norms.
- **Negative symptoms** include a lack of motivation and social interactions and flat affect. Negative symptoms are most frequent in early childhood and later adolescence. Children with high intelligence often show more positive and fewer negative symptoms than children with low intelligence.
- **Disorganization of thoughts and behavior** can cause significant impairment.
- **Cognitive impairment** is common and is perhaps the most disabling feature of schizophrenia, causing marked social and functional impairment.

To meet criteria for diagnosing schizophrenia, clinical symptoms should be present for at least 6 months. If symptoms are present for less than 1 month, the condition is called a **brief psychotic disorder.** If symptoms are present for more than 1 month but less than 6 months, a diagnosis of **schizophreniform disorder** is made. Psychotic symptoms that do not meet full diagnostic criteria for schizophrenia but are clinically significant are diagnosed as an **unspecified schizophrenia spectrum or other psychotic disorder.** Other disorders in the differential diagnosis of a schizophrenia spectrum disorder are ASD, neurocognitive disorders, substance-induced psychosis, bipolar disorders, and organic brain disorders.

There are several disorders that also fall within the spectrum of schizophrenia and other psychotic disorders that should be distinguished from schizophrenia. These include the following:

Schizoaffective disorder is diagnosed when a person has clear symptoms of schizophrenia lasting at least 2 weeks and experiences a major mood episode (major depression/mania) during an uninterrupted period of the illness. These affective syndromes occur at other times, even when psychotic symptoms are present. This condition is very rare in children and has a lifetime prevalence that is much lower than schizophrenia (0.3% lifetime prevalence).

Psychotic disorder due to another medical condition describes psychotic symptoms that are judged to be the direct result of a general medical condition. There are a variety of potential underlying medical etiologies. Some of the most common precipitating illnesses in children are epilepsy, metabolic disorders, and autoimmune disorders.

Substance/medication-induced psychotic disorders have psychotic symptoms related to substance intoxication/withdrawal or following exposure to a medication. While prevalence is not clearly known, estimates suggest that between 7% and 25% of first episodes of psychoses are related to substances.

No diagnostic tests or imaging studies are specific for schizophrenia. It is a clinical diagnosis of exclusion. Obtaining a family history with attention to mental illness is critical. The identification of schizophrenia should include a physical and neurological examination, MRI, electroencephalography (to rule out epilepsy, especially temporal lobe epilepsy), substance/drug screening, and metabolic screening for endocrinopathies. Evaluation to rule out Wilson disease and delirium is also indicated. Psychotic symptoms in younger children must be differentiated from manifestations of normal vivid fantasy life or abuse-related symptoms. Youth with post-traumatic stress disorder often have vivid recollections and nightmares related to abuse but, sometimes, are less specific and can include nightmares with other negative topics. Psychological testing can be helpful in identifying psychotic thought processes.

Treatment is based on a multimodal approach, including the use of antipsychotic medications. First-line drugs are atypical antipsychotics (e.g., risperidone, olanzapine, quetiapine, aripiprazole, ziprasidone, and paliperidone). Second-line medications are typical antipsychotics (e.g., haloperidol, thiothixene, chlorpromazine, trifluoperazine, loxapine, and molindone). It is likely that the newer antipsychotics approved for adults will also work in youth; however, these are not yet all approved in youth by the U.S. Food and Drug Administration. Antipsychotics can be augmented with lithium or another mood stabilizer. Clozapine is generally reserved for resistant cases. Neuroleptic medications also carry the risk of tardive dyskinesia and should be employed cautiously in children. Evidence suggests that prepubertal children are less responsive to antipsychotics and that adolescents, while demonstrating efficacy with the medications, do not reach the level of full efficacy seen in adults.

Psychosocial treatments, including skills training, supportive psychotherapy, behavior modification, and cognitive-behavioral therapy, are all appropriate and should be considered as needed for individual patients. Attention should be paid to psychoeducation for parents and the child about the disease and its treatments. School interventions are needed to ensure that any special learning needs are addressed. Schizophrenia and other psychotic disorders also carry a high risk for suicidality. Co-morbid depressive symptoms increase the risk for suicide. Regular reevaluation of suicidal ideation is necessary throughout treatment.

The course of illness for schizophrenia varies in exacerbations and remissions of psychotic symptoms. The poorest prognosis is seen if the onset is at an age younger than 13 years, with poor premorbid function, when marked negative symptoms are present, and when a family history of schizophrenia exists.

Suggested Readings

American Psychiatric Association (APA). Practice Guidelines. Washington DC: American Psychiatric Association; http://psychiatryonline.org/guidelines.

Baweja R, Mayes SD, Hameed U, et al. Disruptive mood dysregulation disorder: current insights. *Neuropsychiatr Dis Treat.* 2016;12:2115–2124.

Creswell C, Waite P, Cooper PJ. Assessment and management of anxiety disorders in children and adolescents. *Arch Dis Child.* 2014;99(7):674–678.

Lord C, Bishop SL. Recent advances in autism research as reflected in DSM-5 criteria for autism spectrum disorder. *Ann Rev Clin Psychol.* 2015;11:53–70.

Orefici G, Cardona F, Cox CJ, et al. Pediatric autoimmune neuropsychiatric disorders associated with streptococcal infections (PANDAS) 2016 Feb 10. In: Ferretti JJ, Stevens DL, Fischetti VA, eds. *Streptococcus Pyogenes: Basic Biology to Clinical Manifestations.* Oklahoma: University of Oklahoma Health Sciences Center; 2016.

Rapkin AJ, Mikacich JA. Premenstrual dysphoric disorder and severe premenstrual syndrome in adolescents. *Pediatric Drugs.* 2013;15:191–202.

Van Geelen SM, Rydelius PA, Hagquist C. Somatic symptoms and psychological concerns in a general adolescent population: exploring the relevance of DSM-V somatic symptom disorder. *J Psychosom Res.* 2015;9(4):251–258.

Van Meter AR, Burke C, Kowatch RA, et al. Ten-year updated meta-analysis of the clinical characteristics of pediatric mania and hypomania. *Bipolar Disord.* 2016;18(1):19–32.

PEARLS FOR PRACTIONERS

CHAPTER 16

Somatic Symptom and Related Disorders

- Involve physical symptoms (pain, fatigue, or loss of function) that may be medically unexplained or that may accompany diagnosed medical disorders.
- Elevated rates of medical utilization are common (patients repeatedly seek reassurance from family, friends, and medical staff regarding their health).
- In early childhood, symptoms often include recurrent abdominal pain (RAP). Later headaches, neurological symptoms, insomnia, and fatigue are common.
- Screening tools for somatic symptom and related disorders (SSRDs) include the Children's Somatization Inventory, Illness Attitude Scales, Soma Assessment Interview, and the Functional Disability Inventory.
- Selective serotonin reuptake inhibitors (SSRIs) benefit SSRDs involving unexplained headaches, fibromyalgia, body dysmorphic disorder, pain disorder, irritable bowel syndrome, and functional gastrointestinal disorders.
- Tricyclic antidepressants should be avoided in youth with functional abdominal pain (FAP), because they have little proven efficacy and are very dangerous in overdose.
- Stimulants may also be helpful in chronic fatigue syndrome (CFS).
- Therapy, such as cognitive-behavioral therapy (CBT), has demonstrated efficacy in treating recurrent pain, CFS, fibromyalgia, and FAP. Self-management strategies (self-monitoring, relaxation, hypnosis, and biofeedback) have also demonstrated efficacy.
- Home schooling should be avoided; school attendance and performance should be emphasized; parents should limit attention/reinforcement for pain behavior; and normal routines/appropriate schedules (e.g., going to school) should be emphasized.

CHAPTER 17

Anxiety Disorders

- Characterized by uneasiness, excessive rumination, and apprehension about the future.
- Tend to be chronic, recurring, and vary in intensity over time.
- Medical conditions (e.g., hyperthyroidism, medication side effects, substance abuse, or other medical conditions) should be ruled out.
- First-line treatment for mild to moderate anxiety includes evidence-based psychotherapies and psychoeducation. CBT (e.g., systematic desensitization, exposure techniques, operant conditioning, modeling, and cognitive restructuring) can be beneficial in anxiety disorders.
- SSRIs are the medication of choice. The FDA approved SSRIs for children are fluoxetine, sertraline, and fluvoxamine. They

can initially exacerbate anxiety or even panic symptoms. Tricyclic antidepressants have also shown efficacy.
- Benzodiazepines (e.g., clonazepam) include a risk of causing disinhibition in children.
- Alpha-2a-agonists (guanfacine and clonidine) may be useful with autonomic symptoms.
- Anticonvulsant agents (e.g., gabapentin) are used when other agents are ineffective.
- β-Blockers help with performance anxiety.

CHAPTER 18

Depressive Disorders and Bipolar Disorders

Depressive Disorders
- Depressive disorders involve the presence of sad/irritable mood along with physical and cognitive impacts on the child's daily functioning.
- In children, depressed mood often presents as irritability and/or restlessness. Furthermore, many children/adolescents complain of pervasive boredom in major depressive disorder (MDD).
- Many depressive disorders demonstrate genetic predispositions. Anxiety disorders, substance disorders, and conduct/disruptive disorders frequently present as co-morbid with MDD.
- Screening tools such as Kovacs Children's Depression Inventory (CDI) may be helpful.
- SSRIs are first-line pharmacological treatments. Fluoxetine is the only FDA approved medication for treatment of youth. "Off label" medications such as citalopram, escitalopram, paroxetine, and venlafaxine also have positive clinical trial results.
- An antidepressant should be given an adequate trial (6 weeks at therapeutic doses) before switching or discontinuing unless there are serious side effects. For a first episode of depression, treatment for 6-9 months after remission of symptoms is recommended.
- Psychotherapy appears to have good efficacy in mild to moderate depression. In moderate to severe depression, combined treatment with psychotherapy and medication has the greatest rate of response, and CBT and interpersonal therapies have received the most empirical support.
- Suicidal ideation and attempts at suicide are high in depressive disorders. Regular assessment of suicidal ideation should occur.

Bipolar Disorders (BD)
- Consist of distinct periods of mania (elevated, expansive, or irritable mood) and persistent goal-directed activity or energy that may alternate with periods of severe depression.
- Often present with rapid shifts in mood or lability over brief time frames (e.g., shifting between euphoria and dysphoria or irritability). A decreased need for sleep is also common.
- FDA-approved medications in adults (used "off label" in children) include the following: lithium, divalproex sodium, carbamazepine, olanzapine, risperidone, quetiapine, ziprasidone, and aripiprazole. Lithium is often used in acute episodes and as a maintenance treatment in children and adolescents, but this requires periodic monitoring of blood levels.
- Anticonvulsants are used for mixed or rapid cycling cases in adults. They have also been used effectively in youth, but they are not FDA-approved in children for BD.
- Neuroleptics have had positive results in youth with BD; however, the increased risk of tardive dyskinesia should be considered in using such agents.

CHAPTER 19

Obsessive-Compulsive Disorder

- Obsessions (e.g., fears of contamination, fears of dirt/germs, repeated doubts, aggressive thoughts, and orderliness/precision) are recurring intrusive thoughts, images, or impulses.
- Compulsions (e.g., grooming rituals, ordering, checking, requesting reassurance, praying, counting, repeating words silently, and touching rituals) are repetitive nongratifying behaviors that a person feels driven to perform to reduce or prevent distress or anxiety.
- The Yale-Brown Obsessive-Compulsive Scale (Y-BOCS) is regarded as the "gold standard" measure of obsessive-compulsive symptom severity.
- CBT involving exposure and response prevention is considered the treatment of choice in mild to moderate cases.
- SSRIs have demonstrated a favorable risk-to-benefit ratio in obsessive-compulsive disorder (OCD) and are recommended in higher severities of OCD.

CHAPTER 20

Autism Spectrum Disorder and Schizophrenia Spectrum Disorders

Autism Spectrum Disorder (ASD)
- Onset is in infancy and preschool years. Core symptoms reflect impaired communication and impaired social interaction as well as stereotypical behaviors, interests, and activities.
- Intellectual disability is common, and the male to female ratio is 4:1.
- Children with ASD commonly prefer solitary play, are socially withdrawn, struggle to understand nonverbal communication (e.g., eye contact, facial expressions), and do not interact with people as significantly different from objects.
- Communication and speech often are delayed. Intense absorbing interests, ritualistic behavior, and compulsive routines are characteristic.
- Self-injurious behaviors, repetitive motor mannerisms, and hyperreactivity/hyporeactivity to their environment may be noted.
- Screening at 18 and 24 months (e.g., CARS, M-CHAT, GARS, and STAT) and "gold standard" psychological measures (i.e., Autism Diagnostic Observation Schedule [ADOS] and Autism Diagnostic Interview [ADI]-R) are recommended to confirm ASD.
- Nonpharmacological interventions are first line. Therapies have included techniques from applied behavior analysis (ABA), discrete trial training (DTT), functional behavioral analysis (FBA), and structured teaching (TEACCH Model).

- Occupational, speech, and physical therapy are often required.
- There are no pharmacological treatments for the core symptoms of ASDs. Antipsychotics, anticonvulsants, SSRIs, stimulants, and alpha-2 agonists are commonly used to assist with ameliorating secondary and co-morbid symptoms.

Schizophrenia Spectrum and Other Psychotic Disorders

- Childhood-onset schizophrenia is rare and involves the presentation of both positive (hallucinations, delusions) and negative symptoms (poor motivation/social interactions, flat affect).
- No diagnostic tests or imaging studies are specific for schizophrenia. It is a clinical diagnosis of exclusion.
- Work up for schizophrenia should include a physical and neurological examination, MRI, electroencephalography (to exclude epilepsy), drug screening, and metabolic screening for endocrinopathies. Evaluation to exclude Wilson disease and delirium is also indicated.
- First-line pharmacological treatment includes atypical antipsychotics. Second-line medications are typical antipsychotics. Antipsychotics can be augmented with lithium or another mood stabilizer. Neuroleptic medications also carry the risk of tardive dyskinesia and should be employed cautiously in children.
- Prepubertal children are less responsive to antipsychotics and adolescents, while demonstrating efficacy, do not reach the level of full efficacy seen in adults.
- Psychosocial treatments (e.g., skills training, supportive psychotherapy, behavior modification, and CBT) are all appropriate and should be considered as needed.

SECTION 5

PSYCHOSOCIAL ISSUES

Kristine Fortin | Alison H. Downes

CHAPTER 21

Failure to Thrive

Failure to thrive (**FTT**) is a descriptive term given to infants and young children with malnourishment resulting in inadequate growth. To date, there are no universally accepted anthropometric criteria for FTT as different anthropometric indicators and cut points have been used. Commonly used criteria include weight below the 3rd or 5th percentile for age; weight decreasing, crossing two major percentile lines on the growth chart over time; or weight less than 80% of the median weight for the height of the child. Caveats to these definitions exist. According to growth chart standards, 3% of the population naturally falls below the 3rd percentile. These children, who typically have short stature or constitutional delay of growth, usually are proportional (normal weight for height). Additionally, in the first few years of life, large fluctuations in percentile position can occur in normal children. Changes in weight should be assessed in relation to height (length) and head circumference.

Despite these limitations in defining FTT, anthropometric data and growth charts provide important information. Of note, allowances must be made for prematurity; weight corrections are needed until 24 months of age, height corrections until 40 months of age, and head circumference corrections until 18 months of age. Also of note, there are specific growth charts for genetic conditions such as Down syndrome and Turner syndrome that should be used when assessing growth for children with these conditions. Although some growth variants can be difficult to distinguish from FTT, growth velocity and height-for-weight determinations can be useful in distinguishing the cause. In children with FTT, malnutrition initially results in wasting (deficiency in weight gain). Stunting (deficiency in linear growth) generally occurs after months of malnutrition, and head circumference is spared except with chronic, severe malnutrition. FTT that is *symmetric* (proportional weight, height/length, and head circumference) suggests long-standing malnutrition, chromosomal abnormalities, congenital infection, or teratogenic exposures. Short stature with preserved weight suggests an endocrine etiology.

ETIOLOGY

There are multiple possible causes of growth failure (Table 21.1). In the past, etiologies of FTT were sometimes categorized as organic (underlying medical condition diagnosed) and nonorganic (no underlying medical cause). This dichotomous classification can be problematic because, in many cases, the cause of FTT is multifactorial with interaction between multiple biological and psychosocial factors. FTT can be caused by inadequate nutritional intake (e.g., neurological condition impeding feeding, improper mixing of formula, food insecurity), malabsorption (e.g., celiac disease, milk protein allergy), and/or increased metabolic demands (e.g., cardiac disease, chronic infection). Clinical studies suggest that major organic diseases are detected in a minority of patients with FTT. As outlined in Table 21.2, the common causes of FTT vary by age.

DIAGNOSIS AND CLINICAL MANIFESTATIONS

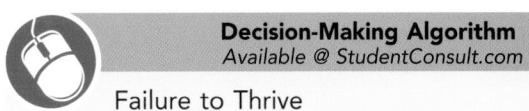

Decision-Making Algorithm
Available @ StudentConsult.com
Failure to Thrive

A careful history and physical examination are the cornerstone of FTT evaluations. A medical history should include prenatal history, gestational age and perinatal history, birth size (weight, length, and head circumference), family, and travel history. Indicators of medical diseases, such as vomiting, diarrhea, fever, respiratory symptoms, and fatigue, should be noted. A careful diet history is essential. Lactation problems in breast-fed infants and improper formula preparation are frequent causes of growth failure early in infancy. It is crucial to evaluate intake of solid foods and liquids for older infants and children. Due to parental dietary beliefs, some children have inappropriately restricted diets; others drink excessive amounts of fruit juice, leading to malabsorption or anorexia. The child's daily meal schedule (timing, frequency, location) should also be noted. Mealtime practices, especially distractions that interfere with completing meals, can influence growth. A complete psychosocial assessment of the child and family is required. Child factors (temperament, development), parental factors (depression, domestic violence, social isolation, cognitive deficits, substance abuse), and environmental and societal factors (poverty, unemployment, illiteracy, lead toxicity) all may contribute to growth failure.

A complete physical examination and developmental screening should assess signs of inflicted injury; oral or dental problems; indicators of pulmonary, cardiac, or gastrointestinal

TABLE 21.1 Causes of Failure to Thrive

ENVIRONMENTAL (COMMON)
Emotional deprivation
Rumination
Child maltreatment
Maternal depression
Poverty
Poor feeding techniques
Improper formula preparation
Improper mealtime environment
Unusual parental nutritional beliefs
GASTROINTESTINAL
Cystic fibrosis and other causes of pancreatic insufficiency
Celiac disease
Other malabsorption syndromes
Gastrointestinal reflux
CONGENITAL/ANATOMIC
Chromosomal abnormalities, genetic syndromes
Congenital heart disease
Gastrointestinal abnormalities (e.g., pyloric stenosis, malrotation)
Vascular rings
Upper airway obstruction
Dental caries
Congenital immunodeficiency syndromes
INFECTIONS
Human immunodeficiency virus
Tuberculosis
Hepatitis
Urinary tract infection, chronic sinusitis, parasitic infection
METABOLIC
Thyroid disease
Adrenal or pituitary disease
Aminoaciduria, organic aciduria
Galactosemia
NEUROLOGICAL
Cerebral palsy
Hypothalamic and other central nervous system tumors
Hypotonia syndromes
Neuromuscular diseases
Degenerative and storage diseases
RENAL
Chronic renal failure
Renal tubular acidosis
Urinary tract infection
HEMATOLOGIC
Sickle cell disease
Iron deficiency anemia

TABLE 21.2 Common Causes of Malnutrition in Early Life

NEONATE
Failed breast-feeding
Improper formula preparation
Congenital syndromes
Prenatal infections
Teratogenic exposures
EARLY INFANCY
Maternal depression
Improper formula preparation
Gastroesophageal reflux
Poverty
Congenital heart disease
Cystic fibrosis
Neurological abnormalities
Child neglect
LATER INFANCY
Celiac disease
Food intolerance
Child neglect
Delayed introduction of age-appropriate foods
Juice consumption
AFTER INFANCY
Acquired diseases
Highly distractible child
Juice consumption
Autonomy struggles
Inappropriate mealtime environment
Inappropriate diet

disease; and dysmorphic features that may suggest a genetic or teratogenic cause for growth failure. A complete neurological examination may reveal spasticity or hypotonia, which can have untoward effects on feeding and growth. Physical findings related to malnutrition include decreased subcutaneous fat, decreased muscle mass, dermatitis, hepatomegaly, cheilosis, or edema (see Chapter 30). Additionally, children with FTT have more otitis media, respiratory, and gastrointestinal infections than age-matched controls; severely malnourished children are at risk for a variety of serious infections. Observation during feeding and home visitation, if possible, is of great diagnostic value in assessing feeding problems, food preferences, mealtime distractions, unusual or disruptive parent-child interactions, and the home environment.

The history and physical examination findings should guide the laboratory evaluation. Routine extensive laboratory and radiology studies are not indicated, but rather tests should be ordered based on findings from the clinical evaluation. Simple screening tests could be used to identify common illnesses that cause growth failure and to search for medical problems resulting from malnutrition. Initial tests may include a complete blood count; screening for iron deficiency anemia and lead toxicity; urinalysis, urine culture, and serum electrolytes to assess renal infection or dysfunction. A review of the child's newborn screen may also be warranted. Additional testing can be ordered as needed, based on the child's signs and symptoms. For example, a stool sample for culture and ova and parasites may be indicated in children with diarrhea, abdominal pain, or malodorous stools.

TREATMENT

Identified biopsychosocial etiologies will inform the treatment plan. Most children with FTT can be treated in the outpatient setting. Children with severe malnutrition, underlying diagnoses that require hospitalization for evaluation or treatment, or whose safety is in jeopardy because of maltreatment require hospitalization. Admitting children to the hospital to induce and document weight gain is not recommended unless intensive outpatient evaluation and intervention has failed or the social circumstances are a contraindication for attempting outpatient management. Potential multidisciplinary treatment team members include pediatricians, nutritionists, developmental specialists, nurses, and social workers.

Nutritional management is the cornerstone of treatment. Children with FTT who are anorexic and picky eaters may have difficulty consuming the amount of calories and protein needed for catch-up growth, and require calorie dense foods. For formula-fed infants, the concentration of formula can be adjusted appropriately (Table 21.3). For toddlers, dietary changes should include increasing the caloric density of favorite foods. High-calorie oral supplements (30 cal/oz) are often well tolerated by toddlers. In some cases, specific carbohydrate, fat, or protein additives are used to boost calories by increasing calories without increasing volume requirements. Additionally, vitamin and mineral supplementation can be required, especially during catch-up growth. In general, the simplest and least costly approach to dietary change is warranted.

Treatment must also address the psychosocial needs of the family. Parents of malnourished children may feel personally responsible and threatened by the diagnosis of FTT. Parents may be so depressed or dysfunctional they cannot focus on their child's needs; they may not recognize the psychosocial and family contributors to malnutrition. These issues can have a profound effect on the success of treatment and need to be addressed.

TABLE 21.3 Infant Formula Preparation*

AMOUNT OF POWDER/ LIQUID	AMOUNT OF WATER (OZ)	FINAL CONCENTRATION (kcal/oz)
1 cup powdered formula	29	20
4 scoops powdered formula	8	20
13 oz liquid concentrate	13	20
1 cup powdered formula	24	24
5 scoops powdered formula	8	24
13 oz liquid concentrate	9	24
1 cup powdered formula	21	27
5.5 scoops powdered formula	8	27
13 oz liquid concentrate	6	27

*Final concentrations are reached by adding formula to water. One scoop of powdered formula = one measuring tablespoon. For healthy infants, formulas are prepared to provide 20 kcal/oz.

From Jew R, ed. Department of Pharmacy Services Pharmacy Handbook and Formulary, 2000–2001. Hudson: Department of Pharmacy Services; 2000:422.

COMPLICATIONS

Malnutrition causes defects in host defenses. Children with FTT may suffer from a **malnutrition-infection cycle**, in which recurrent infections exacerbate malnutrition, leading to greater susceptibility to infection. Children with FTT must be evaluated and treated promptly for infection and followed closely.

During starvation, the body slows metabolic processes and growth to minimize the need for nutrients and uses its stores of glycogen, fat, and protein to maintain normal metabolic requirements. The body also generally maintains homeostasis and normal serum concentrations of electrolytes. With the rapid reinstitution of feeding after starvation, fluid and electrolyte homeostasis may be lost. Changes in serum electrolyte concentrations and the associated complications are collectively termed the **re-feeding syndrome**. These changes typically affect phosphorus, potassium, calcium, and magnesium and can result in life-threatening cardiac, pulmonary, or neurological problems. Infants and children with marasmus, kwashiorkor, and anorexia nervosa and those who experience prolonged fasting are at risk for re-feeding syndrome. Re-feeding syndrome can be avoided by slow institution of nutrition, close monitoring of serum electrolytes during the initial days of feeding, and prompt replacement of depleted electrolytes.

There is concern that FTT could be associated with negative metabolic and neurodevelopmental outcomes in some cases; however, further research is needed to more fully understand long-term health outcomes.

PSYCHOSOCIAL SHORT STATURE

Occasionally, children who live in psychological deprivation develop short stature with or without concomitant FTT or delayed puberty, a syndrome called **psychosocial short stature**. The signs and symptoms include polyphagia, polydipsia, hoarding and stealing of food, gorging and vomiting, and other notable behaviors. Affected children are typically depressed and socially withdrawn. Endocrine dysfunction is often identified in affected children, who may have decreased growth hormone secretion and a muted response to exogenous growth hormone. Removal of the child from the adverse environment typically results in rapid improvement in endocrine function and subsequent rapid somatic and pubertal growth of the child. The prognosis for children with psychosocial short stature depends on the age at diagnosis and the degree of psychological trauma. Early identification and removal from the environment portends a healthy prognosis. Those diagnosed in later childhood or adolescence may not reach their genetic potential for growth and have a poorer psychosocial prognosis.

CHAPTER 22

Child Abuse and Neglect

Child maltreatment is a significant public health concern given its prevalence and potential impact on health not only during childhood but also later in life. Each year in the United States, approximately 3 million reports are made to child welfare agencies. These reports represent only a small proportion of the children who suffer from child maltreatment; surveys of adults about their childhood experiences indicate that many cases never come to the attention of authorities. Child maltreatment can cause short-term physical, mental, and developmental health problems, and in extreme cases can be fatal. Research, including the Adverse Childhood Experiences Study, has shown an association between childhood maltreatment and negative adult health outcomes, including physical health problems such as cardiovascular disease and obesity, as well as psychosocial health problems such as depression and substance abuse. A growing body of research demonstrates how toxic stressors in childhood can influence brain development and epigenetics.

Child maltreatment is an act or failure to act by a parent or caretaker that results in death, harm, sexual abuse, or imminent risk of harm. States define child abuse and neglect in civil and criminal statutes. In every state, physicians are mandated by law to report all cases of *suspected* child abuse and neglect. Child abuse and neglect result from a complex interaction of individual, family, and societal risk factors. Risk factors for maltreatment, such as parental substance abuse, parental depression, and domestic violence in the household, can alert physicians to potential risk and guide development of child maltreatment prevention strategies. However, risk factors should not be used to determine whether a specific patient is a victim of abuse. Child abuse and neglect are often considered in broad categories that include physical abuse, sexual abuse, emotional abuse, and neglect.

NEGLECT

Neglect is the most common form of child maltreatment and is broadly defined as omissions that prevent a child's basic needs from being met. Basic needs include adequate nutrition, shelter, education, emotional needs, adequate supervision, as well as medical and dental care. Neglect can impact child physical, mental, developmental, and behavioral health. Potential physical health consequences include abnormal growth, poor dentition, injuries, or ingestions resulting from lack of supervision or environmental hazards, as well as poorly controlled health problems. Child neglect can contribute to developmental delays, risk-taking behaviors or other behavioral problems, school difficulties, emotional problems, as well as attachment problems. Health care providers play an important role in the multidisciplinary response to neglect. Medical interventions could include treating physical health problems such as growth disturbance or injury, simplifying and clarifying treatment plans for chronic conditions, making referrals to community agencies that can assist with concrete needs such as food or transportation, providing developmental assessments and referrals, as well as referring patients to mental and behavioral health specialists. The approach to neglect involves identification of both factors contributing to the neglect, as well as strengths that can be protective factors. Health care providers can play a role in preventing neglect by screening for potential precipitating factors such as parental depression as well as by providing anticipatory guidance on topics such as supervision and injury prevention tailored to the child's developmental level.

PHYSICAL ABUSE

Decision-Making Algorithms
Available @ StudentConsult.com

Extremity pain
Altered mental status
Alopecia

Physical abuse is second to neglect as the reason for child protective services reports and child maltreatment related fatality. Physical abuse affects children of all ages. In some cases, the diagnosis of physical abuse can be made easily if the child has obvious external abusive injuries or is capable of providing a history of the abuse. In many cases, the diagnosis is not obvious. Abusive injuries are sometimes occult, and children can present with nonspecific symptoms. The history provided by the parent is often inaccurate because the parent is unwilling to provide the correct history or is a nonoffending parent who is unaware of the abuse. The child may be too young or ill to provide a history of the assault. An older child may be too scared to do so or may have a strong sense of loyalty to the perpetrator. History that seems incongruent with the clinical presentation of the child raises concern for physical abuse (Table 22.1).

Although injury to any organ system can occur from physical abuse, some injuries are more common. Bruises are universal findings in healthy ambulatory children but also are among the most common injury identified in abused children. Bruising location, pattern, and the child's age/developmental level are important considerations when evaluating bruising. Bruises suggestive of abuse include those that are patterned, such as a slap mark on the face or looped extension cord marks on

TABLE 22.1 Clues to the Diagnosis of Physical Abuse

A child presents for medical care with significant injuries and a history of trauma is denied, especially if the child is an infant or toddler.
The history provided by the caregiver does not explain the injuries identified.
The history of the injury changes significantly over time.
A history of self-inflicted trauma does not correlate with the child's developmental abilities.
There is an unexpected or unexplained delay in seeking medical care.
Multiple organ systems are injured, including injuries of various ages.
The injuries are pathognomonic for child abuse.

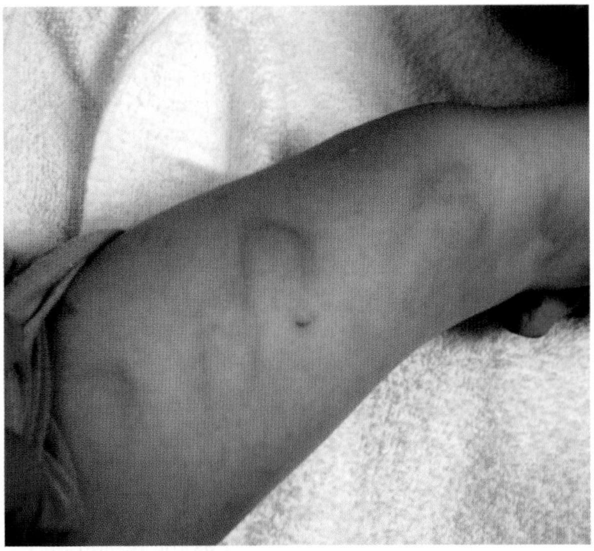

FIGURE 22.1 Multiple looped cord marks on a 2-year-old abused child who presented to the hospital with multiple untreated burns to the back, arms, and feet.

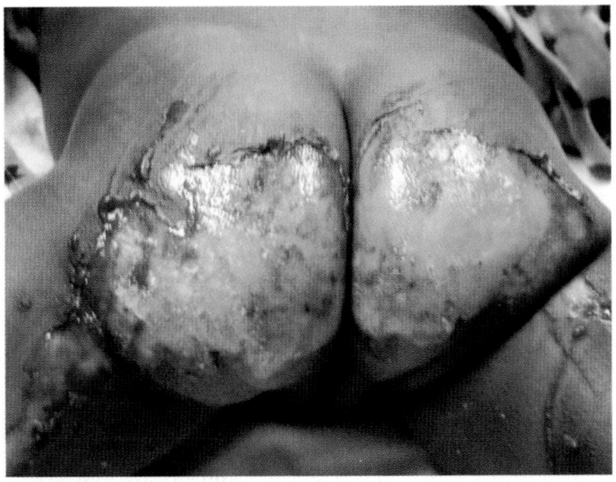

FIGURE 22.2 A 1-year-old child brought to the hospital with a history that she sat on a hot radiator. Suspicious injuries such as this require a full medical and social investigation, including a skeletal survey to look for occult skeletal injuries and a child welfare evaluation.

the body (Fig. 22.1). Bruises in healthy children generally are distributed over bony prominences; bruises that occur in an unusual distribution, such as isolated to the torso, ears, or neck, should raise concern. Bruises in nonambulatory infants are unusual, occurring in less than 2% of healthy infants seen for routine medical care. Occasionally, a subtle bruise may be the only external clue to abuse and can be associated with significant internal injury. Previous sentinel injuries, such as bruising, are common among infants presenting with severe physical abuse. Appropriate evaluation and intervention when non-mobile infants present with unexplained bruising could prevent escalating abuse.

Burns are common pediatric injuries and usually represent preventable unintentional trauma (see Chapter 44). Approximately 10% of children hospitalized with burns are victims of abuse. Thermal burns are the most common type of burn and can result from scalding injuries (Fig. 22.2) or contact with hot objects (irons, radiators, or cigarettes). Features of scald burns that are concerning for inflicted trauma include clear lines of demarcation, uniformity of burn depth and characteristic pattern. Abusive contact burns tend to have distinct margins (branding of the hot object), while accidental contact burns tend to have less distinctive edges.

Inflicted fractures occur more commonly in infants and young children. Although diaphyseal fractures are most common in abuse, they are nonspecific for inflicted injury. Fractures that should raise suspicion for abuse include fractures that are unexplained; occur in young, nonambulatory children; or involve multiple bones. Certain fractures have a high specificity for abuse, such as rib, metaphyseal, scapular, vertebral, or other unusual fractures (Fig. 22.3). Some metabolic diseases can be confused with abuse and should be considered in the differential diagnosis when appropriate.

While abdominal injury is not as common as other forms of child physical abuse such as bruising or fractures, it is associated with a high mortality rate. Abdominal trauma is, therefore, the second leading cause of death from child physical abuse after head injury. Blunt trauma to the abdomen is the primary mechanism of injury; infants and toddlers are the most common victims. Injuries to solid organs, such as the liver or pancreas, predominate and hollow viscus injury occurs more commonly with inflicted trauma than accidental. Even in severe cases of trauma, there may be no bruising to the abdominal wall. The lack of external trauma, along with an inaccurate history, can cause delay in diagnosis. The American Academy of Pediatrics policy statement on diagnostic imaging of child abuse discusses computed tomography (CT) scan as the imaging modality of choice in most settings when abusive abdominal trauma is suspected.

Abusive head trauma is the leading cause of mortality and morbidity from physical abuse. Most victims are young; infants predominate. Shaking and/or blunt impact trauma cause injuries. Caregiver intolerance of infant crying is a common precipitator, and many prevention programs provide education on developmentally normal crying as well as coping techniques. Symptoms at the time of presentation to medical care can range from occult head trauma with no neurological symptoms to irritability, lethargy, vomiting, seizures, apnea, and coma. Unsuspecting physicians misdiagnose approximately one third of infants initially; of these, more than 25% are reinjured before diagnosis. Subdural hemorrhage is a common intracranial injury in children with abusive head trauma (Fig. 22.4). Secondary brain injury can be due to factors such as cerebral edema, hypoxic-ischemic injury, and hypoperfusion. Retinal hemorrhages are seen in many but not all victims. Skeletal trauma, including rib and classic metaphyseal fractures, is sometimes present as well. Victims may present with bruising, but often times there are no external signs of injury. Survivors are at high risk for permanent neurological sequelae.

Work-up for physical abuse includes evaluation for occult injury as well as medical conditions that can mimic physical abuse. Children younger than 2 years with suspected physical abuse should undergo a skeletal survey looking for occult or healing fractures. Infants presenting with extra-cranial injuries may have occult head trauma, and therefore neuroimaging may be indicated for these infants. The extensive **differential diagnosis** of physical abuse depends on the type of injury

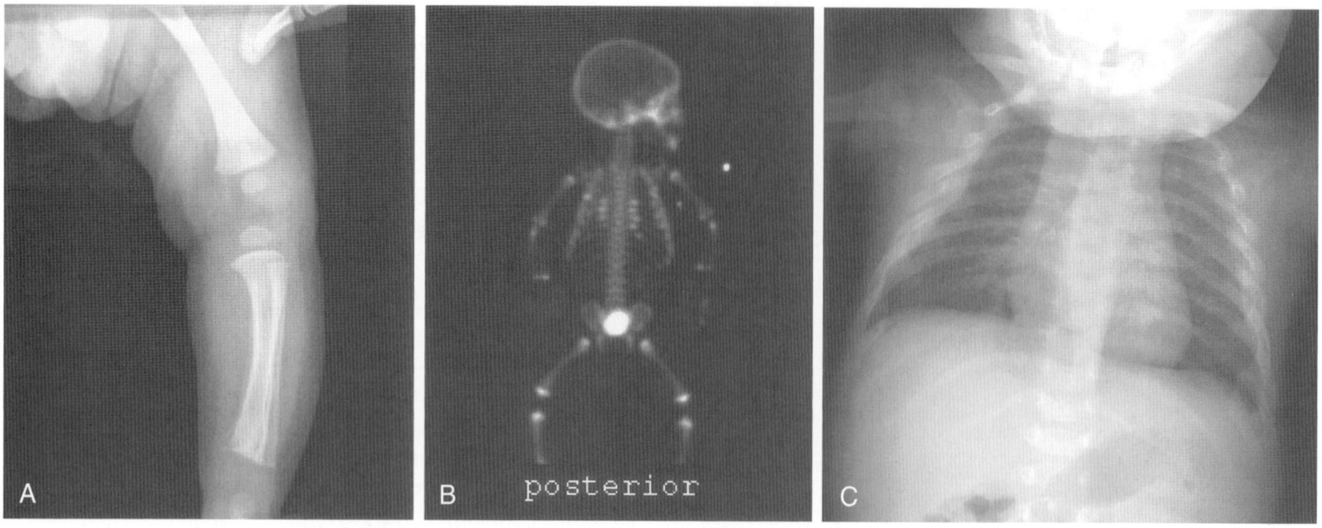

FIGURE 22.3 **A,** Metaphyseal fracture of the distal tibia in a 3-month-old infant admitted to the hospital with severe head injury. There also is periosteal new bone formation of that tibia, perhaps from a previous injury. **B,** Bone scan of the same infant. Initial chest x-ray showed a single fracture of the right posterior fourth rib. A radionuclide bone scan performed 2 days later revealed multiple previously unrecognized fractures of the posterior and lateral ribs. **C,** Follow-up radiographs 2 weeks later showed multiple healing rib fractures. This pattern of fracture is highly specific for child abuse. The mechanism of these injuries is usually violent squeezing of the chest.

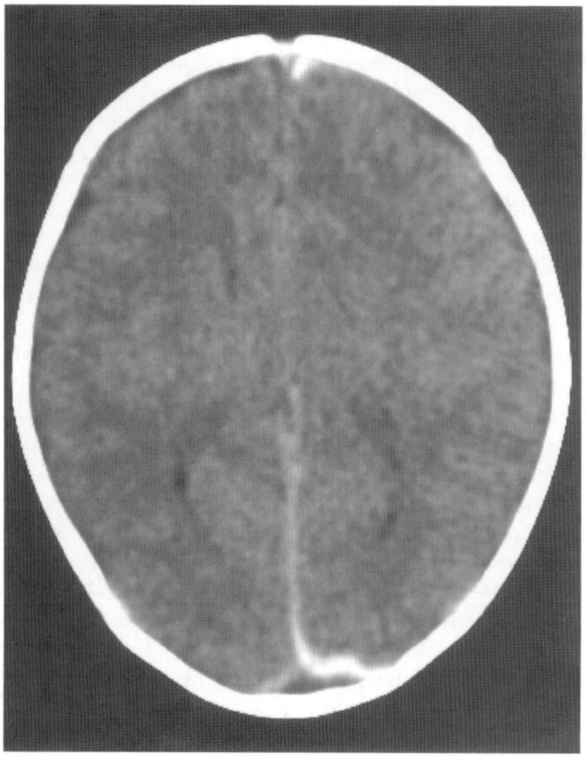

FIGURE 22.4 Acute subdural hemorrhage in the posterior interhemispheric fissure in an abused infant.

(Table 22.2). For children who present with different types of specific injuries to multiple organ systems, an exhaustive search for medical diagnoses is unwarranted. Some medical conditions can be mistaken for abuse, emphasizing the need for careful, objective evaluation of all children.

SEXUAL ABUSE

Child sexual abuse is the involvement of children in sexual activities that they cannot understand, for which they are developmentally unprepared and thus cannot give consent. Sexual abuse can, but does not always, involve physical contact. Examples of abuse not involving physical contact are indecent exposure and deliberately exposing a child to pornography. Sexual abuse can be a single event but is often chronic. Most perpetrators are not strangers but are known to the child through relationships such as family member, neighbor, or member of the community. Most sexual abuse involves manipulation and coercion. Sexual abuse is more common in girls than boys, although sexual abuse of boys is underrecognized and underreported.

Children generally come to attention after they have made a disclosure of their abuse. They may disclose to a nonoffending parent, sibling, relative, friend, teacher, counselor, or other professional. Children commonly delay disclosure for many weeks, months, or years after their abuse. Sexual abuse also should be considered in children who have behavioral problems, although no behavior is pathognomonic. Hypersexual behaviors should raise the possibility of sexual abuse, although alternative considerations include exposure to sexual content, as well as other forms of maltreatment such as neglect. Sexual abuse occasionally is recognized by the discovery of an unexplained vaginal, penile, or anal injury or by the discovery of a sexually transmitted infection. Medical providers may be asked to determine the urgency of medical evaluations. Factors that prompt emergent evaluation include child protection concerns such as ongoing contact with the alleged perpetrator as well as active physical or psychological symptoms such as bleeding or suicidal ideation. Timing of the last possible incident of abuse is also an important consideration, as there are time windows for collecting forensic evidence, administering sexually transmitted

TABLE 22.2 Differential Diagnosis of Physical Abuse*

BRUISES
Accidental injury (common)
Dermatologic disorders
Mongolian spots
Erythema multiforme
Phytophotodermatitis
Hematologic disorders
Idiopathic thrombocytopenic purpura
Leukemia
Hemophilia
Vitamin K deficiency
Disseminated intravascular coagulopathy
Cultural practices
Cao gio (coining)
Quat sha (spoon rubbing)
Infection
Sepsis
Purpura fulminans (meningococcemia)
Genetic diseases
Ehlers-Danlos syndrome
Familial dysautonomia (with congenital indifference to pain)
Vasculitis
Henoch-Schönlein purpura
BURNS
Accidental burns (common)
Infection
Staphylococcal scalded skin syndrome
Impetigo
Dermatologic
Phytophotodermatitis
Stevens-Johnson syndrome
Fixed drug eruption
Epidermolysis bullosa
Severe diaper dermatitis, including Ex-Lax ingestion
Cultural practices
Cupping
Moxibustion
FRACTURES
Accidental injury
Birth trauma
Metabolic bone disease
Osteogenesis imperfecta
Copper deficiency
Rickets
Infection
Congenital syphilis
Osteomyelitis

TABLE 22.2 Differential Diagnosis of Physical Abuse*—cont'd

HEAD TRAUMA
Accidental head injury
Hematologic disorders
Vitamin K deficiency (hemorrhagic disease of the newborn)
Hemophilia
Intracranial vascular abnormalities
Infection
Metabolic diseases
Glutaric aciduria type I, Menkes kinky hair syndrome

The differential diagnosis of physical abuse varies by the type of injury and organ system involved.
From Christian CW. Child abuse physical. In: Schwartz MW, ed. The 5-minute Pediatric Consult. *3rd ed. Philadelphia: Lippincott Williams & Wilkins; 2003.*

infection prophylaxis, HIV post-exposure prophylaxis, and emergency contraception.

In most cases, the diagnosis of sexual abuse is made by the history obtained from the child. In cases in which the sexual abuse has been reported to Child Protective Services (CPS) or the police (or both), and the child has been interviewed before the medical visit, a complete forensic interview at the physician's office is not needed. Many communities have systems in place including Children's Advocacy Centers to ensure quality investigative interviews of sexually abused children. However, children may make spontaneous disclosures to the physician, or physicians may evaluate patients prior to investigative interviews and require information for medical decision making. In these circumstances, open-ended and nonleading questions should be used and carefully documented in the medical record. Information about the medical review of systems, including physical symptoms (examples: genital discharge, pain) and behavioral/emotional health (e.g., suicidal ideation, depression, sleep problems), should also be obtained from the patient and/or the caregiver, as appropriate for the child's developmental level.

The **physical examination** should be complete, with careful external inspection of the genitals and anus. Most sexually abused children have a normal genital examination at the time of the medical evaluation; injuries are diagnosed in only approximately 5% of sexually abused children. Many types of sexual abuse (fondling, vulvar coitus, oral genital contact, exhibitionism) do not injure genital tissue or do not even involve contact with the genital tissue. Genital mucosa heals so rapidly and completely that injuries often heal by the time of the medical examination. For children who present within 72 hours of the most recent assault, special attention should be given to identifying acute injury. Guidelines based on research and expert consensus can assist clinicians in differentiating normal variants or nonspecific findings from findings caused by trauma. Examples of the latter include acute, unexplained lacerations or ecchymosis of the hymen, and complete transection of the hymen. Injuries to other parts of the body such as the oral mucosa, breasts, or thighs should not be overlooked. Forensic evidence collection is also a consideration when children present acutely. Policies vary by jurisdiction. Forensic evidence collection within 72 hours of an assault that could involve transfer of forensic evidence is recommended in many states, although the time frame is longer in some states. Research showing that forensic evidence is rarely recovered from swabs collected from the bodies of prepubertal children 24 hours after assault may also influence local practice.

The **laboratory evaluation** of a sexually abused child is dictated by the child's age, history, and symptoms. Universal screening for sexually transmitted infections for prepubertal children is unnecessary because the risk of infection is low in asymptomatic young children. The type of assault, identity and known medical history of the perpetrator, and the epidemiology of sexually transmitted infections in the community also are considered. Testing methods for *C. trachomatis* and *N. gonorrhea* have evolved with the advent of nucleic acid amplification tests (NAAT) and the declining use of culture, with many labs no longer offering testing by culture. Local experts, such as specialists in infectious diseases and laboratory medicine, can inform protocols for confirmation of positive NAATs. The diagnosis of most sexually transmitted infections in young children requires an investigation for sexual abuse (see Chapter 116).

Pediatric health care providers should also be cognizant of child sex trafficking and commercial sexual exploitation. It can be difficult to identify potential victims, but possible potential indicators include changing demographic information, a child not allowed to speak for himself/herself, a child accompanied by an unrelated adult, history of multiple sexually transmitted infections, tattoos concerning for branding, and signs of inflicted injury. In addition to local resources, there is a National Human Trafficking Resource Center.

MANAGEMENT

The management of child abuse includes medical treatment for injuries and infections, and careful medical documentation of verbal statements and findings. Photographic documentation of physical examination findings can be helpful when possible. Physicians are mandated to report *suspected* child maltreatment to the appropriate authorities (Fig. 22.5). Parents should be informed of the concerns and the need to report to CPS, focusing on the need to ensure the safety and well-being of the child. Crimes that are committed against children also are investigated by law enforcement, so the police become involved in some, but not all, cases of suspected abuse. Physicians should be aware of the potential long-term impacts of maltreatment on child health. Trauma-focused cognitive-behavioral therapy has been shown to improve mental health and behavioral difficulties among children who have experienced trauma. Physicians occasionally are called to testify in court hearings regarding civil issues, such as dependency and custody, or criminal issues. Careful review of the medical records and preparation for court are needed to provide an educated, unbiased account of the child's medical condition and diagnoses.

The prevention of child maltreatment is a great challenge. There are a few partially successful primary prevention programs. Visiting home nursing programs that begin during pregnancy and continue through early childhood may reduce the risk of abuse and neglect. Physician training in screening for risk factors in parents has shown to be supportive of families and reduce child maltreatment in some populations. Ultimately, physicians need to remain cognizant of the diagnosis, aware of their professional mandates, and willing to advocate on behalf of these vulnerable patients.

CHAPTER 23

Homosexuality and Gender Identity

The development of sexuality occurs throughout a child's life. Sexuality includes the interplay of gender roles, gender identity, sexual orientation, and sexual behaviors, and it is influenced by biological and social factors, as well as individual experience. Pediatricians are likely to be consulted if parents have a concern about their child's sexual development or behavior. A pediatrician who provides an open and nonjudgmental environment will also be a valuable resource for an adolescent with questions about sexual behaviors, homosexuality, and/or gender identity (Table 23.1).

DEVELOPMENT OF SEXUALITY

Sexual development begins early on in childhood. Often, parents express concern when their male infant has an erection, or when their child touches his/her genitals during diaper changes or bathing. During the preschool period, masturbation occurs in both sexes. Reassurance from the pediatrician is critical as these behaviors are part of typical child development, represent normal exploration of the body, and should not be treated punitively. However, it is important for children by age 3 years to learn the proper anatomical names for their body parts and that genitals and sexual behaviors are private. It is common for pre-elementary age children to touch their genitals in public. However, showing their genitals to others, "playing doctor," or imitating intercourse or other adult sexual behaviors is unusual at this age. If this behavior is occurring, the child should be evaluated for exposure to inappropriate sexual material and possible sexual abuse (see Chapter 22).

Children in elementary school are typically intrigued by the topics of pregnancy, birth, and gender roles. They often will begin to preferentially play with children of the same gender. Their

TABLE 23.1 Terminology

Term	Definition
Gender identity	Internal sense of one's self as male, female, or other
Cisgender	An individual whose gender identity aligns with physical sex characteristics
Transgender	An individual whose gender identity and expression is not consistent with the sex assigned at birth
Gender role	Culturally derived associations for behaviors and appearance that signal being male or female
Gender expression	Behaviors and appearance used to communicate one's gender identity

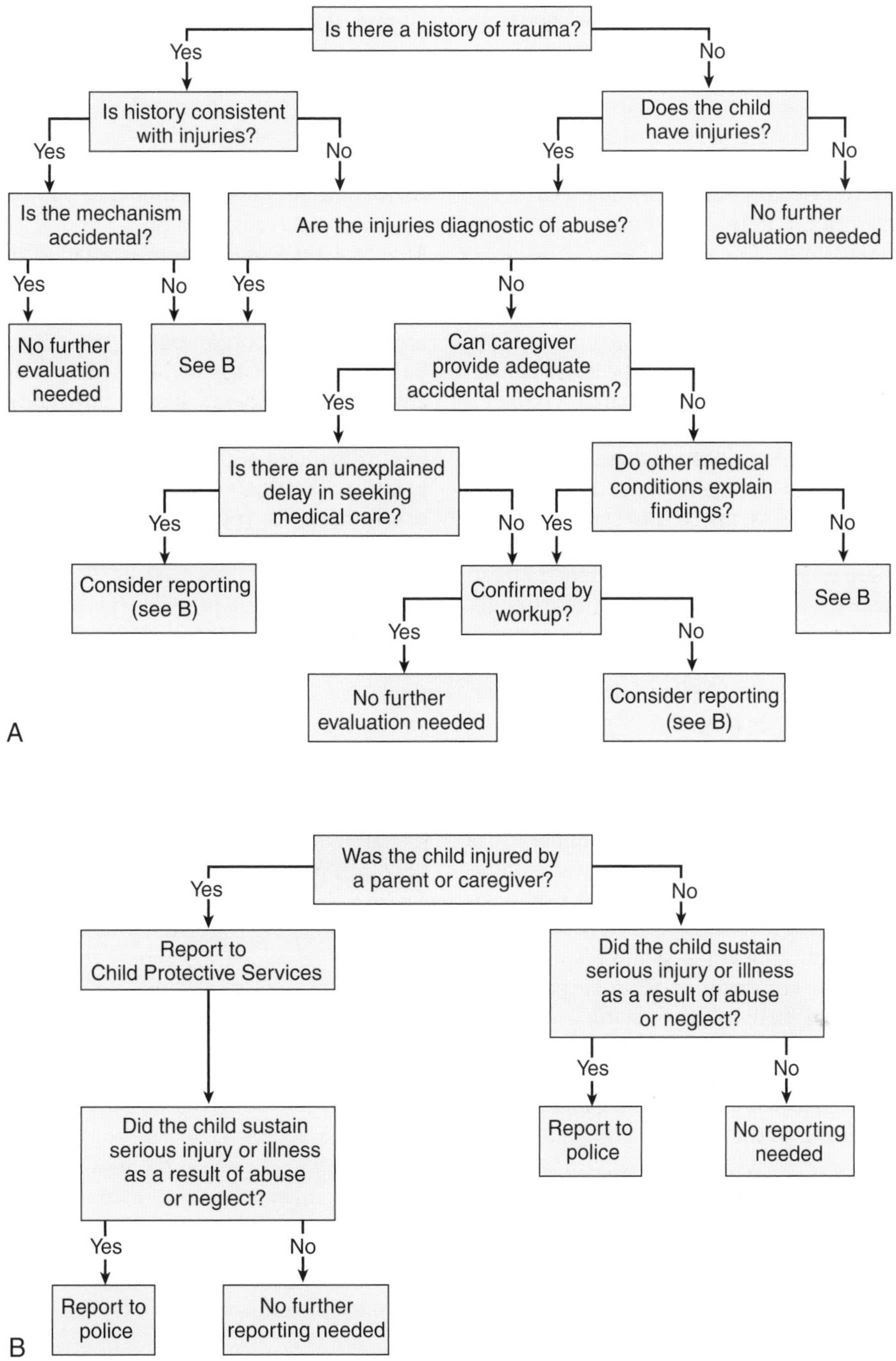

FIGURE 22.5 A, Approach to initiating the civil and criminal investigation of suspected abuse. **B,** Reporting to Child Protective Services (CPS), law enforcement, or both in child abuse cases. CPS reports are required when a child is injured by a parent, by an adult acting as a parent, or by a caregiver of the child. The police investigate crimes against children committed by any person, including parents or other caregivers. (From Christian CW. Child abuse. In: Schwartz MW, ed. *Clinical Handbook of Pediatrics*. 3rd ed. Baltimore: Lippincott Williams & Wilkins; 2003:192–193.)

curiosity and inquiries should be met with accurate information and limited judgment so that future questions will be directed to reliable resources and not answered by peers and the media.

The biological, social, and cognitive changes that occur during adolescence place a focus on sexuality. Puberty can be both scary and exciting. One of the principal developmental tasks of this period is to become comfortable with one's own sexuality. This is often achieved through questioning and experimentation. Some teenagers may try out different sexual practices, including those with members of the same sex, as they explore their own emerging sexuality. Almost half of high school students report ever having had sexual intercourse. The nature of these experiences does not necessarily predict sexual orientation, and similarly, stereotypical masculine and feminine traits do not predict sexual orientation either.

Sexual orientation, the pattern of physical and emotional arousal toward another person, is not always the same as sexual behavior. Typically, an individual's sexual orientation emerges before or early in adolescence. Although many adolescents have sexual experiences with a same-sex partner (10-25%, and more often reported by males than females), fewer will affirm homosexual sexual orientation by late adolescence. By 18 years of age, the majority of individuals endorse certainty around their sexual orientation.

HOMOSEXUALITY

There is no reliable way to predict an individual's sexual orientation. Identical twins (even twins raised in separate families) show a higher concordance rate for sexual orientation than would be expected by chance alone, but nowhere near 100%, as would be expected if genetics were the sole determinant. Attempts to correlate brain imaging or levels of androgens and estrogens with sexual orientation have thus far been inconsistent at best. Although it is well established that parents tend to treat boys and girls differently, there is no evidence that parental behavior alters the developmental trajectory towards a particular sexual orientation.

It is currently estimated that about 10% of adults self-identify as homosexual, meaning they are attracted to people of the same gender. Homosexual children and adolescents face stigmatization derived from homophobia and heterosexism, ostracism, and family rejection. A persistent negative societal attitude toward homosexuality is reflected in the higher rates of social isolation, verbal harassment, and physical assault experienced by sexual minority youth. Additionally, educational and unbiased information about homosexuality is often not available in school and community settings, and homophobic jokes, teasing, and violence are common. Not surprisingly, sexual minority youth are at high risk for having a negative self-esteem, mental health issues, substance abuse, and sexual risk-taking behaviors. Sexual minority youth are more than twice as likely to report considering suicide than their heterosexual peers; rates of legal and illegal substance abuse are significantly higher.

There are also significant health disparities for sexual minority youth related to sexual health outcomes. Although sexual behaviors, not sexual orientation, determine risk of sexually transmitted infections (STI), sexual minority youth are more likely to have had intercourse at a younger age, less likely to use contraception, and report a greater number of sexual partners as compared to heterosexual peers. Rates of STI in the minority group of men who have sex with men (MSM) have not declined along with the downward trend of STI in adolescents overall, including rates of human immunodeficiency virus (HIV). Although education about safe sexual practices should be part of all adolescent well-child visits, Centers for Disease Control and Prevention (CDC) guidelines recommend asking about the gender of all sex partners as part of STI risk assessment. Health care providers should be aware of specific STI screening recommendations for MSM related to anal intercourse (see Chapter 116). Many adolescents who identify as women who have sex with women (WSW) have also had sex with men and will require cervical cancer screening per guidelines. Immunization for human papillomavirus per CDC guidelines is recommended for adolescents regardless of gender or sexual behavior. Additionally, discussions around highly effective birth control methods are prudent with both heterosexual and sexual minority youth.

Acknowledging that one is homosexual and disclosing it to one's parents is often extremely stressful. Although many parents are supportive of their child's sexual orientation, some parents, particularly those who view this behavior as immoral, may reject their child. Adolescents should be counseled that even parents whose initial reaction is one of shock, fear, or grief can come to accept their child's homosexuality. Homosexual youth are at a high risk for homelessness as a consequence of parental rejection. Interventions designed to change sexual orientation are strongly opposed and are not only unsuccessful, but can be detrimental to the mental health of the child or adolescent. Health care providers should provide reassurance to parents feeling guilt or shame by affirming that sexual minority youth are normal and sexual orientation is not related to parenting practices. Evidence supports improved health outcomes for sexual minority youth who experience family connectedness and receive encouragement and positive support for their sexual orientation from their parents. For medical and psychosocial reasons, health care providers need to provide an environment in which adolescents feel comfortable discussing their sexual orientation and families can find the support and resources they need (Table 23.2).

TABLE 23.2 Providing Supportive Health Care Environments for Sexual Minority Youth
Offices should be welcoming to all, regardless of sexual orientation and behavior.
Ensure that office staff and information-gathering forms do not presume heterosexuality of patients or parents (i.e., use gender-neutral language).
All adolescents should have a confidential adolescent psychosocial history including screening and referral for depression, suicidality, other mood disorders, substance abuse, and eating disorders.
Adolescents should have sexual behaviors and risks assessed, with particular attention to sexually transmitted infections testing guidelines affecting sexual minority youths. This should include contraceptive counseling.
Target behavioral interventions to maximize the individual's strengths and resources and minimize risk-taking behaviors.
Be available to answer questions, correct misinformation, and reinforce that minority sexual orientations are normal.
Support and affirm transgender youth and refer as appropriate.
Support parents in working through adjustment issues related to having a child with a minority sexual orientation and encouraging the commitment to a loving and supportive family environment.
Support gay–straight alliances at schools and zero-tolerance policies for bullying and violence.
Provide information about support groups and resources for sexual minority youth and their families.
If a health care provider does not feel competent to provide appropriate care for sexual minority youth, he/she has the responsibility to evaluate and refer families for medically appropriate care.

Data from Levine DA. Committee on adolescence. Office-based care for lesbian, gay, bisexual, transgender, and questioning youth. Pediatrics. *2013;132(1): 198–203.*

DEVELOPMENT OF GENDER IDENTITY

Developing an awareness and appreciation for one's gender identity is an important milestone in psychosocial development. Typically, a child self-identifies as a boy or a girl by age 2 years and begins to demonstrate initial expressions of gender identity. Cross-gendered behaviors, such as stating that one wants to be a member of the opposite sex and/or pretending to be so, are common in preschool years. However, gender constancy, the understanding that one is always a male or always a female, is typically achieved by age 6 years.

Most elementary school–age children show a strong and consistent **gender identity**, and their behaviors **(gender roles)** reflect this. If a child this age is engaging in cross sex gender role behaviors, or playing with toys that are stereotypically associated with the opposite gender, parents may be concerned about teasing/bullying or about the child's eventual sexual orientation. In assessing parental concerns about atypical gender role behaviors, the type of behavior exhibited and its consistency and persistence over time should be considered. Reassurance is appropriate when these behaviors are part of a flexible repertoire of male and female gender roles or in response to a stressor, such as the birth of an infant of the opposite sex or divorce of the parents. In contrast, stating the desire to be, or asserting that one is, of the opposite gender, and demanding clothing, hairstyles, privileges, and/or to be called a name classically used for the opposite gender, is uncommon. A referral for evaluation for **gender dysphoria (GD)** is appropriate when there is a nearly exclusive preference in cross-gender roles in play, playmates, and games/activities stereotypically associated with the opposite gender combined with a dislike of one's sexual anatomy and a desire to be of the other gender persists beyond a period of 6 months and is distressing as it impairs the child's functioning.

GENDER DYSPHORIA

GD is defined as marked distress related to the inconsistency between the way an individual may feel and think of themselves (experienced/expressed gender) and the individual's physical or assigned gender. GD represents a revision of the *Diagnostic and Statistical Manual of Mental Disorders,* fourth edition (DSM-IV), diagnosis of gender identity disorder and embodies an effort to remove the stigmatizing impact of the term "disorder" while maintaining a diagnosis in DSM-V to ensure insurance coverage for medical interventions. According to DSM-V, in children, GD is 2–4.5 times more common among natal boys than among natal girls. By adolescence, the male-to-female ratio is closer to even. There are some associations between gender atypical behavior in young children and the ultimate development of same-sex attraction; many children with GD grow up to be adults who identify as bisexual or homosexual.

In contrast, the term transgender refers to an individual that does not conform to the culturally-derived gender role for the sex they were assigned at birth. A person can have GD, a medical diagnosis, without being considered transgender. The majority of children with GD will not identify as transgender during adolescence and adulthood. There are data to support that children with GD who demonstrate more insistence in affirming their gender identity, use more declarative language, and are more significantly distressed by their body may be more likely to identify as transgender in adolescence or adulthood.

Transgender youth are often faced with rejection from their community and family, leading to rates of depression, anxiety, and suicidality that greatly exceed those in the general population. Evidence is mounting that allowing social transitions for prepubescent transgender children may be linked to improved mental health outcomes. This involves family acceptance and allows the child to present in all aspects as the gender role that aligns with his/her gender identity, and not the gender assigned at birth. In 2009, the Endocrine Society published guidelines that recommend considering reversible suppression of puberty using gonadotropin-releasing hormone analogs. Specialty centers with multidisciplinary teams now exist across the country to address the many needs of transgender children and their families.

CHAPTER 24

Family Structure and Function

A family is a dynamic system of interactions among biologically, socially, or legally related individuals. As such, families have a unique power to influence a child's social, emotional, and physical health, shape their brain development, and impact his/her overall developmental trajectory. When a family functions well, interactions support the physical and emotional needs of all members and the family can serve as a valuable resource for any individual member in need. Alternatively, the problems of an individual member or the negative interactions between members may interfere with the ability of the family system to satisfy the physical and emotional needs of members, and ultimately lead to physical and/or emotional harm. The consequence of a social practice or behavior pattern that undermines the stability of a family unit is referred to as **family dysfunction**.

FAMILY FUNCTIONS

The functions that families carry out in support of their children can be considered within the broad categories of physical needs, emotional support, and education and socialization (Table 24.1). Within these groupings, all families have strengths and weaknesses. The amount of support that an individual child needs in each domain varies with the child's developmental level, personality, temperament, health status, personal experiences, and stressors. In a healthy family, parents can be counted on to provide consistent and appropriate support for their children. Either too much or too little support can interfere with optimal child health and development. In the case of child neglect the family underfunctions, providing inappropriate or inadequate support for the child's basic needs. Further, the violation of basic boundaries of appropriate behavior and infringement on safety is considered child abuse. In contrast, a family that overfunctions may limit a child's opportunity for growth and development of independence skills, creating feelings of helplessness and inadequacy. Parental anxiety and perfectionism creates intense pressure on children around achievement and sets them up to become anxious and fearful themselves.

Toxic stress can accumulate when the child experiences intense, frequent, and prolonged adversity whether it be from

TABLE 24.1	Important Roles Families Play in Supporting Children
PHYSICAL NEEDS	
Safety	
Food	
Shelter	
Health and health care	
EMOTIONAL SUPPORT	
Affection	
Stimulation	
Communication	
Guidance/discipline	
EDUCATION AND SOCIALIZATION	
Values	
Relationships	
Community	
Formal schooling	

physical/emotional abuse, caregiver substance abuse or untreated mental illness, exposure to violence, or the secondary effects of economic hardship. Regardless of the type of family dysfunction, prolonged activation of stress response systems can disrupt the development of vital brain architecture and increase the risk for stress-related disease and cognitive impairment into adulthood.

FAMILY STRUCTURE

The traditional family consists of a married mother and father and their biological children. The diversity in the structure of the family in the United States has increased dramatically; in 2010 only 65% of children were being raised by married parents. Today, children may live with unmarried parents, single parents of either gender, a parent and a stepparent, grandparents, parents living as a same-sex couple, or foster care families. There is little evidence that family structure alone is a significant predictor of child health or development. Regardless of family structure, the best predictor of secure child health and development is the presence of a loving adult or adults serving in a parental role committed to fulfilling a child's basic needs. Stressful life experiences can test a family's ability to promote optimal developmental outcomes, and different family structures face different challenges.

Single-Parent Families

At any one point in time, approximately 30% of children are living in single-parent families, and more than 40% of children are born to unmarried mothers. In some instances, a child is born to a single mother by choice, but oftentimes the child is the result of an unplanned pregnancy. Children may also live in single-parent families as the result of divorce or the death of a parent (see Chapter 26). Although most children in single-parent families are raised by mothers, single-father families are increasing; in 2009 nearly 5% of children lived in single-father families.

Single parents may have limited financial resources and social supports. For single-mother households, the median income is only 40% of the income in two-parent families, and for single-father households, it is only 60% of the income of two parent families. Thus the frequency of children living in poverty is three to five times higher in single-parent families. These parents must also rely to a greater extent on other adults for child care. Although these adults may be sources of support for the single parent, they also may criticize the parent, decreasing confidence in parenting skills. Fatigue associated with working and raising a child independently contributes to parenting difficulties. Single parents are likely to have less time for a social life or other activities, intensifying feelings of isolation and negatively impacting mental health. When the increased burdens of single parenting are associated with exhaustion, isolation, and depression, the evolution of developmental and behavioral problems in the child is more likely.

In the case of a teenage mother in the role of single parent, challenges associated with parenting may be even more impactful (see Section 12). Being a teenage parent is associated with lower educational attainment, lower paying jobs without much opportunity for autonomy or advancement, and lower self-esteem. Teenage mothers are even less likely than adult single mothers to receive any support from the child's father. Children of adolescent mothers are at high risk for cognitive delays, behavioral problems, and difficulties in school. Referral to early intervention services or Head Start programs is imperative in these situations.

However, when a single parent has adequate social supports, is able to collaborate well with other care providers, and has sufficient financial resources, he or she is likely to be successful in raising a child. Pediatricians can improve parental self-esteem through education about child development and behavior, validation of good parenting strategies, positive feedback for compliance, and demonstrating confidence in them as parents. Demonstrating empathy and acknowledging the difficulties faced by single parents can have a healing effect or help a parent feel comfortable to share concerns suggesting the need for a referral to other professionals.

Children Living With Sexual Minority Parents

An estimated 23% of all lesbian/gay/bisexual (LGB)-identified adults (regardless of relationship status) were raising children under age 18 based on the 2013 National Health Interview Survey. Sexual minority adults can build families in a variety of ways. Many children with an LGB parent were conceived in the context of a heterosexual relationship. Alternatively, single LGB parents, as well as same-gender couples, enter into parenthood through adoption, donor insemination, or surrogacy. It is estimated that there are almost 200,000 children being raised by same-sex couples in the United States. Combined with those children being raised by single sexual minority parents, an estimated 2 million children in the United States have LGB parents.

LGB parents and children born from a heterosexual relationship experience unique challenges. Navigating the complex network of past and present, opposite- and same-gender relationships can be stressful for the child who may already have difficulty accepting the change in family structure, living environment, and disclosure of sexual orientation. In general, earlier disclosure of a parent's homosexuality to children, especially before adolescence, is associated with better acceptance. Parents may have concerns that the child will encounter teasing by peers, disapproval from adults, and stress or isolation related to a social stigma associated with having an LGB parent. Although there is some evidence that children of sexual minority parents may have an increased likelihood of being teased at certain stages of development, strong parent-child relationships and a school curriculum addressing acceptance can offer some protection to overall child well-being.

Evidence suggests that there is no causal relationship between having a sexual minority parent and a child's emotional, psychosocial, and behavioral development. Growing up in a same-gender parent family is not associated with academic achievement. Additionally, having an LGB parent does not influence gender role and psychosexual development; the majority of children with an LGB parent identify as heterosexual. Importantly, extensive research has demonstrated that the psychological adjustment of children and adolescents is impacted by the quality of the parent-child relationship, the quality of the relationship between adult caregivers, and the availability of social and economic resources.

Adoption

Adoption is a legal and social process that provides full family membership to a child who is not the adult parent's biological offspring. Most adoptions in the United States involve U.S. parents adopting U.S. children, but shifting cultural trends have increased the diversity in the ways in which adoptions occur; the process can involve biologically related and unrelated children, stepchildren, adoption through private and public agencies, domestic and international adoptions, and independent and informal adoptions. Based on data from the U.S. Department of Health and Human Services, the number of adoptions that are finalized each year has remained relatively stable (between 50,000 and 53,500) over the last decade. Approximately 2% of children in the United States are adopted. In 2009–2011, 13% of adopted children under 18 were internationally adopted. Over that same period, there were 438,000 transracially adopted children under the age of 18 (over a third of whom were foreign born), or 28% of all adopted children under 18. Increasing numbers of same-gender couples or single-LGB adults are raising children via adoption. Each type of adoption raises unique issues for families and health care providers. Data suggests that adopted children live in households that have higher incomes, a lower percentage in poverty, and a higher percentage with a parent with at least a bachelor's degree than stepchildren or biological children. *Open adoptions* in which the biological parents and birth parents agree to interact are occurring with increased frequency and create new issues for the adoption triad (biological parent, adoptive parent, and child).

Pediatricians are in an ideal position to help adoptive parents obtain and evaluate medical information, consider the unique medical needs of the adopted child, and provide a source of advice and counseling from the preadoption period through adolescence. A *preadoption visit* may allow discussion of medical information that the prospective parents have received about the child and identify important missing information such as the medical history of the biological family and the educational and social history of the biological parents. The preadoption period is the time that families are most likely to be able to obtain this information. Depending on the preadoption history, there may be risks of infections, in utero substance exposure, poor nutrition, or inadequate infant care that should be discussed with adoptive parents.

When the adopted child is first seen, screening for medical disorders beyond the typical age-appropriate screening tests should be considered. If the child has not had the standard newborn screening tests, the pediatrician may need to obtain these tests. Documented immunizations should be reviewed and, if needed, a plan developed to complete the needed immunizations (see Chapter 94). Children may be at high risk for infection based on the biological mother's social history or the country from which the child was adopted, including infection with human immunodeficiency virus, hepatitis B, cytomegalovirus, tuberculosis, syphilis, and parasites. A complete blood count may be needed to screen for iron deficiency.

A knowledgeable pediatrician also can be a valuable source of support and advice about psychosocial issues. The pediatrician should help the adoptive parents think about how they will raise the child while helping the child to understand the fact that he or she is adopted. Neither denial of nor intense focus on the adoption is healthy. Parents should use the term *adoption* around their children during the toddler years and explain the simplest facts first. Children's questions should be answered honestly. Parents should expect the same or similar questions repeatedly and that during the preschool period the child's cognitive limitations make it likely the child will not fully understand the meaning of adoption. As children get older, they may have fantasies of being reunited with their biological parents and there may be new challenges as the child begins to interact more with individuals outside of the family. Families may want advice about difficulties created by school assignments such as creating a genealogic chart or teasing by peers. During the teenage years, the child may have questions about his or her identity and a desire to find his or her biological parents. Adoptive parents may need reassurance that these desires do not represent rejection of the adoptive family but the child's desire to understand more about his or her life. Feelings of loss and grief, as well as anger, anxiety, or fear, may occur more often during certain milestones, such as birthdays, graduation, or the death of a parent. In general adopted adolescents should be supported in efforts to learn about their past, but most experts recommend encouraging children to wait until late adolescence before deciding to search actively for the biological parents.

In general, adopted children are within range of nonadopted peers academically and emotionally; however, the likelihood of emotional and academic problems is higher for children adopted after 9 months of age or for children who experienced multiple placements before being adopted. Difficulties in school, learning, and behavioral problems are thought to be more often secondary to biological and social influences that preceded the adoption. The pediatrician can play an important role in helping families distinguish developmental and behavioral variations from problems that may require recommendations for early intervention, counseling, or other services.

Foster Care

The foster care system in the United States is a means of providing care and protection for children who require out-of-home placement due to reasons of abuse and/or neglect. A foster or kinship setting is beholden with the responsibility to promote child well-being by assuring access to health, safety, and stability.

Ultimately, the goal of foster care is to achieve permanency through reunification or an alternative permanent arrangement (adoption, guardianship, or placement with relatives).

From the late 1990s through 2005, over half a million children were in foster care, but between 2005 and 2010, the number of children living in foster care decreased by about 20% as a result of changes in federal and state policies; in 2013, approximately 641,000 children spent some time in foster care placement. The Adoption and Safe Families Act passed by congress in 1997 mandated timely permanency leading to a significant reduction in the length of stay in foster care. In 2008, the enactment of the Fostering Connections to Success and Increasing Adoptions Act increased subsidies and supports to incentivize kinship care, guardianship, and adoption out of foster care. Additional reforms have prioritized the improvement of outcomes for children and youth in foster care by emphasizing monitoring of child development and the availability of mental health supports to ensure emotional well-being.

Children and adolescents in foster care are at extremely high risk for medical, nutritional, developmental, behavioral, and mental health problems. At the time of placement in foster care, most of these children have received incomplete medical care and have had multiple detrimental life experiences. Comprehensive assessments at the time of placement reveal many untreated acute medical problems. Nearly half of foster children have a chronic illness. Developmental delays and serious behavioral or emotional disorders are common.

Ideally foster care provides a healing service for these children and families, leading to reunification or adoption. Too often, children experience multiple changes in placement within the foster care system, further exacerbating challenges in forming a connection between the child and adult caregivers and culminating in child resistance to foster parents' attempts to develop a secure relationship. This detachment from the foster parent may be emotionally difficult for the foster parent to bear, further perpetuating a cycle of placement failures. The history of trauma or neglect that originally led to the need for foster care, in combination with instability of placements, predisposes the foster child to enduring problems. Foster care alumni report rates of anxiety disorders, depression, substance abuse, and post-traumatic stress disorder that are two to six times higher than the general population. Furthermore, although the *protections* of the foster care system often end at 18 years of age, these adolescents rarely have the skills and maturity needed to allow them to be successful living independently. Thus the Fostering Connections to Success and Increasing Adoptions Act of 2008 mandates that effective transition to adulthood planning be done with youth in foster care including the provision of targeted resources for emancipated youths as they enter adulthood.

The challenges for the foster care system are great. However, when children are placed with competent and nurturing foster parents and provided with coordinated care from skilled professionals, significant improvements in child health status, development, and academic achievement typically ensue.

FAMILY DYSFUNCTION: PHYSICAL NEEDS

Failure to meet a child's physical needs for protection or nutrition results in some of the most severe forms of family dysfunction (see Chapters 21 and 22). There are many other ways in which parental behaviors can interfere with a child's access to a healthy and safe environment, such as prenatal and postnatal substance abuse. Prenatal use of alcohol can damage the fetus resulting in a range of adverse effects known as **fetal alcohol spectrum disorders (FASD)**. At the most severe end of the spectrum, this teratogen causes **fetal alcohol syndrome (FAS)**, characterized by in utero and postnatal growth retardation, microcephaly, intellectual disability, and a characteristic dysmorphic facial appearance. Other manifestations of FASD include birth defects and problems with coordination, attention, hyperactivity, impulsivity, learning, or behavior. Children with these difficulties may be diagnosed with *FAS, partial FAS, alcohol-related birth defects (ARBD), alcohol-related neurodevelopmental disorder (ARND),* and *neurobehavioral disorder associated with prenatal alcohol exposure (ND-PAE).* Despite continued efforts to correlate the amount or pattern of alcohol use in pregnancy with the manifestations or likelihood of development of FASD, the only consensus is that the potential for fetal harm increases as maternal alcohol consumption intensifies. Importantly, ARBD and developmental disabilities are entirely preventable with abstinence from alcohol in pregnancy, and the neurocognitive and behavioral problems that can result from prenatal alcohol exposure are enduring.

Other substances may also impact the fetus. Studies of these effects are complicated by the fact that substance use in pregnancy often involves multiple psychoactive substances as well as suboptimal nutrition and prenatal care in women who use these substances. Cigarette smoking during pregnancy is associated with lower birthweight and increased child behavioral problems. Use of cocaine in the perinatal period has been associated with prematurity, impaired fetal growth, intracranial hemorrhages, and placental abruption. Exposure to opiates in utero can result in prematurity and neonatal abstinence syndrome characterized by symptoms of withdrawal (irritability, poor and irregular feeding, tachycardia and tachypnea, vomiting, and hypertonia). Investigations of the effects of cocaine and opiates on cognitive development have produced mixed results. Children with prenatal drug exposure are at increased risk for the development of neurobehavioral disorders, impaired intellectual function and academic achievement, developmental language delays, and executive function deficits, as well as the later development of a substance use disorder themselves.

Parental substance abuse is associated with increased family conflict, decreased organization, increased isolation, and increased family stress related to marital and work problems. Children and adolescents of parents with substance use disorders are also at increased risk for serious medical conditions and injuries. A 2011 study found that 23% of children whose mothers were substance users failed to receive routine child health services during the first 2 years of life. Family discord and violence may be more frequent. Despite the fact that these parents often have difficulty providing discipline and structure, they may expect their children to be independent at a variety of tasks at a younger age as compared to parents who do not use psychoactive substances. This sets the children up for failure and contributes to increased rates of depression, anxiety, and low self-esteem. Academic difficulties are particularly common in children exposed to parental substance use, likely as a result of both prenatal exposure with subsequent cognitive or learning impairments and the unstructured and potentially unsafe home environment. The parental attitude of acceptance toward alcohol and drug use seems to increase the chance that their children will use substances during adolescence.

Parents also may expose children directly to the harmful effects of other substances, such as exposure to *second hand cigarette smoke,* which is consistently associated with increased rates of childhood respiratory illnesses, otitis media, and sudden infant death syndrome. Despite these effects, only a few parents restrict smoking in their homes. There are many other ways in which parents may endanger the health of their children. Failing to immunize children, to childproof the home adequately, and to provide adequate supervision are other examples.

Parents' attempts to provide too much protection for their child can also have deleterious effects. One example of this is the **vulnerable child syndrome** in which a child who is ill early in life continues to be viewed as vulnerable by the parents despite the child having fully recovered. Behavioral difficulties may result if parents are overindulgent and fail to set limits. Parental reluctance to leave the child may contribute to the child having separation anxiety. Parents may be particularly attentive to minor variations in bodily functions, leading them to seek excess medical care. If the physician does not recognize this situation, the child may be exposed to unnecessary medical procedures.

FAMILY DYSFUNCTION: EMOTIONAL SUPPORT, EDUCATION, AND SOCIALIZATION

Failure to meet a child's emotional or educational needs can have a severe and enduring negative impact on child development and behavior. Infants need a consistent adult who learns to understand their signals and meets the infant's needs for attention as well as food. As the adult caregiver learns these signals, he or she responds more rapidly and appropriately to the infant's attempts at communication. Through this process, often referred to as **attachment**, the special relationship between parent and child develops. When affectionate and responsive adults are not consistently available, infants often are less willing to explore the environment and may become unusually clingy, angry, or difficult to soothe.

Appropriate stimulation is also vital for a child's cognitive development. Children whose parents do not read to them and do not play developmentally appropriate games with them have lower scores on intelligence tests and experience more school problems. In these situations, early intervention has been shown to be particularly effective in improving skill development and subsequent academic performance. At the other extreme, there are increasing concerns that some parents may provide too much stimulation and scheduling of the child's day. There may be such emphasis on achievement that children come to feel that parental love is contingent. There are concerns that this narrow definition of success may contribute to problems with anxiety and self-esteem for some children.

CHAPTER 25

Violence

The 2014 National Survey of Children's Exposure to Violence found that close to two thirds of children experienced at least one self- or parent-reported direct exposure to violence in the preceding year. Forms of violence include physical assault, sexual assault, child maltreatment (see Chapter 22), and property crime. Witnessing violence in the family and/or community was also prevalent (approximately one quarter of children). Violence is an important individual and public health concern given its prevalence and impact on well-being.

INTIMATE PARTNER VIOLENCE AND CHILDREN

Intimate partner violence (IPV) is a pattern of purposeful coercive behaviors aimed at establishing control of one partner over the other that may include inflicted physical injury, psychological abuse, sexual assault, progressive social isolation, stalking, deprivation, intimidation, and threats. Although partner violence often occurs between male perpetrators and female victims, it may also occur bidirectionally and may be better conceptualized as family or interpersonal violence. Violence may escalate during the perinatal period.

IPV affects the lives of millions of children each year. Children experience IPV by seeing or hearing the violence and its aftermath. Children may be injured during violent outbursts, sometimes while attempting to intervene on behalf of a parent. Many children are victims of abuse themselves. It is estimated that there is at least a 50% concurrence rate between IPV and child abuse. Exposure to IPV can also impact child development, emotional health, and behavior. There is no particular behavioral consequence or disturbance that is specific to children who witness IPV. Some children are traumatized by fear for their caregiver's safety and feel helpless. Others may blame themselves for the violence. Children may have symptoms of **post-traumatic stress disorder**, depression, anxiety, aggression, or hypervigilance. Older children may have conduct disorders, poor school performance, low self-esteem, or other nonspecific behaviors. Infants and young toddlers are at risk for disrupted attachment and routines around eating and sleeping. Preschoolers may show signs of regression, irritable behavior, or temper tantrums. During school-age years, children may show both externalizing (aggressive or disruptive) and internalizing (withdrawn and passive) behaviors. Because of family isolation, some children have no opportunity to participate in extracurricular activities at school and do not form friendships. Adolescents in homes where IPV is present have higher rates of school failure, substance abuse, and risky sexual behaviors. These adolescents are more likely than their peers to enter into a violent dating relationship.

Because of the high concurrence of IPV and child abuse, asking about IPV is part of the screening for violence against children. Recognizing the importance of IPV screening in pediatric practice, the American Academy of Pediatrics has endorsed screening in this setting and suggests that intervening on behalf of battered women may be one of the most effective means of preventing child abuse. Without standardized screening, pediatricians may underestimate the IPV prevalence in their practices. Parents should not be screened together. Questions about family violence should be direct, nonjudgmental, and done in the context of child safety and anticipatory guidance (Table 25.1).

Intervention is needed for caregivers who disclose IPV. It is appropriate to show concern and to provide available community resources. It is important to assess the safety of the victim and the children. In some states, physicians are mandated to report IPV. Information for families that provides details about community resources and state laws is helpful.

TABLE 25.1 Questions for Adults and Children Related to Family Violence
FOR THE CHILD
How are things at home and at school?
Who lives with you?
How do you get along with your family members?
What do you like to do with them?
What do you do if something is bothering you?
Do you feel safe at home?
Do people fight at home? What do they fight about? How do they fight?
ADDITIONAL QUESTIONS FOR THE ADOLESCENT
Do your friends get into fights often? How about you?
When was your last physical fight?
Have you ever been injured during a fight?
Has anyone you know been injured or killed?
Have you ever been forced to have sex against your will?
Have you ever been threatened with a gun or a knife?
How do you avoid getting in fights?
Do you carry a weapon for self-defense?
FOR THE PARENT
Do you have any concerns about your child?
Who helps with your children?
How do you feel about your neighborhood?
Do you feel safe at home?
Is there any fighting or violence at home?
Does anyone at home use drugs?
Have you been frightened by your partner?
Does your partner ever threaten you or hurt you?

YOUTH VIOLENCE

Rates of juvenile arrests in the United States are approximately 3010 persons between the ages of 10 and 17 per 100,000. Comparison of data from the juvenile justice system and surveys of self-reported behavior highlights that many juveniles commit chargeable offenses and are never arrested. Self-reports of delinquent behavior involvement do not differ much between white and minority adolescents, nor between urban and rural youth. However, urban and minority adolescents are more likely to be arrested. Although boys commit more crimes than girls, this gap has narrowed.

Most violent youth begin to exhibit their delinquent behaviors during early adolescence. The prevalence of delinquent behaviors decreases in the late teens into early adulthood, and most adolescent violence ends by young adulthood. Most violent youth are only intermittently violent. A small proportion of delinquent youth commit frequent, serious crimes; these offenders are more likely to have initiated delinquent activity before puberty. Serious youth violence is not an isolated problem but usually coexists with other adolescent risk-taking behaviors, such as drug use, truancy, school dropout, and early sexual activity as well as with mental health concerns. Gang membership is an important community level factor. Often, these risk factors exist in clusters and tend to be additive. Although understanding risk factors for violence is crucial for developing prevention strategies, the risk factors do not predict whether a particular individual will become violent. It is also important to identify protective factors, which include school connectedness as well as support of nonviolent family members and close friends.

ASSAULT AND BULLYING

The National Survey of Children's Exposure to Violence found that peers and siblings were the most common perpetrators of physical assault on youth. Other perpetrators of physical violence on youth include adults as well as groups or gangs. Assaults sometimes involve a weapon. Assaults can result in significant physical injury. Homicide is one of the leading causes of death among adolescents. Physical assaults can also have psychosocial consequences.

Youth **bullying** is a form of aggression in which a child or group of children repeatedly and intentionally intimidates, harasses, or physically harms another child. Technology-assisted bullying has become a major concern. Bullying peaks in middle school. Psychosocial consequences of being bullied include depression and suicidal ideation. Bullied youth may also experience negative physical, social, and educational outcomes. Prevention strategies include talking to children about bullying as well as how they can stand up to it and how to get help. Strategies at the school level include policies and rules, education, and bullying reporting systems. National resources include stopbullying.gov.

DATING VIOLENCE AND DATE RAPE

Dating violence includes physical violence, emotional abuse (such as name calling or shaming), sexual violence, and stalking. The 2013 National Youth Risk Behavior Survey found that 21% of female and 10% of male students who dated experienced some form of dating violence. Risk factors for dating violence include initiating dating and sexual activity at an early age, prior sexual abuse or victimization, and belief that dating violence is acceptable. Risk factors for perpetrating dating violence include witnessing or experiencing violence in the home, early initiation of sexual activity, and depression or anxiety. Substance use is also a risk factor for harming a partner; alcohol, marijuana, and cocaine may contribute. Flunitrazepam (Rohypnol) and gamma hydroxybutyrate are two commonly implicated drugs that cause sedation and amnesia, especially when used in conjunction with alcohol. Negative health outcomes of experiencing dating violence include depression and anxiety, engaging in unhealthy behaviors, as well as repeat victimization.

Relatively few victims of date rape report the assault to law enforcement. Women who report assaults to the police are more likely to receive timely medical care; it is likely that many sexually assaulted adolescents do not receive medical attention, putting them at risk for physical and mental health consequences. Health care providers can intervene by screening for adolescent dating violence, providing routine sexually transmitted infection evaluation, and identifying counseling resources for teens who are victims or perpetrators of dating violence (see Chapter 116).

VIOLENCE AND TECHNOLOGY

Technology use among youths is prevalent and evolving with the development of new applications and devices. Medical providers, educators, parents, and youth should be aware of the risks for violence through technology. Children can be exposed to violence on television, the internet including social media, and video games. Online sexual solicitation involves requests to engage in sexual activities or talk. In some cases, the solicitor attempts to make contact with the victim offline as well. Cyber bullying or electronic aggression refers to harassment or other aggression perpetrated through technology including text messaging, websites, and social media. Negative outcomes of electronic victimization include emotional distress, school absenteeism, and increased risk for in-person victimization. Anticipatory guidance for technology violence prevention includes setting rules for technology use to regulate content, location of use (i.e., common areas of the home), and amount of time spent with technology. Adults should educate children on steps to take if they are victimized, including informing a trusted adult. Children should be advised not to give out personal information online, friend strangers on social media, or meet someone known from the internet in person without parental supervision.

TRAUMA INFORMED CARE

Traumatic experiences in childhood including directly experiencing or witnessing violence can impact physical and mental health throughout the lifespan. Providing trauma-informed medical care includes realizing the prevalence and impact of trauma, recognizing signs and symptoms of trauma, as well as responding to the medical needs of traumatized patients. Examples of trauma-related symptoms include sleep difficulties, abnormal eating patterns (e.g., hoarding food, loss of appetite), hypervigilance, anxiety, detachment, and decline in school functioning. Anticipatory guidance for caregivers of children with trauma symptoms includes explaining the relationship between symptoms and the trauma experience and reminding the caregiver not to take the behaviors personally. Examples of anticipatory guidance for specific trauma-related symptoms include developing routines for bedtime and eating, remaining calm when children act out, teaching children calming skills such as breathing exercises, as well as helping children to verbalize emotions. Health care providers can also make referrals to trauma-informed mental health providers. Trauma-focused cognitive behavioral therapy is an example of an approach that has been shown to benefit children who have experienced trauma.

CHAPTER 26

Divorce, Separation, and Bereavement

The primary responsibility for ensuring the optimal development and well-being of children lies within the family. A variety of different disruptions can interfere with the family's ability to ensure a child's physical, emotional, social, and academic needs are met. Significant parental conflict can lead to separation or divorce. Parental illness or injury may create a brief or prolonged period of separation, while the death of a parent results in a permanent separation that may be anticipated or unanticipated. All of these disruptions cause significant stress for the child, with the potential for short- and long-term adverse consequences. The child's adaptation to these stresses is affected by the child's developmental stage, temperament, parental behaviors, and the availability of additional support systems.

DIVORCE

Approximately 50% of first marriages in the United States will end in divorce. About half of these divorces occur in the first 10 years of marriage when couples have added children to their family unit prior to the break-up. At least 25% of children experience the divorce or separation of their parents. Few events in childhood are as dramatic and challenging for the child as divorce. Importantly, parental choices and behaviors around a divorce can help promote a healthy emotional adjustment for the child.

Divorce is likely to be accompanied by changes in behavioral and emotional adjustment. In the immediate post-divorce period, many children exhibit anger, noncompliance, anxiety, and depression. Children from divorced families require psychological help two to three times more frequently than children with married parents. Long-term studies suggest that in the absence of ongoing stressors, most children demonstrate good adjustment a few years after the divorce, but some have enduring difficulties. Easygoing temperament and average to above-average cognitive functioning are child characteristics associated with improved coping skills.

Divorce is not a single event but a process that occurs over time. In most cases, marital conflict begins long before the physical or legal separation, but the divorce brings about permanent changes in the family structure. Multiple potential stressors for the child are associated with divorce, including parental discord before and after the divorce, changes in living arrangements and sometimes location, and changes in the child's relationship with both parents. The environmental changes that disturb a child's primary support system as a result of the divorce process further complicate the child's ability to adapt.

The child's relationship with each parent can be affected by the divorce. In the short-term, the parent is likely to experience new burdens and feelings of guilt, anger, or sadness that may disrupt parenting skills and family routines. Contact with the noncustodial parent may decline greatly. Parents may be perceived by their children as being unaware of the child's distress around the time of the divorce. Pediatricians can help parents understand things they can do that will be reassuring to the child. Maintaining contact with both parents, seeing where the noncustodial parent is living, and, in particular, maintaining familiar routines are comforting to the child in the midst of the turmoil of a separation and divorce. The child should attend school and continue to have opportunities to interact with friends. Assistance from extended family can be essential, and so it may be helpful for pediatricians to encourage parents to ask for this support. Pediatricians should look for maladaptive coping responses. Some parents may respond to their increased burdens and distress by treating their children as friends with whom they share their suffering. Alternatively, they may place unnecessary and excessive responsibilities on the child or leave the child unsupervised for longer periods of time. Responses such as these increase the chance that the child will develop behavioral or emotional problems.

Reaction to Divorce at Different Ages

The child's reaction to the divorce is influenced by the child's age and cognitive development. Similarly, warning signs of maladjustment may look different at different stages of child development. Although infants do not comprehend the concept of divorce, their need for a stable daily routine and regular contact with a primary caregiver in order to develop secure attachment requires special considerations in relation to custody and visitation. Separations from a primary caregiver should be brief. Increased infant irritability, changes in sleep and appetite patterns, and withdrawal or listlessness may be indicators of distress. In the worst cases of family stress and neglect, the young child may fail to meet developmental milestones as expected. The developmental phase of **preschool age children** is characterized by magical thinking about cause and effect and an egocentric view of the world. They may believe that something they did caused the divorce, or they may engage in unusual behaviors that they believe will reunite the parents. At this age, parents need to provide a consistent and clear message that the divorce was related to disagreements between the parents, that nothing the child did caused the divorce, and that nothing the child could do would bring the parents back together again. Preschool children may reason that if the parents left each other they also might leave the child. To counteract this fear of abandonment, children may need one-on-one attention and to be reassured that although parents separated, they will not abandon the child and that the child's relationship with both parents will endure.

School-age children have a more concrete understanding of cause and effect; if something bad happened, they understand that something caused it to happen. However, they are less likely to appreciate the subtleties of parental discord or the idea that multiple factors contribute to a conflict. Children at this age may still worry that something they did caused the divorce. They may express more anger than younger children and often feel rejected. Many young school-age children worry about what will happen to one or both parents. School performance often deteriorates. Older elementary school–age children may believe that one parent was wronged by the other. This belief, in conjunction with their concrete understanding of cause and effect, allows children to be easily co-opted by one parent to take sides against the other. Parents need to understand this vulnerability and resist the temptation to support their child in taking sides, while allowing the child to express their feelings openly.

Adolescents may demonstrate difficulty adjusting to divorce by acting out, becoming depressed, or experiencing somatic symptoms. Adolescents are developing a sense of autonomy, a sense of morality, and the capacity for intimacy. Divorce may lead them to question previously held beliefs. They may be concerned about what the divorce means for their future and whether they, too, will experience marital failure. Questioning of previous beliefs, in conjunction with decreased supervision, may set the stage for risk-taking behaviors, such as truancy, sexual behaviors, and alcohol or drug use. Adolescents with divorced parents, in comparison to those with married parents, are at increased risk for internalizing problems like depression and anxiety in addition to the externalizing problems already mentioned. Parents are encouraged to continue to provide consistent behavioral expectations while encouraging an open forum for discussing the adolescent's feelings.

Outcome of Divorce

Regardless of the age or developmental level of the child, children that are exposed to hostility and high levels of stress are at increased risk for emotional, behavioral, and academic struggles in the future. One of the best predictors of children's adaptation to divorce is whether the physical separation is associated with a decrease in the child's exposure to parental discord. In most cases, divorced parents still must interact with each other around the child's schedule, child custody and support, and other parenting issues. These types of issues create the potential for the child to have ongoing exposure to significant discord between the parents. For example, if one parent tends to keep the child up much later than the bedtime at the other parent's house, sleep problems may develop. When children feel caught in the middle of ongoing conflicts between their divorced parents, behavior or emotional problems are much more likely. Regardless of how angry parents are with each other, the parents should be counseled that they must shield their child from this animosity. Clear rules about schedules, discipline, and other parenting roles is ideal, but in cases of conflict, it can also be helpful for the pediatrician to help a parent accept that he or she can only control his or her actions and decisions related to the child. When parents have trouble resolving these issues, mediation may be helpful. Pediatricians need to be wary of parents' attempts to recruit them into custody battles to substantiate claims of poor parenting unless the pediatrician has first-hand knowledge that the concerns are valid.

Although the primary physical residence for most children is still with the mother, the court's bias toward preferring mothers in custody decisions has decreased and there is more emphasis on including both parents in the child's life. In the early 1980s, 50% of children had no contact with their fathers 2 or 3 years after a divorce, whereas today only 20-25% of children have no contact with their father. Most states now allow joint physical or legal custody. In joint physical custody, the child spends a significant amount of time with each parent, and in joint legal custody, parents share authority in decision making. Although joint custody arrangements may promote the involvement of both parents in the child's life, they also can be a vehicle through which parents continue to express their anger at each other. When parents have substantial difficulty working together, joint custody is an inappropriate arrangement and has been associated with deterioration in the child's psychological and social adjustment.

Divorce often leads to financial difficulties. Family income usually declines in the first year after the divorce. Only about half of mothers who have child support awards receive the full amount, and one fourth receive no money at all. These financial changes may have multiple adverse effects on the child. A move to a new house may require the child to attend a new school disrupting peer relationships and other potential supports. The child may spend more time in child care if one or both parents have to increase work hours.

Most men and women remarry within 5 years of divorce, with a slightly higher incidence of men who remarry than women (approximately 60% vs. 50%, respectively). Most spouses in remarried couples already have children, such that at least one third of American children become members of stepfamilies. The adjustment to a parent dating and the transition to a blended family pose additional challenges to the child. Parents are encouraged to be sensitive to the child's reactions and mindful of the importance of maintaining the biological parents as disciplinarians.

Role of the Pediatrician

The pediatrician can be an important voice in helping the parents understand and meet the child's needs (Table 26.1) before, during, and after the divorce. Children should be told of the parents' decision before the physical separation. The separation should be presented as a rational step in managing marital conflict and should prepare the child for the changes that will occur. Parents should be prepared to answer children's questions, and they should expect that the questions will be repeated over the ensuing months. Once parents have told children of the separation, it may be confusing to the child if parents continue to live together and may raise false hopes that the parents will not divorce.

Many parents report feeling like their life did not stabilize until 2-3 years or more after the divorce; for some the divorce remains a painful issue 10 years later. The child's emotional adjustment to divorce is closely predicted by the parents' adjustment. Consequently, parents should be encouraged to seek help for themselves if they are struggling emotionally after a divorce. Although most children ultimately show good adjustment to divorce, some have significant acting-out behaviors or depression that requires referral to a mental health professional. Some parents need the assistance of a mediator or family therapist to help them stay focused on their child's needs. In the most contentious situations, a guardian ad litem can be appointed by the court to investigate and recommend what solutions would be in the "best interests" of a child.

TABLE 26.1 General Recommendations for Pediatricians to Help Children During Separation, Divorce, or Death of a Close Relative
Acknowledge and provide support for grief that the parent/caregiver is experiencing.
Help parent/caregiver consider child's needs and validate his/her feelings.
Encourage parent/caregiver to maintain routines familiar to the child.
Encourage continued contact between child and his or her friends.
If primary residence changes, the child should take transitional objects, familiar toys, and other important objects to the new residence.
Minimize frequent changes in caregivers, and for infants, keep brief the times spent away from primary caregiver.
Have parent/caregiver reassure the child that he or she will continue to be cared for.
Have parent/caregiver reassure the child that he or she did not cause the separation, divorce, or death (especially important in preschool children).
Encourage parent/caregiver to create times or rituals that allow the child to discuss questions and feelings if the child wishes.
Encourage parental self-care. Ensuring that parents are addressing their own mental health needs will have a positive impact on the child's emotional well-being.

SEPARATIONS FROM PARENTS

Children experience separations from their primary caregiver for a variety of reasons. Brief separations, such as those to attend school, camp, or other activities, are nearly a universal experience. Many children experience longer separations for a variety of reasons, including parental business trips, military service, or hospitalization. Child adjustment to separation is affected by child factors (e.g., age of the child and the child's temperament); factors related to the separation (e.g., length of and reason for the separation, whether the separation was planned or unplanned); and factors related to the caregiving environment during the separation (e.g., how familiar the child is with the caregiver and whether the child has access to friends and familiar toys and routines).

Children between 6 months and 3-4 years of age often have the most difficulty adjusting to a separation from their primary caregiver. Older children may be better able to understand the reason for the separation, communicate their feelings, and comprehend the passage of time, allowing them to anticipate the parent's return. For older children, the period immediately before a planned separation may be particularly difficult if the reason for the separation causes significant family tension, as it may in the case of hospitalization or military service.

If parents anticipate a separation, they should provide a clear explanation of the reason for the separation and, to the extent possible, give concrete information about when the parent will be in contact with the child and when they will return home. If the child can remain at home with a familiar and responsive caregiver, this is likely to help adjustment. If children cannot remain at home, they should be encouraged to take transitional objects, such as a favorite blanket, familiar toys, and important objects such as a picture of the parent, with them. Maintenance of familiar family routines and relationships with friends should be encouraged.

DEATH OF A PARENT OR FAMILY MEMBER AND BEREAVEMENT

When a child loses a parent, it is a devastating experience. Unfortunately, this experience is not rare; by 15 years of age, 4% of children in the United States have experienced the death of a parent. The death of a parent is likely to alter forever the child's view of the world as a secure and safe place. The child's developmental level and temperament and the availability of support systems contribute to the child's adjustment following the death of a parent. Many of the recommendations in Table 26.1 are helpful. The death of a parent or close family member also brings up some unique issues.

Explaining Death to a Child

Children's understanding of death changes with their cognitive development and experiences (see Chapter 4). Preschool children often do not view death as permanent and may have magical beliefs about what caused death. As children become older, they understand death as permanent and inevitable, but the concept that death represents the cessation of all bodily functions and has a biological cause may not be fully appreciated until adolescence.

Death should not be hidden from the child. It should be explained in simple and honest terms that are consistent with the family's beliefs. The explanation should help the child to understand that the dead person's body stopped functioning and that the dead person will not return. Preschool children should be reassured that nothing they did caused the individual to die. One should be prepared to answer questions about where the body is and let the child's questions help determine what information the child is prepared to hear. False or misleading information should be avoided. Comparisons of death to sleep may contribute to sleep problems in the child.

There are many possible reactions of children to the death of a parent or close relative. Sadness and a yearning to be with the dead relative are common. Sometimes a child might express a wish to die so that he or she can visit the dead relative, but a plan or desire to commit suicide is uncommon and would necessitate immediate evaluation. A decline in academic functioning, lack of enjoyment with previously preferred activities, and changes in appetite and sleep can occur. Approximately half of children have their most severe grief reactions about 1 month after the death of a loved one; for other children the most severe symptoms of grief do not occur until 6-12 months after the death.

Should the Child Attend the Funeral?

Children often find it helpful to attend the funeral, helping them understand that the death occurred and providing an opportunity to say good-bye. Seeing others express their grief and sadness may help the child to express these feelings. Going to the funeral helps prevent the child from having fears or fantasies about what happened at the funeral. If the child is going to attend the funeral, he or she should be informed of what to expect. If a preschool-age child expresses a desire not to attend the funeral, he or she should not be encouraged to attend. For older children, it may be appropriate to encourage attendance, but a child who feels strongly about not wanting to go to the funeral should not be required to attend.

Suggested Readings

Adams JA, Kellogg ND, Farst KJ, et al. Updated guidelines for the medical assessment and care of children who may have been sexually abused. *J Pediatr Adolesc Gynecol.* 2016;29(2):81–87.

American Academy of Pediatrics, Elk Grove Village, Il. 2016. http://www.aap.org/traumaguide. Accessed October 31, 2016.

Centers for Disease Control and Prevention, Atlanta, GA. https://www.cdc.gov/lgbthealth/index.htm.

Christian CW, Committee on Child Abuse and Neglect, American Academy of Pediatrics. The evaluation of suspected physical abuse. *Pediatrics.* 2015;135(5):e1337–e1354.

Dubowitz H, Giardino A, Gustavson E. Child neglect: guidance for pediatricians. *Pediatr Rev.* 2011;21(4):111–116.

Finkelhor D, Turner HA, Shattuck A, et al. Prevalence of childhood exposure to violence, crime and abuse: results from the National Survey of Children's Exposure to Violence. *JAMA Pediatr.* 2015;169(8):746–754.

Garner AS, Forkey H, Szilagyi M. Translating developmental science to address childhood adversity. *Acad Pediatr.* 2015;15(5):493–502.

Goldberg AE, Gartrell NK. LGB-parent families: the current state of the research and directions for the future. *Adv Child Dev Behav.* 2014;46:57–88.

Greenbaum J, Crawford-Jakubiak JE, Committee on Child Abuse and Neglect. Child sex trafficking and commercial sexual exploitation: health care needs of victims. *Pediatrics.* 2015;135(3):556–574.

Jaffe AC. Failure to thrive: current clinical concepts. *Pediatr Rev.* 2011;32(3):100–107.

Lopez X, Stewart S, Jacobson-Dickman E. Approach to children and adolescents with gender dysphoria. *Pediatr Rev.* 2016;37(3):89–98.

Schonfeld DJ, Demaria T, Committee on Psychosocial Aspects of Child and Family Health, Disaster Preparedness Advisory Council. Supporting the Grieving Child and Family. *Pediatrics.* 2016;138(3):e20162147.

Shonkoff JP, Garner AS, Committee on Psychosocial Aspects of Child and Family Health, Committee on Early Childhood, Adoption, and Dependent Care, Section on Developmental Behavioral Pediatrics. The lifelong effects of early childhood adversity and toxic stress. *Pediatrics.* 2012;129(1):e232–e246.

Smith VC, Wilson CR, Committee on Substance Use and Prevention. Families affected by parental substance use. *Pediatrics.* 2016;138(2):e20161575.

Szilagyi MA, Rosen DS, Rubin D, et al. Health care issues for children and adolescents in foster care and kinship care. *Pediatrics.* 2015;136(4):e1142–e1166.

PEARLS FOR PRACTITIONERS

CHAPTER 21

Failure to Thrive

- There is no single, universally accepted anthropometric criterion for failure to thrive. Commonly used criteria include weight below the 3rd or 5th percentile for age; weight decreasing, crossing two major percentile lines on the growth chart over time; or weight less than 80% of the median weight for the height of the child.
- Failure to thrive can be caused by inadequate intake, malabsorption, or increased metabolic demands.
- History and physical examinations to assess for biological and psychosocial etiologies are the cornerstone of failure to thrive evaluations.

CHAPTER 22

Child Abuse and Neglect

- In every state, physicians are mandated by law to report child abuse and neglect.
- Neglect is the most common form of child maltreatment and can impact physical, mental, developmental and behavioral health in both the short and long term.
- Bruising characteristics that raise concern for inflicted injury include patterned bruising (examples: loop mark, slap mark), unusual location such as ears, neck, or genitals, as well as bruising in nonmobile infants.
- Children with significant internal abdominal injuries may present without any external bruising.

- Abusive head trauma is the leading cause of mortality and morbidity from child physical abuse. Prevention programs often emphasize coping with crying techniques and education.

CHAPTER 23
Homosexuality and Gender Identity

- The vast majority of victims of sexual abuse have normal anogenital examinations.
- Factors to consider when determining the urgency of medical evaluations for victims of sexual abuse include timing of the most recent abuse (i.e., is the child within the window for prophylactic medications against HIV, pregnancy and sexually transmitted infections [STIs], or forensic evidence collection), child safety (i.e., does the child have ongoing contact with the perpetrator), acute physical or mental health symptoms (e.g., active suicidal ideation, genital bleeding).
- Clinical findings that could raise concern for child sex trafficking and commercial sexual exploitation include child not allowed to speak for himself/herself, child accompanied by an unrelated adult, history of multiple STIs, and tattoos concerning for branding.
- There is no reliable way to predict an individual's sexual orientation and no evidence that parental behavior alters the developmental trajectory towards a particular sexual orientation.
- There are significant health disparities for sexual minority youth related to sexual health outcomes. Education about safe sexual practices should be part of all adolescent well-child visits, including asking about the gender of all sex partners as part of STI risk assessment.
- Transgender youth have rates of depression, anxiety, self-destructive choices, and suicide that greatly exceed those in the general population. Connecting with a specialty center with a multidisciplinary team to address the needs of transgender children and their families is vital.

CHAPTER 24
Family Structure and Function

- The accumulation of toxic stress can disrupt brain development in children and increase the risk for stress-related disease and cognitive impairment into adulthood. Supportive nurturing by primary caregivers is crucial to early brain growth and to the physical, emotional, and developmental needs of children.
- Regardless of family structure, the best predictors of secure child health and psychological development are the quality of the parent-child relationship, the quality of the relationship between adult caregivers, and the availability of social and economic resources.
- Children and adolescents in foster care are at extremely high risk for medical, nutritional, developmental, behavioral, and mental health problems.

CHAPTER 25
Violence

- Direct and/or indirect exposure to violence is prevalent among youth. Traumatic experiences impact health outcomes not only in childhood, but also into adulthood. Trauma-informed care includes recognizing and responding to signs/symptoms of trauma including hypervigilance, anxiety, sleep problems, and decline in school functioning.
- Violence through technology such as online solicitation, cyber bullying, or exposure to violent materials is a growing concern. Anticipatory guidance could include setting rules for technology use (e.g., location of use, amount of time of allowable use, social media–related rules), advising children not to give out personal information or meet someone known from the internet in person, and educating children on steps to take if they are bullied.

CHAPTER 26
Divorce, Separation, and Bereavement

- A child's reaction to divorce, separation from a parent, or the death of a loved one is influenced by the child's age, cognitive development, and previous experiences.
- In times of family disruption, it is important that children are assured of continued safety and care, their feelings are validated, any concerns of personal responsibility are nullified, consistency of routine is maintained, and time is appropriated for questions and open communication without punitive judgment.

PEDIATRIC NUTRITION AND NUTRITIONAL DISORDERS

April O. Buchanan | Maria L. Marquez

CHAPTER 27

Diet of the Normal Infant

Proper nutrition in infancy is essential for normal growth, resistance to infections, long-term adult health, and optimal neurologic and cognitive development. Healthy nutrition is especially important during the first 6 months, a period of exceptionally accelerated growth and high nutrient requirements relative to body weight. Breast feeding is associated with a reduced risk of many diseases in infants, children, and mothers (for more details visit http://www.nutrition.gov).

BREAST FEEDING

Human milk and breast feeding are the ideal and normative standards for infant feeding and nutrition. The American Academy of Pediatrics (AAP) recommends human milk as the sole source of nutrition for the first 6 months of life, with continued intake for the first year, and as long as desired thereafter. Breast feeding has short- and long-term advantages for infant neurodevelopment. Pediatric health care providers should approach breast feeding at multiple levels (individual, community, social, and political). The goals of the U.S. Department of Health and Human Services "Healthy People 2020" include 82% of infants with any breast feeding, 25.5% of infants with exclusive breast feeding for the first 6 months of life, and lactation support at work of 38%. In collaboration with national and global organizations, including the AAP, World Health Organization (WHO), United Nations Children's Fund (UNICEF), the Centers for Disease Control and Prevention (CDC), and the Joint Commission, hospitals are asked to promote and facilitate breast feeding.

The first 2 days of breast feeding, and perhaps the first hour of life, may determine the success of breast feeding. The 2011 rate of breast feeding initiation reported by the CDC for the total U.S. population was 79%, which met the target of initiation for "Healthy People 2020"; however, breast feeding did not continue as long as recommended (Fig. 27.1). In response, a multilevel approach has been implemented as described in the following: (1) the federal government is supporting hospitals and health departments to improve the maternity health care practices; (2) state and local governments help hospitals to adapt standards to support breast feeding; (3) hospitals work toward the **Baby-Friendly** designation and work with health care providers and community members to work for hospital policies and create networks for supporting breast feeding in the communities; (4) health care providers can help write hospital policies to support breast feeding and counseling to mothers, promoting continuation of breast feeding at home; and (5) parents can ask questions about breast feeding and their needs. There is greater emphasis to improve and standardize hospital practices with "Baby-Friendly" programs for breast feeding support, utilizing the "Ten Steps to Successful Breastfeeding" recommendations by the UNICEF/WHO; in the United States 29% of the hospitals were "Baby Friendly" in 2007 and 54% in 2013. The percentage of infants born in "Baby-Friendly" hospitals increased from 1% in 2005 to 14% in 2015.

The Department of Health and Human Services and the CDC recognize that breast feeding offers infants, mothers, and society compelling advantages in both industrialized and developing countries. Human-milk feeding decreases the incidence and severity of diarrhea, respiratory illness, otitis media, bacteremia, bacterial meningitis, and necrotizing enterocolitis, as documented by the Agency for Healthcare Research and Quality (AHRQ).

Mothers who breast feed experience both short- and long-term health benefits. Decreased risk of postpartum hemorrhages, more rapid uterine involution, longer period of amenorrhea, and decreased postpartum depression have been observed. Similarly, there is an association between a long lactation of 12-23 months (cumulative lactation of all pregnancies) and a significant reduction of hypertension, hyperlipidemia, cardiovascular disease, and diabetes in the mother. Cumulative lactation of more than 12 months also correlates with reduced risk of ovarian and breast cancer.

Feeding *preterm* infants human milk has beneficial effects on their long-term neurodevelopment (IQ). Preterm breast fed infants also have a lower readmission rate in the first year of life.

Adequacy of milk intake can be assessed by voiding and stooling patterns of the infant. A well-hydrated infant voids 6-8 times a day. Each voiding should soak, not merely moisten, a diaper, and urine should be colorless. By 5-7 days, loose yellow stools should be passed approximately 4 times a day. Rate of weight gain provides the most objective indicator of adequate milk intake. Total weight loss after birth should not exceed 7%, and birth weight should be regained by 10 days. The mean feeding frequency during the early weeks postpartum is 8-12 times per day. An infant may be adequately hydrated while not receiving enough milk to achieve adequate energy and nutrient intake. Telephone follow-up is valuable during the interim between discharge and the first doctor visit to monitor

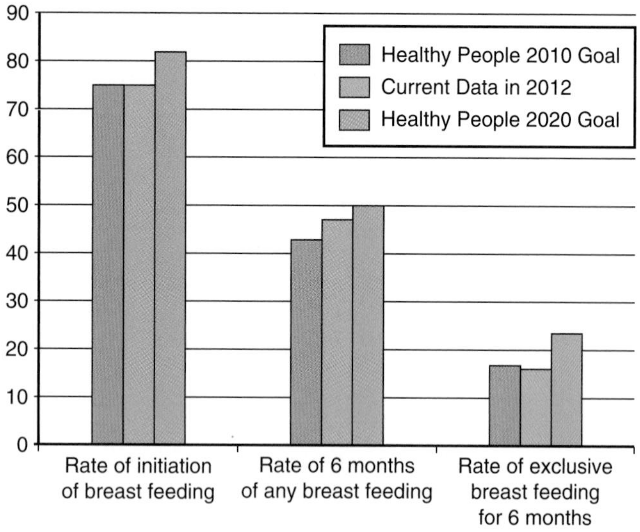

FIGURE 27.1 The 2010 and 2020 Healthy People Targets and the current 2012 rates of breast feeding initiation, 6 months of any breast feeding, and 6 months of exclusive breast feeding in the United States.

the progress of lactation. A follow-up visit should be scheduled by 3-5 days of age and again by 2 weeks of age.

In the newborn period, elevated concentrations of serum bilirubin are present more often in breast fed infants than in formula-fed infants (see Chapter 62). Feeding frequency during the first 3 days of life of breast fed infants is inversely related to the level of bilirubin; frequent feedings stimulate meconium passage and excretion of bilirubin in the stool. Infants who have insufficient milk intake and poor weight gain in the first week of life may have an increase in unconjugated bilirubin secondary to an exaggerated enterohepatic circulation of bilirubin. This is known as **breast feeding jaundice**. Attention should be directed toward improved milk production and intake. The use of water supplements in breast fed infants has no effect on bilirubin levels and is not recommended. After the first week of life in a breast fed infant, prolonged elevated serum bilirubin may be due to the presence of an unknown factor in milk that enhances intestinal absorption of bilirubin. This is termed **breast milk jaundice**, which is a diagnosis of exclusion and should be made only if an infant is otherwise thriving, with normal growth and no evidence of hemolysis, infection, biliary atresia, or metabolic disease (see Chapter 62). Breast milk jaundice usually lasts no more than 1-2 weeks. The AAP recommends vitamin D supplementation (400 IU/day starting soon after birth) for breast fed infants.

Common Breast Feeding Problems

Breast tenderness, engorgement, and cracked nipples are the most common problems encountered by breast feeding mothers. Engorgement, one of the most common causes of lactation failure, should receive prompt attention because milk supply can decrease quickly if the breasts are not adequately emptied. Applying warm or cold compresses to the breasts before nursing and hand expression or pumping of some milk can provide relief to the mother and make the areola easier to grasp by the infant. Nipple tenderness requires attention to proper latch-on and positioning of the infant. Supportive measures include nursing for shorter periods, beginning feedings on the less sore side, air-drying the nipples well after nursing, and applying lanolin cream after each nursing session. Severe nipple pain and cracking usually indicate improper latch-on. Temporary pumping, which is well tolerated, may be needed. Meeting with a lactation consultant may help minimize these problems and allow the successful continuation of breast feeding.

If a lactating woman reports fever, chills, and malaise, **mastitis** should be considered. Treatment includes frequent and complete emptying of the breast and antibiotics. Breast feeding usually should not be stopped because the mother's mastitis commonly has no adverse effects on the breast fed infant. Untreated mastitis may rarely progress to a **breast abscess**. If an abscess is diagnosed, treatment includes incision and drainage, antibiotics, and regular emptying of the breast. Nursing from the contralateral breast can be continued with a healthy infant. If maternal comfort allows, nursing can continue on the affected side.

Maternal infection with human immunodeficiency virus (HIV) is considered a contraindication for breast feeding in developed countries. When the mother has active tuberculosis, syphilis, or varicella, restarting breast feeding may be considered after therapy is initiated. If a woman has herpetic lesions on her breast, nursing and contact with the infant on that breast should be avoided. Women with genital herpes can breast feed. Proper handwashing procedures should be stressed.

There are limited numbers of medical contraindications for breast feeding, including pediatric metabolic disorders such as galactosemia and infants with phenylketonuria, although infants with the latter may alternate breast feeding with special protein-free or modified formulas. Maternal contraindications are shown in Table 27.1.

Maternal Drug Use

Any drug prescribed therapeutically to newborns usually can be consumed via breast milk without ill effect. The factors that determine the effects of maternal drug therapy on the nursing infant include the route of administration, dosage, molecular weight, pH, and protein binding. Few therapeutic drugs are absolutely contraindicated; these include radioactive compounds, antimetabolites, lithium, and certain antithyroid drugs. The mother should be advised against the use of unprescribed drugs, including alcohol, nicotine, caffeine, or "street drugs."

Maternal use of illicit or recreational drugs is a contraindication to breast feeding. If a woman is unable to discontinue drug use, she should not breast feed. Expression of milk for a feeding or two after use of a drug is not acceptable. Breast fed infants of mothers taking methadone (but no alcohol or other drugs) as part of a treatment program generally have not experienced ill effects.

FORMULA FEEDING

Cow's milk–based formulas are the vast majority of commercial formulas. Most milk-based formulas have added iron, which the AAP recommends, and parents should use only iron-fortified formula unless advised otherwise by the primary health care provider. Infant formula manufacturers have begun to examine the benefits of adding a variety of nutrients and biologic factors to infant formula to mimic the composition and quality of breast milk. These include long-chain polyunsaturated fatty

TABLE 27.1 Maternal Contraindications and Recommendations for Breast Feeding

MATERNAL CONTRAINDICATIONS	RECOMMENDATIONS FOR MOTHER
Tuberculosis (active)	Should not breast feed; expressed milk may be provided to child.
Varicella	Should not breast feed; expressed milk may be provided to child.
H1N1 influenza	Should not breast feed; expressed milk may be provided to child. Alternately provide prophylaxis to infant and continue nursing.
Herpes simplex infection of the breast	Should not breast feed; expressed milk may be provided to child.
Human immunodeficiency virus	In industrialized countries, mothers are not recommended to breast feed. In developing countries, women are recommended to combine breast feeding with antiretroviral therapy for 6 months.
Use of phencyclidine (PCP), cocaine, or amphetamines	Recommended to stop use of drugs because they can affect infant neurobehavioral development. Mothers enrolled in supervised methadone programs are encouraged to breast feed.
Alcohol	Limit ingestion to < 0.5 mg of alcohol per kg of body weight due to association with motor development.
Radiopharmaceutical agents	Express milk before exposure to feed infant. Express milk and discard during therapies. Radioactivity may be present in milk from 2-14 days, depending on agent. Consult with nuclear medicine expert.
Antineoplastic and immunosuppressive agents	Substitute formula.

Modified from Eidelman AI, Schanler RJ. American Academy of Pediatrics section on breastfeeding. Breastfeeding and the use of human milk. Pediatrics. 2012;129(3):827–841.

acids, nucleotides, prebiotics, and probiotics. Soy-based formulas, which sometimes have added iron, may be used for newborns who may be allergic to cow's milk. However, some newborns allergic to cow's milk are also allergic to the protein in soy formulas. There are hypoallergenic formulas for infants who cannot tolerate the basic formulas, such as those with allergies to milk or soy proteins. The proteins in these hypoallergenic formulas are broken down to their basic components and are therefore easier to digest (Table 27.2). Specialized formulas are designed for premature, low birth weight babies. The carbohydrate in standard formulas is generally lactose, although lactose-free cow's milk–based formulas are available. The caloric density of formulas is 20 kcal/oz (0.67 kcal/mL), similar to that of human milk. A relatively high-fat and calorically dense diet (human milk or formula) is needed to deliver adequate calories. Formula-fed infants are at higher risk for obesity later in childhood; this may be related to self-regulation of volumes ingested by the newborns and infants.

COMPLEMENTARY FOODS

By approximately 6 months, complementary feeding of semisolid foods is suggested. By this age, an exclusively breast fed infant requires additional sources of several nutrients, including protein, iron, and zinc. Cereals are commonly introduced around 6 months of age, and initially they are mixed with breast milk, formula, or water and later with fruits. By tradition solid cereals are usually introduced first; however, there is no medical evidence that a particular order is better than others for the infants. Baby-cereals are available premixed or dry, to which parents add breast milk, formula, or water. Single-grain iron-fortified cereals (rice, oatmeal, barley) are recommended as starting cereals to help identify possible allergies or food intolerances that may arise, especially when new foods and solids are added to the diet. Infants do not need juices, but if juice is given, it should be started only after 12 months of age, given in a cup (as opposed to a bottle), and limited to 4 oz (for toddlers age 1-3 yr) daily of 100% natural juice, and it should be unsweetened; juices should also be offered only with meals or snacks. If these recommendations are not followed, the infant may have reduced appetite for other more nutritious foods, including breast milk and/or formula. Too much juice may cause diaper rash, diarrhea, and weight gain. An infant should never be put to sleep with a bottle or sippy cup filled with milk, formula, or juice because this can result in **early childhood caries (ECCs)**, formerly known as infant bottle tooth decay (see Chapter 127). For the first 2 months it is important to set the stage for making a distinction between sleeping and feeding time. Healthy infants do not need extra water; breast milk and formula provide all the fluids needed. However, with the introduction of solid foods, water can be added to the infant's diet. If the family lives in an area with fluoridated water, the recommendation is to provide infants the fluoridated water for preventing future tooth decay.

During the 4-6 months of age, starting actively to separate mealtime from bedtime is recommended. After 6 months of age other foods may be introduced as the infant shows signs of readiness to solid feedings. Solid cereals are usually introduced first. Once the infant learns to eat them, parents gradually introduce one food at a time, and they should wait 2-3 days before introducing a new one and watch for signs of an allergic reaction such as diarrhea, rash, or vomiting. In general meats and vegetables have more nutrients per serving than fruits and cereals. Green vegetables bring nutrients, vitamins, minerals, and micronutrients.

The avoidance of foods with high allergic potential in infancy (e.g., fish, tree nuts, peanuts, dairy products, and eggs) is no longer supported, and early introduction may actually help to prevent food allergies. Once the child can sit and bring her hands or other objects to the mouth, parents may provide finger food to help the infant learn to feed themselves. To avoid choking, make sure that anything given to the infant is easy to swallow, soft, and cut in very small pieces. Initially the infant should be eating approximately 4 ounces of solids at each daily meal. If the food fed to the infant is prepared by the adult, it should be prepared without preservatives or high salt. All foods with the potential to obstruct the young infant's main airway should be avoided in general until 4 years of age or older. Honey (risk of infant botulism) should not be given before 1 year of age. Commercially prepared or homemade foods help meet the nutritional needs of the infant. If the introduction of solid foods is delayed, nutritional deficiencies can develop, and oral sensory

TABLE 27.2 Composition of Breast Milk, Breast Milk After Freezing and Pasteurization, and Representative Infant Formulas

COMPONENT	BREAST MILK	BREAST MILK AFTER FREEZING AND PASTEURIZING	STANDARD FORMULA	SOY FORMULA	HYPOALLERGENIC FORMULA
Protein	1.1 per dL	Reduced	1.5 per dL	1.7 per dL	1.9 per d/L
Fat	4.0 per dL	4.0 per dL	3.6 per dL	3.6 per dL	3.8–3.3 per d/L
Carbohydrate	7.2 per dL	7.2 per dL	6.9–7.2 per dL	6.8 per dL	6.9–7.3 per d/L
Calcium	290 mg/L	290 mg/L	420–550 mg/L	700 mg/L	635–777 mg/L
Phosphorus	140 mg/L	140 mg/L	280–390 mg/L	500 mg/L	420–500 mg/L
Sodium	8.0 mg/L	8.0 mg/L	6.5–8.3 mg/L	13 mg/L	14 mg/L
Vitamin D	Variable	Variable	400 per dL	400 per dL	400 per d/L
Vitamin A	100%	100%	—	—	—
Osmolality	253 mOsm/L	253 mOsm/L	230 mOsm/L	200–220 mOsm/L	290 mOSm/L
Renal solute load	75 mOsm/L	75 mOsm/L	100–126 mOsm/L	126–150 mOsm/L	125–175 mOSm/L
IgA and SIgA	Present	Reduced 30%	0	0	0
IgM	Present	Present	0	0	0
IgG	Present	Reduced 30%	0	0	0
Lactoferrin	Present	Reduced 30%	0	0	0
Lysozyme	Present	Reduced 25%	0	0	0
Lipases	Present	0	0	0	0
Monoglycerides	Present	Present	Added to some formulas	Added to some formulas	Added to some formulas
Free fatty acids	Present	Present	Added to some formulas	Added to some formulas	Added to some formulas
Linoleic acid	Present	Present	Added to some formulas	Added to some formulas	Added to some formulas
Alpha-linoleic acid	Present	Present	Added to some formulas	Added to some formulas	Added to some formulas
Bifidus factor	Present	Present	—	—	—
Oligosaccharides	Present	Present	—	—	—

Ig, Immunoglobulin; *SIg*, secretory immunoglobulin.

issues (texture and oral aversion) may occur. General signs of readiness include the ability to hold the head up, big enough (around double the birth weight), opening their mouths wide showing eager anticipation of eating food and interest in foods, sitting unassisted, bringing objects to the mouth, the ability to track a spoon and take food from the spoon, and stopping when they are full. The choice of foods to meet micronutrient needs may be less critical for formula-fed infants because formulas are fortified with those nutrients. With the introduction of solid foods, the infants' stools may have appropriate changes; they become more solid and/or have a stronger odor as new and more sugars may be added. Exposure to different textures and the process of self-feeding are important neurodevelopmental experiences for infants.

Since children will stick anything into their mouths during the "oral stage," take advantage of this and introduce the tooth brush. There are ergonomically designed toothbrushes that are comfortable and safe for infants and used to rub their gums and create the habit of oral hygiene. Children will become accustomed to having a toothbrush in their mouth. Cavities are tooth infections in baby teeth that can lead to problems with adult teeth and health issues. Early caries of childhood are caused by a misbalance of increased sugars and bacteria in the mouth and decreased saliva flow at as early as 6 months of age. Eating a healthy diet and brushing regularly will control the sugar factor and bacteria. Transmission of bacteria from the caretakers can also be prevented by avoiding sharing food or utensils with the infant.

CHAPTER 28

Diet of the Normal Child and Adolescent

For a discussion of nutrient needs for children and adolescents, see https://fnic.nal.usda.gov/lifecycle-nutrition/child-nutrition and https://medlineplus.gov/childnutrition.html.

NUTRITION ISSUES FOR TODDLERS AND OLDER CHILDREN

A healthy diet helps children grow, thrive, and learn. Learning healthy eating behaviors at an early age is an important preventive measure because of the association of diet with several chronic diseases, such as obesity, diabetes, and cardiovascular disease, which account for approximately 63% of all deaths worldwide. These diseases share risk factors that can be modified by lifestyle changes, such as eating less processed food and increasing physical activity. Diets high in fruits and vegetables together with increased physical activity reduce metabolic risk factors. The first 1,000 days of life are an important time to engage in healthy nutrition behaviors that will promote well-being. Accelerated postnatal growth in infants and young children is an important risk factor for obesity. New research is focusing on the human intestinal microbiome starting at birth, suggesting that microbes and their products may function as important modulators in the host immune system. Deviations in the intestinal microbiome have been associated with various diseases, including inflammatory bowel disease, type 2 diabetes, and colorectal cancer.

MILK

The consumption of cow's milk is ideally not introduced until approximately 1 year of age, when it is better tolerated. Low-fat (2%) or whole milk is recommended until 2 years or age, after which fat-free or 1% milk is recommended. Excessive milk intake (more than 24 oz/day) should be avoided in toddlers because larger intakes may reduce the intake of a good variety of nutritionally important solid foods and also result in iron deficiency anemia; large intakes also may contribute to excessive caloric intake.

JUICES

Juice intake for toddlers and young children should be limited to 4 oz, and juice intake for children 7-18 years of age should be limited to 8 oz/day. If juices are provided to children, they should be only natural fruit juices with no added sugar. "Added sugar" refers to sugar, fructose, and honey used in the processing and preparation. Children younger than 2 years should not have any added sugars in their diet. Young people between the ages of 2 and 18 years should get no more than 25 g of added sugar each day, according to the American Heart Association (AHA). This amount of sugar is the equivalent of just six of the white sugar packets or six teaspoons of serving sugar. The typical American child consumes approximately triple the recommended amount of added sugars. Starting in July 2018, food products sold in the United States will have to list the amount of added sugars on the Nutrition Facts Panel. Water and milk are the recommended drinks during the day. Excessive juice with poorly digested carbohydrates may produce toddler diarrhea.

GENERAL RECOMMENDATIONS

"ChooseMyPlate" by the U.S. Department of Agriculture can provide parents with a general guideline for the types of foods to be offered on a regular basis. A child should eat three meals a day and two healthy snacks. A general rule for the quantity of food to offer to a child is one tablespoon per age of each food provided per meal, with more given if the child requests. As a rule of thumb, children should not be eating more than an adult palm per serving. By 1 year of age, infants should be eating meals with the family, have a regular schedule of meals and snacks, and be encouraged to self-feed with appropriate finger foods. The "plate" image is divided into five sections: fruits, grains, vegetables, protein, and dairy (Fig. 28.1; Table 28.1). Half of the "plate" should be vegetables and fruits and the other half grains and proteins, with dairy on the side. The "plate" is simple, organized, and serves as a guide for healthy eating. A weekly recommendation for vegetable intake is also provided (see Table 28.1). Other suggestions include the following: switch to fat-free or low-fat (1%) milk after age 2 years; make at least half of the grains whole instead of refined grains; avoid oversize proportions; compare sodium (salt) in foods such as soup, bread, and frozen meals; choose foods with lower sodium content; and drink water instead of sugary drinks. After 2 years, it is recommended that the fat intake gradually be reduced to approximately 30% and not less than 20% of calories. Replace proteins from red meat with a mix of fish, chicken,

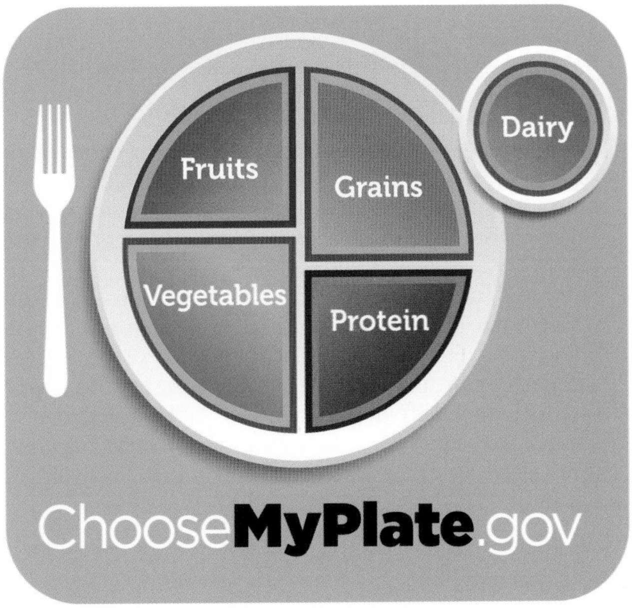

FIGURE 28.1 "ChooseMyPlate" guidelines developed by the U.S. Department of Agriculture. (From www.ChooseMyPlate.gov.)

TABLE 28.1 Recommended Weekly Vegetable Intake (in Cups)

AGE (YR)	GREEN	ORANGE	STARCH	DRY BEANS/ PEAS	OTHER*
2–3	1	½	1½	½	4
4–8	1½	1	2½	5½	4½
>9 Girls	2	1½	2½	2½	5½
>9 Boys	3	2	3	3	6½

*Including cabbage, cauliflower, green beans, lettuce, and zucchini.
From www.ChooseMyPlate.gov.

nuts, and legumes. Power struggles over eating are common between parents and toddlers. The parent's role is to decide the what, when, and where of the meals. The child's role is to decide if, what, and how much to eat.

Recommendations of a nutritious diet for a child are based on the following nutrient-dense foods:

- **Protein.** Provide seafood, lean meat and poultry, eggs, beans, peas, soy products, and unsalted nuts and seeds.
- **Fruits.** Encourage the child to eat a variety of fresh, canned, frozen, or dried fruits—rather than fruit juice. If the child drinks juice, make sure it is 100% juice without added sugars and limit his or her servings. Look for canned fruit that says it is light or packed in its own juice, meaning it is low in added sugar. Keep in mind that one-half cup of dried fruit counts as one cup-equivalent of fruit. When consumed in excess, dried fruits can contribute to extra calories.
- **Vegetables.** Serve a variety of fresh, canned, frozen, or dried vegetables. Aim to provide a variety of vegetables, including dark green, red, and orange, beans and peas, starchy and others, each week. When selecting canned or frozen vegetables, look for options lower in sodium.
- **Grains.** Choose whole grains, such as whole-wheat bread, oatmeal, popcorn, quinoa, or brown or wild rice. Limit refined grains.
- **Dairy.** Encourage the child to eat and drink fat-free or low-fat dairy products, such as milk, yogurt, cheese, or fortified soy beverages.

Aim to limit the child's calories from:

- **Added sugar.** Limit added sugars. Naturally occurring sugars, such as those in fruit, veggies, grains, meat, and milk, are not added sugars. Examples of added sugars include serving sugar, brown sugar, corn sweetener, corn syrup, honey, and others.
- **Saturated and trans-fats.** Limit saturated fats—fats that mainly come from animal sources of food, such as red meat, poultry, and full-fat dairy products. Look for ways to replace saturated fats with vegetable and nut oils, which provide essential fatty acids and vitamin E. Healthier fats are also naturally present in olives, nuts, avocados, and seafood. Limit trans-fats by avoiding foods that contain partially hydrogenated oil.

SALT INTAKE

American children's high salt intake puts them at risk for heart disease later in life. Recommended salt intake for children varies from 1,900-2,300 mg a day, depending on age. Nearly 90% of U.S. kids consume more than the recommended amount of salt for their age. Sodium-heavy breads, pizza, cold cuts, processed snacks, and soups are among the major culprits. Data in 2011–2012 showed that children ages 6-18 years consumed an average of 3,256 mg a day of salt, without including the salt added at the table.

IRON INTAKE

Iron intake may be inadequate in some children between 1 and 3 years of age in the United States. Significant iron deficiency anemia exists in some high-risk minority or low-income populations of young children. Toddlers with excessive milk intakes (>32 oz/day) and/or those who consume little meat, iron-rich green vegetables, or grains are at risk for iron deficiency. Supplemental iron is recommended if the child is iron deficient.

NUTRITION ISSUES FOR ADOLESCENTS

Teen nutrition can be a challenge. Ads for junk food and images of incredibly thin adolescents provide conflicting and unhealthy ideas about what they should eat. Girls ages 14-18 need anywhere from 1,800-2,400 calories per day, depending on their activity level and stage of development. Boys of the same age group need 2,000-3,200 calories daily. Poor eating habits may develop during adolescence. Skipped meals (especially breakfast), binge eating with friends or alone, dieting, and consumption of nutrient-poor, calorically dense foods are common problems. Excessive consumption of sugar from soda, fruit drinks, and specialty coffee and tea drinks may contribute to excess weight gain, as well as tooth decay, and it may displace other needed nutrients. Bones increase in size and mass during periods of growth in childhood and adolescence; peak bone mass is reached around age 30. The greater the peak bone mass, the longer one can delay serious bone loss with aging. Poor calcium intake during adolescence may predispose the adult to future osteoporotic hip fracture. Only 1 of 10 teenage girls and 1 of 4 teenage boys get enough calcium every day. Adolescents ages 9-18 years need 1,300 mg of calcium daily. Good sources include milk, yogurt, fortified orange juice, cheese, soybeans, and tofu.

Inadequate iron intake may result in symptoms of fatigue and iron deficiency anemia. Iron needs increase during growth spurts, which is why teens are more likely to suffer from iron deficiency anemia. Teenage girls are especially prone to anemia from menstrual blood loss. Student athletes are also vulnerable to inadequate iron intakes, severely restrictive eating patterns, and use of inappropriate nutritional and vitamin supplements. Adolescents should be counseled on specific and healthy dietary choices (see Chapter 70).

CHAPTER 29

Obesity

DEFINITIONS

Childhood obesity is an epidemic in the United States. According to the Centers for Disease Control and Prevention (CDC) in 1990, no state in the United States had a prevalence of obesity of 15% or more, but by 2010, no state had a prevalence of obesity less than 20% and a third of the states had a prevalence of 30% or higher. More than one-third of adults (37.9% of the U.S. population) are obese in the United States. **Child and adolescent obesity** was defined as a body mass index (BMI) at or above the gender-specific 95th percentile on the CDC BMI-for-age growth charts. **Childhood extreme obesity** was defined as a BMI at or above 120% of the gender-specific 95th percentile on the CDC BMI-for-age growth chart. **Child and adolescent overweight** was defined as a BMI between the 85th and 95th percentile on the CDC BMI-for-age growth charts. Childhood obesity is associated with a higher risk of premature death and disability in adulthood. Overweight and obese children are more likely to stay obese into adulthood and to develop noncommunicable diseases (NCDs) such as diabetes and cardiovascular diseases (CVDs) at a younger age. For most NCDs resulting from obesity, the risks depend partly on the age of onset and on the duration of obesity. Obese children and adolescents suffer from both short-term and long-term health consequences.

EPIDEMIOLOGY

Many obese children become obese adults, and the risk of remaining obese increases with age of onset and degree of obesity. Obesity may run in families. The main causes of excess weight in youth are similar to those in adults; they include individual causes such as behavior and rarely include genetics. Behavior causes may include dietary patterns, physical activity, inactivity, medication use, and other exposures. Obese children may exercise too little and consume too many calories. The most significant prevalence of obesity in race is in African-American (19.5%) and Hispanic children (21.9%). Individuals with lower income and/or education levels are disproportionally more likely to be obese. American society has become characterized by an environment that promotes decreased consumption of healthy food and physical inactivity. It is hard for children to make the healthy decision when they are exposed to an environment in their home, child care, school, or community that may not be ideally healthy and may be influenced by factors such as advertising, variation in licensure regulations among child-care centers, lack of safe and appealing place to play or be active, limited access to healthy affordable foods, greater availability of high-energy–dense foods and sugar sweetened beverages, increased portion sizes, and lack of breast feeding support. One early major risk factor is maternal obesity during pregnancy. Children born to obese mothers are 3-5 times more likely to be obese in childhood. Children born to women before and after bariatric surgery found that the children born after the surgery were at lower risk for obesity than the children born before the surgery. Women who gain much more weight than recommended during pregnancy have children who have a higher BMI than normal in adolescence. Small gestational age (SGA) newborns have higher risks for abnormal postnatal weight gain and diabetes; they may have long-lasting implications for health, which is possibly because of nutritional effects during the fetal life.

The preventive strategies that are most likely to succeed in a wide-scale population imply a set of very challenging goals of reducing or plateauing the rise in overweight or obesity. These strategies include approaching all the risk factors that can be modified by lifestyle changes and policy making (see Table 29.3), such as eating less processed food, increasing consumption of fruit and vegetables, and increasing physical activity. High BMI increases the risk of metabolic and CVDs and some cancers; it is the most important modifiable risk factor for diabetes.

CLINICAL MANIFESTATIONS

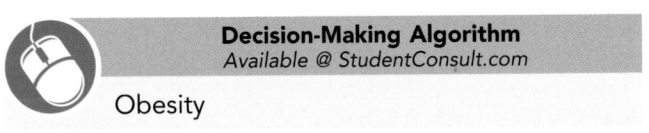

Decision-Making Algorithm
Available @ StudentConsult.com
Obesity

Obesity during childhood can have a harmful effect in a variety of ways. Complications of obesity in children and adolescents can affect every major organ system. High BMI increases the risk of metabolic and CVDs and some cancers; it is also the most important modifiable risk factor for hyperglycemia and diabetes. Children who are obese are at higher risk for (1) high blood pressure and high cholesterol, which are risk factors for CVD; (2) impaired glucose intolerance, insulin resistance, type 2 diabetes; (3) respiratory problems such as sleep apnea and asthma; (4) joint problems and musculoskeletal discomfort; (5) fatty liver disease, gallstones, and gastroesophageal reflux; (6) psychologic stress such as depression, behavioral problems, and bullying issues at school; (7) low self-esteem and low self-reported quality of life; and (8) impaired social, physical, and emotional functioning. Children who are obese are more likely to become obese adults. Adult obesity is associated with a number of serious health conditions including heart disease, metabolic syndrome, and cancer. If children were obese, obesity and these risk factors in adulthood are likely to be more severe. The history and physical examination should screen for many potential complications noted among obese patients (Table 29.1) in addition to specific diseases associated with obesity (Table 29.2). Medical complications usually are related to the degree of obesity and usually decrease in severity or resolve with weight reduction.

The diagnosis of obesity depends on the measurement of excess body fat. Actual measurement of body composition is not practical in most clinical situations. BMI may be an imperfect measure of body fat and real health risk. There are racial and ethnic differences in body fat at the same BMI level. Among children and adolescents, the definition of obesity is statistical. Children and adolescents are compared with a group of U.S. children in the 1960s to early 1990s, so the prevalence of obesity is dependent on the characteristics of the age-specific population during that period. BMI is a convenient screening tool that correlates fairly strongly with body fatness in children and adults. BMI age-specific and gender-specific percentile curves (for 2-20 year olds) allow an assessment of BMI percentile

TABLE 29.1 Complications of Obesity

COMPLICATION	EFFECTS
Psychosocial	Peer discrimination, teasing, reduced college acceptance, isolation, depression, eating disorders (binge eating), reduced job promotion*
Growth	Advance bone age, increased height, early menarche
Central nervous system	Pseudotumor cerebri
Respiratory	Obstructive sleep apnea
Cardiovascular	Hypertension, cardiac hypertrophy, arrhythmias, ischemic heart disease,* sudden death*
Orthopedic	Slipped capital femoral epiphysis, Blount disease
Metabolic	Insulin resistance, type 2 diabetes mellitus, hypertriglyceridemia, hypercholesterolemia, gout,* hepatic steatosis, polycystic ovary disease, cholelithiasis

**Complications unusual until adulthood.*

TABLE 29.2 Endocrine and Genetic Causes of Obesity

DISEASE	SYMPTOMS	LABORATORY
ENDOCRINE		
Cushing syndrome	Central obesity, hirsutism, moon face, hypertension	Dexamethasone suppression test
GH deficiency	Short stature, slow linear growth	Evoked GH response, IGF-1
Hyperinsulinism	Nesidioblastosis, pancreatic adenoma, hypoglycemia, Mauriac syndrome	Insulin level
Hypothyroidism	Short stature, weight gain, fatigue, constipation, cold intolerance, myxedema	TSH, FT_4
Pseudohypoparathyroidism	Short metacarpals, subcutaneous calcifications, dysmorphic facies, mental retardation, short stature, hypocalcemia, hyperphosphatemia	Urine cAMP after synthetic PTH infusion
GENETIC		
Alstrom syndrome	Cognitive impairment, retinitis pigmentosa, diabetes mellitus, hearing loss, hypogonadism, retinal degeneration	*ALMS1* gene
Bardet-Biedl syndrome	Retinitis pigmentosa, renal abnormalities, polydactyly, hypogonadism	*BBS1* gene
Biemond syndrome	Cognitive impairment, iris coloboma, hypogonadism, polydactyly	
Carpenter syndrome	Polydactyly, syndactyly, cranial synostosis, mental retardation	Mutations in the *RAB23* gene, located on chromosome 6 in humans
Cohen syndrome	Mid-childhood-onset obesity, short stature, prominent maxillary incisors, hypotonia, mental retardation, microcephaly, decreased visual activity	Mutations in the *VPS13B* gene (often called the *COH1* gene) at locus 8q22
Deletion 9q34	Early-onset obesity, mental retardation, brachycephaly, synophrys, prognathism, behavior and sleep disturbances	Deletion 9q34
Down syndrome	Short stature, dysmorphic facies, mental retardation	Trisomy 21
ENPP1 gene mutations	Insulin resistance, childhood obesity	Gene mutation on chromosome 6q
Fröhlich syndrome	Hypothalamic tumor	—
FTO gene polymorphism	Dysregulation of orexigenic hormone acyl-ghrelin, poor postprandial appetite suppression	Homozygous for *FTO* AA allele
Leptin or leptin receptor gene deficiency	Early-onset severe obesity, infertility (hypogonadotropic hypogonadism)	Leptin
Melanocortin 4 receptor gene mutation	Early-onset severe obesity, increased linear growth, hyperphagia, hyperinsulinemia Most common known genetic cause of obesity Homozygous worse than heterozygous	*MC4R* mutation
Prader-Willi syndrome	Neonatal hypotonia, slow infant growth, small hands and feet, mental retardation, hypogonadism, hyperphagia leading to severe obesity, paradoxically elevated ghrelin	Partial deletion of chromosome 15 or loss of paternally expressed genes
Proopiomelanocortin deficiency	Obesity, red hair, adrenal insufficiency, hyperproinsulinemia	Loss-of-function mutations of the *POMC* gene
Rapid-onset obesity with hypothalamic dysfunction, hypoventilation, and autonomic dysregulation	Often confused with congenital central hypoventilation syndrome, presentation ≥1.5 years with weight gain, hyperphagia, hypoventilation, cardiac arrest, central diabetes insipidus, hypothyroidism, growth hormone deficiency, pain insensitivity, hypothermia, precocious puberty, neural crest tumors	Unknown genes May be a paraneoplastic disorder
Turner syndrome	Ovarian dysgenesis, lymphedema, web neck, short stature, cognitive impairment	XO chromosome

cAMP, Cyclic adenosine monophosphate; *FT_4*, free thyroxine; *GH*, growth hormone; *IGF*, insulin-like growth factor; *PTH*, parathyroid hormone; *TSH*, thyroid-stimulating hormone.

From Gahagan S. Overweight and obesity. In: Kliegman RM, Stanton BF, St. Geme JW, Schor NF, eds. Nelson Textbook of Pediatrics. *20th ed. Philadelphia: Elsevier; 2016. Table 47.1.*

(available online at http://www.cdc.gov/growthcharts). Table 29.3 provides BMI interpretation guidelines. For children younger than 2 years of age, weight-for-length measurements greater than 95th percentile may indicate overweight and warrant further assessment. Child and adolescent obesity was defined as a BMI at or above the gender-specific 95th percentile on the CDC BMI-for-age growth charts. A BMI for age and gender above the 95th percentile is strongly associated with excessive body fat and co-morbidities. Extreme obesity was defined as a BMI at or above 120% of the gender-specific 95th percentile on the CDC BMI-for-age growth chart.

ASSESSMENT

Early recognition of excessive rates of weight gain, overweight, or obesity in children is essential because the earlier the interventions, the more likely they are to be successful.

Routine evaluation at well child visits should include the following:

1. **Anthropometric data**, including weight, height, and calculation of BMI. Data should be plotted on age-appropriate and gender-appropriate growth charts and assessed for BMI trends (see Table 29.3).
2. **Dietary and physical activity history** (Table 29.4). Assess patterns and potential targets for behavioral change.
3. **Physical examination.** Assess blood pressure, adiposity distribution (central versus generalized), markers of co-morbidities (acanthosis nigricans, hirsutism, hepatomegaly, orthopedic abnormalities), and physical stigmata of a genetic syndrome (explains fewer than 5% of cases).
4. **Laboratory studies.** These are generally reserved for children who are obese (BMI >95th percentile), who have evidence of co-morbidities, or both. All 9-11 year olds should be screened for high cholesterol levels. Other useful laboratory tests may include hemoglobin A1c, fasting lipid profile, fasting glucose levels, liver function tests, and thyroid function tests (if there is a faster increase in weight than height).

PREVENTION

Obesity and its associated co-morbidities have emerged as a major health problem. In fact, obese children are becoming affected by diseases and health problems previously observed only in adults. The main reason to target childhood obesity is that many obese children have a high probability to become an obese adult with all the short- and long-term co-morbidities, and it is more challenging for adults to lose excess weight if they are obese. Prevention is the key to success for obesity control. Behavioral and lifestyle modifications are the primary tools for reducing obesity. However, if the environment contributes to the unhealthy eating practices and sedentary lifestyle, strategies and interventions relying only on individual "self-control" will not be very effective. Children are less equipped to make informed choices about what is healthy and what is not, making it imperative to concentrate on modifying the environment. Prevention of childhood obesity on the other hand can be more rewarding, providing better chances for reducing long-term complications. There are three levels of prevention in dealing with childhood obesity: (1) primordial prevention as it deals with keeping a healthy weight and a normal BMI through childhood and into teens; (2) primary prevention aiming to prevent overweight children from becoming obese; and (3) secondary prevention directed toward the treatment of obesity so as to reduce the co-morbidities and reverse overweight and obesity if possible. The approach to therapy and aggressiveness of treatment should be based on risk factors including age, severity of overweight and obesity and co-morbidities, and family history and support. The primary goal for all children with uncomplicated obesity and fast-rising weight-for-height is to achieve a healthy balance of energy consumption as a caloric intake, **healthy eating, with the number of calories used with the activities and activity**

TABLE 29.3 Body Mass Index Interpretation

BMI/AGE PERCENTILE	INTERPRETATION
<5th	Underweight
5th-85th	Normal
85th-95th	Overweight
>95th	Obese

BMI, Body mass index.
From *www.cdc.gov/healthyweight.*

TABLE 29.4 Eating and Activity Habits for Overweight/Obesity Prevention

	ACTIVITIES FOR OVERWEIGHT/OBESITY PREVENTION
INDIVIDUAL	1. Be physically active >1 hr per day 2. Limit screen time (television, computer games/Internet, video games) to <1–2 hr per day (no TV for child <2 yr of age) 3. Consume five or more servings of fruits and vegetables per day 4. Minimize consumption of sugar-sweetened beverages 5. Consume a healthy breakfast every day
FAMILY	1. Eat at table, as a family, at least five to six times per week 2. Prepare more meals at home rather than purchasing restaurant food 3. Allow child to self-regulate his or her meals and avoid overly restrictive feeding behaviors 4. Do not reward children with food or drinks 5. Have only healthy foods available for snacking 6. Encourage outdoor activity
COMMUNITY	Schools 1. Serve healthy foods 2. Limit what is available in vending machines 3. Have physical activity daily 4. Have outdoor recess daily 5. Teach healthy eating Health Care Providers 1. Take a nutrition history 2. Speak to patients about healthy weight and good nutrition 3. Advise exercise
GOVERNMENT	1. Increase access to healthy food and eliminate food deserts 2. Regulate food ads or serving sizes 3. Add more sidewalks and parks 4. Emphasize safety

TABLE 29.5 Setting Explicit Goals to Prevent or Treat Obesity

FIGHT OBESITY EFFECTIVELY	AMBIGUOUS GOALS	SPECIFIC GOALS
Keep it simple	Walk or bike more	Walk or bike to school 2 days a week
Countable goals/unambiguous	Watch less TV	Watch no TV on school days
Two short-term goals/time	—	—
Be able to count	Decrease size of serving	Small bowls (parent palm)
Aim to change behaviors	—	Avoid eating from the box
Do not focus on consumption of carbohydrates, fat, protein	Decrease to 20 g of fat	Eat fish once a week
Focus on specific categories	Decrease sugars	Avoid sweetened foods
Focus on healthier preparation methods	—	Avoid frying
Focus on eating patterns	—	Avoid double dinner
Focus on portion size	—	Portion parent's palm size
Eating fast food	Eat less junk food	Limit trips to McDonalds to once a week
Sweetened beverages	Avoid soda/juices	No soda or juices
Healthy beverages	—	Drink only milk or water
Fruits	Buy fewer juices	Have no juices in the refrigerator
	Increase eating fruits	Keep a bowl of fruits in the kitchen
Vegetables	Increase eating veggies	Have a bowl of veggies in the refrigerator
		Cooperation, competition, and social interaction such as building a house of veggies
Physical activities	Walk more	Family hikes every Sunday
		Specific activity time for activities and sedentary behavior
	Increase walking from school	Parents picking up from school 2 days a week

patterns. For children with a secondary complication, improvement of the complication is an important goal. Childhood and adolescent obesity treatment programs can lead to sustained weight loss and decreases in BMI when treatment focuses on behavioral changes and is family centered. Concurrent changes in dietary and physical activity patterns are most likely to provide success (Table 29.5). All of the previously mentioned strategies should be put into practice sequentially from the perinatal period to adolescence. In the **perinatal** period this includes adequate prenatal nutrition with optimal maternal weight gain, good blood sugar control in diabetes, and postpartum weight loss with healthy nutrition and exercises. During **infancy**, early initiation of breast feeding, exclusive breast feeding for 6 months followed by inclusion of solid foods, providing a balanced diet with avoidance of unhealthy calorie-rich snacks, and close monitoring of weight gain should be emphasized. The transition to complementary and table foods and the importance of regularly scheduled meals and snacks, versus grazing behavior, should be emphasized. During the **preschool** age period, putting these strategies into practice includes providing nutritional education and guidance to parents and children so as to develop healthy eating practices, offering healthy food preferences by giving early experiences of different food and flavors, and following closely the rate of weight gain to prevent early adiposity rebound. In school-aged children, this includes monitoring both weight and height, preventing excessive prepubertal adiposity, providing nutritional counseling, and emphasizing daily physical activity should be emphasized. In **adolescence** preventing the increase in weight after a growth spurt, maintaining healthy eating behavior, and reinforcing the need for daily exercise are most important. Furthermore, advocate for specific and attainable goal settings and positive reinforcement of target behavior. The **traffic light diet** may be useful in promoting nutritional goals with the following categories: (1) green-GO includes foods that are low in calories and can be eaten without any restrictions; (2) yellow-CAUTION includes food items with moderate to high calorie content that can be eaten only in moderation; and (3) Red-STOP includes high-calorie food items that should be avoided or eaten rarely. Physical activity is the key component for prevention and management of obesity. Preschool children require unstructured activities and thus will benefit from outdoor play and games. On the other hand, school children and adolescents require at least 60 minutes of daily physical activities, so instead of recommending a wide open schedule to walk or bike to school more, suggest walking or biking to school two or more days a week. Rather than recommending that a child watch less television, suggest watching no television on school days. It is important to keep it simple and set one or two short-term goals at a time. In addition, behavioral risk factors need to be identified, such as going to get fast food when family life gets hectic. Helping the family think of fast, healthy alternatives is important.

Age-appropriate **portion sizes** for meals and snacks should be encouraged. Children should be taught to recognize hunger and satiety cues, guided by reasonable portions and healthy food choices by parents. Smaller bowls should be used; children should never eat directly from a bag or box. No juices or soda should be the rule. Children should never be forced to eat when they are not willing, and overemphasis on food as a reward should be avoided. ChooseMyPlate.gov by the U.S. Department of Agriculture can provide parents with a general guideline for the types of foods to be offered on a regular basis, including fruits, vegetables, grains, protein, and dairy.

The importance of physical activity should be emphasized. For some children, organized sports and school-based activities provide opportunities for vigorous activity and fun, whereas for others a focus on activities of daily living, such as increased walking, using stairs, and more active play may be better received. Children should have an hour of activity a day. Time spent in **sedentary behavior**, such as television viewing and video/computer games, should be limited. Television in children's rooms is associated with more television time and with higher rates of overweight, and the risks of this practice should be discussed with parents. Clinicians may need to help families identify alternatives to sedentary activities, especially for families with deterrents to activity, such as unsafe neighborhoods or lack of supervision after school. Obesity is challenging to treat and can cause significant medical and psychosocial issues for young children and adolescents (see Table 29.1).

We as a society need to ensure the convenient access to healthy food and safe places for physical activities. Preschools, schools, clubs, and social gathering places need to curb available junk food and sodas and provide healthy and nutritious foods for children and adolescents. Fast food restaurants need to continue to offer healthy menu items and strive to reduce calories and fat in all of the products they provide. Communities need to work to provide playgrounds, sports activities, bike trails, and other opportunities for physical activities for all children, especially those in certain ethnic groups known to be at the highest risk for obesity.

TREATMENT

More aggressive therapies are considered only for those who have not responded to other interventions. The initial interventions include a systematic approach that promotes multidisciplinary brief, office-based interventions for obese children and promotes reducing weight. Before enrolling any patient in a weight-loss program, the clinician must have a clear idea of that individual's expectations. Patients with unrealistic expectations should not be enrolled until these are changed to realistic and attainable goals. Using the pneumonic described, the clinician should guide the patient who seeks weight reduction to create **SMART** goals: Specific, Measurable, Attainable, Realistic, and Timely.

Pediatric experiences with drugs are limited. Anorectic drugs are not recommended for routine use, and the efficiency and safety of these drugs have to be established by controlled clinical trial.

In the context of a general lack of effective tools for primary prevention or behavioral treatment of obesity, **surgical treatment** may be advocated as a preferred and cost-effective solution for certain children and adolescents. However, the role of bariatric surgery in the treatment of obese children or adolescents is controversial. The concerns about surgery to treat obesity in young populations include whether or not surgery is cost-effective, how to ensure healthy growth through to adulthood, what support services are needed after surgery, compliance with the postoperative nutrition regimen, and attendance at appointments for long-term follow-up and care. There is very limited evidence available to adequately estimate long-term safety, effectiveness, cost-effectiveness, or durability of bariatric surgery in growing children. Although based on methodologically limited and underpowered studies, the existing evidence suggests that bariatric surgery in severely obese adolescents results in significant weight loss and improvements in comorbidities and quality of life. Postoperative complications (both physical and psychological), compliance, and follow-up may be more problematic in adolescents than adults, and long-term data on safety, effectiveness, and cost remain largely unavailable.

CHAPTER 30

Pediatric Undernutrition

Pediatric undernutrition is usually the result of inadequate food supply, access, or utilization; poor access to health and sanitation; chronic health conditions; and/or inappropriate feeding or child-care practices. The greatest risk of undernutrition is in utero through age 2 years. Various guidelines can be used to classify pediatric malnutrition (Table 30.1). International references are established that allow normalization of anthropometric measures in terms of *z* scores. Other measurements include height and weight for age, weight for height, BMI, and mid-upper arm circumference. The greatest consequence of undernutrition is death, but significant intellectual and physical disability exists in many who survive.

Protein-energy malnutrition (PEM) is a spectrum of conditions caused by varying levels of protein and calorie deficiencies. Primary PEM is caused by social or economic factors that result in a lack of food. Secondary PEM occurs in children with various conditions associated with increased caloric requirements (infection, trauma, cancer; Fig. 30.1), increased caloric loss (malabsorption), reduced caloric intake (anorexia, cancer, oral intake restriction, social factors), or a combination of these three variables. Protein and calorie malnutrition may be associated with other nutrient deficiencies, which may be evident on physical examination (Table 30.2).

FAILURE TO THRIVE

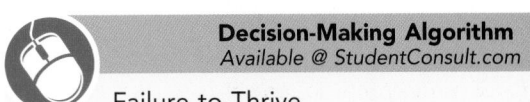

Decision-Making Algorithm
Available @ StudentConsult.com
Failure to Thrive

Pediatric **undernutrition** in the United States is often termed **failure to thrive** and describes circumstances in which a child fails to gain weight appropriately or, in more severe cases, experiences failure in linear growth or head circumference. The terms **organic** and **nonorganic** failure to thrive have lost favor in recognition of the frequent interplay between underlying medical conditions that may cause maladaptive behaviors. Similarly, social and behavioral factors that initially may have been associated with feeding problems (see Chapter 21) and poor growth may also be associated with medical problems, including frequent minor acute illnesses.

TABLE 30.1 Definitions of Malnutrition

CLASSIFICATION	DEFINITION	GRADING	
Gomez	Weight below % median WFA	Mild (grade 1)	75-90% WFA
		Moderate (grade 2)	60-74% WFA
		Severe (grade 3)	<60% WFA
Waterlow	*z* scores (SD) below median WFH	Mild	80-90% WFH
		Moderate	70-80% WFH
		Severe	<70% WFH
WHO (wasting)	*z* scores (SD) below median WFH	Moderate	−3 ≤ *z* score <−2
		Severe	*z* score <−3
WHO (stunting)	*z* scores (SD) below median HFA	Moderate	−3 ≤ *z*-score <−2
		Severe	*z* score <−3
Kanawati	MUAC divided by occipitofrontal head circumference	Mild	<0.31
		Moderate	<0.28
		Severe	<0.25
Cole	*z* scores of BMI for age	Grade 1	BMI for age *z* score <−1
		Grade 2	BMI for age *z* score <−2
		Grade 3	BMI for age *z* score <−3

BMI, Body mass index; *HFA*, height for age; *MUAC*, mid-upper arm circumference; *NCHS*, U.S. National Center for Health Statistics; *SD*, standard deviation; *WFA*, weight for age; *WFH*, weight for height; *WHO*, World Health Organization.
From Grover Z, Ee LC. Protein energy malnutrition. Pediatr Clin North Am. *2009;56:1055–1068.*

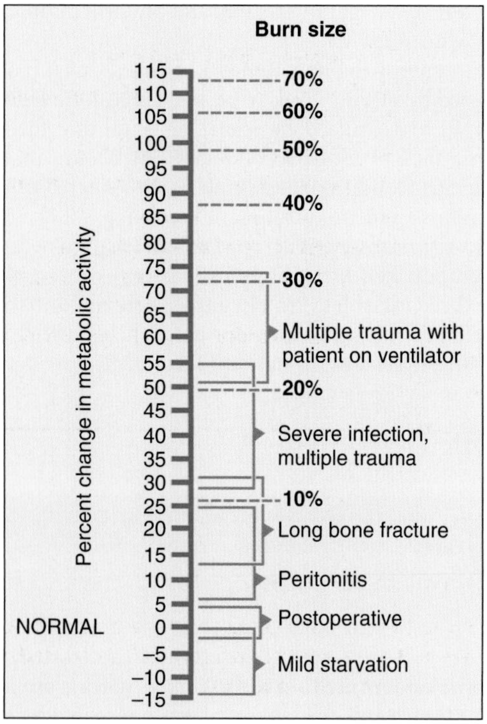

FIGURE 30.1 Increased energy needs with stress. (Modified from Wilmore D. *The Metabolic Management of the Critically Ill.* New York: Plenum Publishing; 1977. Revised in Walker W, Watkins J, eds. *Nutrition in Pediatrics: Basic Science and Clinical Application.* Boston: Little, Brown; 1985.)

MARASMUS

Marasmus results from the body's physiologic response to inadequate calories and nutrients. Loss of muscle mass and subcutaneous fat stores can be confirmed by inspection or palpation and quantified by anthropometric measurements. The head may appear large but generally is proportional to the body length. Edema usually is absent. The skin is dry and thin, and the hair may be thin, sparse, and easily pulled out. Marasmic children may be apathetic and weak and may be irritable when touched. Bradycardia and hypothermia signify severe and life-threatening malnutrition. Inappropriate or inadequate weaning practices and chronic diarrhea are common findings in developing countries. **Stunting** (impaired linear growth) results from a combination of malnutrition, especially micronutrients, and recurrent infections.

KWASHIORKOR

Kwashiorkor results from inadequate protein intake in the presence of fair to good caloric intake. The hypoalbuminemic state results in pitting edema that starts in the lower extremities and ascends with increasing severity. Other factors, such as acute infection, toxins, and possibly specific micronutrient or amino acid imbalances, are likely to contribute to the etiology. The major **clinical manifestation** of kwashiorkor is that the body weight is near normal for age; weight alone does not accurately reflect the nutritional status because of edema. **Physical examination** reveals a relative maintenance of subcutaneous adipose tissue and a marked atrophy of muscle mass. Edema varies from a minor pitting of the dorsum of the foot to generalized edema with involvement of the eyelids and scrotum. The hair is sparse, easily plucked, and appears dull brown, red, or yellow-white. Nutritional repletion restores hair

TABLE 30.2 Physical Signs of Nutritional Deficiency Disorders

SYSTEM	SIGN	DEFICIENCY
General appearance	Reduced weight for height	Calories
Skin and hair	Pallor	Anemias (iron, vitamin B_{12}, vitamin E, folate, and copper)
	Edema	Protein, thiamine
	Nasolabial seborrhea	Calories, protein, vitamin B_6, niacin, riboflavin
	Dermatitis	Riboflavin, essential fatty acids, biotin
	Photosensitivity dermatitis	Niacin
	Acrodermatitis	Zinc
	Follicular hyperkeratosis (sandpaper-like)	Vitamin A
	Depigmented skin	Calories, protein
	Purpura	Vitamins C, K
	Scrotal, vulval dermatitis	Riboflavin
	Alopecia	Zinc, biotin, protein
	Depigmented, dull hair, easily pluckable	Protein, calories, copper
Subcutaneous tissue	Decreased	Calories
Eye (vision)	Adaptation to dark	Vitamins A, E, zinc
	Color discrimination	Vitamin A
	Bitot spots, xerophthalmia, keratomalacia	Vitamin A
	Conjunctival pallor	Nutritional anemias
	Fundal capillary microaneurysms	Vitamin C
Face, mouth, and neck	Moon facies	Kwashiorkor
	Simian facies	Marasmus
	Angular stomatitis	Riboflavin, iron
	Cheilosis	Vitamins B_6, niacin, riboflavin
	Bleeding gums	Vitamins C, K
	Atrophic papillae	Riboflavin, iron, niacin, folate, vitamin B_{12}
	Smooth tongue	Iron
	Red tongue (glossitis)	Vitamins B_6, B_{12}, niacin, riboflavin, folate
	Parotid swelling	Protein
	Caries	Fluoride
	Anosmia	Vitamins A, B_{12}, zinc
	Hypogeusia	Vitamin A, zinc
	Goiter	Iodine
Cardiovascular	Heart failure	Thiamine, selenium, nutritional anemias
Genital	Hypogonadism	Zinc
Skeletal	Costochondral beading	Vitamins D, C
	Subperiosteal hemorrhage	Vitamin C, copper
	Cranial bossing	Vitamin D
	Wide fontanel	Vitamin D
	Epiphyseal enlargement	Vitamin D
	Craniotabes	Vitamin D, calcium
	Tender bones	Vitamin C
	Tender calves	Thiamine, selenium, vitamin C
	Spoon-shaped nails (koilonychia)	Iron
	Transverse nail line	Protein
Neurologic	Sensory, motor neuropathy	Thiamine, vitamins E, B_6, B_{12}
	Ataxia, areflexia	Vitamin E
	Ophthalmoplegia	Vitamin E, thiamine
	Tetany	Vitamin D, Ca^{2+}, Mg^{2+}
	Retardation	Iodine, niacin
	Dementia, delirium	Vitamin E, niacin, thiamine
	Poor position sense, ataxia	Thiamine, vitamin B_{12}

color, leaving a band of hair with altered pigmentation followed by a band with normal pigmentation (flag sign). Skin changes are common and range from hyperpigmented hyperkeratosis to an erythematous macular rash (pellagroid) on the trunk and extremities. In the most severe form of kwashiorkor, a superficial desquamation occurs over pressure surfaces ("flaky paint" rash). Angular cheilosis, atrophy of the filiform papillae of the tongue, and monilial stomatitis are common. Enlarged parotid glands and facial edema result in moon facies; apathy and disinterest in eating are typical of kwashiorkor. Examination of the abdomen may reveal an enlarged, soft liver with an indefinite edge. Lymph node and tonsils are commonly atrophic. Chest examination may reveal basilar rales. The abdomen is distended, and bowel sounds tend to be hypoactive.

MIXED MARASMUS-KWASHIORKOR

These children often have concurrent wasting and edema in addition to stunting. These children exhibit features of dermatitis, neurologic abnormalities, and fatty liver.

TREATMENT OF MALNUTRITION

The basal metabolic rate and immediate nutrient needs decrease in cases of malnutrition. When nutrients are provided, the metabolic rate increases, stimulating anabolism and increasing nutrient requirements. The body of the malnourished child may have compensated for micronutrient deficiencies with lower metabolic and growth rates, and refeeding may unmask these deficiencies. Nutritional rehabilitation should be initiated and advanced *slowly* to minimize these complications. The initial approach involves correction of dehydration and antiinfective (bacteria, parasites) therapy if indicated. Oral rehydration is recommended over intravenous fluid to avoid excessive fluid and solute load and resultant heart or renal failure.

When nutritional rehabilitation is initiated, calories can be safely started at 20% above the child's recent intake. If no estimate of the caloric intake is available, 50-75% of the normal energy requirement is safe. High-calorie oral solutions or ready-to-use therapeutic foods (a mixture of powdered milk, peanuts, sugar, vitamins, and minerals) are frequently used in developing countries. Nutritional rehabilitation can be complicated by **refeeding syndrome**, which is characterized by fluid retention, hypophosphatemia, hypomagnesemia, and hypokalemia. Careful monitoring of laboratory values and clinical status with severe malnutrition is essential.

When nutritional rehabilitation has begun, caloric intake can be increased 10-20% per day, monitoring for electrolyte imbalances, poor cardiac function, edema, or feeding intolerance. If any of these occurs, further caloric increases are not made until the child's status stabilizes. Caloric intake is increased until appropriate regrowth or catch-up growth is initiated. Catch-up growth refers to gaining weight at greater than 50th percentile for age and may require 150% or more of the recommended calories for an age-matched, well-nourished child. A general rule of thumb for infants and children up to 3 years of age is to provide 100-120 kcal/kg based on *ideal* weight for height. Protein needs also are increased as anabolism begins and are provided in proportion to the caloric intake. Vitamin and mineral intake in excess of the daily recommended intake is provided to account for the increased requirements; this is frequently accomplished by giving an age-appropriate daily multiple vitamin with other individual micronutrient supplements as warranted by history, physical examination, or laboratory studies. Iron supplements are not recommended during the acute rehabilitation phase, especially for children with kwashiorkor, for whom ferritin levels are often high. Additional iron may pose an oxidative stress; iron supplementation at this time is associated with higher morbidity and mortality.

In most cases, cow's milk–based formulas are tolerated and provide an appropriate mix of nutrients. Other easily digested foods, appropriate for the age, also may be introduced slowly. If feeding intolerance occurs, lactose-free or semi-elemental formulas should be considered.

COMPLICATIONS OF MALNUTRITION

Malnourished children are more susceptible to **infection,** especially sepsis, pneumonia, and gastroenteritis. Hypoglycemia is common after periods of severe fasting but may also be a sign of sepsis. Hypothermia may signify infection or, with bradycardia, may signify a decreased metabolic rate to conserve energy. Bradycardia and poor cardiac output predispose the malnourished child to heart failure, which is exacerbated by acute fluid or solute loads. **Micronutrient deficiencies** also can complicate malnutrition. Vitamin A and zinc deficiencies are common in the developing world and are an important cause of altered immune response and increased morbidity and mortality. Depending on the age at onset and the duration of the malnutrition, malnourished children may have permanent growth stunting (from malnutrition in utero, infancy, or adolescence) and delayed development (from malnutrition in infancy or adolescence). Environmental (social) deprivation may interact with the effects of the malnutrition to impair further development and cognitive function.

CHAPTER 31

Vitamin and Mineral Deficiencies

Micronutrients include vitamins and trace elements. In industrialized societies, frank clinical deficiencies are unusual in healthy children, but they can and do occur in certain high-risk circumstances. Risk factors include diets that are consistently limited in variety (especially with the exclusion of entire food groups), malabsorption syndromes, and conditions causing high physiologic requirements. Various common etiologies of vitamin and nutrient deficiency states are highlighted in Table 31.1, and characteristics of vitamin deficiencies are outlined in Table 31.2. Treatment is noted in Table 31.3.

WATER-SOLUBLE VITAMINS

Water-soluble vitamins are not *stored* in the body except for vitamin B_{12}; intake therefore alters tissue levels. Absorption from the diet is usually high, and the compounds exchange readily between intracellular and extracellular fluids; excretion is via the urine. Water-soluble vitamins typically function as coenzymes in energy, protein, amino acid, and nucleic acid metabolism; as cosubstrates in enzymatic reactions; and as structural components.

Ascorbic Acid

Decision-Making Algorithm
Available @ StudentConsult.com
Anemia

The principal forms of vitamin C are ascorbic acid and the oxidized form, dehydroascorbic acid. Ascorbic acid accelerates hydroxylation reactions in many biosynthetic reactions, including hydroxylation of proline in the formation of collagen. The needs of full-term infants for ascorbic acid and dehydroascorbic acid are calculated by estimating the availability in human milk.

A deficiency of ascorbic acid results in the clinical manifestation of **scurvy**. Infantile scurvy is manifested by irritability, bone tenderness with swelling, and pseudoparalysis of the legs. The disease may occur if infants are fed unsupplemented cow's milk in the first year of life or if the diet is devoid of fruits and vegetables. Subperiosteal hemorrhage, bleeding gums and petechiae, hyperkeratosis of hair follicles, and a succession of mental changes characterize the progression of the illness. Anemia secondary to bleeding, decreased iron absorption, or abnormal folate metabolism are also seen in chronic scurvy. Treatment is noted in Table 31.3.

TABLE 31.1 Etiology of Vitamin and Nutrient Deficiency States

ETIOLOGY	DEFICIENCY
DIET	
Vegans (strict)	Protein, vitamins B_{12}, D, riboflavin, iron
Breast fed infant	Vitamins K, D
Cow's milk–fed infant	Iron
Bulimia, anorexia nervosa	Electrolytes, other deficiencies
Parenteral alimentation	Essential fatty acids, trace elements
Alcoholism	Calories, vitamin B_1, B_6, folate
MEDICAL PROBLEMS	
Malabsorption syndromes	Vitamins A, D, E, K, zinc, essential fatty acids
Cholestasis	Vitamins E, D, K, A, zinc, essential fatty acids
MEDICATIONS	
Sulfonamides	Folate
Phenytoin, phenobarbital	Vitamins D, K, folate
Mineral oil	Vitamins A, D, E, K
Antibiotics	Vitamin K
Isoniazid	Vitamin B_6
Antacids	Iron, phosphate, calcium
Digitalis	Magnesium, calcium
Penicillamine	Vitamin B_6
SPECIFIC MECHANISMS	
Transcobalamin II or intrinsic factor deficiency	Vitamin B_{12}
Other digestive enzyme	Carbohydrate, fat, protein deficiencies
Menkes kinky hair syndrome	Copper
Acrodermatitis enteropathica	Zinc
Reduced exposure to direct sunlight	Vitamin D

B Vitamins

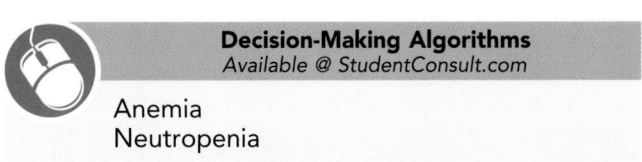

Decision-Making Algorithms
Available @ StudentConsult.com

Anemia
Neutropenia

The B vitamins thiamine, riboflavin, and niacin are routinely added to enriched grain products; deficiencies in normal hosts are rare in the United States. Levels from human milk reflect maternal intake, and deficiency can develop in breast fed infants of deficient mothers.

Thiamine

Vitamin B_1 functions as a coenzyme in biochemical reactions related to carbohydrate metabolism, decarboxylation of α-ketoacids and pyruvate, and transketolase reactions of the pentose pathway. Thiamine also is involved in the decarboxylation of branched-chain amino acids. Thiamine is lost during milk pasteurization and sterilization.

Thiamine deficiency occurs in alcoholics and has been reported in adolescents who have undergone bariatric surgery for severe obesity. **Infantile beriberi** occurs between 1 and 4 months of age in breast fed infants whose mothers have a thiamine deficiency (alcoholism), in infants with protein-calorie malnutrition, in infants receiving unsupplemented hyperalimentation fluid, and in infants receiving boiled milk. Acute **wet beriberi** with cardiac symptoms and signs predominates in infantile beriberi. Anorexia, apathy, vomiting, restlessness, and pallor progress to dyspnea, cyanosis, and death from heart failure. Infants with beriberi have a characteristic aphonic cry; they appear to be crying, but no sound is uttered. Other signs include peripheral neuropathy and paresthesias. For treatment see Table 31.3.

Riboflavin

Vitamin B_2 is a constituent of two coenzymes, riboflavin 5′-phosphate and flavin-adenine dinucleotide, essential components of glutathione reductase and xanthine oxidase, which are involved in electron transport. A deficiency of riboflavin affects glucose, fatty acid, and amino acid metabolism. Riboflavin and its phosphate are decomposed by exposure to light and by strong alkaline solutions.

Ariboflavinosis is characterized by an angular stomatitis; glossitis; cheilosis; seborrheic dermatitis around the nose and mouth; and eye changes that include reduced tearing, photophobia, corneal vascularization, and the formation of cataracts. Subclinical riboflavin deficiencies have been found in diabetic subjects, children in families with low socioeconomic status, children with chronic cardiac disease, and infants undergoing prolonged phototherapy for hyperbilirubinemia.

Niacin

Niacin consists of the compounds nicotinic acid and nicotinamide (niacinamide). Nicotinamide, the predominant form of the vitamin, functions as a component of the coenzymes nicotinamide adenine dinucleotide (NAD) and nicotinamide adenine dinucleotide phosphate (NADP). Niacin is involved in multiple metabolic processes, including fat synthesis, intracellular respiratory metabolism, and glycolysis.

In determining the needs for niacin, the content of tryptophan in the diet must be considered because tryptophan is converted to niacin. Niacin is stable in foods and withstands heating and prolonged storage. Approximately 70% of the total niacin equivalents in human milk are derived from tryptophan. **Pellagra**, or niacin deficiency disease, is characterized by weakness, lassitude, dermatitis, photosensitivity, inflammation of mucous membranes, diarrhea, vomiting, dysphagia, and, in severe cases, dementia.

Vitamin B_6

Vitamin B_6 refers to three naturally occurring pyridines: pyridoxine (pyridoxol), pyridoxal, and pyridoxamine. The phosphates of the latter two pyridines are metabolically and functionally related and are converted in the liver to the coenzyme form, pyridoxal phosphate. The metabolic functions of vitamin B_6 include interconversion reactions of amino acids, conversion of tryptophan to niacin and serotonin, metabolic reactions in

TABLE 31.2 Characteristics of Vitamin Deficiencies

VITAMIN	PURPOSE	DEFICIENCY	COMMENTS	SOURCE
WATER SOLUBLE				
Thiamine (B_1)	Coenzyme in ketoacid decarboxylation (e.g., pyruvate→acetyl-CoA transketolase reaction)	*Beriberi:* polyneuropathy, calf tenderness, heart failure, edema, ophthalmoplegia	Inborn errors of lactate metabolism; boiling milk destroys B_1	Liver, meat, milk, cereals, nuts, legumes
Riboflavin (B_2)	FAD coenzyme in oxidation-reduction reactions	Anorexia, mucositis, anemia, cheilosis, nasolabial seborrhea	Photosensitizer	Milk, cheese, liver, meat, eggs, whole grains, green leafy vegetables
Niacin (B_3)	NAD coenzyme in oxidation-reduction reactions	*Pellagra:* photosensitivity, dermatitis, dementia, diarrhea, death	Tryptophan is a precursor	Meat, fish, liver, whole grains, green leafy vegetables
Pyridoxine (B_6)	Cofactor in amino acid metabolism	Seizures, hyperacusis, microcytic anemia, nasolabial seborrhea, neuropathy	Dependency state: deficiency secondary to drugs	Meat, liver, whole grains, peanuts, soybeans
Pantothenic acid	CoA in Krebs cycle	None reported	—	Meat, vegetables
Biotin	Cofactor in carboxylase reactions of amino acids	Alopecia, dermatitis, hypotonia, death	Bowel resection, inborn error of metabolism,* and ingestion of raw eggs	Yeast, meats; made by intestinal flora
B_{12}	Coenzyme for 5-methyltetrahydrofolate formation; DNA synthesis	Megaloblastic anemia, peripheral neuropathy, posterior lateral spinal column disease, vitiligo	Vegans; fish tapeworm; short gut syndrome; transcobalamin or intrinsic factor deficiencies	Meat, fish, cheese, eggs
Folate	DNA synthesis	Megaloblastic anemia; neural tube defects	Goat milk deficient; drug antagonists; heat inactivates	Liver, greens, vegetables, cereals, cheese
Ascorbic acid (C)	Reducing agent; collagen metabolism	*Scurvy:* irritability, purpura, bleeding gums, periosteal hemorrhage, aching bones	May improve tyrosine metabolism in preterm infants	Citrus fruits, green vegetables; cooking destroys it
FAT SOLUBLE				
A	Epithelial cell integrity; vision	Night blindness, xerophthalmia, Bitot spots, follicular hyperkeratosis; immune defects	Common with protein-calorie malnutrition; malabsorption	Liver, milk, eggs, green and yellow vegetables, fruits
D	Maintain serum calcium, phosphorus levels	*Rickets:* reduced bone mineralization	Prohormone of 25- and 1,25-vitamin D	Fortified milk, cheese, liver; sunlight
E	Antioxidant	Hemolysis in preterm infants; areflexia, ataxia, ophthalmoplegia	May benefit patients with G6PD deficiency	Seeds, vegetables, germ oils, grains
K	Posttranslation carboxylation of clotting factors II, VII, IX, X and proteins C, S	Prolonged prothrombin time; hemorrhage; elevated protein induced in vitamin K absence (PIVKA)	Malabsorption; breast fed infants	Liver, green vegetables; made by intestinal flora

**Biotinidase deficiency.*

CoA, Coenzyme A; *FAD,* flavin adenine dinucleotide; *G6PD,* glucose-6-phosphate dehydrogenase; *NAD,* nicotinamide adenine dinucleotide.

the brain, carbohydrate metabolism, immune development, and the biosynthesis of heme and prostaglandins. The pyridoxal and pyridoxamine forms of the vitamin are destroyed by heat; heat treatment was responsible for vitamin B_6 deficiency and seizures in infants fed improperly processed formulas. Goat's milk is deficient in vitamin B_6.

Dietary deprivation or malabsorption of vitamin B_6 in children results in hypochromic microcytic anemia, vomiting, diarrhea, failure to thrive, listlessness, hyperirritability, and seizures. Children receiving isoniazid or penicillamine may require additional vitamin B_6 because the drug binds to the vitamin. Vitamin B_6 is unusual as a water-soluble vitamin, in that very large doses (≥500 mg/day) have been associated with a sensory neuropathy.

Folate

Decision-Making Algorithms
Available @ StudentConsult.com

Anemia
Neutropenia

A variety of chemical forms of folate are nutritionally active. Folate functions in transport of single-carbon fragments in synthesis of nucleic acids and for normal metabolism of certain amino acids and in conversion of homocysteine to methionine. Food sources include green leafy vegetables, oranges, and whole

TABLE 31.3 Treatment of Vitamin Deficiencies

	CLINICAL FEATURES	SUGGESTED DOSES
Vitamin A	Severe deficiency with xerophthalmia	Infants: 7,500-15,000 U/day IM, followed by oral 5,000-10,000 U/day for 10 days. Children 1-8 yr of age: oral 5,000-10,000 U/kg/day for 5 days or until recovery. Children >8 yr of age and adults: oral 500,000 U/day for 3 days; then 50,000 U/day for 14 days; then 10,000-20,000 U/day for 2 mo.
	Deficiency without corneal changes	Infants <1 yr of age: 100,000 U/day orally, q4-6 mo. Children 1-8 yr of age: 200,000 U/day orally, q4-6 mo. Children >8 yr and adults: 100,000 U/day for 3 days, followed by 50,000 U/day for 10 days.
	Deficiency	IM given only to those patients with malabsorption in whom oral dosing is not possible. Infants: 7,500-15,000 U/day for 10 days. Children 1-8 yr of age: 17,500-35,000 U/day for 10 days. Children >8 yr of age and adults: 100,000 U/day for 3 days, then 50,000 U/day for 14 days. Give follow-up oral multivitamin that contains vitamin A: LBW infants: no dose established, children ≤8 yr of age: 5,000-10,000 U/day, children >8 yr of age and adults: 10,000-20,000 U daily.
	Malabsorption syndrome (prophylaxis)	Children >8 yr of age and adults: oral 10,000-50,000 U/day of water-miscible product.
	Cystic fibrosis	1,500-10,000 U/day prophylaxis (CF Foundation).
	Measles	WHO recommendations: single dose, repeating the dose next day and at 4 wk for children with eye findings: 6 mo to 1 yr of age: 100,000 U; >1 yr of age: 200,000 U.
Vitamin D	Liver disease	4,000-8,000 U/day ergocalciferol.
	Malabsorption	1000 U/day ergocalciferol
	Nutritional rickets and osteomalacia	Ergocalciferol: children and adults with normal absorption: 1,000-5,000 U/day. Children with malabsorption: 10,000-25,000 U/day. Adults with malabsorption: 10,000-300,000 U/day.
	Renal disease and failure	Ergocalciferol: child: 4,000-40,000 U/day; adults: 20,000 U/day.
	Cystic fibrosis	Ergocalciferol: 400-800 U/day PO (CF Foundation).
	Hypoparathyroidism	Children: 50,000-200,000 U/day ergocalciferol and calcium supplements. Adults: 25,000-200,000 U/day ergocalciferol and calcium supplements.
	Vitamin D-dependent rickets	Children: 3,000-5,000 U/day ergocalciferol; max: 60,000 U/day. Adults: 10,000-60,000 U/day ergocalciferol.
	Vitamin D-resistant rickets	Children: initial 40,000-80,000 U/day with phosphate supplements, daily dosage is increased at 3-4 mo intervals in 10,000-20,000 U increments. Adults: 10,000-60,000 U/day with phosphate supplements.
Vitamin E	Premature infant, neonates, infants of low birth weight	D-α-tocopherol: 25-50 U/day for 1 wk orally.
	Fat malabsorption and liver disease	10-25 U/kg/day of water-miscible vitamin E preparation.
	Cystic fibrosis	<1 yr of age: 25-50 U/day; 1-2 yr of age: 100 U/day; >2 yr of age: 100 U/day bid or 200 U daily orally (CF Foundation).
	Sickle cell disease	450 U/day orally.
	β-Thalassemia	750 U/day orally.
Vitamin K	Hemorrhagic disease of the newborn	Phytonadione: 0.5-1.0 mg SC or IM as prophylaxis within 1 hr of birth, may repeat 6-8 hr later; 1-2 mg/day as treatment.
	Deficiency	Infants and children: 2.5-5 mg/day orally, or 1-2 mg/dose SC, IM, IV as a single dose; adults: 5-25 mg/day or 10 mg IM, IV.
	Cystic fibrosis	2.5 mg, twice a week (CF Foundation).
Folate, folic acid, and folacin	Deficiency	Infants: 50 µg daily. Children 1-10 yr of age: 1 mg/day initially, then 0.1-0.4 mg/day as maintenance. Children >11 yr of age and adults: 1 mg/day initially, then 0.5 mg/day as maintenance.
	Hemolytic anemia	May require higher doses than those listed previously.
Niacin	Pellagra	Children: 50-100 mg tid. Adults: 50-100 mg/day, max 100 mg/day.

Continued

TABLE 31.3 Treatment of Vitamin Deficiencies—cont'd

	CLINICAL FEATURES	SUGGESTED DOSES
Pyridoxine (B_6)	Seizures	Neonates and infants: initial 50-100 mg/day orally, IM, IV, SC.
	Drug-induced deficiencies	Children: 10-50 mg/day as treatment, 1-2 mg/kg/day as prophylaxis.
		Adults: 100-200 mg/day as treatment, 25-100 mg/day as prophylaxis.
	Dietary deficiency	Children: 5-25 mg/day for 3 wk, then 1.5-2.5 mg/day in a multivitamin product.
		Adults: 10-20 mg/day for 3 wk.
Riboflavin (B_2)		Children: 2.5-10 mg/day in divided doses.
		Adults: 5-30 mg/day in divided doses.
Thiamine (B_1)	Beriberi: critically ill	Children: 10-25 mg/day IM or IV.
		Adults: 5-30 mg/dose IM, IV tid, then 5-30 mg/day orally in a single or three divided doses for 1 mo.
	Beriberi: not critically ill	Children: 10-50 mg/day orally for 2 wk, then 5-10 mg/day for 1 mo.
	Metabolic disease	Adults: 10-20 mg/day orally.
	Wernicke encephalopathy	Adults: initially 100 mg IV, then 50-100 mg/day IM/IV until eating a balanced diet.
Cyanocobalamin (B_{12})	Nutritional deficiency	Intranasal gel: 500 μg once a week.
		Orally: 25-250 μg/wk.
	Anemia	Give IM or deep SC; oral route not recommended because of poor absorption and IV route not recommended because of more rapid elimination.
	Pernicious anemia	If evidence of neurologic involvement in neonates and infants (congenital), 1,000 μg/day IM, SC, for at least 2 wk, and then maintenance, 50-100 μg/mo or 100 μg/day for 6-7 days. If clinical improvement, give 100 μg every other day for 7 doses, then every 3-4 days for 2-3 wk, followed by 100 μg/mo for life. Administer with folic acid if needed (1 mg/day for 1 mo concomitantly).
		Children: 30-50 μg/day for 2 or more wk (total dose of 1000 μg) IM, SC, then 100 μg/mo as maintenance.
		Adults: 100 μg/day for 6-7 days; if improvement, administer same dose on alternate days for 7 doses, then every 3-4 days for 2-3 wk. Once hematologic values are normal, give maintenance doses of 100 μg/mo parenterally.
	Hematologic remission	No evidence of neurologic involvement: use intranasal gel: 500 μg per wk.
	Vitamin B_{12} deficiency	Children with neurologic signs: 100 μg/day for 10-15 days (total dose of 1-1.5 mg), then 1-2/wk for several mo and taper to 60 μg/mo.
		Children with hematologic signs: 10-50 μg/day for 5-10 days, followed by 100-250 μg/day every 2-4 wk.
		Adults: 30 μg/day for 5-10 days, followed by maintenance doses of 100-200 μg/mo.
Ascorbic acid	Scurvy	Children: 100-300 mg/day in divided doses orally, IM, IV, or SC for several days.
		Adults: 100-250 mg/day 1-2 times/day.

bid, Two times per day; *CF,* cystic fibrosis; *IM,* intramuscular; *IV,* intravenous; *LBW,* low birth weight; *PO,* by mouth; *q,* every; *SC,* subcutaneous; *tid,* three times per day; *WHO,* World Health Organization.

Data from Lexi-Comp Inc., Hudson, Ohio, 2004; table from Kronel S, Mascarenhas. Vitamin deficiencies and excesses. In: Burg FD, Ingelfinger JR, Polin RA, Gershon AA, eds. Current Pediatric Therapy. *Philadelphia: Elsevier; 2006, Table 3:104–105.*

grains; folate fortification of grains is now routine in the United States.

Folate deficiency, characterized by **hypersegmented neutrophils**, **macrocytic anemia**, and glossitis, may result from a low dietary intake, malabsorption, or vitamin-drug interactions. Deficiency can develop within a few weeks of birth because infants require 10 times as much folate as adults relative to body weight but have scant stores of folate in the newborn period. Folate is particularly heat labile. Heat-sterilizing home-prepared formula can decrease the folate content by half. Evaporated milk and goat's milk are low in folate. Patients with chronic hemolysis (sickle cell anemia, thalassemia) may require extra folate to avoid deficiency because of the relatively high requirement of the vitamin to support erythropoiesis. Other conditions with risk of deficiency include pregnancy, alcoholism, and treatment with anticonvulsants (phenytoin) or antimetabolites (methotrexate). First occurrence and recurrence of **neural tube defects** are reduced significantly by maternal supplementation during embryogenesis. Because closure of the neural tube occurs before usual recognition of pregnancy, all women of reproductive age are recommended to have a folate intake of at least 400 μg/day as prophylaxis.

Vitamin B_{12}

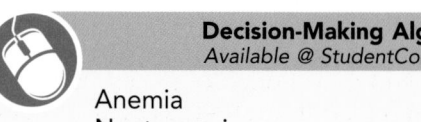

Decision-Making Algorithms
Available @ StudentConsult.com

Anemia
Neutropenia

Vitamin B_{12} is one of the most complex vitamin molecules, containing an atom of cobalt held in a *corrin ring* (similar to that of iron in hemoglobin). The cobalt ion is at the active center of the ring and serves as the site for attachment of alkyl groups during their transfer. The vitamin functions in single-carbon transfers and is intimately related to folate function and interconversions. Vitamin B_{12} is essential for normal lipid and carbohydrate metabolism in energy production and in protein biosynthesis and nucleic acid synthesis.

In contrast to other water-soluble vitamins, absorption of vitamin B_{12} is complex, involving cleavage of the vitamin from dietary protein and binding to a glycoprotein called *intrinsic factor*, which is secreted by the gastric mucosa (parietal cells). The cobalamin–intrinsic factor complex is efficiently absorbed from the distal ileum.

As vitamin B_{12} is absorbed into the portal circulation, it is transported bound to a specific protein, transcobalamin II. Its large stores in the liver also are unusual for a water-soluble vitamin. Efficient enterohepatic circulation normally protects from deficiency for months to years. Dietary sources of the vitamin are animal products only. Strict vegetarians should take a vitamin B_{12} supplement.

Vitamin B_{12} deficiency in children is rare. Early diagnosis and treatment of this disorder in childhood are important because of the danger of irreversible neurologic damage. Most cases in childhood result from a specific defect in absorption (see Table 31.2). Such defects include **congenital pernicious anemia** (absent intrinsic factor), **juvenile pernicious anemia** (autoimmune), and deficiency of transcobalamin II transport. Gastric or intestinal resection and small bowel bacterial overgrowth also cause vitamin B_{12} deficiency. Exclusively breast fed infants ingest adequate vitamin B_{12} unless the mother is a strict vegetarian without supplementation.

Depression of serum vitamin B_{12} and the appearance of hypersegmented neutrophils and macrocytosis (indistinguishable from folate deficiency) are early clinical manifestations of deficiency. Vitamin B_{12} deficiency also causes **neurologic manifestations**, including depression, peripheral neuropathy, posterior spinal column signs, dementia, and eventual coma. The neurologic signs do not occur in folate deficiency, but administration of folate may mask the hematologic signs of vitamin B_{12} deficiency, while the neurologic manifestations progress. Patients with vitamin B_{12} deficiency also have increased urine levels of methylmalonic acid. Most cases of vitamin B_{12} deficiency in infants and children are not of dietary origin and require treatment throughout life. Maintenance therapy consists of repeated monthly intramuscular injections, although a form of vitamin B_{12} is administered intranasally.

FAT-SOLUBLE VITAMINS

Fat-soluble vitamins generally have stores in the body, and dietary deficiencies generally develop more slowly than for water-soluble vitamins. Absorption of fat-soluble vitamins depends on normal fat intake, digestion, and absorption. The complexity of normal fat absorption and the potential for perturbation in many disease states explains the more common occurrence of deficiencies of these vitamins.

Vitamin A

Decision-Making Algorithms
Available @ StudentConsult.com

Hepatomegaly
Hypercalcemia

The basic constituent of the vitamin A group is retinol. Ingested plant carotene or animal tissue retinol esters release retinol after hydrolysis by pancreatic and intestinal enzymes. Chylomicron-transported retinol esters are stored in the liver as retinol palmitate. Retinol is transported from the liver to target tissues by retinol-binding protein, releasing free retinol to the target tissues. The kidney then excretes the retinol-binding protein. Diseases of the kidney diminish excretion of retinol-binding protein, whereas liver parenchymal disease or malnutrition lowers the synthesis of retinol-binding protein. Specific cellular binding proteins facilitate the uptake of retinol by target tissues. In the eye, retinol is metabolized to form **rhodopsin**; the action of light on rhodopsin is the first step of the visual process. Retinol also influences the growth and differentiation of epithelia. The clinical manifestations of vitamin A deficiency in humans appear as a group of ocular signs termed **xerophthalmia**. The earliest symptom is **night blindness**, which is followed by **xerosis** of the conjunctiva and cornea. Untreated, xerophthalmia can result in ulceration, necrosis, keratomalacia, and a permanent corneal scar. Clinical and subclinical vitamin A deficiencies are associated with **immunodeficiency**; increased risk of infection, especially measles; and increased risk of mortality, especially in developing nations. Xerophthalmia and vitamin A deficiency should be urgently treated. Hypervitaminosis A also has serious sequelae, including headaches, pseudotumor cerebri, hepatotoxicity, and teratogenicity.

Vitamin E

Eight naturally occurring compounds have vitamin E activity. The most active of these, α-tocopherol, accounts for 90% of the vitamin E present in human tissues and is commercially available as an acetate or succinate. Vitamin E acts as a biologic **antioxidant** by inhibiting the peroxidation of polyunsaturated fatty acids present in cell membranes. It scavenges free radicals generated by the reduction of molecular oxygen and by the action of oxidative enzymes.

Vitamin E deficiency occurs in children with fat malabsorption secondary to liver disease, untreated celiac disease, cystic fibrosis, and abetalipoproteinemia. In these children, without vitamin E supplementation, a syndrome of progressive **sensory and motor neuropathy** develops; the first sign of deficiency is loss of deep tendon reflexes. Deficient preterm infants at 1-2 months of age have hemolytic anemia characterized by an elevated reticulocyte count, an increased sensitivity of the erythrocytes to hemolysis in hydrogen peroxide, peripheral edema, and thrombocytosis. All the abnormalities are corrected after oral, lipid, or water-soluble vitamin E therapy.

Vitamin D

Decision-Making Algorithms
Available @ StudentConsult.com

Hypertension
Hypocalcemia

Cholecalciferol (vitamin D_3) is the mammalian form of vitamin D and is produced by ultraviolet irradiation of inactive precursors in the skin. Ergocalciferol (vitamin D_2) is derived from plants. Vitamin D_2 and vitamin D_3 require further metabolism to become active. They are of equivalent potency. Clothing, lack of sunlight exposure, and skin pigmentation decrease generation of vitamin D in the epidermis and dermis.

Vitamin D (D_2 and D_3) is metabolized in the liver to calcidiol, or 25-hydroxyvitamin D (25-[OH]-D); this metabolite, which has little intrinsic activity, is transported by a plasma-binding globulin to the kidney, where it is converted to the most active metabolite calcitriol, or 1,25-dihydroxyvitamin D (1,25-$[OH]_2$-D). The action of 1,25-$(OH)_2$-D results in a decrease in the concentration of messenger RNA (mRNA) for collagen in bone and an increase in the concentration of mRNA for vitamin D–dependent calcium-binding protein in the intestine (directly mediating increased intestinal calcium transport). The antirachitic action of vitamin D probably is mediated by provision of appropriate concentrations of calcium and phosphate in the extracellular space of bone and by enhanced intestinal absorption of these minerals. Vitamin D also may have a direct anabolic effect on bone. 1,25-$(OH)_2$-D has direct feedback to the parathyroid gland and inhibits secretion of parathyroid hormone.

Vitamin D deficiency appears as **rickets** in children and as **osteomalacia** in postpubertal adolescents. Inadequate direct sun exposure and vitamin D intake are sufficient causes, but other factors, such as various drugs (phenobarbital, phenytoin) and malabsorption, may increase the risk of development of vitamin-deficiency rickets. Breast fed infants, especially those with dark-pigmented skin, are at risk for vitamin D deficiency.

The pathophysiology of rickets results from defective bone growth, especially at the epiphyseal cartilage matrix, which fails to mineralize. The uncalcified osteoid results in a wide, irregular zone of poorly supported tissue, the rachitic metaphysis. This soft, rather than hardened, zone produces many of the skeletal deformities through compression and lateral bulging or flaring of the ends of bones.

The **clinical manifestations** of rickets are most common during the first 2 years of life and may become evident only after several months of a vitamin D–deficient diet. **Craniotabes** is caused by thinning of the outer table of the skull, which when compressed feels like a Ping-Pong ball to the touch. Enlargement of the costochondral junction (**rachitic rosary**) and thickening of the wrists and ankles may be palpated. The anterior fontanelle is enlarged, and its closure may be delayed. In advanced rickets, scoliosis and exaggerated lordosis may be present. Bowlegs or knock-knees may be evident in older infants, and greenstick fractures may be observed in long bones.

The **diagnosis** of rickets is based on a history of poor vitamin D intake and little exposure to direct ultraviolet sunlight. The serum calcium usually is normal but may be low; the serum phosphorus level usually is reduced, and serum alkaline phosphatase activity is elevated. When serum calcium levels decline to less than 7.5 mg/dL, tetany may occur. Levels of 24,25-$(OH)_2$-D are undetectable, and serum 1,25-(OH)2-D levels are commonly less than 7 ng/mL, although 1,25-$(OH)_2$-D levels also may be normal. The best measure of vitamin D status is the level of 25-(OH)-D. Characteristic **radiographic** changes of the distal ulna and radius include widening; concave cupping; and frayed, poorly demarcated ends. The increased space seen between the distal ends of the radius and ulna and the metacarpal bones is the enlarged, nonossified metaphysis.

Breast fed infants born of mothers with adequate vitamin D stores usually maintain adequate serum vitamin D levels for at least 2 months, but rickets may develop subsequently if these infants are not exposed to the sun or do not receive supplementary vitamin D. The American Academy of Pediatrics recommends vitamin D supplementation of all breast fed infants in the amount of 400 IU/day, started soon after birth and given until the infant is taking more than 1,000 mL/day of formula or vitamin D–fortified milk (for age >1 yr). Toxic effects of excessive chronic vitamin D may include hypercalcemia, muscle weakness, polyuria, and nephrocalcinosis.

Vitamin K

Decision-Making Algorithm
Available @ StudentConsult.com

Bleeding

The plant form of vitamin K is phylloquinone, or vitamin K_1. Another form is menaquinone, or vitamin K_2, one of a series of compounds with unsaturated side chains synthesized by intestinal bacteria. Plasma factors II (prothrombin), VII, IX, and X in the cascade of blood coagulation factors depend on vitamin K for synthesis and for posttranslational conversion of their precursor proteins. The posttranslational conversion of glutamyl residues to carboxyglutamic acid residues of a prothrombin molecule creates effective calcium-binding sites, making the protein active.

Other vitamin K–dependent proteins include proteins C, S, and Z in plasma and γ-carboxyglutamic acid–containing proteins in several tissues. Bone contains a major vitamin K–dependent protein, osteocalcin, and lesser amounts of other glutamic acid–containing proteins.

Phylloquinone is absorbed from the intestine and transported by chylomicrons. The rarity of dietary vitamin K deficiency in humans with normal intestinal function suggests that the absorption of menaquinones is possible. Vitamin K deficiency has been observed in subjects with impaired fat absorption caused by obstructive jaundice, pancreatic insufficiency, and celiac disease; often these problems are combined with the use of antibiotics that change intestinal flora.

Hemorrhagic disease of the newborn, a disease more common among breast fed infants, occurs in the first few weeks of life. It is rare in infants who receive prophylactic intramuscular vitamin K on the first day of life. Hemorrhagic disease of the newborn usually is marked by generalized ecchymoses, gastrointestinal hemorrhage, or bleeding from a circumcision or umbilical stump; intracranial hemorrhage can occur, but is uncommon. The American Academy of Pediatrics recommends that parenteral vitamin K (0.5-1 mg) be given to all newborns shortly after birth.

MINERALS

The major minerals are those that require intakes of more than 100 mg/day and contribute at least 0.1% of total body weight. There are seven essential major minerals: calcium, phosphorus, magnesium, sodium, potassium, chloride, and sulfur. Ten trace minerals, which constitute less than 0.1% of body weight, have essential physiologic roles. Characteristics of trace mineral deficiencies are listed in Table 31.4.

Calcium

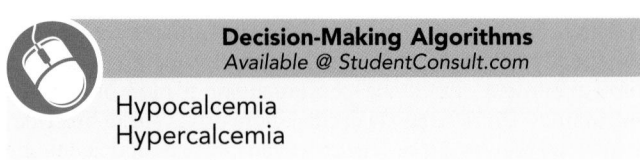

Decision-Making Algorithms
Available @ StudentConsult.com

Hypocalcemia
Hypercalcemia

Calcium is the most abundant major mineral. Ninety-nine percent of calcium is in the skeleton; the remaining 1% is in extracellular fluids, intracellular compartments, and cell membranes. The nonskeletal calcium has a role in nerve conduction, muscle contraction, blood clotting, and membrane permeability. There are two distinct bone calcium phosphate pools—a large, crystalline form and a smaller, amorphous phase. Bone calcium constantly turns over, with concurrent bone reabsorption and formation. Approximately half of **bone mineral accretion** occurs during adolescence. Bone mineral density peaks in early adulthood and is influenced by prior and concurrent dietary calcium intake, exercise, and hormone status (testosterone, estrogen).

Calcium intake can come from a variety of sources, with dairy products providing the most common and concentrated source. The calcium equivalent of 1 cup of milk (about 300 mg of calcium) is $\frac{3}{4}$ cup of plain yogurt, 1.5 oz of cheddar cheese, 2 cups of ice cream, $\frac{4}{5}$ cup of almonds, or 2.5 oz of sardines. Other sources of calcium include some leafy green vegetables (broccoli, kale, collards); lime-processed tortillas; calcium-precipitated tofu; and calcium-fortified juices, cereals, and breads.

There is no classic calcium deficiency syndrome because blood and cell levels are closely regulated. The body can mobilize skeletal calcium and increase the absorptive efficiency of dietary calcium. **Osteoporosis** that occurs in childhood is related to protein-calorie malnutrition, vitamin C deficiency, steroid therapy, endocrine disorders, immobilization and disuse, osteogenesis imperfecta, or calcium deficiency (in premature infants). It is believed that the primary method of prevention of **postmenopausal osteoporosis** is to ensure maximum peak bone mass by providing optimal calcium intake during childhood and adolescence. Bone mineral status can be monitored by dual-energy x-ray absorptiometry.

TABLE 31.4 Characteristics of Trace Mineral Deficiencies

MINERAL	FUNCTION	MANIFESTATIONS OF DEFICIENCY	COMMENTS	SOURCES
Iron	Heme-containing macromolecules (e.g., hemoglobin, cytochrome, and myoglobin)	Anemia, spoon nails, reduced muscle and mental performance	History of pica, cow's milk, gastrointestinal bleeding	Meat, liver, grains, legumes
Copper	Redox reactions (e.g., cytochrome oxidase)	Hypochromic anemia, neutropenia, osteoporosis, hypotonia, hypoproteinemia	Inborn error, Menkes kinky hair syndrome	Liver, nuts, grains, legumes, chocolate
Zinc	Metalloenzymes (e.g., alkaline phosphatase, carbonic anhydrase, DNA polymerase); wound healing	*Acrodermatitis enteropathica:* poor growth, acro-orificial rash, alopecia, delayed sexual development, hypogeusia, infection	Protein-calorie malnutrition; weaning; malabsorption syndromes	Meat, grains, legumes
Selenium	Antioxidant; glutathione peroxidase	Keshan cardiomyopathy in China	Endemic areas; long-term TPN without Se	Meat, vegetables
Chromium	Insulin cofactor	Poor weight gain, glucose intolerance, neuropathy	Protein-calorie malnutrition, long-term TPN without Cr	Yeast, breads
Fluoride	Strengthening of dental enamel	Caries	Supplementation during tooth growth, narrow therapeutic range, fluorosis may cause staining of the teeth	Seafood, fortified water
Iodine	Thyroxine, triiodothyronine production	Simple endemic goiter *Myxedematous cretinism:* congenital hypothyroidism *Neurologic cretinism:* mental retardation, deafness, spasticity, normal thyroxine level at birth	Endemic in New Guinea, the Congo; endemic in Great Lakes area before use of iodized salt	Seafood, iodized salt

TPN, Total parenteral nutrition.

No adverse effects are observed in adults with dietary calcium intakes of 2.5 g/day. There is concern that higher intakes may increase the risk of urinary stone formation, constipation, and decreased renal function and may inhibit intestinal absorption of other minerals (iron, zinc).

Iron

Decision-Making Algorithms
Available @ StudentConsult.com

Gastrointestinal Bleeding
Anemia
Failure to Thrive

Iron, the most abundant trace mineral, is used in the synthesis of hemoglobin, myoglobin, and enzyme iron. Body iron content is regulated primarily through modulation of iron absorption, which depends on the state of body iron stores, the form and amount of iron in foods, and the mixture of foods in the diet. There are two categories of iron in food. The first is *heme iron,* present in hemoglobin and myoglobin, which is supplied by meat and rarely accounts for more than one fourth of the iron ingested by infants. The absorption of heme iron is relatively efficient and is not influenced by other constituents of the diet. The second category is **nonheme iron**, which represents the preponderance of iron intake consumed by infants and exists in the form of iron salts. The absorption of nonheme iron is influenced by the composition of consumed foods. Enhancers of nonheme iron absorption are ascorbic acid, meat, fish, and poultry. Inhibitors are bran, polyphenols (including the tannates in tea), and phytic acid, a compound found in legumes and whole grains. The percent intestinal absorption of the small amount of iron in human milk is 10%; 4% is absorbed from iron-fortified cow's milk formula and from iron-fortified infant dry cereals.

In a normal term infant, there is little change in total body iron and little need for exogenous iron before 4 months of age. Iron deficiency is rare in term infants during the first 4 months, unless there has been substantial blood loss (see Chapter 62). After about 4 months of age, iron reserves become marginal, and, unless exogenous sources of iron are provided, the infant becomes progressively at risk for anemia as the iron requirement to support erythropoiesis and growth increases (see Chapter 150). Premature or low birth weight infants have a lower amount of stored iron because significant amounts of iron are transferred from the mother in the third trimester. In addition, their postnatal iron needs are greater because of rapid rates of growth and when frequent phlebotomy occurs. Iron needs can be met by supplementation (ferrous sulfate) or by iron-containing complementary foods. Under normal circumstances, iron-fortified formula should be the only alternative to breast milk in infants younger than 1 year of age. Premature infants fed human milk may develop iron deficiency anemia earlier unless they receive iron supplements. Formula-fed preterm infants should receive iron-fortified formula.

In older children, iron deficiency may result from inadequate iron intake with excessive cow's milk intake or from intake of foods with poor iron bioavailability. Iron deficiency also can result from blood loss from such sources as menses, gastric ulceration, or inflammatory bowel disease. Iron deficiency affects many tissues (muscle and central nervous system) in addition to producing anemia. **Iron deficiency** and **anemia** have been associated with lethargy and decreased work capacity and **impaired neurocognitive development**, the deficits of which may be irreversible when onset is in the first 2 years of life.

The diagnosis of iron deficiency anemia is established by the presence of a microcytic hypochromic anemia, low serum ferritin levels, low serum iron levels, reduced transferrin saturation, normal to elevated red blood cell width distribution, and enhanced iron-binding capacity. The mean corpuscular volume and red blood cell indices are reduced, and the reticulocyte count is low. Iron deficiency may be present without anemia. Clinical manifestations are noted in Table 31.4.

Treatment of iron deficiency anemia includes changes in the diet to provide adequate iron and the administration of 3–6 mg iron/kg per 24 hours (as ferrous sulfate) divided tid. Reticulocytosis is noted within 3-7 days of starting treatment. Oral treatment should be continued for 5 months. Rarely, intravenous iron therapy is needed if oral iron cannot be given. Parenteral therapy carries the risk of anaphylaxis and should be administered according to a strict protocol, including a test dose.

Zinc

Decision-Making Algorithms
Available @ StudentConsult.com

Diarrhea
Vesicles and Bullae

Zinc is the second most abundant trace mineral and is important in protein metabolism and synthesis, in nucleic acid metabolism, and in stabilization of cell membranes. Zinc functions as a cofactor for more than 200 enzymes and is essential to numerous cellular metabolic functions. Adequate zinc status is especially crucial during periods of growth and for tissue proliferation (immune system, wound healing, skin, and gastrointestinal tract integrity); physiologic functions for which zinc is essential include normal growth, sexual maturation, and immune function.

Dietary zinc is absorbed (20-40%) in the duodenum and proximal small intestine. The best dietary sources of zinc are animal products, including human milk, from which it is readily absorbed. Whole grains and legumes also contain moderate amounts of zinc, but phytic acid inhibits absorption from these sources. On a global basis, poor bioavailability secondary to phytic acid is thought to be a more important factor than low intake in the widespread occurrence of zinc deficiency. Excretion of zinc occurs from the gastrointestinal tract. In the presence of ongoing losses, such as in chronic diarrhea, requirements can drastically increase.

Zinc deficiency dwarfism syndrome was first described in a group of children in the Middle East with low levels of zinc in their hair, poor appetite, diminished taste acuity, hypogonadism, and short stature. Zinc supplementation reduces morbidity and mortality from **diarrhea** and **pneumonia** and enhances growth in developing countries. Mild to moderate zinc deficiency is considered to be highly prevalent in developing countries, particularly in populations with high rates of **stunting**. Mild zinc deficiency occurs in older breast fed infants without adequate zinc intake from complementary foods or in young children with poor total or bioavailable zinc intake in the general diet. A high infectious burden also may increase the risk of zinc deficiency in developing countries. Acute, acquired severe zinc deficiency occurs in patients receiving total parenteral nutrition without zinc supplementation and in premature infants fed human milk without fortification. **Clinical manifestations** of mild zinc deficiency include anorexia, growth faltering, and immune impairment. Moderately severe manifestations include delayed sexual maturation, rough skin, and hepatosplenomegaly. The signs of severe deficiency include acral and periorificial erythematous, scaling dermatitis; growth and immune impairment; diarrhea; mood changes; alopecia; night blindness; and photophobia.

Diagnosis of zinc deficiency is challenging. Plasma zinc concentration is most commonly used, but levels are frequently normal in conditions of mild deficiency; levels in moderate to severe deficiency are typically less than 60 μg/dL. Acute infection also can result in depression of circulating zinc levels. The standard for the diagnosis of deficiency is response to a trial of supplementation, with outcomes such as improved linear growth or weight gain, improved appetite, and improved immune function. Because there is no pharmacologic effect of zinc on these functions, a positive response to supplementation is considered evidence of a preexisting deficiency. Clinically an empirical trial of zinc supplementation (1 μg/kg per day) is a safe and reasonable approach in situations in which deficiency is considered possible.

Acrodermatitis enteropathica is an autosomal recessive disorder that begins within 2-4 weeks after infants have been weaned from breast milk. It is characterized by an acute perioral and perianal dermatitis, alopecia, and failure to thrive. The disease is caused by severe zinc deficiency from a specific defect of intestinal zinc absorption. Plasma zinc levels are markedly reduced, and serum alkaline phosphatase activity is low. **Treatment** is with high-dose oral zinc supplements. A relatively uncommon condition associated with presentation of severe zinc deficiency is due to a defect in the secretion of zinc from the mammary gland, resulting in abnormally low milk zinc concentrations. Breast fed infants, especially those born prematurely, present with classic signs of zinc deficiency: growth failure, diarrhea, and dermatitis. Because there is no defect in the infant's ability to absorb zinc, treatment consists of supplementing the infant with zinc for the duration of breast feeding, which can be successfully continued. Subsequent infants born to the mother will also need zinc supplementation if breast fed. Zinc is relatively nontoxic. Excess intake produces nausea, emesis, abdominal pain, headache, vertigo, and seizures.

Fluoride

Dental enamel is strengthened when fluoride is substituted for hydroxyl ions in the hydroxyapatite crystalline mineral matrix of the enamel. The resulting fluoroapatite is more resistant to chemical and physical damage. Fluoride is incorporated into the enamel during the mineralization stages of tooth formation and by surface interaction after the tooth has erupted. Fluoride is similarly incorporated into bone mineral and may protect against osteoporosis later in life.

Because of concern about the risk of **fluorosis**, infants should not receive fluoride supplements before 6 months of age. Commercial formulas are made with defluoridated water and contain small amounts of fluoride. The fluoride content of human milk is low and is not influenced significantly by maternal intake. Practitioners should evaluate all potential fluoride sources and conduct a caries risk assessment before prescribing fluoride supplementation.

Suggested Readings

Baby Friendly, USA. http://www.babyfriendlyusa.org.

Batool R, Butt MS, Sultan MT, et al. Protein-energy malnutrition: a risk factor for various ailments. *Crit Rev Food Sci Nutr.* 2015;55(2): 242–253.

Boschert S, Robinson T. Fight obesity with specific, countable goals. *Pediatr News.* October 2012.

Centers for Disease Control and Prevention. Racial and ethnic differences in breastfeeding initiation and duration, by state National Immunization Survey, United States, 2004-2008. *MMWR Morb Mortal Wkly Rep.* 2010;59(11):327–334.

Children's Aid Society. http://www.childrensaidsociety.org.

Gartner LM, Morton J, Lawrence RA, et al. Breastfeeding and the use of human milk. *Pediatrics.* 2005;115(2):496–506.

Gribble JN, Murray NJ, Menotti EP. Reconsidering childhood undernutrition: can birth spacing make a difference? An analysis of the 2002–2003 El Salvador National Family Health Survey. *Matern Child Nutr.* 2009;5:49–63.

Grover Z, Ee LC. Protein energy malnutrition. *Pediatr Clin North Am.* 2009;56:1055–1068.

Hylander MA, Strobino DM, Dhanireddy R. Human milk feedings and infection among very low birth weight infants. *Pediatrics.* 1998;102(3):e38.

Kliegman RM, Stanton BF, St. Geme JW, et al, eds. *Nelson Textbook of Pediatrics.* 20th ed. Philadelphia: Elsevier; 2016.

Krebs NF, Hambidge KM. Trace elements. In: Duggan C, Watkins JB, Walker WA, eds. *Nutrition in Pediatrics: Basic Science and Clinical Applications.* 4th ed. Hamilton, Ontario: BC Decker; 2008:67–82.

National Agricultural Library. http://www.nal.usda.gov.

National Center for Biotechnology Information. https://ncbi.nlm.nih.gov.

Ogden CL, Carroll MD, Lawman HG, et al. Trends in obesity prevalence among children and adolescents in the United States, 1988–1994 through 2013-2014. *JAMA.* 2016;315(21):2292–2299.

Penny ME. Protein-energy malnutrition: pathophysiology, clinical consequences, and treatment. In: Duggan C, Watkins JB, Walker WA, eds. *Nutrition in Pediatrics: Basic Science and Clinical Applications.* 4th ed. Hamilton, Ontario: BC Decker; 2008:127–142.

Quader ZS, Gillespie C, Sliwa SA, et al. Sodium intake among US school-aged children: National survey and nutrition examination survey, 2011–2012. *J Acad Nutr Diet.* 2017;117(1):39–47.e5. http://dx.doi.org/10.1016/j.jand.2016.09.010.

The National Health and Nutrition Examination Surveys (NHANES). https://www.cdc.gov/nchs/nhanes/.

USDA Center for Nutrition Policy and Promotion. http://www.cnpp.esda.org.

USDA Child Nutrition. http://fnic.nal.usda.gov/lifecycle-nutrition/child-nutrition.

USDA Choose My Plate. http://www.choosemyplate.gov.

Wagner CL, Greer FR; Section on Breastfeeding and Committee on Nutrition, American Academy of Pediatrics. Prevention of rickets and vitamin D deficiency: new guidelines for vitamin D intake. *Pediatrics.* 2008;122:1142–1152.

de Vos WM. Microbial biofilms and the human intestinal microbiome. NPJ Biofilms and Microbiomes. www.nature.com/npjbiofilms. [25.03.15].

PEARLS FOR PRACTITIONERS

CHAPTER 27

Diet of the Normal Infant

- Proper nutrition is essential for normal growth, healthy immune system, appropriate eating habits, and optimal neurological and cognitive development.
- Healthy nutrition is especially important in the first 6 months of life, as it is the period of exceptionally accelerated growth and brain development.
- Breast feeding offers many benefits to infants and is the ideal nutrition for infant feeding and nutrition.
- The American Academy of Pediatrics recommends human milk as the sole source of nutrition for the first 6 months of life, with continued intake for the first year, and as long as desire thereafter.
- The first 2 days of life is important for the future successes of breast feeding.
- A multilevel approach is necessary to promote and support breast feeding: federal and state government policy making, hospital policies, health care providers contributing to policy making, and parental guidance and support. The Baby Friendly initiative has been beneficial in enhancing breast feeding.
- Breast feeding has protective effects for the well-being of children and adults.
- There are few contraindications for breast feeding such as metabolic disorders, certain infections, and pharmacological therapies.
- All breast fed infants need 400 IU/day of vitamin D supplementation.
- Breast tenderness, engorgement, and cracked nipples are the most common problems encountered by breast feeding mothers.
- Feeding frequency during the first 3 days of life of breast fed infants is inversely related to the level of bilirubin; frequent feedings stimulate meconium passage and excretion of bilirubin in the stool.
- Breast milk jaundice is an indirect hyperbilirubinemia that is usually benign and peaks at 1-2 weeks of age. Kernicterus is very rare.
- Complementary foods are recommended by approximately 6 months of age.
- Healthy infants do not need supplements with water or juice.
- Honey (risk of infant botulism) should not be given before 1 year of age.
- Early caries of childhood are caused by a misbalance of increased sugars and bacteria in the mouth and decrease saliva flow, as early as 6 months of age. Eating a healthy diet and regular brushing will control the sugar factor and bacteria.

CHAPTER 28

Diet of the Normal Child and Adolescent

- A healthy diet helps children grow, thrive, and learn and helps prevent obesity and weight-related diseases, such as diabetes.
- Learning healthy eating behaviors at an early age is an important preventive measure.
- The intestinal microbial biofilms and human microbiome start happening at birth. These microbes and biofilms in the intestinal track may have a great impact on human health and diseases.
- Cow's milk should be introduced at 12 months of age. Low-fat (2%) or whole milk is recommended until 2 years or age, after which fat-free or 1% milk is recommended.
- Excessive milk intake (more than 24 oz/day) should be avoided in toddlers, as it may result in iron deficiency anemia from poor iron intake and intestinal blood loss secondary to milk protein–induced colitis.
- The avoidance of foods with high allergic potential in infancy (e.g., fish, tree nuts, peanuts, dairy products, and eggs) is no longer supported, and early introduction may actually help prevent food allergies.
- No juice is recommended during infancy (<1 yr), 4 oz after 2 years, and 6 oz after 7 years.
- Excessive juice consumption may produce toddler diarrhea.
- ChooseMyPlate by the U.S. Department of Agriculture can provide parents with a general guideline for the types of healthy food to feed their child.
- American children are eating a high salt intake. Daily salt intake recommended is 1,900-2,300 mg.
- Poor calcium intake during adolescence has significant consequences for bone health. Good sources include milk, yogurt, fortified orange juice, cheese, soybeans, and tofu.
- Iron deficiency may reappear in menstruating teens.

CHAPTER 29

Obesity

- Childhood obesity is an epidemic in the United States with 17% of children obese.
- The definition of obesity above 2 years is a body mass index (BMI) higher than the 95 percentile on the Center for Disease Control BMI-for-age growth chart.
- Overweight and obese children are more likely to stay obese into adulthood and to develop chronic diseases.

- The National Health and Nutrition Examination Surveys (NHANES) reported in 2016 that the largest significant differences in the prevalence of obesity between 2011 and 2014 were seen mainly in the Hispanic race/ethnicity origin and education level of the household head.
- Fewer than 5% of obese children have a specific obesity producing syndrome or genetic mutation.
- Sixty minutes of physical activities are recommended every day.
- A healthy diet is emphasized, especially eating high nutrient dense foods.
- Obesity during childhood can have a harmful effect on the body in a variety of ways and can affect virtually every major organ system. Prevention is the key to success for obesity control.
- The clinician should guide the patient who seeks weight reduction to create **SMART** goals: Specific, Measurable, Attainable, Realistic, and Timely.
- More aggressive therapies are considered only for those who have no response to other intervention and preventions. These methods include bariatric surgery for excessively obese adolescents.

CHAPTER 30

Pediatric Undernutrition

- Pediatric undernutrition is usually the result of inadequate food supply, access, or utilization; poor access to health and sanitation; chronic health conditions; and/or inappropriate feeding or child-care practices.
- International references are established that allow normalization of anthropometric measures in terms of *z* scores.
- Primary protein-energy malnutrition (PEM) is caused by social or economic factors that result in a lack of food.
- Secondary PEM occurs in children with various conditions associated with increased caloric requirements (infection, trauma, cancer), increased caloric loss (malabsorption), reduced caloric intake (anorexia, cancer, oral intake restriction, social factors), or a combination of these three variables.
- *Marasmus* results from the body's physiologic response to inadequate calories and nutrients.
- Kwashiorkor results from inadequate protein intake in the presence of fair to good caloric intake.
- Adequate weight does not always signify appropriate nutrition, as the weight may be due to edema caused by a state of malnutrition.
- Vitamin A and zinc deficiency often accompany malnutrition.
- Dermatitis may be seen with protein-calorie malnutrition as well as riboflavin, biotin, and essential fatty acid deficiencies.
- Neuropathy may be seen in thiamin and vitamin B_6, B_{12}, and E deficiencies.
- Treatment for iron deficiency should be delayed until full nutritional rehabilitation.

CHAPTER 31

Vitamin and Mineral Deficiencies

- Risk factors for micronutrient deficiencies in developed countries include exclusion of entire food groups, malabsorption syndromes, and conditions causing high physiologic requirements.
- Exclusively breast fed term infants are at higher risk for vitamin D and K deficiencies. The American Academy of Pediatrics recommends vitamin D supplementation for all breast fed infants in the amount of 400 IU/day, started soon after birth and continued until the infant is taking more than 1,000 mL/day of formula or vitamin D-fortified milk after age 1 year. The American Academy of Pediatrics recommends that parenteral vitamin K (0.5-1 mg) be given to all newborns shortly after birth to prevent hemorrhagic disease of the newborn.
- Niacin (vitamin B_3) deficiency results in pellagra: a combination of weakness, photosensitivity, dermatitis, vomiting, diarrhea, and dementia.
- Deficiency of vitamin B_{12} results in megaloblastic anemia, peripheral neuropathy, posterior column disease, and vitiligo.
- Folate deficiency results in hypersegmented neutrophils, macrocytic anemia, and neural tube defects.
- Scurvy: a combination of irritability, purpura, bleeding gums, periosteal hemorrhage, and aching bones, results from a deficiency of ascorbic acid (vitamin C).
- The fat-soluble vitamins are A, D, E, and K.
- Vitamin D deficiency appears as rickets in children and osteomalacia in postpubertal adolescents. The clinical manifestations of rickets include craniotabes, rachitic rosary, and enlarged anterior fontanelle in younger infants and bowlegs or knock-knees in older infants.
- The diagnosis of iron deficiency anemia is established by the presence of a microcytic hypochromic anemia, low serum ferritin levels, low serum iron levels, reduced transferrin saturation, normal to elevated red blood cell width distribution, and enhanced iron-binding capacity.
- Because of concern about the risk of **fluorosis**, infants should not receive fluoride supplements before 6 months of age.

FLUIDS AND ELECTROLYTES

Alana M. Karp | Larry A. Greenbaum

CHAPTER 32

Maintenance Fluid Therapy

BODY COMPOSITION

Water is the most plentiful constituent of the human body. **Total body water (TBW)** as a percentage of body weight varies with age. The fetus has a high TBW, which gradually decreases to about 75% of birth weight for a term infant; TBW is higher in premature infants. During the first year of life, TBW decreases to about 60% of body weight and basically remains at this level until puberty. At puberty, the fat content of females increases more than that of males, who acquire more muscle mass than females. Because fat has low water content and muscle has high water content, by the end of puberty, TBW in males remains at 60%, but it decreases to 50% of body weight in females. During dehydration, TBW decreases and is a smaller percentage of body weight.

TBW has two main compartments: **intracellular fluid (ICF)** and **extracellular fluid (ECF)**. In the fetus and newborn, the ECF volume is larger than the ICF volume. The normal postnatal diuresis causes an immediate decrease in the ECF volume. This decrease in ECF volume is followed by continued expansion of the ICF volume because of cellular growth. By 1 year of age, the ratio of the ICF volume to the ECF volume approaches adult levels. The ECF volume is 20-25% of body weight, and the ICF volume is 30-40% of body weight (Fig. 32.1). With puberty, the increased muscle mass of males results in a higher ICF volume than in females.

The ECF is divided further into **plasma water** and **interstitial fluid** (see Fig. 32.1). Plasma water is about 5% of body weight. The blood volume, given a hematocrit of 40%, is usually 8% of body weight, although it is higher in newborns and young infants. The interstitial fluid, normally 15% of body weight, can increase dramatically in diseases associated with edema, such as heart failure, protein-losing enteropathy, liver failure, and nephrotic syndrome.

The composition of solutes in the ICF and ECF is different. Sodium and chloride are the dominant cation and anion in the ECF. Potassium is the most abundant cation in the ICF, and proteins, organic anions, and phosphate are the most plentiful anions in the ICF. The dissimilarity between the anions in the ICF and the ECF is determined largely by the presence of intracellular molecules that do not cross the cell membrane, the barrier separating the ECF and the ICF. In contrast, the difference in the distribution of cations—sodium and potassium—is due to the activity of the Na^+,K^+-ATPase pump, which extrudes sodium from cells in exchange for potassium.

REGULATION OF INTRAVASCULAR VOLUME AND OSMOLALITY

Proper cell functioning requires close regulation of plasma osmolality and intravascular volume; these are controlled by independent systems for water balance which determines osmolality, and sodium balance which determines volume status. Maintenance of a normal **osmolality** depends on control of water balance. Control of **volume status** depends on regulation of sodium balance.

The plasma osmolality is tightly controlled between 285 and 295 mOsm/kg through regulation of water intake and urinary water losses. A small increase in the plasma osmolality stimulates thirst. Urinary water losses are regulated by the secretion of **antidiuretic hormone (ADH)**, which increases in response to an increasing plasma osmolality. ADH, by stimulating renal tubular reabsorption of water, decreases urinary water losses. Control of osmolality is subordinate to maintenance of an adequate intravascular volume. When significant volume depletion is present, ADH secretion and thirst are stimulated, regardless of the plasma osmolality.

Volume depletion and volume overload may cause significant morbidity and mortality. Because sodium is the principal extracellular cation and is restricted to the ECF, adequate body sodium is necessary for maintenance of intravascular volume. The kidney determines sodium balance because there is little homeostatic control of sodium intake, although salt craving occasionally occurs, typically in children with chronic renal salt loss or adrenal insufficiency. The kidney regulates sodium balance by altering the percentage of filtered sodium that is reabsorbed along the nephron. The **renin-angiotensin system** is an important regulator of renal sodium reabsorption and excretion. The juxtaglomerular apparatus produces renin in response to decreased *effective* intravascular volume. Renin cleaves angiotensinogen, producing angiotensin I, which angiotensin-converting enzyme converts into angiotensin II. The actions of angiotensin II include direct stimulation of the proximal tubule to increase sodium reabsorption and stimulation of the adrenal gland to increase aldosterone secretion, which increases sodium reabsorption in the distal nephron. In contrast, volume expansion stimulates the synthesis of **atrial natriuretic peptide**, which increases urinary sodium excretion.

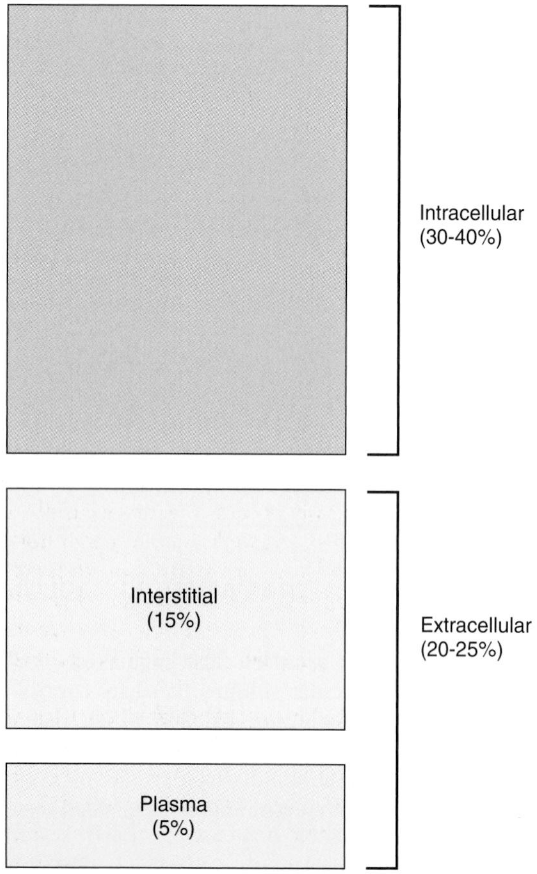

FIGURE 32.1 Compartments of total body water, expressed as percentage of body weight, in an older child or adult. (From Greenbaum LA. Pathophysiology of body fluids and fluid therapy. In: Kliegman RM, Stanton BF, St Geme JW, Schor NF, Behrman RE, Nelson WE, eds. *Nelson Textbook of Pediatrics*. 20th ed. Philadelphia: Saunders; 2016:347.)

MAINTENANCE FLUIDS

Maintenance intravenous (IV) fluids are used in children who cannot be fed enterally. Along with maintenance fluids, children may require concurrent **replacement fluids** if they have excessive **ongoing losses**, such as may occur with diarrhea, vomiting, or drainage from a nasogastric tube. In addition, if dehydration is present, the patient also needs to receive deficit replacement (see Chapter 33).

Maintenance fluids are composed of a solution of water, glucose, sodium, potassium, and chloride. This solution replaces electrolyte losses from the urine and stool, as well as water losses from the urine, stool, skin, and lungs. The glucose in maintenance fluids provides approximately 20% of normal caloric needs. This is enough to prevent the development of starvation ketoacidosis and diminishes the protein degradation that would occur if the patient received no calories.

Maintenance fluids do not provide adequate calories, protein, fat, minerals, or vitamins. Patients should not remain on maintenance therapy indefinitely; parenteral nutrition (see Chapter 34) should be used for children who cannot be fed enterally for more than a few days.

Daily water losses are measurable (urine and stool) and not measurable (*insensible losses* from the skin and lungs). Failure to replace these losses leads to a thirsty child and, ultimately, a dehydrated child. Table 32.1 provides a system for calculating **24-hour maintenance water** needs based on the patient's weight.

TABLE 32.1 Body Weight Method for Calculating Maintenance Fluid Volume and Rate

BODY WEIGHT (kg)	VOLUME PER DAY	HOURLY RATE
0-10	100 mL/kg	4 mL/kg/hr
11-20	1,000 mL + 50 mL/kg for each 1 kg >10 kg	40 mL/hr + 2 mL/kg/hr × (wt–10)
>20	1,500 mL + 20 mL/kg for each 1 kg >20 kg*	60 mL/hr + 1 mL/kg/hr × (wt–20)†

*The maximum total fluid per day is normally 2,400 mL.
†The maximum fluid rate is normally 100 mL/hr.

After calculation of water needs and electrolyte needs, children typically receive D5 in ½ NS plus 20 mEq/L of KCl as a maintenance solution. This assumes that there is no disease process present that would require an adjustment in either the volume or the electrolyte composition of maintenance fluids. Children with renal insufficiency may be hyperkalemic or unable to excrete potassium and may not tolerate 20 mEq/L of KCl. In children with complicated pathophysiological derangements, it may be necessary to adjust the electrolyte composition and rate of maintenance fluids empirically based on electrolyte measurements and assessment of fluid balance.

CHAPTER 33

Dehydration and Replacement Therapy

REPLACEMENT THERAPY

There are three sources of normal water loss—the components of maintenance water (see Chapter 32): urine (60%), **insensible losses** from the skin and lungs (35%), and stool (5%) (Table 33.1). Sweating is not insensible and, in contrast to evaporative losses, sweat contains water and electrolytes.

A variety of clinical situations modify normal maintenance water balance (Table 33.2). Evaporative skin water losses can be higher in neonates, especially premature infants who are under radiant warmers or undergoing phototherapy. Burns can result in massive losses of water and electrolytes (see Chapter 44). Fever increases insensible losses. Tachypnea or a tracheostomy increases evaporative losses from the lungs.

The gastrointestinal tract is potentially a source of considerable water and electrolyte losses. A child who has large amounts

TABLE 33.1 Components of Maintenance Water

Urine	60%
Insensible losses (skin and lungs)	35%
Stool	5%

TABLE 33.2 Adjustments in Maintenance Water

SOURCE	CAUSES OF INCREASED WATER NEEDS	CAUSES OF DECREASED WATER NEEDS
Skin	Radiant warmer Phototherapy Fever Sweat Burns	Incubator (premature infants)
Lungs	Tachypnea Tracheostomy	Humidified ventilator
Gastrointestinal	Diarrhea Emesis Nasogastric suction	
Renal	Polyuria	Oliguria/anuria
Miscellaneous	Surgical drain Third space losses	Hypothyroidism

TABLE 33.3 Adjusting Fluid Therapy for Gastrointestinal Losses

AVERAGE COMPOSITION	APPROACH TO REPLACEMENT
DIARRHEA	**REPLACEMENT OF ONGOING STOOL LOSSES**
Sodium: 55 mEq/L	Solution: 5% dextrose in ¼ normal saline + 20 mEq/L sodium bicarbonate + 20 mEq/L potassium chloride Replace stool mL/mL every 1-6 hr
Potassium: 25 mEq/L	
Bicarbonate: 15 mEq/L	
GASTRIC FLUID	**REPLACEMENT OF ONGOING GASTRIC LOSSES**
Sodium: 60 mEq/L	Solution: normal saline + 10 mEq/L potassium chloride Replace output mL/mL every 1-6 hr
Potassium: 10 mEq/L	
Chloride: 90 mEq/L	

of gastrointestinal losses should have these losses measured and replaced with an appropriate **replacement solution** (Table 33.3).

Urine output is normally the largest cause of *water* loss. Diseases such as renal failure and the syndrome of inappropriate antidiuretic hormone (SIADH) can lead to a decrease in urine volume. Maintenance fluids in a patient with oliguria or anuria may produce fluid overload if the cause is acute kidney injury. In contrast, other conditions produce an increase in urine volume; these include the polyuric phase of acute kidney injury, diabetes mellitus, and diabetes insipidus. When the urine output is excessive, the patient must receive more than standard maintenance fluids to prevent dehydration.

The approach to decreased or increased urine output is similar (Table 33.4). Insensible losses are replaced by a solution that

TABLE 33.4 Adjusting Fluid Therapy for Altered Renal Output

OLIGURIA/ANURIA	POLYURIA
Place the patient on insensible fluids (⅓ maintenance)	Place the patient on insensible fluids (⅓ maintenance)
Replace urine output mL/mL with half normal saline	Measure urine electrolytes
	Replace urine output mL/mL with a solution that is based on the measured urine electrolytes

is administered at a rate one third of the normal maintenance rate. Placing the **anuric** child on "insensibles" theoretically maintains an even fluid balance, with the caveat that one third of maintenance fluid is only an *estimate* of insensible losses. This rate may need to be adjusted based on monitoring of the patient's weight and hydration status. An **oliguric** child needs to receive a urine replacement solution. Most children with **polyuria** (except for children with diabetes mellitus [see Chapter 171]) should be placed on insensible fluids plus urine replacement.

Output from surgical drains and chest tubes, when significant, should be measured and replaced. **Third space losses** manifest with edema and ascites and are due to a shift of fluid from the intravascular space into the interstitial space. Third space losses cannot be quantitated. Nonetheless, these losses can be large and lead to intravascular volume depletion, despite weight gain from edema or ascites. Replacement of third space fluid is empirical but should be anticipated in patients who are at risk, such as children who have sepsis, shock, burns, or abdominal surgery. Third space losses and chest tube output are isotonic and usually require replacement with an **isotonic fluid,** such as normal saline (NS) or Ringer lactate. Adjustments in the amount of replacement fluid for third space losses are based on continuing assessment of the patient's intravascular volume status.

DEHYDRATION

Dehydration, most often due to gastroenteritis, is common in children. The first step in caring for a dehydrated child is to assess the degree of dehydration. The degree of dehydration dictates the urgency of the situation and the volume of fluid needed for rehydration. Table 33.5 summarizes the clinical features that are present with varying degrees of dehydration.

A patient with **mild dehydration** has few clinical signs or symptoms. The history may describe decreased intake but more often increased fluid losses. An infant with **moderate dehydration** has demonstrable physical signs and symptoms. The patient needs fairly prompt intervention. A patient with **severe dehydration** is gravely ill. The decrease in blood pressure indicates that vital organs may be receiving inadequate perfusion (shock) (see Chapter 40). Such a patient should receive immediate and aggressive intravenous (IV) therapy. Clinical assessment of dehydration is only an estimate; the patient must be continually re-evaluated during therapy. The degree of dehydration is underestimated in hypernatremic dehydration because the osmotically driven shift of water from the

TABLE 33.5 Assessment of Degree of Dehydration

	MILD	MODERATE	SEVERE
Infant	5%	10%	15%
Adolescent	3%	6%	9%
Infants and young children	Thirsty, alert; restless	Thirsty; restless or lethargic; irritable	Drowsy; limp, cold, sweaty, cyanotic extremities; may be comatose
Older children	Thirsty, alert	Thirsty, alert (usually)	Usually conscious (but at reduced level), apprehensive; cold, sweaty, cyanotic extremities; wrinkled skin on fingers and toes; muscle cramps
SIGNS AND SYMPTOMS			
Tachycardia	Absent	Present	Present
Palpable pulses	Present	Present (weak)	Decreased
Blood pressure	Normal	Orthostatic hypotension	Hypotension
Cutaneous perfusion	Normal	Normal	Reduced and mottled
Skin turgor	Normal	Slight reduction	Reduced
Fontanelle	Normal	Slightly depressed	Sunken
Mucous membrane	Moist	Dry	Very dry
Tears	Present	Present or absent	Absent
Respirations	Normal	Deep, may be rapid	Deep and rapid
Urine output	Normal	Oliguria	Anuria and severe oliguria

Data from World Health Organization.

intracellular space to the extracellular space helps to preserve the intravascular volume.

Laboratory Evaluation

Serum blood urea nitrogen (BUN) and creatinine concentrations are useful in assessing a child with dehydration. Volume depletion without renal insufficiency may cause a disproportionate increase in the BUN, with little or no change in the creatinine concentration. This is secondary to increased passive reabsorption of urea in the proximal tubule caused by appropriate renal conservation of sodium and water. This increase in the BUN may be absent or blunted in a child with poor protein intake because urea production depends on protein degradation. Conversely, the BUN may be disproportionately increased in a child with increased urea production, as occurs in a child with a gastrointestinal bleed or a child who is receiving glucocorticoids. A significant elevation of the creatinine concentration suggests renal injury.

The urine specific gravity is usually elevated (≥1.025) in cases of significant dehydration but decreases after rehydration. With dehydration, a urinalysis may show hyaline and granular casts, a few white blood cells and red blood cells, and 30-100 mg/dL of proteinuria. These findings usually are not associated with significant renal pathology, and they remit with therapy. Hemoconcentration from dehydration increases the hematocrit and hemoglobin.

Calculation of Fluid Deficit

A child with dehydration has lost water; there is usually a concurrent loss of sodium and potassium. The fluid deficit is the percentage of dehydration multiplied by the patient's weight (for a 10-kg child, 10% of 10 kg = 1 L deficit).

Approach to Dehydration

The child with dehydration requires acute intervention to ensure that there is adequate tissue perfusion (see Chapter 40). This resuscitation phase requires rapid restoration of the circulating intravascular volume, which should be done with an isotonic solution, such as NS or Ringer lactate. Blood is an appropriate fluid choice for a child with acute blood loss but is not always available at the start of fluid resuscitation. The child is given a fluid bolus, usually 20 mL/kg of the isotonic solution, over about 20 minutes. A child with severe dehydration may require multiple fluid boluses and may need to receive fluid at a faster rate. The initial resuscitation and rehydration is complete when signs of intravascular volume depletion resolve. The child typically becomes more alert and has a lower heart rate, normal blood pressure, and improved perfusion.

With adequate intravascular volume, it is now appropriate to plan the fluid therapy for the next 24 hours (Table 33.6). To ensure that the intravascular volume is restored, the patient receives an additional 20 mL/kg bolus of isotonic fluid over 2 hours. The child's total fluid needs are added together (maintenance + deficit). The volume of isotonic fluids the patient has received as acute resuscitation is subtracted from this total. The remaining fluid volume is then administered over 24 hours. Potassium usually is not included in the IV fluids until the patient voids, unless significant hypokalemia is present. *Children with significant ongoing losses need to receive an appropriate replacement solution.*

TABLE 33.6 Fluid Management of Dehydration

Restore intravascular volume
Normal saline: 20 mL/kg over 20 min
Repeat as needed
Rapid volume repletion: 20 mL/kg normal saline (maximum = 1 L) over 2 hr
Calculate 24-hr fluid needs: maintenance + deficit volume
Subtract isotonic fluid already administered from 24-hr fluid needs
Administer remaining volume over 24 hr using D5 ½ normal saline + 20 mEq/L KCl
Replace ongoing losses as they occur

TABLE 33.7 Monitoring Therapy

Vital signs
Pulse
Blood pressure
Intake and output
Fluid balance
Urine output and specific gravity
Physical examination
Weight
Clinical signs of fluid volume depletion or overload
Electrolytes

MONITORING AND ADJUSTING THERAPY

Decision-Making Algorithms
Available @ StudentConsult.com

Hypernatremia
Hyponatremia

All calculations in fluid therapy are only approximations. Thus the patient needs to be monitored during treatment with therapy modifications based on the clinical situation (Table 33.7).

Hyponatremic dehydration occurs in children who have diarrhea and consume a hypotonic fluid (water or diluted formula). Volume depletion stimulates secretion of antidiuretic hormone, preventing the water excretion that should correct the hyponatremia. Some patients develop symptoms, predominantly neurological, from the hyponatremia (see Chapter 35). Most patients with hyponatremic dehydration do well with the same general approach outlined in Table 33.6. Overly rapid correction of hyponatremia (>12 mEq/L per 24 hour) should be avoided because of the remote risk of **central pontine myelinolysis**.

Hypernatremic dehydration is usually a consequence of an inability to take in fluid because of a lack of access, a poor thirst mechanism (neurological impairment), intractable emesis, or anorexia. The movement of water from the intracellular space to the extracellular space during hypernatremic dehydration partially protects the intravascular volume losses. Urine output may be preserved longer, and there may be less tachycardia. Children with hypernatremic dehydration are often lethargic and irritable. Hypernatremia may cause fever, hypertonicity, hyperreflexia, and seizures. More severe neurological symptoms may develop if cerebral bleeding or dural sinus thrombosis occurs.

Overly rapid treatment of hypernatremic dehydration may cause significant morbidity and mortality. **Idiogenic osmoles** are generated within the brain during the development of hypernatremia. Idiogenic osmoles increase the osmolality within the cells of the brain, providing protection against brain cell shrinkage secondary to movement of water out of cells into the hypertonic extracellular fluid. These idiogenic osmoles dissipate slowly during correction of hypernatremia. With rapid lowering of the extracellular osmolality during correction of hypernatremia, a new gradient may be created that causes water movement from the extracellular space into the cells of the brain, producing **cerebral edema**. Possible manifestations of the resultant cerebral edema include headache, altered mental status, seizures, and potentially lethal brain herniation.

To minimize the risk of cerebral edema during correction of hypernatremic dehydration, the serum sodium concentration should not decrease more than 12 mEq/L every 24 hours (Fig. 33.1). The choice and rate of fluid replacement are not nearly as important as vigilant monitoring of the serum sodium concentration and adjustment of the therapy based on the result (see Fig. 33.1). Nonetheless, the initial resuscitation-rehydration phase of therapy remains the same as for other types of dehydration.

Oral Rehydration

Mild to moderate dehydration from diarrhea of any cause can be treated effectively using a simple, oral rehydration solution (ORS) containing glucose and electrolytes (see Chapter 112). The ORS relies on the coupled transport of sodium and glucose in the intestine. Oral rehydration therapy has significantly reduced the morbidity and mortality from acute diarrhea but is underused in developed countries. It should be attempted for most patients with mild to moderate diarrheal dehydration. Oral rehydration therapy is less expensive than IV therapy and has a lower complication rate. IV therapy may still be required for patients with severe dehydration; patients with uncontrollable vomiting; patients unable to drink because of extreme fatigue, stupor, or coma; or patients with gastric or intestinal distention. Rapidly absorbed ondansetron may be used to treat vomiting, thus facilitating oral rehydration.

As a guideline for oral rehydration, 50 mL/kg of the ORS should be given within 4 hours to patients with mild dehydration, and 100 mL/kg should be given over 4 hours to patients with moderate dehydration. Supplementary ORS is given to replace ongoing losses from diarrhea or emesis. An additional 10 mL/kg of ORS is given for each stool. Fluid intake should be decreased if the patient appears fully hydrated earlier than expected or develops periorbital edema. After rehydration, patients should resume their usual diet (breast milk, formula).

When rehydration is complete, maintenance therapy should be started, using 100 mL of ORS/kg in 24 hours until the diarrhea stops. Breast feeding or formula feeding should be maintained and not delayed for more than 24 hours. Patients with more severe diarrhea require continued supervision. The volume of ORS ingested should equal the volume of stool losses. If stool volume cannot be measured, an intake of 10-15 mL of ORS/kg per hour is appropriate.

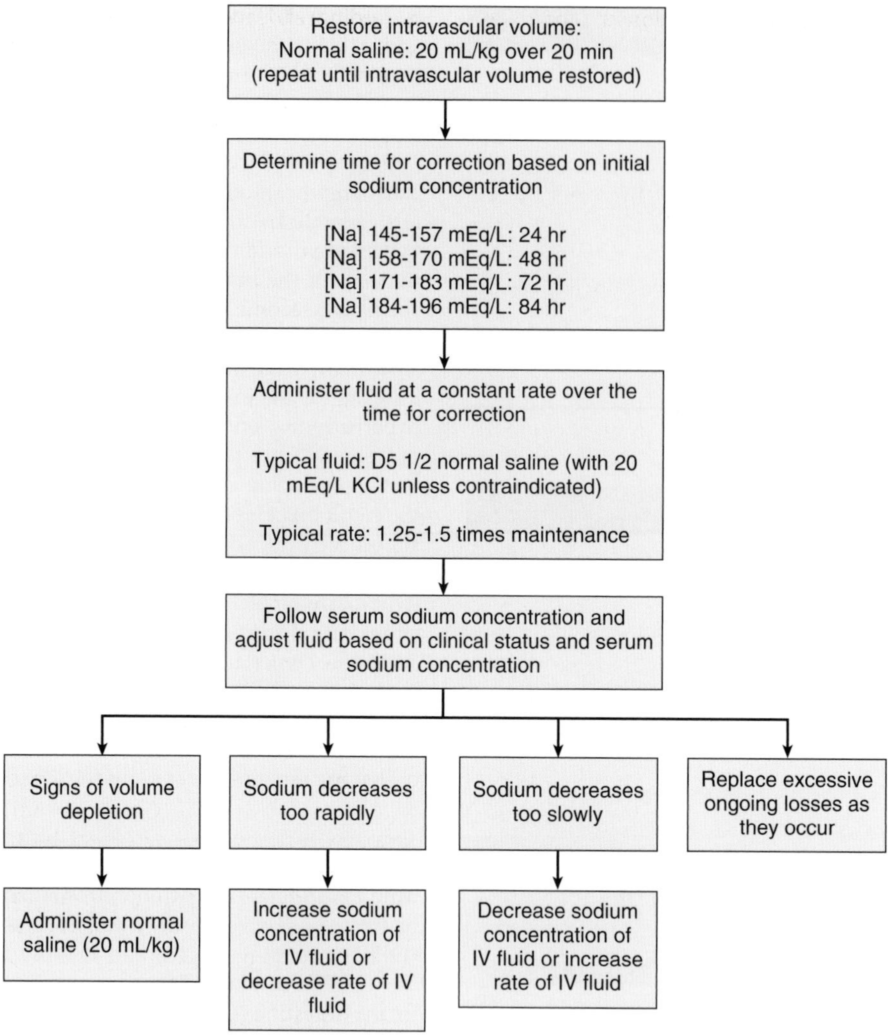

FIGURE 33.1 Strategy for correcting hypernatremic dehydration.

CHAPTER **34**

Parenteral Nutrition

Parenteral nutrition (PN) is necessary when enteral feeding is inadequate to meet the nutritional needs of a patient. Enteral nutrition is always preferred because it is more physiological, less expensive, and associated with fewer complications. Fewer complications are expected if at least some nutrition can be provided enterally.

INDICATIONS

A variety of clinical situations necessitate PN (Table 34.1). Acute PN is frequently given in an intensive care unit when there is poor tolerance of enteral feeds, potentially secondary to a transient ileus, concerns regarding bowel ischemia, or the risk of aspiration pneumonia. **Short bowel syndrome** is the most common indication for long-term PN; it may be caused by a congenital gastrointestinal anomaly or acquired after necrotizing enterocolitis (see Chapter 63). Some patients with a chronic

TABLE **34.1** Indications for Parenteral Nutrition
ACUTE
Prematurity
Trauma
Burns
Bowel surgery
Multiorgan system failure
Bone marrow transplantation
Malignancy
CHRONIC
Short bowel
Intractable diarrhea syndromes
Intestinal pseudo-obstruction
Inflammatory bowel disease
Immunodeficiency

indication for PN eventually may be transitioned to partial or full enteral feedings.

ACCESS FOR PARENTERAL NUTRITION

PN can be given via either a peripheral intravenous (IV) line or a central venous line (CVL). Long-term PN should be given via a CVL. Acute PN may be given peripherally, although a temporary CVL is often used. Most children with cancer or receiving a bone marrow transplant have a CVL. A **peripherally inserted central catheter** is an excellent source of central access for acute PN because of the lower risk for complications than with a standard CVL.

A peripheral IV line has two major limitations. First, it frequently fails, necessitating interruption of PN and potentially painful placement of a new line. Second, high-osmolality solutions cause **phlebitis** of peripheral veins; this limits the dextrose and amino acid content of peripheral PN. The dextrose content of peripheral PN cannot be greater than 12%, with a lower limit if the amino acid concentration is high. Lipid emulsion has a low osmolality; therefore it can be administered peripherally via the same IV line as the dextrose and amino acid solution. Patients can receive adequate nutrition via a peripheral IV line, but the volume of PN needs to be higher than is necessary when central access is available because of the limitations on dextrose and amino acid concentration. This situation may be problematic in patients who cannot tolerate larger fluid volumes.

COMPOSITION OF PARENTERAL NUTRITION

PN can provide calories, amino acids, electrolytes, minerals, essential fatty acids, vitamins, iron, and trace elements. The **calories** in PN are from dextrose and fat. The amino acids in PN are a potential source of calories, but they should be used predominantly for protein synthesis. PN is given as two separate solutions: a dextrose plus amino acid solution and a 20% lipid emulsion. The dextrose solution has all of the other components of PN except for fat.

The dextrose concentration of peripheral PN is typically 10-12%, whereas central PN has a concentration of about 20%, although it may be increased to 25-30% in patients who are fluid restricted. To avoid hyperglycemia, the dextrose delivery is increased gradually when starting PN. Protein delivery in PN is via amino acids in the dextrose solution. The goal is 0.8-2 g protein/kg per 24 hour for older children, 1.5-3 g/kg per 24 hour for full-term and older infants, and 2.5-3.5 g/kg per 24 hour for preterm infants.

The electrolyte and mineral composition of PN depends on the age and the underlying illness. The 20% lipid emulsion provides essential fatty acids and calories. The lipid emulsion is started at a rate of 0.5-1 g/kg per 24 hour, gradually increasing the rate so that the patient receives adequate calories; this typically requires 2.5-3.5 g/kg per 24 hour. The lipid emulsion usually provides 30-40% of the required calories; it should not exceed 60%. The serum triglyceride concentration is monitored as the rate of lipid emulsion is increased, with reduction of the lipid emulsion rate if significant hypertriglyceridemia develops.

COMPLICATIONS

There are many potential complications of PN. CVLs are associated with complications during insertion (pneumothorax or bleeding) and long-term issues (thrombosis). **Catheter-related sepsis**, most commonly due to coagulase-negative staphylococci, is common and, on occasion, necessitates catheter removal. Other potential pathogens are *Staphylococcus aureus*, gram-negative bacilli, and fungi. Electrolyte abnormalities, nutritional deficiencies, hyperglycemia, and complications from excessive protein intake (azotemia or hyperammonemia) can be detected with careful monitoring.

The most concerning complication of long-term PN is **cholestatic liver disease**, which can lead to jaundice, cirrhosis, and occasionally liver failure. Current PN decreases the risk of liver disease by including reduced amounts of hepatotoxic amino acids. The best preventive strategy is early use of the gastrointestinal tract, even if only trophic feeds are tolerated.

CHAPTER 35

Sodium Disorders

The kidney regulates sodium balance and is the principal site of sodium excretion. Sodium is unique among electrolytes because **water balance,** not sodium balance, usually determines its concentration. When the sodium concentration increases, the resultant higher plasma osmolality causes increased thirst and increased secretion of antidiuretic hormone (ADH), which leads to renal conservation of water. Both of these mechanisms increase the water content of the body, and the sodium concentration returns to normal. During hyponatremia, the fall in plasma osmolality decreases ADH secretion, and consequent renal water excretion leads to an increase in the sodium concentration. Although water balance is usually regulated by osmolality, volume depletion also stimulates thirst, ADH secretion, and renal conservation of water. In fact, volume depletion takes precedence over osmolality; volume depletion stimulates ADH secretion, even if a patient has hyponatremia.

The excretion of sodium by the kidney is not determined by the plasma osmolality. The patient's effective plasma volume regulates the amount of sodium in the urine through a variety of regulatory systems, including the renin-angiotensin-aldosterone system. In hyponatremia or hypernatremia, the underlying pathophysiology determines the urinary sodium concentration, not the serum sodium concentration.

HYPONATREMIA

Decision-Making Algorithm
Available @ StudentConsult.com

Hyponatremia

Etiology

Different mechanisms can cause hyponatremia (Fig. 35.1). **Pseudohyponatremia** is a laboratory artifact that is present when the plasma contains high concentrations of protein or lipid. It does not occur when a direct ion-selective electrode determines the sodium concentration, a technique that is increasingly used in clinical laboratories. In true hyponatremia,

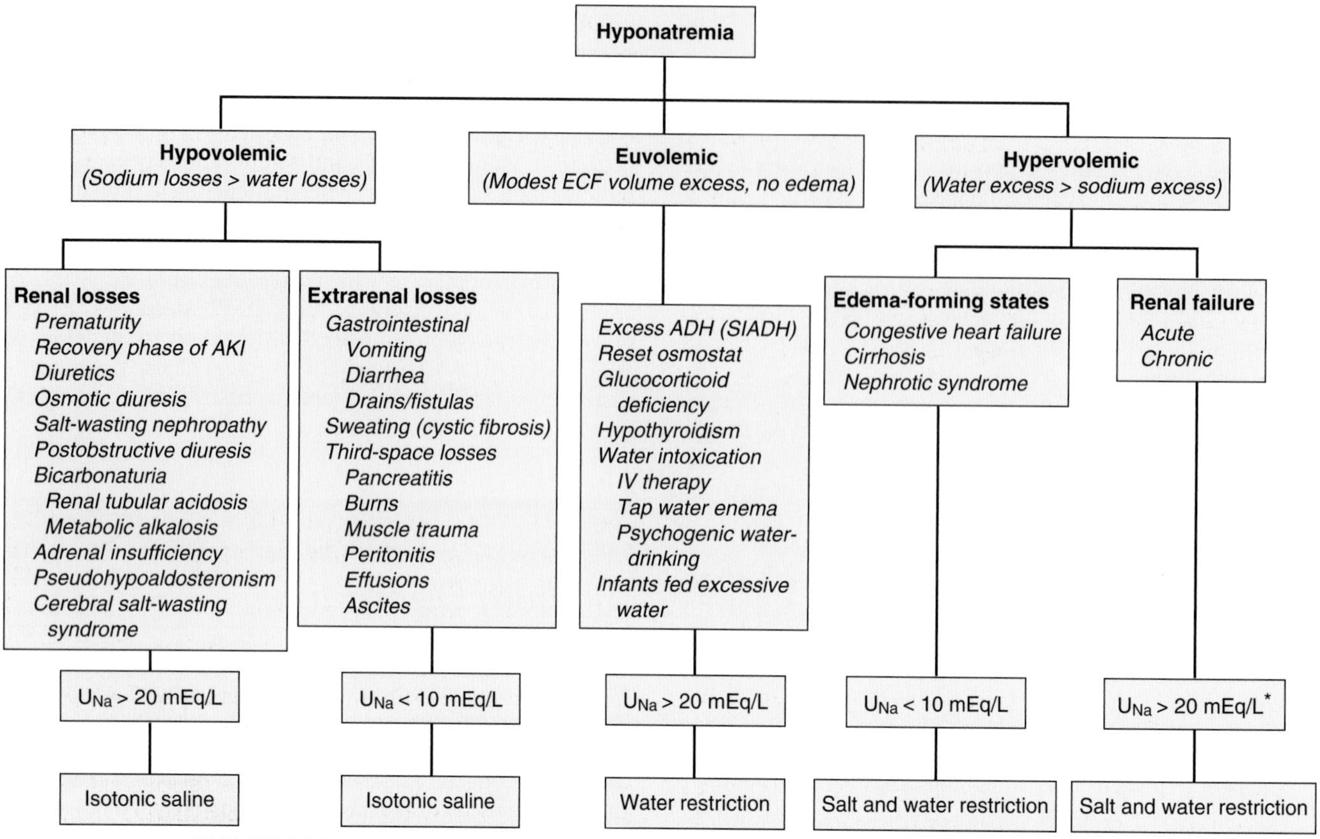

FIGURE 35.1 Classification, diagnosis, and treatment of hyponatremic states. *In water intoxication the urine sodium is often <20 mEq/L. †Urinary sodium is <10 mEq/L in acute renal failure secondary to glomerular disease. *ADH*, Antidiuretic hormone; *AKI*, acute kidney injury; *ECF*, extracellular fluid; *IV*, intravenous; *SIADH*, syndrome of inappropriate antidiuretic hormone secretion. (Modified from Berl T, Anderson RJ, McDonald KM, Schrier RW. Clinical disorders of water metabolism. *Kidney Int.* 1976;10:117–132. Fig 2.)

the *measured* osmolality is low, whereas it is normal in pseudohyponatremia. **Hyperosmolality**, resulting from mannitol infusion or hyperglycemia, causes a low serum sodium concentration, because water moves down its osmotic gradient from the intracellular space into the extracellular space, diluting the sodium concentration. For every 100 mg/dL increment of the serum glucose, the serum sodium decreases by 1.6 mEq/L. Because the manifestations of hyponatremia are due to the low plasma osmolality, patients with hyponatremia caused by hyperosmolality do not have symptoms of hyponatremia and do not require the correction of hyponatremia.

Classification of true hyponatremia is based on the patient's volume status (see Fig. 35.1). In **hypovolemic hyponatremia,** the child has lost sodium from the body. Water balance may be positive or negative, but there has been a higher net sodium loss than water loss; this is often due to oral or intravenous (IV) water intake, with water retention by the kidneys to compensate for the intravascular volume depletion. If the sodium loss is due to a nonrenal disease (e.g., diarrhea), the urine sodium concentration is very low, as the kidneys attempt to preserve the intravascular volume by conserving sodium. In renal diseases, the urine sodium is inappropriately elevated.

Patients with hyponatremia and no evidence of volume overload or volume depletion have **euvolemic hyponatremia.** These patients typically have an excess of total body water and a slight decrease in total body sodium. Some of these patients have an increase in weight, implying that they are volume overloaded. Nevertheless, they usually appear normal or have only subtle signs of fluid overload. In the **syndrome of inappropriate ADH (SIADH),** there is secretion of ADH that is not inhibited by either low serum osmolality or expanded intravascular volume. Retention of water causes hyponatremia, and the expansion of the intravascular volume results in an increase in renal sodium excretion. SIADH is associated with stress, pneumonia, mechanical ventilation, meningitis, and other central nervous system disorders (trauma). Ectopic (tumor) production of ADH is rare in children. Infants can develop euvolemic hyponatremia as a result of excessive water consumption or inappropriately diluted formula.

In **hypervolemic hyponatremia,** there is an excess of total body water and sodium, although the increase in water is greater than the increase in sodium. In renal failure, there is an inability to excrete sodium or water; the urine sodium may be low or high, depending on the cause of the renal insufficiency. In other causes of hypervolemic hyponatremia, there is a decrease in the effective blood volume because of either third space fluid loss or poor cardiac output (see Chapter 145). In response to the low effective blood volume, ADH causes renal water retention, and the kidneys also retain sodium, which leads to a low urine sodium concentration. The patient's serum sodium concentration decreases when water intake exceeds sodium intake, and ADH prevents the normal loss of excess water.

Clinical Manifestations

Hyponatremia causes a fall in the osmolality of the extracellular space. Because the intracellular space then has a higher osmolality, water moves from the extracellular space to the intracellular space to maintain osmotic equilibrium. The increase in intracellular water may cause cells to swell. **Brain cell swelling** is responsible for most of the symptoms of hyponatremia. Neurological symptoms of hyponatremia include anorexia, nausea, emesis, malaise, lethargy, confusion, agitation, headache, seizures, coma, and decreased reflexes. Patients may develop hypothermia, Cheyne-Stokes respirations, muscle cramps, and weakness. Symptoms are more severe when hyponatremia develops rapidly; chronic hyponatremia can be asymptomatic because of a compensatory decrease in brain cell osmolality, which limits cerebral swelling.

Treatment

Rapid correction of hyponatremia can produce **central pontine myelinolysis.** Avoiding more than a 12-mEq/L increase in the serum sodium every 24 hours is prudent, especially in chronic hyponatremia. Treatment of hypovolemic hyponatremia requires administration of IV fluids with sodium to provide maintenance requirements and deficit correction, and to replace ongoing losses (see Chapter 33). For children with SIADH, water restriction is the cornerstone of therapy, although vaptans, which are ADH antagonists, have a role in some patients. Children with hyponatremia secondary to hypothyroidism or cortisol deficiency need specific hormone replacement. **Acute water intoxication** rapidly self-corrects with the transient restriction of water intake, which is followed by introduction of a normal diet. Treatment of hypervolemic hyponatremia centers on restriction of water and sodium intake, but disease-specific measures, such as dialysis in renal failure, may also be necessary.

Emergency treatment of **symptomatic hyponatremia,** such as seizures, uses IV hypertonic saline to rapidly increase the serum sodium concentration, which leads to a decrease in brain edema. One milliliter per kilogram of 3% sodium chloride increases the serum sodium by approximately 1 mEq/L. A child often improves after receiving 4-6 mL/kg of 3% sodium chloride.

HYPERNATREMIA

Decision-Making Algorithm
Available @ StudentConsult.com

Hypernatremia

Etiology

There are three basic mechanisms of hypernatremia (Fig. 35.2). **Sodium intoxication** is frequently iatrogenic in a hospital setting, resulting from correction of metabolic acidosis with sodium bicarbonate. In hyperaldosteronism, there is renal retention of sodium and resultant hypertension; the hypernatremia is mild.

Hypernatremia resulting from water losses develops only if the patient does not have access to water or cannot drink adequately because of neurological impairment, emesis, or anorexia. Infants are at high risk because of their inability to control their own water intake. Ineffective breast feeding, often in a primiparous mother, can cause severe hypernatremic dehydration. High insensible losses of water are especially common in premature infants; the losses increase further as a result of radiant warmers or phototherapy for hyperbilirubinemia. Children with extrarenal causes of water loss have high levels of ADH and very concentrated urine.

Children with diabetes insipidus have inappropriately diluted urine. Hereditary **nephrogenic diabetes insipidus** causes

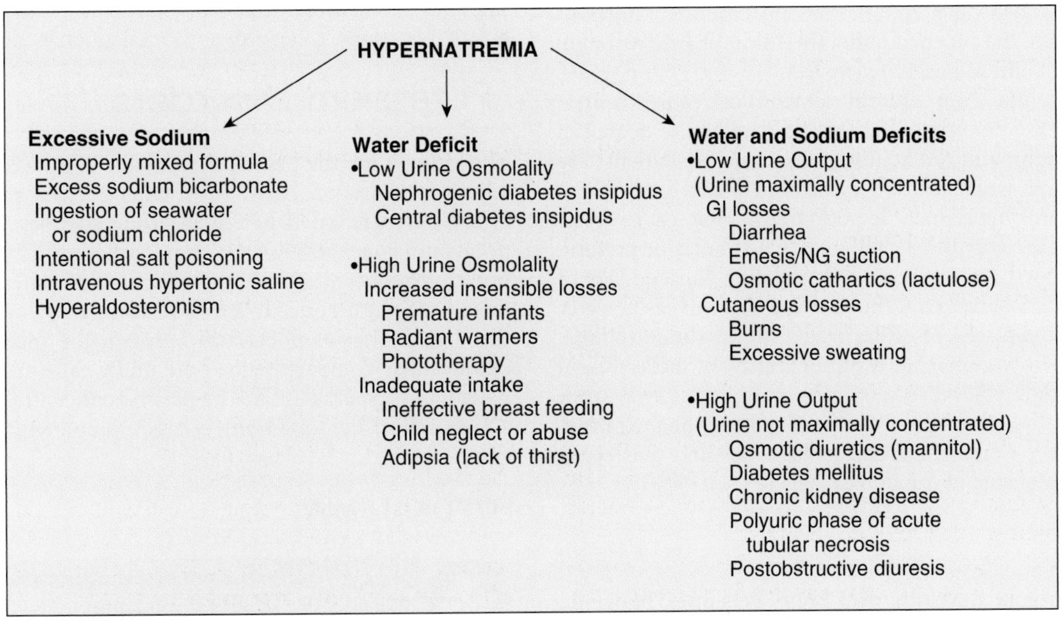

FIGURE 35.2 Differential diagnosis of hypernatremia by mechanism. *GI*, Gastrointestinal; *NG*, nasogastric.

massive urinary water losses. Because it is most commonly an X-linked disorder due to a mutation in the gene for the ADH receptor, it usually occurs in boys, who may have episodes of severe hypernatremic dehydration and failure to thrive. *Acquired nephrogenic diabetes insipidus* may be secondary to interstitial nephritis, sickle cell disease, hypercalcemia, hypokalemia, or medications (lithium). If the defect is due to **central diabetes insipidus,** urine output decreases and urine osmolality increases in response to administration of an ADH analog. Central causes of ADH deficiency include tumor, infarction, or trauma. There is no response to an ADH analog in a child with nephrogenic diabetes insipidus.

Diarrhea results in sodium and water depletion. Most children with gastroenteritis do not develop hypernatremia because they drink enough hypotonic fluid to compensate at least partially for stool water losses. Hypernatremia is most likely in a child with diarrhea who has inadequate intake because of emesis, lack of access to water, or anorexia. Some renal diseases, including obstructive uropathy, renal dysplasia, and juvenile nephronophthisis, can cause losses of sodium and water, potentially producing hypernatremia if the patient consumes insufficient water.

In situations with combined sodium and water deficits, analysis of the urine differentiates renal and nonrenal etiologies. When the losses are extrarenal, the kidney responds to volume depletion with low urine volume, a concentrated urine, and sodium retention (urine sodium <10 mEq/L). With renal causes, the urine volume is usually high, the urine is not maximally concentrated, and the urine sodium may be inappropriately elevated.

Clinical Manifestations

Most children with hypernatremia are dehydrated and have the typical signs and symptoms of dehydration (see Chapter 33). Children with hypernatremic dehydration tend to have better preservation of intravascular volume owing to the shift of water from the intracellular space to the extracellular space. Hypernatremic infants potentially become more dehydrated before seeking medical attention. Probably because of intracellular water loss, the pinched abdominal skin of a dehydrated, hypernatremic infant has a *doughy* feel.

Hypernatremia, even without dehydration, causes central nervous system symptoms that tend to parallel the degree of sodium elevation and the acuity of the increase. Patients are irritable, restless, weak, and lethargic. Some infants have a high-pitched cry and hyperpnea; hypernatremia may cause fever. Alert patients are very thirsty, although nausea may be present.

Brain hemorrhage is the most devastating consequence of hypernatremia. As the extracellular osmolality increases, water moves out of brain cells, resulting in a decrease in brain volume. This decrease in volume can result in tearing of intracerebral veins and bridging blood vessels as the brain moves away from the skull and the meninges. Patients may have subarachnoid, subdural, and parenchymal hemorrhage. Seizures and coma are possible sequelae of the hemorrhage.

Treatment

As hypernatremia develops, the brain generates idiogenic osmoles to increase the intracellular osmolality and prevent the loss of brain water. This mechanism is not instantaneous and is most prominent when hypernatremia has developed gradually. If the serum sodium concentration is lowered rapidly, there is movement of water from the serum into the brain cells to equalize the osmolality in the two compartments. The resultant brain swelling manifests as seizures or coma. Because of these dangers, hypernatremia should be corrected slowly. The goal is to decrease the serum sodium by less than 12 mEq/L every 24 hours (see Fig. 33.1). The most important components of correcting moderate or severe hypernatremia are restoring the effective intravascular volume and then frequently monitoring the serum sodium to allow adjustment of fluid therapy and to provide adequate correction that is neither too slow nor too fast.

In a child with hypernatremic dehydration, as in any child with dehydration, the first priority is restoration of intravascular volume with isotonic fluid. Fig. 33.1 outlines a general approach for correcting hypernatremic dehydration secondary to gastroenteritis. If the hypernatremia and dehydration are secondary to water loss, as occurs with diabetes insipidus, a more hypotonic IV fluid is appropriate. A child with central diabetes insipidus should receive an ADH analog to prevent further excessive water loss. A child with nephrogenic diabetes insipidus requires a urine replacement solution to offset ongoing water losses. Chronically, reduced sodium intake, thiazide diuretics, and nonsteroidal antiinflammatory drugs can decrease water losses in nephrogenic diabetes insipidus.

Acute, severe hypernatremia, usually secondary to sodium administration, can be corrected more rapidly because idiogenic osmoles have not had time to accumulate; this balances the high morbidity and mortality from severe, acute hypernatremia with the dangers of overly rapid correction. When hypernatremia is due to sodium intoxication, and the hypernatremia is severe, it may be impossible to administer enough water to rapidly correct the hypernatremia without worsening volume overload. Some patients require the use of a loop diuretic or dialysis.

CHAPTER 36

Potassium Disorders

The kidneys are the principal regulator of potassium balance, adjusting excretion based on intake. Factors affecting renal potassium excretion include aldosterone, acid-base status, serum potassium concentration, and renal function. The intracellular potassium concentration is approximately 30 times the extracellular potassium concentration. A variety of conditions alter the distribution of potassium between the intracellular and extracellular compartments, potentially causing either hypokalemia or hyperkalemia. The plasma concentration does not always reflect the total body potassium content.

HYPOKALEMIA

Decision-Making Algorithm
Available @ StudentConsult.com

Hypokalemia

Etiology

Hypokalemia is common in children, with most cases related to gastroenteritis. Spurious hypokalemia occurs in patients with leukemia and elevated white blood cell counts if plasma for analysis is left at room temperature, permitting the white blood cells to take up potassium from the plasma. There are four basic mechanisms of hypokalemia (Table 36.1). Low intake, nonrenal losses, and renal losses all are associated with total body potassium depletion. With a **transcellular shift**, total body potassium is normal unless there is concomitant potassium depletion secondary to other factors.

The transcellular shift of potassium after initiation of insulin therapy in children with diabetic ketoacidosis (see Chapter 171) can be dramatic. These patients have reduced total body potassium because of urinary losses, but they often have a normal serum potassium level before insulin therapy from a transcellular shift into the extracellular space secondary to insulin deficiency and metabolic acidosis. Children receiving aggressive doses of β-adrenergic agonists (albuterol) for asthma can develop hypokalemia resulting from the intracellular movement of potassium. Poor intake is an unusual cause of hypokalemia, unless it is also associated with significant weight loss (anorexia nervosa).

Diarrhea has a high concentration of potassium, and the resulting hypokalemia is usually associated with a metabolic acidosis secondary to stool losses of bicarbonate. With emesis or nasogastric suction, there is gastric loss of potassium, but this is fairly minimal given the low potassium content of gastric fluid (~10 mEq/L). More important is the gastric loss of hydrochloride, leading to a metabolic alkalosis and a state of volume depletion. Metabolic alkalosis and volume depletion increase urinary losses of potassium.

Urinary potassium wasting may be accompanied by a metabolic acidosis (proximal or distal renal tubular acidosis; see Chapter 37). Loop and thiazide diuretics lead to hypokalemia and a metabolic alkalosis. **Bartter syndrome** and **Gitelman syndrome** are autosomal recessive disorders resulting from defects in tubular transporters, and are associated with hypokalemia and a metabolic alkalosis. Bartter syndrome is usually associated with hypercalciuria, often with nephrocalcinosis; children with Gitelman syndrome have low urinary calcium

TABLE 36.1 Causes of Hypokalemia

Spurious	With metabolic alkalosis
High white blood cell count	Low urine chloride
Transcellular shifts	Emesis/nasogastric suction
Alkalemia	Pyloric stenosis
Insulin	Chloride-losing diarrhea
β-Adrenergic agonists	Cystic fibrosis
Drugs/toxins (theophylline, barium, toluene)	Low-chloride formula
Hypokalemic periodic paralysis	Posthypercapnia
Refeeding syndrome	Previous loop or thiazide diuretic use
Decreased intake	High urine chloride and normal blood pressure
Extrarenal losses	Gitelman syndrome
Diarrhea	Bartter syndrome
Laxative abuse	Loop and thiazide diuretics
Sweating	High urine chloride and high blood pressure
Renal losses	Adrenal adenoma or hyperplasia
With metabolic acidosis	Glucocorticoid-remediable aldosteronism
Distal RTA	Renovascular disease
Proximal RTA	Renin-secreting tumor
Ureterosigmoidostomy	17α-Hydroxylase deficiency
Diabetic ketoacidosis	11β-Hydroxylase deficiency
Without specific acid-base disturbance	Cushing syndrome
Tubular toxins (amphotericin, cisplatin, aminoglycosides)	11β-Hydroxysteroid dehydrogenase deficiency
Interstitial nephritis	Licorice ingestion
Diuretic phase of acute tubular necrosis	Liddle syndrome
Postobstructive diuresis	
Hypomagnesemia	
High urine anions (e.g., penicillin or penicillin derivatives)	

RTA, Renal tubular acidosis.

TABLE 36.2 Bartter and Gitelman Syndromes

	TYPE I BARTTER SYNDROME	TYPE II BARTTER SYNDROME	TYPE III BARTTER SYNDROME	TYPE IV BARTTER SYNDROME	TYPE V BARTTER SYNDROME	GITELMAN SYNDROME
Inheritance	AR	AR	AR	AR	AD	AR
Affected tubular region	TAL	TAL + CCD	TAL + DCT	TAL + DCT	TAL	DCT
Gene	*SLC12A2*	*KCNJ1*	*CLCBRK*	*BSND*	*CASR*	*SLC12A3* Few have *CLCNKB*
Onset	Prenatal, postnatal	Prenatal, postnatal	Variable	Prenatal, postnatal	Variable	Adolescent, adult
Urine PGE2	Very high	Very high	Slightly elevated	Elevated	Elevated	Normal
Hypokalemic metabolic alkalosis	Present	Present	Present	Present	Present	Present
Features	Polyhydramnios, prematurity, nephrocalcinosis, dehydration, hyposthenuria, polyuria, failure to thrive	Same as type I	Failure to thrive, dehydration, salt craving, low serum magnesium in 20%, mildest form	Same as type I, with sensorineural hearing loss and no nephrocalcinosis	Hypocalcemia, low parathyroid hormone levels, hypercalciuria, uncommon cause of Bartter syndrome	Hypomagnesemia in 100%, mild dehydration, occasional growth retardation, tetany

AD, Autosomal dominant; *AR*, autosomal recessive; *CCD*, cortisol collecting duct; *DCT*, descending convoluted tubule; *PGE2*, prostaglandin E2; *TAL*, thick ascending loop of Henle.
From Sreedharan R, Avner ED. Bartter syndrome. In: Kliegman RM, Stanton BF, St. Geme JW, Schor NF, eds. Nelson Textbook of Pediatrics. *20th ed. Philadelphia: Elsevier; 2016, Table 531.1.*

losses, but hypomagnesemia secondary to urinary losses (Table 36.2).

In the presence of a high aldosterone level, there is urinary loss of potassium, hypokalemia, and a metabolic alkalosis. There also is renal retention of sodium, leading to hypertension. A variety of genetic and acquired disorders can cause high aldosterone levels. **Liddle syndrome**, an autosomal dominant disorder caused by constitutively active sodium channels, has the same clinical features as hyperaldosteronism, but the serum aldosterone level is low.

Clinical Manifestations

The heart and skeletal muscle are especially vulnerable to hypokalemia. **Electrocardiographic (ECG) changes** include a flattened T wave, a depressed ST segment, and the appearance of a U wave, which is located between the T wave (if still visible) and P wave. Ventricular fibrillation and torsades de pointes may occur, although usually only in the context of underlying heart disease. Hypokalemia makes the heart especially susceptible to digitalis-induced arrhythmias.

The clinical consequences in skeletal muscle include muscle weakness and cramps. **Paralysis** is a possible complication (generally only at potassium levels <2.5 mEq/L). Paralysis usually starts with the legs, followed by the arms. Respiratory paralysis may require mechanical ventilation.

Some hypokalemic patients develop **rhabdomyolysis**, especially following exercise. Hypokalemia slows gastrointestinal motility; potassium levels less than 2.5 mEq/L may cause an ileus. Hypokalemia impairs bladder function, potentially leading to urinary retention. Hypokalemia causes polyuria by producing secondary nephrogenic diabetes insipidus. Chronic hypokalemia may cause kidney damage, including interstitial nephritis and renal cysts. In children, chronic hypokalemia, as in Bartter syndrome, leads to poor growth.

Diagnosis

It is important to review the child's diet, history of gastrointestinal losses, and medications. Emesis and diuretic use can be surreptitious. The presence of hypertension suggests excess mineralocorticoids. Concomitant electrolyte abnormalities are useful clues. The combination of hypokalemia and metabolic acidosis is characteristic of diarrhea, and proximal or distal renal tubular acidosis. A concurrent metabolic alkalosis is characteristic of gastric losses, aldosterone excess, diuretics, Bartter syndrome, or Gitelman syndrome.

Treatment

Factors that influence the therapy of hypokalemia include the potassium level, clinical symptoms, renal function, presence of transcellular shifts of potassium, ongoing losses, and the patient's ability to tolerate oral potassium. Severe, symptomatic hypokalemia requires aggressive treatment. Supplementation is more cautious if renal function is decreased because of the kidney's limited ability to excrete excessive potassium. The plasma potassium level does not always provide an accurate estimation of the total body potassium deficit because there may be shifts of potassium from the intracellular space to the plasma. Clinically, this shift occurs most commonly with metabolic acidosis and as a result of the insulin deficiency of diabetic ketoacidosis; the plasma potassium underestimates the degree of total body potassium depletion. When these problems are corrected, potassium moves into the intracellular space, and these patients require more potassium supplementation to correct the hypokalemia. Patients who have ongoing losses of potassium need correction of the deficit and replacement of the ongoing losses.

Because of the risk of hyperkalemia, intravenous (IV) potassium should be used cautiously. Oral potassium is safer in nonurgent situations. The dose of IV potassium is 0.5-1 mEq/kg, usually given over 1 hour. The adult maximum dose is 40 mEq. Conservative dosing is generally preferred. For patients with excessive urinary losses, potassium-sparing diuretics are effective. When hypokalemia, metabolic alkalosis, and volume depletion are present, restoration of intravascular volume decreases urinary potassium losses.

HYPERKALEMIA

Decision-Making Algorithm
Available @ StudentConsult.com

Hyperkalemia

Etiology

Three basic mechanisms cause hyperkalemia (Table 36.3). In the individual patient, the etiology is sometimes multifactorial. **Factitious hyperkalemia** is usually due to hemolysis during phlebotomy, but it can be the result of prolonged tourniquet application or fist clenching during phlebotomy, which causes local potassium release from muscle. Falsely elevated serum potassium levels can occur when serum levels are measured in patients with markedly elevated white blood cell or platelet counts; a promptly analyzed plasma sample usually provides an accurate result.

Because of the kidney's ability to excrete potassium, it is unusual for excessive intake, by itself, to cause hyperkalemia. This mechanism can occur in a patient who is receiving large quantities of IV or oral potassium for excessive losses that are no longer present. Frequent or rapid blood transfusions can increase the potassium level acutely secondary to the high potassium content of stored blood. Increased intake may precipitate hyperkalemia if there is an underlying defect in potassium excretion.

The intracellular space has a high potassium concentration, so a **shift of potassium from the intracellular space** to the

TABLE 36.3 Causes of Hyperkalemia

Causes of Hyperkalemia
Spurious laboratory value
Hemolysis
Tissue ischemia during blood drawing
Thrombocytosis
Leukocytosis
Increased intake
IV or PO
Blood transfusions
Transcellular shifts
Acidemia
Rhabdomyolysis
Tumor lysis syndrome
Tissue necrosis
Hemolysis/hematomas/gastrointestinal bleeding
Succinylcholine
Digitalis intoxication
Fluoride intoxication
β-Adrenergic blockers
Exercise
Hyperosmolality
Insulin deficiency
Malignant hyperthermia
Hyperkalemic periodic paralysis
Decreased excretion
Renal failure
Primary adrenal disease
Acquired Addison disease
21-hydroxylase deficiency
3β-hydroxysteroid-dehydrogenase deficiency
Lipoid congenital adrenal hyperplasia
Adrenal hypoplasia congenita
Aldosterone synthase deficiency
Adrenoleukodystrophy
Hyporeninemic hypoaldosteronism
Urinary tract obstruction
Sickle cell disease
Kidney transplant
Lupus nephritis
Renal tubular disease
Pseudohypoaldosteronism type 1
Pseudohypoaldosteronism type 2
Urinary tract obstruction
Sickle cell disease
Kidney transplant
Medications
ACE inhibitors
Angiotensin II blockers
Potassium-sparing diuretics
Cyclosporine
NSAIDs
Trimethoprim

ACE, Angiotensin-converting enzyme; *IV*, intravenous; *NSAIDs*, nonsteroidal antiinflammatory drugs; *PO*, oral.

extracellular space can have a significant impact on the plasma potassium. This shift occurs with acidosis, cell destruction (rhabdomyolysis or tumor lysis syndrome), insulin deficiency, medications (succinylcholine, β-blockers), malignant hyperthermia, and hyperkalemic periodic paralysis.

Hyperkalemia secondary to decreased excretion occurs with renal insufficiency. The risk of hyperkalemia secondary to medications that decrease renal potassium excretion is greatest in patients with underlying renal insufficiency.

Aldosterone deficiency or unresponsiveness to aldosterone causes hyperkalemia, often with associated metabolic acidosis (see Chapter 37) and hyponatremia. A form of congenital adrenal hyperplasia, **21-hydroxylase deficiency,** is the most frequent cause of aldosterone deficiency in children. Untreated patients have hyperkalemia, metabolic acidosis, hyponatremia, and volume depletion.

Renin, via angiotensin II, stimulates aldosterone production. A deficiency in renin, resulting from kidney damage, can lead to decreased aldosterone production. These patients typically have hyperkalemia and a metabolic acidosis, without hyponatremia. Some patients have impaired renal function, partially accounting for the hyperkalemia, but the impairment in potassium excretion is more extreme than expected for the degree of renal insufficiency.

Children with **pseudohypoaldosteronism (PHA) type 1** have hyperkalemia, metabolic acidosis, and salt wasting, leading to hyponatremia and volume depletion; aldosterone levels are elevated. In the autosomal recessive variant, there is a defect in the renal sodium channel that is normally activated by aldosterone. In the autosomal dominant form, patients have a defect in the aldosterone receptor, and the disease is milder, often remitting in adulthood. PHA type 2, also called **Gordon syndrome,** is an autosomal dominant disorder characterized by hypertension secondary to salt retention and impaired excretion of potassium and acid, leading to hyperkalemia and metabolic acidosis. PHA type 2 responds to a thiazide diuretic.

Clinical Manifestations

The most import effects of hyperkalemia are due to the role of potassium in membrane polarization. The cardiac conduction system is usually the dominant concern. **ECG changes** begin with peaking of the T waves. As the potassium level increases, an increased P-R interval, flattening of the P wave, and widening of the QRS complex occur; this eventually can progress to ventricular fibrillation. Asystole also may occur. Some patients have paresthesias, weakness, and tingling, but cardiac toxicity usually precedes these clinical symptoms.

Diagnosis

The etiology of hyperkalemia is often readily apparent. Spurious hyperkalemia is common in children, so a repeat potassium level is often appropriate. If there is a significant elevation of the white blood cells or platelets, the repeat sample should be from plasma that is evaluated promptly. Initially, the history should focus on potassium intake, risk factors for transcellular shifts of potassium, medications that cause hyperkalemia, and the presence of signs of renal insufficiency, such as oliguria or an abnormal urinalysis. Initial laboratory evaluation should include serum creatinine and assessment of acid-base status. Many causes of hyperkalemia, such as renal insufficiency and aldosterone insufficiency or resistance, cause a metabolic acidosis. Cell destruction, as seen in rhabdomyolysis or tumor lysis syndrome, can cause concomitant hyperphosphatemia, hyperuricemia, and an elevated serum lactate dehydrogenase.

TABLE 36.4 Treatment of Hyperkalemia

Rapidly decrease the risk of life-threatening arrhythmias
Shift potassium intracellularly
Sodium bicarbonate administration (IV)
Insulin and glucose (IV)
β-agonist (albuterol via nebulizer)
Cardiac membrane stabilization
IV calcium
Remove potassium from the body
Loop diuretic (IV or PO)
Sodium polystyrene (PO or rectal)
Dialysis

IV, Intravenous; *PO*, oral.

Treatment

The plasma potassium level, the ECG, and the risk of the problem worsening determine the aggressiveness of the therapeutic approach. A high serum potassium level with ECG changes requires more vigorous treatment. An additional source of concern is a patient with increasing plasma potassium despite minimal intake. This situation can occur if there is cellular release of potassium (tumor lysis syndrome), especially in the setting of diminished excretion (renal failure).

The first action in a child with a concerning elevation of plasma potassium is to stop all sources of additional potassium (oral and IV). If the potassium level is greater than 6.5 mEq/L, an ECG should be obtained to help assess the urgency of the situation. Therapy of hyperkalemia has two basic goals:

1. Prevent life-threatening arrhythmias
2. Remove potassium from the body (Table 36.4)

Treatments that acutely prevent arrhythmias all work quickly (within minutes), but do not remove potassium from the body.

Long-term management of hyperkalemia includes reducing intake via dietary changes, and eliminating or reducing medications that cause hyperkalemia. Some patients require medications, such as sodium polystyrene sulfonate and loop or thiazide diuretics, to increase potassium losses. The disorders that are due to a deficiency in aldosterone respond to replacement therapy with fludrocortisone, which is a mineralocorticoid.

CHAPTER 37

Acid-Base Disorders

Close regulation of pH is necessary for cellular enzymes and other metabolic processes, which function optimally at a normal pH (7.35-7.45). Chronic, mild derangements in acid-base status may interfere with normal growth and development, whereas acute, severe changes in pH can be fatal. Control of acid-base balance depends on the kidneys, the lungs, and the intracellular and extracellular buffers.

The lungs and kidneys maintain a normal acid-base balance. Carbon dioxide (CO_2) generated during normal metabolism is a weak acid. The lungs prevent an increase in the partial pressure of CO_2 (P_{CO_2}) in the blood by excreting the CO_2. Production of CO_2 varies depending on the body's metabolic needs. The rapid pulmonary response to changes in CO_2 concentration occurs via central sensing of the P_{CO_2}, and a subsequent increase or decrease in ventilation to maintain a normal P_{CO_2} (35-45 mm Hg).

The kidneys excrete endogenous acids. An adult normally produces about 1-2 mEq/kg per day of hydrogen ions, whereas a child produces 2-3 mEq/kg per day. The hydrogen ions from endogenous acid production are neutralized by bicarbonate, potentially causing the bicarbonate concentration to fall. The kidneys regenerate this bicarbonate by secreting hydrogen ions, maintaining the serum bicarbonate concentration in the normal range (20-28 mEq/L).

CLINICAL ASSESSMENT OF ACID-BASE DISORDERS

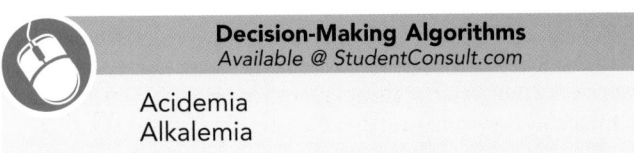

Decision-Making Algorithms
Available @ StudentConsult.com

Acidemia
Alkalemia

Acidemia is a pH below normal (<7.35), and **alkalemia** is a pH above normal (>7.45). **Acidosis** is a pathological process that causes an increase in the hydrogen ion concentration, and **alkalosis** is a pathological process that causes a decrease in the hydrogen ion concentration. A **simple acid-base disorder** is a single primary disturbance. During a simple metabolic disorder, there is respiratory compensation; the P_{CO_2} decreases during metabolic acidosis and increases during metabolic alkalosis. With metabolic acidosis, the decrease in the pH increases the ventilatory drive, causing a decrease in the P_{CO_2}. The fall in the CO_2 concentration leads to an increase in the pH. This **appropriate respiratory compensation** for a metabolic process happens quickly and is complete within 12–24 hours.

During a primary respiratory process, there is metabolic compensation mediated by the kidneys. The kidneys respond to a respiratory acidosis by increasing hydrogen ion excretion, increasing bicarbonate generation, and raising the serum bicarbonate concentration. The kidneys increase bicarbonate excretion to compensate for a respiratory alkalosis; the serum bicarbonate concentration decreases. In contrast to a rapid respiratory compensation, it takes 3-4 days for the kidneys to complete **appropriate metabolic compensation.** However, there is a small and rapid compensatory change in the bicarbonate concentration during a primary respiratory process. The expected appropriate metabolic compensation for a respiratory disorder depends on whether the process is acute or chronic.

A **mixed acid-base disorder** is present when there is more than one primary acid-base disturbance. An infant with bronchopulmonary dysplasia may have respiratory acidosis from chronic lung disease and metabolic alkalosis from a diuretic used to treat the chronic lung disease. Formulas are available for calculating the appropriate metabolic or respiratory compensation for the six primary simple acid-base disorders (Table 37.1). Appropriate compensation is expected in a simple disorder; it is not optional. If a patient does not have appropriate compensation, a mixed acid-base disorder is present.

METABOLIC ACIDOSIS

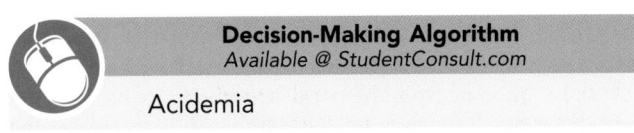

Decision-Making Algorithm
Available @ StudentConsult.com

Acidemia

Metabolic acidosis occurs frequently in hospitalized children; diarrhea is the most common cause. For a patient with an unknown medical problem, the presence of metabolic acidosis is often diagnostically helpful because it suggests a relatively narrow differential diagnosis (Table 37.2).

TABLE 37.1 Appropriate Compensation During Simple Acid-Base Disorders

DISORDER	EXPECTED COMPENSATION*
Metabolic acidosis	$P_{CO_2} = 1.5 \times [HCO_3^-] + 8 \pm 2$
Metabolic alkalosis	P_{CO_2} increases by 7 mm Hg for each 10 mEq/L increase in the serum $[HCO_3^-]$
Respiratory acidosis	
Acute	$[HCO_3^-]$ increases by 1 for each 10 mm Hg increase in the P_{CO_2}
Chronic	$[HCO_3^-]$ increases by 3.5 for each 10 mm Hg increase in the P_{CO_2}
Respiratory alkalosis	
Acute	$[HCO_3^-]$ falls by 2 for each 10 mm Hg decrease in the P_{CO_2}
Chronic	$[HCO_3^-]$ falls by 4 for each 10 mm Hg decrease in the P_{CO_2}

*$[HCO_3^-]$ is expressed in mEq/L.

TABLE 37.2 Causes of Metabolic Acidosis

NORMAL ANION GAP
Diarrhea
Renal tubular acidosis
Urinary tract diversions
Posthypocapnia
Ammonium chloride intake
INCREASED ANION GAP
Lactic acidosis (shock)
Ketoacidosis (diabetic, starvation, or alcoholic)
Kidney failure
Poisoning (e.g., ethylene glycol, methanol, or salicylates)
Inborn errors of metabolism

Etiology

The plasma **anion gap** is useful for evaluating patients with metabolic acidosis. It divides patients into two diagnostic groups: normal anion gap and increased anion gap. The following formula determines the anion gap:

$$\text{Anion Gap} = Na^+ - (Cl^- + HCO_3^-)$$

A normal anion gap is 12 ± 2 mEq/L.

Normal anion gap metabolic acidosis occurs in the setting of diarrhea and renal tubular acidosis (RTA). Diarrhea causes a loss of bicarbonate from the body. The amount of bicarbonate lost in the stool depends on the volume of diarrhea and the bicarbonate concentration of the stool, which tends to increase with more severe diarrhea. Diarrhea often causes volume depletion because of losses of sodium and water, potentially exacerbating the acidosis by causing hypoperfusion (shock) and a lactic acidosis.

There are three forms of RTA:

1. Distal (type I)
2. Proximal (type II)
3. Hyperkalemic (type IV)

In **distal RTA (dRTA),** children may have accompanying hypokalemia, hypercalciuria, nephrolithiasis, and nephrocalcinosis; rickets is a less common finding. Failure to thrive, resulting from chronic metabolic acidosis, is the most common presenting complaint. Autosomal dominant (relatively mild) and autosomal recessive (more severe) forms of dRTA exist. Autosomal recessive dRTA is often associated with deafness secondary to a defect in the gene for a H^+-ATPase that is present in the kidney and the inner ear. dRTA also may be secondary to medications or congenital or acquired renal disease. Patients with dRTA cannot acidify their urine and have a urine pH greater than 5.5, despite metabolic acidosis.

Proximal RTA is rarely present in isolation. In most patients, proximal RTA is part of **Fanconi syndrome**, a generalized dysfunction of the proximal tubule. Along with renal wasting of bicarbonate, Fanconi syndrome causes glycosuria, aminoaciduria, and excessive urinary losses of phosphate and uric acid. The chronic hypophosphatemia is more clinically significant because it ultimately leads to rickets in children. Rickets or failure to thrive may be the presenting complaint. Fanconi syndrome is rarely an isolated genetic disorder, with pediatric cases usually secondary to an underlying genetic disorder, most commonly **cystinosis.** Medications, such as ifosfamide or valproate, may cause Fanconi syndrome. The ability to acidify the urine is intact in proximal RTA, and untreated patients have a urine pH less than 5.5.

In **hyperkalemic RTA,** renal excretion of acid and potassium is impaired because of either an absence of aldosterone or an inability of the kidney to respond to aldosterone. In severe aldosterone deficiency, as occurs with congenital adrenal hyperplasia secondary to 21α-hydroxylase deficiency, the hyperkalemia and metabolic acidosis are accompanied by hyponatremia and volume depletion from renal salt wasting. Incomplete aldosterone deficiency causes less severe electrolyte disturbances; children may have isolated hyperkalemic RTA, hyperkalemia without acidosis, or isolated hyponatremia.

Distal and hyperkalemic RTA are similar in that distal tubular acidification is impaired. Conversely, in proximal RTA, distal tubular acidification is intact, but leads to metabolic acidosis due to bicarbonate wasting.

Increased anion gap metabolic acidosis occurs with lactic acidosis, ketoacidosis, chronic renal failure, and toxic ingestions. Lactic acidosis most commonly occurs when inadequate oxygen delivery to the tissues leads to anaerobic metabolism and excess production of lactic acid. Lactic acidosis may be secondary to shock, severe anemia, or hypoxemia. Inborn errors of carbohydrate metabolism produce a severe lactic acidosis (see Chapter 52). In diabetes mellitus, inadequate insulin leads to hyperglycemia and diabetic ketoacidosis (see Chapter 171). Renal failure (see Chapter 165) causes metabolic acidosis because the kidneys are unable to excrete the acid produced by normal metabolism.

A variety of **toxic ingestions** cause metabolic acidosis. Acute **salicylate** intoxication occurs after a large overdose. Chronic salicylate intoxication is possible because of the gradual buildup of the drug. Patients may also have a respiratory alkalosis. Other symptoms of salicylate intoxication include fever, seizures, lethargy, and coma. Hyperventilation may be particularly marked. Tinnitus, vertigo, and hearing impairment are more likely with chronic salicylate intoxication. **Ethylene glycol,** a component of antifreeze, is converted in the liver to glyoxylic and oxalic acids, causing a severe metabolic acidosis. Excessive oxalate excretion causes calcium oxalate crystals to appear in the urine, and calcium oxalate precipitation in the kidney tubules can cause renal failure. The toxicity of **methanol** ingestion also depends on liver metabolism; formic acid is the toxic end product that causes the metabolic acidosis and other sequelae, which include damage to the optic nerve and central nervous system.

There are many **inborn errors of metabolism** that may cause metabolic acidosis (see Section 10). Metabolic acidosis may be due to excessive production of ketoacids, lactic acid, or other organic anions. Some patients may have accompanying hyperammonemia. In most patients, acidosis occurs only episodically during acute decompensations, which may be precipitated by the ingestion of specific dietary substrates (proteins), the stress of a mild illness (fasting, catabolism), or poor adherence with dietary or medical therapy.

Clinical Manifestations

The underlying disorder usually produces most of the signs and symptoms in children with a mild or moderate metabolic acidosis. The clinical manifestations of the acidosis are related to the degree of acidemia; patients with appropriate respiratory compensation and less severe acidemia have fewer manifestations than patients with a concomitant respiratory acidosis. At a serum pH less than 7.20, there is impaired cardiac contractility and an increased risk of arrhythmias, especially if underlying heart disease or other predisposing electrolyte disorders are present. With acidemia, there is a decrease in the cardiovascular response to catecholamines, potentially exacerbating hypotension in children with volume depletion or shock. Acidemia causes vasoconstriction of the pulmonary vasculature, which is especially problematic in neonates with primary pulmonary hypertension of the newborn (see Chapter 61). The normal respiratory response to metabolic acidosis—compensatory hyperventilation—may be subtle with mild metabolic acidosis, but it causes discernible increased respiratory effort with worsening acidemia. Chronic metabolic acidosis causes failure to thrive.

Diagnosis

Calculating the anion gap can help narrow the differential diagnosis for acidosis. However, the anion gap should not be interpreted in dogmatic isolation; consideration of other laboratory abnormalities and the clinical history improves its diagnostic utility. A decrease in the albumin concentration of 1 g/dL decreases the anion gap by roughly 4 mEq/L. Similarly, albeit less commonly, an increase in unmeasured cations, such as calcium, potassium, or magnesium, decreases the anion gap. Conversely, a decrease in unmeasured cations is a rare cause of an increased anion gap. Because of these variables, the broad range of a normal anion gap, and other factors, the presence of a normal or increased anion gap is not always reliable in differentiating the causes of a metabolic acidosis, especially when the metabolic acidosis is mild. Some patients have more than one explanation for their metabolic acidosis, such as a child with diarrhea and lactic acidosis secondary to shock.

Treatment

The most effective therapeutic approach for patients with a metabolic acidosis is correction of the underlying disorder, if possible. The administration of insulin in diabetic ketoacidosis or restoration of adequate perfusion in lactic acidosis from shock eventually results in normalization of acid-base balance. The use of bicarbonate therapy is indicated when the underlying disorder is irreparable; examples include RTA and chronic renal failure. In salicylate poisoning, alkali administration increases renal clearance of salicylate and decreases the amount of salicylate in brain cells. Short-term base therapy is often necessary in other poisonings and inborn errors of metabolism.

METABOLIC ALKALOSIS

Etiology

The causes of a metabolic alkalosis are divided into two categories based on the urinary chloride (Table 37.3). The alkalosis in patients with a low urinary chloride is maintained by volume depletion. They are called **chloride responsive** because volume repletion with fluid containing sodium chloride and potassium chloride is necessary to correct the metabolic alkalosis. Emesis, which causes loss of hydrochloride and volume depletion, is the most common cause of a metabolic alkalosis. Diuretic use increases chloride excretion in the urine. Consequently, while a patient is receiving diuretics, the urinary chloride is typically high (>20 mEq/L). After the diuretic effect resolves, the urinary chloride is low (<15 mEq/L) because of appropriate renal chloride retention in response to volume depletion. Categorization of diuretics based on urinary chloride depends on the timing of the measurement. The metabolic alkalosis from diuretics is clearly chloride responsive; it corrects after adequate volume repletion. This is the rationale for including it among the chloride-responsive causes of a metabolic alkalosis.

The **chloride-resistant** causes of metabolic alkalosis can be subdivided based on blood pressure. Patients with the rare disorders that cause metabolic alkalosis and hypertension either have increased aldosterone or act as if they have increased aldosterone. Patients with Bartter syndrome or Gitelman syndrome (Chapter 36) have metabolic alkalosis, hypokalemia, and normal blood pressure secondary to renal tubular defects, which cause continuous urinary losses of chloride.

TABLE 37.3 Causes of Metabolic Alkalosis

CHLORIDE RESPONSIVE (URINARY CHLORIDE <15 mEq/L)
Gastric losses (emesis or nasogastric suction)
Pyloric stenosis
Diuretics (loop or thiazide)
Chloride-losing diarrhea
Chloride-deficient formula
Cystic fibrosis (sweat losses of chloride)
Posthypercapnia (chloride loss during respiratory acidosis)
CHLORIDE RESISTANT (URINARY CHLORIDE >20 mEq/L)
High Blood Pressure
Adrenal adenoma or hyperplasia
Glucocorticoid-remediable aldosteronism
Renovascular disease
Renin-secreting tumor
17α-hydroxylase deficiency
11β-hydroxylase deficiency
Cushing syndrome
11 β-hydroxysteroid dehydrogenase deficiency
Licorice ingestion
Liddle syndrome
Normal Blood Pressure
Gitelman syndrome
Bartter syndrome
Base administration

Clinical Manifestations

The symptoms in patients with metabolic alkalosis often are related to the underlying disease and associated electrolyte disturbances. Hypokalemia is often present and occasionally severe (see Chapter 36). Children with chloride-responsive causes of metabolic alkalosis often have symptoms related to volume depletion (see Chapter 33). In contrast, children with chloride-unresponsive causes may have symptoms related to hypertension. Severe alkalemia may cause arrhythmias, hypoxia secondary to hypoventilation, or decreased cardiac output.

Diagnosis

Measurement of the urinary chloride concentration is the most helpful test in differentiating among the causes of metabolic alkalosis. The history usually suggests a diagnosis, although no obvious explanation may be present in the patient with bulimia, surreptitious diuretic use, or an undiagnosed genetic disorder, such as Bartter syndrome or Gitelman syndrome.

Treatment

The approach to therapy of metabolic alkalosis depends on the severity of the alkalosis and the underlying etiology. In children with mild metabolic alkalosis ($[HCO_3^-] < 32$ mEq/L), intervention is often unnecessary. Patients with chloride-responsive

TABLE 37.4 Causes of Respiratory Acidosis
Central nervous system depression (encephalitis or narcotic overdose)
Disorders of the spinal cord, peripheral nerves, or neuromuscular junction (botulism or Guillain-Barré syndrome)
Respiratory muscle weakness (muscular dystrophy)
Pulmonary disease (pneumonia or asthma)
Upper airway disease (laryngospasm)

TABLE 37.5 Causes of Respiratory Alkalosis
Hypoxemia or tissue hypoxia (carbon monoxide poisoning or cyanotic heart disease)
Lung receptor stimulation (pneumonia or pulmonary embolism)
Central stimulation (anxiety or brain tumor)
Mechanical ventilation
Hyperammonemias

metabolic alkalosis respond to the correction of hypokalemia and volume repletion with sodium and potassium chloride, but aggressive volume repletion may be contraindicated if mild volume depletion is medically necessary in the child receiving diuretic therapy. In children with chloride-resistant causes of metabolic alkalosis that are associated with hypertension, volume repletion is contraindicated because it exacerbates the hypertension and does not repair the metabolic alkalosis. Treatment focuses on eliminating or blocking the action of the excess mineralocorticoid. In children with Bartter syndrome or Gitelman syndrome, therapy includes oral sodium and potassium supplementation and potassium-sparing diuretics.

RESPIRATORY ACID-BASE DISTURBANCES

During respiratory acidosis, there is a decrease in the effectiveness of CO_2 removal by the lungs. The causes of respiratory acidosis are either pulmonary or nonpulmonary (Table 37.4). A respiratory alkalosis is an inappropriate reduction in the blood CO_2 concentration. A variety of stimuli can increase the ventilatory drive and cause respiratory alkalosis (Table 37.5). Treatment of respiratory acid-base disorders focuses on correction of the underlying disorder. Mechanical ventilation may be necessary in a child with refractory respiratory acidosis.

Suggested Readings

Colletti JE, Brown KM, Sharieff GQ, et al. ACEP Pediatric Emergency Medicine Committee. The management of children with gastroenteritis and dehydration in the emergency department. *J Emerg Med.* 2010;38:686–698.
Friedman A. Fluid and electrolyte therapy: a primer. *Pediatr Nephrol.* 2010;25:843–846.
Gennari FJ. Pathophysiology of metabolic alkalosis: a new classification based on the centrality of stimulated collecting duct ion transport. *Am J Kidney Dis.* 2011;58:626–636.
Greenbaum LA. Pathophysiology of body fluids and fluid therapy. In: Kliegman RM, Stanton BF, St. Geme JW, et al, eds. *Nelson Textbook of Pediatrics.* 20th ed. Philadelphia: Elsevier Science; 2016:346–391.
Kraut JA, Madias NE. Differential diagnosis of nongap metabolic acidosis: value of a systematic approach. *Clin J Am Soc Nephrol.* 2012;7:671–679.
Pepin J, Shields C. Advances in diagnosis and management of hypokalemic and hyperkalemic emergencies. *Emerg Med Pract.* 2012;14:1–17.
Simpson JN, Teach SJ. Pediatric rapid fluid resuscitation. *Curr Opin Pediatr.* 2011;23:286–292.
Unwin RJ, Luft FC, Shirley DG. Pathophysiology and management of hypokalemia: a clinical perspective. *Nat Rev Nephrol.* 2011;7:75–84.

PEARLS FOR PRACTITIONERS

CHAPTER 32

Maintenance Fluid Therapy

- Maintenance of normal plasma osmolality within the extracellular compartment depends on the regulation of water balance, which is controlled by antidiuretic hormone (ADH); water intake due to thirst has an important role when the osmolality is elevated.
- Control of osmolality is subordinate to the maintenance of an adequate intravascular volume. When significant volume depletion is present, ADH secretion and thirst are stimulated, regardless of the plasma osmolality.
- Sodium is the dominant extracellular fluid space cation and usually reflects extracellular fluid status.
- Control of volume status depends on the regulation of sodium balance. Excretion of sodium by the kidneys is driven by effective plasma volume rather than by serum osmolality or sodium.
- Maintenance intravenous (IV) fluids in patients who cannot be fed enterally replace insensible, stool, and urinary losses of water, and urinary and stool losses of electrolytes.
- The glucose in maintenance fluids provides approximately 20% of normal caloric needs to prevent the development of starvation ketoacidosis and diminish the protein degradation that would occur if the patient received no calories, but maintenance fluids are not a long-term replacement for nutrition.
- Maintenance solutions are usually D5 in ½ NS plus 20 mEq/L KCl.

CHAPTER 33

Dehydration and Replacement Therapy

- Insensible water losses from the skin and lungs are about 35% of normal water losses.

- An anuric child who is not dehydrated and is not being fed enterally only requires normal insensible fluids to maintain euvolemia.
- Children with excessive losses (stool, urine, other) may need a replacement solution to avoid volume depletion.
- A 20 mL/kg bolus of an isotonic fluid (normal saline, Ringer's lactate) is given over approximately 20 minutes in a child with significant dehydration.
- The blood urea nitrogen (BUN) is elevated out of proportion to the serum creatinine in patients with volume depletion.
- Hyponatremic dehydration occurs when hypotonic fluids such as water or diluted formula are given to a child with gastroenteritis.
- Hypernatremic dehydration occurs in children with poor thirst, poor fluid intake, or excessive urine water losses (diabetes insipidus).
- Too rapid correction of hypernatremic dehydration may produce cerebral edema.
- Mild to moderate diarrheal dehydration can be treated with oral rehydration solution.

CHAPTER 34

Parenteral Nutrition

- Parenteral nutrition (PN) is necessary when enteral feeding is inadequate to meet nutritional needs.
- Short bowel syndrome is a common disorder requiring PN.
- Calories from PN are predominantly from dextrose and fat. Amino acids should mostly be used for protein synthesis.
- Complications of PN include thrombosis and line infection.
- The most concerning complication of long-term PN is cholestatic liver disease, but the risk is reduced by utilization of the gastrointestinal (GI) tract even if just for trophic feeds.

CHAPTER 35

Sodium Disorders

- Most disorders of sodium are secondary to abnormalities in water balance.
- The symptoms of hyponatremia, such as seizures, are principally due to water movement into brain cells.
- The symptoms of hypernatremia are due water movement out of brain cells, which may lead to brain hemorrhage if the hypernatremia is severe.
- Symptoms of hyponatremia are much more likely if the hyponatremia develops rapidly.
- Diagnosing the etiology of hyponatremia should begin by assessing a patient's volume status (hypovolemic, euvolemic, or hypervolemic).
- Most cases of hyponatremia are due to gastroenteritis, but the syndrome of inappropriate antidiuretic hormone secretion (SIADH) or hypervolemic causes (heart failure, cirrhosis) should be considered.
- Most cases of hypernatremia are due to gastroenteritis, but diabetes insipidus must be considered.
- Overly rapid correction of hyponatremia can lead to central pontine myelinolysis; it is optimal to increase the serum sodium less than 12 mEq/L per 24 hours.
- Due to the presence of idiogenic osmoles, overly rapid correction of hypernatremia can lead to cerebral edema, and thus the target decrease in serum sodium is <12 mEq/L per 24 hours.
- Acute water intoxication producing hyponatremia often self-corrects once excessive water intake has stopped.
- The emergency treatment of symptomatic hyponatremia involves the use of IV hypertonic saline to decrease brain edema.

CHAPTER 36

Potassium Disorders

- The kidneys are the principal regulator of potassium balance.
- Hypokalemia is secondary to renal losses, nonrenal losses (diarrhea), low intake, or transcellular shifts.
- Transcellular potassium shifts are seen in treated diabetic ketoacidosis and patients with asthma treated with albuterol.
- Severe hypokalemia causes muscle cramps and muscle weakness, which may proceed to paralysis.
- Hypokalemia with a metabolic acidosis suggests renal tubular acidosis.
- Hypokalemia with a metabolic alkalosis is most commonly due to emesis or NG losses, but may also be due to Bartter or Gitelman syndromes or diuretic use.
- Arrhythmias, which may be fatal, are often the initial clinical manifestation of hyperkalemia.
- Peaked T waves are a sign of hyperkalemia.
- Hyperkalemia is most commonly due to decreased excretion or a transcellular shift, although increased intake may cause or contribute.
- Hyperkalemia may be seen in disorders with decreased renin, decreased aldosterone (congenital adrenal hyperplasia) or lack response to aldosterone (decreased aldosterone effect).
- Hyperkalemia may produce paresthesia and muscle weakness.
- The two goals of treating hyperkalemia, which require different therapeutic approaches, are to prevent cardiac toxicity and to decrease total body potassium.
- Total body potassium may be reduced by loop or thiazide diuretics, dialysis, or potassium-binding resins.

CHAPTER 37

Acid-Base Disorders

- Acute, severe changes in pH can be fatal, while chronic, mild derangements may interfere with growth and development.
- The lungs and the kidneys maintain normal acid-base balance. The lungs (respiratory) regulate CO_2 concentration, and the kidneys (metabolic) regulate bicarbonate concentration.
- During a primary respiratory process, the kidneys compensate, but full compensation takes a few days.
- During a primary metabolic process, the lungs compensate, and this compensation occurs rapidly.

- Appropriate compensation is expected in a simple acid-base disorder; it is not optional. If a patient does not have appropriate compensation, a mixed acid-base disorder is present.
- The plasma anion gap divides patients with metabolic acidosis into two categories: normal anion gap and increased anion gap.
- Normal anion gap metabolic acidosis occurs in the setting of diarrhea and renal tubular acidosis.
- Increased anion gap metabolic acidosis occurs with lactic acidosis, ketoacidosis, chronic renal failure, and toxic ingestions.
- The differential diagnosis of metabolic alkalosis begins by measuring the urine chloride and separating patients based on whether the urinary chloride is low or high.
- Patients with a metabolic alkalosis and a low urine chloride are volume depleted, and the alkalosis responds to administration of sodium or potassium chloride (chloride responsive).
- Patients with chloride-resistant metabolic alkalosis (urine chloride not low) are subdivided based on the presence of a normal or elevated blood pressure.

ACUTELY ILL OR INJURED CHILD

Tara L. Petersen | K. Jane Lee

CHAPTER 38

Assessment and Resuscitation

INITIAL ASSESSMENT

Initial assessment (the **ABCs—airway, breathing, and circulation**) of an acutely ill or injured child includes rapid identification of physiological derangements in **tissue perfusion and oxygenation.** Once identified, immediate resuscitation must be implemented before pursuing the usual information needed to develop a differential diagnosis. Initial resuscitation measures are directed at achieving and maintaining adequate tissue perfusion and oxygenation. **Oxygen delivery** depends on cardiac output, hemoglobin concentration, and hemoglobin-oxygen saturation. The latter depends on air movement, alveolar gas exchange, pulmonary blood flow, and hemoglobin-oxygen binding characteristics.

HISTORY

In the initial assessment of an acutely ill or traumatically injured child, access to historical information may be limited. Characterization of the onset of symptoms, event details, and a brief identification of underlying medical problems should be sought by members of the team not actively involved in the resuscitation. The mnemonic AMPLE can be employed to help direct a focused history during this time: A, Allergies; M, Medications; P, Past medical history; L, Last meal; and E, Events leading up to patient presentation. Attempts at identifying historical issues that affect the ABCs are useful but should not delay intervention if tissue oxygenation and perfusion are markedly impaired.

PHYSICAL EXAMINATION

Initial examination must focus on the responsiveness of a patient followed by assessment of the **ABCs** (Table 38.1) to systematically address the issues of oxygen delivery to tissues. Assessment of airway patency should also include evaluation of the neurologically injured child's ability to protect the airway. Protection of the cervical spine should be initiated at this step in any child with traumatic injury or who presents with altered mental status of uncertain etiology. Assessment of breathing includes observation of respiratory effort, rate, and chest rise, plus the auscultation of air movement and the application of a pulse oximeter (when available) to identify current oxygenation status. Circulatory status is assessed by palpation for distal and central pulses, focusing on the presence and quality of the pulses. Bounding pulses and a wide pulse pressure are often the first sign of the vasodilatory phase of shock and require immediate resuscitation measures. Weak, thready, or absent pulses are indicators for fluid resuscitation, initiation of chest compressions, or both. When assessment of the **ABCs** is complete and measures have been taken to achieve an acceptable level of tissue oxygenation, a more complete physical examination is performed. The sequence of this examination depends on whether the situation involves an acute medical illness or trauma. In trauma patients, the examination follows the **ABCDE pathway. D** stands for disability and prompts assessment of the neurological system and evaluation for major traumatic injuries. **E** stands for exposure; the child is disrobed and examined for evidence of any life-threatening or limb-threatening problems. For the acutely ill and the injured child, the physical examination should identify evidence of organ dysfunction, starting with areas suggested in the chief complaint and progressing to a thorough and systematic investigation of the entire patient.

COMMON MANIFESTATIONS

The physiological responses to acute illness and injury are mechanisms that attempt to correct inadequacies of tissue oxygenation and perfusion. When initial changes, such as increasing heart and respiratory rates, fail to meet the body's needs, other manifestations of impending cardiopulmonary failure occur (Table 38.2). **Respiratory failure**, the most common cause of acute deterioration in children, may result in inadequate tissue oxygenation and in respiratory acidosis. Signs and symptoms of respiratory failure (tachypnea, tachycardia, increased work of breathing, abnormal mentation) progress as tissue oxygenation becomes more inadequate. Inadequate perfusion (shock) leads to inadequate oxygen delivery and a resulting metabolic acidosis. **Shock** is characterized by signs of inadequate tissue perfusion (pallor, cool skin, poor pulses, delayed capillary refill, oliguria, and abnormal mentation). The presence of any of these symptoms demands careful assessment and intervention to correct the abnormality and to prevent further deterioration.

INITIAL DIAGNOSTIC EVALUATION

Screening Tests

During the initial phase of resuscitation, monitoring vital signs and physiological status is the key screening activity. Continuous monitoring with attention to changes may indicate response to therapy or further deterioration requiring additional

TABLE 38.1 Rapid Cardiopulmonary Assessment

AIRWAY PATENCY
Able to be maintained independently
Maintainable with positioning, suctioning
Unmaintainable, requires assistance
BREATHING
Rate
Mechanics
• Retractions
• Grunting
• Use of accessory muscles
• Nasal flaring
Air movement
• Chest expansion
• Breath sounds
• Stridor
• Wheezing
• Paradoxical chest motion
Color
CIRCULATION
Heart rate
Peripheral and central pulses
• Present/absent
• Volume/strength
Skin perfusion
• Capillary refill time
• Skin temperature
• Color
• Mottling
Blood pressure
CENTRAL NERVOUS SYSTEM PERFUSION
Responsiveness (AVPU)
Recognition of parents or caregivers
Pupillary response to light Posturing

AVPU, **A**lert, responds to **v**oice, responds to **p**ain, **u**nresponsive.

intervention. During the initial rapid assessment, diagnostic evaluation often is limited to pulse oximetry and bedside measurement of glucose levels. The latter is important in any child with altered mental status or at risk for inadequate glycogen stores (infants, malnourished patients). After resuscitation measures, further diagnostic tests and imaging are often necessary.

Diagnostic Tests and Imaging

The choice of appropriate diagnostic tests and imaging is determined by the mechanism of disease and the results of evaluation after initial resuscitation. The initial evaluation of major trauma patients is focused on identifying evidence of hemorrhage and organ and tissue injury. For an acutely ill child with respiratory distress, a chest x-ray is important. Appropriate cultures should be obtained when sepsis is suspected. Children with historical or physical evidence of inadequate intravascular volume should have serum electrolyte levels obtained, including bicarbonate, blood urea nitrogen, and creatinine.

TABLE 38.2 Warning Signs and Symptoms Suggesting the Need for Resuscitation*

SYSTEM	SIGNS AND SYMPTOMS
Central nervous system	Lethargy, agitation, delirium, obtundation, confusion
Respiratory	Apnea, grunting, nasal flaring, dyspnea, retracting, tachypnea, poor air movement, stridor, wheezing
Cardiovascular	Arrhythmia, bradycardia, tachycardia, weak pulses, poor capillary refill, hypotension
Skin and mucous membranes	Mottling, pallor, cyanosis, diaphoresis, poor membrane turgor, dry mucous membranes

**Action would seldom be taken if only one or two of these signs and symptoms were present, but the occurrence of several in concert foreshadows grave consequences. Intervention should be directed at the primary disorder.*

RESUSCITATION

Resuscitation is focused on correcting identified abnormalities of oxygenation and perfusion and preventing further deterioration. **Oxygen supplementation** may improve oxygen saturation but may not completely correct tissue oxygenation. When oxygen supplementation is insufficient or air exchange is inadequate, assisted ventilation must be initiated. Inadequate perfusion is usually best managed initially by providing a fluid bolus. **Isotonic crystalloids** (normal saline, lactated Ringer solution) are the initial fluid of choice. A bolus of 10-20 mL/kg should be delivered in monitored conditions. Improvement, but not correction, after an initial bolus should prompt repeated boluses until circulation has been re-established. Because most children with shock have noncardiac causes, fluid administration of this magnitude is well tolerated. If hemorrhage is known or highly suspected, administration of packed red blood cells is appropriate. Monitoring for deteriorating physiological status during fluid resuscitation (increase in heart rate, decrease in blood pressure) identifies children who may have diminished cardiac function. In these cases, as fluid resuscitation increases the preload, impaired cardiac function may worsen and pulmonary edema can result. If deterioration occurs, fluid administration should be interrupted and further resuscitation should be aimed at improving cardiac function.

When respiratory support and fluid resuscitation are insufficient, introduction of **vasoactive substances** is the next step. The choice of which agent to use depends on the type of shock present. Hypovolemic shock (when further volume is contraindicated) and distributive shock benefit from drugs that increase systemic vascular resistance (drugs with α-agonist activity, such as epinephrine or norepinephrine). The treatment of cardiogenic shock is more complex. To improve cardiac output by increasing the heart rate, drugs with positive chronotropy are used (epinephrine, norepinephrine, and dopamine). Afterload reduction, using drugs such as dobutamine, nitroprusside, or milrinone, also may be needed. Measuring central mixed venous oxygen saturation, central venous pressure, and regional oxygen saturations helps guide therapy.

CARDIOPULMONARY ARREST

The outcome of cardiopulmonary arrest in children is poor; survival to hospital discharge is about 6% for out-of-hospital arrest and about 27% for in-hospital arrest, with most survivors having some degree of permanent neurological disability. The ability to anticipate or recognize precardiopulmonary arrest conditions and initiate prompt and appropriate therapy is not only lifesaving but also preserves the quality of life (see Table 38.2).

Children who need cardiopulmonary resuscitation (CPR) usually have a primary respiratory arrest. Hypoxia usually initiates the cascade leading to arrest and also produces organ dysfunction or damage (Table 38.3). The approach to cardiopulmonary arrest extends beyond CPR and includes efforts to preserve vital organ function. The goal in resuscitating a pediatric patient following a cardiopulmonary arrest should be to optimize **cardiac output** and tissue oxygen delivery, which may be accomplished by using artificial ventilation and chest compression, and by the judicious administration of pharmacological agents.

Pediatric Advanced Life Support and Cardiopulmonary Resuscitation

In 2010, the American Heart Association revised the recommendations for resuscitation of adults, children, and infants. The biggest change was the recommendation to start chest compressions immediately, rather than beginning with airway and breathing (C[compressions]-A[airway]-B[breathing/ventilation]).

Circulation

Chest compressions should be initiated if a pulse cannot be palpated or if the heart rate is less than 60 beats/min with concurrent signs of poor systemic perfusion. Chest compressions should be performed immediately by one person while a second person prepares to begin ventilation. **Ventilation** is extremely important in pediatric arrests given the high likelihood of a primary respiratory cause; however, ventilation requires equipment and is therefore sometimes delayed. For this reason, the recommendation is to start chest compressions first while preparing for ventilation.

For optimal chest compressions, the child should be supine on a flat, hard surface. Effective CPR requires a compression depth of one-third to one-half of the anterior-posterior diameter of the chest with complete recoil after each compression. The compression rate should be at least 100/min with breaths delivered 8-10 times/min. If an advanced airway is in place, compressions should not pause for ventilation; both should continue simultaneously.

TABLE 38.3 Target Organs for Hypoxic-Ischemic Damage

ORGAN	EFFECT
Brain	Seizures, cerebral edema, infarction, herniation, anoxic damage, SIADH, diabetes insipidus
Cardiovascular	Heart failure, myocardial infarct
Lung and pulmonary vasculature	Acute respiratory distress syndrome, pulmonary hypertension
Liver	Infarction, necrosis, cholestasis
Kidney	Acute tubular necrosis, acute cortical necrosis
Gastrointestinal tract	Gastric ulceration, mucosal damage
Hematological	Disseminated intravascular coagulation

SIADH, Syndrome of inappropriate secretion of antidiuretic hormone.

Airway

Ventilation requires a **patent airway**. In children, airway patency often is compromised by a loss of muscle tone, allowing the mandibular block of tissue, including the tongue, bony mandible, and the soft surrounding tissues, to rest against the posterior pharyngeal wall. The head tilt–chin lift maneuver should be used to open the airway in children with no sign of head or neck trauma. In children with signs of head or neck trauma, the jaw thrust maneuver should be used.

Bag-mask ventilation can be as effective as, and possibly safer than, endotracheal intubation for short periods of time in an out-of-hospital setting. If skilled personnel and proper equipment are available, pediatric patients requiring resuscitation should be endotracheally intubated. Before intubation, the patient should be ventilated with 100% oxygen using a bag and mask. Cricoid pressure should be used to minimize inflation of the stomach. Many conscious patients may benefit from the use of induction medications (sedatives, analgesics, and paralytics) to assist intubation, but caution is necessary to prevent further cardiovascular compromise from vasodilating effects of many sedatives. The correct size of the tube may be estimated according to the size of the child's mid-fifth phalanx or the following formula: 4 + (patient age in years/4).

When the endotracheal tube is in place, the adequacy of ventilation and the position of the tube must be assessed. Use of both clinical assessment and confirmatory devices is recommended. Clinical assessment may include looking for adequate chest wall movement and auscultation of the chest to detect bilateral and symmetric breath sounds. Confirmatory devices, such as end-tidal carbon dioxide (CO_2) monitoring devices, are useful for the validation of endotracheal placement, but low levels of detected CO_2 may be seen secondary to lack of pulmonary circulation. If the patient's condition fails to improve or deteriorates, consider the possibilities of tube **D**isplacement or **O**bstruction, **P**neumothorax, or **E**quipment failure (mnemonic DOPE).

Breathing

The major role of endotracheal intubation is to protect or maintain the airway and ensure the delivery of adequate oxygen to the patient. Because hypoxemia is the final common pathway in pediatric cardiopulmonary arrests, providing oxygen is more important than correcting the respiratory acidosis. The clinician should deliver 100% oxygen at a rate of 8-10 breaths/min during CPR, or 12-20 breaths/min for a patient who has a perfusing

TABLE 38.4 Drug Doses for Cardiopulmonary Resuscitation

DRUG	INDICATION	DOSE
Adenosine	Supraventricular tachycardia	IV: 0.1 mg/kg (maximum 6 mg); second dose: 0.2 mg/kg (maximum 12 mg)
Amiodarone	Pulseless VF/VT	IV/IO: 5 mg/kg; may repeat twice up to 15 mg/kg; maximum single dose 300 mg
	Perfusing tachyarrhythmias	Dose as above but administer slowly over 20-60 min. Expert consultation strongly recommended
Atropine	Supraventricular or junctional bradycardia	IV/IO/IM: 0.02 mg/kg; ET: 0.04-0.06 mg/kg; maximum single dose: 0.5 mg; higher doses needed in organophosphate poisoning
Bicarbonate	Hyperkalemia, some toxidromes	IV/IO: 1 mEq/kg bolus; ensure adequate ventilation; monitor ABGs; can repeat every 10 min
Calcium chloride (10%)	Hypocalcemia, calcium channel blocker overdose, hypermagnesemia, hyperkalemia	IV/IO: 20 mg/kg; maximum single dose 2 g; administer slowly
Dextrose	Hypoglycemia	IV/IO: Newborns: 5-10 mL/kg of 10% dextrose; infants and children: 2-4 mL/kg of 25% dextrose; adolescents: 1-2 mL/kg of 50% dextrose
Epinephrine	Hypotension, chronotropy, inotropy	IV/IO: 0.01 mg/kg (0.1 mL/kg 1:10,000); ET: 0.1 mg/kg (0.1 mL/kg 1:1,000); may repeat every 3-5 min; may promote arrhythmias
Fluid	Hypovolemia, sepsis	IV/IO: Administer crystalloid in 20 mL/kg boluses titrated to patient's physiological needs
Lidocaine	VT	IV/IO: 1 mg/kg/bolus followed by 20-50 μg/kg/min continuous infusion; ET: Loading dose: 2-3 mg/kg/dose; flush with 5 mL of NS and follow with 5 assisted manual ventilations

ABG, Arterial blood gas; *ET*, endotracheal tube; *IM*, intramuscular; *IO*, intraosseous; *IV*, intravenous; *VF*, ventricular fibrillation; *VT*, ventricular tachycardia.
Data from the American Heart Association. Web-based Integrated Guidelines for Cardiopulmonary and Emergency Cardiovascular Care—Part 12. Pediatric advanced life support. Available at https://eccguidelines.heart.org/index.php/circulation/cpr-ecc-guidelines-2/part-12-pediatric-advanced-life-support/.

rhythm. Use only the tidal volume necessary to produce visible chest rise. Care should be taken not to hyperventilate the patient.

Drugs

When mechanical means fail to re-establish adequate circulation, pharmacological intervention is essential (Table 38.4). If intravascular access is not present or rapidly established, administration through an intraosseous route is recommended. Some drugs can also be administered effectively through the endotracheal tube or intramuscularly.

Epinephrine, a catecholamine with mixed α-agonist and β-agonist properties, constitutes the mainstay of drug therapy for CPR. The α-adrenergic effects are most important during acute phases of resuscitation, causing an increase in systemic vascular resistance that improves coronary blood flow. Standard dose therapy is recommended for the first and subsequent boluses. There is no benefit offered by high-dose epinephrine. Vasopressin, an endogenous hormone, causes constriction of capillaries and small arterioles and may be useful. Insufficient data support its routine use, but vasopressin may be considered in children failing standard medication administration.

The routine use of **sodium bicarbonate** is currently not recommended. Sodium bicarbonate may be judiciously used to treat toxidromes or hyperkalemic arrest; however, oxygen delivery and elimination of CO_2 must be established first. Side effects include hypernatremia, hyperosmolality, hypokalemia, metabolic alkalosis (shifting the oxyhemoglobin curve to the left and impairing tissue oxygen delivery), reduced ionized calcium level, and impaired cardiac function.

Routine administration of **calcium** is not recommended. It may be useful in cases of documented hypocalcemia, calcium channel blocker overdose, hypermagnesemia, or hypokalemia, but is otherwise not beneficial and is potentially harmful.

TABLE 38.5 Recommendations for Defibrillation and Cardioversion in Children

DEFIBRILLATION
Place self-adhesive defibrillation pads or paddles with electrode gel at the apex of the heart and the upper right side of the chest • Use infant paddles or self-adhesive pads for children <10 kg; adult size for children >10 kg
Notify all participating personnel before discharging paddles so that no one is in contact with patient or bed
Begin with 2 J/kg; resume chest compressions immediately
If unsuccessful, increase to 4 J/kg and repeat
Higher energy levels may be considered, not to exceed 10 J/kg or the adult maximum dose
CARDIOVERSION
Consider sedation if possible
For symptomatic supraventricular tachycardia* or ventricular tachycardia with a pulse, synchronize signal with ECG
Choose paddles, position pads, and notify personnel as above
Begin with 0.5-1 J/kg
If unsuccessful, use 2 J/kg

*Consider adenosine first (see Table 38.4).
ECG, Electrocardiogram.

Hypoglycemia is not uncommon in infants and children who sustain cardiac arrest. Blood glucose should be checked, and hypoglycemia should be promptly treated with **glucose**.

Prompt electrical **defibrillation** is indicated when ventricular fibrillation or pulseless ventricular tachycardia is noted (Table 38.5). CPR should continue until immediately before defibrillation and resume immediately afterward, minimizing interruptions in compressions. If a second attempt at defibrillation is necessary, it should be followed by a dose of epinephrine. Children failing two episodes of defibrillation may benefit from administration of amiodarone. Defibrillation should be distinguished from **cardioversion** of supraventricular tachycardias, which also may compromise cardiac output. Cardioversion requires a lower starting dose and synchronization of the discharge to the electrocardiogram to prevent discharging during a susceptible period, which may convert supraventricular tachycardia to ventricular tachycardia or fibrillation.

CHAPTER 39

Respiratory Failure

ETIOLOGY

Acute respiratory failure occurs when the pulmonary system is unable to maintain adequate gas exchange to meet metabolic demands. The resulting failure can be classified as hypercarbic ($Paco_2$ >50 mm Hg in previously healthy children), hypoxemic (Pao_2 <60 mm Hg in previously healthy children without an intracardiac shunt), or both. **Hypoxemic respiratory failure** is frequently caused by ventilation-perfusion mismatch (perfusion of lung that is not adequately ventilated) and shunting (deoxygenated blood bypasses ventilated alveoli). **Hypercarbic respiratory failure** results from inadequate alveolar ventilation secondary to decreased minute ventilation (tidal volume × respiratory rate) or an increase in dead space ventilation (ventilation of areas receiving no perfusion).

Respiratory failure may occur with **acute respiratory distress syndrome (ARDS)**. The pediatric-specific definition for acute respiratory distress syndrome (PARDS) builds on the adult-based Berlin Definition, but has been modified to account for differences between adults and children with ARDS. Pediatric ARDS, and its severity, is defined by (1) timing: onset within 7 days of known clinical insult; (2) respiratory failure not fully explained by cardiac failure or fluid overload; (3) chest imaging findings of new infiltrate(s) consistent with acute pulmonary parenchymal disease; and (4) impairment in oxygenation (as described in Table 39.1). Pediatric ARDS can be triggered by a variety of insults, including sepsis, pneumonia, shock, burns, or traumatic injury, all resulting in inflammation and increased vascular permeability leading to pulmonary edema. Numerous mediators of inflammation (tumor necrosis factor, interferon-γ, nuclear factor κB, and adhesion molecules) may be involved in the development of ARDS. Surfactant action also may be affected.

EPIDEMIOLOGY

Respiratory failure is frequently caused by bronchiolitis (often caused by respiratory syncytial virus), asthma, pneumonia, upper airway obstruction, and systemic inflammation resulting in ARDS. Respiratory failure requiring mechanical ventilation develops in 7-21% of patients hospitalized for respiratory syncytial virus.

Asthma is increasing in prevalence and is the most common reason for unplanned hospital admissions in children 3-12 years of age in the United States. Environmental factors (exposure to cigarette smoke) and prior disease characteristics (severity of asthma, exercise intolerance, delayed start of therapy, and previous intensive care unit admissions) affect hospitalization and near-fatal episodes. The mortality rate of asthma for children younger than 19 years of age has increased by nearly 80% since 1980. Deaths are more common in African American children.

Chronic respiratory failure (with acute exacerbations) is often due to chronic lung disease (bronchopulmonary dysplasia, cystic fibrosis), neurological or neuromuscular abnormalities, and congenital anomalies.

CLINICAL MANIFESTATIONS

Early signs of hypoxic respiratory failure include **tachypnea and tachycardia** in an attempt to improve minute ventilation and cardiac output and to maintain delivery of oxygenated blood to the tissues. Further progression of disease may result in dyspnea, nasal flaring, grunting, use of accessory muscles of respiration, and diaphoresis. Late signs of inadequate oxygen delivery include **cyanosis** and **altered mental status** (initially confusion and agitation). Signs and symptoms of hypercarbic respiratory failure include attempts to increase minute ventilation (tachypnea and increased depth of breathing) and altered mental status (somnolence).

LABORATORY AND IMAGING STUDIES

A chest radiograph may show evidence of the etiology of respiratory failure. The detection of atelectasis, hyperinflation,

TABLE 39.1 Pediatric Acute Respiratory Distress Syndrome Severity Based on Oxygenation

NONINVASIVE MECHANICAL VENTILATION PARDS (no severity stratification)	INVASIVE MECHANICAL VENTILATION PARDS (severity per OI or OSI)
Full face mask: bi-level positive airway pressure or continuous positive airway pressure ≥5 H_2O: PF ratio ≤300 SF ratio ≤264	Mild: $4 \le OI < 8$; $5 \le OSI < 7.5$ Moderate: $8 \le OI < 16$; $7.5 \le OSI < 12.3$ Severe: OI >16; OSI ≥12.3

PF ratio = Pao_2:Fio_2; if Pao_2 is not available, wean Fio_2 to maintain Spo_2 ≤97% to calculate the SF ratio = Spo_2: Fio_2.
OI = oxygenation index = [Fio_2 × mean airway pressure × 100]/Pao_2; if Pao_2 is not available, wean Fio_2 to maintain Spo_2 ≤97% to calculate the oxygen saturation index (OSI; [Fio_2 × mean airway pressure × 100]/Spo_2).
PARDS, Pediatric acute respiratory distress syndrome.
Modified from Khemani RG, Smith LS, Zimmerman JJ, Erickson S; Pediatric Acute Lung Injury Consensus Conference Group. Pediatric acute respiratory distress syndrome: definition, incidence and epidemiology: proceeding from the Pediatric Acute Lung Injury Consensus Conference. Pediatr Crit Care Med. *2015;16(5 suppl 1):S23–S40. Fig. 2.*

infiltrates, or pneumothoraces assists with ongoing management. Diffuse infiltrates or pulmonary edema may suggest ARDS. The chest radiograph may be normal when upper airway obstruction or impaired respiratory controls are the etiology. In patients presenting with stridor or other evidence of upper airway obstruction, a lateral neck film or computed tomography (CT) may delineate anatomical defects. Direct visualization through flexible bronchoscopy allows the identification of dynamic abnormalities of the anatomical airway. Helical CT helps diagnose a pulmonary embolus.

Pulse oximetry allows noninvasive, continuous assessment of oxygenation but is unable to provide information about ventilation abnormalities. Determination of CO_2 levels requires a blood gas measurement (venous, capillary or arterial). An **arterial blood gas** is the gold standard for measurement of serum CO_2 levels and allows for analysis of the severity of oxygenation defect through calculation of an alveolar-arterial oxygen difference. A normal $Paco_2$ in a patient who is hyperventilating should heighten concern about the risk of further deterioration.

DIFFERENTIAL DIAGNOSIS

Hypoxic respiratory failure resulting from impairment of alveolar-capillary function is seen in ARDS; cardiogenic pulmonary edema; interstitial lung disease; aspiration pneumonia; bronchiolitis; bacterial, fungal, or viral pneumonia; and sepsis. It also can be due to intracardiac or intrapulmonary shunting seen with atelectasis and embolism.

Hypercarbic respiratory failure can occur when the respiratory center fails as a result of drug use (opioids, barbiturates, anesthetic agents), neurological or neuromuscular junction abnormalities (cervical spine trauma, demyelinating diseases, anterior horn cell disease, botulism), chest wall injuries, or diseases that cause increased resistance to airflow (croup, vocal cord paralysis, postextubation edema). Maintenance of ventilation requires adequate function of the chest wall and diaphragm. Disorders of the neuromuscular pathways, such as muscular dystrophy, myasthenia gravis, and botulism, result in inadequate chest wall movement, development of atelectasis, and respiratory failure. Scoliosis rarely results in significant chest deformity that leads to restrictive pulmonary function. Similar impairments of air exchange may result from distention of the abdomen (postoperatively or due to ascites, obstruction, or a mass) and thoracic trauma (flail chest).

Mixed forms of respiratory failure are common and occur when disease processes result in more than one pathophysiological change. Increased secretions seen in asthma often lead to atelectasis and hypoxia, whereas restrictions of expiratory airflow may lead to hypercarbia. Progression to respiratory failure results from peripheral airway obstruction, extensive atelectasis, and resultant hypoxemia and retention of CO_2.

TREATMENT

Initial treatment of patients in respiratory distress includes addressing the ABCs (see Chapter 38). **Bag/mask ventilation** must be initiated for patients with apnea. In other patients, oxygen therapy is administered using appropriate methods (e.g., simple mask). Administration of oxygen by nasal cannula allows the patient to entrain room air and oxygen, making it an insufficient delivery method for most children in respiratory failure. Delivery methods, including intubation and mechanical ventilation, should be escalated if there is an inability to increase oxygen saturation appropriately.

Patients presenting with hypercarbic respiratory failure are often hypoxic as well. When oxygenation is established, measures should be taken to address the underlying cause of hypercarbia. Patients who are hypercarbic without signs of respiratory fatigue or somnolence may not require intubation based on the Pco_2 alone; however, patients with marked increase in the work of breathing or inadequate respiratory effort may require assistance with ventilation.

After identification of the etiology of respiratory failure, specific interventions and treatments are tailored to the needs of the patient. External support of oxygenation and ventilation may be provided by **noninvasive ventilation** methods (heated humidified high-flow nasal cannula, continuous positive airway pressure, biphasic positive airway pressure, or negative pressure ventilation) or through invasive methods (traditional **mechanical ventilation,** high-frequency oscillatory ventilation, or extracorporeal membrane oxygenation). Elimination of CO_2 is achieved through manipulation of minute ventilation (tidal volume and respiratory rate). Oxygenation is improved by altering variables that affect oxygen delivery (fraction of inspired oxygen) or mean airway pressure (positive end-expiratory pressure [PEEP], peak inspiratory pressure, inspiratory time, gas flow).

COMPLICATIONS

The major complication of hypoxic respiratory failure is the development of organ dysfunction. **Multiple organ dysfunction** includes the development of two or more of the following: respiratory failure, cardiac failure, renal insufficiency/failure, gastrointestinal or hepatic insufficiency, disseminated intravascular coagulation, and hypoxic-ischemic brain injury. Mortality rates increase with increasing numbers of involved organs (see Table 38.3).

Complications associated with mechanical ventilation include pressure-related and volume-related lung injury. Both overdistention and insufficient lung distention (loss of functional residual capacity) are associated with lung injury. Pneumomediastinum and pneumothorax are potential complications of the disease process and overdistention. Inflammatory mediators may play a role in the development of chronic fibrotic lung diseases in ventilated patients.

PROGNOSIS

Prognosis varies with the etiology of respiratory failure. Less than 1% of previously healthy children with bronchiolitis die. Asthma mortality rates, although still low, have increased. Population-based studies report a variable mortality rate for pediatric ARDS from 18-35% depending on the study population.

PREVENTION

Prevention strategies are explicit to the etiology of respiratory failure. Some infectious causes can be prevented through active immunization against organisms causing primary respiratory disease (pertussis, pneumococcus, *Haemophilus influenzae* type

b) and sepsis (pneumococcus, *H. influenzae* type b). Passive immunization with respiratory syncytial virus immunoglobulins prevents severe illness in highly susceptible patients (prematurity, bronchopulmonary dysplasia). Primary prevention of traumatic injuries may decrease the incidence of pediatric ARDS. Compliance with appropriate therapies for asthma may decrease the number of episodes of respiratory failure (see Chapter 78).

CHAPTER 40

Shock

ETIOLOGY AND EPIDEMIOLOGY

Shock is the inability to provide sufficient perfusion of oxygenated blood and substrate to tissues to meet metabolic demands. **Oxygen delivery** is directly related to the arterial oxygen content (oxygen saturation and hemoglobin concentration) and to cardiac output (stroke volume and heart rate). Changes in metabolic needs are met primarily by adjustments in cardiac output. Stroke volume is related to myocardial end-diastolic fiber length (preload), myocardial contractility (inotropy), and resistance of blood ejection from the ventricle (afterload; see Chapter 145). In a young infant whose myocardium possesses relatively less contractile tissue, increased demand for cardiac output is met primarily by a neurally mediated increase in heart rate. In older children and adolescents, cardiac output is most efficiently augmented by increasing stroke volume through neurohormonally mediated changes in vascular tone, resulting in increased venous return to the heart (increased preload), decreased arterial resistance (decreased afterload), and increased myocardial contractility.

Once the initial assessment of an acutely ill child is completed, the constellation of clinical characteristics can suggest one of the five broad classifications of shock: hypovolemic, distributive, cardiogenic, obstructive, and dissociative.

TABLE 40.1 Classification of Shock and Common Underlying Causes

TYPE	PRIMARY CIRCULATORY DERANGEMENT	COMMON CAUSES
Hypovolemic	Decreased circulating blood volume	Hemorrhage
		Diarrhea
		Diabetes insipidus, diabetes mellitus
		Burns
		Adrenogenital syndrome
		Capillary leak
Distributive	Vasodilation → venous pooling → decreased preload	Sepsis
	Maldistribution of regional blood flow	Anaphylaxis
		CNS/spinal injury
		Drug intoxication
Cardiogenic	Decreased myocardial contractility	Congenital heart disease
		Arrhythmia
		Hypoxic/ischemic injuries
		Cardiomyopathy
		Metabolic derangements
		Myocarditis
		Drug intoxication
		Kawasaki disease
Obstructive	Mechanical obstruction to ventricular filling or outflow	Cardiac tamponade
		Massive pulmonary embolus
		Tension pneumothorax
		Cardiac tumor
Dissociative	Oxygen not appropriately bound or released from hemoglobin	Carbon monoxide poisoning
		Methemoglobinemia

CNS, Central nervous system.

HYPOVOLEMIC SHOCK

Acute hypovolemia is the most common cause of shock in children. It results from loss of fluid from the intravascular space secondary to inadequate intake or excessive losses (vomiting and diarrhea, blood loss, capillary leak syndromes, or pathological renal fluid losses) (Table 40.1). Reduced blood volume decreases preload, stroke volume, and cardiac output. Hypovolemic shock results in increased sympathoadrenal activity, producing an increased heart rate and enhanced myocardial contractility. Neurohormonally mediated constriction of the arterioles and capacitance vessels maintains blood pressure, augments venous return to the heart to improve preload, and redistributes blood flow from nonvital to vital organs. If hypovolemic shock remains untreated, the increased heart rate may impair coronary blood flow and ventricular filling, while elevated systemic vascular resistance increases myocardial oxygen consumption, resulting in worsening myocardial function. Ultimately, intense systemic vasoconstriction and hypovolemia produce tissue ischemia, impairing cell metabolism and releasing potent vasoactive mediators from injured cells. Cytokines and other vasoactive peptides can change myocardial contractility and vascular tone and promote release of other inflammatory mediators that increase capillary permeability and impair organ function further.

DISTRIBUTIVE SHOCK

Abnormalities in the distribution of blood flow may result in profound inadequacies in tissue perfusion, even in the presence of a normal or high cardiac output. This maldistribution of flow usually results from abnormalities in vascular tone. Septic shock is the most common type of distributive shock in children. Other causes include anaphylaxis, neurological injury, and drug-related causes (see Table 40.1).

Distributive shock may present with the **systemic inflammatory response syndrome** (SIRS), defined as two or more of the following: temperature greater than 38°C or less than 36°C; heart rate greater than 90 beats/min or more than two standard deviations above normal for age; tachypnea; or white blood cell count that is greater than 12,000 cells/

mm^3, less than 4,000 cells/mm^3, or has greater than 10% immature forms.

CARDIOGENIC SHOCK

Cardiogenic shock is caused by an abnormality in myocardial function and is expressed as depressed myocardial contractility and cardiac output with poor tissue perfusion. Compensatory mechanisms may contribute to the progression of shock by depressing cardiac function further. Neurohormonal vasoconstrictor responses increase afterload and add to the work of the failing ventricle. Tachycardia may impair coronary blood flow, which decreases myocardial oxygen delivery. Increased central blood volume caused by sodium and water retention and by incomplete emptying of the ventricles during systole results in elevated left ventricular volume and pressure, which impair subendocardial blood flow. As compensatory mechanisms are overcome, the failing left ventricle produces increased ventricular end-diastolic volume and pressure, which leads to increased left atrial pressure, resulting in pulmonary edema. This sequence also contributes to right ventricular failure because of increased pulmonary artery pressure and increased right ventricular afterload.

Primary cardiogenic shock may occur in children who have congenital heart disease. Cardiogenic shock also may occur in previously healthy children secondary to viral myocarditis, dysrhythmias, or toxic or metabolic abnormalities or after hypoxic-ischemic injury (see Chapters 142, 145, and 147, as well as Table 40.1).

OBSTRUCTIVE SHOCK

Obstructive shock results from mechanical obstruction of ventricular outflow. Causes include congenital lesions, such as coarctation of the aorta, interrupted aortic arch, and severe aortic valvular stenosis, along with acquired diseases (e.g., hypertrophic cardiomyopathy) (see Table 40.1). For neonates presenting in shock, obstructive lesions must be considered.

DISSOCIATIVE SHOCK

Dissociative shock refers to conditions in which tissue perfusion is normal, but cells are unable to use oxygen because the hemoglobin has an abnormal affinity for oxygen, preventing its release to the tissues (see Table 40.1).

CLINICAL MANIFESTATIONS

All forms of shock produce evidence that tissue perfusion and oxygenation are insufficient (increased heart rate, abnormal blood pressure, alterations of peripheral pulses). The etiology of shock may alter the initial presentation of these signs and symptoms.

Hypovolemic Shock

Hypovolemic shock is distinguished from other causes of shock by history and the absence of signs of heart failure or sepsis. In addition to the signs of sympathoadrenal activity (tachycardia, vasoconstriction), clinical manifestations include signs of dehydration (dry mucous membranes, decreased urine output) or blood loss (pallor). Recovery depends on the degree of hypovolemia, the patient's pre-existing status, and rapid diagnosis and treatment. The prognosis is good, with a low mortality in uncomplicated cases.

Distributive Shock

Patients with distributive shock usually have tachycardia and alterations of peripheral perfusion. In early stages, when cytokine release results in vasodilation, pulses may be bounding and vital organ function may be maintained (an alert patient, with rapid capillary refill and some urine output in *warm shock*). As the disease progresses untreated, extremities become cool and mottled with a delayed capillary refill time. At this stage, the patient has hypotension and vasoconstriction. If the etiology of distributive shock is sepsis, the patient often has fever, lethargy, petechiae, or purpura, and he or she may have an identifiable source of infection.

Cardiogenic Shock

Cardiogenic shock results when the myocardium is unable to supply the cardiac output required to support tissue perfusion and organ function. Because of this self-perpetuating cycle, heart failure progressing to death may be rapid. Patients with cardiogenic shock have tachycardia and tachypnea. The liver is usually enlarged, a gallop is often present, and jugular venous distention may be noted. Because renal blood flow is poor, sodium and water are retained, resulting in oliguria and peripheral edema.

Obstructive Shock

Restriction of cardiac output results in an increase in heart rate and an alteration of stroke volume. The pulse pressure is narrow (making pulses harder to feel), and capillary refill is delayed. The liver is often enlarged, and jugular venous distention may be evident.

Dissociative Shock

The principal abnormality in dissociative shock is the inability to deliver oxygen to tissues. Symptoms include tachycardia, tachypnea, alterations in mental status, and, ultimately, cardiovascular collapse.

LABORATORY AND IMAGING STUDIES

Shock requires immediate resuscitation before obtaining laboratory or diagnostic studies. Following initial stabilization (including glucose administration if hypoglycemia is present), the type of shock dictates the necessary laboratory studies. All patients with shock may benefit from the determination of a baseline arterial blood gas and blood lactate level to assess the impairment of tissue oxygenation. Measurement of central **mixed venous oxygen saturation** aids in the assessment of the adequacy of oxygen delivery. In contrast to other forms of shock, patients with sepsis often have high mixed venous saturation values because of impairment of mitochondrial function and inability of tissues to extract oxygen. A complete blood count can potentially assess intravascular blood volume after equilibration following a hemorrhage. Electrolyte measurements in patients with hypovolemic shock may identify abnormalities from losses.

Patients presenting in distributive shock require appropriate bacterial and viral cultures to identify a cause of infection. If cardiogenic or obstructive shock is suspected, an echocardiogram assists with the diagnosis and, in the case of tamponade, assists with placement of a pericardial drain to relieve the fluid. Patients with dissociative shock require detection of the causative agent (carbon monoxide, methemoglobin). The management of shock also requires monitoring of arterial blood gases for oxygenation, ventilation (CO_2), and acidosis and frequently assessing the levels of serum electrolytes, calcium, magnesium, phosphorus, and blood urea nitrogen (BUN).

DIFFERENTIAL DIAGNOSIS

See Table 40.1.

TREATMENT

General Principles

The key to therapy is the recognition of shock in its early, partially compensated state, when many of the hemodynamic and metabolic alterations may be reversible. Initial therapy for shock follows the ABCs of resuscitation. Later therapy can then be directed at the underlying cause. Therapy should minimize cardiopulmonary work, while ensuring cardiac output, blood pressure, and gas exchange. Intubation, combined with mechanical ventilation with oxygen supplementation, improves oxygenation and decreases or eliminates the work of breathing but may impede venous return if distending airway pressures (positive end-expiratory pressure [PEEP] or peak inspiratory pressure) are excessive. Blood pressure support is crucial because the vasodilation in sepsis may reduce perfusion despite supranormal cardiac output.

Monitoring a child in shock requires maintaining access to the arterial and central venous circulation to record pressure measurements, perform blood sampling, and measure systemic blood pressure continuously. These measurements facilitate the estimation of preload and afterload. Regional monitoring with near infrared spectroscopy may allow early, noninvasive detection of alterations in perfusion.

Organ-Directed Therapeutics

Fluid Resuscitation

Alterations in preload have a dramatic effect on cardiac output. In hypovolemic and distributive shock, decreased preload significantly impairs cardiac output. In these cases, early and aggressive fluid resuscitation is important and greatly affects outcome. In cardiogenic shock, an elevated preload contributes to pulmonary edema.

Selection of fluids for resuscitation and ongoing use is dictated by clinical circumstances. Crystalloid volume expanders are generally recommended as initial choices because they are effective and inexpensive. Most acutely ill children with signs of shock may safely receive, and usually benefit greatly from, rapid administration of a 20-mL/kg bolus of an isotonic crystalloid. This dose may be repeated until a response is noted. Colloids contain larger molecules that may stay in the intravascular space longer than crystalloid solutions and exert oncotic pressure, drawing fluid out of the tissues into the vascular compartment. However, the long-term risks of colloids may exceed the benefits. Care must be exercised in treating cardiogenic shock with volume expansion because the ventricular filling pressures may rise without improvement or with deterioration of cardiac performance. Carefully monitoring cardiac output or central venous pressure guides safe volume replacement.

Cardiovascular Support

In an effort to improve cardiac output after volume resuscitation, or when further volume replacement may be dangerous, a variety of inotropic and vasodilator drugs may be useful (Table 40.2). Therapy is directed first at increasing myocardial contractility, then at decreasing left ventricular afterload. The hemodynamic status of the patient dictates the choice of the agent.

Therapy may be initiated with dopamine at 5-20 μg/kg per minute; however, epinephrine or norepinephrine may be preferable in patients with decompensated shock. In addition to improving contractility, certain catecholamines cause an increase in systemic vascular resistance. The addition of a vasodilator drug may improve cardiac performance by decreasing the resistance against which the heart must pump (afterload). Afterload reduction may be achieved with dobutamine, milrinone, amrinone, nitroprusside, nitroglycerin, and angiotensin-converting enzyme inhibitors. The use of these drugs may be particularly important in late shock, when vasoconstriction is prominent.

Respiratory Support

The lung is a target organ for inflammatory mediators in shock and SIRS. Respiratory failure may develop rapidly and become progressive. Intervention requires endotracheal intubation and mechanical ventilation accompanied by the use of supplemental oxygen and PEEP. Care must be taken with the process of intubation because a child with compensated

TABLE 40.2 Medications Used to Improve Cardiac Output

	POSITIVE INOTROPE	POSITIVE CHRONOTROPE	DIRECT PRESSOR	VASOCONSTRICTOR	VASODILATOR
Dopamine	++	+	±	++ (high dose)	+ (low dose)
Dobutamine	++	±	–	–	+
Epinephrine	+++	+++	+++	++ (high dose)	+ (low dose)
Norepinephrine	+++	+++	+++	+++	–
Milrinone	+	–	–	–	+

shock may suddenly decompensate on administration of sedative medications that reduce systemic vascular resistance. Severe cardiopulmonary failure may be managed with inhaled nitric oxide and, if necessary, extracorporeal membrane oxygenation.

Renal Salvage

Poor cardiac output accompanied by decreased renal blood flow may cause prerenal azotemia and oliguria/anuria. Severe hypotension may produce **acute tubular necrosis** and **acute renal failure.** Prerenal azotemia is corrected when blood volume deficits are replaced or myocardial contractility is improved, but acute tubular necrosis does not improve immediately when shock is corrected. Prerenal azotemia is associated with a serum BUN-to-creatinine ratio of greater than 10:1 and a urine sodium level less than 20 mEq/L; acute tubular necrosis has a BUN-to-creatinine ratio of 10:1 or less and a urine sodium level between 40 and 60 mEq/L (see Chapter 165). Aggressive fluid replacement is often necessary to improve oliguria associated with prerenal azotemia. Because the management of shock requires administering large volumes of fluid, maintaining urine output greatly facilitates patient management.

Prevention of acute tubular necrosis and the subsequent complications associated with acute renal failure (hyperkalemia, acidosis, hypocalcemia, fluid overload) is important. The use of pharmacological agents to augment urine output is indicated when the intravascular volume has been replaced. The use of loop diuretics, such as furosemide, or combinations of a loop diuretic and a thiazide agent may enhance urine output. Infusion of low-dose dopamine, which produces renal artery vasodilation, also may improve urine output. Nevertheless, if hyperkalemia, refractory acidosis, hypervolemia, or altered mental status associated with uremia occurs, dialysis or hemofiltration should be initiated.

COMPLICATIONS

Shock results in impairment of tissue perfusion and oxygenation and activation of inflammation and cytokine pathways. The major complication of shock is multiple organ system failure, defined as the dysfunction of more than one organ, including respiratory failure, renal failure, liver dysfunction, coagulation abnormalities, or cerebral dysfunction. Patients with shock and multiple organ failure have a higher mortality rate and, for survivors, a longer hospital stay.

PROGNOSIS

Early recognition and **goal-directed intervention** in patients with shock improve survival. However, delays in treatment of hypotension increase the incidence of multiple organ failure and mortality. Goal-directed therapy focused on maintaining mixed venous oxygen saturation may improve survival.

PREVENTION

Prevention strategies for shock are focused, for the most part, on shock associated with sepsis and hypovolemia. Some forms of septic shock can be prevented through the use of immunizations (*Haemophilus influenzae* type b, meningococcal, pneumococcal vaccines). Decreasing the risk of sepsis in a critically ill patient requires adherence to strict hand washing, isolation practices, and minimizing the duration of indwelling catheters. Measures to decrease pediatric trauma do much to minimize hemorrhage-induced shock.

CHAPTER 41

Injury Prevention

EPIDEMIOLOGY AND ETIOLOGY

Unintentional injury is the leading cause of death in children aged 1-18 years. In the United States, between 2009 and 2015, the unintentional injury death rate for children younger than 19 years of age declined by 12% (from 11.0 to 9.7 per 100,000). This decline has been attributed to increased use of child safety seats and seat belts, reduction in drunk driving, increased use of child-resistant packaging, enhanced safety awareness, and improved medical care.

The most common causes of fatal injuries differ among age groups. For instance, suffocation is the most common type of fatal injury among infants (83% in 2012); however, it accounts for only 1% of unintentional fatalities among 15-19 year olds. Conversely, motor vehicle collisions account for 6% of fatal injuries among infants, whereas they account for 66% of adolescent fatal injuries. Drowning is the most common cause of fatal injury among children ages 1-4 years (31%), while it accounts for 7% of fatal injuries among adolescents. Notably, differences in geography, climate, population density (access to care), and population traits affect the frequency, etiology, and severity of these injuries.

Injury occurs through interaction of the **host** (child) with the **agent** (e.g., car and driver) through a vector and an **environment** (e.g., roadways, weather) that is conducive to exposure. The age of the child may determine the exposure to various agents and environments. For example, most injuries in infants and toddlers occur in the home as the result of exposure to agents found there (water heaters, bathtubs, soft bedding). Gender affects exposure to injury, with boys having a fatal injury rate greater than that of girls.

EDUCATION FOR PREVENTING INJURIES

The recognition that much of the morbidity and mortality are determined at the scene of an injury has stimulated the development of prevention measures. The **Haddon matrix** combines the epidemiological components (host, agent, physical and social environments) with time factors (before, during, and after the event) to identify effective interventions focused on different aspects of the injury event. Primary strategies (preventing the event), secondary strategies (minimizing the severity of injury), and tertiary strategies (minimizing long-term impact) can be targeted for each epidemiological component. Such strategies typically fall into one of three areas: education, enforcement, and environment (including engineering).

Education is often the first strategy considered, but it requires behavioral change and action on the part of people. Most educational strategies are not well evaluated.

Despite the reliance on an action by the individuals involved, some active strategies benefit from enforcement. Children wearing bicycle helmets experience a significantly lower incidence of traumatic brain injury and death. The enforcement of seatbelt laws increases seatbelt use and may decrease injuries.

Automatic strategies require no action on the part of the population and often change the environment (speed bumps) or involve engineering (child-resistant pill bottles, air bags). Automatic strategies have more consistently resulted in a significant reduction in injuries. The most successful approaches to preventing injury have combined strategies (education, environmental changes, and engineering changes focused on the host, agent, and environment in all three time phases).

CHAPTER 42

Major Trauma

ASSESSMENT AND RESUSCITATION

The general goal of **prehospital trauma care** is rapid assessment, support of the ABCs, immobilization, and transportation. Outcomes of patients with major or life-threatening trauma are significantly improved in a pediatric trauma center or in an adult center with pediatric trauma certification compared with level I or II adult trauma centers.

Once the injured child arrives at the emergency department, the trauma team must initiate an organized and synchronized response. The initial assessment of a seriously injured child should involve a systematic approach, including a primary survey, resuscitation, secondary survey, post-resuscitation monitoring, and definitive care. The **primary survey** focuses on the **ABCDEs** of emergency care, as modified for trauma from the ABCs of cardiopulmonary resuscitation (see Chapter 38). The assessment of the airway and breathing components should include control of the cervical spine (especially if the patient has an altered mental status), evaluation for injuries that could impair air entry or gas exchange, and consideration of the likelihood of a full stomach (risk of aspiration pneumonia). Circulation can be assessed via observation (heart rate, skin color, mental status) and palpation (pulse quality, capillary refill, skin temperature) and restored (via two large peripheral intravenous lines, when possible) while control of bleeding is accomplished through the use of direct pressure. Assessment for **disabilities** (D), including neurologic status, includes examination of pupil size and reactivity, a brief mental status assessment (*AVPU—a*lert; responds to *v*oice; responds to *p*ain; *u*nresponsive), and examination of extremity movement to assess for spinal cord injury. The **Glasgow Coma Scale** can direct decisions regarding the initiation of cerebral resuscitation in patients with suspected closed head injuries (Table 42.1). **E,** which stands for *exposure,* requires a full assessment by completely disrobing the child for a detailed examination of the entire body. The examiner should ensure a neutral thermal environment to prevent hypothermia.

On completion of the primary survey, a more detailed head-to-toe examination (the **secondary survey**) should ensue, along with efforts to obtain a more complete history. The purpose of this careful re-examination is to identify life-threatening and limb-threatening injuries, as well as less serious injuries. Coincident with the secondary survey and depending, in part, on the assessed physiological status of the patient, certain procedures and resuscitative measures are initiated. The prioritization of definitive care needs is determined by the injury findings collected from the primary and secondary surveys, the child's physiological response to resuscitation, and the data from continuous monitoring. A **tertiary survey,** including repeat primary and secondary surveys along with a review of the laboratory tests and radiological studies, should be performed within 24 hours.

TABLE 42.1 Glasgow Coma Scales

ACTIVITY	BEST RESPONSE	SCORE
Eye opening	Spontaneous	4
	To verbal stimuli	3
	To pain	2
	None	1
Verbal	Oriented • Infant: coos, babbles	5
	Confused • Infant: irritable, cries	4
	Inappropriate words • Infant: cries to pain	3
	Nonspecific sounds • Infant: moans to pain	2
	None	1
Motor	Follows commands • Infant: spontaneous movement	6
	Localizes pain • Infant: withdraws to touch	5
	Withdraws to pain	4
	Flexion to pain • Infant: abnormal flexion	3
	Extension to pain • Infant: abnormal extension	2
	None	1

ETIOLOGY AND EPIDEMIOLOGY

See Chapter 41.

LABORATORY AND IMAGING STUDIES

Screening laboratory studies during the initial resuscitation often includes the tests listed in Table 42.2. Radiographic studies are determined by the pattern of injuries. A head computed tomography (CT) scan should be obtained in patients with evidence of head trauma or a history of loss of consciousness. Patients with obvious injury to the thorax or abdomen or who have pulmonary or abdominal symptoms may benefit from a CT scan. The focused assessment with sonography for trauma (FAST) is gaining popularity because of concerns about radiation exposure. Diagnostic peritoneal lavage has limited utility. A helical CT scan should be performed if there is concern about thoracic arterial injuries.

TABLE 42.2 Initial Laboratory Evaluation of the Major Trauma Patient

HEMATOLOGY
Complete blood count
Platelet count
Type and cross match
URINALYSIS
Gross
Microscopic
CLINICAL CHEMISTRY
Amylase/lipase
Aspartate aminotransferase/alanine aminotransferase
RADIOLOGY
Cervical spine films
Anteroposterior chest radiograph
Radiographs of all apparent fractures
Computed tomography scans where indicated for head, chest, and abdominal trauma

CLINICAL MANIFESTATIONS AND TREATMENT

Head injuries and injuries to the limbs are the most common. Multiple organ involvement is also common, and penetrating trauma is becoming more frequent. After the initial evaluation and stabilization, the team focuses on the involved organ systems.

Head Trauma

See Chapter 184.

Spinal Cord Trauma

Although spinal cord injury is not common in pediatric trauma patients, it is potentially devastating when it occurs. Cervical spine immobilization should be maintained until a spinal cord injury is ruled out. Cervical spine radiographs are not sufficient to rule out a spinal cord injury because the immature vertebral column in children may allow stretching of the cord or nerve roots with no radiological abnormality (spinal cord injury without radiological abnormality [SCIWORA]). SCIWORA may occur in a significant percentage of children with a spinal cord injury; when it is suspected, magnetic resonance imaging should be performed.

Thoracic Trauma

Thoracic injury is the second leading cause of trauma death. Pulmonary contusion, pneumothorax, and rib fractures occur most commonly, and patients may present without external signs of trauma. Patients with pulmonary parenchymal injury should receive supportive treatment to ensure adequate oxygenation and ventilation. Most pediatric blunt thoracic injuries can be managed without surgery. Injury to the heart and great vessels is rare but requires urgent diagnosis and treatment. Great vessel injury should be suspected if a widened mediastinum is seen on chest radiograph.

Abdominal Trauma

The relative size and closer proximity of intraabdominal organs in children increase the risk of significant injury after blunt trauma. Penetrating trauma may result in a child who is asymptomatic or who presents in hypovolemic shock.

Imaging studies such as abdominal CT and serial physical examinations are the primary methods of obtaining information on which to base decisions regarding operative intervention. Abdominal wall bruising is an important physical examination finding and is associated with significant intraabdominal injury in more than 10% of patients. Operative intervention may be required in patients whose vital signs are persistently unstable in the face of aggressive fluid resuscitation, even in the absence of extravascular volume loss or an enlarging abdomen.

Most blunt solid organ injury is handled nonoperatively. Clinical observation is important because most failures with nonoperative management occur in the first 12 hours.

Injury to the Spleen

The most frequently injured abdominal organ in children is the spleen. Suspicion of a splenic injury should be heightened if there are left upper quadrant abrasions or tenderness. A positive *Kehr sign* (pressure on the left upper quadrant eliciting left shoulder pain) is due to diaphragmatic irritation by the ruptured spleen and strongly suggests splenic injury. CT scans are used to identify and grade splenic injury.

Nonoperative management is the treatment of choice for most serious splenic injuries unless there is continued large blood loss or hemodynamic instability. If a splenectomy is performed, patients should receive penicillin prophylaxis and should receive pneumococcal and *Haemophilus influenzae* vaccines to decrease the increased risk of overwhelming sepsis.

Liver Trauma

Major trauma to the liver is a serious cause of morbidity. Severe hemorrhage is more common in patients with liver injury than with other abdominal injuries because of its dual blood supply. Without significant vascular injury, hepatic injury presents and behaves clinically like a splenic injury. Nonoperative management is recommended but requires close clinical observation for signs of ongoing blood loss or hemodynamic instability. As with splenic injury, there is a grading system based on the pattern of injury.

Renal Injury

The kidney is less frequently injured than the liver or spleen, and when injured it is often associated with other injuries. A young child's kidney is more vulnerable to trauma than an adult's because of a more compliant rib cage and relatively immature abdominal muscle development. The diagnosis of renal injury is based on history and physical examination coupled with urinalysis showing blood and increased protein levels. An ultrasound or CT may also be useful. Low-grade renal injury is usually managed conservatively, with bed rest, catheter drainage, and monitoring for resolution of the injury by ultrasound or

CT. Surgery may be required for falling hemoglobin levels, refractory shock, or urinary obstruction caused by clots.

Pancreatic Injury

Injuries of the pancreas are less common in children than in adults but are seen in bicycle handlebar injuries, motor vehicle crashes, and nonaccidental trauma. The diagnosis is difficult unless there is obvious injury to overlying structures, such as the stomach or duodenum. Diffuse abdominal tenderness, pain, and vomiting may be accompanied by elevations of amylase and lipase but may not occur until several days after the injury. Hemodynamic instability secondary to retroperitoneal hemorrhage may be the presenting sign. Abdominal CT is useful but may not be sufficient to evaluate ductal injury. Nonoperative management is appropriate for contusions, but surgical intervention may be required in patients with ductal injuries. Drainage of pseudocysts, in patients who develop them, may be required if they are unresponsive to bowel rest and parenteral nutrition.

Intestinal Injury

Injury to the intestine occurs less frequently than injury to solid intraabdominal organs and varies with the amount of intestinal contents. A full bowel is likely to shear more easily than an empty bowel. Shearing occurs at points of fixation (the ligament of Treitz, the ileocecal valve, and the ascending and descending peritoneal reflections). Pneumoperitoneum should prompt surgical exploration. Serial physical examinations are useful when the clinical picture is uncertain.

Duodenal hematoma can occur in the absence of perforation. Duodenal hematomas result from blunt injury to the abdomen. Affected patients often present with persistent pain and bilious emesis. Most hematomas respond to nonoperative management with gastric decompression and parenteral nutrition.

COMPLICATIONS

Patients requiring hospitalization for multiple trauma are at risk for a variety of complications based on the type and severity of injury. Sepsis and multiple organ failure may occur in children with multiple trauma. Delays in enteral nutrition because of an ileus may further increase the risk of sepsis secondary to translocation of bacteria across the intestinal mucosa.

Renal failure secondary to myoglobinuria may be seen in children who sustain crushing or electrical injuries and burns. Deep venous thrombosis is less common in the pediatric population, but prophylaxis for children who will be immobilized because of injury should be provided.

PROGNOSIS

Unintentional injury is the leading cause of death for children aged 1-18; however, many of these deaths occur in the field immediately after the injury. Once admitted to the hospital, mortality rates are much lower. Morbidities are numerous and include hypoxic-ischemic brain injury, loss of limbs, and psychological dysfunction.

PREVENTION

See Chapter 41.

CHAPTER 43

Drowning

ETIOLOGY

Drowning, as defined by the World Congress on Drowning in 2002, is the process of experiencing respiratory impairment from submersion/immersion in liquid. Outcomes may be categorized as death, morbidity, or no morbidity. Other terms such as near drowning, secondary drowning, or dry drowning should be abandoned.

Initially, submersion or immersion results in aspiration of small amounts of fluid into the larynx, triggering breath holding or laryngospasm. In many cases, the laryngospasm resolves, and larger volumes of water or gastric contents are aspirated into the lungs, destroying surfactant and causing alveolitis and dysfunction of the alveolar-capillary gas exchange. The resulting hypoxemia leads to hypoxic brain injury that is exacerbated by ischemic injury after circulatory collapse.

EPIDEMIOLOGY

Drowning deaths overall have decreased; however, drowning is still a significant cause of morbidity and mortality and is the second leading cause of injury death for children ages 1-14 years. Boys are four times more likely than girls to drown. The most common location of drowning varies by age, with drowning in natural bodies of water becoming more frequent in older age groups.

CLINICAL MANIFESTATIONS

Hypoxemia is the result of laryngospasm and aspiration during drowning. Victims may also develop respiratory distress secondary to **pulmonary endothelial injury, increased capillary permeability,** and **destruction of surfactant.** Clinical manifestations include tachypnea, tachycardia, increased work of breathing, and decreased breath sounds with or without crackles. The hypoxic-ischemic injury that may occur can lead to depressed myocardial function resulting in tachycardia, impaired perfusion, and, potentially, cardiovascular collapse. After resuscitation, acute respiratory distress syndrome is common. Altered mental status may be present and requires frequent monitoring of neurological status. Following submersion in cold water, hypothermia may result in relative bradycardia and hypotension and place the child at risk for cardiac dysrhythmias.

LABORATORY AND IMAGING STUDIES

After resuscitation, arterial blood gas measurement assists in assessing pulmonary gas exchange. A chemistry profile may reveal elevated liver enzymes if hypoxemia and ischemia were of long duration and provide baseline renal functions. Electrolytes are often obtained, although alterations of serum electrolytes are minimal, even in freshwater drowning.

TREATMENT

Resuscitation of a drowning victim includes the basic ABCs (see Chapter 38). Victims of unwitnessed drowning require stabilization of the cervical spine because of the possibility of a fall or diving injury. Optimizing oxygenation and maintaining cerebral perfusion are two of the major foci of treatment. Rewarming the hypothermic patient requires careful attention to detail, including acid-base and cardiac status. Further treatment is based on the patient response to initial resuscitation. Some children begin breathing spontaneously and awaken before arrival at an emergency department. If the episode was significant, these children still require careful observation for pulmonary complications over the subsequent 6-12 hours. Children who have evidence of lung injury, cardiovascular compromise, or neurological compromise should be monitored in an intensive care unit. Pulmonary dysfunction often results in hypoxemia. Oxygen supplementation should be implemented to maintain normal oxygen saturations. Mechanical ventilation may be needed in patients with significant pulmonary or neurological dysfunction. Cardiovascular compromise is often the result of impaired contractility because of hypoxic-ischemic injury. The use of intracranial pressure monitoring devices and medical management with hypothermia and sedation is controversial and has not been shown to improve outcomes. Prophylactic antibiotics have not been shown to be beneficial and may increase the selection of resistant organisms.

PROGNOSIS

The outcome of drowning is determined by the success of immediate resuscitation efforts and the severity of the **hypoxic-ischemic injury** to the brain. Patients who have regained consciousness on arrival at the hospital will likely survive with intact neurological function. Unfavorable prognostic markers include the need for continued cardiopulmonary resuscitation (CPR) at the hospital, Glasgow Coma Scale of 5 or less, fixed and dilated pupils, seizures, and coma for more than 72 hours.

PREVENTION

Despite the decreased incidence of drowning since the 1990s, few prevention strategies have been shown to be effective. Exceptions include implementation of mandatory four-sided fencing around pools (decreasing the number of children <5 years of age who drown) and immediate provision of CPR to children who drown. The use of safety flotation devices in older children during water sport activities may be beneficial. Enhanced supervision is required to reduce the incidence of infants drowning in bathtubs.

CHAPTER 44

Burns

ETIOLOGY

The pathophysiology of burn injury is caused by disruption of the three key functions of the skin: regulation of heat loss, preservation of body fluids, and barrier to infection. Burn injury releases inflammatory and vasoactive mediators resulting in increased capillary permeability, decreased plasma volume, and decreased cardiac output. The body then becomes hypermetabolic with increased resting energy expenditure and protein catabolism. This hypermetabolic state may continue for up to a year after injury.

Burns usually are classified based on four criteria:

- Depth of injury
- Percent of body surface area involved
- Location of the burn
- Association with other injuries

EPIDEMIOLOGY

More than 100,000 children sustain a burn injury each year. Fatalities from burns are decreasing, but burns remain a significant cause of morbidity. Boys are more likely to sustain a burn injury, as are children age 4 and under. Scald burns are more common in younger children as compared with older children. Overall, thermal burns secondary to scald or flame are much more common than electrical or chemical burns. Most fire-related childhood deaths and injuries occur in homes.

CLINICAL MANIFESTATIONS

The depth of injury should be assessed by the clinical appearance. Categories of first-degree, second-degree, and third-degree are commonly used; however, classification by depth (superficial, superficial partial-thickness, deep partial-thickness, and full-thickness) conveys more information about the structures injured and the likely need for surgical treatment and may be more clinically useful.

Superficial (first-degree) burns are red, painful, and dry. They are commonly seen with sun exposure or mild scald injuries, and these burns involve injury to the epidermis only. They heal in 2-5 days without scarring and are not included in burn surface area calculations. **Superficial partial-thickness** (second-degree) burns involve the entire epidermis and superficial dermis. These burns have fluid-containing blisters. After debridement, the underlying dermis appears erythematous and wet, is painful, and blanches under pressure. Healing is dependent on the uninjured dermis and usually occurs within 7–21 days without the need for skin grafting and without scarring. **Deep partial-thickness** (also second-degree) burns involve the entire epidermis and deeper portions of the dermis. These burns may also have blistering, but the dermal base is less blanching, mottled pink or white, and less painful than superficial partial-thickness burns. They behave more like full-thickness burns and often require excision and grafting. **Full-thickness** (third-degree and fourth-degree) burns involve all skin layers. They appear dry, white, dark red, brown, or black in color. They do not blanch and are usually insensate. Full-thickness burns require surgical management. Fourth-degree burns involve underlying fascia, muscle, or bone and may require reconstruction in addition to grafting. **Inhalation injuries** should be suspected if there are facial burns, singed nasal hairs, or carbonaceous sputum. Hoarseness on vocalization also is consistent with a supraglottic injury. Inhalation injuries may result in bronchospasm, airway inflammation, and impaired pulmonary function.

There are multiple methods and charts available for calculating the percentage of skin surface involved in a burn. One method that may be used for children of various ages is presented in Fig. 44.1. The extent of skin involvement of older adolescent and adult patients may be estimated as follows: each upper

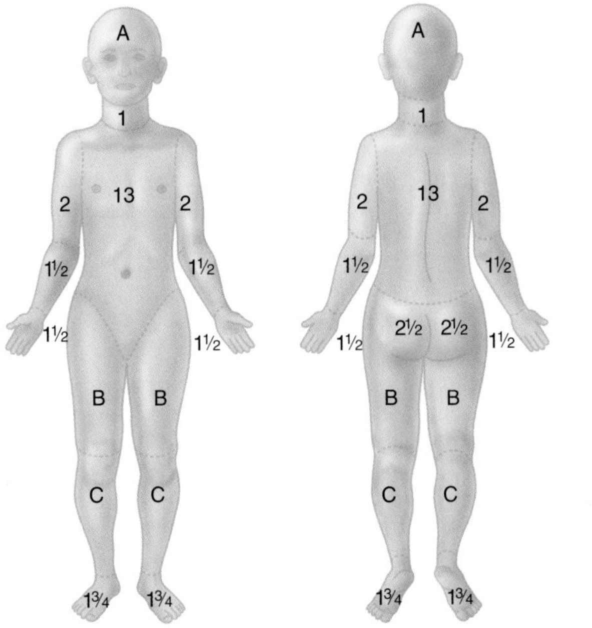

PERCENTAGE OF SURFACE AREA OF HEAD AND LEGS AT VARIOUS AGES

AREA IN DIAGRAM	AGE IN YEARS 0	1	5	10	15
A = ½ of head	9½	8½	6½	5½	4½
B = ½ of one thigh	2¾	3¼	4	4¼	4½
C = ½ of one lower leg	2½	2½	2¾	3	3¼

FIGURE 44.1 This chart of body areas, together with the table inserted in the figure showing the percentage of surface area of head and legs at various ages, can be used to estimate the surface area burned in a child. (From Solomon JR. Pediatric burns. *Crit Care Clin.* 1985;1:159–174.)

extremity, 9%; each lower extremity, 18%; anterior trunk, 18%; posterior trunk, 18%; head, 9%; and perineum, 1%.

The location of the burn is important in assessing the risk of disability. The risk is greatest when the face, eyes, ears, feet, perineum, or hands are involved. Inhalation injuries not only cause respiratory compromise but also may result in difficulty in eating and drinking.

LABORATORY AND IMAGING STUDIES

Initial laboratory testing, including complete blood count, type and cross match for blood, coagulation studies, basic chemistry profile, arterial blood gas, and chest radiograph, can be helpful for patients with major burns. A carboxyhemoglobin assessment should be performed for any suspected inhalation exposure (a house or closed-space fire or a burn victim who requires cardiopulmonary resuscitation). Cyanide levels should be considered in children who sustain smoke inhalation and have altered mental status. Unusual patterns of burns may increase suspicion of child abuse and result in appropriate evaluation to assess for nonaccidental trauma to the skeleton or central nervous system.

TREATMENT

For severe burns care is best managed by a multidisciplinary team in a qualified burn center. The American Burn Association criteria for patients who should be transferred to a burn center are as follows: partial-thickness burns greater than 10% total body surface area (TBSA); partial and full-thickness burns involving the face, hands, feet, genitalia, perineum, or major joints; full-thickness burns in any age group; electrical burns (including lightning injury); chemical burns; inhalation injury; burn injury in patients with preexisting medical conditions that could complicate management, prolong recovery, or affect mortality; any burn with concomitant trauma in which the burn injury poses the greatest risk; burn injury in children admitted to hospitals without qualified personnel or equipment for pediatric care; burn injury in patients requiring special social, emotional, or rehabilitative support, including child abuse cases.

Initial treatment should follow the ABCs of resuscitation (see Chapter 38). **Airway management** should include assessment for the presence of airway or inhalation injury, with early intubation if such an injury is suspected. Smoke inhalation may be associated with carbon monoxide toxicity; 100% humidified oxygen should be given if hypoxia or inhalation is suspected.

The systemic capillary leak that occurs after a serious burn makes initial fluid and electrolyte support of a burned child crucial. The first priority is to support the circulating blood volume, which requires the administration of intravenous fluids to provide maintenance fluid and electrolyte requirements and to replace ongoing burn-related losses. Formulas exist to help guide **fluid management**; however, no formula accurately predicts the fluid needs of every burn patient. Children with a significant burn should receive a rapid bolus of 20 mL/kg of lactated Ringer solution. Thereafter, the resuscitation formula for fluid therapy is determined by the percent of body surface burned. Total fluids are 2-4 mL/kg per percent burn per 24 hours, with half the estimated burn requirement administered during the first 8 hours. (If resuscitation is delayed, half of the fluid replacement should be completed by the end of the eighth hour post-injury.) Fluids should be titrated to achieve adequate perfusion, and one marker of which is urine output greater than 1 mL/kg per hour. Controversy exists over whether and when to administer colloid during fluid resuscitation, but colloid therapy may be needed for patients with extensive burns.

Because burn injury produces a **hypermetabolic** response, children with significant burns require immediate nutritional support. Enteral feeds should be started early unless there is a specific contraindication. Children with critical burn injury may require parenteral nutrition if unable to tolerate full enteral feeds. Consider supplementation of vitamins and trace elements. Other factors that may improve the hypermetabolic state include pain control, blood glucose control, and the use of medications including anabolic steroids such as oxandrolone and β blockers such as propranolol.

Wound care starts with cleaning and debriding the wound. Effective pain control is important to allow for complete debridement. Topical agents and dressings are then applied to control bacterial colonization, decrease evaporative losses, and aid in pain control. Various grafts, such as cadaver allografts, porcine xenografts, or skin substitutes, have been used initially to cover wounds. For full-thickness burns, skin autografting and skin substitutes are required for eventual closure.

COMPLICATIONS

See Table 44.1.

TABLE 44.1 Complications of Burns

PROBLEM	TREATMENT
Sepsis	Monitor for infection, avoid prophylactic antibiotics
Hypovolemia	Fluid replacement
Hypothermia	Adjust ambient temperature: dry blankets in field
Laryngeal edema	Endotracheal intubation, tracheostomy
Carbon monoxide poisoning	100% oxygen, hyperbaric oxygen
Cyanide poisoning	100% O_2 plus amyl nitrate, sodium nitrate, and sodium thiosulfate
Cardiac dysfunction	Inotropic agents, diuretics
Gastric ulcers	H_2-receptor antagonist, antacids
Compartment syndrome	Escharotomy incision
Contractures	Physical therapy
Hypermetabolic state	Enteral and parenteral nutritional support, pain control, glucose control, consider β blockers and anabolic steroids
Renal failure	Supportive care, dialysis
Transient antidiuresis	Expectant management
Anemia	Transfusions as indicated
Psychological trauma	Psychological rehabilitation
Pulmonary infiltrates	PEEP, ventilation, oxygen
Pulmonary edema	Avoid overhydration, give diuretics
Pneumonia	Antibiotics
Bronchospasm	β-Agonist aerosols

PEEP, Positive end-expiratory pressure.

PROGNOSIS

Most children who sustain burns recover without significant disability, but estimation of morbidity is difficult to ascertain from databases. Physical scarring and emotional impact of disfiguring burns are long-term consequences of burn injuries.

PREVENTION

Most burns occur in the home. Prevention is possible by using smoke and fire alarms, having identifiable escape routes and a fire extinguisher, and reducing hot water temperature to 49°C (120°F). Immersion full-thickness burns develop after 1 second at 70°C (158°F), after 5 seconds at 60°C (140°F), after 30 seconds at 54.5°C (130°F), and after 10 minutes at 49°C (120°F).

CHAPTER 45

Poisoning

ETIOLOGY AND EPIDEMIOLOGY

The most common agents ingested by young children include cosmetics, personal care products, cleaning solutions, and analgesics. In 2014 fatal childhood poisonings were most commonly caused by analgesics, fumes/gases/vapors, and cough and cold preparations.

More than 2 million human exposures are called into poison control centers in the United States each year. More than half of all exposures are in children (62% in 2014) with a male predominance in children under 13, but a female predominance in adolescence. Most ingestions in young children are unintentional, with intentional ingestions becoming more common in children 13 and older.

CLINICAL MANIFESTATIONS

Any child who presents with unexplained symptoms including altered mental status, seizure, cardiovascular compromise, or metabolic abnormality should be considered to have ingested a poison until proven otherwise. A history and physical examination by someone who understands the signs and symptoms of various ingestions often provide sufficient clues to distinguish between toxic ingestion and organic disease (Table 45.1). Determination of all substances that the child was exposed to, type of medication, amount of medication, and time of exposure is crucial in directing interventions. Available data often are incomplete or inaccurate, requiring a careful physical examination and laboratory approach. A complete physical examination, including vital signs, is necessary. Certain complexes of symptoms and signs are relatively specific to a given class of drugs (toxidrome; Table 45.2).

COMPLICATIONS

A poisoned child can exhibit any one of six basic clinical patterns: coma, toxicity, metabolic acidosis, heart rhythm aberrations, gastrointestinal symptoms, and seizures.

Coma

Coma is perhaps the most striking symptom of a poison ingestion, but it also may be seen as a result of several other causes including trauma, a cerebrovascular accident, asphyxia, or meningitis. A careful history and clinical examination are needed to distinguish among these alternatives.

Direct Toxicity

Hydrocarbon ingestion occasionally may result in systemic toxicity, but more often it leads to pulmonary toxicity. Hydrocarbons with low viscosity, low surface tension, and high volatility pose the greatest risk of producing aspiration pneumonia; however, when swallowed, they pose no risk unless emesis is induced. Emesis or lavage should *not* be initiated in a child who has ingested volatile hydrocarbons.

Caustic ingestions may cause dysphagia, epigastric pain, oral mucosal burns, and low-grade fever. Patients with esophageal lesions may have no oral burns or may have significant signs and symptoms. Treatment depends on the agent ingested and the presence or absence of esophageal injury. Alkali agents may be solid, granular, or liquid. Liquid agents are tasteless and produce full-thickness liquefaction necrosis of the esophagus or oropharynx. When the esophageal lesions heal, strictures form. Ingestion of these agents also creates a long-term risk of esophageal carcinoma. Treatment includes antibiotics if there

TABLE 45.1 Historical and Physical Findings in Poisoning

ODOR	
Bitter almonds	Cyanide
Acetone	Isopropyl alcohol, methanol, paraldehyde, salicylate
Alcohol	Ethanol
Wintergreen	Methyl salicylate
Garlic	Arsenic, thallium, organophosphates, selenium
Violets	Turpentine
OCULAR SIGNS	
Miosis	Narcotics (except propoxyphene, meperidine, and pentazocine), organophosphates, muscarinic mushrooms, clonidine, phenothiazines, chloral hydrate, barbiturates (late)
Mydriasis	Atropine, cocaine, amphetamines, antihistamines, cyclic antidepressants, PCP, LSD
Nystagmus	Phenytoin, barbiturates, ethanol, carbamazepine, PCP, ketamine, dextromethorphan
Lacrimation	Organophosphates, irritant gas or vapors
Retinal hyperemia	Methanol
Poor vision	Methanol, botulism, carbon monoxide
CUTANEOUS SIGNS	
Needle tracks	Heroin, PCP, amphetamine
Dry, hot skin	Anticholinergic agents, botulism
Diaphoresis	Organophosphates, muscarinic mushrooms, aspirin, cocaine
Alopecia	Thallium, arsenic, lead, mercury
Erythema	Boric acid, mercury, cyanide, anticholinergics
ORAL SIGNS	
Salivation	Organophosphates, salicylate, corrosives, strychnine, ketamine
Dry mouth	Amphetamine, anticholinergics, antihistamine
Burns	Corrosives, oxalate-containing plants
Gum lines	Lead, mercury, arsenic
Dysphagia	Corrosives, botulism
INTESTINAL SIGNS	
Diarrhea	Antimicrobials, arsenic, iron, boric acid, cholinergics
Constipation	Lead, narcotics, botulism
Hematemesis	Corrosives, iron, salicylates, NSAIDs
CARDIAC SIGNS	
Tachycardia	Atropine, aspirin, amphetamine, cocaine, cyclic antidepressants, theophylline
Bradycardia	Digitalis, narcotics, clonidine, organophosphates, β blockers, calcium channel blockers
Hypertension	Amphetamine, LSD, cocaine, PCP
Hypotension	Phenothiazines, barbiturates, cyclic antidepressants, iron, β blockers, calcium channel blockers, clonidine, narcotics
RESPIRATORY SIGNS	
Depressed respiration	Alcohol, narcotics, barbiturates
Increased respiration	Amphetamines, aspirin, ethylene glycol, carbon monoxide, cyanide
Pulmonary edema	Hydrocarbons, organophosphates
CENTRAL NERVOUS SYSTEM SIGNS	
Ataxia	Alcohol, barbiturates, anticholinergics, narcotics
Coma	Sedatives, narcotics, barbiturates, salicylate, cyanide, carbon monoxide, cyclic antidepressants, alcohol
Hyperpyrexia	Anticholinergics, salicylates, amphetamine, cocaine
Muscle fasciculation	Organophosphates, theophylline
Muscle rigidity	Cyclic antidepressants, PCP, phenothiazines, haloperidol
Peripheral neuropathy	Lead, arsenic, mercury, organophosphates
Altered behavior	LSD, PCP, amphetamines, cocaine, alcohol, anticholinergics

LSD, Lysergic acid diethylamide; *MSG*, monosodium glutamate; *NSAID*, nonsteroidal antiinflammatory drug; *PCP*, phencyclidine.

TABLE 45.2 Toxic Syndromes

AGENT	MANIFESTATIONS
Acetaminophen	Nausea, vomiting, pallor, delayed jaundice–hepatic failure (72-96 hr)
Amphetamine, cocaine, and sympathomimetics	Tachycardia, hypertension, hyperthermia, psychosis and paranoia, seizures, mydriasis, diaphoresis, piloerection, aggressive behavior
Anticholinergics	Mania, delirium, fever, red dry skin, dry mouth, tachycardia, mydriasis, urinary retention
Carbon monoxide	Headache, dizziness, coma, other systems affected
Cyanide	Coma, convulsions, hyperpnea, bitter almond odor
Ethylene glycol (antifreeze)	Metabolic acidosis, hyperosmolarity, hypocalcemia, oxalate crystalluria
Iron	Vomiting (bloody), diarrhea, hypotension, hepatic failure, leukocytosis, hyperglycemia, radiopaque pills on KUB, late intestinal stricture, *Yersinia* sepsis
Narcotics	Coma, respiratory depression, hypotension, pinpoint pupils, bradycardia
Cholinergics (organophosphates, nicotine)	Miosis, salivation, urination, diaphoresis, lacrimation, bronchospasm (bronchorrhea), muscle weakness and fasciculations, emesis, defecation, coma, confusion, pulmonary edema, bradycardia
Salicylates	Tachypnea, fever, lethargy, coma, vomiting, diaphoresis, alkalosis (early), acidosis (late)
Cyclic antidepressants	Coma, convulsions, mydriasis, hyperreflexia, arrhythmia (prolonged Q-T interval), cardiac arrest, shock

KUB, Kidney-ureter-bladder radiograph.

are signs of infection and dilation of late-forming (2-3 weeks later) strictures.

Ingested button batteries also may produce a caustic mucosal injury. Batteries that remain in the esophagus may cause esophageal burns and erosion and should be removed with an endoscope. In addition, acid agents can injure the lungs (with hydrochloric acid fumes), oral mucosa, esophagus, and stomach. Because acids taste sour, children usually stop drinking the solution, limiting the injury. Acids produce a coagulation necrosis, which limits the chemical from penetrating into deeper layers of the mucosa and damages tissue less severely than alkali. The signs, symptoms, and therapeutic measures are similar to those for alkali ingestion.

Metabolic Acidosis

A poisoned child may also have a high anion gap metabolic acidosis (mnemonic *MUDPILES*; Table 45.3), which is assessed easily by measuring arterial blood gases, serum electrolyte levels, and urine pH. An osmolar gap, if present, strongly suggests the presence of an unmeasured component, such as methanol or ethylene glycol. These ingestions require thorough assessment and prompt intervention.

TABLE 45.3 Screening Laboratory Clues in Toxicological Diagnosis

ANION GAP METABOLIC ACIDOSIS (MNEMONIC = MUDPILES)
Methanol,* metformin
Uremia*
Diabetic ketoacidosis*
Paraldehyde,* phenformin
Isoniazid, iron
Lactic acidosis (cyanide, carbon monoxide)
Ethanol,* ethylene glycol*
Salicylates, starvation, seizures
HYPOGLYCEMIA
Ethanol
Isoniazid
Insulin
Propranolol
Oral hypoglycemic agents
HYPERGLYCEMIA
Salicylates
Isoniazid
Iron
Phenothiazines
Sympathomimetics
HYPOCALCEMIA
Oxalate
Ethylene glycol
Fluoride
RADIOPAQUE SUBSTANCE ON KUB (MNEMONIC = CHIPPED)
Chloral hydrate, calcium carbonate
Heavy metals (lead, zinc, barium, arsenic, lithium, bismuth as in Pepto-Bismol)
Iron
Phenothiazines
Play-Doh, potassium chloride
Enteric-coated pills
Dental amalgam

*Indicates hyperosmolar condition.
KUB, Kidney-ureter-bladder radiograph.

Dysrhythmias

Dysrhythmias may be prominent signs of a variety of toxic ingestions, although ventricular arrhythmias are rare. Prolonged Q-T intervals may suggest phenothiazine or antihistamine ingestion, and widened QRS complexes are seen with ingestions of cyclic antidepressants and quinidine. Because many drug and chemical overdoses may lead to sinus tachycardia, this is not a useful or discriminating sign; however, sinus bradycardia suggests digoxin, cyanide, a cholinergic agent, or β blocker ingestion (Table 45.4).

TABLE 45.4 Drugs Associated With Major Modes of Presentation

COMMON TOXIC CAUSES OF CARDIAC ARRHYTHMIA	Hypoglycemic agents
Amphetamine	Lead
Antiarrhythmics	Lithium
Anticholinergics	Methemoglobinemia*
Antihistamines	Methyldopa
Arsenic	Narcotics
Carbon monoxide	Phencyclidine
Chloral hydrate	Phenothiazines
Cocaine	Salicylates
Cyanide	**COMMON AGENTS CAUSING SEIZURES (MNEMONIC = CAPS)**
Cyclic antidepressants	**C**amphor
Digitalis	Carbamazepine
Freon	Carbon monoxide
Phenothiazines	Cocaine
Physostigmine	Cyanide
Propranolol	**A**minophylline
Quinine, quinidine	Amphetamine
Theophylline	Anticholinergics
CAUSES OF COMA	Antidepressants (cyclic)
Alcohol	**P**b (lead) (also lithium)
Anticholinergics	Pesticide (organophosphate)
Antihistamines	Phencyclidine
Barbiturates	Phenol
Carbon monoxide	Phenothiazines
Clonidine	Propoxyphene
Cyanide	**S**alicylates
Cyclic antidepressants	Strychnine

Causes of methemoglobinemia: amyl nitrite, aniline dyes, benzocaine, bismuth subnitrate, dapsone, primaquine, quinones, spinach, sulfonamides.

Gastrointestinal Symptoms

Gastrointestinal symptoms of poisoning include emesis, nausea, abdominal cramps, and diarrhea. These symptoms may be the result of direct toxic effects on the intestinal mucosa or of systemic toxicity after absorption.

Seizures

Seizures are the sixth major mode of presentation for children with toxic ingestions, but poisoning is an uncommon cause of afebrile seizures. When seizures do occur with intoxication, they may be life-threatening and require aggressive therapeutic intervention.

LABORATORY AND IMAGING STUDIES

Laboratory studies helpful in initial management include specific toxin-drug assays; measurement of arterial blood gases and electrolytes, osmoles, and glucose; and calculation of the anion or osmolar gap. A full 12-lead electrocardiogram should be part of the initial evaluation in all patients suspected of ingesting toxic substances. Urine screens for drugs of abuse or to confirm suspected ingestion of medications in the home may be revealing.

Quantitative toxicology assays are important for some agents (Table 45.5), not only for identifying the specific drug, but also for providing guidance for therapy, anticipating complications, and estimating the prognosis.

TREATMENT

The four foci of treatment for poisonings are supportive care, decontamination, enhanced elimination, and specific antidotes.

Supportive Care

Supportive care is the mainstay of treatment in most cases. Prompt attention must be given to protecting and maintaining the airway, establishing effective breathing, and supporting the circulation. This management sequence takes precedence over other diagnostic or therapeutic procedures. If the level of consciousness is depressed and a toxic substance is suspected, glucose (1 g/kg intravenously), 100% oxygen, and naloxone should be administered.

Gastrointestinal Decontamination

The intent of gastrointestinal decontamination is to prevent the absorption of a potentially toxic ingested substance and, in theory, to prevent the poisoning. There has been great controversy about which methods are the safest and most efficacious. Recommendations from the American Academy of Clinical Toxicology (AACT) and the European Association of Poison Centres and Clinical Toxicologists (EAPCCT) follow. **Syrup of ipecac** should not be administered routinely to poisoned patients because of potential complications and lack of evidence that it improves outcome. Likewise, **gastric lavage** should not be used routinely, if ever, in the management of poisoned patients because of the lack of efficacy and potential complications. **Single-dose activated charcoal** decreases drug absorption when used within 1 hour of ingestion; however, it has not been shown to improve outcome. Thus it should be used selectively in the management of a poisoned patient. Charcoal is ineffective against caustic or corrosive agents, hydrocarbons, heavy metals (arsenic, lead, mercury, iron, lithium), glycols, and water-insoluble compounds.

The administration of a cathartic (sorbitol or magnesium citrate) alone has no role in the management of the poisoned patient. The AACT has stated that based on available data, the use of a cathartic in combination with activated charcoal is not recommended.

Whole-bowel irrigation using polyethylene glycol (GoLYTELY) as a nonabsorbable cathartic may be effective for toxic ingestion of sustained-release or enteric-coated drugs. The AACT does not recommend the routine use of whole-bowel irrigation. However, there is theoretical benefit in its use for potentially toxic ingestions of iron, lead, zinc, or packets of illicit drugs.

TABLE 45.5 Drugs Amenable to Therapeutic Monitoring for Drug Toxicity

ANTIBIOTICS
Aminoglycosides—gentamicin, tobramycin, and amikacin
Chloramphenicol
Vancomycin
IMMUNOSUPPRESSION
Methotrexate
Cyclosporine
ANTIPYRETICS
Acetaminophen
Salicylate
OTHER
Digoxin
Lithium
Theophylline
Anticonvulsant drugs
Serotonin uptake inhibitor agent

Enhanced Elimination

Multiple-dose activated charcoal should be considered only if a patient has ingested a life-threatening amount of carbamazepine, dapsone, phenobarbital, quinine, or theophylline. **Alkalinization of urine** may be helpful for salicylate or methotrexate ingestion. **Dialysis** may be used for substances that have a low volume of distribution, low molecular weight, low protein binding, and high degree of water solubility, such as methanol, ethylene glycol, salicylates, theophylline, bromide, and lithium.

Specific Antidotes

See Table 45.6.

For recommendations on specific therapy, contact one of the U.S. Poison Control Centers at 1-800-222-1222.

TABLE 45.6 Specific Antidotes

POISON	ANTIDOTE	DOSAGE	COMMENTS
Acetaminophen	N-Acetylcysteine	140 mg/kg PO initial dose, then 70 mg/kg PO q4hr × 17 doses 150 mg/kg IV over 1 hr, followed by 50 mg/kg IV over 4 hr, followed by 100 mg/kg IV over 16 hr	Most effective within 16 hr of ingestion
Benzodiazepine	Flumazenil	0.2 mg IV, may repeat to 1 mg max	Possible seizures, arrhythmias, DO NOT USE FOR UNKNOWN INGESTIONS
β-Blocking agents	Glucagon	0.15 mg/kg IV, followed by infusion of 0.05-0.15 mg/kg/hr	
Carbon monoxide	Oxygen	100%; hyperbaric O_2	Half-life of carboxyhemoglobin is 5 hr in room air but 1.5 hr in 100% O_2
Cyclic antidepressants	Sodium bicarbonate	1-2 mEq/kg IV, followed by continuous infusion; titrated to produce pH of 7.5-7.55	Follow potassium levels and replace as needed
Iron	Deferoxamine	Infusion of 5-15 mg/kg/hr IV (max 6 g/24 hr)	Hypotension (worse with rapid infusion rates)

TABLE 45.6 Specific Antidotes—cont'd

POISON	ANTIDOTE	DOSAGE	COMMENTS
Lead	Edetate calcium disodium (EDTA)	35-50 mg/kg/day IV × 5 days; continuous infusion or divided q12hr	
	British anti-Lewisite (BAL; dimercaprol)	4 mg/kg/dose IM q4hr × 2-7 days	May cause sterile abscesses Prepared in peanut oil, do not use in patients with peanut allergy
	Succimer (2,3-dimercaptosuccinic acid ([DMSA])	10 mg/kg/dose PO tid × 5 days, then 10 mg/kg/dose PO bid × 14 days	Few toxic effects, requires lead-free home plus compliant family
Nitrites/ methemoglobinemia*	Methylene blue	1-2 mg/kg IV, repeat q 30-60 min if needed; treat for levels >30%	Exchange transfusion may be needed for severe methemoglobinemia; methylene blue overdose also causes methemoglobinemia
Opiates	Naloxone	0.1 mg/kg IV, ET, SC, IM for children, up to 2 mg, repeat as needed	Naloxone causes no respiratory depression
Organophosphates	Atropine	0.02-0.05 mg/kg IV/IO, repeat every 20-30 min as needed	Physiological: blocks acetylcholine
	Pralidoxime (2 PAM; Protopam)	25-50 mg/kg IV over 5-10 min (max 2000 mg/dose); may repeat after 1-2 hr, then q10-12hr as needed	Specific: disrupts phosphate-cholinesterase bond

*See Table 45.4 for causes of methemoglobinemia.
ET, Endotracheal; *IM*, intramuscular; *IV*, intravenous; *PO*, oral; *SC*, subcutaneous.
From Kliegman RM, Stanton BF, St. Geme JW, et al., eds. Nelson Textbook of Pediatrics. *19th ed. Philadelphia: Saunders; 2011: 256–257.*

PROGNOSIS

Most poisonings result in minimal or no toxicity, or have minor effects. Intentional ingestions result in a much higher rate (5.2%) of major effects or death compared with unintentional ingestions (0.2%). Adolescents are more likely to have a moderate, major, or fatal effect from ingestion compared to younger children (17.3% of teens compared with 1.1% of children under 6 years).

PREVENTION

Properly educating parents regarding safe storage of medications and household toxins is necessary for preventing ingestions. If a child has ingested poison, a poison control center should be called.

CHAPTER 46

Sedation and Analgesia

An acutely ill pediatric patient may have pain, discomfort, and anxiety resulting from injury, surgery, and invasive procedures (intubation, bone marrow aspiration, venous access placement) or during mechanical ventilation. Clear goals should be identified to allow provision of optimal analgesia or sedation without compromising the physiological status of the patient. Anxiolysis, cooperation, amnesia, immobility, and lack of awareness all are goals of sedation and can be accomplished with various drugs (Table 46.1). Many of these goals can be achieved with behavioral techniques (preprocedural teaching), but sedation is often a necessary adjunct for painful procedures. Pain may be expressed by verbal or visible discomfort, crying, agitation, tachycardia, hypertension, and tachypnea. A variety of scales have been developed in an attempt to quantify pain and allow more directed therapy. Few of these scales are well validated, especially in populations of acutely ill children with physiological derangements secondary to the underlying pathology. Pain caused by procedural interventions should always be treated with analgesics in addition to sedation (Table 46.2).

ASSESSMENT

Procedural Sedation

A medical evaluation must be performed for any patient receiving procedural sedation to identify underlying medical conditions that may affect the choice of sedative agents. Specific attention must be paid to assessment of the airway (for ability to maintain a patent airway) and respiratory system (asthma, recent respiratory illness, loose teeth), cardiovascular status (especially adequacy of volume status), factors affecting drug metabolism (renal or liver disease), and risk of aspiration (adequate nothing-by-mouth status, gastroesophageal reflux). During the administration of procedural sedation, assessment of status must include monitoring of oxygen saturation, heart rate, and respiratory rate, as well as some assessment of effectiveness of ventilation. This assessment must be performed by someone who is not involved in the procedure; this person is also responsible for recording vital signs and drugs administered on a time-based graph. Monitoring must be continued until the child has returned to baseline. Patients who are receiving long-term sedation (e.g., to maintain endotracheal tube placement) may need only local anesthesia for painful procedures but may benefit from additional sedation or analgesia as well.

TABLE 46.1 Agents that Produce Sedation

SEDATIVES	EFFECT	CONCERNS
Midazolam	Anxiolysis, sedation, muscle relaxation, amnesia	Tolerance is possible; apnea, hypotension, depressed myocardial function; short action
Lorazepam	Anxiolysis, sedation, muscle relaxation, amnesia	Same as midazolam; longer action
Dexmedetomidine	Sedation without respiratory depression	May cause bradycardia
Ketamine	Anesthesia, analgesia, amnesia	Dissociative reactions, tachycardia, hypertension, increased bronchial secretions, emergent delirium, hallucinations; increases intracranial pressure
Chloral hydrate	Sedative	Emesis, hypotension, arrhythmias, hepatic dysfunction
Propofol	Rapid-onset sedative for induction and maintenance of anesthesia	Metabolic acidosis in children; may depress cardiac function

TABLE 46.2 Agents that Produce Analgesia

ANALGESIC	EFFECT	COMPLICATIONS
Acetaminophen and NSAIDs	Moderate analgesia, antipyresis	Ceiling effect NSAIDs—gastrointestinal bleed, ulceration
Opioids		No ceiling effect; respiratory depression, sedation, pruritus, nausea/vomiting, decreased gastric motility, urinary retention, tolerance with abuse potential
Morphine	Analgesia	May cause myocardial depression
Codeine	Analgesia	Nausea/vomiting
Fentanyl, alfentanil, sufentanil	Analgesia, sedation	No adverse effects on cardiovascular system; stiff chest syndrome
Methadone	Analgesia	

NSAIDs, Nonsteroidal antiinflammatory drugs.

Nonprocedural Sedation

Many ventilated pediatric patients require sedation and some analgesia while intubated. Dexmedetomidine, a centrally-acting selective α(2)-receptor agonist, is becoming increasingly popular due to its ability to provide sedation without respiratory depression. Longer acting benzodiazepine and opioids are also commonly used. Avoidance of oversedation is important. Use of appropriate pain and sedation scores allows for titration of medications to achieve goals of the sedation plan. Long-term use of benzodiazepines and opioids leads to tolerance, a problematic occurrence that must be considered as medications are added and weaned. Medications used for sedation and analgesia may also contribute to delirium, a phenomenon that is being increasingly recognized in critically ill patients.

PAIN AND ANALGESIA

The subjective aspect of pain requires that self-reporting be used for assessment. Visual analog scales, developed for adult patients (allowing patients to rate pain on a scale of 1 to 10), have been used for older children. Pain scales for younger children often incorporate behavioral and physiological parameters, despite the imprecision of physiological responses.

Local anesthetics, such as lidocaine, can be used for minor procedures. However, lidocaine requires subcutaneous or intradermal injection. The use of EMLA, a cream containing lidocaine and prilocaine, is less effective than intradermal lidocaine but is preferred by many patients.

Patient-controlled analgesia is an effective method for providing balanced analgesia care in older children and adolescents. Children using patient-controlled analgesia have better pain relief and experience less sedation than patients receiving intermittent, nurse-controlled, bolus analgesics. Analgesics can be administered through the patient-controlled analgesia pump with continuous basal infusions, bolus administration, or both. Morphine is the most frequent opioid used for patient-controlled analgesia. Monitoring of oxygen saturations and respiratory rate are crucial with continuous opioid infusions because of the shift in CO_2 response curve and potential to decrease ventilatory response to hypoxia.

Epidural analgesia decreases the need for inhalation anesthetics during surgery and can provide significant analgesia without sedation in the postoperative period. Decreased costs and length of stay also may be benefits of epidural analgesic approaches. Medications used in epidurals include bupivacaine and morphine. Adverse effects include nausea and vomiting, motor blockade, and technical problems requiring catheter removal. Infection and permanent neurological deficits are rare.

Suggested Readings

American Heart Association. CPR and first aid emergency cardiovascular care guidelines. Available at https://eccguidelines.heart.org/index.php/circulation/cpr-ecc-guidelines-2/part-11-pediatric-basic-life-support-and-cardiopulmonary-resuscitation-quality/.

Kliegman RM, Stanton B, St. Geme J, et al. *Nelson Textbook of Pediatrics*. 20th ed. Philadelphia: Elsevier; 2016.

PEARLS FOR PRACTITIONERS

CHAPTER 38

Assessment and Resuscitation

- Initial assessment focuses on the ABCs—airway, breathing, and circulation of an acutely ill or injured child.
- Respiratory failure is the most common cause of acute deterioration in children.
- In cardiopulmonary arrest:
  - The goal should be to optimize cardiac output and tissue oxygen delivery.
  - Begin chest compressions immediately, followed by support of the airway and breathing/ventilation (C-A-B).
- Monitoring vital signs and physiological status is the key screening activity.
  - The choice of appropriate diagnostic tests and imaging is determined by the mechanism of disease and results of evaluation after initial resuscitation.

CHAPTER 39

Respiratory Failure

- Acute respiratory failure occurs when the pulmonary system is unable to maintain adequate gas exchange to meet metabolic demands.
- Respiratory failure
  - Can be classified as hypercarbic, hypoxemic, or both.
  - Is frequently caused by bronchiolitis, asthma, pneumonia, upper airway obstruction, and/or systemic inflammation resulting in acute respiratory distress syndrome (ARDS).
- Pediatric ARDS and its severity are defined by: (1) onset within 7 days of known clinical insult; (2) respiratory failure not fully explained by cardiac failure or fluid overload; (3) chest imaging findings of new infiltrate(s); and (4) impairment in oxygenation.
- Pulse oximetry allows noninvasive, continuous assessment of oxygenation but is unable to provide information about ventilation abnormalities

CHAPTER 40

Shock

- Shock is the inability to provide sufficient perfusion of oxygenated blood and substrate to tissues to meet metabolic demands.
  - Acute hypovolemia is the most common cause of shock in children.
  - Other forms of shock include distributive shock, cardiogenic shock, hemorrhagic shock, obstructive shock, and dissociative shock
- Shock requires immediate resuscitation before obtaining laboratory or diagnostic studies.
- The key to therapy is the recognition of shock in its early, partially compensated state, when many of the hemodynamic and metabolic alterations may be reversible.

CHAPTER 41

Injury Prevention

- Injury occurs through interaction of the host with an agent through a vector and an environment that is conducive to exposure.
- Unintentional injury is the leading cause of death in children 1-18 years of age.
- The most common causes of fatal injuries differ among age groups.
- The Haddon matrix combines the epidemiological components with time factors to identify effective interventions focused on different aspects of the injury event.

CHAPTER 42

Major Trauma

- Injury is the leading cause of death in children ages 1-18 years.
- Primary Survey is focused on assessment of ABCDE—Airway, Breathing, Circulation, Disability (including neurological status), and Exposure (including disrobing the child and performing a detailed assessment of the entire body).
- Secondary Survey is focused on a more detailed head-to-toe examination along with obtaining more history.
- Resuscitative measures are performed concurrently with primary and secondary survey.
- The leading causes of death in trauma are head injury (first) and thoracic injury (second).
- Most blunt abdominal organ injury is managed nonoperatively.

CHAPTER 43

Drowning

- Drowning is defined as respiratory impairment from submersion/immersion in liquid and is the second leading cause of death for children ages 1-14 years.
- Other terms, including near drowning, secondary drowning, and dry drowning, should not be used.
- Outcomes are categorized as death, morbidity, or no morbidity and closely linked to the degree of hypoxic-ischemic brain injury.
- Treatment is focused on optimizing oxygenation and perfusion, especially cerebral perfusion.

CHAPTER 44

Burns

- Classification by depth (superficial, superficial partial-thickness, deep partial-thickness, and full-thickness) conveys more information about the structures injured and the likely need for surgical treatment than the commonly used first-degree, second-degree, and third-degree burn designation.
- For severe burns, care is best managed by a multidisciplinary team in a qualified burn center.
- Severe burn injury results in a hypermetabolic state.

CHAPTER 45

Poisoning

- Consider poisoning in any child who presents with unexplained altered mental status, seizure, cardiovascular compromise, or metabolic abnormality.
- A poisoned child can exhibit any one of six basic clinical patterns: coma, toxicity, metabolic acidosis, heart rhythm aberrations, gastrointestinal symptoms, and/or seizures.
- The four foci of treatment for poisonings are supportive care, decontamination, enhanced elimination, and specific antidotes.

CHAPTER 46

Sedation and Analgesia

- Sedation and analgesia are necessary to treat the pain, discomfort, and anxiety experienced by many acutely ill and injured pediatric patients.
- Clear goals should be identified to allow provision of optimal analgesia or sedation without compromising the physiological status of the patient.
- Long-term use of benzodiazepines and opioids leads to tolerance.

HUMAN GENETICS AND DYSMORPHOLOGY

Robert W. Marion | Paul A. Levy

CHAPTER 47

Patterns of Inheritance

TYPES OF GENETIC DISORDERS

Among infants born in the United States, 2-4% have **congenital malformations**, abnormalities of form or function identifiable at birth. At 1 year of age, the number approaches 7%, because some anomalies may not be identifiable until after the neonatal period. The prevalence of congenital malformations is much greater in inpatient pediatric populations; 30-50% of hospitalized children have congenital anomalies or genetic disorders.

The clinical geneticist attempts to identify the etiology, mode of inheritance, and risk that a disorder might occur in the affected child's siblings. In evaluating children with congenital malformations, the condition's etiology may be classified into one of five different categories:

1. Single-gene mutations, occurring in 6% of children with congenital anomalies
2. Chromosomal disorders, accounting for approximately 7.5%
3. Multifactorially inherited conditions, accounting for 20%
4. Disorders that show an unusual pattern of inheritance, accounting for 2-3%
5. Conditions caused by exposure to teratogens, accounting for 6%

In most cases, the etiology cannot be classified into one of these categories. In these individuals, the etiology remains unknown.

INTRODUCTION TO GENETICS AND GENOMICS

DNA is composed of four nucleotide building blocks: adenine, guanine, cytosine, and thymine. Each nucleotide is linked to other nucleotides, forming a chain. The DNA molecule consists of two chains of nucleotides held together by hydrogen bonds. The purine nucleotides, adenine and guanine, cross link by hydrogen bonds to the pyrimidines, thymine and cytosine. Because of this cross linking, the nucleotide sequence of one strand sets the other strand's sequence. Separating the two strands permits complementary nucleotides to bind to each DNA strand; this copies the DNA and replicates the sequence.

DNA exists as multiple fragments that, together with a protein skeleton (chromatin), form chromosomes. Human cells have 23 pairs of chromosomes, with one copy of each chromosome inherited from each parent. Twenty-two pairs of chromosomes are **autosomes**; the remaining pair consists of **sex chromosomes**. Females have two X chromosomes; males have one X and one Y.

Spread along the chromosomes like beads on a string, DNA sequences form **genes,** the basic units of heredity. A typical gene contains a promoter sequence, an untranslated region, and an open reading frame. In the open reading frame, every three nucleotides represent a single **codon**, coding for a particular amino acid. In this way, the sequence of bases dictates the sequence of amino acids in the corresponding protein. Some codons, rather than coding for specific amino acids, act as "start" signals, whereas others serve as "stop" signals. Between the start and stop codons, genes consist of two major portions: **exons**, regions containing the code that ultimately corresponds to a sequence of amino acids, and **introns** (intervening sequence), which do not become part of the amino acid sequence.

Genes are **transcribed** into messenger RNA (mRNA) then **translated** into proteins. During transcription, RNA is processed to remove introns. The mRNA serves as a template to construct the protein.

Human genetic material contains 3 billion bases. Less than 2% of the DNA codes for proteins, comprising the genome's 19,000-20,000 genes. Through a mechanism called **alternative splicing**, these genes may create more than 100,000 proteins. The remainder of the DNA, the portion not involved in protein formation, was once termed *junk DNA*, but a project called ENCODE (Encyclopedia of DNA Elements) found that much of this presumed *junk DNA* is functional and likely serves regulatory functions.

Disease may be caused by changes or **mutations** in the DNA sequence, with the **point mutation**, a change in a single DNA base, being the most common type. A point mutation that changes a codon and the resulting amino acid that goes into the protein is referred to as a **missense mutation.** A **nonsense mutation** is a point mutation that changes the codon to a "stop" signal so that transcription ends prematurely. A **frameshift mutation** often stems from the loss or addition of one or more bases; this causes a shift in how the DNA is transcribed and generally leads to premature stop codons.

Pedigree Drawing

To identify specific patterns of inheritance, geneticists construct and analyze pedigrees, pictorial representations of a family history. Males are represented by squares and females by circles. Matings are connected with a solid line between each partner's symbols. Children from a couple are represented below their parents and are the next generation.

Grandparents, uncles, aunts, and cousins are added in similar fashion. Ages or birthdays may be written next to or underneath each symbol. The proband (the patient who is the initial contact) is indicated with an arrow. Affected individuals are indicated by shading or some other technique, which should be explained in a key. Carriers for a disorder (e.g., sickle cell disease) usually are indicated by a dot in the center of their symbol (Fig. 47.1).

To be useful, pedigrees should include representatives of at least three generations of family members.

Autosomal Dominant Disorders

If a single copy of a gene bearing a mutation is sufficient to cause disease and that gene is not on one of the sex chromosomes, that condition is inherited in an autosomal dominant (AD) fashion (Table 47.1). In AD disorders, each child of an affected parent has a 50% chance of inheriting the mutated gene (Fig. 47.2; Table 47.2). Possessing one *working* gene and one *nonworking* gene is termed **heterozygous.** If both copies are the same, they are referred to as **homozygous**.

Some people who are obligate carriers of a mutation known to cause an AD disorder do not show clinical signs of the condition, while other such individuals manifest symptoms. This phenomenon is referred to as **penetrance.** If all individuals who carry a mutation for an AD disorder show signs of that disorder, the gene is said to have complete penetrance. Many AD disorders show decreased penetrance.

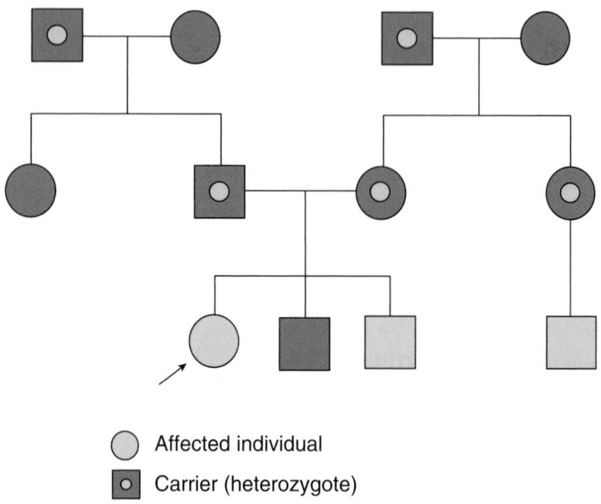

FIGURE 47.1 Pedigree showing affected individuals and carriers.

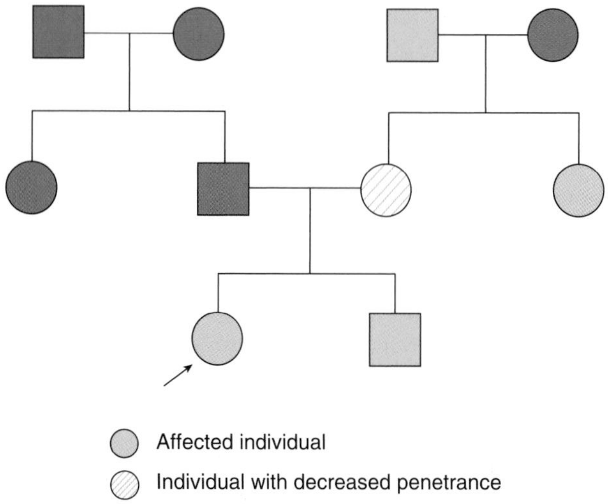

FIGURE 47.2 Pedigree showing decreased penetrance for an autosomal dominant disorder. Proband *(arrow)* is affected. Maternal grandfather also is affected. The individual's mother is presumed to be the carrier of the gene, even though she may show only slight symptoms of disease.

TABLE 47.1 Autosomal Dominant Diseases

DISEASE	FREQUENCY	COMMENTS
Achondroplasia Thanatophoric dysplasia Crouzon syndrome with acanthosis nigricans Nonsyndromic craniosynostosis	~1:25,000	Mutations are in the gene for *fibroblast growth factor receptor-3* on chromosome 4p16.3. 40% of cases are new mutations (different mutations in the same gene cause achondroplasia, thanatophoric dysplasia, Crouzon syndrome with acanthosis, and nonsyndromic craniosynostosis)
Neurofibromatosis 1	1:3,500	About 50% of cases result from new mutations in the gene for neurofibromin, a tumor suppressor gene located at 17q11.2. Expression is quite variable
Neurofibromatosis 2 (NF2)	Genotype at birth, 1:33,000 Phenotype prevalence, 1:200,000	The *NF2* gene is a tumor suppressor gene located at 22q12.2. The protein is called "Merlin." Associated with bilateral acoustic neuromas
Huntington disease (HD)	Variable in populations, 1:5,000-1:20,000	The disease is caused by a (CAG) repeat expansion in the "Huntington" protein gene on chromosome 4p16.3
Myotonic dystrophy (DM, Steinert disease)	1:500 in Quebec 1:25,000 Europeans	The disease is caused by a (CTG) repeat expansion in the DM protein kinase gene at chromosome 19q13.2. The condition shows genetic anticipation with successive generations
Marfan syndrome	1:10,000	The syndrome is caused by mutations in the fibrillin 1 *(FBN1)* gene on chromosome 15q21.1; there is variable expression
Hereditary angioedema (HAE; C-1 esterase inhibitor that regulates the C-1 component of complement)	1:10,000	The gene is located on chromosome 11q11-q13.2. The phenotype of episodic and variable subcutaneous and submucosal swelling and pain is caused by diminished or altered esterase inhibitor protein, which can result from any one of many mutations in the gene

TABLE 47.2 Rules of Autosomal Dominant Inheritance
Trait appears in every generation
Each child of an affected parent has a one in two chance of being affected
Males and females are equally affected
Male-to-male transmission occurs
Traits generally involve mutations in genes that code for regulatory or structural proteins (collagen)

Often, AD disorders show variability in symptoms expressed in different individuals carrying the same mutated gene. Some individuals have only mild clinical symptoms, whereas others have more severe disease. This phenomenon is referred to as **variable expressivity.**

AD disorders sometimes appear in a child of unaffected parents because of a **spontaneous mutation.** Known in some cases to be associated with advanced paternal age (>35 years of age), spontaneous mutations may account for most individuals with some disorders. For instance, 80% of children born with achondroplasia (ACH) have a spontaneous mutation in the fibroblast growth factor receptor type 3 *(FGFR3)* gene. The following are examples of AD disorders.

Achondroplasia

Caused by a defect in cartilage-derived bone, ACH is the most common skeletal dysplasia in humans. The bony abnormalities lead to short stature, macrocephaly, a flat midface with a prominent forehead, and rhizomelic ("root of the limb") shortening of the limbs. The disorder occurs in approximately 1 in 25,000 births.

ACH is caused by a mutation in *FGFR3*. Early in development, this gene is expressed during endochondral bone formation. More than 95% of cases of ACH are caused by one of two mutations in the same base pair (site 1138). This site, extremely active for mutations, is known as a mutational **hot spot.**

As they grow, children with ACH often develop associated medical and psychological problems. Hydrocephalus and central apnea may occur because of narrowing of the foramen magnum and compression of the brainstem and may present a life-threatening complication in infancy. Bowing of the legs may occur later in childhood because of unequal growth of the tibia and fibula. Dental malocclusion, obstructive apnea, and hearing loss due to middle ear dysfunction are common in later childhood. During later childhood and adolescence, the psychological effects of the short stature may manifest. In adulthood, further complications include compression of nerve roots and sciatica. People with ACH have normal life spans and normal intelligence.

The diagnosis of ACH is made on the basis of clinical findings, and characteristic x-ray abnormalities confirm the diagnosis. Molecular testing is available, and prenatal diagnosis is possible using fetal cells obtained through amniocentesis or chorionic villus sampling.

Neurofibromatosis Type 1

One of the most common AD disorders, neurofibromatosis type 1 (NF1) is present in 1 in 3,500 individuals. The condition is caused by a mutation in the *NF1* gene, which codes for the protein neurofibromin.

Although the penetrance of NF1 is 100%, the expression is extremely variable, and many affected individuals have features so mild that they are never diagnosed.

See Chapter 186.

Marfan Syndrome

A condition that occurs in approximately 1 in 10,000 individuals, Marfan syndrome (MFS) shows pleiotropy, a condition in which abnormalities in multiple organ systems are caused by a mutation in a single gene. Caused by a mutation in *FBN1*, clinical symptoms mainly involve three systems: **cardiac, ophthalmological**, and **skeletal**. Skeletal findings include dolichostenomelia (a tall, thin body habitus, spider-like fingers and toes (arachnodactyly), abnormalities of the sternum (pectus excavatum or carinatum), scoliosis, pes planus, and joint laxity. Eye findings include high myopia, which can lead to vitreoretinal degeneration; an abnormal suspensory ligament of the lens, which can lead to ectopia lentis (dislocation of the lens); and cataracts. Cardiac findings include progressive dilatation of the aortic root, and aortic insufficiency followed by aortic dissection is a common complication. Other clinical features include dural ectasia, abnormal pulmonary septation, and striae. Diagnostic criteria for MFS are summarized in Table 47.3.

New mutations in *FBN1* account for 25% of cases of MFS. The gene is large and complex, and more than 1,300 mutations have been identified in affected individuals. Many of the symptoms of MFS are caused not by the defect in the fibrillin protein itself but rather by an excess in transforming growth factor-beta (TGF-β), a protein usually bound by fibrillin.

Autosomal Recessive Disorders

Disorders that are inherited in an autosomal recessive (AR) manner manifest only when *both* copies of a gene pair located on a non-sex chromosome have a mutation (Tables 47.4 and 47.5). Children affected with AR disorders are usually born to unaffected parents, each of whom carries one copy of the mutation. If both members of a couple are carriers (or heterozygotes) for this mutation, each of their offspring has a 25% chance of being affected (Fig. 47.3).

Sickle Cell Disease

See Chapter 150.

Tay-Sachs Disease

See Chapters 56 and 185.

X-Linked Disorders

Approximately 2,000 genes have been identified on the X chromosome, whereas only 200 are believed to be present on the Y chromosome. Females, whose cells have two copies of an X chromosome, possess two copies of each of these genes, whereas males, who have one X chromosome and one Y chromosome, have only one copy. Early in female development, one X chromosome is randomly inactivated in each cell. There are many X-linked disorders (colorblindness, Duchenne muscular dystrophy, hemophilia A) in which heterozygous (carrier) females show some manifestations of the disorder due to skewed X chromosome inactivation.

TABLE 47.3 Revised Ghent Nosology for the Diagnosis of Marfan Syndrome

AORTIC ROOT DILATATION* (Z ≥ 2SD) OR AORTIC DISSECTION	ECTOPIA LENTIS	SYSTEMIC ≥7 POINTS	*FBN1* MUTATION	DIAGNOSIS
WITHOUT FAMILY HISTORY				
+	+	– or +		MFS[†]
+			+	MFS
+	–	+	(unknown or neg)	MFS[†]
–	+		+	MFS
–	+			Ectopia Lentis syndrome
–	–	≥5		MASS
Mitral valve prolapse	–	<5		MVPS
WITH FAMILY HISTORY				
	+			MFS
		+		MFS[†]
+ (Z ≥2, if >20 yr) (Z ≥3, if <20 yr)				MFS[†]
SCORING SYSTEM FOR SYSTEMIC FEATURES[‡]				
Thumb AND Wrist Sign			3	
Thumb OR Wrist Sign			1	
Pectus Carinatum			2	
Pectus Excavatum or Chest Asymmetry			1	
Hindfoot Deformity			2	
Pes Planus			1	
Pneumothorax (History)			2	
Dural Ectasia			2	
Protrusio acetabuli			2	
Decreased US/LS ratio AND increased arm/height BUT NO SCOLIOSIS			1	
Scoliosis or Thoracolumbar kyphosis			1	
Reduced Elbow Extension			1	
Facial features (3 of 5)[§]			1	
Skin Striae			1	
Myopia >3 diopters			1	
Mitral valve prolapse			1	

Aortic root dilatation (measured at the Sinuses of Valsalva).
[†]*Loeys-Dietz syndrome (LDS), Shprintzen-Goldberg syndrome (SGS), and the vascular form of Ehlers Danlos (vEDS) should be excluded. If clinical features are suggestive, then DNA testing for* TGFBR1, TGFBR2 *(LDS),* COL3A1 *(vEDS) or collagen biochemistry should be done to help rule out these disorders.*
[‡]*Maximum Total: 20 points; more than 7 points indicates systemic involvement.*
[§]*Facial Features: Dolichocephaly, enophthalmos, downslanting palpebral fissures, malar hypoplasia, retrognathia.*
FBN1, Fibrillin-1; *MASS*, myopia, mitral valve prolapse, borderline aortic root dilatation (Z < 2), striae, skeletal findings; *MFS*, Marfan syndrome; *MVPS*, mitral valve prolapse syndrome; *US/LS*, upper segment/lower segment.
Data from Loeys BL, Dietz HC, Braverman AC, et al. The revised Ghent nosology for the Marfan syndrome. J Med Genet. *2010;47:476–485.*

X-Linked Recessive Inheritance

Most disorders involving the X chromosome show recessive inheritance. With only one copy of the X chromosome, males are more likely to manifest these diseases than females. Each son born to a female carrier of an X-linked recessive trait has a 50% chance of inheriting the trait, but none of this woman's daughters would be expected to be affected (each daughter has a 50% chance of being a carrier). An affected father transmits the mutation to all his daughters, who are carriers, but not to his sons; having received their father's Y chromosome, they would not be affected (thus there is no male-to-male transmission; Tables 47.6 and 47.7; Fig. 47.4).

Duchenne Muscular Dystrophy

See Chapter 182.

Hemophilia A

See Chapter 151.

TABLE 47.4 Autosomal Recessive Diseases

DISEASE	FREQUENCY	COMMENTS
Adrenal hyperplasia, congenital (CAH, 21-hydroxylase deficiency, CA21H, CYP21, cytochrome P450, subfamily XXI)	1:5,000	Phenotype variation corresponds roughly to allelic variation. A deficiency causes virilization in females. The gene is located at 6p21.3 within the human leukocyte antigen (HLA) complex and within 0.005 centimorgans (cM) of HLA B.
Phenylketonuria (PKU, phenylalanine hydroxylase deficiency, *PAH*)	1:12,000-1:17,000	There are hundreds of disease-causing mutations in the PAH gene located on chromosome 12q22–q24.1. The first population-based newborn screening was a test for PKU because the disease is treatable by diet. Women with elevated phenylalanine have infants with damage to the central nervous system because high phenylalanine is neurotoxic and teratogenic.
Cystic fibrosis (CF)	1:2,500 whites	The gene *CF transmembrane conductance regulator* (CFTR) is on chromosome 7q31.2.
Friedreich ataxia (FA, frataxin)	1:25,000	Frataxin is a mitochondrial protein involved with iron metabolism and respiration. The gene is on chromosome 9q13-q21, and the common mutation is a GAA expanded triplet repeat located in the first *intron* of the gene. FA does not show anticipation.
Gaucher disease, all types (glucocerebrosidase deficiency, acid β-glucosidase deficiency; a lysosomal storage disease)	1:2,500 Ashkenazi Jews	The gene is located on chromosome 1q21. There are many mutations; some mutations lead to neuropathic disease, but most are milder in expression. The phenotypes correspond to the genotypes, but the latter are difficult to analyze.
Sickle cell disease (hemoglobin beta locus, beta 6 glu → val mutation)	1:625 African Americans	This is the first condition with a defined molecular defect (1959). A single base change results in an amino acid substitution of valine for glutamic acid at position 6 of the beta chain of hemoglobin, with resulting hemolytic anemia. The gene is on chromosome 11p15.5. Penicillin prophylaxis reduces death from pneumococcal infections in affected persons, especially in infants.

TABLE 47.5 Rules of Autosomal Recessive Inheritance

Trait appears in siblings, not in their parents or their offspring
On average, 25% of siblings of the proband are affected (at the time of conception, each sibling has a 25% chance of being affected)
A *normal* sibling of an affected individual has a two-thirds chance of being a carrier (heterozygote)
Males and females are likely to be affected equally
Rare traits are likely to be associated with parental consanguinity
Traits generally involve mutations in genes that code for enzymes (e.g., phenylalanine hydroxylase–deficient in PKU) and are associated with serious illness and shortened life span

PKU, Phenylketonuria.

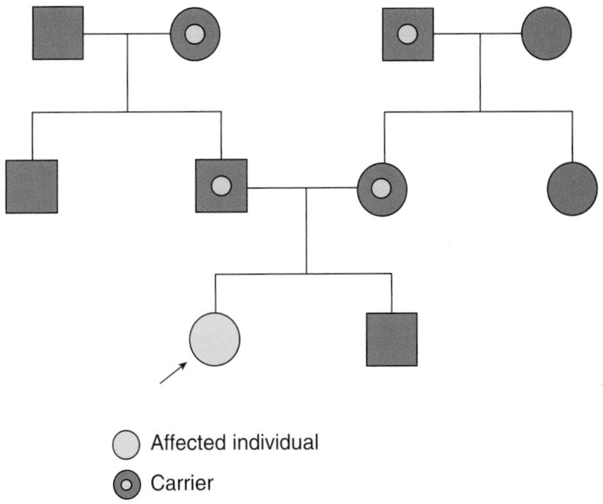

FIGURE 47.3 Pedigree of family showing autosomal recessive inheritance.

X-Linked Dominant Inheritance

Only a few examples of X-linked dominantly inherited disorders have been described. Both males and females are affected by this group of disorders, but females have less severe symptoms due to X-chromosome inactivation. This is the case for **X-linked vitamin D–resistant rickets** (hypophosphatemic rickets), a disorder in which the kidney's ability to reabsorb phosphate is impaired. Phosphate levels and resulting rickets are not as severe in females as in males.

Some X-linked dominant disorders are lethal in males, with death occurring before birth. Affected mothers can have affected or normal daughters but only normal sons. This is the case in **incontinentia pigmenti**, caused by a mutation in the *NEMO* or *IKBKG* gene, which has a characteristic swirling skin pattern of hyperpigmentation that develops after a perinatal skin rash with blistering. Affected females also have variable involvement of the central nervous system, hair, nails, teeth, and eyes. In **Rett syndrome**, caused by mutations in the *MECP2* gene, females are normal at birth but later in the first year of life develop microcephaly, developmental regression, and often a seizure disorder. Girls often are diagnosed with autism and, by 2 years of age, adopt a *handwashing* posture that causes them to lose all purposeful hand movements.

OTHER TYPES OF GENETIC DISORDERS

Multifactorial Disorders

Also known as **polygenic inheritance**, multifactorially inherited disorders result from the interplay of genetic and environmental factors. In addition to 20% of congenital malformations,

TABLE 47.6 X-Linked Recessive Diseases

DISEASE	FREQUENCY	COMMENTS
Fragile X syndrome (FRAX; numerous other names)	1:4,000 males	The gene is located at Xq27.3. The condition is attributable to a CGG triplet expansion that is associated with localized methylation (inactivation) of distal genes. Females may have some expression. Instability of the site may lead to tissue mosaicism; lymphocyte genotype and phenotype may not correlate.
Duchenne muscular dystrophy (DMD, pseudohypertrophic progressive MD, dystrophin, Becker variants)	1:4,000 males	The gene is located at Xp21. The gene is relatively large, with 79 exons, and mutations and deletions may occur anywhere. The gene product is called *dystrophin*. Dystrophin is absent in DMD but abnormal in Becker MD.
Hemophilia A (factor VIII deficiency, classic hemophilia)	1:5,000-1:10,000; males	The gene is located at Xq28. Factor VIII is essential for normal blood clotting. Phenotype depends on genotype and the presence of any residual factor VIII activity.
Color blindness (partial deutan series, green color blindness [75%]; partial protan series, red color blindness [25%])	1:12; males	The gene is located at Xq28 (proximal) for deutan color blindness and at Xq28 (distal) for protan color blindness.
Adrenoleukodystrophy (ALD, XL-ALD, Addison disease, and cerebral sclerosis)	Uncommon	The gene is located at Xq28. The disease involves a defect in peroxisome function relating to *very long-chain fatty acid CoA synthetase* with accumulation of C-26 fatty acids. Phenotype is variable, from rapid childhood progression to later onset and slow progression.
Glucose-6-phosphate dehydrogenase deficiency (G6PD)	1:10 African Americans 1:5 Kurdish Jews A heteromorphism in these and other populations	The gene is located at Xq28. There are numerous variants in which oxidants cause hemolysis. Variants can confer partial resistance to severe malaria.

TABLE 47.7 Rules of X-Linked Recessive Inheritance

Incidence of the trait is higher in males than in females
Trait is passed from carrier females, who may show mild expression of the gene, to half of their sons, who are more severely affected
Each son of a carrier female has a one in two chance of being affected
Trait is transmitted from affected males to all their daughters; it is never transmitted father to son
Because the trait can be passed through multiple carrier females, it may *skip* generations

including cleft lip and palate and spina bifida, most common disorders of childhood and adult life, such as asthma, atherosclerosis, diabetes, and cancer, result from an interaction between genes and the environment. Though these disorders do not follow simple mendelian modes of inheritance, affected individuals tend to cluster in families. The disorders occur more often in first- and second-degree relatives than would be expected by chance, and they are more likely to be concordant (although not 100%) in monozygotic twins than in dizygotic twins.

Hypertrophic Pyloric Stenosis

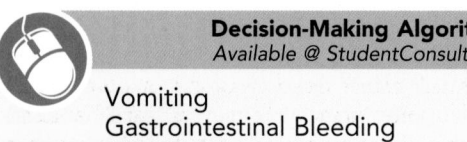

Decision-Making Algorithms
Available @ StudentConsult.com

Vomiting
Gastrointestinal Bleeding
Alkalemia

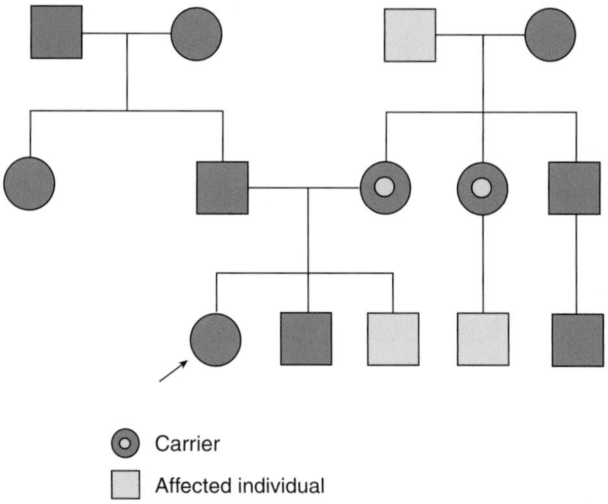

FIGURE 47.4 Pedigree showing X-linked recessive inheritance.

Occurring in about 1 in 300 children, hypertrophic pyloric stenosis (HPS) is five times more likely to occur in males than in females. When a child with HPS is born, the recurrence risk in future progeny is 5-10% for males and 1.5-2% for females. In adulthood, the risk of an affected male having an affected child is markedly increased over the general population; 4% of sons and 1% of daughters of such men would be likely to be affected. Even more striking is the risk to children born to affected females; 17-20% of sons and 7% of daughters are affected.

The thickness of the pyloric muscle may be distributed across a bell-shaped curve; the position on the bell-shaped curve is determined by many factors, including the expression of multiple, unknown genes. HPS may result when an individual's genetic and environmental influences cause him or her to fall to an extreme position on this curve, past a certain point called a **threshold**. In HPS this threshold is farther to the left for males than it is for females.

Neural Tube Defects, Including Myelomeningocele

Before 1998 myelomeningocele affected 1 in 1,000 liveborn infants in the United States. Anencephaly occurred with a similar frequency, although most anencephalic infants were either stillborn or died in the neonatal period. Since 1998, because of the supplementation of food staples with folic acid, the incidence of both conditions has decreased by 70%. Multiple genetic and nongenetic factors dictate the speed with which the neural tube closes, as follows:

1. The frequency of neural tube defects (NTDs) varies greatly in different ethnic groups. They are more common in the British Isles, where, in 1990, they occurred in 1 in 250 live births, and are far less common in Asia, where the frequency was 1 in 4,000. These ethnic differences suggest a **genetic** component.
2. Couples from the British Isles who move to the United States have a risk intermediate between the risks in the United Kingdom and the United States, suggesting an **environmental** component.
3. The occurrence of NTDs exhibits seasonality. In the United States affected infants are more likely to be born during late fall and early winter, again suggesting an **environmental** component or a folate responsive gene effect.
4. Periconceptual supplementation with folic acid has significantly lowered the risk of having an infant with an NTD. This nutritional influence suggests an **environmental** or gene modifying component.
5. Parents who have one child with an NTD are 20-40 times more likely to have a second affected child; this provides further evidence of a **genetic** component.

Disorders With Unusual Patterns of Inheritance

Mitochondrial Inheritance

Human cells contain nonnuclear DNA; a single chromosome is present in each mitochondrion, and mutations within this DNA are associated with a group of diseases.

Mitochondrial DNA (mtDNA), which is circular and 16.5 kb in length, replicate independently of nuclear DNA. Involved in energy production used to run the cell, mtDNA codes for a few respiratory chain proteins (most mitochondrial proteins are coded on **nuclear** DNA) and for a set of transfer RNAs unique to mitochondrial protein synthesis. Virtually all mitochondria are supplied by the oocyte, which means that mtDNA is maternally derived. A woman with a mutation in mtDNA passes this mutation to all her children. More than one population of mitochondria may be present in the oocyte, a phenomenon called **heteroplasmy**. The mtDNA mutation may be present in a few or many mitochondria. When the fertilized egg divides, mitochondria are distributed randomly. The presence of symptoms in the offspring, and their severity, depends on the ratio of mutant to wild-type mtDNA present in a particular tissue. If an abundance of mutant mitochondria exists in tissue that has high energy requirements (brain, muscle, and liver), clinical symptoms occur. If fewer mutant mitochondria are present, few clinical symptoms may be seen.

Mitochondrial encephalomyopathy with lactic acidosis and strokelike episodes (MELAS) is an example of a mitochondrial disorder. Normal in early childhood, individuals affected with MELAS develop episodic vomiting, seizures, and recurrent cerebral insults that resemble strokes between 5 and 10 years of age. In 80% of cases, analysis of the mtDNA reveals a specific mutation (A3242G) in *MTTL1,* a gene that codes for a mitochondrial transfer RNA.

In families in which MELAS occurs, a range of symptoms is seen in first-degree relatives, including **progressive external ophthalmoplegia**, hearing loss, cardiomyopathy, and diabetes mellitus. Although all offspring of a woman who carries a mutation would be affected, because of heteroplasmy the severity of disease varies depending on the percentage of mitochondria bearing the mutation that are present.

Uniparental Disomy

Evaluation of a child with uniparental disomy (UPD) reveals a normal karyotype. However, chromosomal markers for one particular chromosome are identical to the markers found on the chromosomes of the patient's mother or father (but not both as is normal). In UPD, the individual inherits two copies of one parent's chromosome and no copy from the other parent.

UPD probably occurs through a few mechanisms, but the most common results from a spontaneous *rescue* mechanism. At the time of conception, through nondisjunction, the fertilized egg is trisomic for a particular chromosome, with two copies of one parent's chromosome and one copy of the other parent's chromosome; conceptuses with trisomy often miscarry early in development. Fetuses with UPD survive because they spontaneously lose one of three copies of the affected chromosome. If the single chromosome from one parent is lost, the patient has UPD.

An alternate explanation involves monosomy for a chromosome rather than trisomy. Had the conceptus, at the time of conception, inherited only a single copy of a chromosome, spontaneous duplication of the single chromosome would lead to UPD.

Prader-Willi and Angelman Syndromes

Decision-Making Algorithms
Available @ StudentConsult.com

Hypotonia and Weakness
Short Stature
Pubertal Delay
Obesity
Polyuria

Prader-Willi syndrome (PWS), which occurs in 1 in 15,000 infants, is characterized by neonatal hypotonia; postnatal growth delay; a characteristic appearance, including almond-shaped eyes and small hands and feet; developmental disability; hypogonadotropic hypogonadism; and obesity after infancy. Early in life, affected infants are so hypotonic that they cannot consume enough calories to maintain their weight. Nasogastric feeding is invariably necessary, and failure to thrive is common. During the first year of life, muscle tone improves and children develop a voracious appetite with resulting obesity. Between 60% and 70% of individuals with PWS have a small deletion of chromosome 15 (15q11). In individuals without a deletion, 20% have UPD of chromosome 15.

Angelman syndrome (AS) is a condition with moderate to severe intellectual disability, absence of speech, ataxic movements of the arms and legs, a characteristic craniofacial appearance, and a seizure disorder that is characterized by inappropriate laughter. AS is also characterized by a deletion in the 15q11 region in 70% of affected individuals; UPD for chromosome 15 can be demonstrated in approximately 10% of AS patients.

If the deletion occurs in paternal chromosome 15, the affected individual will develop PWS, whereas AS results from a deletion occurring only in the maternal chromosome 15. When UPD is responsible, maternal UPD results in PWS, whereas paternal UPD results in AS. To summarize, if a copy of paternal chromosome 15q11.2 is lacking, PWS occurs; if maternal chromosome 15q11.2 is lacking, AS results.

This phenomenon is explained by **genomic imprinting**. Imprinting is an **epigenetic** phenomenon, a nonheritable change in the DNA that causes an alteration in gene expression based on parental origin of the gene. PWS is caused by deficiency of the protein product of the gene *SNRPN* (small nuclear ribonucleoprotein). Although present on both maternally and paternally derived chromosome 15, *SNRPN* is expressed only in the paternally derived chromosome. Expression is blocked in the maternal chromosome because the bases of the open reading frame are methylated; this physical change in the DNA prevents gene expression. PWS results whenever a paternal chromosome 15 is missing, either through deletion or through UPD.

AS results from a lack of expression of ubiquitin-protein ligase E3A *(UBE3A)*, a second gene in the chromosome 15q11.2 region. *UBE3A* is normally expressed only in the maternally derived chromosome 15. Although present in paternal chromosome 15, *UBE3A* is methylated, and gene expression is blocked. Therefore if either the critical region of maternal chromosome 15 is deleted, or paternal UPD occurs, the individual will manifest symptoms of AS.

Expansion of a Trinucleotide Repeat

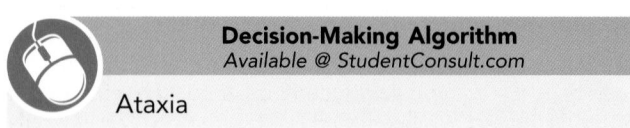

Decision-Making Algorithm
Available @ StudentConsult.com

Ataxia

More than 50% of human DNA appears as repeat sequences, two or three bases repeated over and over again. Disorders caused by expansion of trinucleotide repeats include **fragile X syndrome (FRAX)**, **Huntington disease**, **myotonic dystrophy**, **Friedreich ataxia**, and the **spinocerebellar ataxias**. Although an increase in the number of the three repeated bases is at the heart of each disorder, the molecular mechanism differs.

FRAX, which occurs with a frequency of approximately 1 in 2,000 children, is the most common cause of inherited intellectual disability. Features include characteristic craniofacial findings (large head; prominent forehead, jaw, and ears); macroorchidism with testicular volume twice normal in adulthood; a mild connective tissue disorder, including joint laxity, patulous eustachian tubes, and mitral valve prolapse; and a characteristic neurobehavioral profile, including intellectual disability (ranging from mild to profound) and autism spectrum disorders.

Positional cloning in the Xq27 region identified a triplet repeat region composed of one cytosine and two guanine residues (CGG). These repeats occur in the promoter region of the gene *FMR1*. Unaffected individuals who have no family history of FRAX have 0-45 CGG repeats (most have 25-35). In individuals with FRAX, the number of repeats is greater than 200; such people are said to have a *full mutation*. Between these two categories, a third group has 56-200 repeats; these individuals, known as **premutation carriers,** have typical development.

FRAX results from a failure to express FMRP, the protein product of the *FMR1* gene, which is expressed primarily in the central nervous system and testes during early embryonic development. Although FMRP is produced in unaffected individuals and premutation carriers, in those with the full mutation, FMRP transcription of the protein is blocked because the large number of CGG repeats become methylated (an epigenetic phenomenon). Thus FRAX occurs as a consequence of a **loss-of-function mutation**—the failure of expression of FMRP because of methylation of the promoter sequence.

In female premutation carriers, an expansion in the number of repeats from the premutation to the full mutation range may occur during gametogenesis. The cause of this expansion is not understood. Although premutation carriers do not show symptoms and signs of FRAX, women may manifest primary ovarian insufficiency and early menopause, and men and women may develop a movement disorder, known as fragile X tremor/ataxia syndrome later in life.

TERATOGENIC AGENTS

Approximately 6.5% of all birth defects are attributed to teratogens—chemical, physical, or biological agents that have the potential to damage embryonic tissue and result in congenital malformations. Agents known to be teratogenic include drugs (prescription and nonprescription); intrauterine infections (rubella); maternal diseases, such as diabetes mellitus; and environmental substances, such as alcohol and heavy metals. Knowledge of teratogenic agents and their effect on the developing fetus is important because limiting exposure to these agents is an effective way to prevent birth defects (see Chapter 59).

Maternal Infections

Rubella was the first maternal infection known to cause a pattern of malformations in fetuses affected in utero. Cytomegalovirus, *Toxoplasma gondii*, herpes simplex, Zika virus, and varicella are additional potentially teratogenic in utero infections (see Chapter 66).

Maternal Disease

Maternal diabetes mellitus and maternal phenylketonuria can result in congenital anomalies in the fetus. Strict control of these disorders before and during pregnancy protects the developing child (see Chapter 59).

Medications and Chemicals

Fetal alcohol spectrum disorder, which occurs in 10-20 per 1,000 children, may be the most common teratogenic syndrome.

Features include prenatal and postnatal growth deficiency, developmental disabilities, microcephaly, skeletal and cardiac anomalies, and a characteristic facial appearance. To cause the full-blown fetal alcohol syndrome, pregnant women must drink alcohol throughout the pregnancy. Lesser consumption during all or part of the gestation will lead to milder symptoms.

Warfarin, retinoic acid, and phenytoin are additional teratogenic agents (see Chapter 59).

Radiation

High-dose radiation exposure during pregnancy in Hiroshima and Nagasaki, Japan, was shown to increase the rate of spontaneous abortion and result in children born with microcephaly, mental retardation, and skeletal malformations. Estimates of exposure to cause these effects were approximately 25 rad. *The dose from routine radiological diagnostic examinations is in the millirad range.*

CHAPTER 48
Genetic Assessment

Individuals referred to a geneticist because of suspicion of a genetic disorder are called **probands**; individuals who come for genetic counseling are **consultands**. Referral for genetic evaluation may be made for a wide variety of reasons and at different stages of life (fetus, neonate, childhood, pregnancy, adulthood).

PRECONCEPTION AND PRENATAL COUNSELING

Familial Factors

Families with relatives affected with genetic disorders may have questions about how a disorder is inherited and whether their progeny may be at risk. The inheritance pattern and the risk of having an affected child can be discussed with a geneticist.

In some cultures, it is common, even desirable, for relatives to marry. This relatedness or **consanguinity** increases the likelihood that offspring may be born with a rare autosomal recessive (AR) condition, as both parents may be carriers of the same mutated gene. Generally, the closer the relation between the partners, the greater the chance that the couple shares one or more mutated genes in common, increasing the risk that offspring will have an AR disorder. The risk of first cousins having a child with an AR disorder is 1 in 64. In evaluating these couples, it is important to determine which ethnic group they belong to and to test for conditions commonly found in that group (see later).

Screening

It is common for couples to be screened for disorders that may occur more commonly in their particular ethnic group. People of Ashkenazi Jewish background may choose to be screened for heterozygosity for an expanding panel of AR disorders, including Tay-Sachs and Niemann-Pick diseases, Bloom and Gaucher syndromes, Canavan disease, cystic fibrosis, Fanconi anemia, and familial dysautonomia. People of African ancestry may choose to be screened for sickle cell disease. People whose ancestors originated in the Mediterranean basin may be screened for thalassemia.

Historically, prenatal screening has involved invasive and noninvasive testing. Invasive testing includes amniocentesis and chorionic villus sampling (CVS). Noninvasive testing includes sonography, which is utilized routinely throughout pregnancies, and the use of a series of biochemical markers present in the mother's blood. The first such marker identified was elevated maternal serum alpha-fetoprotein (MS AFP) and is now used to identify pregnancies in which the fetus was affected with neural tube defects, omphalocele, or gastroschisis. An additional association between low levels of MS AFP and fetal aneuploidy is known. Approximately 50% of fetuses with autosomal trisomies (Down syndrome, trisomy 18, trisomy 13) can be detected by low levels of MS AFP.

Additional proteins—unconjugated estriol (uE3), inhibin A, and human chorionic gonadotropin (HCG), each of which has been shown to be associated with varying risks of fetal aneuploidy—have been added to MS AFP to create a biochemical profile known as the **quad screen.** The addition of these compounds increased the detection rate to about 80%.

The quad screen is performed in the second trimester. During the first trimester, measurement of the fetal nuchal fold by sonogram can be used to identify risk for aneuploidy; increase in the nuchal thickness is a marker not only for fetal chromosomal anomalies, but for certain genetic and structural abnormalities as well. Once standardized, the detection rate for aneuploidy approached using this technique rose to 70%. The addition of testing for abnormalities in free β-HCG and PAPP-A (pregnancy associated plasma protein) has enhanced first trimester screening to a detection rate of almost 90%.

Although the risk of nondisjunction resulting in aneuploidy rises with maternal age, all pregnant women should be individually counseled as to their risk for aneuploidy and other fetal abnormalities. A combination of first and second trimester screening together with the women's age produces an individualized risk factor. **It is important to emphasize that both first and second trimester screening tests are just that—screening tests used to identify individuals who are at increased risk.** If the risk is high or if concerns exist about the presence of a fetal anomaly, a more definitive test, either CVS or amniocentesis, has been offered as further testing. Fetal cells are usually tested for chromosomal abnormalities by cytogenetic techniques, but the use of chromosomal microarray is becoming more common. Biochemical testing for a known family history of an inherited metabolic disorder and molecular screening for known familial mutations can also be performed on fetal cells.

Prenatal diagnosis using cell-free fetal DNA in maternal blood offers the ability to detect trisomies in fetuses using a maternal blood sample without an invasive test (amniocentesis, CVS). Noninvasive prenatal testing (NIPT) use has been increasing in popularity. Because of its low risk and high accuracy, it is expected that NIPT will eventually replace all other forms of prenatal genetic testing.

Maternal Factors

The presence of either acute or chronic maternal illness during pregnancy may lead to complications in the developing fetus.

Chronic conditions may expose the fetus to maternal medications that are potentially teratogenic. Acute illnesses, especially from the TORCH agents (toxoplasmosis, rubella, cytomegalovirus, herpes virus, and "other," including syphilis, varicella, and Zika virus), expose the fetus to infectious agents that may cause birth defects. Other factors, such as maternal smoking, alcohol use, and maternal exposure to radiation or chemicals, also may necessitate genetic counseling.

Postnatal—Newborn and Infant

Between 2% and 4% of newborns have a genetic abnormality or congenital malformation (see Chapter 47). The broad definition of malformations includes not only visible abnormalities but also functional defects that might not be apparent at birth.

Congenital malformations and genetic disorders have a significant impact on childhood morbidity and mortality. Almost 11% of childhood deaths can be traced to a genetic cause. If contributing genetic factors related to childhood deaths are considered, this increases to nearly 25%. Consultation with a geneticist for a newborn or infant may be prompted by many different findings, including the presence of a malformation, abnormal results on a routine newborn screening test, abnormalities in growth (e.g., failure to gain weight, increase in length, or abnormal head growth), developmental delay, blindness or deafness, and the knowledge of a family history of a genetic disorder or chromosomal abnormality or (as a result of prenatal testing) the presence of a genetic disorder or chromosomal abnormality in the infant.

Adolescent and Adult

Adolescents and adults may be seen by a geneticist for evaluation of a genetic disorder that has late onset. Some neurodegenerative disorders, such as Huntington disease and adult-onset spinal muscular atrophy, present later in life. Some forms of hereditary blindness (retinal degenerative diseases) and deafness (Usher syndrome, neurofibromatosis type 2) may not show significant symptoms until adolescence or early adulthood. Similarly, inherited cardiac disorders such as hypertrophic cardiomyopathy and long QT syndrome may not be identifiable until adulthood. Genetic consultation also may be prompted for a known family history of a **hereditary cancer syndrome** (breast, thyroid, colon, and ovarian cancers). Individuals may wish to have testing done to determine if they carry a mutation for these syndromes and would be at risk for developing certain types of cancers. A known family history or personal history of a genetic disorder or chromosomal abnormality might prompt testing in anticipation of pregnancy planning.

GENERAL APPROACH TO PATIENTS

Family History

A pedigree usually is drawn to help visualize various inheritance patterns. Answers to questions about the family help determine if there is an autosomal dominant (AD), AR, X-linked, or sporadic disorder segregating in the family. When a child is affected with the new onset of an AD disorder, it is necessary to closely examine the parents to check for the presence of manifestations. If the parents are unaffected, the child's condition is most likely the result of a new mutation, in which case, the risk of recurrence is extremely low (although not 0, because of the possibility of gonadal mosaicism in one of the parents). When one parent is affected (even mildly so, due to varying expressivity), the recurrence risk rises to 50% for each subsequent pregnancy. With X-linked disorders, the focus is on the maternal family history to determine if there is a significant enough risk to warrant testing.

Questions about the couple's age are important to ascertain the risk related to maternal age for chromosome abnormalities and paternal age for new mutations leading to AD and X-linked disorders. A history of more than two spontaneous abortions increases the risk that one of the parents carries a balanced translocation and the spontaneous abortions are due to chromosomal abnormalities in the fetus.

Pregnancy

During a genetic consultation, it is important to gather information about the pregnancy (see Chapters 58, 59, and 60). A maternal history of a chronic medical condition, such as a seizure disorder or diabetes, has known consequences in the fetus. Medication used in pregnancy can be teratogenic; the pregnant woman's exposure to toxic chemicals (work related) or use of alcohol, cigarettes, or drugs of abuse can have serious effects on the developing fetus. Maternal infection during pregnancy with TORCH agents (see earlier), among others, has been found to cause malformations in the fetus.

Information about the pregnancy may provide clues as to the health of the fetus. For more information about this, please see Chapter 50.

Follow-up is needed if prenatal testing revealed abnormal results.

Delivery and Birth

An infant born prematurely is likely to have more complications than a term infant. An infant can be small, appropriate, or large for his or her gestational age; each of these has implications for the child (see Chapters 58 and 60).

Medical History

Children with inborn errors of metabolism who have intermittent symptoms often have a history of multiple hospitalizations for dehydration or vomiting. Children with neuromuscular disorders may have a normal period followed by increasing weakness or ataxia. Children with lysosomal storage diseases, such as the mucopolysaccharidoses, often have recurrent ear infections and can develop sleep apnea.

Development

Many genetic disorders are associated with developmental disabilities. However, the onset of the disability may not always be present from the newborn period; many inborn errors of metabolism, including storage disorders, cause developmental manifestations after a period of normal development (see Chapters 7 and 8). Some adult-onset disorders have no symptoms until the teens or later. Assessing school problems is important. The type of learning problem, age at onset, and whether there is improvement with intervention or continued decline all are important for proper assessment.

Physical Examination

A careful and thorough physical examination is necessary for all patients with signs, symptoms, or suspicion of genetic disease. Sometimes subtle clues may lead to an unsuspected diagnosis. Features suggestive of a syndrome are discussed in more detail in Chapter 50.

Laboratory Evaluation

Chromosome Analysis

An individual's chromosome complement, known as the karyotype, can be analyzed using cells capable of dividing. In pediatrics, lymphocytes obtained from peripheral blood are the usual source for such cells, but cells obtained from bone marrow aspiration, skin biopsy (fibroblasts), or, prenatally, from amniotic fluid or chorionic villi also can be used. Cells are placed in culture medium and stimulated to grow using a mitogen; their division is arrested in either metaphase or prophase using a spindle poison; slides are made, the chromosomes are stained with Giemsa or other dyes, and the chromosomes are examined and analyzed under a microscope.

In metaphase, chromosomes are short, squat, and easy to count. Metaphase analysis should be ordered in children whose features suggest a known aneuploidy syndrome, such as a trisomy or monosomy. Chromosomes analyzed in prophase are long, thin, and drawn out; analysis gives far more details than are seen in metaphase preparations. Prophase analysis is ordered in individuals with multiple congenital anomalies without an obvious disorder.

Fluorescent In Situ Hybridization

Fluorescent in situ hybridization (FISH) allows the identification of the presence or absence of a specific region of DNA. A complementary DNA probe specific for the region in question is generated, and a fluorescent marker is attached. The probe is incubated with cells from the subject and viewed under a microscope. The bound probe fluoresces, allowing the number of copies of the DNA segment in question to be counted. This technique is useful in Prader-Willi syndrome and Angelman syndrome, in which a deletion in a segment of 15q11.2 occurs, in Williams syndrome, known to be associated with a deletion in 7q11.2, in velocardiofacial (DiGeorge) syndrome, which is associated with a deletion of 22q11.2, and in other disorders in which a small duplication or deletion is known to occur.

Microarray Comparative Genomic Hybridization

Microarray comparative genomic hybridization (array CGH) has essentially supplanted prophase analysis in cases in which a subtle copy number variant **(chromosomal deletion or duplication)** is suspected. DNA from the individual being studied and a normal control are labeled with fluorescent markers and hybridized to thousands of FISH-like probes for sequences spread around the genome. The probes are derived from known genes and noncoding regions. By analyzing the ratio of intensity of the fluorescent marker at each site, it is possible to determine whether the individual has any difference in copy number compared with the control DNA.

Direct DNA Analysis

Direct DNA analysis allows identification of mutations in a growing number of genetic disorders. Using polymerase chain reaction, the specific gene in question can be amplified and analyzed. The websites http://www.genetests.org and https://www.ncbi.nlm.nih.gov/gtr/ list disorders in which direct DNA analysis is available and identifies laboratories performing such testing.

Whole Exome Sequencing

Whole exome sequencing (WES) represents a major change in the approach to individuals with suspected genetic disorders. Rather than looking for mutations in a single gene or group of genes, as is done in direct DNA analysis, WES permits examination of all 20,000-21,000 genes that compose the genome. Using polymerase chain reaction and other techniques developed during the Human Genome Project, WES isolates DNA from an individual, looks for variations in the exomes or coding sequences of the genes, and compares identified variation with the DNA from the individual's parents. Variation found in the subject that is not present in either parent suggests a spontaneous mutation; two copies of a mutation in an individual whose parents are each found to be carriers of the mutation suggests that the subject is affected with an autosomal recessively inherited disorder.

Though there exist several shortcomings in WES (it is expensive, the interpretation is complicated as thousands of variations are often identified, the vast majority of which are benign), its benefit as a diagnostic tool is incredible. WES and the related whole genome sequencing will revolutionize the way clinical genetics, and in fact all of pediatrics, is practiced.

CHAPTER 49

Chromosomal Disorders

Errors that occur in meiosis during the production of gametes can lead to abnormalities of chromosome structure or number. Syndromes caused by chromosomal abnormalities include trisomy 21 (Down syndrome [DS]), trisomy 13, trisomy 18, Turner syndrome (TS), and Klinefelter syndrome (KS), as well as rarer chromosomal duplications, deletions, or inversions.

Chromosomal abnormalities occur in approximately 8% of fertilized ova but in only 0.6% of liveborn infants. Fifty percent of spontaneous abortuses have a chromosomal abnormality, the most common being 45,X (TS); an estimated 99% of 45,X fetuses are spontaneously aborted. The fetal loss rate for DS, the most viable of the autosomal aneuploidies, approaches 80%. Most other chromosomal abnormalities also adversely affect fetal viability. In newborns and older children, features that suggest the presence of a chromosome anomaly include low birth weight (small for gestational age), failure to thrive, developmental disability, and the presence of three or more congenital malformations.

ABNORMALITIES IN NUMBER (ANEUPLOIDY)

During meiosis or mitosis, failure of a chromosomal pair to separate properly results in nondisjunction. **Aneuploidy** is a change in the number of chromosomes that results from nondisjunction. A cell may have one **(monosomy)** or three **(trisomy)** copies of a particular chromosome.

Trisomies

Down Syndrome

Decision-Making Algorithms
Available @ StudentConsult.com

Stiff or Painful Neck
Hypotonia and Weakness
Pancytopenia

DS is the most common abnormality of chromosomal number in liveborn infants. It occurs in approximately 1 of every 800 births. Most cases (92.5%) are due to nondisjunction; in 68%, the nondisjunctional event occurs in maternal meiosis phase I. As a result of nondisjunction, the fertilized egg contains three copies of chromosome 21 (trisomy 21); using standard cytogenetic nomenclature, trisomy 21 is designated 47,XX,+21 or 47,XY,+21. In 4.5% of cases, the extra chromosome is part of a **robertsonian translocation**, which occurs when the long arms (q) of two acrocentric chromosomes (numbers 13, 14, 15, 21, or 22) fuse at the centromeres, and the short arms (p), containing copies of ribosomal RNA, are lost. The most common robertsonian translocation leading to DS involves chromosomes 14 and 21; standard nomenclature is 46,XX,t(14q21q) or 46,XY,t(14q21q). The parents of infants with DS who have translocations should have a karyotype to exclude a balanced translocation.

In 1-2% of children with DS, **mosaicism** occurs. These individuals have two populations of cells: one with trisomy 21 and one with a normal chromosome complement. Mosaicism results either from a nondisjunctional event that occurs sometime after fertilization or from **trisomic rescue**. The loss of this aneuploidy returns the cell to 46,XX or 46,XY. In either case the individual is referred to as a mosaic for these two populations of cells and is designated 47,XX, +21/46XX or 47,XY,+21/46,XY. Although it is widely believed that individuals with mosaic DS are more mildly affected, there are wide variations in clinical findings.

Children with DS are usually diagnosed in the newborn period. They tend to have normal birth weight and length, but they are hypotonic. The characteristic facial appearance, with brachycephaly, flattened occiput, hypoplastic midface, flattened nasal bridge, upslanting palpebral fissures, epicanthal folds, and large protruding tongue, is often apparent at birth. Infants also have short broad hands, often with a single transverse palmar crease, and a wide gap between the first and second toes. Hypotonia may cause feeding problems and decreased activity. Intellectual disability is noted in almost all patients with DS.

Almost half of all children with DS have **congenital heart disease**, including atrioventricular canal, ventriculoseptal or atrioseptal defects, and valvular disease. Between 5% and 10% of newborns with DS have **gastrointestinal tract anomalies**. The three most common defects are duodenal atresia, annular pancreas, and imperforate anus.

Four percent to 18% of infants with DS are found to have congenital hypothyroidism, which is identified as part of the newborn screening program. Acquired hypothyroidism is a more common problem. Thyroid function must be monitored periodically during the child's life.

Polycythemia at birth (hematocrit levels >70%) is common and may require treatment. Some infants with DS show a leukemoid reaction, with markedly elevated white blood cell counts. Although this resembles congenital leukemia, it is a self-limited condition, resolving on its own over the first month of life. Nonetheless, children with DS also have an increased risk of **leukemia**, with a 10- to 20-fold increase in risk compared with individuals without DS. In children with DS who are younger than 2 years of age, the type is generally acute megakaryoblastic leukemia; in individuals older than 3 years of age, the types of leukemia are similar to those of other children, with acute lymphoblastic leukemia being the predominant type.

Children with DS are more susceptible to infection, more likely to develop cataracts, and between 5% and 10% have atlantoaxial instability, an increased distance between the first and second cervical vertebrae that may predispose to spinal cord injury. Many individuals older than 35 years of age develop Alzheimer-like features.

The recurrence risk for parents who have had a child with DS depends on the child's cytogenetic findings. If the child has trisomy 21, the empiric recurrence risk is 1% (added to the age-specific risk for women up to 40 years of age; after 40, the age-specific risk alone is used for subsequent pregnancies). If the child has a robertsonian translocation, chromosomal analysis of both parents must be performed. In approximately 65% of cases, the translocation is found to have arisen de novo (i.e., spontaneously, with both parents having normal karyotypes), and in 35% of cases, one parent has a balanced translocation. The recurrence risk depends on which parent is the carrier: if the mother is the carrier, the risk is 10-15%; if the father is the carrier, the recurrence risk is 2-5%.

Trisomy 18

Trisomy 18 (47,XX,+18 or 47,XY,+18) is the second most common autosomal trisomy, occurring in approximately 1 in 7,500 live births. Virtually all cases of trisomy 18 are due to nondisjunction. More than 95% of conceptuses with trisomy 18 are lost as spontaneous abortuses in the first trimester; females are far more likely to survive to term than males; the ratio of male to female liveborns with trisomy 18 is 1 : 4. Infants with trisomy 18 rarely survive; fewer than 10% will reach their first birthdays. Most infants with trisomy 18 are small for gestational age. Clinical features include hypertonia, prominent occiput, micrognathia, low-set and malformed ears, short sternum, rocker-bottom feet, hypoplastic nails, and characteristic clenching of fists—the second and fifth digits overlap the third and fourth digits (Table 49.1).

Trisomy 13

The third of the common trisomies, trisomy 13 (47,XX,+13 or 47,XY,+13), occurs in 1 in 12,000 live births. As in trisomy 18, trisomy 13 is usually fatal in the first year of life, with only 8.6% of infants surviving beyond their first birthday.

As in DS, trisomy 13 can be caused by nondisjunction (seen in 75% of cases) or a robertsonian translocation (in 20%). The most common translocation involves chromosomes 13 and 14. Counseling regarding recurrence risk for future progeny is similar to that described above for trisomy 21.

Infants with trisomy 13 have numerous malformations (see Table 49.1). They are small for gestational age and microcephalic. Midline facial defects such as cyclopia (single orbit), cebocephaly (single nostril), and cleft lip and palate are common, as are midline central nervous system anomalies, such as alobar holoprosencephaly. The forehead is generally sloping, ears are often small and malformed, and microphthalmia or anophthalmia

TABLE 49.1 Possible Clinical Findings in Trisomy 13 and Trisomy 18

	TRISOMY 13	TRISOMY 18
Head and face	Scalp defects (e.g., cutis aplasia) Microphthalmia, corneal abnormalities Cleft lip and palate in 60-80% of cases Microcephaly Sloping forehead Holoprosencephaly (arrhinencephaly) Capillary hemangiomas Deafness	Small and premature appearance Tight palpebral fissures Narrow nose and hypoplastic nasal alae Narrow bifrontal diameter Prominent occiput Micrognathia Cleft lip or palate
Chest	Congenital heart disease (e.g., VSD, PDA, and ASD) in 80% of cases Thin posterior ribs (missing ribs)	Congenital heart disease (e.g., VSD, PDA, and ASD) Short sternum, small nipples
Extremities	Overlapping of fingers and toes (clinodactyly) Polydactyly Hypoplastic nails, hyperconvex nails	Limited hip abduction Clinodactyly and overlapping fingers; index over third, fifth over fourth Rocker-bottom feet Hypoplastic nails
General	Severe developmental delays and prenatal and postnatal growth retardation Renal abnormalities Nuclear projections in neutrophils Only 5% live >6 months	Severe developmental delays and prenatal and postnatal growth retardation Premature birth, polyhydramnios Inguinal or abdominal hernias Only 5% live >1 year

ASD, Atrial septal defect; *PDA*, patent ductus arteriosus; *VSD*, ventricular septal defect.

may occur. Postaxial polydactyly of the hands is common, as is clubfeet or rocker-bottom feet. Hypospadias and cryptorchidism are common in boys, whereas girls generally have hypoplasia of the labia minora. In addition, most infants with trisomy 13 have congenital heart disease. **Many infants with trisomy 13 have a punched-out scalp lesion over the occiput called aplasia cutis congenita;** when seen in conjunction with polydactyly and some or all the facial features, this finding is essentially pathognomonic for the diagnosis of trisomy 13.

Klinefelter Syndrome

Decision-Making Algorithms
Available @ StudentConsult.com

Short Stature
Pubertal Delay
Gynecomastia

Occurring in 1 in 1,000 births (1 in 500 males), KS is the most common genetic cause of hypogonadism and infertility in men. It is caused by the presence of an extra X chromosome (47,XXY). The extra chromosome arises from nondisjunction in either the sperm or egg. About 15% of boys with features of KS are found to be mosaic, with 46,XY/47,XXY mosaicism being the most common. Before puberty, boys with KS are phenotypically indistinguishable from the rest of the population.

The diagnosis is often made in adolescence when the hallmark of the condition, under androgenation in the presence of testes that remain infantile in volume, should alert the clinician. Young adults with KS tend to be tall with long limbs. During adolescence or adulthood, gynecomastia may occur.

Because of failure of growth and maturation of the testes, males with KS have hypergonadotropic hypogonadism and failure to produce viable sperm. Low production of testicular testosterone results in failure to develop later secondary sexual characteristics, such as facial hair, deepening of the voice, and libido. In adulthood, osteopenia and osteoporosis develop. Because of these findings, testosterone supplementation is indicated.

Most men with KS are infertile because they produce few viable sperm. Through the use of microdissection testicular sperm extraction, a technique in which viable sperm are isolated from testicular tissue, coupled with in vitro fertilization and intracytoplasmic sperm injection, it is possible for men with KS to father children; all children born to these men using this technology have had a normal chromosome complement.

Monosomies

Turner Syndrome

Decision-Making Algorithms
Available @ StudentConsult.com

Amenorrhea
Short Stature
Pubertal Delay
Obesity

TS is the only condition in which a monosomic conceptus survives to term; however, 99% of embryos with 45,X are spontaneously aborted. The most common aneuploidy found in conceptuses (accounting for 1.4%), 45,X is seen in 13% of first-trimester pregnancy losses. Occurring in 1 in 3,200 liveborn females, TS is notable for its relatively mild phenotype. Affected women tend to have typical intelligence and normal life expectancy.

Females with TS typically have a characteristic facial appearance with low-set, mildly malformed ears, triangular face, flattened nasal bridge, and epicanthal folds. There is webbing of the neck, with or without cystic hygroma, a shield-like chest with widened internipple distance, and puffiness of the hands and feet. Internal malformations may include congenital heart defect (in 45%; coarctation of the aorta is the most common anomaly, followed by bicuspid aortic valve; later in life, poststenotic aortic dilation with aneurysm may develop). Renal anomalies, including horseshoe kidney, are seen in more than 50% of patients. Short stature is a cardinal feature of this condition, and acquired hypothyroidism is estimated to occur five times more frequently in women with TS than in the general population.

The presence of streak gonads (gonadal dysgenesis) instead of well-developed ovaries leads to estrogen deficiency, which prevents these women from developing secondary sexual characteristics and results in amenorrhea. Although 10% of women with TS may have normal pubertal development and are even fertile, most affected women require estrogen replacement to complete secondary sexual development.

Infertility in these women is not corrected by estrogen replacement. Assisted reproductive technology using donor ova has permitted women with TS to bear children. During pregnancy, these women must be followed carefully because poststenotic dilatation of the aorta, leading to dissecting aneurysm, may occur.

Many girls with TS escape detection during the newborn period because phenotypic features are subtle. One third of girls with TS are diagnosed in the newborn period because of the presence of physical features; another 33% are diagnosed in childhood, often during a work-up for short stature (for which, they may receive growth hormone therapy); the final one third are diagnosed during adolescence or adulthood when they fail to develop secondary sexual characteristics or during work-ups for infertility.

The karyotypic spectrum in girls with TS is wide. Only 50% have a 45,X karyotype; 15% have an isochromosome Xq [46,X,i(Xq)], in which one X chromosome is represented by two copies of the long arm (leading to a trisomy of Xq and a monosomy of Xp); and approximately 25% are mosaic (45,X/46,XX or 45,X/46,XY). Deletions involving the short (p) arm of the X chromosome (Xp22) produce short stature and congenital malformations, whereas deletions of the long arm (Xq) cause gonadal dysgenesis.

Although monosomy X is caused by nondisjunction, TS is not associated with advanced maternal age. Rather, it is believed that the 45,X karyotype results from a loss of either an X or a Y chromosome after conception; that is, it is a postconceptual mitotic (rather than meiotic) nondisjunctional event.

SYNDROMES INVOLVING CHROMOSOMAL DELETIONS

Cri du Chat Syndrome

A deletion in the short arm of chromosome 5 is responsible for cri du chat syndrome, with its characteristic catlike cry during infancy, the result of tracheal hypoplasia. Other clinical features include low birth weight, postnatal failure to thrive, hypotonia, developmental disability, microcephaly, and craniofacial dysmorphism, including ocular hypertelorism, epicanthal folds, downward obliquity of the palpebral fissures, and low-set malformed ears. Clefts of the lip and palate, congenital heart disease, and other malformations may be seen.

The clinical severity of cri du chat syndrome depends on the size of the deletion, with larger deletions associated with more severe expression. Most cases arise de novo, with rare cases related to a balanced reciprocal chromosome translocation in a parent. When it arises de novo, the deletion is usually in the chromosome 5 inherited from the father.

Williams Syndrome

Decision-Making Algorithm
Available @ StudentConsult.com
Hypercalcemia

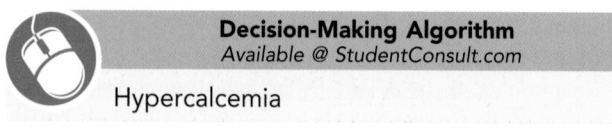

Caused by a 1.55 megabase deletion in chromosome 7q11.2 that contains at least 28 genes, Williams syndrome is associated with a unique phenotype. Features associated with the condition include congenital heart disease (in 80%), with supravalvar aortic and pulmonic stenosis being the most common anomalies; growth delay with short stature; a distinctive facial appearance, with median flare of the eyebrows, fullness of the perioral and periorbital region, blue irides with a stellate pattern of pigment, and depressed nasal bridge with anteversion of the nares; moderate intellectual disability (average IQ 57) with strengths in personal social skills and deficiencies in cognitive areas; and hypercalcemia (in ~20%).

Individuals with Williams syndrome often have a striking personality. Loquacious and gregarious, they are often described as having a *cocktail party* personality. However, at least 10% of children with Williams syndrome have features of autism spectrum disorder. Patients occasionally have unusual musical ability. Most children with Williams syndrome have a de novo deletion. In rare cases, the deletion is inherited from a parent in an autosomal dominant pattern.

Aniridia Wilms Tumor Association

WAGR syndrome (**W**ilms tumor, **a**niridia, **g**enitourinary anomalies, and mental **r**etardation) is caused by a deletion of 11p13. The deletion usually arises de novo, with rare cases being associated with a balanced translocation in one of the parents. Genitourinary abnormalities include cryptorchidism and hypospadias. Patients often have short stature, and 50% have microcephaly. Wilms tumor develops in 50% of patients with aniridia, genitourinary abnormalities, and mental retardation (see Chapter 159).

Prader-Willi Syndrome

See Chapter 47.

Angelman Syndrome

See Chapter 47.

Chromosome 22q11.2 Deletion Syndromes (22q11DS)

Decision-Making Algorithm
Available @ StudentConsult.com
Hypocalcemia

Deletions of chromosome 22q11.2 are responsible for a group of findings that have been called by several names, including **velocardiofacial syndrome**, **conotruncal anomaly face syndrome**, **Shprintzen syndrome**, and **DiGeorge syndrome**. These conditions represent a continuum of findings, and virtually all of which are due to the same chromosomal deletion.

Although 22q11DS can be inherited in an autosomal dominant fashion, most cases arise de novo. Common features include clefting of the palate with velopharyngeal insufficiency; conotruncal cardiac defects (including truncus arteriosus, ventriculoseptal defect, tetralogy of Fallot, and right-sided aortic arch); and a characteristic facial appearance, characterized by a prominent nose and broad nasal root. Speech and language difficulties are common, as is mild intellectual impairment. More than 200 additional abnormalities have been identified in individuals with these conditions. About 70% have immunodeficiency, largely related to T-cell dysfunction. A wide spectrum of psychiatric disturbances, including schizophrenia and bipolar disorder, has been seen in at least one third of affected adults.

Damage to the third and fourth pharyngeal pouches, embryonic structures that form parts of the cranial portion of the developing embryo, leads to abnormalities in the developing face (clefting of the palate, micrognathia), the thymus gland, the parathyroid glands, and the conotruncal region of the heart. This spectrum of findings, called the **DiGeorge malformation** sequence, is an important part of 22q11DS.

Confirmation of the deletion requires either fluorescence in situ hybridization (FISH) or chromosomal microarray analysis. The region, composed of about 3 million bases, contains between 30 and 40 genes. Although many of these deleted genes probably contribute to the phenotype, special attention has been focused on *TBX1* and *COMT*, which are believed to be responsible for many of the features of the condition.

SYNDROMES INVOLVING CHROMOSOME DUPLICATION

Duplications and deletions occur secondary to misalignment and unequal crossing over during meiosis. Small extra chromosomes are found in a small percentage of the population (0.06%). These "marker" chromosomes may be associated with intellectual disabilities and other abnormalities, but they often have no apparent phenotypic effects.

Inverted Duplication Chromosome 15

Chromosome 15 is the most common of all marker chromosomes, and its inverted duplication accounts for almost 40% of this group of chromosomal abnormalities. Features seen in children with 47,XX,+inv dup (15q) or 47,XY,inv dup(15q) depend on the size of the extra chromosomal material present: the larger the region, the worse the prognosis. Common features seen include varying degrees of developmental disability, autism spectrum disorders, seizures, and behavioral issues. Minimal dysmorphic features may be seen, including a sloping forehead, short and downward-slanting palpebral fissures, a prominent nose with a broad nasal bridge, a long and well-defined philtrum, a midline crease in the lower lip, and micrognathia.

Cat Eye Syndrome

Named for the iris coloboma that gives patients' eyes a catlike appearance, cat eye syndrome is caused by the presence of a small, extra chromosome composed of an inversion duplication of 22q11. The two copies of 22q11 on this extra chromosome plus the two normal copies of chromosome 22 result in four copies of this region. Although the colobomas name the syndrome, they occur in fewer than 50% of individuals with the marker chromosome. Other clinical features include mild intellectual disability, behavioral disturbances, ocular hypertelorism, downward-slanting palpebral fissures, micrognathia, auricular pits and/or tags, anal atresia with rectovestibular fistula, and renal agenesis.

CHAPTER 50

Approach to the Dysmorphic Child

Dysmorphology is the study of congenital malformation and the recognition of patterns of malformations that occur in syndromes (Table 50.1).

Syndromes are collections of abnormalities, including **malformations**, **deformations**, dysmorphic features, and abnormal behaviors that result from a unifying, identifiable etiology. This etiology may be the presence of a mutation in a

TABLE 50.1 Glossary of Selected Terms Used in Dysmorphology

TERMS PERTAINING TO THE FACE AND HEAD
Brachycephaly: Condition in which head shape is shortened from front to back along the sagittal plane; the skull is rounder than normal
Canthus: The lateral or medial angle of the eye formed by the junction of the upper and lower lids
Columella: The fleshy tissue of the nose that separates the nostrils
Glabella: Bony midline prominence of the brows
Nasal alae: The lateral flaring of the nostrils
Nasolabial fold: Groove that extends from the margin of the nasal alae to the lateral aspects of the lips
Ocular hypertelorism: Increased distance between the pupils of the two eyes
Palpebral fissure: The shape of the eyes based on the outline of the eyelids
Philtrum: The vertical groove in the midline of the face between the nose and the upper lip
Plagiocephaly: Condition in which head shape is asymmetric in the sagittal or coronal planes; can result from asymmetry in suture closure or from asymmetry of brain growth
Scaphocephaly: Condition in which the head is elongated from front to back in the sagittal plane; most normal skulls are scaphocephalic
Synophrys: Eyebrows that meet in the midline
Telecanthus: A wide space between the medial canthi
TERMS PERTAINING TO THE EXTREMITIES
Brachydactyly: Condition of having short digits
Camptodactyly: Condition in which a digit is bent or fixed in the direction of flexion (a "trigger finger"–type appearance)
Clinodactyly: Condition in which a digit is crooked and curves toward or away from adjacent digits
Hypoplastic nail: An unusually small nail on a digit
Melia: Suffix meaning "limb" (e.g., amelia—missing limb; brachymelia—short limb)
Polydactyly: The condition of having six or more digits on an extremity
Syndactyly: The condition of having two or more digits at least partially fused (can involve any degree of fusion, from webbing of skin to full bony fusion of adjacent digits)

single gene, as is the case in **Rett syndrome**, a disorder caused by a mutation in *MECP2,* a gene on Xq28; by the deletion or duplication of genetic material, as in **Prader-Willi syndrome**, caused by the deletion of the paternal copy of the *SNRPN* gene on chromosome 15q11.2; or by exposure to a teratogenic substance during embryonic development, as in fetal alcohol spectrum disorder.

DEFINITIONS

Congenital **malformations** are defined as clinically significant abnormalities in either form or function that are identifiable at birth. They result from localized **intrinsic** defects in morphogenesis, which were caused by an event that occurred in embryonic or early fetal life. This event may have been a disturbance of development from some unknown cause, but often mutations in developmental genes lead to the abnormality. **Extrinsic** factors may cause **disruptions** of development resulting from disturbances to the development of apparently normal tissues. These disruptions may include amniotic bands, disruption of blood supply to developing tissues, or exposure to teratogens. A **malformation sequence** is a spectrum of abnormalities, including malformations, deformations, and disruptions that result from the effects of a single malformation. For instance, in the **Pierre Robin sequence,** a primary malformation, the failure of growth of the mandible during the first weeks of gestation results in micrognathia, which forces the normal-sized tongue into an unusual position. The abnormally-positioned tongue blocks the fusion of the palatal shelves, which normally come together in the midline to produce the hard and soft palate; this leads to the presence of a U-shaped cleft palate. After delivery, the normal-sized tongue in the smaller-than-normal sized oral cavity leads to airway obstruction, a potentially life-threatening complication. So, the triad of features comprising the Pierre Robin sequence (micrognathia, U-shaped cleft palate, and obstructive apnea) all result from the failure of the jaw to grow at a critical time during gestation.

Malformation sequences can occur alone or may be part of a multiple malformation syndrome. For instance, individuals with Pierre Robin sequence may have it as part of **Stickler syndrome**, an autosomal dominant disorder caused by mutations in collagen genes. Stickler syndrome also manifests with ocular and musculoskeletal abnormalities.

Deformations arise as a result of environmental forces acting on normal structures. They occur later in pregnancy or after delivery. For instance, **plagiocephaly** (rhomboid shaped head) may result from intrauterine positioning or from torticollis experienced in the newborn period. Deformations often resolve with minimal intervention, but malformations often require surgical and medical management.

Minor malformations, variants of normal that occur in less than 3% of the population, include findings such as single transverse palmar creases, low-set ears, or ocular hypertelorism (wide-spaced eyes); when isolated, they have no clinical significance. A **multiple malformation syndrome** is the recognizable pattern of anomalies that results from a single identifiable underlying cause. It may involve a series of malformations, malformation sequences, and deformations. These syndromes often prompt a consultation with a clinical geneticist.

An **association** differs from a syndrome in that in the former, no single underlying etiology explains the recognizable pattern of anomalies that occur together more often than would be expected by chance alone. The **VACTERL** association (**v**ertebral anomalies, **a**nal atresia, **c**ardiac defects, **t**racheo**e**sophageal fistula, **r**enal anomalies, and **l**imb anomalies) is an example of a group of malformations that occur more commonly together than might be expected by chance. No single unifying etiology explains this condition, so it is considered an association.

In approximately 50% of children noted to have one or more congenital malformations, only a single malformation is identifiable; in the other 50%, multiple malformations are present. About 6% of infants with congenital malformations have chromosomal defects, 7.5% have a single gene disorder, 20% have conditions that are due to multifactorial effects (an interplay between genetic and environmental factors), and approximately 7% are due to exposure to a teratogen. In more than 50% of cases, no cause can be identified.

HISTORY AND PHYSICAL EXAMINATION

Pregnancy History

In attempting to solve the puzzle, the history of the pregnancy and birth can reveal multiple factors that may prove helpful to the dysmorphologist. Infants who are small for gestational age may have a chromosome anomaly or may have been exposed to a teratogen. Large for gestational age infants may be infants of diabetic mothers or have an overgrowth syndrome, such as Beckwith-Wiedemann syndrome. When evaluating an older child with intellectual disabilities, complications of extreme prematurity may account for the child's problems. Postmaturity also is associated with some chromosome anomalies (e.g., trisomy 18) and anencephaly. Infants born from breech presentation are more likely to have congenital malformations than those born from vertex.

As a woman gets older, there is increased risk of nondisjunction leading to trisomies. Advanced paternal age may be associated with the risk of a new mutation leading to an autosomal dominant trait. Maternal medical problems and exposures (medications, drugs, cigarette smoking, and alcohol use) are associated with malformations (see Chapters 48 and 59).

An increased amount of amniotic fluid may be associated with intestinal obstruction or a central nervous system anomaly that leads to poor swallowing. A decreased amount of fluid may be the result of a chronic amniotic fluid leak or point to a urinary tract abnormality that results in a failure to produce urine.

Family History

A pedigree comprising at least three generations should be constructed, searching for similar or dissimilar abnormalities in first- and second-degree relatives. A history of pregnancy or neonatal losses should be documented. For a more detailed discussion of pedigrees, see Chapter 47.

Physical Examination

When examining children with dysmorphic features, the following approach should be used.

Growth

The height (length), weight, and head circumference should be measured carefully and plotted on appropriate growth curves. Small size or growth restriction may be secondary to a chromosomal abnormality, skeletal dysplasia, or exposure to toxic or teratogenic agents. Larger than expected size suggests an **overgrowth syndrome** (Sotos or Beckwith-Wiedemann syndrome) or, in the newborn period, might suggest a diabetic mother.

The clinician should note if the child is proportionate. Limbs that are too short for the head and trunk imply the presence of a short-limbed bone dysplasia, such as achondroplasia. A trunk and head that are too short for the extremities suggest a disorder affecting the vertebrae, such as spondyloepiphyseal dysplasia.

Craniofacial

Decision-Making Algorithm
Available @ StudentConsult.com
Abnormal Head Size, Shape, and Fontanels

Careful examination of the head and face is crucial for the diagnosis of many congenital malformation syndromes. Head shape should be carefully assessed; if the head is not normal in size and shape (normocephalic), it may be long and thin **(dolichocephalic)**, short and wide **(brachycephalic)**, or asymmetrical or lopsided **(plagiocephalic)**.

Any asymmetry of facial features should be noted. Asymmetry may be due to a deformation related to intrauterine position or a malformation of one side of the face. The face should be divided into four regions, which are evaluated separately. The **forehead** may show overt prominence (achondroplasia) or deficiency (often described as a sloping appearance, which occurs in children with primary microcephaly). The **midface,** extending from the eyebrows to the upper lip and from the outer canthi of the eyes to the commissures of the mouth, is especially important. Careful assessment of the distance between the **eyes** (inner canthal distance) and the pupils (interpupillary distance) may confirm the impression of hypotelorism (eyes that are too close together), which suggests a defect in midline brain formation, or **hypertelorism** (eyes that are too far apart). The length of the palpebral fissure should be noted and may help define whether the opening for the eye is short, as is found with fetal alcohol syndrome, or excessively long, as in **Kabuki syndrome** (short stature, intellectual disability, long palpebral fissures with eversion of lateral portion of lower lid).

Other features of the eyes should be noted. The obliquity (slant) of the palpebral fissures may be upward (as seen with Down syndrome) or downward (as in Treacher Collins syndrome). The presence of epicanthal folds (Down syndrome and fetal alcohol syndrome) is also important. Features of the **nose**—especially the nasal bridge, which can be flattened in Down syndrome, fetal alcohol syndrome, and many other syndromes, or prominent as in velocardiofacial syndrome—should be noted.

The **malar** region of the face is examined next. It extends from the ear to the midface. The ears should be checked for size (measured and checked against appropriate growth charts), shape, position (low-set ears are below a line drawn from the outer canthus to the occiput), and orientation (posterior rotation is where the ear appears turned toward the rear of the head). Ears may be low set because they are small (or microtic) or because of a malformation of the mandibular region.

The **mandibular region** is the area from the lower portion of the ears bounded out to the chin by the mandible. In most newborns, the chin is often slightly retruded (that is, slightly behind the vertical line extending from the forehead to the philtrum). If this retrusion is pronounced, the child may have the Pierre Robin malformation sequence. In addition, the mouth should be examined. The number and appearance of the teeth should be noted, the tongue should be observed for abnormalities, and the palate and uvula checked for defects.

Neck

Examination of the neck may reveal webbing, a common feature in Turner syndrome and Noonan syndrome, or shortening, as is seen occasionally in some skeletal dysplasias and in conditions in which anomalies of the cervical spine occur, such as Klippel-Feil syndrome. The position of the posterior hairline also should be evaluated. The size of the thyroid gland should be assessed.

Trunk

The chest may be examined for shape (shield-like chest in Noonan syndrome and Turner syndrome) and for symmetry. The presence of a pectus deformity should be noted and is common in Marfan syndrome. The presence of scoliosis should be assessed; it is common in Marfan syndrome and many other syndromes.

Extremities

Many congenital malformation syndromes are associated with anomalies of the extremities. All joints should be examined for range of motion. The presence of single or multiple joint contractures suggests either intrinsic neuromuscular dysfunction, as in some forms of muscular dystrophy, or external deforming forces that limited motion of the joint in utero. Multiple contractures also are found with **arthrogryposis multiplex congenita** and are due to a variety of causes. **Radioulnar synostosis**, an inability to pronate or supinate the elbow, occurs in fetal alcohol spectrum disorder and in some X chromosome aneuploidy syndromes.

Examination of the hands is important. **Polydactyly** (the presence of extra digits) usually occurs as an isolated autosomal dominant trait but also can be seen in trisomy 13. **Oligodactyly** (a deficiency in the number of digits) is seen in Fanconi anemia (anemia, leukopenia, thrombocytopenia, and associated heart, renal, and limb anomalies—usually radial aplasia and thumb malformation or aplasia), in which it is generally part of a more severe limb reduction defect, or secondary to intrauterine amputation, which may occur with amniotic band disruption sequence. **Syndactyly** (a joining of two or more digits) is common to many syndromes, including Smith-Lemli-Opitz syndrome.

Dermatoglyphics include palmar crease patterns. A transverse palmar crease, indicative of hypotonia during early fetal life, is seen in approximately 50% of children with Down syndrome (and 10% of individuals in the general population). A characteristic palmar crease pattern is also seen in fetal alcohol spectrum disorder.

Genitalia

Decision-Making Algorithm
Available @ StudentConsult.com
Ambiguous Genitalia

Genitalia should be examined closely for abnormalities in structure. In boys, if the penis appears short, it should be measured and compared with known age-related data. Ambiguous genitalia often are associated with endocrinological disorders, such as congenital adrenal hyperplasia (girls have masculinized external genitalia, but male genitalia may be unaffected), or chromosomal disorders such as 45,X/46,XY mosaicism or possibly secondary to a multiple congenital anomaly syndrome (see Chapter 177). Although hypospadias, which occurs in 1 in 300 newborn boys, is a common congenital malformation that often occurs as an isolated defect, if it is associated with other anomalies, especially cryptorchidism, there is a strong possibility of a syndrome.

LABORATORY EVALUATION

Chromosome analysis should be ordered for children with multiple congenital anomalies, the involvement of one major organ system and the presence of multiple dysmorphic features, or the presence of mental retardation. **Microarray comparative genomic hybridization has supplanted routine or high-resolution chromosome analysis in most situations.** For a complete discussion of chromosome analysis, see Chapter 48.

Direct DNA analysis can be performed to identify specific mutations. It is necessary to use web-based resources to keep up to date. An extremely helpful website is http://www.genetests.org, which provides information about the availability of testing for specific conditions and identifies laboratories performing the testing.

Whole exome sequencing (WES) has begun to supplant direct DNA analysis for identification of mutations associated with an individual's specific phenotype. In this technique, analysis of all coding sequences (exomes) of all genes within the genome is performed. For a description of this technique, please see discussion in Chapter 48.

Radiological imaging plays an important role in the evaluation of children with dysmorphic features. Individuals found to have multiple external malformations should have a careful evaluation to search for the presence of internal malformations. Testing includes **ultrasound exams** of the head and abdomen to look for anomalies in the brain, kidney, bladder, liver, and spleen. **Skeletal radiographs** should be performed if there is concern about a possible skeletal dysplasia. The presence of a heart murmur should trigger a cardiology consultation; an **electrocardiogram** and **echocardiogram** may be indicated. **Magnetic resonance imaging** may be indicated in children with neurological abnormalities or a spinal defect. The presence of craniosynostosis may indicate a **computed tomography scan** of the head.

For those patients for whom testing does not yield a diagnosis, whole exome sequencing or whole genome sequencing is becoming a powerful tool.

DIAGNOSIS

Although the presence of characteristic findings may make the diagnosis of a multiple malformation syndrome straightforward, in most cases no specific diagnosis is immediately evident. Some constellations of findings are rare, and finding a "match" may prove difficult. In many cases, all laboratory tests are normal, and confirmation relies on subjective findings. Clinical geneticists have attempted to resolve this difficulty by developing scoring systems, cross-referenced tables of anomalies that help in the development of a differential diagnosis, and computerized diagnostic programs. An accurate diagnosis is important for the following reasons:

1. It offers an explanation to the family why their child was born with congenital anomalies. This may help allay guilt for parents, who often believe they are responsible for their child's problem.
2. With well-described natural histories of many disorders, a diagnosis allows anticipation of medical problems associated with a particular syndrome and appropriate screening. It also provides reassurance that other medical problems are no more likely to occur than they might with other children who do not have the diagnosis.
3. It permits genetic counseling to be done to identify the risk to future children and permits prenatal testing to be done for the disorders for which it is available.

Diagnosis enables the clinician to provide the family with educational materials about the diagnosis and facilitate contact with support groups for particular disorders. The Internet has become an important source for such information. Care should be exercised, as information on the Internet is not subject to editorial control and may be inaccurate. A good site is the National Organization for Rare Disorders (http://www.rarediseases.org), a clearinghouse for information about rare diseases and their support groups. Genetic testing information is available at the GeneTests website (http://www.genetests.org). This site provides information on available clinical and research testing for many diseases.

Suggested Readings

Brent RL. Environmental causes of human congenital malformations. *Pediatrics.* 2004;113:957–968.

Crissman BG, Worley G, Roizen N, et al. Current perspectives on Down syndrome: selected medical and social issues. *Am J Med Genet C Semin Med Genet.* 2006;142C:127–130.

Encode Project Consortium. An integrated encyclopedia of DNA elements in the human genome. *Nature.* 2012;489:57–74.

Hobbs CA, Cleves MA, Simmons CJ. Genetic epidemiology and congenital malformations: from the chromosome to the crib. *Arch Pediatr Adolesc Med.* 2002;156:315–320.

Holmes LB, Westgate MN. Inclusion and exclusion criteria for malformations in newborns exposed to potential teratogens. *Birth Defects Res A.* 2011;91:807–812.

Kliegman RM, Stanton B, St. Geme J, et al. *Nelson Textbook of Pediatrics.* 19th ed. Philadelphia: Saunders; 2016.

Online Mendelian Inheritance in Man (website). http://www.ncbi.nlm.nih.gov/sites/entrez?db=omim.

PEARLS FOR PRACTITIONERS

CHAPTER 47

Patterns of Inheritance

DNA Basics

- The four DNA nucleotides—adenine, guanine, thymine, and cytosine—are linked together to form a DNA strand.
- Two strands form a DNA molecule.
- Pyrimidines (thymine and cytosine) are cross linked to purines (adenosine and guanine) by hydrogen bonds.
- Chromosomes are strands of DNA wound tightly with a protein skeleton (chromatin) and histones.
- Human cells have 23 pairs of chromosomes, one set of 23 from each parent.
- Twenty-two of the chromosomes are autosomes, and the 23rd pair are the sex chromosomes. Females have two X chromosomes (46,XX), and males have a Y chromosome (46,XY).
- Genes are stretches of DNA that code for a protein. A typical gene has a promoter sequence, an untranslated region, and an open reading frame.
- Every three nucleotides represent a single codon that codes for a particular amino acid.
- Some codons act as a start signal and others as a stop signal for transcription.
- Within the gene there are regions—exons—that code for the sequence of the protein, and introns, which are not incorporated into the transcribed messenger RNA (mRNA).
- Less than 2% of the 3.1 million DNA bases code for proteins. These regions represent about 21,000 genes. Alternative splicing of the transcribed mRNA can generate a possible 100,000 proteins.
- Changes in the DNA sequence can lead to changes in the amino acid in a protein (missense mutations) or to a premature stop codon (nonsense mutation).
- A third change in the DNA is frameshift mutation, which is the result of the addition or deletion of one or more DNA bases that "shifts" the reading from of the codons usually resulting in production of a new stop codon that is before the end of the gene and is considered "premature."

Pedigrees

- Pedigrees are symbolic depictions of a family's history with symbols for males (squares) and females (circles).
- Pedigrees permit a quick visual determination of an inheritance pattern in a family.

Autosomal Dominant Disorders

- A single copy of a mutation not on a sex chromosome that results in disease.
- Affected parents have a 50% chance of passing mutation on to each child.
- The phenomenon where some patients with the mutation show clinical symptoms and others may not is called penetrance. Many autosomal dominant (AD) disorders can show decreased penetrance.
- Variable expressivity describes the phenomenon where different family members may vary in the severity of clinical symptoms and which clinical symptoms are manifest.
- Often, patients with an AD disorder may be new mutations (they have unaffected parents).

Autosomal Recessive Disorders

- Both copies of gene on a non-sex chromosome have a mutation.
- Affected patients usually have unaffected parents, each of whom is a carrier for the disorder.

X-linked Disorders (General)

- Females have two copies of the X-chromosome; males have one X-Chromosome and a Y chromosome.
- The X-chromosome has approximately 2,000 genes, the Y about 200.
- Females randomly inactivate one of their X-chromosomes (Lyonization).

X-linked Recessive Inheritance

- Most X chromosome disorders show recessive inheritance.
- Males, having one X-chromosome, are more likely to manifest disease than females.
- Sons of carrier females have a 50% chance of being affected; daughters have a 50% chance of being a carrier.
- Daughters of affected males have a 50% chance of being a carrier; all sons are unaffected.

X-linked Dominant

- Females with these disorders show symptoms.
- Females are usually less affected than males due to X-chromosome inactivation.
- Some X-linked dominant disorders are lethal in males with death before birth.

Mitochondrial Inheritance

- Mitochondrial DNA (mtDNA) replicates independently from nuclear DNA.
- Virtually all mitochondria are supplied by the oocyte.
- mtDNA has a few genes that code for respiratory complex proteins (most are coded on the nuclear DNA) and a set of tRNAs that are needed for protein synthesis within the mitochondria.
- Disorders involving the mtDNA are maternally inherited.
- There are many mitochondria in each cell. If the DNA is different in some of these mitochondria (two populations), this is referred to as **heteroplasmy**.
- There are some disorders due to loss or deficiency of mitochondria. This is referred to as **mitochondrial depletion.**

Uniparental Disomy

- Patients with **Uniparental Disomy** have a normal karyotype with a normal number of chromosomes.
- The affected chromosome will be identical—two copies of one parent's chromosome—without a copy from the other parent.
- Some genes are methylated ("inactivated") depending on their parental origin. Having uniparental disomy might result in both copies of the gene being inactivated.

Multifactorial Inheritance

- Result from the interplay of genetic and environmental factors.
- About 20% of congenital malformations are due to multifactorial inheritance.

- Disorders such as asthma, atherosclerosis, diabetes, and cancer.
- Do not follow mendelian rules of inheritance, but are more likely to occur in first and second degree relatives more frequently than would be expected by chance and are more likely to be concordant in monozygotic twins than dizygotic twins.

Nucleotide Repeats

- Much of human DNA consists of two or three DNA bases repeated over and over.
- Some disorders are due to expansion of trinucleotide repeats (fragile-X, Huntington disease, myotonic dystrophy, Friedreich ataxia, and the spinocerebellar ataxias).

Exposure to Teratogenic Agents

- Approximately 6.5% of birth defects can be attributed to exposure to teratogens.
- Teratogens can be chemical, physical, or biological.
- Examples include alcohol, infections, and lead.

CHAPTER 48

Genetic Assessment

- Individuals referred to a geneticist because of suspicion of a genetic disease are called **probands.**
- **Consultands** are individuals referred for genetic counseling.
- There are many reasons for referral to genetics. Referral may occur at different stages of life (fetus, neonate, childhood, pregnancy, or adulthood).

Preconception and Prenatal Counseling

- Families with relatives affected with a genetic disorder may wonder if their children are at risk.
- A family history may uncover a pattern of inheritance. A known disorder will have a pattern of inheritance that can be discussed with a geneticist or genetic counselor.
- **Consanguinity** is when couples are related. This increases the likelihood that offspring could be born with a rare autosomal recessive condition.
- Couples may be screened for disorders that affect their particular ethnic group (African ancestry may suggest screening for sickle cell, Mediterranean ancestry screening for thalassemia, Ashkenazi Jewish ancestry screening for Tay-Sachs, Gaucher).
- Next generation sequencing has made screening for whole panels of genes relatively inexpensive.

Prenatal Screening and Prenatal Testing

- Screening helps identify an increased risk for an abnormality.
- Many pregnant women are screened to see if they are carriers for sickle cell disease, cystic fibrosis, and increasingly, spinal muscular atrophy (SMA).
- First trimester screening—a maternal blood test to measure PAPP-A (pregnancy associated plasma protein-A) and human chorionic gonadotropin (hCG) together with measurement of the fetus' nuchal (neck) fold by ultrasound—can be used to assess risk for chromosomal abnormality (Down syndrome) and possible cardiac abnormalities.
- Second trimester maternal serum screening (Quad Screen) measures AFP (alpha fetoprotein), uE3 (unconjugated estriol), inhibin A, and hCG.
- Abnormal first and second trimester screening reveals and increased risk. Diagnostic testing on cells from an amniocentesis may be suggested as follow up.
- If the parents are found to be carriers of a recessive disease, testing of the amniocytes can determine if the fetus is affected.
- The use of cell free fetal DNA (cfDNA) from a maternal blood sample is quickly replacing other screening tests for chromosomal aneuploidy.
- Confirmation of noninvasive prenatal screening (NIPS) with cfDNA from a maternal blood sample requires confirmation by amniocentesis.
- Screening for fetal malformations by ultrasound is performed in the second trimester.

Postnatal—Newborn and Infant

- Two percent to 4% of newborns may have a genetic abnormality or "birth defect."
- This includes malformations (2-3%), inherited disorders (1%), and chromosomal abnormalities (0.5%).
- Consultation with a geneticist may be prompted by the presence of a malformation, abnormal newborn screening results, abnormalities of growth (poor weight gain, poor linear growth, poor head growth), developmental delay, blindness or deafness, or a family history of a genetic disorder.

Adolescent and Adult

- Adolescent and adults may be referred for evaluation of a later onset genetic disorder. Many neurodegenerative disorders have onset later in life (e.g., Huntington disease, spinocerebellar ataxia, and spinal muscular atrophy).
- A family history of a hereditary cancer (breast, colon, thyroid) may also prompt an evaluation by a geneticist.

General Approach to Patients

- Family History
  - Pedigree is drawn to look for a pattern of inheritance.
  - If there is suspected new onset of an autosomal disorder, examine the parents carefully for signs of the disorder.
  - If a new mutation, recurrence risk is about 1% due to gonadal mosaicism.
  - If one of the parents is even mildly affected, the recurrence risk is 50%.
  - For prenatal counseling, the age of the couple is important.
    - Increased paternal age has an increased risk for AD and X-linked disorders.
    - Increased maternal age has an increased risk for chromosomal disorders.
- Pregnancy History
  - Exposure to teratogens (medications, alcohol, infections) can lead to malformations.
  - Poor fetal movement may suggest neurological abnormalities.
  - A history of low or absent amniotic fluid (oligohydramnios) or high levels of amniotic fluid (polyhydramnios) may suggest neurological, pulmonary, or renal problems for the infant.
- Birth History
  - Premature infants have more complications than term infants.
  - The size of the infant—small for gestational age, or large for gestational age has implications for different genetic disorders.

- Underlying disorders may predispose to difficult a delivery.
- Resuscitation in the delivery room has implications for growth and development.
- Medical History
  - Children with recurrent hospitalizations for vomiting and dehydration may suggest an inborn error of metabolism.
  - Children with neuromuscular disorders may have a normal period followed by increasing weakness or ataxia.
  - Children with lysosomal storage disorders will have worsening symptoms with increasing age, often having a history of frequent otitis media and may develop sleep apnea.
  - Evaluation of growth may reveal poor prenatal and postnatal growth, good prenatal and poor postnatal, or acquired microcephaly or macrocephaly, all of which suggest different underlying genetic disorders.
- Development
  - Many genetic disorders are associated with delays in development.
  - Sometimes development is normal for a period of time, then slows, and is then followed by regression that can suggest a lysosomal storage disorder.
- Physical Exam
  - A careful physical exam is necessary for all patients with signs, symptoms, or suspicion of genetic disease.
  - Anomalous (dysmorphic) features may suggest an underlying genetic syndrome.

Laboratory Evaluation

- Chromosome Analysis
  - Routine chromosome analysis during prophase was the standard way of analyzing chromosome number and large chromosome aberrations.
  - It remains the only way to identify balanced chromosome rearrangements.
  - Chromosomal microarray (array CGH) has supplanted routine cytogenetic techniques for chromosome analysis.
  - Fluorescence in situ hybridization (FISH) uses small DNA probes to identify copy number of common chromosome deletions. It is also helpful to determine complex chromosomal rearrangements.
- Direct DNA Analysis
  - Sequencing of genes involved in many genetic disorders is now often possible. Several websites offer assistance to find labs that can do specific gene tests.
- Whole Exome Sequencing
  - Next generation sequencing has enabled the sequencing of a patient's exome relatively inexpensively.
  - Helps identify potential cause for undiagnosed genetic disorders.
  - Analysis and interpretation is complex.

CHAPTER 49

Chromosomal Disorders

- Errors in meiosis lead to abnormalities of chromosome structure or number (aneuploidy).
- Common syndromes caused by abnormalities of chromosome number include the following:
  - Down syndrome, Trisomy 13, Trisomy 18, Turner syndrome, Klinefelter syndrome.

Down Syndrome

- Most common chromosome abnormality in liveborn infants.
- About 92.5% are due to nondisjunction, 4.5% are due to Robertsonian translocations—a fusion of two acrocentric chromosomes (most commonly chromosomes 21 and 14).
- Characteristic facial features, hypotonia, and congenital heart disease (40%) are noted in the neonatal period.

Trisomy 18

- Second most common autosomal trisomy.
- Most trisomy 18 conceptions end in spontaneous abortion.
- 10% of those born will survive to 1 year of age.

Trisomy 13

- Usually fatal in the first year of life (less than 10% survive)
- Small for gestational age, midline facial defects, postaxial polydactyly, clubfeet, scalp lesions (cutis aplasia).

Klinefelter

- 1:500 males.
- Most common cause of infertility in men.
- Hypogonadism results in lack of secondary sexual characteristics.

Turner Syndrome

- Turner syndrome is the only monosomy that survives to term.
- Most common chromosomal abnormality in conceptuses.
- Somewhat characteristic facial features, with webbed neck, shield-like chest, and short stature.
- Coarctation of the aorta, horseshoe kidney, hypothyroidism, and infertility.

Cri du chat

- Due to the partial deletion of the short arm of chromosome 5.
- Larger deletions are more severe.
- "Cat-like" cry.

Williams Syndrome

- Deletion of 7q11.2.
- Supravalvar aortic stenosis.
- Distinctive facial appearance, moderate intellectual disability, verbal skills above their deficiencies in other areas.

22q Del Syndrome (DiGeorge, Velocardiofacial Syndrome)

- Cleft palate, velopharyngeal insufficiency.
- Conotruncal cardiac defects (truncus arteriosus, ventricular septal defect [VSD], tetralogy of Fallot).

CHAPTER 50

Approach to the Dysmorphic Child

- Dysmorphology is the study of congenital malformations and the patterns of malformations that occur in syndromes.
- Syndromes are collections of abnormalities (malformations, deformations, dysmorphic features, and abnormal behaviors) that are associated with an identifiable etiology.
- Syndromes may be due to a mutation, a deletion or duplication of a chromosome, or by exposure to a teratogen.

- Congenital **malformations** that are the result of intrinsic defects in morphogenesis are identifiable at birth.
- **Deformations** are due to environmental forces acting on normal structures.
- An **Association** is a pattern of anomalies with no clear underlying etiology that occurs more frequently than by chance alone.

History and Physical Examination

Elements of the history and physical often provide information that leads to a diagnosis.

- Pregnancy
  - Growth of fetus (small or large for gestational age), premature or postmature, fetal movement, amount of amniotic fluid (oligohydramnios or polyhydramnios), exposure to drug, and environmental toxins, maternal age.
- Family History
  - Important clues about a pattern of inheritance can be determined from the family history.
- Physical Exam
  - Growth
    - Height, weight, and head circumference should be plotted on age appropriate growth curves.
    - Is the child small or large? Is the child proportional?
  - Craniofacial
    - Assess head shape, asymmetry.
    - Face can be divided into four regions (forehead, midface, malar, and mandibular), each which requires close examination.
  - Neck
    - Length, webbing, posterior hairline, thyroid gland should be assessed.
  - Trunk
    - Chest shape—shield like, pectus deformity.
    - Scoliosis.
  - Extremities
    - Joints should be assessed for range of motion, contractures.
    - Number of fingers and toes, their size, and shape (polydactyly, oligodactyly, syndactyly).
  - Genitalia
    - Normal male or female, ambiguous.
    - Size, presence of testicles in males, and their size.

Laboratory Evaluation

- Chromosome Analysis
  - Today this is usually by chromosomal microarray.
- DNA Analysis (Sequencing)
  - For individual genes or sometimes panels of genes related to a family of disorders.
- Whole Exome Sequencing
  - Useful for undiagnosed disorders.
- Radiological Imaging
  - Individuals with external malformations need a careful evaluation for internal malformations.
  - Ultrasound (head in neonates, abdomen, kidneys).
  - Skeletal radiographs for possible skeletal dysplasias, lysosomal storage disorders.
  - MRI for children with possible neurological abnormalities or spinal defects.
  - CT of the skull for craniofacial abnormalities.

A genetic diagnosis is important for the following reasons:

- Allays guilt of parents.
- Diagnosis with a particular disorder may permit screening for medical problems.
- May permit treatment for disorder.
- Permits genetic counseling for future pregnancies.

SECTION 10

METABOLIC DISORDERS

David Dimmock

CHAPTER 51

Metabolic Assessment

Optimal outcomes for children with inborn errors of metabolism (IEMs) depend upon recognition of the signs and symptoms of metabolic disease and prompt evaluation and referral to a center familiar with their management. Delay in diagnosis may result in end-organ damage including progressive neurological injury or death.

With the exception of phenylketonuria (PKU), and medium-chain acyl-CoA dehydrogenase (MCAD) deficiency, most metabolic disorders are individually rare, having an incidence of less than 1 per 100,000 births in the United States. When considered collectively, the incidence may approach 1 in 800 to 2,500 births (Table 51.1) with the prevalence of a confirmed metabolic disorder detected by newborn screening in 1 in 4,000 live births (about 12,500 diagnoses each year) in the United States. This is comparable with the 1 in 1,000 infants who have early-onset bacterial sepsis and the 1 in 3,000 infants who have invasive group B streptococcal infections.

IEMs are frequent causes of sepsis-like presentations, intellectual disability, seizures, sudden infant death, and neurological impairment. Indeed there are 89 identified IEMs that are amenable to therapy targeted to the underlying cause, which present with intellectual disability as a prominent feature.

Single gene disorders are estimated to account for up to 35% of neonatal intensive care unit (NICU) admissions and 20% of general admissions to a regional children's hospital. Congenital anomalies and single gene disorders are the leading cause of death in the NICU and pediatric intensive care unit (PICU).

Metabolic disorders can be classified using a variety of schemes based on the clinical presentation, including the age of onset, the tissues or organ systems involved, the defective metabolic pathways, or the subcellular localization of the underlying defect. These classification schemes have differing utility when considering approach to diagnosis, management, and screening strategies. The clinical presentation and long-term prognosis have the most bearing on management of children with genetic metabolic disorders.

Genetic metabolic disorders result from the deficiency of an enzyme, its cofactors, or biochemical transporters that lead to the deficiency of a required metabolite, the buildup of a toxic compound, or a combination of both processes (Fig. 51.1, Table 51.2). Understanding which of these mechanisms is involved and if the effects are systemic or restricted to the local tissue enables a rational approach to diagnosis, therapy, and management.

SIGNS AND SYMPTOMS

Decision-Making Algorithms
Available @ StudentConsult.com

Seizures and Other Paroxysmal Disorders
Altered Mental Status
Irritable Infant

The signs and symptoms of an inborn error are diverse and can involve any organ system. The presentation varies among age groups. IEMs often present a few hours to weeks after birth, often mimicking late-onset sepsis. Infants who survive the neonatal period without developing recognized symptoms often experience intermittent illness separated by periods of being well. While pursuing the evaluation of the specific clinical presentations (e.g., the approach to the sick newborn, irritable child, or child with liver dysfunction), the hypoglycemic and intoxicating (encephalopathy) metabolic disorders should be considered in all neonates presenting with lethargy, poor tone, poor feeding, hypothermia, irritability, or seizures. In most cases these should be evaluated by assessment of plasma ammonia, blood glucose, and anion gap (Fig. 51.2). Significant ketosis in the neonate is unusual and suggests an organic acid disorder. Similarly, specific metabolic disorders predispose to cardiomyopathy, myopathy, hepatopathy, developmental delay, sepsis, and developmental regression; appropriate evaluation should be tailored to the clinical presentation.

Introduction of new foods or metabolic stress associated with fasting or fever may unmask an inborn error of metabolism during infancy or in older children. The introduction of fructose or sucrose in the diet may lead to decompensation in hereditary fructose intolerance. In older children, increased protein intake may unmask disorders of ammonia detoxification.

TYPES OF CLINICAL PRESENTATION OF INBORN ERRORS

Toxic Presentation

Decision-Making Algorithms
Available @ StudentConsult.com

Vomiting
Altered Mental Status
Acidemia

TABLE 51.1 Estimates of Incidence of Various Classes of Disorders Diagnosed or Followed at Specialized Clinics per 100,000 Population*

	BRITISH COLUMBIA 1969–1996	WEST MIDLANDS 1999–2003
Amino acid disorders (excluding phenylketonuria)	7.5	19
Lysosomal storage diseases	7.5	19
Phenylketonuria	7.5	8
Organic acidemias	4	12.5
Peroxisomal disorders	3.5	7.5
Mitochondrial diseases	3	20
Glycogen storage diseases	2	7
Urea cycle diseases	2	4.5

Populations in British Columbia, Canada (a predominantly white population), between 1969 and 1996, and in the West Midlands of the United Kingdom (which has a diverse ethnic breakdown) between 1999 and 2003.

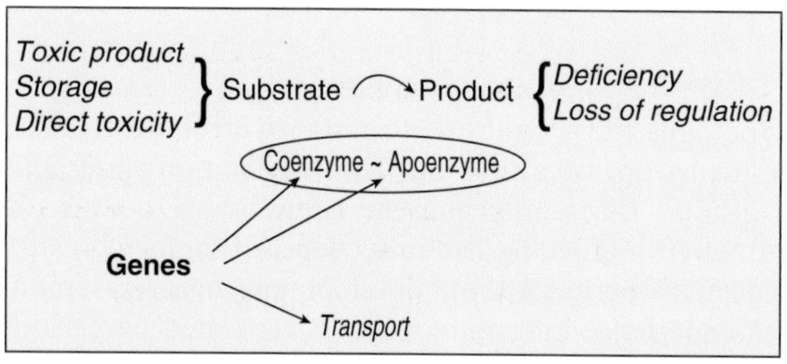

FIGURE 51.1 Depiction of the basic paradigm in inherited disorders of metabolism. Deficiency of an enzyme complex results in accumulation of metabolites proximal to the blocked metabolism and deficiency of the product of the reaction. Sites of genetic control are indicated.

The toxic presentation often presents as an **encephalopathy.** Fever, infection, fasting, or other catabolic stresses may precipitate the symptom complex. A **metabolic acidosis**, vomiting, lethargy, and other neurological findings may be present. Diagnostic testing is most effective when metabolites are present in highest concentration in blood and urine at presentation. Abnormal metabolism of amino acids, organic acids, ammonia, or carbohydrates may be at fault. **Hyperammonemia** is an important diagnostic possibility if an infant or child presents with features of toxic encephalopathy (see Fig. 51.2). Symptoms and signs depend on the underlying cause of the hyperammonemia, the age at which it develops, and its degree. The severity of hyperammonemia may provide a clue to the etiology (Tables 51.3 and 51.4).

Severe Neonatal Hyperammonemia

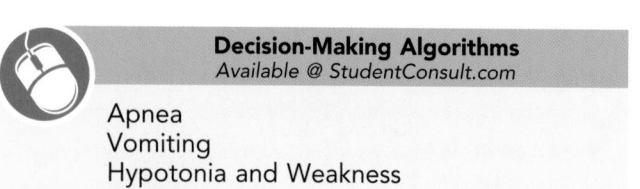

Decision-Making Algorithms
Available @ StudentConsult.com

Apnea
Vomiting
Hypotonia and Weakness
Alkalemia

Infants with genetic defects in urea synthesis, transient neonatal hyperammonemia, and impaired synthesis of urea and glutamine secondary to genetic disorders of organic acid metabolism can have levels of blood ammonia (>1,000 μmol/L) more than 10 times normal in the neonatal period. Poor feeding, hypotonia, apnea, hypothermia, and vomiting rapidly give way to **coma** and occasionally to intractable seizures. *Respiratory alkalosis is common.* Death occurs in hours to days if the condition remains untreated.

Moderate Neonatal Hyperammonemia

Decision-Making Algorithms
Available @ StudentConsult.com

Vomiting
Altered Mental Status

Moderate neonatal hyperammonemia (range, 200-400 μmol/L) is associated with depression of the central nervous system, poor feeding, and vomiting. Seizures are not characteristic. Respiratory alkalosis may occur. This type of hyperammonemia may be caused by partial or more distal blocks in urea synthesis and commonly is caused by disorders of organic acid metabolism (producing a metabolic acidosis) that secondarily interfere with the elimination of nitrogen.

Clinical Hyperammonemia in Later Infancy and Childhood

Infants who are affected by defects in the urea cycle may continue to do well while receiving the low-protein intake of breast milk, developing clinical hyperammonemia when dietary protein is increased or when catabolic stress occurs. Vomiting and lethargy may progress to coma. Seizures are not typical. During a crisis, the plasma ammonia level is usually 200-500 μmol/L. However, as the ammonia level decreases with decreased protein intake, the condition may go unrecognized for years, especially in the absence of specific central nervous system symptoms. If a crisis occurs during an epidemic of influenza, the child may be mistakenly thought to have **Reye syndrome**. Older children may have neuropsychiatric or behavioral abnormalities (see Fig. 51.2).

Specific Organ Presentation

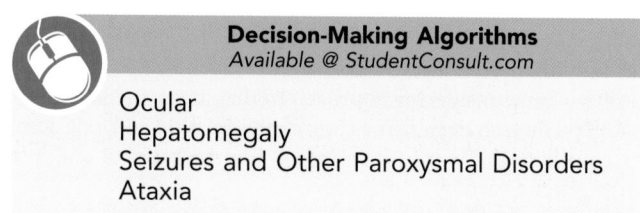

Decision-Making Algorithms
Available @ StudentConsult.com

Ocular
Hepatomegaly
Seizures and Other Paroxysmal Disorders
Ataxia

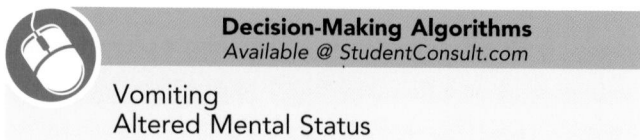

Any organ or system can be injured by toxic accumulation of any of the metabolites involved in inborn errors. Symptoms relate to organ-specific or system-specific toxicity and injury. Examples include nervous system (seizures, coma, ataxia), liver

TABLE 51.2 Primary Underlying Pathophysiological Mechanisms for Select Metabolic Disorders

DISORDER	DEFICIENCY OF A REQUIRED COMPOUND	ACCUMULATION OF TOXIC COMPOUND	RESULT
HYPOGLYCEMIC DISORDERS			
Medium-chain fatty acid oxidation defects	Fat for energy		Use of glucose with consequent hypoglycemia
Long-chain fatty acid oxidation defects	Fat for energy	Long-chain fats	Use of glucose with consequent hypoglycemia; mitochondrial dysfunction in liver, heart, etc., leading to organ dysfunction
Glycogen storage disease	Glucose to prevent fasting hypoglycemia	Glycogen resulting in storage in liver, muscle, heart	Risk of hypoglycemic brain injury and dysfunction of tissue with storage
Ketone utilization disorders	Fat for energy	Ketones	Risk of hypoglycemic brain injury; profound metabolic acidosis and reversible neurological dysfunction Cyclic vomiting
Galactosemia		Galactose	Elevated galactose leads to severe hepatic dysfunction, neurological injury, and impaired immune response
INTOXICATING DISORDERS (ENCEPHALOPATHY)			
Urea cycle defects		Ammonia	Central nervous system dysfunction, probably mediated through glutamine
Propionic acidemia, methymalonic acidemia, other organic acidemias		Organic acids	Systemic or local impairment of mitochondrial function; impaired neurotransmission; impairment of urea cycle
Phenylketonuria	Tyrosine	Phenylalanine	Impairment of tryptophan metabolism leading to serotonin deficiency; defective neurotransmission and white matter damage
Maple syrup urine disease		Leucine	Leucine toxicity leading to cerebral edema
CELLULAR COMPARTMENT DISORDERS			
Mitochondrial disease	Deficiency of ATP (energy) in affected tissues		Failure of affected tissues to carry out normal functions (e.g., muscle weakness, failure of relaxation of blood vessel muscles); failure of Cori cycle leading to lactate accumulation; cardiomyopathy
Peroxisomal disorders	Defect in peroxisomal β-oxidation. Deficiency of steroid hormones necessary for signaling	Accumulation of the saturated very-long-chain fatty acids	Aberrant embryonic patterning and hormone deficiency, defects in maintenance of myelin and white matter
Lysosomal storage disorders		Tissue-specific accumulation of compound not metabolized by lysosome	Cell type–specific damage and dysfunction as a result of lysosomal failure and reaction to waste product buildup
OTHER			
Disorders of creatine biosynthesis	Deficiency of cerebral creatine	Accumulation of guanidinoacetate in AGAT deficiency leads to seizures	Global brain energy defect leads to severe cognitive delays
Cholesterol biosynthesis disorders	Deficiency of steroid hormones		Endocrinopathies; disordered cellular signaling leading to aberrant organogenesis

AGAT, Arginine:glycine amidinotransferase deficiency.

(hepatocellular damage), eye (cataracts, dislocated lenses), renal (tubular dysfunction, cysts), and heart (cardiomyopathy, pericardial effusion) (Table 51.5).

Energy Deficiency

Disorders whose pathophysiology results in energy deficiency (e.g., disorders of fatty acid oxidation, mitochondrial function/oxidative phosphorylation, or carbohydrate metabolism) may manifest with myopathy; central nervous system dysfunction, including intellectual disability and seizures; cardiomyopathy; vomiting; hypoglycemia; or renal tubular acidosis.

Ketosis and Ketotic Hypoglycemia

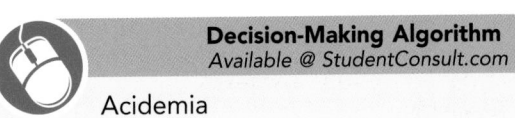

Decision-Making Algorithm
Available @ StudentConsult.com

Acidemia

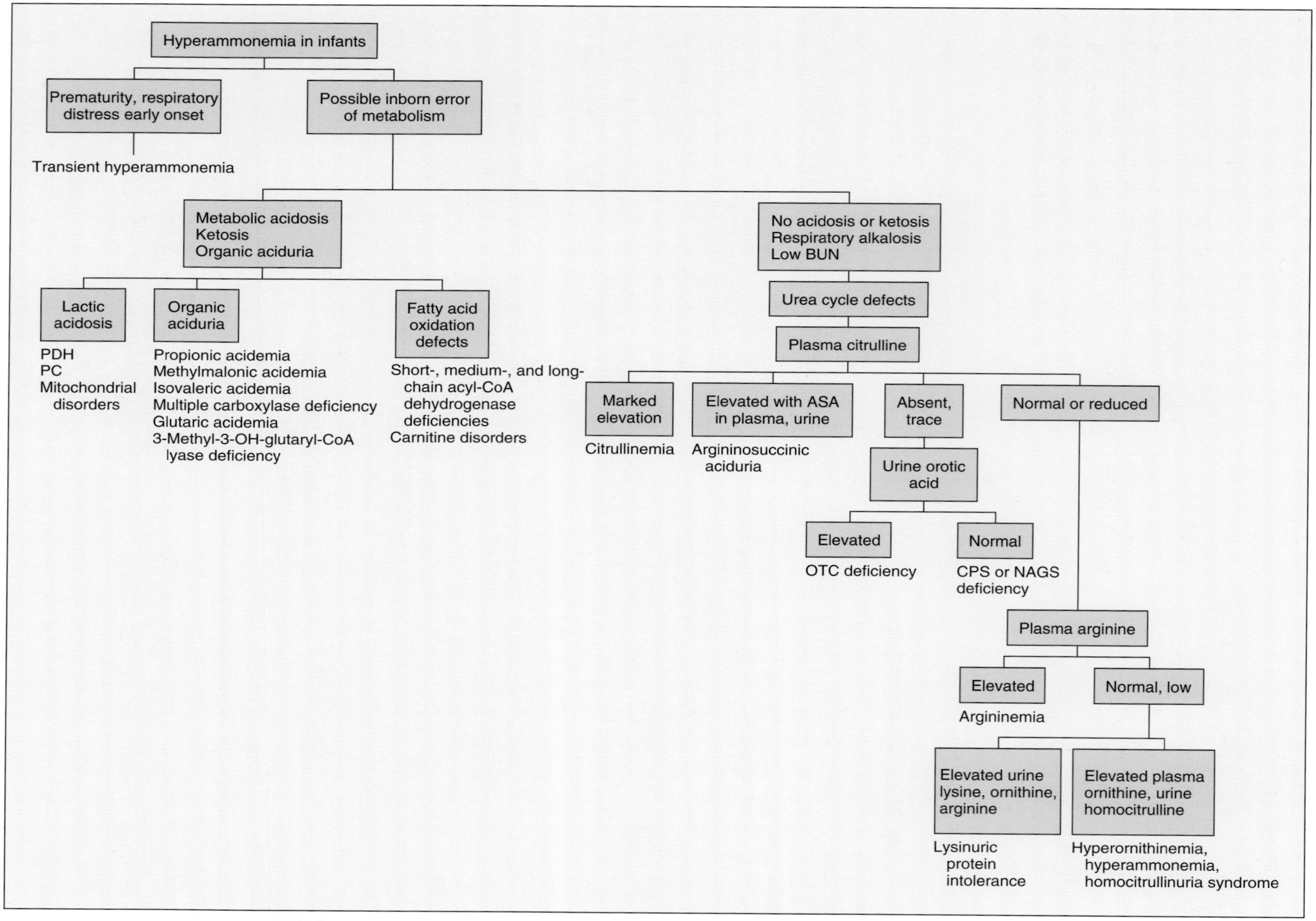

FIGURE 51.2 Algorithm for the approach to hyperammonemia infants. *ASA*, Argininosuccinic acid; *BUN*, blood urea nitrogen; *CoA*, coenzyme A; *CPS*, carbamylphosphate synthase; *NAGS*, N-acetylglutamate synthase; *OTC*, ornithine transcarbamylase; *PC*, pyruvate carboxylase deficiency; *PDH*, pyruvate dehydrogenase deficiency.

Acidosis is often found in children without metabolic diseases and may be due to fasting associated with anorexia, vomiting, diarrhea, and dehydration in the course of a viral illness. In this normal result of fasting, the blood glucose is relatively low; a mild acidosis and ketonuria may be present. Administration of carbohydrate restores balance. Severe ketosis may also be the result of disorders of ketone utilization such as ketothiolase deficiency or succinyl-CoA:3 ketoacid CoA transferase (SCOT) deficiency. In these conditions, which frequently present in the context of fasting, infection with fever, or decreased intake secondary to vomiting and diarrhea, hypoglycemia may be profound; the ketosis resolves slowly. As ketone bodies accumulate, cyclic vomiting may ensue.

Ketotic hypoglycemia is a common condition in which tolerance for fasting is impaired. Symptomatic hypoglycemia with seizures or coma occurs when the child encounters a catabolic stress. The hypoglycemia may occur with significant stress (e.g., viral infection with vomiting) or less commonly after minor stress (e.g., a prolongation by several hours of the normal overnight fast). Ketotic hypoglycemia first appears in the second year of life and occurs in otherwise healthy children. It is treated by frequent snacks and the provision of glucose during periods of stress. The pathophysiology is poorly understood (see Chapter 172). Although ketonuria is a normal response to prolonged (not overnight) fasting in older infants and children, it should prompt investigation for metabolic disease in neonates. **A high anion gap metabolic acidosis with or without ketosis** suggests a metabolic disorder (Table 51.6). Although ketone production may be reduced in some fatty acid oxidation disorders, the presence of ketonuria does not exclude this group of disorders.

Disorders Associated With Dysmorphic Findings

Congenital malformations or dysmorphic features are not intuitively thought of as symptoms and signs of inborn errors.

TABLE 51.3 Inborn Errors of Metabolism Presenting With Neurological Signs in Infants Less Than 3 Months of Age

GENERALIZED SEIZURES	ENCEPHALOPATHIC COMA WITH OR WITHOUT SEIZURES
All disorders that cause hypoglycemia: • Most hepatic glycogen storage diseases • Galactosemia, hereditary fructose intolerance • Fructose-1,6-bisphosphatase deficiency • Disorders of fatty acid β-oxidation • Glucose transporter deficiency	Mitochondrial disease: • *POLG* deficiency • Iron-sulfur cluster disease Maple syrup urine disease Nonketotic hyperglycinemia Diseases producing extreme hyperammonemia: • Disorders of the urea cycle • Disorders of the propionate pathway Disorders of β-oxidation Congenital lactic acidoses
Disorders of the propionate pathway	
HMG-CoA lyase deficiency	
Menkes disease	
Pyruvate carboxylase deficiency (PCD)	
Maple syrup urine disease	
SEIZURES AND/OR POSTURING	
Nonketotic hyperglycinemia	
Maple syrup urine disease	

HMG-CoA, 3-hydroxy-3-methylglutaryl-CoA.

TABLE 51.4 Etiologies of Hyperammonemia in Infants

ETIOLOGY OF HYPERAMMONEMIA	COMMENTS
Disorders of the urea cycle	Lethal hyperammonemia is common
Disorders of the propionate pathway	Severe hyperammonemia may precede acidosis
Disorders of fatty acid catabolism and of ketogenesis	Reye-like syndrome possible
Transient neonatal hyperammonemia	Idiopathic, self-limited
Portal-systemic shunting	Thrombosis of portal vein, cirrhosis, hepatitis
Mitochondrial DNA depletion	Typically associated with elevated lactate level
Drug intoxication: salicylate, valproic acid, acetaminophen	Obtain drug levels
Hyperinsulinism/hyperammonemia syndrome	Clinical hypoglycemia, subclinical hyperammonemia
Nonmetabolic liver disease including infections such as herpes, cytomegalovirus	Ensure evaluation of hepatic function and appropriate infectious disease work-up

TABLE 51.5 Inborn Errors of Metabolism Presenting With Hepatomegaly or Hepatic Dysfunction in Infants

HEPATOMEGALY	HEPATIC FAILURE	JAUNDICE
GSD I	Citrin deficiency Galactosemia	Citrin deficiency Galactosemia
GSD III	Hereditary fructose intolerance	Hereditary fructose intolerance
Mucopolysaccharidosis I and II	Tyrosinemia type 1 (fumarylacetoacetate hydrolase deficiency)	Infantile tyrosinemia (fumarylacetoacetate hydrolase deficiency)
Gaucher and Niemann-Pick diseases	GSD IV (slowly evolving) Mitochondrial hepatopathies	Crigler-Najjar disease Rotor, Dubin-Johnson syndromes

GSD, Glycogen storage disease.

TABLE 51.6 Etiologies of Metabolic Acidosis Caused by Inborn Errors of Metabolism in Infants

DISORDER	COMMENT
Methylmalonic acidemia (MMA)	Hyperammonemia, ketosis, neutropenia, thrombocytopenia
Propionic acidemia	Similar to MMA
Isovaleric acidemia	Odor of *sweaty feet*
Pyruvate dehydrogenase deficiency	Lactic acidosis, hyperammonemia
Pyruvate carboxylase deficiency	Lactic acidosis, hypoglycemia, and ketosis
Respiratory chain (mitochondrial) disorders	Lactic acidosis, ketosis occasionally seen
Medium-chain acyl-CoA dehydrogenase deficiency (MCAD)	Moderate acidosis, hypoglycemia, decreased ketones, possible hyperammonemia
Other fatty acid oxidation defects	Similar to MCAD, with potential hepatic and cardiac disease
Galactosemia	Renal tubular acidosis, *Escherichia coli* neonatal sepsis, hypoglycemia
3-Hydroxy-3-methyl-glutaryl-CoA lyase deficiency	Severe lactic acidosis, hyperammonemia, hypoglycemia
Multiple acyl-CoA dehydrogenase deficiency (glutaric aciduria 2)	Metabolic acidosis, hypoglycemia, lethal renal malformations

Conditions that cause congenital malformations include carbohydrate-deficient glycoprotein syndrome, disorders of cholesterol biosynthesis (e.g., Smith-Lemli-Opitz syndrome), disorders of copper transport (e.g., Menkes syndrome, occipital horn syndrome), maternal PKU syndrome, glutaric aciduria II (also called multiple acyl-coenzyme A [CoA] dehydrogenase deficiency), Aicardi-Goutieres syndrome (mimics congenital infection), and several storage diseases.

Storage Disorders

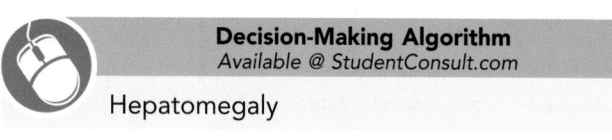

Decision-Making Algorithm
Available @ StudentConsult.com

Hepatomegaly

Storage disorders are caused by accumulation of incompletely metabolized macromolecules. This storage often occurs in subcellular organelles, such as lysosomes. The glycogen storage diseases (GSDsII), Niemann-Pick disease, and mucopolysaccharide disorders are examples of storage disorders.

CLINICAL ASSESSMENT AND LABORATORY TESTING

The assessment begins with a careful history (family and individual) and clinical evaluation. Clinical laboratory testing can define the metabolic derangement (Table 51.7). The results

TABLE 51.7 Initial Diagnostic Evaluation for a Suspected Inborn Error of Metabolism*

BLOOD AND PLASMA	URINE
Arterial blood gas	Glucose
Electrolytes—anion gap	pH
Glucose	Ketones
Ammonia	Reducing substances
Liver enzymes	Organic acids
Complete blood count, differential,† and platelet count	Acylglycines
Lactate, pyruvate	Orotic acid
Organic acids	
Amino acids	
Acylcarnitines	
Carnitine	

**Organ-specific evaluation is indicated for specific symptoms (e.g., cranial magnetic resonance imaging for coma or seizures; echocardiography for cardiomyopathy/poor perfusion; quantitative paired plasma/cerebrospinal fluid amino acids if nonketotic hyperglycemia is suspected).*

†Thrombocytopenia and neutropenia are seen in organic acidurias; vacuolated lymphocytes and metachromatic granules are seen in lysosomal disorders.

generate a differential diagnosis and a list of more specific laboratory testing to confirm the diagnosis.

The combination of symptoms and abnormal clinical laboratory findings demands urgent metabolic evaluation. A metabolic emergency often presents with vomiting, acidosis, hypoglycemia, ketosis (or *lack of appropriate ketosis*), intercurrent infection, anorexia/failure to feed, lethargy proceeding to coma, seizures, and hyperventilation or hypoventilation. Clinical evaluation should focus on the cardiac, renal, neurological, and developmental assessment as well as looking for changes in mental status, seizures, abnormal tone, visual symptoms, poor developmental progress, global developmental delay, loss of developmental milestones (regression), cardiomyopathy, cardiac failure, cystic renal malformation, and renal tubular dysfunction.

Clinical laboratory testing should begin with tests that are available in most hospital clinical laboratories. Care in the collection and handling of laboratory specimens is crucial to obtaining accurate results. Plasma measurements of lactate and ammonia are particularly subject to spurious results if not handled correctly. Significant ketosis in the neonate is unusual and suggests an organic acid disorder. Ketosis out of proportion to fasting status in an older child occurs in disorders of ketone utilization. Lack of severe ketosis in an older child under conditions of metabolic stress is a feature of fatty acid oxidation disorders or hyperinsulinemic hypoglycemia syndromes. In some disorders, such as urea cycle disorders, ketone utilization disorders, milder forms of fatty acid oxidation defects, and intermittent maple syrup urine disease (MSUD), the laboratory abnormalities may be absent aside from during an acute presentation. Therefore normal testing in the well state does not rule out a metabolic disorder.

GENETIC ASPECTS OF INBORN ERRORS

Mechanisms of Inheritance

Although all of the classic mechanisms of inheritance are represented, most IEMs are autosomal recessive. Isolation or founder effect may make a specific recessive condition common in some populations (e.g., MSUD in the Old Order Mennonite population in Pennsylvania). X-linked conditions exhibit increased presentation in males. In general, carriers of recessive or X-linked diseases are usually asymptomatic. However, in ornithine transcarbamylase (OTC; also known as ornithine carbamoyltransferase) deficiency or Fabry disease, females can be symptomatic if they have a low proportion of unaffected cells (unfavorable X-inactivation). Most mitochondrial disorders in children are a result of pathogenic variants in autosomal genes, although there are X-linked forms. Pathogenic variants in the mitochondrial DNA also lead to mitochondrial disease. In this situation the type and severity of the presentation depend on the specific defects and the tissue-specific ratio of normal to abnormal copies of the mitochondrial DNA *(the degree of heteroplasmy)*.

Identification of Molecular Pathology

If the molecular basis of an inborn error of metabolism is known (i.e., the gene or genes have been mapped and disease-causing variants defined), specific genetic testing may be clinically available. In some disorders there is a good correlation between specific disease-causing variants and clinical outcome. Genetic testing in other at-risk family members can provide important genetic information for them, potentially enabling presymptomatic therapy and alternate decision making throughout the rest of the family.

IDENTIFICATION OF INBORN ERRORS BY NEONATAL SCREENING

Disorders Identified by Neonatal Screening

In the United States the majority of infants diagnosed with a treatable metabolic disorder will be identified as a result of an abnormal newborn screen. Most states use tandem mass spectrometry to screen for a core panel of metabolic disorders (Table 51.8). Proposed additions or removal of conditions recommended for screening are evaluated by the federal advisory committee on heritable disorders in the newborn and child (ACHDNC). Approved conditions are then included in the "recommended uniform screening panel" (RUSP). In most states, biotinidase deficiency and galactosemia are typically screened for by evaluating enzyme function. Two storage disorders (mucopolysaccharidosis type 1[MPS1], Hurler, Hurler-Schei, and Schei diseases) and Pompe disease (GSDII) as well as one disorder of peroxisomal function (ALD) have been added to the RUSP. The lysosomal storage disorders may be detected by enzymatic function with degradation products detected through colorimetry or tandem mass spectrometry. The peroxisomal disorder is detected by looking for an analyte detected using a tandem mass spectrometer in a different mode.

Strategy of Neonatal Screening

The purpose of neonatal screening is the early detection and rapid treatment of disorders before the onset of symptoms, thus preventing morbidity and mortality. In most states, infants are tested at 24-48 hours (see Chapter 58). A positive test demands prompt evaluation. Specific follow-up testing and treatment of an affected child depends on the disorder. Consistent with most screening tests, a significant proportion of infants who have a positive neonatal screening test do not have a metabolic disorder.

Confirmatory Testing Principles

Neonatal screening is designed to maximize detection of affected infants but is not diagnostic. "Cutoff values" for each test are established carefully to identify infants with an elevated concentration of the substance or decreased activity of an enzyme with an acceptable number of false-positive results. A positive screening test must be followed by prompt clinical assessment as recommended by the screening program and/or metabolic specialist. In many cases children will also be provided therapy until the completion of definitive testing.

A positive screening test result causes anxiety for new parents; management of such anxiety is essential to minimize the harm of the program. In addition, definitive testing must be carried out promptly and accurately. If an inborn error of metabolism is excluded, parents need a thorough explanation of the results and reassurance that the infant is well. Such explanations will frequently require the expertise of a metabolic specialist or genetic counselor in the newborn period but may require reassessment of parental understanding by the primary care physician in the long term.

Specialized Laboratory and Clinical Testing

Specialized testing for inherited disorders of metabolism is effective in confirming a diagnosis suspected on the basis of an abnormal newborn screening result or on the basis of clinical suspicion. The tests that are helpful and examples of diagnoses made using these measurements depend on the deficient pathway in the disorder under consideration (Table 51.9).

Amino acid analysis is performed in plasma, urine, and cerebrospinal fluid (CSF). The plasma amino acid profile is most useful in identifying disorders of amino acid catabolism. Amino acids may also be abnormal in specific disorders of organic acid degradation, but often they are normal or not diagnostic.

The urine amino acid profile is helpful in diagnosing primary disorders of renal tubular function, such as Lowe syndrome and cystinuria, as well as secondary disorders of renal tubular function, such as cystinosis and Fanconi syndrome of any cause. The test may also be useful in screening for several disorders of amino acid transport such as the detection of urinary homocitrulline in hyperornithinemia-hyperammonemia-homocitrullinuria (HHH) syndrome. The urine amino acid profile is not the test of choice for diagnosing disorders of amino acid or organic acid metabolism.

Markers of disordered fatty acid oxidation are measured in urine and plasma. Excessive intermediates of fatty acid oxidation and organic acid catabolism are conjugated with glycine and carnitine. The **urine acylglycine profile** and the **plasma acylcarnitine profile** reflect this accumulation. In organic acid disorders and fatty acid oxidation disorders, measurement of plasma carnitine may reveal a secondary deficiency of carnitine and abnormal distribution of free and acylated carnitine. The plasma free fatty acid (nonesterified fatty acid) to 3-OH-butyrate ratio is helpful in the diagnosis of disorders of fatty acid oxidation. Excess 3-OH-butyrate suggests a disorder of ketone metabolism; absence of ketones or decreased 3-OH-butyrate suggests a fatty acid oxidation disorder. Profiling of fatty acid intermediates in cultured skin fibroblasts may be informative.

Disorders of organic acid metabolism, such as propionic acidemia and methylmalonic acidemia, have typical urine organic acid profiles. Although analysis of blood and urine

TABLE 51.8 Disorders Identified by Newborn Screening Programs in the United States

DISORDER	METHODS	FOLLOW ON TESTING
AMINO ACID		
Argininosuccinic aciduria	MS/MS	Plasma amino acid profile, look for elevated citrulline and argininosuccinic acid
Citrullinemia, type I	MS/MS	Plasma amino acid profile, look for elevated citrulline without argininosuccinic acid
Maple syrup urine disease (MSUD)	MS/MS	Plasma amino acid profile, look for alloisoleucine
Homocystinuria	MS/MS	Total plasma homocysteine, plasma amino acid profile
Phenylketonuria (PKU)	MS/MS	Plasma phenylalanine, DNA testing
Tyrosinemia	MS/MS	Plasma amino acid profile, urine succinylacetone
ORGANIC ACID		
Propionic acidemia	MS/MS	Urine organic acid profile
Methylmalonic acidemias including methylmalonyl-CoA mutase and cobalamin disorders	MS/MS	Urine organic acid profile, plasma amino acid profile, plasma homocysteine B12 and B12 binding levels in mother and child
Isovaleric acidemia	MS/MS	Urine organic acid profile
3-Methylcrotonyl-CoA carboxylase deficiency	MS/MS	Urine organic acid profile
3-Hydroxy-3-methylglutaric aciduria	MS/MS	Urine organic acid profile
Holocarboxylase synthase deficiency	MS/MS	Urine organic acid profile
Biotinidase deficiency	Enzyme measurement	Quantitative biotinidase measurement, DNA testing
FATTY ACID		
Medium-chain acyl-CoA dehydrogenase deficiency (MCAD)	MS/MS	Urine organic acid profile, urine acylglycine profile, plasma acylcarnitine profile
Long-chain 3-hydroxyacyl-CoA dehydrogenase deficiency (LCHAD)	MS/MS	Urine organic acid profile, urine acylglycine profile, plasma acylcarnitine profile
Very-long-chain acyl-CoA dehydrogenase deficiency (VLCAD)	MS/MS	Urine organic acid profile, urine acylglycine profile, plasma acylcarnitine profile
Carnitine uptake defect/carnitine transport defect	MS/MS	Blood free and total carnitine levels
CARBOHYDRATE		
Galactosemia	GALT enzyme measurement	GALT enzyme measurement, DNA testing, galactose-1-P measurement
STORAGE DISORDERS		
Glycogen storage disease Type II (Pompe)	Acid alpha-glucosidase (GAA) enzyme activity	GAA enzyme activity, DNA testing
Mucopolysaccharidosis type 1	α-L-iduronidase enzyme activity	α-L-iduronidase enzyme activity, DNA testing
Peroxisomal disorders		
X-linked adrenoleukodystrophy	MS/MS for C26:0	HPLC-MS/MS, DNA testing

MS/MS, Tandem mass spectrometry; *HPLC*, high-performance liquid chromatography.

usually suggest the specific diagnosis, more targeted testing by measuring enzymatic activity in the pathway or establishing DNA changes in the gene is typically needed to identify the specific enzymatic defect.

Disorders of creatine biosynthesis are suggested by a reduction in creatine in CSF and, in one form, an increase in guanidinoacetic acid in blood and urine. Disorders of purine and pyrimidine metabolism are suggested by the presence of an abnormal urinary profile of purines, such as xanthine, hypoxanthine, inosine, guanosine, adenosine, adenine, or succinyladenosine. Similarly, disorders of pyrimidine metabolism are identified by an abnormal profile of pyrimidines, including uracil, uridine, thymine, thymidine, orotic acid, orotidine, dihydrouracil, dihydrothymine, pseudouridine, *N*-carbamoyl-β-alanine, or *N*-carbamoyl-β-aminoisobutyrate, in the urine.

Some storage disorders show abnormalities in urine mucopolysaccharides (glycosaminoglycans, glycoproteins), sialic acid, heparan sulfate, dermatan sulfate, or chondroitin sulfate. In several disorders, CSF is the most helpful specimen, including glycine encephalopathy (CSF amino acid profile when compared to concurrent plasma amino acids), disorders of neurotransmitter synthesis (biogenic amine profile), glucose transporter (GLUT1) deficiency (plasma-to-CSF glucose ratio), and serine synthesis defect (amino acid profile).

TABLE 51.9 Specialized Metabolic Testing

TEST	ANALYTES MEASURED	TEST HELPFUL IN IDENTIFYING DISORDERS
Plasma amino acid profile	Amino acids, including alloisoleucine	PKU, urea cycle defects, tyrosinemias, MSUD, homocystinuria
Plasma total homocysteine	Protein-bound and free homocysteine	Homocystinuria, some forms of methylmalonic acidemia
Urine amino acid profile	Amino acids	Disorders of amino acid renal transport
Plasma acylcarnitine profile	Acylcarnitine derivatives of organic and fatty acid catabolism	Organic acid disorders, fatty acid oxidation disorders
Urine acylglycine profile	Acylglycine derivatives of organic and fatty acid catabolism	Organic acid disorders, fatty acid oxidation disorders
Plasma carnitines	Free, total, and acylated carnitine	Primary and secondary carnitine deficiency; abnormal in many organic acid and fatty acid disorders
Urine organic acid profile	Organic acids	Organic acid, mitochondrial and fatty acid disorders
Urine or blood succinylacetone	Succinylacetone	Tyrosinemia I
Urine oligosaccharide chromatography	Glycosaminoglycans, mucopolysaccharides	Lysosomal storage disorders

MSUD, Maple syrup urine disease; *PKU*, phenylketonuria.

The correct tissue for enzymatic confirmation depends on the disorder, and in many cases may be measured on white blood cells or cultured skin fibroblasts. Consequently, such samples should only be collected after review of the testing laboratory's requirements.

In many disorders, an abnormal metabolic profile is consistently present during illness and when the child is well. In some cases, it is only diagnostic during an episode of illness.

OVERVIEW OF TREATMENT

There are several basic principles for treatment of IEMs. Syndromes with toxicity often present with encephalopathy; removal of toxic compounds is the first goal of therapy. Strategies include hemodialysis, hemovenovenous filtration, and administration of alternate pathway agents (see Chapter 53). A second strategy is to enhance deficient enzyme activity through administration of enzyme cofactors (e.g., pyridoxine in homocystinuria, tetrahydrobiopterin in PKU). If deficiency of a pathway product plays an important role, providing missing products is helpful (e.g., tyrosine in the treatment of PKU). A further principle is to decrease flux through the deficient pathway by restricting precursors in the diet. Examples include the restriction of protein in disorders of ammonia detoxification, phenylalanine in PKU, and of amino acid precursors in the organic acid disorders.

CHAPTER 52

Carbohydrate Disorders

GLYCOGEN STORAGE DISEASES

Many glycogen storage diseases are characterized by **hypoglycemia** and **hepatomegaly** (Table 52.1). Glycogen, the storage form of glucose, is found most abundantly in the liver (where it modulates blood glucose levels) and in muscles (where it facilitates anaerobic work). Glycogen is synthesized from uridine diphosphoglucose through the concerted action of glycogen synthetase and brancher enzyme (Fig. 52.1). The accumulation of glycogen is stimulated by insulin. Glycogenolysis occurs through a cascade initiated by epinephrine or glucagon. It results in rapid phosphorolysis of glycogen to yield glucose 1-phosphate, accompanied by, to a lesser degree, hydrolysis of glucose residues from the branch points in glycogen molecules. In the liver and kidneys, glucose 1-phosphate is converted to glucose 6-phosphate through the actions of phosphoglucomutase; glucose 6-phosphatase hydrolyses glucose 6-phosphate to produce glucose. The latter enzyme is not present in muscles. Glycogen storage diseases fall into the following four categories:

1. Diseases that predominantly affect the liver and have a direct influence on blood glucose (types I, VI, and VIII)
2. Diseases that predominantly involve muscles and affect the ability to do anaerobic work (types V and VII)
3. Diseases that can affect the liver and muscles and directly influence blood glucose and muscle metabolism (type III)
4. Diseases that affect various tissues but have no direct effect on blood glucose or on the ability to do anaerobic work (types II and IV)

The **diagnosis** of type I or type III glycogen storage disease is suggested by elevated uric acid, lactate, and triglycerides in blood. For all forms, a diagnosis can normally be confirmed by DNA testing. When this is feasible, invasive procedures, such as muscle and liver biopsy, can be avoided. When DNA testing is not available or is inconclusive, enzyme measurements in tissue from the affected organ confirm the diagnosis. If the diagnosis cannot be established, metabolic challenge and exercise testing may be needed. **Treatment** of hepatic glycogen storage disease is aimed at maintaining satisfactory blood glucose levels or supplying alternative energy sources to muscle. In glucose-6-phosphatase deficiency (type I), the treatment usually requires nocturnal intragastric feedings of glucose during the first 1 or 2 years of life. Thereafter, snacks and uncooked cornstarch may be satisfactory; however, many centers also use nocturnal intragastric feedings. Hepatic tumors (sometimes malignant) are a threat in adolescence and adult life. No specific treatment exists for the diseases of muscle that impair skeletal muscle ischemic

TABLE 52.1 Glycogen Storage Diseases*

DISEASE	AFFECTED ENZYME	ORGANS AFFECTED	CLINICAL SYNDROME	NEONATAL MANIFESTATIONS	PROGNOSIS
Type 1a: von Gierke	Glucose 6-phosphatase	Liver, kidney, GI tract, platelets	Hypoglycemia, lactic acidosis, ketosis, hepatomegaly, hypotonia, slow growth, diarrhea, bleeding disorder, gout, hypertriglyceridemia, xanthomas	Hypoglycemia, lactic acidemia, liver may not be enlarged	Early death from hypoglycemia, lactic acidosis; do well with early diagnosis and strict adherence to dietary therapy; hepatomas may occur in late childhood
Type 1b	Glucose-6-phosphate translocase	Liver, kidney, GI tract, platelets, white blood cells	As type 1a, but in addition have clinically significant neutropenia	As type 1a but also may present with infections	In addition to risks for type 1a, children have significant IBD-like symptoms. Historically, death due to infections has occurred in the second decade.
Type II: Pompe	Lysosomal α-glucosidase	All; notably striated muscle, nerve cells	Symmetrical profound muscle weakness, cardiomegaly, heart failure, shortened P-R interval	May have muscle weakness, cardiomegaly, or both	Very poor in neonatal form; death in the first year of life is usual; variants exist; therapy with recombinant human α-glucosidase is promising
Type III: Forbes	Debranching enzyme	Liver, muscles	Early in course hypoglycemia, ketonuria, hepatomegaly that resolves with age; may show muscle fatigue	Usually none	Very good for hepatic disorder; if myopathy present, it tends to be like that of type I and V
Type IV: Andersen	Branching enzyme	Liver, other tissues	Hepatic cirrhosis beginning at several months of age; early liver failure	Usually none	Very poor; death from hepatic failure in first decade is typical
Type V: McArdle	Muscle phosphorylase	Muscle	Muscle fatigue beginning in adolescence	None	Good, with sedentary lifestyle
Type VI: Hers	Liver phosphorylase	Liver	Mild hypoglycemia with hepatomegaly, ketonuria	Usually none	Probably good
Type VII: Tarui	Muscle phosphofructokinase	Muscle	Clinical findings similar to type V	None	Similar to that of type V
Type VIII	Phosphorylase kinase	Liver	Clinical findings similar to type III, without myopathy	None	Good

**Except for one form of hepatic phosphorylase kinase, which is X-linked, these disorders are autosomal recessive.*
GI, Gastrointestinal; *IBD*, inflammatory bowel disease.

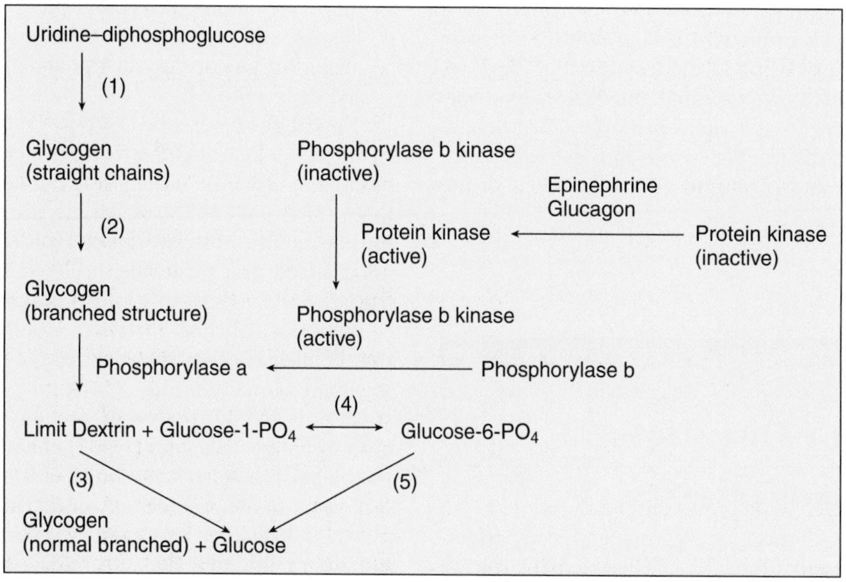

FIGURE 52.1 Glycogen synthesis and degradation. (1) Glycogen synthetase, (2) brancher enzyme, (3) debrancher enzyme, (4) phosphoglucomutase, (5) glucose 6-phosphatase.

exercise. Enzyme replacement early in life is effective in Pompe disease (type II), which involves cardiac and skeletal muscle.

GALACTOSEMIA

Decision-Making Algorithms
Available @ StudentConsult.com

Visual Impairment and Leukocoria
Jaundice
Hepatomegaly
Alkalemia

Galactosemia is an autosomal recessive disease caused by deficiency of galactose-1-phosphate uridyltransferase (Fig. 52.2). Clinical manifestations are most striking in a neonate who, when fed milk, generally exhibits evidence of **liver failure** (hyperbilirubinemia, disorders of coagulation, hypoglycemia), disordered **renal tubular function** (acidosis, glycosuria, aminoaciduria), and **cataracts**. The neonatal screening test must have a rapid turnaround time because affected infants may die in the first week of life. Affected infants are at increased risk for severe neonatal *Escherichia coli* sepsis. Major effects on liver and kidney function and the development of cataracts are limited to the first few years of life; older children may have learning disorders despite dietary compliance. Girls usually develop premature ovarian failure despite treatment.

Laboratory manifestations of galactosemia depend on dietary galactose intake. When galactose is ingested (as lactose), levels of plasma galactose and erythrocyte galactose 1-phosphate are elevated. Hypoglycemia is frequent, and albuminuria is present. Galactose frequently is present in the urine and can be detected by a positive reaction for reducing substances without a reaction with glucose oxidase on urine strip tests. The absence of urinary reducing substances cannot be relied on to exclude the diagnosis. The diagnosis is made by showing extreme reduction in erythrocyte galactose-1-phosphate uridyltransferase activity. DNA testing for pathogenic variants in galactose-1-phosphate uridyltransferase confirms the diagnosis and may be useful in predicting prognosis. Renal tubular dysfunction may be evidenced by a normal anion-gap hyperchloremic metabolic acidosis. **Treatment** by the elimination of dietary galactose results in rapid correction of abnormalities, but infants who are extremely ill before treatment may die before therapy is effective.

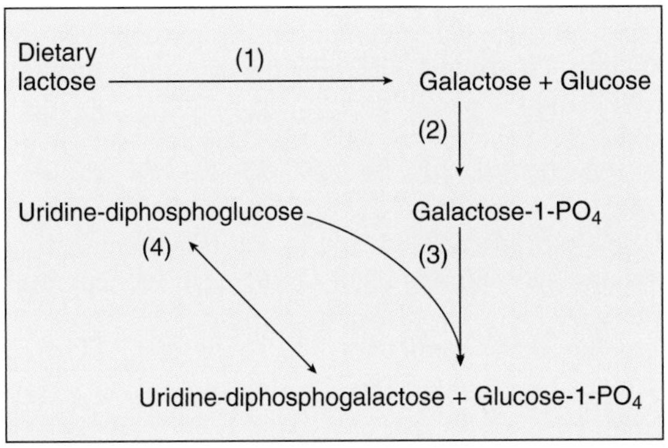

FIGURE 52.2 Pathway of galactose metabolism. (1) Lactase (intestinal), (2) galactokinase, (3) galactose-1-phosphate uridyltransferase, (4) uridine diphosphoglucose 4-epimerase.

Galactokinase deficiency, an autosomal recessive disorder, also leads to the accumulation of galactose in body fluids (see Fig. 52.2), which results in the formation of galactitol (dulcitol) through the action of aldose reductase. Galactitol, acting as an osmotic agent, can be responsible for cataract formation and, rarely, for increased intracranial pressure. These are the only clinical manifestations. Individuals homozygous for galactokinase deficiency usually develop cataracts after the neonatal period, whereas heterozygous individuals may be at risk for cataracts as adults.

Hereditary fructose intolerance, in many ways, is analogous to galactosemia. When fructose is ingested, deficiency of fructose-1-phosphate aldolase leads to the intracellular accumulation of fructose 1-phosphate with resultant emesis, hypoglycemia, and severe liver and kidney disease. Elimination of fructose and sucrose from the diet prevents clinical disease. **Fructosuria** is caused by fructokinase deficiency, but its deficiency is not associated with clinical consequences.

CHAPTER 53

Amino Acid Disorders

DISORDERS OF AMINO ACID METABOLISM

Disorders of amino acid metabolism are the result of the inability to catabolize specific amino acids derived from protein. Usually a single amino acid pathway is involved. This amino acid accumulates in excess and is toxic to various organs, such as the brain, eyes, skin, or liver. Treatment is directed at the specific pathway and usually involves dietary restriction of the offending amino acid and supplementation with special medical foods (formulas) that provide the other amino acids and other nutrients. Confirmatory testing includes quantitative specific plasma amino acid profiles along with specific pathogenic variant testing and sometimes enzymology.

PHENYLKETONURIA

Phenylketonuria (PKU), an autosomal recessive disease, primarily affects the brain and occurs in 1 in 10,000 persons. Classic PKU is the result from a defect in the hydroxylation of phenylalanine to form tyrosine (Fig. 53.1); the activity of phenylalanine hydroxylase in the liver is absent or greatly reduced. Affected infants are normal at birth, but if untreated, severe intellectual disability (IQ 30) develops in the first year of life. A positive newborn screening test must be followed up by performing quantitative plasma amino acid analysis. A plasma phenylalanine value of greater than 360 μM (6 mg/dL) is consistent with the diagnosis of one of the hyperphenylalaninemias and demands prompt evaluation and treatment. Untreated, classic PKU is characterized by blood phenylalanine concentrations higher than 600 μM. Milder forms of hyperphenylalaninemia are indicated by values of plasma phenylalanine lower than this but higher than 360 μM. A significant percentage of premature infants and a few full-term infants have transient elevations in phenylalanine. Short-term follow-up usually

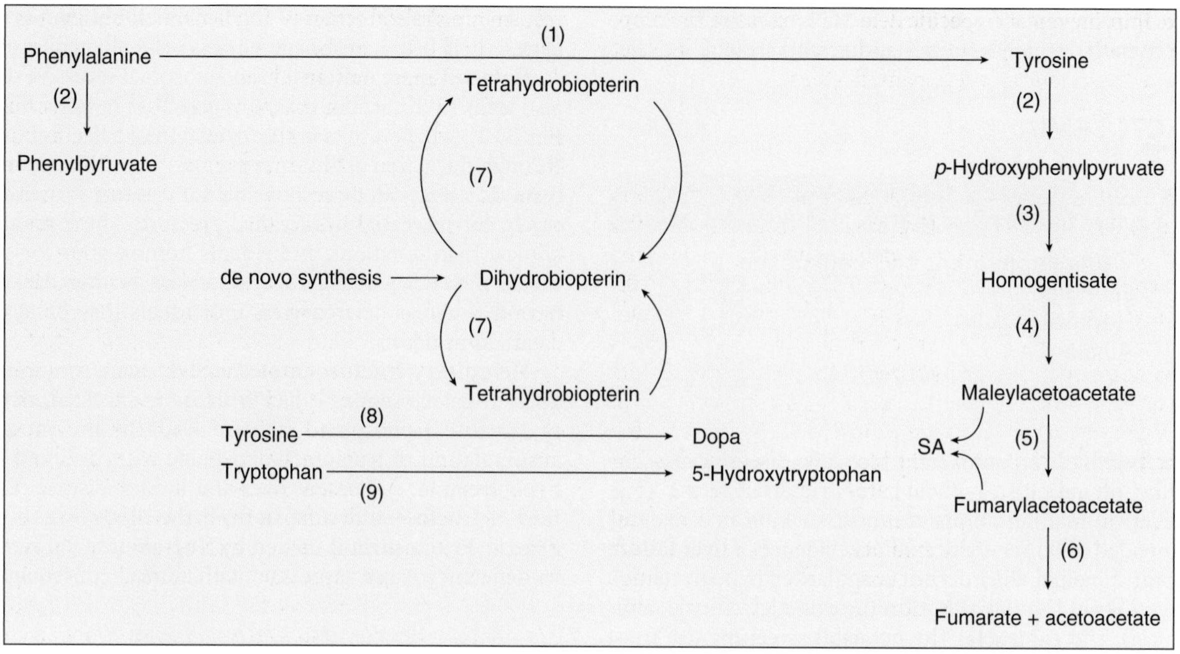

FIGURE 53.1 Metabolism of aromatic amino acids. (1) Phenylalanine hydroxylase, (2) transaminase, (3) *p*-hydroxyphenylpyruvate oxidase, (4) homogentisate oxidase, (5) maleylacetoacetate isomerase, (6) fumarylacetoacetate hydrolase, (7) dihydrobiopterin reductase, (8) tyrosine hydroxylase, (9) tryptophan hydroxylase. *SA*, Succinylacetone.

identifies these infants promptly. A small percentage of infants diagnosed with PKU (≤2% in the United States) have a defect in the synthesis or metabolism of tetrahydrobiopterin, the cofactor for phenylalanine hydroxylase and for other enzymes involved in the intermediary metabolism of aromatic amino acids. Such disorders in biopterin metabolism are diagnosed by measuring dihydrobiopterin reductase in erythrocytes and by analyzing biopterin metabolites in urine. This testing should be carried out in all hyperphenylalaninemic infants.

Treatment is designed to maintain plasma phenylalanine values in the therapeutic range of 120-360 mM using a diet specifically restricted in phenylalanine but otherwise nutritionally complete. Since the early 1980s, treatment for life is recommended to reduce the risks of long-term neuropsychiatric problems and reduce the risk of maternal PKU syndrome.

Outcome of treatment in classic PKU is excellent. Most infants with classic PKU who are treated within the first 10 days of life achieve normal intelligence. However, learning problems and problems with executive function are more frequent than in unaffected peers. The safe concentration of phenylalanine in older children and adults with PKU has not been clearly established. Reversible cognitive dysfunction is associated with acute elevations of plasma phenylalanine in adults and children with PKU. If the elevated level has been sustained, the dysfunction may not be reversible. Treatment with modified preparation of tetrahydrobiopterin has shown good responses in some individuals with PKU.

Females with PKU and their families must be educated on the risks and prevention of maternal PKU syndrome. **Maternal hyperphenylalaninemia** requires rigorous management before conception and throughout pregnancy to prevent fetal brain damage, congenital heart disease, and microcephaly.

TYROSINEMIAS

Tyrosinemia is identified in neonatal screening programs using tandem mass spectrometry methods to detect elevated tyrosine and/or succinylacetone. Elevated tyrosine levels also occur as a nonspecific consequence of severe liver disease or transient tyrosinemia of the newborn, which responds to ascorbic acid treatment. The inherited disorders of tyrosine metabolism are a target of neonatal screening. **Tyrosinemia type I,** which is due to fumarylacetoacetate hydrolase deficiency (see Fig. 53.1), is a rare disease in which accumulated metabolites produce severe liver disease associated with bleeding disorder, hypoglycemia, hypoalbuminemia, elevated transaminases, and defects in renal tubular function. Hepatocellular carcinoma may eventually occur. Quantitative measurement of plasma tyrosine and blood or urine succinylacetone is performed after a positive neonatal screen. The **diagnosis** of tyrosinemia I is confirmed by an increased concentration of succinylacetone; DNA testing is available. **Treatment** with nitisinone (NTBC; an inhibitor of the oxidation of parahydroxyphenylpyruvic acid) effectively eliminates the production of the toxic succinylacetone. A low-phenylalanine, low-tyrosine diet may also play a role. These treatments have obviated the immediate need for liver transplantation in children identified by neonatal screening. Whether they completely eliminate the occurrence of hepatocellular carcinoma is the focus of ongoing studies.

Tyrosinemias II and **III** are more benign forms of hereditary tyrosinemia. Blocked metabolism of tyrosine at earlier steps in the pathway is responsible, and succinylacetone is not produced. The clinical features include **hyperkeratosis** of palms and soles and **keratitis**, which can cause severe visual disturbance. Significant elevations of tyrosine levels are associated with mild cognitive impairment and specific defects in executive function. Treatment with a phenylalanine- and tyrosine-restricted diet is effective in preventing these complications.

HOMOCYSTINURIA

Homocystinuria, an autosomal recessive disease (1:200,000 live births) involving connective tissue, the brain, and the vascular system, is caused by a deficiency of cystathionine β-synthase. In the normal metabolism of the sulfur amino acids, methionine gives rise to cystine; homocysteine is a pivotal intermediate (Fig. 53.2). When cystathionine β-synthase is deficient, homocysteine accumulates in the blood and appears in the urine. Another result is enhanced reconversion of homocysteine to methionine, resulting in an increase in the concentration of methionine in the blood. The neonatal screening test most commonly used evaluates for elevated methionine. An excess of homocysteine produces a slowly evolving **clinical syndrome** that includes dislocated ocular lenses; long, slender extremities; malar flushing; and livedo reticularis. Arachnodactyly, scoliosis, pectus excavatum or carinatum, and genu valgum are skeletal features. Intellectual disability, psychiatric illness, or both may be present. Major arterial or venous thromboses are a constant threat.

Confirmation of the **diagnosis** requires demonstration of elevated total homocysteine in the blood. A plasma amino acid profile reveals hypermethioninemia. Measurement of cystathionine β-synthase is not clinically available, but numerous pathogenic variants in the gene are known and can be tested.

There are two clinical forms of homocystinuria. In one form, activity of the deficient enzyme can be enhanced by the administration of large doses of pyridoxine (100-500 mg/day). Folate supplementation is added to overcome folate deficiency if folate is trapped in the process of remethylation of homocysteine to methionine. This pyridoxine-responsive form comprises approximately 50% of cases and is the form more likely to be missed by neonatal screening because the methionine concentrations are not always above the screening cutoff. The second form is not responsive to pyridoxine therapy. The use of supplemental betaine (trimethylglycine), a donor of methyl groups for remethylation of homocysteine to methionine, also has a role in the management of pyridoxine-unresponsive patients. Some cases may benefit from B12 and folate supplementation. Consequently, diet and betaine are sometimes required to control plasma homocysteine, even in pyridoxine-responsive patients. The prognosis is good for infants whose plasma homocysteine concentration is controlled.

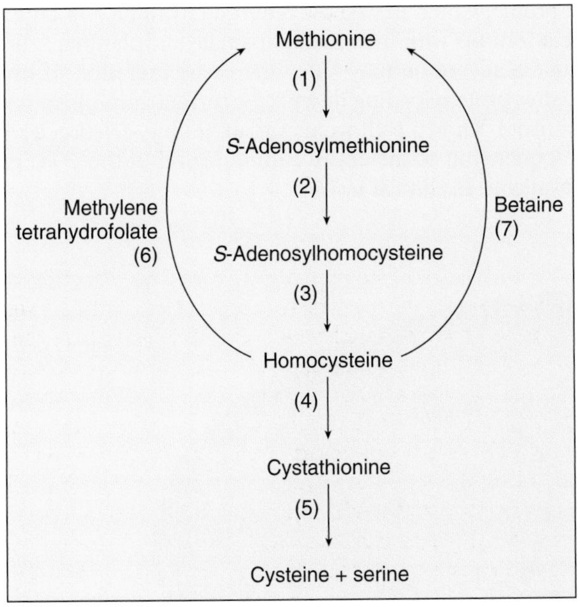

FIGURE 53.2 Metabolism of methionine and homocysteine. (1) Methionine adenosyltransferase, (2) *S*-methyltransferase, (3) *S*-adenosylhomocysteine hydrolase, (4) cystathionine β-synthase, (5) cystathionase, (6) homocysteine methyltransferase, (7) betaine-homocysteine methyltransferase.

MAPLE SYRUP URINE DISEASE

Maple syrup urine disease (MSUD) is an autosomal recessive disease, also called **branched chain ketoaciduria**. It is caused by a deficiency of the decarboxylase that initiates the degradation of the ketoacid analogs of the three branched chain amino acids—leucine, isoleucine, and valine (Fig. 53.3). Classic MSUD is rare (1:250,000) in the general population but much more common in some population isolates (Pennsylvania Mennonites 1:150). The recommended uniform screening panel (RUSP) includes MSUD.

Although MSUD does have intermittent-onset and late-onset forms, **clinical manifestations** of the classic form typically occur within 1-4 weeks of birth. Poor feeding, vomiting, and tachypnea commonly are noted, but the hallmark of the disease is profound depression of the central nervous system, associated with alternating hypotonia and hypertonia **(extensor spasms)**, opisthotonos, and seizures. The urine may have the odor of maple syrup.

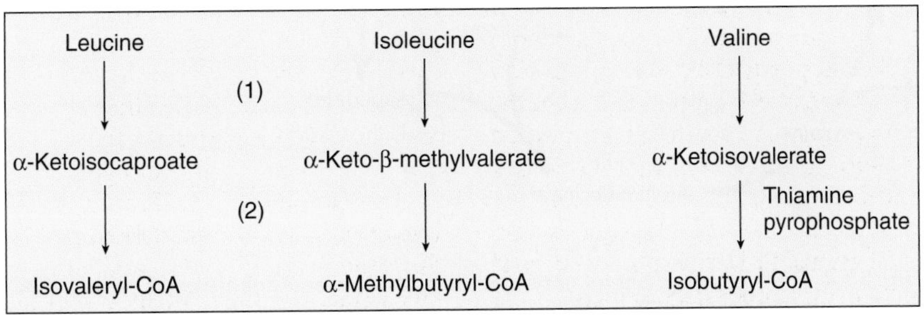

FIGURE 53.3 Metabolism of the branched chain amino acids. (1) Aminotransferases, (2) α-ketoacid dehydrogenase complex.

Laboratory manifestations of MSUD include hypoglycemia and a variable presence of metabolic acidosis, with elevation of the undetermined anions; the acidosis is caused in part by plasma branched-chain organic acids. MSUD should be strongly suspected in a child with positive urine ketones on dipstick with no or low β-hydroxybutyrate. A rapid, more specific test demonstrates the rapid formation of copious, white precipitate when 2,4-dinitrophenylhydrazine is added to the urine sample. This is because branched-chain ketoacids in urine (but not β-hydroxybutyrate or acetoacetate) specifically react with 2,4-dinitrophenylhydrazine.

The **definitive diagnosis** of MSUD generally is made by showing large increases in plasma leucine with less increases in isoleucine, and valine concentrations and identification of excess alloisoleucine in the plasma. The urinary organic acid profile is usually abnormal and shows the ketoacid derivatives of the branched-chain amino acids. The diagnosis can be substantiated by detection of pathogenic variants in one of the three genes BCKDHA, encoding BCKA decarboxylase (E1) alpha subunit (MSUD type 1A); BCKDHB, encoding BCKA decarboxylase (E1) beta subunit (MSUD type 1B); and DBT, encoding dihydrolipoyl transacylase (E2) subunit (MSUD type 2)

Provision of adequate calories and protein, **with restriction of leucine**, is crucial for acute and chronic management. Ordinary catabolic stresses, such as moderate infections or labor and delivery in a pregnant mother with MSUD, can precipitate clinical crises. The most feared complication of metabolic decompensation is brain edema. This requires careful management in an intensive care setting. Liver transplantation effectively treats MSUD.

DISORDERS OF AMMONIA DISPOSAL

Inherited enzymatic deficiencies have been described for each of the steps of urea synthesis (Fig. 53.4). Neonatal screening does not currently detect all of the disorders in the urea cycle. Clinically the two most frequent disorders in the United States are ornithine carbamoyltransferase (OTC) deficiency and argininosuccinate lyase (ASL) deficiency.

OTC deficiency is X-linked. Pathogenic variants range from whole gene deletions to single nucleotide substitutions. If the enzyme is nonfunctional, there is no OTC activity in affected males, who are likely to die in the neonatal period. Affected females are heterozygous and, because of lyonization, may have a significant degree of enzyme deficiency; they may become clinically affected at any time in life. **Clinical manifestations** range from lethal disease in the male (coma, encephalopathy) to clinical normalcy in a high percentage of females. Late-onset forms in males also occur. Manifestations in clinically affected females include recurrent emesis, lethargy, seizures, developmental delay, psychosis, or episodic confusion. Affected females may spontaneously limit their protein intake.

Confirmatory testing for OTC includes a plasma amino acid profile, which may show reduced citrulline and arginine concentrations with increased glutamate and alanine. A urine organic acid profile may show increased excretion of orotic acid after protein loading or with concurrent administration of allopurinol. Known pathogenic variant testing, deletion testing, and sequencing of the entire coding region of the OTC gene are available as clinical testing.

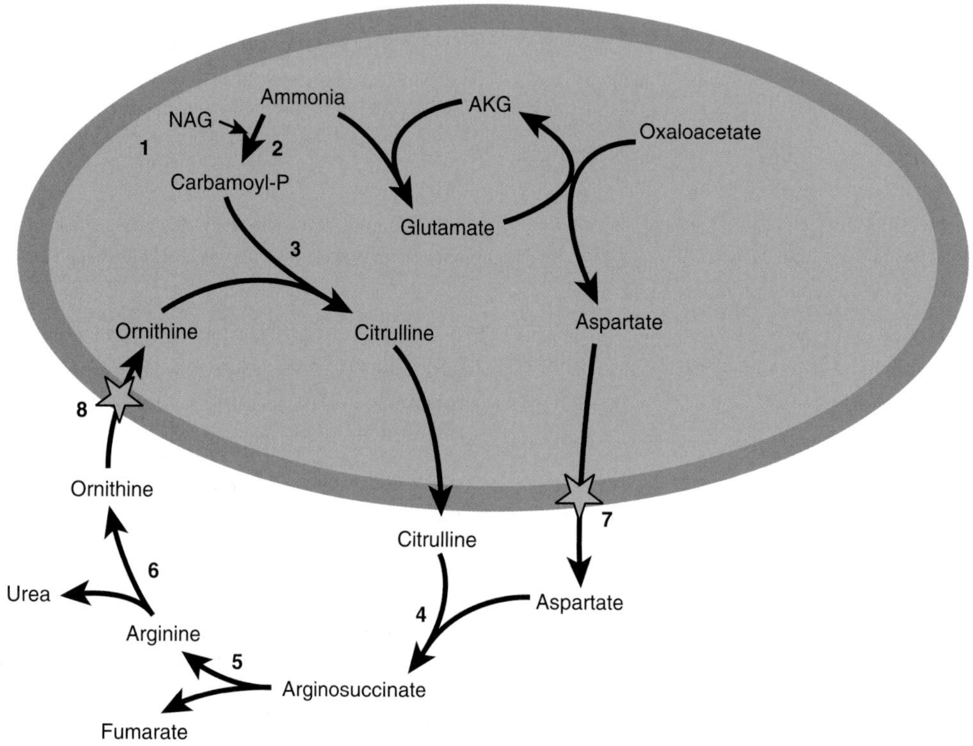

FIGURE 53.4 The urea cycle. Site of enzymatic defects: (1) *N*-acetylglutamate synthase *(NAG)*, (2) carbamoylphosphate synthetase, (3) ornithine carbamoyltransferase, (4) argininosuccinate acid synthetase, (5) argininosuccinate acid lyase, (6) arginase. Transporters *(star)*: (7) citrin, (8) ornithine translocator *(star)*. *AKG*, Alpha ketoglutarate.

ASL deficiency is autosomal recessive, and most children in the United States are detected as a result of an elevated citrulline on newborn screening. The diagnosis is confirmed by the detection of elevated argininosuccinic acid in the urine.

Treatment of Hyperammonemia

During episodes of symptomatic hyperammonemia, protein intake is reduced, and intravenous glucose is given in sufficient quantity to suppress catabolism of endogenous protein. Ammonia can be eliminated by use of the **alternate pathway** agents, **sodium benzoate** and **sodium phenylacetate**, which are excreted in the urine as conjugates of glycine and glutamine. Arginine, which is usually deficient, is supplied. When ammonia levels are very high (>1,000 μM) or refractory to therapy, direct removal of ammonia using hemodialysis or hemofiltration, but not peritoneal dialysis, is required. The neurological status must be followed closely and cerebral edema treated promptly. Despite successful management of hyperammonemic crises, the long-term outcome for males with severe neonatal OTC deficiency and all children with severe ASL deficiency is guarded. Early liver transplantation has increased survival, especially in males with severe OTC deficiency.

Restriction of dietary protein intake to daily needs is the mainstay of ongoing treatment for urea cycle defects. Crystalline essential amino acids can be supplied in amounts just sufficient to support protein synthesis. Arginine is an essential amino acid when arginine synthesis via the urea cycle is grossly impaired; thus arginine or citrulline must be supplied except in the case of arginase deficiency. Ongoing maintenance treatment with phenylbutyrate (which is metabolized to phenylacetate) prevents accumulation of ammonia.

DISORDERS OF AMINO ACID TRANSPORT THAT AFFECT SPECIFIC TRANSPORT MECHANISMS IN THE KIDNEY AND INTESTINE

Cystinuria is a disorder of renal tubular transport of cystine, lysine, arginine, and ornithine. Although intestinal transport is affected in some genetic forms, the symptoms are largely due to the renal transport abnormality. The concentration of cystine exceeds its solubility product and results in significant renal stones. Evaluation and diagnosis are based on the pattern of amino acid excretion in the urine. DNA testing is likely to be informative. **Treatment** is based on increasing the solubility of cystine by complexing it with compounds such as penicillamine.

Intestinal transport of tryptophan is impaired in **Hartnup syndrome**; pellagra-like symptoms result from this deficiency. Diagnosis is based on the amino acid pattern in urine. Treatment with tryptophan improves outcomes.

CHAPTER 54

Organic Acid Disorders

DISORDERS OF ORGANIC ACID METABOLISM

Organic acid disorders result from a block in the pathways of amino acid catabolism. Occurring after the amino moiety has been removed, they result in the accumulation of specific organic acids in the blood and urine. Treatment is directed at the specific abnormality, with restriction of precursor substrates and administration of enzyme cofactors, when available. Outcome is generally poor for children with neonatal-onset propionic or methylmalonic acidemia but is influenced by frequency and severity of crises and is optimal when diagnosis is made before the onset of the first episode. Liver transplantation has been used in some patients with early indicators of success. Confirmatory testing begins with a urine organic acid profile and plasma amino acid profile. More specific testing often requires enzyme measurements in appropriate tissues. When abnormal results suggest a specific disorder, DNA testing may identify the pathogenic variants involved.

PROPIONIC ACIDEMIA AND METHYLMALONIC ACIDEMIA

Propionic acidemia and methylmalonic acidemia result from defects in a series of reactions called the propionate pathway (Fig. 54.1). Defects in these steps produce **ketosis** and **hyperglycinemia**. Propionic acidemia and methylmalonic acidemia are identified by neonatal screening with tandem mass spectrometry methods. The **clinical manifestations** of both of these disorders in the neonatal period consist of tachypnea, vomiting, lethargy, coma, intermittent ketoacidosis, hyperglycinemia, neutropenia, thrombocytopenia, hyperammonemia, and hypoglycemia. If these disorders are not identified by neonatal screening, intermittent episodes of metabolic acidosis occur. Crises occur during periods of catabolic stress, such as fever, vomiting, and diarrhea; they also may occur without an apparent precipitating event. During periods of neutropenia, the risk of serious bacterial infection is increased. Failure to thrive and impaired development are common.

Propionic acidemia results from deficiency in propionyl coenzyme A (CoA)-carboxylase, an enzyme that has two pairs of identical subunits. All forms of propionic acidemia are inherited in an autosomal recessive manner and are due to pathogenic variants in one of the subunits. **Methylmalonic acidemia** results from deficiency in methylmalonyl mutase; this may be caused by pathogenic variants in the gene for the mutase protein itself or in one of the steps of the synthesis of the cobalamin (B12) cofactors for the enzyme. A complex set of defects in cobalamin metabolism results in other forms of methylmalonic acidemia, some of which are associated with hyperhomocystinemia. **Treatment** with large doses of hydroxocobalamin (the active form of vitamin B12) is helpful in some cases of methylmalonic acidemia.

For propionic acidemia and the vitamin B12–unresponsive forms of methylmalonic acidemia, management includes the restriction of dietary protein and addition of a medical food deficient in the specific amino acid precursors of propionyl-CoA (isoleucine, valine, methionine, and threonine). Carnitine supplementation is often needed because it is lost in the urine as acylcarnitines. Intestinal bacteria produce a significant quantity of propionate; thus antibacterial treatment to reduce the population of bacteria in the gut has some beneficial effect in propionic acidemia and vitamin B12–unresponsive methylmalonic acidemia.

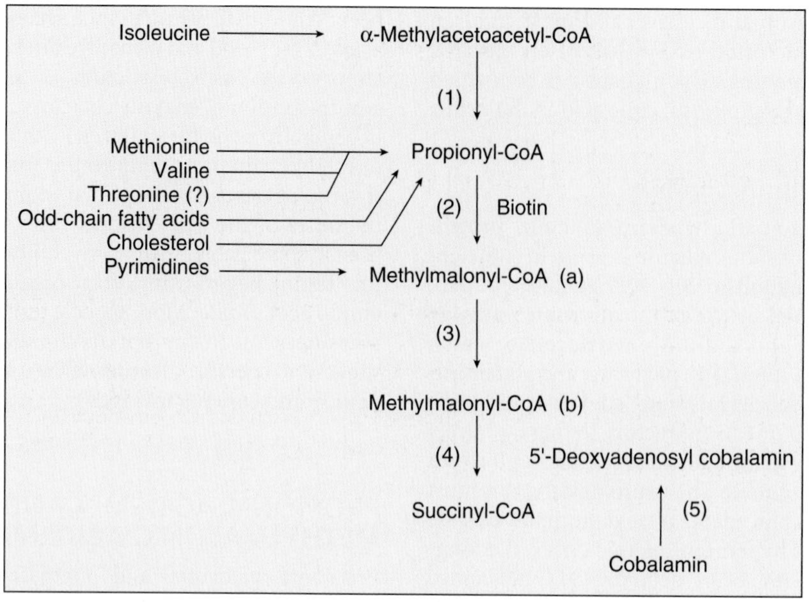

FIGURE 54.1 The propionate pathway. (1) β-Ketothiolase, (2) propionyl-CoA carboxylase, (3) methylmalonyl-CoA isomerase, (4) methylmalonyl-CoA mutase, (5) cobalamin metabolic pathway. *CoA*, Coenzyme A.

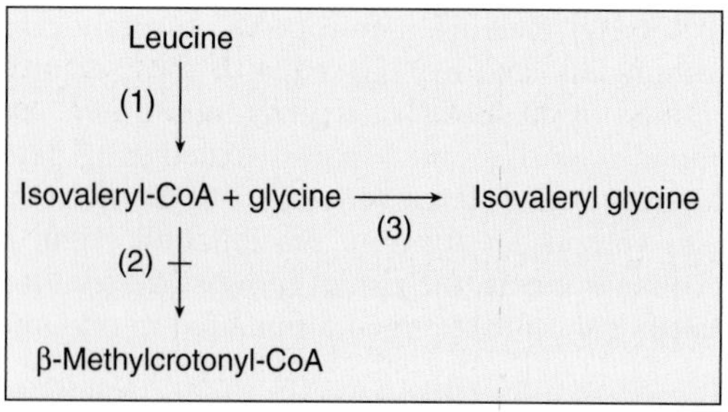

FIGURE 54.2 Metabolism in isovaleric acidemia. (1) Leucine catabolic pathway (transamination and decarboxylation), (2) isovaleryl-CoA dehydrogenase, (3) glycine acyltransferase. *CoA*, Coenzyme A.

ISOVALERIC ACIDEMIA

Isovaleric acidemia results from a block in the catabolism of leucine. Its clinical manifestations are similar to those of defects in the propionate pathway. The strong odor of isovaleric acid results in **sweaty feet odor** in untreated infants. Therapy involves restricting the intake of leucine and providing glycine as an alternate pathway therapy that conjugates isovaleric acid (Fig. 54.2) and is then excreted in the urine.

GLUTARIC ACIDEMIA I

Glutaric acidemia I results from a deficiency at the end of the lysine catabolic pathway. It is an autosomal recessive disease produced by deficiency of glutaryl-CoA dehydrogenase activity (Fig. 54.3). **Clinical manifestations** include **macrocephaly** (although head circumference may be in the normal range), which may be present at birth. Before the advent of newborn screening, more than 70% of children had *metabolic strokelike episodes* associated with infarction of the basal ganglia and **dystonia**, which characteristically develops after an episode of intercurrent illness, although it may reflect birth stress or prenatal insults. **Treatment** includes a protein-restricted diet accompanied by a medical food deficient in lysine and aggressive management of intercurrent illness. Despite this treatment, as many as one third of children still develop neurological symptoms.

BIOTINIDASE DEFICIENCY AND HOLOCARBOXYLASE DEFICIENCY

Biotin is a ubiquitous vitamin that is covalently linked to many carboxylases and cannot be recycled from its attachment to the carboxylases. Thus inherited biotinidase deficiency greatly increases the dietary requirement for biotin. Affected individuals become biotin deficient while consuming normal diets. Clinical disease can appear in the neonatal period or be delayed until later infancy, depending on the degree of deficiency.

Clinical manifestations of biotin deficiency vary greatly (seizures, hypotonia, sensory neural deafness, alopecia, skin rash, metabolic acidosis, immune deficits) and depend on which enzymes in which tissues have the most biotin depletion. Carboxylation is a crucial reaction in the metabolism of organic acids; most patients with biotinidase deficiency excrete abnormal amounts of several organic acids, among which β-methylcrotonylglycine is prominent. In addition to biotinidase deficiency, an inherited deficiency of holocarboxylase synthetase gives rise to severe disease and to similar patterns of organic aciduria. Both conditions respond well to **treatment** with large doses of biotin (5–20 mg/day). Confirmatory testing is accomplished with quantitative measurement of biotinidase activity.

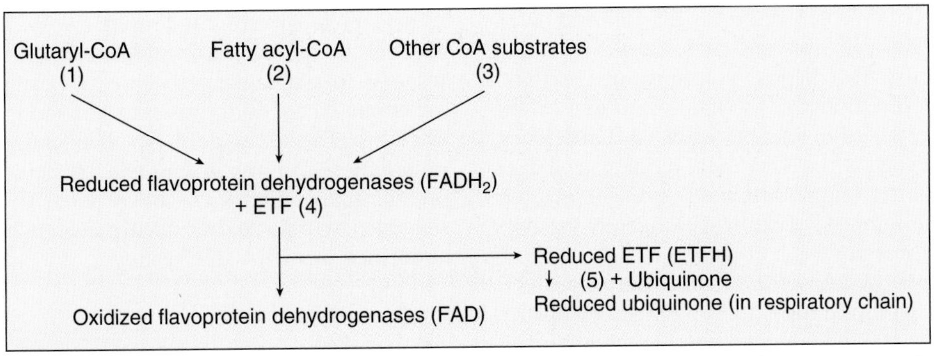

FIGURE 54.3 Scheme of flavoprotein metabolism with reference to glutaric aciduria types I and II. (1) Glutaryl-CoA dehydrogenase (deficient in glutaric aciduria type1), (2) fatty acyl-CoA dehydrogenases, (3) other flavoprotein dehydrogenases, (4) ETF (deficiency results in glutaric aciduria type II), (5) ETF-ubiquinone oxidoreductase (deficiency results in glutaric aciduria type II). *CoA*, Coenzyme A; *ETF*, electron transfer flavoprotein.

CHAPTER 55

Disorders of Fat Metabolism

DISORDERS OF FATTY ACID OXIDATION

Fatty acids are derived from hydrolysis of triglycerides and catabolism of fat. The catabolism of fatty acids (Fig. 55.1) proceeds through the serial, oxidative removal of two carbons at a time as acetyl groups (each as acetyl-coenzyme A [CoA]). The reactions are catalyzed by a group of enzymes that exhibit specificities related to the chain length and other properties of the fatty acids: very-long-chain acyl-CoA dehydrogenase (VLCAD), long-chain hydroxyacyl-CoA dehydrogenase (LCHAD) or trifunctional protein, medium-chain acyl-CoA dehydrogenase (MCAD), and short-chain acyl-CoA dehydrogenase (SCAD).

MCAD deficiency is the most common inborn error of β-oxidation. Hypoketotic hypoglycemia is a common

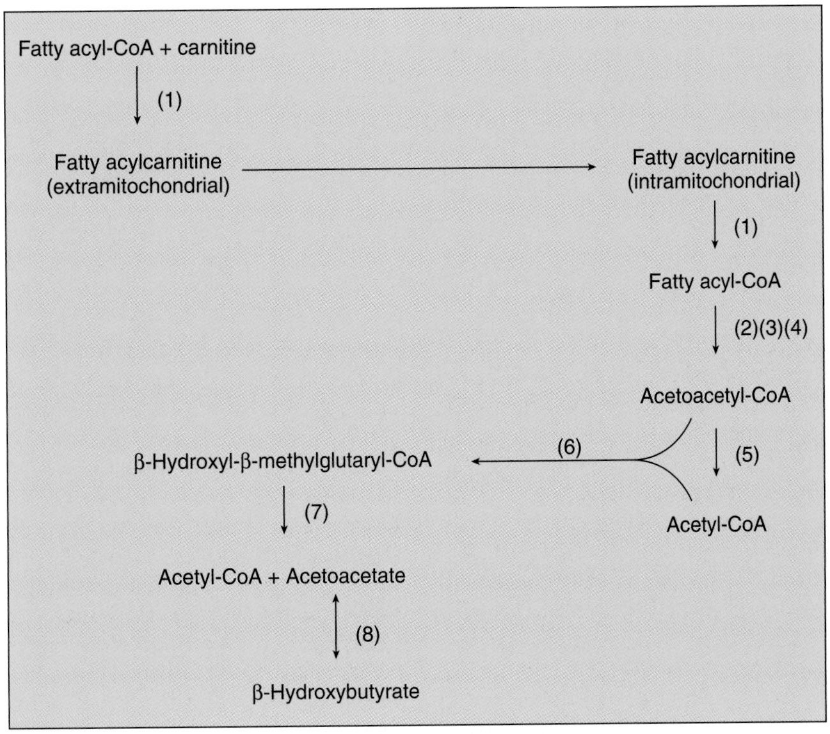

FIGURE 55.1 Scheme of fatty acid and catabolism and ketone body formation. (1) Carnitine acyl-CoA dehydrogenases, (2) long-chain fatty acyl-CoA dehydrogenase (trifunctional protein), (3) medium-chain fatty acyl-CoA dehydrogenase, (4) short-chain fatty acyl-CoA dehydrogenase, (5) β-ketothiolase, (6) β-hydroxy-β-methylglutaryl-CoA synthase, (7) β-hydroxy-β-methylglutaryl-CoA lyase, (8) β-hydroxybutyrate dehydrogenase. *CoA*, Coenzyme A.

manifestation, as is a Reye syndrome–like illness with hypoglycemia and elevated liver enzymes. Fatty infiltration of the liver also occurs. True hepatic failure is rare. Episodes may be recurrent in the patient or the family. **Sudden infant death syndrome** is reported in infants with MCAD deficiency, perhaps related to hypoglycemia. **Treatment** requires avoidance of fasting and provision of calories with fever or other metabolic stress. In a vomiting infant or child, this frequently requires parenteral (intravenous) provision of dextrose.

VLCAD deficiency and LCHAD (trifunctional protein) deficiency result in significant myopathy and cardiomyopathy. This cardiomyopathy may be rapidly reversed with appropriate dietary treatment. LCHAD deficiency is accompanied by a retinopathy in later childhood. In all of the disorders of β-oxidation, carnitine depletion can occur through excessive urinary excretion of carnitine esters of the incompletely oxidized fatty acids. Measurement of plasma carnitine is helpful in monitoring for this deficiency, which results in weakness and muscle pain, along with myoglobinuria in some people.

Hydroxymethylglutaryl-CoA lyase deficiency, although not a disorder of β-oxidation, interferes profoundly with hepatic adaptation to fasting by impairing ketogenesis (see Fig. 55.1). The clinical manifestations are those of MCAD deficiency, except that carnitine depletion is less prominent.

The diagnosis of disorders involving a deficiency of β-oxidation is suggested by the clinical picture and by **hypoketotic hypoglycemia.** The diagnosis is suggested by abnormal urinary organic acid and acylglycine profiles, along with plasma acylcarnitine and free fatty acid profiles. Enzyme measurements and/or DNA testing are required to confirm the diagnosis. The profile of acylcarnitines in cultured skin fibroblasts may be helpful if other testing is not conclusive. In MCAD deficiency a single pathogenic variant c.985 A→G accounts for a significant percentage of cases, especially among children of Northern European ancestry. **Treatment** includes avoidance of fasting, as well as fluid and calorie supplementation during periods of metabolic stress, such as fever. In MCAD deficiency, medium-chain triglycerides must be avoided. In the long-chain fatty acid metabolic disorders, provision of medium-chain fatty acids improves muscle energy metabolism.

GLUTARIC ACIDURIA TYPE II

Glutaric aciduria type II (multiple acyl-CoA dehydrogenase deficiency) is a clinical disease produced by a defect in the transfer of electrons from flavine adenine nucleotides to the electron transport chain (electron transfer flavoprotein [ETF], or ETF dehydrogenase); this defect results in a deficiency of multiple fatty acyl-CoA dehydrogenases (see Fig. 55.1). It should not be confused with glutaric acidemia type I (see Chapter 54). When the enzyme essentially is nonfunctional, congenital anomalies are common, including renal cysts, facial abnormalities, rocker-bottom feet, and hypospadias. Severely affected infants have nonketotic hypoglycemia, metabolic acidosis, and the odor of sweaty feet soon after birth; these infants may die within the neonatal period. Less severely affected infants may have a more episodic, Reye syndrome–like illness. Skeletal and cardiac myopathy can be prominent in this complex, multisystemic disease. Onset in later childhood may be marked by recurrent hypoglycemia and myopathy. **Treatment** has not been effective in infants with complete deficiency. Milder forms respond to avoidance of fasting and caloric support during metabolic stress. Some patients respond to administration of riboflavin. Glutaric aciduria type II exhibits autosomal recessive inheritance. Clinical testing will typically include abnormal organic acid and acylcarnitine profiles. The diagnosis may be suggested by abnormal fatty acid oxidation studies. It is typically confirmed through DNA testing.

CARNITINE DEFICIENCY

Carnitine is a crucial cofactor in the transport of long-chain fatty acids across the mitochondrial inner membrane (see Fig. 55.1). It is synthesized from lysine by humans and is present in dietary red meat and dairy products. Carnitine deficiency is either primary (caused by failure of intake, synthesis, or transport of carnitine) or secondary (caused by the excretion of excessive amounts of carnitine as carnityl esters in patients with other inborn errors of metabolism; treatment with drugs that complex carnitine, such as valproic acid; or as a result of renal replacement therapy). Primary systemic carnitine deficiency is rare and results from inadequate renal reabsorption of carnitine secondary to pathogenic variants in the sodium-dependent carnitine transporter. It responds well to carnitine supplementation. There are numerous examples of secondary carnitine deficiency among the organic acidurias, most prominently in disorders of the propionate pathway and in disorders of the β-oxidation of long-chain and medium-chain fatty acids. Clinical manifestations of carnitine deficiency include hypoketotic hypoglycemia, lethargy, lassitude, muscle weakness, sudden death, and cardiomyopathy.

CHAPTER 56 Lysosomal and Peroxisomal Disorders

PEROXISOMAL DISORDERS

Peroxisomes are subcellular organelles involved in metabolism and biosynthesis of bile acids, membrane phospholipids, and some β-oxidation of long-chain fatty acids. Disorders include conditions caused by abnormal peroxisomal enzyme function and abnormal peroxisomal biogenesis. **Clinical symptoms** are diverse and frequently include **developmental delay** and **dysmorphic features** that can involve the skeleton and the head. Zellweger syndrome, neonatal adrenoleukodystrophy, and infantile Refsum disease are examples of disorders of peroxisome biogenesis. **Zellweger syndrome,** an autosomal recessive disease (1 : 100,000 births), is also called *cerebrohepatorenal syndrome.* Peroxisomes are virtually absent, as are normal peroxisomal functions, which include the oxidation of very-long-chain fatty acids (VLCFAs). Affected infants have high foreheads, flat orbital ridges, widely open fontanelles, hepatomegaly, and hypotonia. Other anomalies are common. Failure to thrive, seizures, and nystagmus develop early, and death occurs within the first year. Refsum disease, neonatal adrenoleukodystrophy, and malonic aciduria are examples of peroxisomal single-enzyme disorders. Diagnostic testing includes measurement of VLCFAs in plasma and pipecolic acid in urine. Specific molecular testing, particularly for the disorders involving one in the series of *PEX* genes, is available for some disorders. Most of these conditions are untreatable; however, bone marrow transplant can be helpful in X-linked adrenoleukodystrophy (X-ALD) before the onset of severe symptoms.

X-ALD has been added to the recommended uniform screening panel (RUSP). This disorder, which affects 1 : 20,000 males, is caused by a defect in a peroxisomal membrane protein. There are three main phenotypes seen in males with pathogenic variants in this gene: Childhood onset cerebral form, adrenomyeloneuropathy (AMN), and "Addison disease." Approximately 20% of carrier females will develop a milder form of the AMN phenotype. The phenotype of affected males cannot be predicted by analyte (VLCFA) levels or by genotype. The childhood cerebral form is a severe progressive disease that typically presents with inattentive symptoms and can progress to total disability within 6 months. Hematopoietic stem cell transplantation (HSCT) should be considered for boys in the early stages of the cerebral form who have evidence of brain involvement on MRI. Because of the significant risks, HSCT is recommended for individuals with evidence of brain involvement by MRI and minimal neuropsychological findings (performance IQ >80) with a normal clinical neurological examination. Corticosteroid replacement therapy can be lifesaving in individuals with AMN or Addison only presentation. The most sensitive indicators of adrenal dysfunction are elevated plasma ACTH and impaired cortisol response to ACTH challenge.

LYSOSOMAL STORAGE DISORDERS

Lysosomes are subcellular organelles that contain degradative enzymes for complex **glycosaminoglycans**, also called **mucopolysaccharides**. Glycosaminoglycans are macromolecules that play a number of roles within cells. Genetic disorders result from abnormal formation of the lysosome itself or from deficiency in specific hydrolytic enzymes, in the mechanisms that protect intralysosomal enzymes from hydrolytic destruction, or in the transport of materials into the lysosome and of metabolites out of the lysosome. These materials are stored in cells and ultimately result in their destruction, especially in the nervous system. The clinical disorders are diverse, reflecting tissue specificity of lysosomal function and the intrinsic turnover rates of the compounds whose cycling is affected (Table 56.1). Some disorders are apparent only during adult life. Storage in solid organs results in hepatosplenomegaly. Some disorders affect many tissues but spare the brain, with some having almost exclusive involvement of the musculoskeletal system. In many of these disorders, developmental delay, corneal clouding, and limitation of joint mobility are common features. Storage in tissues of the upper and lower airways may result in respiratory compromise. Nonimmune hydrops fetalis occurs in several lysosomal disorders.

DIAGNOSTIC TESTING

Most cases of Pompe (see Chapter 52) and MPS1 will be detected on newborn blood spot screening, in states that have adopted this testing. However, this testing has a significant false-positive rate. Diagnostic testing includes measurement of glycosaminoglycans in urine and specific assays for lysosomal enzyme activity in white blood cells. If the urine test is positive, it helps direct specific enzyme measurement. If it is negative, it does not exclude a lysosomal storage disorder, and other testing modalities are needed if clinical signs are convincing. In disorders in which specific pathogenic variants are known, molecular testing refines the diagnosis and is an important way to resolve disease status in infants with a positive newborn screen. Specific diagnosis, carrier testing, and evaluation of at-risk family members often require a multipronged approach to testing. Making a specific diagnosis is assuming increasing importance because specific treatment for some lysosomal disorders is most effective when started early in the disease course.

TREATMENT STRATEGIES

Specific treatment directed at the metabolic abnormality is available for some lysosomal disorders. In specific disorders (e.g., Gaucher disease), oral medication may be successful in reducing the accumulation of the metabolite that cannot be catabolized. For some disorders, bone marrow (stem cell) transplantation is the most efficacious mechanism to restore lysosomal function. For others, replacement of the missing hydrolytic enzyme by systemic administration of the enzyme allows degradation of stored material. The disorders caused by deficient α-L-iduronidase (MPS1, Hurler syndrome, Scheie syndrome, and their variants) respond to treatment with intravenous human recombinant α-L-iduronidase (laronidase). Other disorders for which enzyme therapy is available include MPS VI (Maroteaux-Lamy syndrome), Gaucher disease, Fabry disease, and MPS II (Hunter syndrome). Stem cell transplantation or ex vivo gene therapy has been helpful or are under investigation in the following disorders: MPS type IH (Hurler syndrome), MPS type VI (Maroteaux-Lamy syndrome), MPS type VII (Sly syndrome), metachromatic leukodystrophy, alpha-fucosidosis, alpha-mannosidosis, Gaucher disease, and Niemann-Pick disease type B. A discussion of appropriate target therapeutic strategies should be held with patients and their relevant caregivers by an expert in the specific disorder. Nonetheless, treatment for many of these conditions is supportive, with careful attention to respiratory status and physical therapy. As a result of the rapidly changing diagnostic and therapeutic options, providers with a special interest in these disorders should be consulted when a diagnosis is suspected. Treatment decisions should be made by the family in the light of the potential therapeutic benefits and burdens of therapy and typically should be resolved before the onset of central nervous system manifestations, which are typically not improved by these approaches.

TABLE 56.1 Lysosomal Storage Diseases

DISEASE (EPONYM)	ENZYME DEFICIENCY	CLINICAL ONSET	DYSOSTOSIS MULTIPLEX	CORNEA	RETINA	LIVER, SPLEEN	CNS FINDINGS	STORED MATERIAL IN URINE	WBC/ BONE MARROW	COMMENT	MULTIPLE FORMS
MUCOPOLYSACCHARIDOSES (MPS)											
MPS I (Hurler)	α-L-Iduronidase	~1 yr	Yes	Cloudy	—	Both enlarged	Profound loss of function	Acid mucopolysaccharide	Alder-Reilly bodies (WBC)	Kyphosis On RUSP	Yes—Scheie and compounds
MPS II (Hunter)	Iduronate-2-sulfatase	1-2 yr	Yes	Clear	Retinal degeneration, papilledema	Both enlarged	Slow loss of function	Acid mucopolysaccharide	Alder-Reilly bodies (WBC)	X-linked	Yes
MPS III (Sanfilippo)	One of several degrading heparan SO_4s	2-6 yr	Mild	Clear	—	Liver ± enlarged	Rapid loss of function	Acid mucopolysaccharide	Alder-Reilly bodies (WBC)	—	Several types biochemically
MPS IV (Morquiro)	Galactose-6-sulfatase or β-galactosidase	2 yr	No, dwarfism deformities	Faint clouding	—	–	Normal	Acid mucopolysaccharide	Alder-Reilly bodies (WBC)	—	Yes
MPS VI (Maroteaux-Lamy)	*N*-Acetylgalactosamine-4-sulfatase	2 yr	Yes	Cloudy	—	Normal in size	Normal	Acid mucopolysaccharide	Alder-Reilly bodies (WBC)	—	Yes
MPS VII (Sly)	β-Glucuronidase	Variable neonatal	Yes	± Cloudy	—	Both enlarged	± Affected	Acid mucopolysaccharide	Alder-Reilly bodies (WBC)	Nonimmune hydrops	Yes
LIPIDOSES											
Glucosylceramide lipidosis (Gaucher 1)	Glucocerebrosidase	Any age	No	Clear	Normal	Both enlarged	Normal	No	Gaucher cells in marrow	Bone pain fractures	Variability is the rule
Glucosylceramide lipidosis 2 (Gaucher 2)	Glucocerebrosidase	Fetal life-2nd yr	No	Clear	Normal	Both enlarged	Profound loss of function	No	Gaucher cells in marrow	—	Yes
Sphingomyelin lipidosis A (Niemann-Pick A)	Sphingomyelinase	1st mo	No	Clear	Cherry red spots (50%)	Both enlarged	Profound loss of function	No	Foam cells in marrow	—	No
Sphingomyelin lipidosis B (Niemann-Pick B)	Sphingomyelinase	1st mo or later	No	Clear	Normal	Both enlarged	Normal	No	Foam cells in marrow	—	Yes
Niemann-Pick C	Lysosomal cholesterol; trafficking (*NPC1* gene)	Fetal life to adolescence	No	Clear	Normal	Enlarged	Vertical ophthalmoplegia, dystonia, cataplexy, seizures	No	Foam cells and sea-blue histiocytes in marrow	Pathogenesis not as for NP-A and NP-B	Lethal neonatal to adolescent onset

Continued

GM_2 gangliosidosis (Tay-Sachs)	Hexosaminidase A	3-6 mo	No	Clear	Cherry red spots	Normal	Profound loss of function	No		Normal	Sandhoff disease related	Yes
Generalized gangliosidosis (infantile) (GM_1)	β-Galactosidase	Neonatal to 1st mo	Yes	Clear	Cherry red spots (50%)	Both enlarged	Profound loss of function	No		Inclusion in WBC	—	Yes
Metachromatic leukodystrophy	Arylsulfatase A	1-2 yr	No	Clear	Normal	Normal	Profound loss of function	No		Normal	—	Yes
Fabry disease	α-Galactosidase A (cerebrosidase)	Childhood, adolescence	No	Cloudy by slit lamp	—	Liver may be enlarged	Normal	No		Normal	X-linked	No
Galactosyl-ceramide lipidosis (Krabbe)	Galactocerebroside β-galactosidase	Early months	No	Clear	Optic atrophy	Normal	Profound loss of function	No		Normal	Storage not lysosomal	Yes
Wolman disease	Acid lipase	Neonatal	No	Clear	Normal	Both enlarged	Profound loss of function	No		Inclusion in WBC	New therapy recently approved	Yes
Farber lipogranulomatosis	Acid ceramidase	1st 4 mo	No	Usually clear	Cherry red spots (12%)	May be enlarged	Normal or impaired	Usually not		—	Arthritis, nodules	Yes
MUCOLIPIDOSES (ML) AND CLINICALLY RELATED DISEASE												
Sialidosis II (formerly ML I)	Neuraminidase	Neonatal	Yes	Cloudy	Cherry red spot	Both enlarged	Yes		Oligosaccharides	Vacuolated lymphocytes	—	Yes (also see galactosiali-dosis)
Sialidosis I (formerly ML I)	Neuraminidase	Usually second decade	No	Fine opacities	Cherry red spot	Normal	Myoclonus, seizures		Oligosaccharides	Usually none	Cherry red spot/ myoclonus syndrome	Severity varies
Galactosialidosis	Absence of PP/CathA causes loss of neuraminidase and β-galactosidase	Usually second decade	Frequent	Clouding	Cherry red spot	Occasionally enlarged	Myoclonus, seizures Mental retardation		Oligosaccharides	Foamy lymphocytes	Onset from 1 to 40 yr	Congenital and infantile forms such as sialidosis 2
ML II (I-cell disease)	Mannosyl phosphotransferase	Neonatal	Yes	Clouding	—	Liver often enlarged	Profound loss of function		Oligosaccharides	No	Gingival hyperplasia	No
ML III (pseudo-Hurler polydystrophy)	Mannosyl phosphotransferase	2-4 yr	Yes	Late clouding	Normal	Normal in size?	Modest loss of function		Oligosaccharides	No	—	No

Continued

TABLE 56.1 Lysosomal Storage Diseases—cont'd

DISEASE (EPONYM)	ENZYME DEFICIENCY	CLINICAL ONSET	DYSOSTOSIS MULTIPLEX	CORNEA	RETINA	LIVER, SPLEEN	CNS FINDINGS	STORED MATERIAL IN URINE	WBC/ BONE MARROW	COMMENT	MULTIPLE FORMS
Multiple sulfatase deficiency	Many sulfatases	1-2 yr	Yes	Usually clear	Usually normal	Both enlarged	Profound loss of function	Acid mucopolysaccharide	Alder-Reilly bodies (WBC)	Ichthyosis	Yes
Aspartylglyco-saminuria	Aspartylglucos-aminidase	6 mo	Mild	Clear	Normal	Early, not late	Profound loss of function	Aspartylgluco-samine	Inclusions in lymphocytes	Develop cataracts	No
Mannosidosis	α-Mannosidase	1st mo	Yes	Cloudy	—	Liver enlarged	Profound loss of function	Generally no	Inclusions in lymphocytes	Cataracts	Yes
Fucosidosis	α-L-Fucosidase	1st mo	Yes	Clear	May be pigmented	Both enlarged commonly	Profound loss of function	Oligosaccharides	Inclusions in lymphocytes	—	Yes
STORAGE DISEASES CAUSED BY DEFECTS IN LYSOSOMAL PROTEOLYSIS											
Neuronal ceroid lipofuscinosis (NCL), Batten disease	Impaired lysosomal proteolysis—various specific etiologies	6 mo-10 yr, adult form	No	Normal	May have brown pigment	Normal, distinct	Optic atrophy, seizures, dementia			Clinical picture consistent, time course variable	Etiologies for age-related forms
STORAGE DISEASES CAUSED BY DEFECTIVE SYNTHESIS OF THE LYSOSOMAL MEMBRANE											
Cardiomyopathy, myopathy, mental retardation, Danon disease	Lamp-2, a structural protein of lysosomes, is deficient	Usually 5-6 yr	No	Normal	Normal	Hepatomegaly	Delayed development, seizures			X-linked pediatric disease in males only	Variability in time course of signs
STORAGE DISEASES CAUSED BY DYSFUNCTION OF LYSOSOMAL TRANSPORT PROTEINS											
Nephropathic cystinosis	Defect in cystine transport from lysosome to cytoplasm	6 mo-1 yr	No	Cystine crystals	Pigmentary retinopathy	Hepatomegaly common	Normal CNS function	Generalized aminoaciduria	Elevated cystine in WBCs	Treatment with cysteamine is effective	Yes
Salla disease	Defect in sialic acid transport from lysosome to cytoplasm	6-9 mo	No	Normal	Normal	Normal	Delayed development, ataxia, nystagmus, exotropia	Sialic aciduria	Vacuolated lymphocytes may be found	Growth retarded in some	Lethal infantile form

CNS, Central nervous system; *RUSP*, recommended uniform screening panel; *WBC*, white blood cell.

CHAPTER 57

Mitochondrial Disorders

MITOCHONDRIAL FUNCTION

Mitochondria are very complex organelles located in virtually all cells of the body. They perform a variety of functions such as intracellular signaling of oxygen tension and key roles in programmed cell death. From a biochemical perspective, mitochondria are the key site of energy production in the cell. Indeed they are the site of β-oxidation (see Chapter 55), the Krebs cycle, and parts of the urea cycle (see Fig. 53.4). This complexity requires more than 1,000 proteins localized specifically to the mitochondrion. Only 13 of these are encoded by the mitochondrial DNA (mtDNA); the remainder are nuclear encoded (on the chromosomes) and require import into the mitochondrion. In addition, the mtDNA needs its own set of proteins to allow for its maintenance, transcription, and translation.

Mitochondrial disorders are typically defined as defects in the ability to generate energy from oxidative phosphorylation to produce adenosine triphosphate (ATP) by transferring electrons formed by glycolysis and the Krebs cycle to a cascade that generates NADH and $FADH_2$ (Fig. 57.1) and are also known as phosphorylation disorders or respiratory chain disorders. The more dependent on energy production an organ is, the more profound the symptoms of deficiency of mitochondrial function in that organ. Certain proteins are only expressed in specific tissues, and defects in these will lead to differing patterns of disease. Taken together, mitochondrial disorders may affect as many as 1 in 2,500 people.

SIGNS AND SYMPTOMS OF GENETIC DISORDERS OF MITOCHONDRIAL FUNCTION

The signs and symptoms of mitochondrial disorders are varied. Symptoms depend on how an organ is affected by energy deficiency. Muscle function that is compromised will result in muscle fatigue and weakness. Myopathy is common and may show **ragged red fibers** on a muscle biopsy. **Rhabdomyolysis** can occur. Brain dysfunction may be expressed as seizures, loss of intellectual function, headache, or signs consistent with stroke. Spastic paraplegia may occur. Ataxia and basal ganglia symptoms are features of some disorders. Vision and eye muscle movement

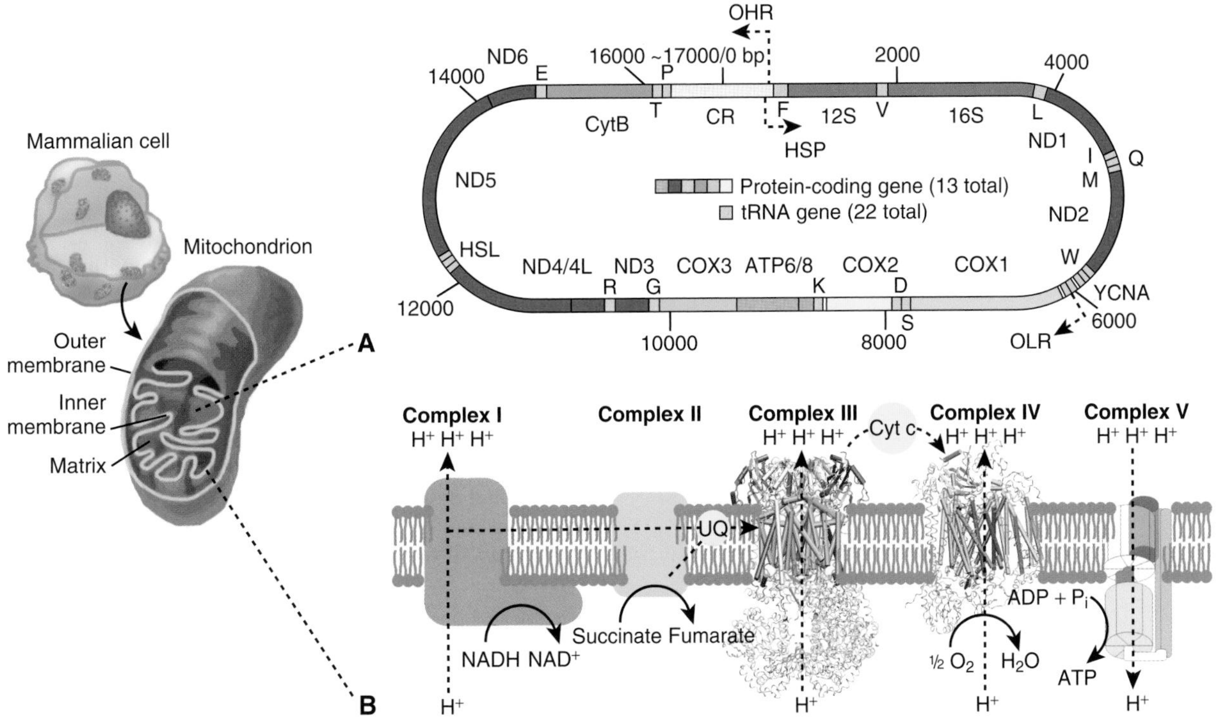

FIGURE 57.1 The mammalian mitochondrial genome and its protein-coding gene repertoire involved in the oxidative phosphorylation pathway. (A) Schematic representation of genes within mammalian mitochondrial genome (~7,000 bp). Genes on the outer circle are transcribed from the light strand. Location of the tRNAs *(red boxes)* conforms to the canonical placental mammalian arrangement. (B) Simplified view of the mitochondrial oxidative phosphorylation machinery. Complexes I (NADH dehydrogenase) and II (succinate dehydrogenase) receive electrons from either NADH or FADH2. Electrons are then carried between complexes by the carrier molecules coenzyme Q/ubiquinone (UQ) and cytochrome c (CYC). The potential energy of these electron transfer events is used to pump protons against the gradient, from the mitochondrial matrix into the intermembrane space (complexes I and III [cytochrome bc_1] and IV [CYC oxidase]). ATP synthesis by complex V (ATP synthase) is driven by the proton gradient and occurs in the mitochondrial matrix. *HSP*, Putative heavy-strand promoter; *IM*, intermembrane space; *MM*, mitochondrial matrix; *OHR*, origin of heavy-strand replication; *OLR*, origin of light-strand replication. (From da Fonseca RR, Johnson WE, O'Brien SJ, et al. The adaptive evolution of the mammalian mitochondrial genome. *BMC Genomics*. 2008;9:119.)

may be compromised, with **progressive external ophthalmoplegia** being almost diagnostic of an oxidative phosphorylation defect. **Cardiomyopathy** is frequent, and cardiac rhythm disturbances occur. Liver dysfunction may be expressed as both synthetic deficiencies and frank liver failure. Diabetes may signal pancreatic involvement. Renal tubular abnormalities and renal failure both occur. Gastrointestinal symptoms include both diarrhea and constipation that are difficult to treat. **Alper disease** (cerebral degeneration and liver disease) and **Leigh disease** (subacute necrotizing encephalomyelopathy) show similar brain lesions but in distinctly different areas of the brain. Because the signs and symptoms may involve multiple organs and may seem nonspecific, physicians may not suspect a mitochondrial disorder until significant progression has occurred. Conversely, because there are no reliable tests to exclude a mitochondrial diagnosis, a high degree of confidence should be required before labeling a child as having a mitochondrial disease.

BIOCHEMICAL ABNORMALITIES IN MITOCHONDRIAL FUNCTION

Defects in the mitochondrial respiratory chain may produce **lactic acidosis**. Given the complexity of the respiratory chain, it is not surprising that the described defects are varied as to cause, intensity, and tissues affected. The metabolism of glucose to carbon dioxide and water, with pyruvate as an intermediate (Fig. 57.2), occurs as part of the energy cycle in many tissues. Interference with mitochondrial oxidative metabolism may result in the accumulation of pyruvate. Because lactate dehydrogenase is ubiquitous, and because the equilibrium catalyzed by this enzyme greatly favors lactate over pyruvate, the accumulation of pyruvate results in lactic acidosis. The most common cause of such lactic acidosis is end-organ oxygen deficiency caused by hypoxia or poor perfusion. Lactic acidosis also occurs when specific reactions of pyruvate are impaired. In the liver, pyruvate undergoes carboxylation to form oxaloacetate using the enzyme pyruvate carboxylase; deficiency in this enzyme causes severe lactic acidosis. In many tissues, lactate is catabolized to form acetyl-coenzyme A (CoA) by the pyruvate dehydrogenase complex; deficiency in pyruvate dehydrogenase also can cause lactic acidosis. Because these reactions also play a role in gluconeogenesis, hypoglycemia can be a feature of these disorders. These disorders comprise forms of **primary lactic acidosis**. They frequently present as intractable, lethal acidosis in the first days or weeks of life and are difficult to treat. Some of the enzymes in this pathway can be measured and specific diagnosis can be made. This may require white blood cells or tissue biopsy.

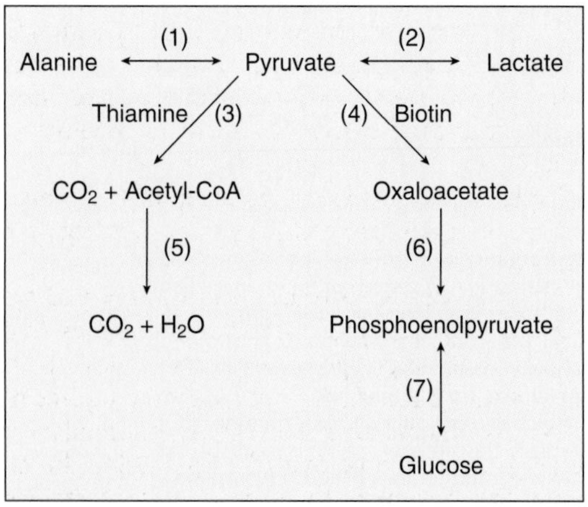

FIGURE 57.2 Metabolism of pyruvate and lactate. *(1)* Alanine aminotransferase, *(2)* lactate dehydrogenase, *(3)* pyruvate dehydrogenase, *(4)* pyruvate carboxylase, *(5)* Krebs cycle, *(6)* phosphoenolpyruvate carboxykinase, *(7)* reverse glycolysis. *CoA*, Coenzyme A.

GENETICS OF MITOCHONDRIAL DISORDERS

Mitochondrial function is carried out by proteins that are coded for by both nuclear and mitochondrial genes. These enzymes are extremely complicated, and several are quite large. The mitochondrial genome encodes 13 subunits of the enzymes involved in mitochondrial oxidative phosphorylation. More than 85 autosomal genes code for the rest of the subunits of these enzymes. In children, only about 15% of cases of mitochondrial disease are caused by pathogenic variants in mtDNA; the rest are due to pathogenic variants in nuclear genes. The most frequent cases in several large series have been pathogenic variants that lead to a reduction in the ability of the mtDNA to maintain itself. Large population studies show carrier rates of about 2% of the population for pathogenic variants in polymerase (DNA directed), gamma *(POLG)*, and deoxyguanosine kinase *(DGUOK)*. Most disorders show autosomal recessive inheritance. A few are X-linked or caused by pathogenic variants in the mtDNA inherited from the mother, such as mitochondrial encephalopathy with lactic acidosis **(MELAS)** and mitochondrial encephalopathy with ragged red fibers **(MERRF)**, or deletions such as maternally inherited diabetes and deafness **(MIDD)**.

TREATMENT OF MITOCHONDRIAL DISORDERS

Repairing the basic energy deficit and getting the appropriate drugs and cofactors to the appropriate location within the mitochondrion are difficult. Nevertheless, a number of strategies are used, including judicious physical therapy and exercise with adequate rest, adequate nutrition, and cofactors for the deficient pathway. Specific treatment is limited for most mitochondrial defects. Vitamin cofactors for the respiratory chain, such as riboflavin and pharmaceutical forms of coenzyme Q, are often used. When a single organ bears most of the damage, organ transplant may be effective. Identification of family members at risk may allow earlier diagnosis and treatment.

Suggested Readings

Ah Mew N, Lanpher BC, Gropman A, et al. Urea cycle disorders consortium urea cycle disorders overview. In: Pagon RA, Adam MP, Ardinger HH, et al, eds. *GeneReviews® [Internet]*. Seattle, WA: University of Washington; April 29, 2003:1993–2016. https://www.ncbi.nlm.nih.gov/books/NBK1217/. (Updated April 9, 2015).

Bali DS, Chen YT, Austin S, et al. Glycogen storage disease type I. In: Pagon RA, Adam MP, Ardinger HH, et al, eds. *GeneReviews® [Internet]*. Seattle, WA: University of Washington; April 19, 2006:1993–2016. https://www.ncbi.nlm.nih.gov/books/NBK1312/. (Updated August 25, 2016).

Carrillo N, Adams D, Venditti CP. Disorders of intracellular cobalamin metabolism. In: Pagon RA, Adam MP, Ardinger HH, et al, eds. *GeneReviews® [Internet]*. Seattle, WA: University of Washington; February 25, 2008:1993–2016. https://www.ncbi.nlm.nih.gov/books/NBK1328/. (Updated November 21, 2013).

Clarke LA. Mucopolysaccharidosis type I. In: Pagon RA, Adam MP, Ardinger HH, et al, eds. *GeneReviews® [Internet]*. Seattle, WA: University of Washington; October 31, 2002:1993–2016. https://www.ncbi.nlm.nih.gov/books/NBK1162/. (Updated February 11, 2016).

Matern D, Rinaldo P. Medium-chain acyl-coenzyme A dehydrogenase deficiency. In: Pagon RA, Adam MP, Ardinger HH, et al, eds. *GeneReviews® [Internet]*. Seattle, WA: University of Washington; April 20, 2000:1993–2016. https://www.ncbi.nlm.nih.gov/books/NBK1424/. (Updated March 5, 2015).

Steinberg SJ, Moser AB, Raymond GV. X-linked adrenoleukodystrophy. In: Pagon RA, Adam MP, Ardinger HH, et al, eds. *GeneReviews® [Internet]*. Seattle, WA: University of Washington; March 26, 1999:1993–2016. https://www.ncbi.nlm.nih.gov/books/NBK1315/. (Updated April 9, 2015).

Strauss KA, Puffenberger EG, Morton DH. Maple syrup urine disease. In: Pagon RA, Adam MP, Ardinger HH, et al, eds. *GeneReviews® [Internet]*. Seattle, WA: University of Washington; January 30, 2006:1993–2016. https://www.ncbi.nlm.nih.gov/books/NBK1319/. (Updated May 9, 2013).

PEARLS FOR PRACTITIONERS

CHAPTER 51

Metabolic Assessment

- Metabolic inborn errors of metabolism (IEMs) disorders are individually uncommon but as a group account for a significant disease burden.
- IEMs are frequent causes of sepsis-like presentations, mental retardation, seizures, sudden infant death, and neurological impairment.
- There are 89 identified IEMs that are amenable to therapy targeted to the underlying cause and that present with intellectual disability as a prominent feature.
- Genetic metabolic disorders result from the deficiency of an enzyme, its cofactors, or biochemical transporters that lead to the deficiency of a required metabolite, the buildup of a toxic compound, or a combination of both processes.
- Hypoglycemic and intoxicating (encephalopathy) metabolic disorders should be considered in all neonates presenting with lethargy, poor tone, poor feeding, hypothermia, irritability, or seizures.
- All children presenting with altered levels of consciousness, irritability, neurological impairment, or apparent sepsis-like episodes should have a plasma ammonia, blood glucose, and anion gap tested.
- Significant ketosis in the neonate is unusual and suggests an organic acid disorder.
- In general diagnostic testing for disorders of small molecule metabolism is most effective when metabolites are present in highest concentration in blood and urine. This is typically at times of catabolism such as during intercurrent illness or prolonged starvation.
- Testing for urea cycle defects, intermittent maple syrup urine disease (MSUD), or fatty acid oxidation defects may be normal in affected children if the child is not under significant catabolic stress.
- Respiratory alkalosis is frequently seen in the early stages of a hyperammonemic crisis, but this may give way to respiratory failure as the ammonia level increases.
- General clinical laboratory testing can define the metabolic derangement and refine the differential diagnosis in a child suspected to have an inborn error of metabolism.
- In the United States the majority of infants diagnosed with a treatable metabolic disorder will be identified as a result of an abnormal newborn screen.
- The "recommended uniform screening panel" (RUSP) is defined by the Federal Advisory Committee on Heritable Disorders in the Newborn and Child (ACHDNC). In order to be added to the RUSP, conditions must have a proven benefit of identification through newborn screening in terms of reducing mortality or improving long-term neurocognitive outcomes.
- For many disorders the success of newborn screening is dependent on the blood sample being drawn at the correct time and analyzed in a timely fashion.
- For the newborn screening system to protect babies it must include prompt return of results to families and mechanisms for rapid institution of therapy.
- Newborn screening tests have a wide range of specificity, with some tests having close to 90% false positive rate. Therefore it is essential to perform appropriate confirmatory testing.
- Therapy for metabolic disease may focus on reducing the intake of specific substances that lead to buildup of toxic compounds for example restricting protein intake to prevent phenylalanine buildup in phenylketonuria (PKU). In addition, specific medications may prevent the buildup of toxic substances (e.g., miglustat in Gaucher disease). Therapy may provide supraphysiological cofactors that enhance residual enzymatic function for example tetrahydrobiopterin in PKU.
- In most metabolic disorders caused by the accumulation of toxic small molecules, catabolism increases the rate of production of these toxic metabolites. Consequently adequate and, at times, supraphysiological provision of sources of energy (e.g., parenteral dextrose) is used to drive the patient to an anabolic state where less of this compound can be produced.
- In many metabolic disorders, compounds that would otherwise be nonessential need to be provided (e.g., tyrosine in PKU).
- In specific metabolic disorders the primary pathology is driven by a deficiency of essential compounds (e.g., the inability to undergo glyconeogenesis leads to fasting hypoglycemia). In these disorders ongoing replacement of such factors is essential for prevention of secondary injury.
- Several disorders can be treated by providing the missing enzyme. This may be in the form of enzyme replacement therapy, organ transplant (e.g., liver transplant in ornithine transcarbamylase [OTC] deficiency), or cell-based therapy (e.g., HSCT in MPS1).

CHAPTER 52

Carbohydrate Disorders

- Glycogen storage disease type I manifests with hypoglycemia, hepatomegaly, lactic acidosis, and hypertriglyceridemia.
- Enzyme replacement therapy improves the outcome of Pompe disease (glycogen storage disease type II), which presents with cardiomyopathy.
- Patients with galactosemia present with hepatic failure, renal tubular dysfunction, cataracts, and *Escherichia coli* sepsis.

CHAPTER 53

Amino Acid Disorders

- PKU is an autosomal recessive disorder and will result in severe intellectual disability; patients are normal at birth.
- Tyrosinemia type I manifests with severe hepatic dysfunction, coagulopathy, hypoglycemia, and renal tubular dysfunction.
- Homocystinuria resembles a connective tissue disorder and manifests with dislocated lens, long slender fingers, scoliosis, and arterial or venous thrombosis.
- MSUD presents 1-4 weeks after birth with poor feeding, emesis, coma, and hypotonia alternating with extensor spasms.

CHAPTER 54

Organic Acid Disorders

- Propionic and methylmalonic acidemias may present with tachypnea, emesis, lethargy, coma, neutropenia, thrombocytopenia, ketosis, hypoglycemia, and hyperglycinemia.
- Glutaric academia I presents with macrocephaly, dystonia, and metabolic strokes.

CHAPTER 55

Disorders of Fat Metabolism

- Medium-chain acyl-CoA dehydrogenase (MCAD) deficiency is the most common disorder of fatty acid oxidation and presents with hypoketotic hypoglycemia, sudden death, and a Reye-like syndrome.
- Glutaric academia II may present with congenital anomalies, nonketotic hypoglycemia, and myopathy.

CHAPTER 56

Lysosomal and Peroxisomal Disorders

- Peroxisomal disorders often present with developmental delay and dysmorphic features affecting the skeleton or skin.

CHAPTER 57

Mitochondrial Disorders

- Most mitochondrial disorders are due to mutations in nuclear genes.
- Mitochondrial DNA mutations are maternally inherited.
- Mitochondrial disorders can produce myopathy, cardiomyopathy, central nervous system dysfunction, or hepatopathy, with or occasionally without lactic acidosis.

FETAL AND NEONATAL MEDICINE

Clarence W. Gowen Jr.

CHAPTER 58

Assessment of the Mother, Fetus, and Newborn

ASSESSMENT OF THE MOTHER

Pregnancies associated with perinatal morbidity or mortality are considered high risk. Identification of high-risk pregnancies is essential to the care of the infant because they may result in intrauterine fetal death, intrauterine growth restriction (IUGR), congenital anomalies, excessive fetal growth, birth asphyxia and trauma, prematurity (birth at <38 weeks) or postmaturity (birth at ≥42 weeks), neonatal disease, or long-term risks of cerebral palsy, intellectual disability, and chronic sequelae of neonatal intensive care. Ten percent to 20% of women may be high risk at some time during their pregnancy. Although some obstetric complications are first seen during labor and delivery and cannot be predicted, more than 50% of perinatal mortality and morbidity results from problems identified before delivery as high risk. After a high-risk pregnancy is identified, measures can be instituted to prevent complications, provide intensive fetal surveillance, and initiate appropriate treatments of the mother and fetus.

A history of previous premature birth, intrauterine fetal death, multiple gestation, IUGR, congenital malformation, explained or unexplained neonatal death (e.g., group B streptococcal sepsis), birth trauma, preeclampsia, gestational diabetes, grand multipara status (five or more pregnancies), or cesarean section is associated with additional risk in subsequent pregnancies.

Pregnancy complications that increase the risk of a poor outcome can be secondary to maternal or fetal causes or both. Complications include placenta previa; abruptio placentae; preeclampsia; diabetes; oligohydramnios or polyhydramnios; multiple gestation; blood group sensitization; abnormal levels of unconjugated estriols, chorionic gonadotropin, or alpha-fetoprotein; abnormal fetal ultrasound; hydrops fetalis; maternal trauma or surgery; abnormal fetal presentation (breech); exposure to prescribed or illicit drugs; prolonged labor; cephalopelvic disproportion; prolapsed cord; fetal distress; prolonged or premature rupture of membranes; short cervical length (<25 mm) and the presence of fetal fibronectin in cervical secretions at less than 35 weeks' gestation (a predictor of preterm labor); cervical infections and vaginosis; and congenital infections, including rubella, cytomegalovirus, herpes simplex, human immunodeficiency virus (HIV), toxoplasmosis, syphilis, and gonorrhea.

Maternal medical complications associated with increased risk of maternal and fetal morbidity and mortality include diabetes, chronic hypertension, congenital heart disease (especially with right-to-left shunting and Eisenmenger complex), glomerulonephritis, collagen vascular disease (especially systemic lupus erythematosus with or without antiphospholipid antibodies), lung disease (cystic fibrosis), severe anemia (sickle cell anemia), hyperthyroidism, myasthenia gravis, idiopathic thrombocytopenic purpura, inborn errors of metabolism (maternal phenylketonuria), and malignancy.

Obstetric complications often are associated with increased fetal or neonatal risk. Vaginal bleeding in the first trimester or early second trimester may be caused by a threatened or actual spontaneous abortion and is associated with increased risk of congenital malformations or chromosomal disorders. Painless vaginal bleeding that is not associated with labor and occurs in the late second or (more likely) third trimester often is the result of **placenta previa**. Bleeding develops when the placental mass overlies the internal cervical os; this may produce maternal hemorrhagic shock, necessitating transfusions. Bleeding also may result in premature delivery. Painful vaginal bleeding is often the result of retroplacental hemorrhage or **placental abruption**. Associated findings may be advanced maternal age and parity, maternal chronic hypertension, maternal cocaine use, preterm rupture of membranes, polyhydramnios, twin gestation, and preeclampsia. Fetal asphyxia ensues as the retroplacental hematoma causes placental separation that interferes with fetal oxygenation. Both types of bleeding are associated with fetal blood loss. Neonatal anemia may be more common with placenta previa.

Abnormalities in the volume of amniotic fluid, resulting in oligohydramnios or polyhydramnios, are associated with increased fetal and neonatal risk. **Oligohydramnios** (amniotic ultrasound fluid index ≤2 cm) is associated with IUGR and major congenital anomalies, particularly of the fetal kidneys, and with chromosomal syndromes. Bilateral renal agenesis results in diminished production of amniotic fluid and a specific deformation syndrome **(Potter syndrome)**, which includes clubfeet, characteristic compressed facies, low-set ears, scaphoid abdomen, and diminished chest wall size accompanied by pulmonary hypoplasia and, often, pneumothorax. Uterine compression in the absence of amniotic fluid retards lung growth, and patients with this condition die of respiratory failure rather than renal insufficiency. Twin-to-twin transfusion syndrome (donor) and complications from amniotic fluid leakage also are associated with oligohydramnios. Oligohydramnios increases the risk of fetal distress during labor (meconium-stained fluid and variable decelerations); the risk may be reduced by saline amnioinfusion during labor.

Polyhydramnios may be acute and associated with premature labor, maternal discomfort, and respiratory compromise. More often, polyhydramnios is chronic and is associated with diabetes, immune or nonimmune hydrops fetalis, multiple gestation, trisomy 18 or 21, and major congenital anomalies. Anencephaly, hydrocephaly, and meningomyelocele are associated with reduced fetal swallowing of amniotic fluid. Esophageal and duodenal atresia as well as cleft palate interfere with swallowing and gastrointestinal fluid dynamics. Additional causes of polyhydramnios include Werdnig-Hoffmann and Beckwith-Wiedemann syndromes, conjoined twins, chylothorax, cystic adenomatoid lung malformation, diaphragmatic hernia, gastroschisis, sacral teratoma, placental chorioangioma, and myotonic dystrophy. **Hydrops fetalis** may be a result of Rh or other blood group incompatibilities and anemia caused by intrauterine hemolysis of fetal erythrocytes by maternal IgG-sensitized antibodies crossing the placenta. Hydrops is characterized by fetal edema, ascites, hypoalbuminemia, and congestive heart failure. Causes of **nonimmune hydrops** include fetal arrhythmias (supraventricular tachycardia, congenital heart block), fetal anemia (bone marrow suppression, nonimmune hemolysis, or twin-to-twin transfusion), severe congenital malformation, intrauterine infections, congenital neuroblastoma, inborn errors of metabolism (storage diseases), fetal hepatitis, nephrotic syndrome, and pulmonary lymphangiectasia. Twin-to-twin transfusion syndrome (recipient) also may be associated with polyhydramnios. Polyhydramnios is often the result of unknown causes. If severe, polyhydramnios may be managed with bed rest, indomethacin, or serial amniocenteses.

Premature rupture of the membranes, which occurs in the absence of labor, and **prolonged rupture of the membranes** (>24 hours) are associated with an increased risk of maternal or fetal infection (chorioamnionitis) and preterm birth. In the immediate newborn period, group B streptococcus and *Escherichia coli* are the two most common pathogens associated with sepsis. *Listeria monocytogenes* is a less common cause. *Mycoplasma hominis, Ureaplasma urealyticum, Chlamydia trachomatis*, and anaerobic bacteria of the vaginal flora also have been implicated in infection of the amniotic fluid. Infection with community-acquired methicillin-resistant *Staphylococcus aureus* must be considered for infants with skin infections or with known exposures. The risk of serious fetal infection increases as the duration between rupture and labor (latent period) increases, especially if the period is greater than 24 hours. Intrapartum antibiotic therapy decreases the risk of neonatal sepsis.

Multiple gestations are associated with increased risk resulting from polyhydramnios, premature birth, IUGR, abnormal presentation (breech), congenital anomalies (intestinal atresia, porencephaly, and single umbilical artery), intrauterine fetal demise, birth asphyxia, and twin-to-twin transfusion syndrome. **Twin-to-twin transfusion syndrome** is associated with a high mortality and is seen only in monozygotic twins who share a common placenta and have an arteriovenous connection between their circulations. The fetus on the arterial side of the shunt serves as the blood donor, resulting in fetal anemia, growth retardation, and oligohydramnios for this fetus. The recipient, or venous-side twin, is larger or discordant in size, is plethoric and polycythemic, and may show polyhydramnios. Weight differences of 20% and hemoglobin differences of 5 g/dL suggest the diagnosis. Ultrasonography in the second trimester reveals discordant amniotic fluid volume with oliguria/oligohydramnios and hypervolemia/polyuria/polyhydramnios with a distended bladder, with or without hydrops and heart failure. Treatment includes attempts to ablate the arteriovenous connection (using a laser). The birth order of twins also affects morbidity by increasing the risk of the second-born twin for breech position, birth asphyxia, birth trauma, and respiratory distress syndrome.

Overall, twinning is observed in 1 of 80 pregnancies; 80% of all twin gestations are dizygotic twins. The diagnosis of the type of twins can be determined by placentation, sex, fetal membrane structure, and, if necessary, tissue and blood group typing or DNA analysis.

Toxemia of pregnancy, or **preeclampsia/eclampsia**, is a disorder of unknown but probably vascular etiology that may lead to maternal hypertension, uteroplacental insufficiency, IUGR, intrauterine asphyxia, maternal seizures, and maternal death. Toxemia is more common in nulliparous women and in women with twin gestation, chronic hypertension, obesity, renal disease, positive family history of toxemia, or diabetes mellitus. A subcategory of preeclampsia, the *HELLP* syndrome (**h**emolysis, **e**levated **l**iver enzyme levels, **l**ow **p**latelets), is more severe and is often associated with a fetal inborn error of fatty acid oxidation (long-chain hydroxyacyl–coenzyme A dehydrogenase of the trifunctional protein complex).

FETUS AND NEWBORN

The late fetal–early neonatal period has the highest mortality rate of any age interval. **Perinatal mortality** refers to fetal deaths occurring from the 20th week of gestation until the 28th day after birth and is expressed as number of deaths per 1,000 live births. Intrauterine fetal death accounts for 40-50% of the perinatal mortality rate. Such infants, defined as **stillborn**, are born without a heart rate and are apneic, limp, pale, and cyanotic. Many stillborn infants exhibit evidence of maceration; pale, peeling skin; corneal opacification; and soft cranial contents.

Mortality rates around the time of birth are expressed as number of deaths per 1,000 live births. The **neonatal mortality rate** includes all infants dying during the period from after birth to the first 28 days of life. Modern neonatal intensive care allows many newborns with life-threatening diseases to survive the neonatal period, only to die of their original diseases or of complications of therapy after 28 days of life. This delayed mortality and mortality caused by acquired illnesses occur during the **postneonatal period**, which begins after 28 days of life and extends to the end of the first year of life.

The **infant mortality rate** encompasses the neonatal and the postneonatal periods. In the United States, it declined to 5.8 : 1,000 in 2015. The rate for African American infants was approximately 11.0 : 1,000. The most common causes of perinatal and neonatal death are listed in Table 58.1. Overall, congenital anomalies and diseases of the premature infant are the most significant causes of neonatal mortality.

Low birth weight (LBW) infants, defined as infants having birth weights of less than 2,500 g, represent a disproportionately large component of the neonatal and infant mortality rates. Although LBW infants make up only about 6-7% of all births, they account for more than 70% of neonatal deaths. IUGR is the

TABLE 58.1 Major Causes of Perinatal and Neonatal Mortality
FETUS
Abruptio placentae
Chromosomal anomalies
Congenital malformations (heart, CNS, renal)
Hydrops fetalis
Intrauterine asphyxia*
Intrauterine infection*
Maternal underlying disease (chronic hypertension, autoimmune disease, diabetes mellitus)
Multiple gestation*
Placental insufficiency*
Umbilical cord accident
PRETERM INFANT
Respiratory distress syndrome/bronchopulmonary dysplasia (chronic lung disease)*
Severe immaturity*
Congenital anomalies
Infection
Intraventricular hemorrhage*
Necrotizing enterocolitis
FULL-TERM INFANT
Birth asphyxia*
Birth trauma
Congenital anomalies*
Infection*
Macrosomia
Meconium aspiration pneumonia
Persistent pulmonary hypertension

*Common.
CNS, Central nervous system.

most common cause of LBW in developing countries, whereas prematurity is the cause in developed countries.

Very low birth weight (VLBW) infants, weighing less than 1,500 g at birth, represent about 1% of all births but account for 50% of neonatal deaths. Compared with infants weighing 2,500 g or more, LBW infants are 40 times more likely to die in the neonatal period; VLBW infants have a 200-fold higher risk of neonatal death. The LBW rate has not improved in recent years and is one of the major reasons that the U.S. infant mortality rate is high compared with other large, modern, industrialized countries.

Maternal factors associated with a LBW caused by premature birth or IUGR include a previous LBW birth, low socioeconomic status, low level of maternal education, no antenatal care, maternal age younger than 16 years or older than 35 years, short interval between pregnancies, cigarette smoking, alcohol and illicit drug use, physical (excessive standing or walking) or psychological (poor social support) stresses, unmarried status, low prepregnancy weight (<45 kg), poor weight gain during pregnancy (<10 lb), and African American race. LBW and VLBW rates for African American women are twice the rates for white women. The neonatal and infant mortality rates are nearly twofold higher among African American infants. These racial differences are only partly explained by poverty.

ASSESSMENT OF THE FETUS

Fetal size can be determined accurately by ultrasound techniques. **Fetal growth** can be assessed by determining the fundal height of the uterus through bimanual examination of the gravid abdomen. Ultrasound measurements of the fetal biparietal diameter, femur length, and abdominal circumference are used to estimate fetal growth. A combination of these measurements predicts fetal weight. Deviations from the normal fetal growth curve are associated with high-risk conditions.

IUGR is present when fetal growth stops and, over time, declines to less than the 5th percentile of growth for gestational age or when growth proceeds slowly, but absolute size remains less than the 5th percentile. Growth restriction may result from fetal conditions that reduce the innate growth potential, such as fetal rubella infection, primordial dwarfing syndromes, chromosomal abnormalities, and congenital malformation syndromes. Reduced fetal production of insulin and insulin-like growth factor I is associated with fetal growth restriction. Placental causes of IUGR include villitis (congenital infections), placental tumors, chronic abruptio placentae, twin-to-twin transfusion syndrome, and placental insufficiency. Maternal causes include severe peripheral vascular diseases that reduce uterine blood flow (chronic hypertension, diabetic vasculopathy, and preeclampsia/eclampsia), reduced nutritional intake, alcohol or drug abuse, cigarette smoking, and uterine constraint (noted predominantly in mothers of small stature with a low prepregnancy weight) and reduced weight gain during pregnancy. The outcome of IUGR depends on the cause of the reduced fetal growth and the associated complications after birth (Table 58.2). Fetuses subjected to chronic intrauterine hypoxia as a result of uteroplacental insufficiency are at an increased risk for the comorbidities of birth asphyxia, polycythemia, and hypoglycemia. Fetuses with reduced tissue mass due to chromosomal, metabolic, or multiple congenital anomaly syndromes have poor outcomes based on the prognosis for the particular syndrome. Fetuses born to small mothers and fetuses of mothers with poor nutritional intake usually show catch-up growth after birth.

Fetal size does not always correlate with functional or structural maturity. Determining **fetal maturity** is crucial when making a decision to deliver a fetus because of fetal or maternal disease. Fetal gestational age may be determined accurately on the basis of a correct estimate of the last menstrual period. Clinically relevant landmark dates can be used to determine gestational age; the first audible heart tones by fetoscope are detected at 18-20 weeks (12-14 weeks by Doppler methods), and quickening of fetal movements usually is perceived at 18-20 weeks. However, it is not always possible to determine fetal maturity by such dating, especially in a high-risk situation, such as preterm labor or a diabetic pregnancy.

Surfactant, a combination of surface-active phospholipids and proteins, is produced by the maturing fetal lung and eventually is secreted into the amniotic fluid. The amount of surfactant in amniotic fluid is a direct reflection of surface-active material in the fetal lung and can be used to predict the presence or absence of **pulmonary maturity**. Because phosphatidylcholine, or lecithin, is a principal component of

TABLE 58.2 Problems of Intrauterine Growth Restriction and Small for Gestational Age

PROBLEM*	PATHOGENESIS
Intrauterine fetal demise	Placental insufficiency, hypoxia, acidosis, infection, lethal anomaly
Temperature instability	Cold stress, ↓ fat stores, hypoxia, hypoglycemia
Perinatal asphyxia	↓ Uteroplacental perfusion during labor with or without chronic fetal hypoxia-acidosis, meconium aspiration syndrome
Hypoglycemia	↓ Tissue glycogen stores; ↓ gluconeogenesis, hyperinsulinism, ↑ glucose needs of hypoxia, hypothermia, relatively large brain
Polycythemia-hyperviscosity	Fetal hypoxia with ↑ erythropoietin production
Reduced oxygen consumption/ hypothermia	Hypoxia, hypoglycemia, starvation effect, poor subcutaneous fat stores
Dysmorphology	Syndrome anomalads, chromosomal-genetic disorders, oligohydramnios-induced deformations
Pulmonary hemorrhage	Hypothermia, polycythemia, hypoxia

*Other problems are common to the gestational age–related risks of prematurity if born before 37 weeks.
Modified from Carlo WA. The high-risk infant. In: Kliegman RM, Stanton BF, St. Geme JW, et al., eds. Nelson Textbook of Pediatrics. *19th ed. Philadelphia: Elsevier Science; 2011.*

surfactant, the determination of lecithin in amniotic fluid is used to predict a mature fetus. Lecithin concentration increases with increasing gestational age, beginning at 32-34 weeks.

Methods used to assess **fetal well-being** before the onset of labor are focused on identifying a fetus at risk for asphyxia or a fetus already compromised by uteroplacental insufficiency. The **oxytocin challenge test** simulates uterine contractions through an infusion of oxytocin sufficient to produce three contractions in a 10-minute period. The development of periodic fetal bradycardia out of phase with uterine contractions (late deceleration) is a positive test result and predicts an at-risk fetus.

The **nonstress test** examines the heart rate response to fetal body movements. Heart rate increases of more than 15 beats/min lasting 15 seconds are reassuring. If two such episodes occur in 30 minutes, the test result is considered reactive (versus nonreactive), and the fetus is not at risk. Additional signs of fetal well-being are fetal breathing movements, gross body movements, fetal tone, and the presence of amniotic fluid pockets more than 2 cm in size, detected by ultrasound. The **biophysical profile** combines the nonstress test with these four parameters and offers the most accurate fetal assessment.

Doppler examination of the fetal aorta or umbilical arteries permits identification of decreased or reversed diastolic blood flow associated with increased peripheral vascular resistance, fetal hypoxia with acidosis, and placental insufficiency. **Cordocentesis** (percutaneous umbilical blood sampling) can provide fetal blood for Pa_{O_2}, pH, lactate, and hemoglobin measurements to identify a hypoxic, acidotic, or anemic fetus that is at risk for intrauterine fetal demise or birth asphyxia. Cordocentesis also can be used to determine fetal blood type, platelet count, microbial testing, antibody titer, and rapid karyotype.

In a high-risk pregnancy, the fetal heart rate should be monitored continuously during labor, as should uterine contractions. Fetal heart rate abnormalities may indicate baseline tachycardia (>160 beats/min as a result of anemia, β-sympathomimetic drugs, maternal fever, hyperthyroidism, arrhythmia, or fetal distress), baseline **bradycardia** (<120 beats/min as a result of fetal distress, complete heart block, or local anesthetics), or reduced beat-to-beat variability (flattened tracing resulting from fetal sleep, tachycardia, atropine, sedatives, prematurity, or fetal distress). Periodic changes of the heart rate relative to uterine pressure help determine the presence of hypoxia and acidosis caused by uteroplacental insufficiency or maternal hypotension (late or type II decelerations) or by umbilical cord compression (variable decelerations). In the presence of severe decelerations (late or repeated prolonged variable), a fetal scalp blood gas level should be obtained to assess **fetal acidosis**. A scalp pH of less than 7.20 indicates fetal hypoxic compromise. A pH between 7.20 and 7.25 is in a borderline zone and warrants repeat testing.

Fetal anomalies may be detected by ultrasonography. Emphasis should be placed on visualization of the genitourinary tract; the head (for anencephaly or hydrocephaly), neck (for thickened nuchal translucency), and back (for spina bifida); skeleton; gastrointestinal tract; and heart. Four-chamber and great artery views are required for detection of heart anomalies. **Chromosomal anomaly syndromes** are often associated with an abnormal "quadruple test" (low unconjugated estriols, low maternal serum alpha-fetoprotein levels, high inhibin A, and elevated placental chorionic gonadotropin levels). Fetal genetic and chromosomal disorders can also be detected by analyzing free fetal DNA that is present in the maternal circulation. If a fetal abnormality is detected, fetal therapy or delivery with therapy in the neonatal intensive care unit may be lifesaving.

ASSESSMENT OF THE NEWBORN

The approach to the birth of an infant requires a detailed history (Table 58.3). Knowing the mother's risk factors enables the delivery room team to anticipate problems that may occur after birth. The history of a woman's labor and delivery can reveal events that might lead to complications affecting either the mother or the neonate, even when the pregnancy was previously considered low risk. Anticipating the need to resuscitate a newborn as a result of fetal distress increases the likelihood of successful resuscitation.

The **transition from fetal to neonatal physiology** occurs at birth. Oxygen transport across the placenta results in a gradient between the maternal and fetal Pa_{O_2}. Although fetal oxygenated blood has a low Pa_{O_2} level compared with that of adults and infants, the fetus is not anaerobic. Fetal oxygen uptake and consumption are similar to neonatal rates, even though the thermal environments and activity levels of fetuses and neonates differ. The oxygen content of fetal blood is almost equal to the oxygen content in older infants and children because fetal blood has a much higher concentration of hemoglobin.

Fetal hemoglobin (two alpha and two gamma chains) has a higher affinity for oxygen than adult hemoglobin, facilitating oxygen transfer across the placenta. The fetal hemoglobin-oxygen dissociation curve is shifted to the left of the adult curve (Fig. 58.1); at the same Pa_{O_2} level, fetal hemoglobin is more saturated than adult hemoglobin. Because fetal hemoglobin functions on the steep, lower end of the oxygen saturation curve (Pa_{O_2},

TABLE 58.3 Components of the Perinatal History

DEMOGRAPHIC SOCIAL INFORMATION	Fetal surveillance (OCT, NST, biophysical profile)
Age	Ultrasonography (anomalies, hydrops)
Race	Amniotic fluid analysis (L/S ratio)
Sexually transmitted infections, hepatitis, AIDS	Oligohydramnios-polyhydramnios
Illicit drugs, cigarettes, ethanol, cocaine, opiates	Vaginal bleeding
Immune status (syphilis, rubella, hepatitis B, HIV, blood group)	Preterm labor
Occupational exposure	Premature (prolonged) rupture of membranes (duration)
PAST MEDICAL DISEASES	Preeclampsia
Chronic hypertension	Urinary tract infection
Heart disease	Colonization status (herpes simplex, group B streptococcus)
Diabetes mellitus	Medications/drugs
Thyroid disorders	Acute medical illness/exposure to infectious agents
Hematological/malignancy	Fetal therapy
Collagen-vascular disease (SLE)	**LABOR AND DELIVERY**
Genetic history—inborn errors of metabolism, bleeding, jaundice	Duration of labor
Drug therapy	Presentation—vertex, breech
PRIOR PREGNANCY	Vaginal versus cesarean section
Abortion/stillbirths	Spontaneous labor versus augmented or induced with oxytocin (Pitocin)
Intrauterine fetal demise	Forceps delivery
Congenital malformation	Presence of meconium-stained fluid
Incompetent cervix	Maternal fever/amnionitis
Birth weight	Fetal heart rate patterns (distress)
Prematurity	Scalp pH
Twins	Maternal analgesia, anesthesia
Blood group sensitization/neonatal jaundice	Nuchal cord
Hydrops	Apgar score/methods of resuscitation
Infertility	Gestational age assessment
PRESENT PREGNANCY	Growth status (AGA, LGA, SGA)
Current gestational age	
Method of assessing gestational age	

AGA, Average for gestational age; *AIDS*, acquired immunodeficiency syndrome; *HIV*, human immunodeficiency virus; *LGA*, large for gestational age; *L/S*, lecithin-to-sphingomyelin ratio; *NST*, nonstress test; *OCT*, oxytocin challenge test; *SGA*, small for gestational age; *SLE*, systemic lupus erythematosus.

20-30 mm Hg), however, oxygen unloading to the tissue is not deficient. In contrast, at the higher oxygen concentrations present in the placenta, oxygen loading is enhanced. In the last trimester, fetal hemoglobin production begins to decrease as adult hemoglobin production begins to increase, becoming the only hemoglobin available to the infant by 3-6 months of life. At this time, the fetal hemoglobin dissociation curve has shifted to the adult position.

A portion of well-oxygenated umbilical venous blood returning to the heart from the placenta perfuses the liver. The remainder bypasses the liver through a shunt (the **ductus venosus**) and enters the inferior vena cava. This oxygenated blood in the vena cava constitutes 65-70% of venous return to the right atrium. The crista dividens in the right atrium directs one third of this blood across the patent foramen ovale to the left atrium, where it subsequently is pumped to the coronary, cerebral, and upper extremity circulations by the left ventricle. Venous return from the upper body combines with the remaining two thirds of the vena caval blood in the right atrium and is directed to the right ventricle. This mixture of venous low-oxygenated blood from the upper and lower body enters the pulmonary artery. Only 8-10% of it is pumped to the pulmonary circuit; the remaining 80-92% of the right ventricular output bypasses the lungs through a **patent ductus arteriosus** and enters the descending aorta. The amount of blood flowing to the pulmonary system is low because vasoconstriction produced by medial muscle hypertrophy of the pulmonary arterioles and fluid in the fetal lung increases resistance to blood flow. Pulmonary artery tone also responds to hypoxia, hypercapnia, and acidosis with vasoconstriction, a response that may increase pulmonary vascular resistance further. The ductus arteriosus remains patent in the fetus because of low Pa_{O_2} levels and dilating prostaglandins. In utero, the right ventricle is the dominant ventricle, pumping 65% of the combined ventricular output,

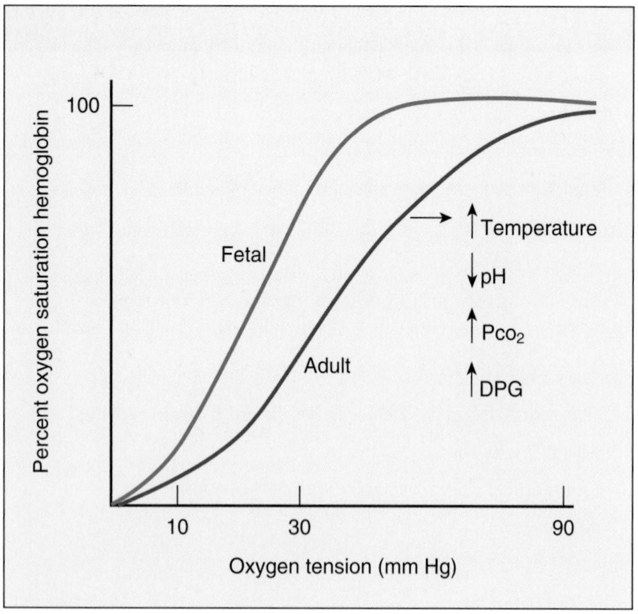

FIGURE 58.1 Hemoglobin-oxygen dissociation curves. The position of the adult curve depends on the binding of adult hemoglobin to 2,3-diphosphoglycerate (DPG), temperature, P_{CO_2}, and hydrogen ion concentration (pH).

which is a high volume (450 mL/kg/min) compared with that pumped by an older infant's right ventricle (200 mL/kg/min).

The **transition of the circulation**, occurring between the fetal and neonatal periods, involves the removal of the low-resistance circulation of the placenta, the onset of breathing, reduction of pulmonary arterial resistance, and closure of in utero shunts. Clamping the umbilical cord eliminates the low-pressure system of the placenta and increases systemic blood pressure. Decreased venous return from the placenta decreases right atrial pressure. As breathing begins, air replaces lung fluid, maintaining the functional residual capacity. Fluid leaves the lung, in part, through the trachea; it is either swallowed or squeezed out during vaginal delivery. The pulmonary lymphatic and venous systems reabsorb the remaining fluid.

Most normal infants require little pressure to spontaneously open the lungs after birth (5-10 cm H_2O). With the onset of breathing, pulmonary vascular resistance decreases, partly a result of the mechanics of breathing and partly a result of the elevated arterial oxygen tensions. The increased blood flow to the lungs increases the volume of pulmonary venous blood returning to the left atrium; left atrial pressure now exceeds right atrial pressure, and the foramen ovale closes. As the flow through the pulmonary circulation increases and arterial oxygen tensions rise, the ductus arteriosus begins to constrict. In a term infant, this constriction functionally closes the ductus arteriosus within 1 day after birth. A permanent closure requires thrombosis and fibrosis, a process that may take several weeks. In a premature infant, the ductus arteriosus is less sensitive to the effects of oxygen; if circulating levels of vasodilating prostaglandins are elevated, the ductus arteriosus may remain patent. This patency is a common problem in a premature infant with respiratory distress syndrome.

Ventilation, oxygenation, and normal pH and P_{CO_2} levels immediately reduce pulmonary artery vasoconstriction by causing smooth muscle relaxation. Remodeling of the medial muscle hypertrophy begins at birth and continues for the next 3 months, resulting in a further reduction of pulmonary vascular resistance and a further increase of pulmonary blood flow. Persistence or aggravation of pulmonary vasoconstriction caused by acidosis, hypoxia, hypercapnia, hypothermia, polycythemia, asphyxia, shunting of blood from the lungs, or pulmonary parenchymal hypoplasia results in **persistent pulmonary hypertension of the newborn (PPHN)**. Failure to replace pulmonary alveolar fluid completely with air can lead to respiratory distress **(transient tachypnea of the newborn)**.

Routine Delivery Room Care and Resuscitation

Silver nitrate (1%) instilled into both eyes without being washed out is an indicated effective therapy for the prevention of neonatal gonococcal ophthalmia, which can result in severe panophthalmitis and subsequent blindness. Silver nitrate may produce a chemical conjunctivitis with a mucopurulent discharge and is not effective against *C. trachomatis.* Many hospitals use erythromycin drops to prevent neonatal gonococcal and chlamydial eye disease.

Bacterial colonization of a newborn may begin in utero if the fetal membranes have been ruptured. Most infants undergo colonization after birth and acquire the bacteria present in the mother's genitourinary system, such as group B streptococci, staphylococci, *E. coli*, and clostridia. Antiseptic skin or cord care is routine in most nurseries to prevent the spread of pathological bacteria from one infant to another and to prevent disease in the individual infant. Staphylococcal bullous impetigo, omphalitis, diarrhea, and systemic disease may result from colonization with virulent *S. aureus.* Triple antibiotic ointment (polymyxin B, neomycin, and bacitracin) or bacitracin may be applied to the umbilical cord to reduce its colonization with gram-positive bacteria. Epidemics of *S. aureus* nursery infections are managed with strict infectious disease control measures (cohorting, hand washing, and monitoring for colonization).

Vitamin K prophylaxis (intramuscular) should be given to all infants to prevent hemorrhagic disease of the newborn. Before discharge, infants should receive the hepatitis B vaccine and be screened for various diseases (Tables 58.4 and 58.5).

Fetal or neonatal hypoxia, hypercapnia, poor cardiac output, and a metabolic acidosis can result from numerous conditions affecting the fetus, the placenta, or the mother. Whether in utero or after birth, asphyxia-caused **hypoxic-ischemic brain injury** is the result of reduced gaseous exchange through the placenta or through the lungs. Asphyxia associated with severe bradycardia or cardiac insufficiency reduces or eliminates tissue blood flow, resulting in ischemia. The fetal and neonatal circulatory systems respond to reduced oxygen availability by shunting the blood preferentially to the brain, heart, and adrenal glands and away from the intestine, kidneys, lungs, and skin.

Metabolic acidosis during asphyxia is caused by the combined effects of poor cardiac output secondary to hypoxic depression of myocardial function, systemic hypoxia, and tissue anaerobic metabolism. With severe or prolonged intrauterine or neonatal asphyxia, multiple vital organs are affected (Table 58.6).

Many conditions that contribute to **fetal or neonatal asphyxia** are the same medical or obstetric problems associated with high-risk pregnancy (Table 58.7). Maternal diseases that interfere with uteroplacental perfusion (chronic hypertension, preeclampsia, and diabetes mellitus) place the fetus at risk for intrauterine asphyxia. Maternal epidural anesthesia and the development of the vena caval compression syndrome may produce maternal

TABLE 58.4 Core Disorders Recommended for Screening by American College of Medical Genetics

DISORDER	ACRONYM	PRIMARY MARKER
METABOLIC DISORDERS DETECTED USING TANDEM MASS SPECTROMETRY		
Organic Acid Disorders		
Beta-ketothiolase deficiency (mitochondrial acetoacetyl coenzyme A [CoA] thiolase deficiency)	BKT	C5:1/C5OH
Cobalamin defects A, B	CBL (A,B)	C3
Isovaleric academia*	IVA	C5
Glutaric aciduria I	GA-I	C5DC
3-Hydroxy 3-methylglutaryl-CoA lyase deficiency*	HMG	C5OH/C5-3M-DC
Multiple carboxylase deficiency*	MCD	C3/C5OH
3-Methylcrotonyl-CoA carboxylase deficiency	3MCC	C5OH
Methylmalonic aciduria (mutase)*	MMA	C3
Propionic academia*	PA	C3
Fatty Acid Oxidation Defects		
Carnitine uptake defect (carnitine transporter defect)	CUD	C0
Long-chain hydroxyacyl-CoA dehydrogenase deficiency*	LCHAD/D	C16OH/C18:1OH
Medium-chain acyl-CoA dehydrogenase deficiency	MCAD/D	C8
Trifunctional protein deficiency*	TFP	C16OH/C18:1OH
Very-long-chain acyl-CoA dehydrogenase deficiency	VLCAD/D	C14:1/C14
Amino Acid Disorders		
Argininosuccinic aciduria (argininosuccinate lyase deficiency)*	ASA	ASA
Citrullinemia I (argininosuccinate synthase deficiency)*	CIT-I	Citrulline
Phenylketonuria	PKU	Phenylalanine
Maple syrup urine disease*	MSUD	Leucine
Homocystinuria	HCY	Methionine
Tyrosinemia type I	TYR-I	Tyrosine
OTHER METABOLIC DISORDERS		
Biotinidase deficiency	BIOT	Biotinidase activity
Galactosemia*	GALT	Total galactose, GALT activity
ENDOCRINE DISORDERS		
Congenital adrenal hyperplasia*	CAH	17-Hydroxyprogesterone
Congenital hypothyroidism	CH	T_4, TSH
HEMOGLOBIN DISORDERS		
Sickle cell anemia	HbSS	Hb variants
Sickle cell disorder	HbS/C	Hb variants
Hemoglobin S/β-thalassemia	HbS/betaTh	Hb variants
OTHER DISORDERS		
Cystic fibrosis	CF	Immunoreactive trypsinogen
Hearing	HEAR	

*Can manifest acutely in the first week of life.
From Sahai I, Levy H. Newborn screening. In: Gleason C, Devasker D, eds. Avery's Diseases of the Newborn. *9th ed. Philadelphia: Saunders; 2012.*

hypotension, which decreases uterine perfusion. Maternal medications given to relieve pain during labor may cross the placenta and depress the infant's respiratory center, resulting in apnea at the time of birth.

Fetal conditions associated with asphyxia usually do not become manifested until delivery, when the infant must initiate and sustain ventilation. In addition, the upper and lower airways must be patent and unobstructed. Alveoli must be free from foreign material, such as meconium, amniotic fluid debris, and infectious exudates, which increases airway resistance, reduces lung compliance, and leads to respiratory distress and hypoxia. Some extremely immature infants weighing less than 1,000 g at birth may be unable to expand their lungs, even in the absence of other pathology. Their compliant chest walls and surfactant

TABLE 58.5 Abnormal Newborn Screening Results: Possible Implications and Initial Action to Be Taken

NEWBORN SCREENING FINDING	DIFFERENTIAL DIAGNOSIS	INITIAL ACTION
↑ Phenylalanine	PKU, non-PKU hyperphenylalaninemia, pterin defect, galactosemia, transient hyperphenylalaninemia	Repeat blood specimen
↓ T_4, ↑ TSH	Congenital hypothyroidism, iodine exposure	Repeat blood specimen or thyroid function testing, begin thyroxine treatment
↓ T_4, normal TSH	Maternal hyperthyroidism, thyroxine-binding globulin deficiency, secondary hypothyroidism, congenital hypothyroidism with delayed TSH elevation	Repeat blood specimen
↑ Galactose (1-P) transferase	Galactosemia, liver disease, reducing substance, repeat deficiency variant (Duarte), transient	Clinical evaluation, urine for blood specimen. If reducing substance positive, begin lactose-free formula
↓ Galactose-1-phosphate uridyltransferase	Galactosemia, transferase deficiency variant (Duarte), transient	Clinical evaluation, urine for reducing substance, repeat blood specimen. If reducing substance positive, begin lactose-free formula
↑ Methionine	Homocystinuria, isolated liver dysfunction, tyrosinemia type I, transient hypermethioninemia	Repeat blood and urine specimen
↑ Leucine	Maple syrup urine disease, transient elevation	Clinical evaluation including urine for ketones, acid-base status, amino acid studies, immediate neonatal ICU care if urine ketones positive
↑ Tyrosine	Tyrosinemia type I or type II, transient tyrosinemia, liver disease	Repeat blood specimen
↑ 17α-Hydroxyprogesterone	Congenital adrenal hyperplasia, prematurity, transient (residual fetal adrenal cortex), stress in neonatal period, early specimen collection	Clinical evaluation including genital examination, serum electrolytes, repeat blood specimen
S-hemoglobin	Sickle cell disease, sickle cell trait	Hemoglobin electrophoresis
↑ Trypsinogen	Cystic fibrosis, transient, intestinal anomalies, perinatal stress, trisomies 13 and 18, renal failure	Repeat blood specimen, possible sweat test and DNA testing
↑ Creatinine phosphokinase	Duchenne muscular dystrophy, other type of muscular dystrophy, birth trauma, invasive procedure	Repeat blood test
↓ Biotinidase	Biotinidase deficiency	Serum biotinidase assay, biotin therapy
↓ G6PD	G6PD deficiency	Complete blood count, bilirubin determination
↓ α_1-Antitrypsin	α_1-Antitrypsin deficiency	Confirmatory test
Toxoplasma antibody (IgM)	Congenital toxoplasmosis	Infectious disease consultation
HIV antibody (IgG)	Maternally transmitted HIV, possible AIDS	Infectious disease consultation
↑ Organic acids	Fatty acid oxidation defects (medium-chain acyl-CoA dehydrogenase deficiency)	Perform specific assay (tandem mass spectroscopy); frequent feeds

AIDS, Acquired immunodeficiency syndrome; *G6PD*, glucose-6-phosphate dehydrogenase; *HIV*, human immunodeficiency virus; *ICU*, intensive care unit; *PKU*, phenylketonuria; T_4, thyroxine; *TSH*, thyroid-stimulating hormone.
From Kim SZ, Levy HL. Newborn screening. In: Taeusch HW, Ballard RA, eds. Avery's Diseases of the Newborn. *7th ed. Philadelphia: Saunders; 1998.*

TABLE 58.6 Effects of Asphyxia

SYSTEM	EFFECT
Central nervous system	Hypoxic-ischemic encephalopathy, IVH, PVL, cerebral edema, seizures, hypotonia, hypertonia
Cardiovascular	Myocardial ischemia, poor contractility, tricuspid insufficiency, hypotension
Pulmonary	Persistent pulmonary hypertension, respiratory distress syndrome
Renal	Acute tubular or cortical necrosis
Adrenal	Adrenal hemorrhage
Gastrointestinal	Perforation, ulceration, necrosis
Metabolic	Inappropriate ADH, hyponatremia, hypoglycemia, hypocalcemia, myoglobinuria
Integument	Subcutaneous fat necrosis
Hematology	Disseminated intravascular coagulation

ADH, Antidiuretic hormone; *IVH*, intraventricular hemorrhage; *PVL*, periventricular leukomalacia.

TABLE 58.7 Etiology of Birth Asphyxia

TYPE	EXAMPLE
INTRAUTERINE	
Hypoxia-ischemia	Uteroplacental insufficiency, abruptio placentae, prolapsed cord, maternal hypotension, unknown
Anemia-shock	Vasa previa, placenta previa, fetomaternal hemorrhage, erythroblastosis
INTRAPARTUM	
Birth trauma	Cephalopelvic disproportion, shoulder dystocia, breech presentation, spinal cord transection
Hypoxia-ischemia	Umbilical cord compression, tetanic uterine contraction, abruptio placentae
POSTPARTUM	
Central nervous system	Maternal medication, trauma, previous episodes of fetal hypoxia-acidosis
Congenital neuromuscular disease	Congenital myasthenia gravis, myopathy, myotonic dystrophy
Infection	Consolidated pneumonia, shock
Airway disorder	Choanal atresia, severe obstructing goiter or tumor, laryngeal webs
Pulmonary disorder	Severe immaturity, pneumothorax, pleural effusion, diaphragmatic hernia, pulmonary hypoplasia
Renal disorder	Pulmonary hypoplasia, pneumothorax

TABLE 58.8 Apgar Score

	POINTS		
SIGNS	0	1	2
Heart rate	0	<100/min	>100/min
Respiration	None	Weak cry	Vigorous cry
Muscle tone	None	Some extremity flexion	Arms, legs well flexed
Reflex irritability	None	Some motion	Cry, withdrawal
Color of body	Blue	Pink body, blue extremities	Pink all over

deficiency may result in poor air exchange, retractions, hypoxia, and apnea.

The newborn (particularly a preterm infant) responds paradoxically to hypoxia with apnea rather than tachypnea as occurs in adults. Episodes of intrauterine asphyxia also may depress the neonatal central nervous system. If recovery of the fetal heart rate occurs as a result of improved uteroplacental perfusion, fetal hypoxia and acidosis may resolve. Nonetheless, if the effect on the respiratory center is more severe, a newborn may not initiate an adequate ventilatory response at birth and may undergo another episode of asphyxia.

The **Apgar examination**, a rapid scoring system based on physiological responses to the birth process, is a good method for assessing the need to resuscitate a newborn (Table 58.8). At intervals of 1 and 5 minutes after birth, each of the five physiological parameters is observed or elicited by a qualified examiner. Full-term infants with a normal cardiopulmonary adaptation should score 8-9 at 1 and 5 minutes. Apgar scores of 4-7 warrant close attention to determine whether the infant's status will improve and to ascertain whether any pathological condition is contributing to the low Apgar score.

By definition, an Apgar score of 0-3 represents either a cardiopulmonary arrest or a condition caused by severe bradycardia, hypoventilation, or central nervous system depression. Most low Apgar scores are caused by difficulty in establishing adequate ventilation and not by primary cardiac pathology. In addition to an Apgar score of 0-3, most infants with asphyxia severe enough to cause neurological injury also manifest fetal acidosis (pH <7); seizures, coma, or hypotonia; and multiorgan dysfunction. Low Apgar scores may be caused by fetal hypoxia or other factors listed in Table 58.7. Most infants with low Apgar scores respond to assisted ventilation by face mask or by endotracheal intubation and usually do not need emergency medication.

Resuscitation of a newborn with a low Apgar score follows the same systematic sequence as that for resuscitation of older patients, but in the newborn period this simplified *ABCD* approach requires some qualification (Fig. 58.2). In the ABCD approach, **A** stands for securing a patent airway by clearing amniotic fluid or meconium by suctioning; **A** is also a reminder of *anticipation* and the need for knowing the events of pregnancy, labor, and delivery. Evidence of a diaphragmatic hernia and a low Apgar score indicate that immediate endotracheal intubation is required. If a mask and bag are used, gas enters the lung and the stomach, and the latter may act as an expanding mass in the chest that compromises respiration. If fetal hydrops has occurred with pleural effusions, bilateral thoracentesis to evacuate the pleural effusions may be needed to establish adequate ventilation.

B represents **breathing**. If the neonate is apneic or hypoventilating and remains cyanotic, artificial ventilation should be initiated. Ventilation should be performed with a well-fitted mask attached to an anesthesia bag and a manometer to prevent extremely high pressures from being given to the newborn; 100% oxygen should be administered through the mask. If the infant does not revive, an endotracheal tube should be placed, attached to the anesthesia bag and manometer, and 100% oxygen should be administered. The pressure generated should begin at 20-25 cm H_2O, with a rate of 40-60 breaths/minute. An adequate response to ventilation includes good chest rise, return of breath sounds, well-oxygenated color, heart rate returning to the normal range (120-160 beats/min), normal end-tidal carbon dioxide, and, later, increased muscle activity and wakefulness. The usual recovery after a cardiac arrest first involves a return to a normal heart rate, followed by disappearance of cyanosis and noticeably improved perfusion.

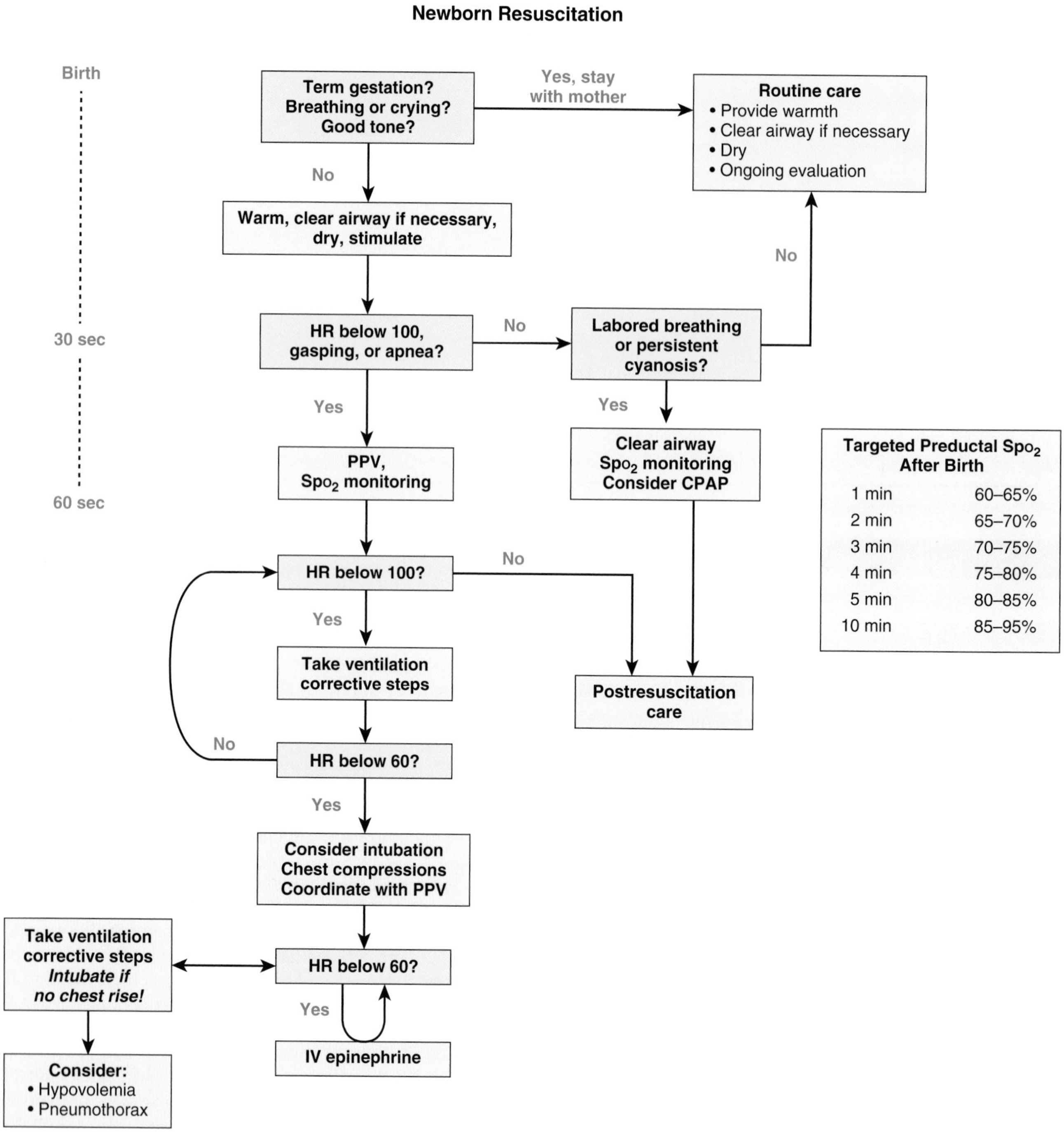

FIGURE 58.2 New guidelines and algorithm for neonatal resuscitation. *CPAP*, Continuous positive airway pressure; *IV*, intravenous; *HR*, heart rate; *PPV*, positive pressure ventilation; *Spo*$_2$, blood oxygen saturation. (From Kattwinkel J, Perlman JM, Aziz K, et al. Special report—neonatal resuscitation: 2010 American Heart Association guidelines for cardiopulmonary resuscitation and emergency cardiovascular care. *Pediatrics.* 2010;126[5]:e1400–e1413. Erratum in Neoreviews 2011;128[1]:176.)

An infant may remain limp and be apneic for a prolonged time after return of cardiac output and correction of acidosis.

Breathing initially should be briefly delayed if meconium-stained amniotic fluid is present to avoid dissemination of meconium into the lungs, producing severe aspiration pneumonia. If meconium is noted in the amniotic fluid, the oropharynx should be suctioned when the head is delivered. After the birth of a **depressed infant**, the oral cavity should be suctioned again; the vocal cords should be visualized and the infant intubated.

C represents **circulation** and external cardiac massage. If artificial ventilation does not improve bradycardia, if asystole is present, or if peripheral pulses cannot be palpated, external cardiac massage should be performed at a rate of 120 compressions/minute with compressions and breaths given at a ratio of 3:1. External cardiac massage usually is not

TABLE 58.9 Life-Threatening Congenital Anomalies

NAME	MANIFESTATIONS
Choanal atresia (stenosis)	Respiratory distress in delivery room, apnea, unable to pass nasogastric tube through nares
Pierre Robin syndrome	Micrognathia, cleft palate, airway obstruction
Diaphragmatic hernia	Scaphoid abdomen, bowel sounds present in left chest, heart shifted to right, respiratory distress, polyhydramnios
Tracheoesophageal fistula	Polyhydramnios, aspiration pneumonia, excessive salivation, unable to place nasogastric tube in stomach
Intestinal obstruction: volvulus, duodenal atresia, ileal atresia	Polyhydramnios, bile-stained emesis, abdominal distention
Gastroschisis/omphalocele	Polyhydramnios; intestinal obstruction
Renal agenesis/Potter syndrome	Oligohydramnios, anuria, pulmonary hypoplasia, pneumothorax
Hydronephrosis	Bilateral abdominal masses
Neural tube defects: anencephaly, meningomyelocele	Polyhydramnios, elevated α-fetoprotein; decreased fetal activity
Down syndrome (trisomy 21)	Hypotonia, congenital heart disease, duodenal atresia
Ductal-dependent congenital heart disease	Cyanosis, murmur, shock

needed because most infants in the delivery room respond to ventilation.

D represents the **administration of drugs**. If bradycardia is unresponsive to ventilation or if asystole is present, epinephrine should be administered. Intravenous (IV) epinephrine (1 : 10,000), 0.1-0.3 mL/kg, should be given through an umbilical venous line or injected into the endotracheal tube. However, when epinephrine is administered through the endotracheal tube, the result is often unpredictable. Before medications are administered in the presence of electrical cardiac activity with poor pulses, it is important to determine whether there is a **pneumothorax**. Transillumination of the thorax, involving the use of a bright light through each side of the thorax and over the sternum, may suggest pneumothorax if one side transmits more light than the other. Breath sounds may be decreased over a pneumothorax and there may be a shift of the heart tones away from the side of a tension pneumothorax.

If central nervous system depression in the infant may be due to a narcotic medication given to the mother, 0.1 mg/kg of naloxone (Narcan) can be given to the infant intravenously or endotracheally. Before this drug is administered, the ABCs should be followed carefully. Naloxone should not be given to a newborn of a mother who is suspected of being addicted to narcotics or is on methadone maintenance because the newborn may experience severe withdrawal seizures.

In babies of more than 35 weeks' gestation suffering moderate to severe hypoxic-ischemic injury at birth, induced therapeutic **hypothermia** (33.0-34.0°C) for 72 hours has been shown in clinical studies to be efficacious in reducing the severity of brain injury. Brain hypothermia, whether induced by whole-body or selective head cooling, provides neuroprotection against encephalopathy presumably due to hypoxic ischemia.

Physical Examination and Gestational Age Assessment

The first physical examination of a newborn may be a general physical examination of a well infant or an examination to confirm fetal diagnoses or to determine the cause of various manifestations of neonatal diseases. Problems in the transition from fetal to neonatal life may be detectable immediately in the delivery room or during the first day of life. Physical examination also may reveal effects of the labor and delivery resulting from asphyxia, drugs, or birth trauma. The first newborn examination is an important way to detect congenital malformations or deformations (Table 58.9). Significant congenital malformations may be present in 1-3% of all births.

Appearance

Signs such as cyanosis, nasal flaring, intercostal retractions, and grunting suggest pulmonary disease. Meconium staining of the umbilical cord, nails, and skin suggest fetal distress and the possibility of aspiration pneumonia. The level of spontaneous activity, passive muscle tone, quality of the cry, and apnea are useful screening signs to evaluate the state of the nervous system.

Vital Signs

The examination should proceed with an assessment of vital signs, particularly heart rate (normal rate, 120-160 beats/min), respiratory rate (normal rate, 30-60 breaths/min), temperature (usually done per rectum and later as an axillary measurement), and blood pressure (often reserved for sick infants). Length, weight, and head circumference should be measured and plotted on growth curves to determine whether growth is normal, accelerated, or retarded for the specific gestational age.

Gestational Age

Gestational age is determined by an assessment of various physical signs (Fig. 58.3) and neuromuscular characteristics (Fig. 58.4) that vary according to fetal age and maturity. **Physical criteria** mature with advancing fetal age, including increasing firmness of the pinna of the ear; increasing size of the breast tissue; decreasing fine, immature lanugo hair over the back; and decreasing opacity of the skin. **Neurological criteria** mature with gestational age, including increasing flexion of the legs, hips, and arms; increasing tone of the flexor muscles of the neck; and decreasing laxity of the joints. These signs are determined during the first day of life and are assigned scores.

Physical maturity	−1	0	1	2	3	4	5
Skin	Sticky, friable, transparent	Gelatinous, red, translucent	Smooth, pink, visible veins	Superficial peeling or rash, few veins	Cracking, pale areas, rare veins	Parchment, deep cracking, no vessels	Leathery, cracked, wrinkled
Lanugo	None	Sparse	Abundant	Thinning	Bald areas	Mostly bald	
Plantar surface	Heel–toe 40-50 mm: −1 Less than 40 mm: −2	<50 mm, no crease	Faint red marks	Anterior transverse crease only	Creases on anterior 2/3	Creases over entire sole	
Breast	Impercep-tible	Barely perceptible	Flat areola–no bud	Stripped areola, 1-2 mm bud	Raised areola, 3-4 mm bud	Full areola, 5-10 mm bud	
Eye/ear	Lids fused, loosely (−1), tightly (−2)	Lids open, pinna flat, stays folded	Slightly curved pinna; soft, slow recoil	Well-curved pinna, soft but ready recoil	Formed and firm; instant recoil	Thick cartilage, ear stiff	
Genitals male	Scrotum flat, smooth	Scrotum empty, faint rugae	Testes in upper canal, rare rugae	Testes descending, few rugae	Testes down, good rugae	Testes pendulous, deep rugae	
Genitals female	Clitoris prominent, labia flat	Prominent clitoris, small labia minora	Prominent clitoris, enlarging minora	Majora and minora equally prominent	Majora large, minora small	Majora cover clitoris and minora	

FIGURE 58.3 Physical criteria for assessment of maturity and gestational age. Expanded New Ballard Score includes extremely premature infants and has been refined to improve accuracy in more mature infants. (From Ballard JL, Khoury JC, Wedig K, et al. New Ballard Score, expanded to include extremely premature infants. *J Pediatr.* 1991;119:417–423.)

The cumulative score is correlated with a gestational age, which is usually accurate to within 2 weeks (Fig. 58.5).

Gestational age assessment permits the detection of abnormal fetal growth patterns, aiding in predicting the neonatal complications of largeness or smallness for gestational age (Fig. 58.6). Infants born at a weight greater than the 90th percentile for age are considered **large for gestational age**. Among the risks associated with being large for gestational age are all the risks of the infant of a diabetic mother and risks associated with postmaturity. Infants born at a weight less than 10th percentile for age (some growth curves use <2 standard deviations or the 5th percentile) are **small for gestational age** and have IUGR. Problems associated with small for gestational age infants include congenital malformations, in addition to the problems listed in Table 58.2.

Skin

The skin should be evaluated for pallor, plethora, jaundice, cyanosis, meconium staining, petechiae, ecchymoses, congenital nevi, and neonatal rashes. Vasomotor instability with cutis marmorata, telangiectasia, phlebectasia (intermittent mottling with venous prominence), and acrocyanosis (feet and hands) is normal in a premature infant. Acrocyanosis also may be noted in a healthy term infant in the first days after birth.

The skin is covered with lanugo hair, which disappears by term gestation. **Hair tufts** over the lumbosacral spine suggest a spinal cord defect. **Vernix caseosa**, a soft, white, creamy layer covering the skin in preterm infants, disappears by term. Post-term infants often have peeling, parchment-like skin. **Mongolian spots** are transient, dark blue to black pigmented macules seen over the lower back and buttocks in 90% of African American, Indian, and Asian infants. **Nevus simplex** *(salmon patch)*, or pink macular hemangioma, is common, usually transient, and noted on the back of the neck, eyelids, and forehead. **Nevus flammeus**, or **port-wine stain**, is seen on the face and should cause the examiner to consider Sturge-Weber syndrome (trigeminal angiomatosis, convulsions, and ipsilateral intracranial *tram-line* calcifications).

Congenital melanocytic nevi are pigmented lesions of varying size noted in 1% of neonates. **Giant pigmented nevi** are uncommon but have malignant potential. **Capillary hemangiomas** are raised, red lesions, whereas **cavernous hemangiomas** are deeper, blue masses. Both lesions increase in size after birth then resolve when the child is 1-4 years of age. When enlarged, these hemangiomas may produce high-output heart failure or platelet trapping and hemorrhage. **Erythema toxicum** is an erythematous, papular-vesicular rash common in neonates that develops after birth and involves

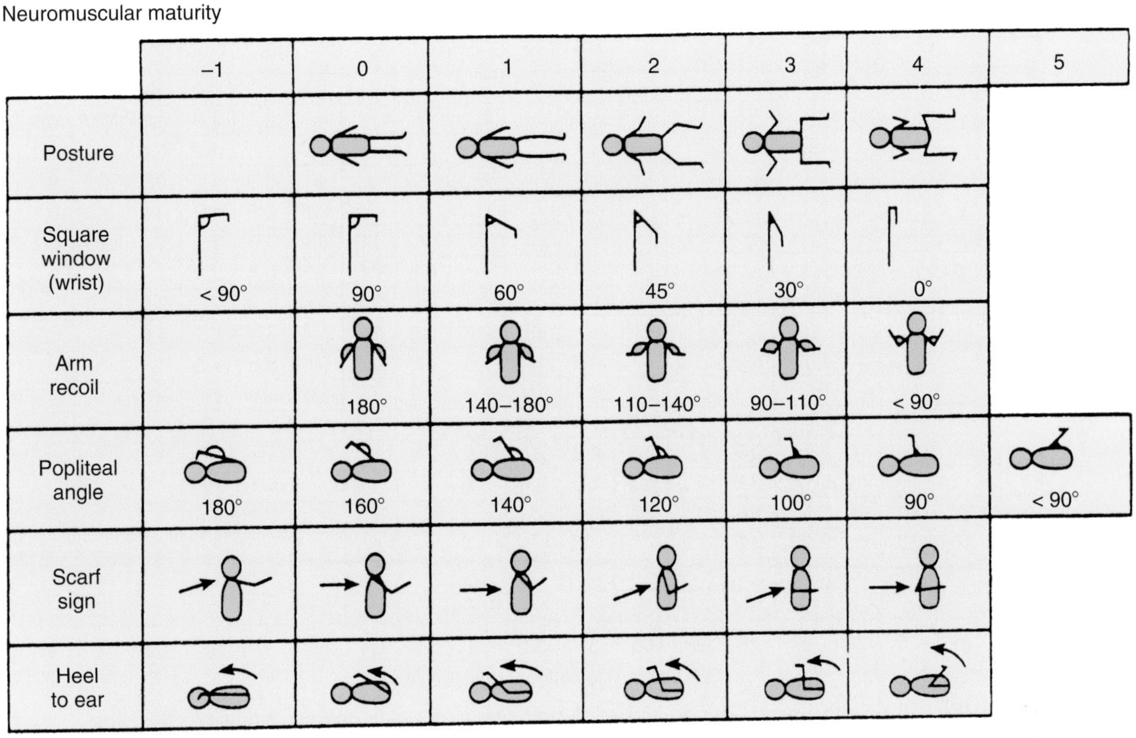

Neuromuscular maturity
-1
0
1
2
3
4
5
Posture
Square window (wrist)
< 90°
90°
60°
45°
30°
0°
Arm recoil
180°
140–180°
110–140°
90–110°
< 90°
Popliteal angle
180°
160°
140°
120°
100°
90°
< 90°
Scarf sign
Heel to ear

FIGURE 58.4 Neuromuscular criteria for assessment of maturity and gestational age. Expanded New Ballard Score includes extremely premature infants and has been refined to improve accuracy in more mature infants. (From Ballard JL, Khoury JC, Wedig K, et al. New Ballard Score, expanded to include extremely premature infants. *J Pediatr.* 1991;119:417–423.)

Maturity rating

Score	Weeks
−10	20
−5	22
0	24
5	26
10	28
15	30
20	32
25	34
30	36
35	38
40	40
45	42
50	44

FIGURE 58.5 Maturity rating as calculated by adding the physical and neurological scores, calculating the gestational age. (From Ballard JL, Khoury JC, Wedig K, et al. New Ballard Score, expanded to include extremely premature infants. *J Pediatr.* 1991;119:417–423.)

eosinophils in the vesicular fluid. **Pustular melanosis**, more common in African American infants, may be seen at birth and consists of a small, dry vesicle on a pigmented brown macular base. Erythema toxicum and pustular melanosis are benign lesions but may mimic more serious conditions, such as the vesicular rash of disseminated herpes simplex or the bullous eruption of *S. aureus* impetigo. Tzanck smear, Gram stain, Wright stain, direct fluorescent antibody stain, polymerase chain reaction for herpes DNA, and appropriate cultures may be needed to distinguish these rashes. Other common characteristic rashes are **milia** (yellow-white epidermal cysts of the pilosebaceous follicles that are noted on the nose) and **miliaria** (prickly heat), which is caused by obstructed sweat glands. **Edema** may be present in preterm infants, but also suggests hydrops fetalis, sepsis, hypoalbuminemia, or lymphatic disorders.

Skull

The skull may be elongated and molded after a prolonged labor; this resolves 2-3 days after birth. The sutures should be palpated to determine the width and the presence of premature fusion or cranial synostosis. The anterior and posterior fontanelles should be soft and nonbulging, with the anterior larger than the posterior. A large fontanelle is associated with hydrocephalus, hypothyroidism, rickets, and other disorders. Soft areas away from the fontanelle are **craniotabes**; these lesions feel like a Ping-Pong ball when they are palpated. They may be a result of in utero compression. The skull should be examined carefully for signs of trauma or lacerations from internal fetal electrode sites or fetal scalp pH sampling; abscesses may develop in these areas.

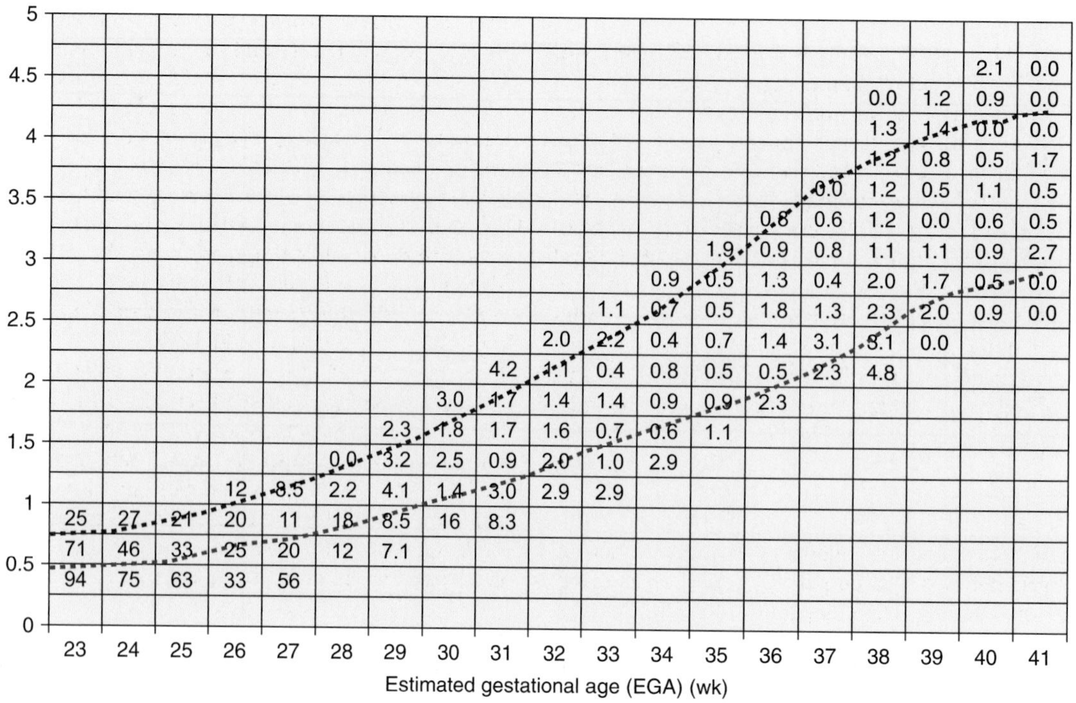

FIGURE 58.6 Birth weight–specific and estimated gestational age–specific mortality rates. The dashed lines of the figure represent the 10th and 90th percentile weights. The grid lines are plotted by each gestational age and in 250-g weight increments. Each number in the box is the percent mortality rate for the grid defined by gestational age and birth weight range. (From Thomas P, Peabody J, Turnier V, et al. A new look at intrauterine growth and impact of race, attitude, and gender. *Pediatrics.* 2000;106:E21.)

Face, Eyes, and Mouth

The face should be inspected for dysmorphic features, such as epicanthal folds, hypertelorism, preauricular tags or sinuses, low-set ears, long philtrum, and cleft lip or palate. Facial asymmetry may be a result of seventh nerve palsy; head tilt may be caused by torticollis.

The eyes should open spontaneously, especially in an upright position. Before 28 weeks' gestational age, the eyelids may be fused. Coloboma, megalocornea, and microphthalmia suggest other malformations or intrauterine infections. A cloudy cornea greater than 1 cm in diameter also may be seen in congenital glaucoma, uveal tract dysgenesis, and storage diseases. Conjunctival and retinal hemorrhages are common and usually of no significance. The pupillary response to light is present at 28 weeks of gestation. The **red reflex** of the retina is shown easily. A white reflex, or **leukokoria**, is abnormal and may be the result of cataracts, ocular tumor, severe chorioretinitis, persistent hyperplastic primary vitreous, or retinopathy of prematurity.

The mouth should be inspected for the presence of natal teeth, clefts of the soft and hard palate and uvula, and micrognathia. A bifid uvula suggests a submucosal cleft. White, shiny, multiple transient epidermal inclusion cysts (Epstein pearls) on the hard palate are normal. Hard, marble-sized masses in the buccal mucosa are usually transient idiopathic fat necrosis. The **tympanic membranes** are dull, gray, opaque, and immobile in the first 1-4 weeks. These findings should not be confused with otitis media.

Neck and Chest

The neck appears short and symmetrical. Abnormalities include midline clefts or masses caused by thyroglossal duct cysts or by goiter and lateral neck masses (or sinuses), which are the result of branchial clefts. Cystic hygromas and hemangiomas may be present. Shortening of the sternocleidomastoid muscle with a fibrous tumor over the muscle produces head tilt and asymmetrical facies (neonatal torticollis). Arnold-Chiari malformation and cervical spine lesions also produce torticollis. Edema and webbing of the neck suggest Turner syndrome. Both clavicles should be palpated for fractures.

Examination of the **chest** includes inspection of the chest wall to identify asymmetry resulting from absence of the pectoralis muscle and inspection of the breast tissue to determine gestational age and detect a breast abscess. Boys and girls may have breast engorgement and produce milk; milk expression should not be attempted. **Supernumerary nipples** may be bilateral and may be associated with renal anomalies.

Lungs

Examination of the lungs includes observations of the rate, depth, and nature of intercostal or sternal retractions. Breath sounds should be equal on both sides of the chest, and rales should not be heard after the first 1-2 hours of life. Diminished or absent breath sounds on one side suggest pneumothorax, collapsed lung, pleural effusion, or diaphragmatic hernia. Shift of the cardiac impulse away from a tension pneumothorax and diaphragmatic hernia and toward the collapsed lung is a helpful physical finding for differentiating these disorders. Subcutaneous emphysema of the neck or chest also suggests a pneumothorax or pneumomediastinum, whereas bowel sounds auscultated in the chest in the presence of a scaphoid abdomen suggest a diaphragmatic hernia.

Heart

The position of the heart in infants is more midline than in older children. The first heart sound is normal, whereas the second heart sound may not be split in the first day of life. Decreased splitting of the second heart sound is noted in PPHN, transposition of the great vessels, and pulmonary atresia. Heart murmurs in newborns are common in the delivery room and during the first day of life. Most of these murmurs are transient and are due to closure of the ductus arteriosus, peripheral pulmonary artery stenosis, or a small ventral septal defect. Pulses should be palpated in the upper and lower extremities (over the brachial and femoral arteries). Blood pressure in the upper and lower extremities should be measured in all patients with a murmur or heart failure. An upper-to-lower extremity gradient of more than 10-20 mm Hg suggests coarctation of the aorta.

Abdomen

The liver may be palpable 2 cm below the right costal margin. The spleen tip is less likely to be palpable. A left-sided liver suggests situs inversus and asplenia syndrome. Both kidneys should be palpable in the first day of life with gentle, deep palpation. The first urination occurs during the first day of life in more than 95% of normal term infants.

Abdominal masses usually represent hydronephrosis or dysplastic-multicystic kidney disease. Less often, masses indicate ovarian cysts, intestinal duplication, neuroblastoma, or mesoblastic nephroma. Masses should be evaluated immediately with ultrasound. Abdominal distention may be caused by intestinal obstructions, such as ileal atresia, meconium ileus, midgut volvulus, imperforate anus, or Hirschsprung disease. Meconium stool is passed normally within 48 hours of birth in 99% of term infants. The anus should be patent. An imperforate anus is not always visible; the first temperature taken with a rectal thermometer should be taken carefully. The abdominal wall musculature may be absent, as in prune-belly syndrome, or weak, resulting in diastasis recti. **Umbilical hernias** are common in African American infants. The umbilical cord should be inspected to determine the presence of two arteries and one vein and the absence of an urachus or a herniation of abdominal contents, as occurs with an **omphalocele**. The latter is associated with extraintestinal problems, such as genetic trisomies and hypoglycemia (Beckwith-Wiedemann syndrome). Bleeding from the cord suggests a coagulation disorder, and a chronic discharge may be a granuloma of the umbilical stump or, less frequently, a draining omphalomesenteric cyst or urachus. Erythema around the umbilicus is **omphalitis** and may cause portal vein thrombophlebitis and subsequent extrahepatic portal hypertension. The herniation of bowel through the abdominal wall 2-3 cm lateral to the umbilicus is a **gastroschisis**.

Genitalia

Decision-Making Algorithm
Available @ StudentConsult.com

Ambiguous Genitalia

At term, the testes should be descended into a well-formed pigmented and rugated scrotum. The testes occasionally are in the inguinal canal; this is more common among preterm infants, as is cryptorchidism. Scrotal swelling may represent a hernia, transient hydrocele, in utero torsion of the testes, or, rarely, dissected meconium from meconium ileus and peritonitis. Hydroceles are clear and readily seen by transillumination, whereas testicular torsion in the newborn may present as a painless, dark swelling. The urethral opening should be at the end of the penis. Epispadias or hypospadias alone should not raise concern about pseudohermaphroditism. However, if no testes are present in the scrotum and hypospadias is present, problems of sexual development should be suspected. Circumcision should be deferred with hypospadias because the foreskin is often needed for the repair. The normal prepuce is often too tight to retract in the neonatal period.

The female genitalia normally may reveal a milky white or blood-streaked vaginal discharge as a result of maternal hormone withdrawal. Mucosal tags of the labia majora are common. Distention of an imperforate hymen may produce hydrometrocolpos and a lower midline abdominal mass as a result of an enlarged uterus. Clitoral enlargement with fusion of the labial-scrotal folds (labia majora) suggests adrenogenital syndrome or exposure to masculinizing maternal hormones.

Extremities

Examination of the extremities should involve assessment of length, symmetry, and presence of hemihypertrophy, atrophy, polydactyly, syndactyly, simian creases, absent fingers, overlapping fingers, rocker-bottom feet, clubfoot, congenital bands, fractures, and amputations.

Spine

The spine should be examined for evidence of sacral hair tufts, a dermal sinus tract above the gluteal folds, congenital scoliosis (a result of hemivertebra), and soft tissue masses such as lipomas or meningomyeloceles.

Hips

The hips should be examined for congenital dysplasia (dislocation). Gluteal fold asymmetry or leg length discrepancy is suggestive of dysplasia, but the examiner should perform the Barlow test and the Ortolani maneuver to evaluate the stability of the hip joint. These tests determine whether the femoral head can be displaced from the acetabulum **(Barlow test)** and then replaced **(Ortolani maneuver)**.

NEUROLOGICAL ASSESSMENT

The neurological examination should include assessment of active and passive tone, level of alertness, primary neonatal (primitive) reflexes, deep tendon reflexes, spontaneous motor activity, and cranial nerves (involving retinal examination, extraocular muscle movement, masseter power as in sucking, facial motility, hearing, and tongue function). The Moro reflex, present at birth and gone in 3-6 months, is one of the primary newborn reflexes. It is elicited by sudden, slight dropping of the supported head from a slightly raised supine position, which should elicit opening of the hands and extension and abduction of the arms, followed by upper extremity flexion and a cry. The palmar grasp is present by 28 weeks' gestation and gone by 4 months of age. Deep tendon reflexes may be brisk in a normal newborn; 5-10 beats of ankle clonus are normal. The Babinski sign is extensor (upgoing). The sensory examination can be evaluated by withdrawal of an extremity, grimace, and cry in response to painful stimuli. The rooting reflex (turning of the

TABLE 58.10 Differential Diagnosis of Neonatal Cyanosis

SYSTEM/DISEASE	MECHANISM
PULMONARY	
Respiratory distress syndrome	Surfactant deficiency
Sepsis, pneumonia	Inflammation, pulmonary hypertension, ARDS
Meconium aspiration pneumonia	Mechanical obstruction, inflammation, pulmonary hypertension
Persistent pulmonary hypertension of the newborn	Pulmonary hypertension
Diaphragmatic hernia	Pulmonary hypoplasia, pulmonary hypertension
Transient tachypnea	Retained lung fluid
CARDIOVASCULAR	
Cyanotic heart disease with decreased pulmonary blood flow	Right-to-left shunt as in pulmonary atresia, tetralogy of Fallot
Cyanotic heart disease with increased pulmonary blood flow	Mixing lesion as in single ventricle or truncus arteriosus
Cyanotic heart disease with congestive heart failure	Pulmonary edema and poor cardiac output as in hypoplastic left heart and coarctation of aorta
Heart failure alone	Pulmonary edema and poor cardiac contractility as in sepsis, myocarditis, supraventricular tachycardia, or complete heart block; high-output failure as in PDA or vein of Galen or other arteriovenous malformations
CENTRAL NERVOUS SYSTEM (CNS)	
Maternal sedative drugs	Hypoventilation, apnea
Asphyxia	CNS depression
Intracranial hemorrhage	CNS depression, seizure
Neuromuscular disease	Hypotonia, hypoventilation, pulmonary hypoplasia
HEMATOLOGICAL	
Acute blood loss	Shock
Chronic blood loss	Heart failure
Polycythemia	Pulmonary hypertension
Methemoglobinemia	Low-affinity hemoglobin or red blood cell enzyme defect
METABOLIC	
Hypoglycemia	CNS depression, congestive heart failure
Adrenogenital syndrome	Shock (salt-losing)

ARDS, Acute respiratory distress syndrome; *CNS*, central nervous system; *PDA*, patent ductus arteriosus.

head toward light tactile stimulation of the perioral area) is present by 32 weeks' gestation.

Special Conditions Requiring Resuscitation in the Delivery Room

Cyanosis

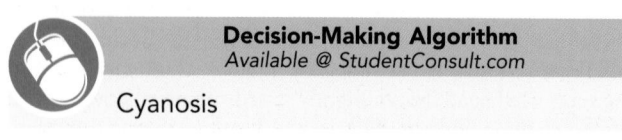

Decision-Making Algorithm
Available @ StudentConsult.com

Cyanosis

Acrocyanosis (blue color of the hands and feet with pink color of the rest of the body) is common in the delivery room and is usually normal. **Central cyanosis** of the trunk, mucosal membranes, and tongue can occur at any time after birth and is always a manifestation of a serious underlying condition. Cyanosis is noted with 4-5 g/dL of deoxygenated hemoglobin. Central cyanosis can be caused by problems in many different organ systems, although cardiopulmonary diseases are the most common (Table 58.10). Respiratory distress syndrome, sepsis, and cyanotic heart disease are the three most common causes of cyanosis in infants admitted to a neonatal intensive care unit. A systematic evaluation of these and other causes of cyanosis is required for every cyanotic infant after prompt administration of oxygen, with or without assisted ventilation.

Life-Threatening Congenital Malformations

Various congenital anomalies can interfere with vital organ function after birth (see Table 58.9). Some malformations, such as choanal atresia and other lesions obstructing the airway, may complicate ventilation. Intrathoracic lesions, such as cysts or diaphragmatic hernia, interfere with respiration. Other malformations that obstruct the gastrointestinal system at the level of the esophagus, duodenum, ileum, or colon may lead to aspiration pneumonia, intestinal perforation, or gangrene. Gastroschisis and omphalocele are associated with exposed bowel on the abdominal wall. Omphalocele is often associated with other malformations, whereas intestinal necrosis is more common in gastroschisis.

Shock

Shock in the delivery room is manifested by pallor, poor capillary refill time, lack of palpable pulses, hypotonia, cyanosis, and eventually cardiopulmonary arrest. Blood loss before or during labor and delivery is a common cause of shock in the delivery room. Blood loss may be caused by fetal-maternal hemorrhage, placenta previa, vasa previa, twin-to-twin transfusion syndrome, or displacement of blood from the fetus to the placenta as during asphyxia *(asphyxia pallida)*. Hemorrhage into a viscus, such as the liver or spleen, may be noted in macrosomic infants, and hemorrhage into the cerebral ventricles may produce shock and apnea in preterm infants. Anemia, hypoalbuminemia, hypovolemia, and shock at birth are common manifestations of Rh immune hydrops.

Severe intrauterine bacterial sepsis may present with shock in the delivery room or immediately after the infant is transferred to the nursery. Typically these infants are mottled, hypotonic, and cyanotic and have diminished peripheral pulses. They have a normal hemoglobin concentration but may manifest neutropenia, thrombocytopenia, and disseminated intravascular coagulation. Peripheral symmetrical gangrene (purpuric rash) often is a sign of hypotensive shock in infants with severe congenital bacterial infections. Congenital left ventricular cardiac obstruction (critical aortic stenosis or hypoplastic left heart syndrome) also produces shock, although not usually in the delivery room.

Treatment of newborn infants with shock should involve the management approaches used for the sick infant. Problems may be anticipated through knowledge of the infant's immune status, evidence of hydrops, or suspicion of intrauterine infection or anomalies. Stabilization of the airway and institution of respiratory support are essential. Hypovolemic shock should be managed with repeated boluses of 10-15 mL/kg of normal saline or lactated Ringer solution. If severe immune hemolysis is predicted, blood typed against the mother's blood should be available in the delivery room and should be given to the newborn if signs of anemia and shock are present. Thereafter, all blood should be crossmatched with the infant's and mother's blood before transfusion. Drugs such as dopamine, epinephrine, or cortisol may improve cardiac output and tissue perfusion.

Birth Injury

Birth injury refers to avoidable and unavoidable injury to the fetus during the birth process. **Caput succedaneum** is a diffuse, edematous, often dark swelling of the soft tissue of the scalp that extends across the midline and suture lines. In infants delivered from a face presentation, soft tissue edema of the eyelids and face is an equivalent phenomenon. Caput succedaneum may be seen after prolonged labor in full-term and preterm infants. Molding of the head often is associated with caput succedaneum and is the result of pressure that is induced from overriding the parietal and frontal bones against their respective sutures.

A **cephalhematoma** is a subperiosteal hemorrhage that does not cross the suture lines surrounding the respective bones. A linear skull fracture rarely may be seen underlying a cephalhematoma. With time, the cephalhematoma may organize, calcify, and form a central depression.

Infants with cephalhematoma and caput succedaneum require no specific treatment. Occasionally a premature infant may develop a massive scalp hemorrhage. This **subgaleal bleeding** and the bleeding noted from a cephalhematoma may cause indirect hyperbilirubinemia requiring phototherapy. **Retinal and subconjunctival hemorrhages** are common but usually are small and insignificant; no treatment is necessary.

Spinal cord or **spine injuries** may occur in the fetus as a result of the hyperextended *star gazing* posture. Injuries also may occur in infants after excessive rotational (at C3-4) or longitudinal (at C7-T1) force is transmitted to the neck during vertex or breech delivery. Fractures of vertebrae are rare; trauma may cause direct damage to the spinal cord, leading to transection and permanent sequelae, hemorrhage, edema, and neurological signs. Rarely, a snapping sound indicating cord transection rather than vertebral displacement is heard at the time of delivery. Neurological dysfunction usually involves complete flaccid paralysis, absence of deep tendon reflexes, and absence of responses to painful stimuli below the lesion. Painful stimuli may elicit reflex flexion of the legs. Infants with spinal cord injury often are flaccid, apneic, and asphyxiated, all of which may mask the underlying spinal cord transection.

Injury to the nerves of the **brachial plexus** may result from excessive traction on the neck, producing paresis or complete paralysis. The mildest injury (neurapraxia) is edema; axonotmesis is more severe and consists of disrupted nerve fibers with an intact myelin sheath; neurotmesis, or complete nerve disruption or root avulsion, is most severe. **Erb-Duchenne paralysis** involves the fifth and sixth cervical nerves and is the most common and usually mildest injury. The infant cannot abduct the arm at the shoulder, externally rotate the arm, or supinate the forearm. The usual picture is one of painless adduction, internal rotation of the arm, and pronation of the forearm. The **Moro reflex** is absent on the involved side, and the hand grasp is intact. **Phrenic nerve palsy** (C3, C4, and C5) may lead to diaphragmatic paralysis and respiratory distress. Elevation of the diaphragm caused by nerve injury must be differentiated from elevation caused by eventration resulting from congenital weakness or absence of diaphragm muscle. **Klumpke paralysis** is caused by injury to the seventh and eighth cervical nerves and the first thoracic nerve, resulting in a paralyzed hand and, if the sympathetic nerves are injured, an ipsilateral **Horner syndrome** (ptosis, miosis). Complete arm and hand paralysis is noted with the most severe form of damage to C5, C6, C7, C8, and T1. **Treatment** of brachial plexus injury is supportive and includes positioning to avoid contractures. Active and passive range of motion exercises also may be beneficial. If the deficit persists, nerve grafting may be beneficial.

Facial nerve injury may be the result of compression of the seventh nerve between the facial bone and the mother's pelvic bones or the physician's forceps. This peripheral nerve injury is characterized by an asymmetric crying face whose normal side, including the forehead, moves in a regular manner. The affected side is flaccid, the eye does not close, the nasolabial fold is absent, and the side of the mouth droops at rest. If there is a central injury to the facial nerve, only the lower two thirds of the face (not the forehead) are involved. Complete agenesis of the facial nucleus results in a central facial paralysis; when this is bilateral, as in **Möbius syndrome**, the face appears expressionless.

Skull fractures are rare, are usually linear, and require no treatment other than observation for very rare, delayed (1-3 months) complications (e.g., leptomeningeal cyst). Depressed skull fractures are unusual but may be seen with complicated forceps delivery and may need surgical elevation. Fractures of the **clavicle** usually are unilateral and are noted in macrosomic infants after shoulder dystocia. Often a snap is heard after a difficult delivery, and the infant exhibits an asymmetrical Moro response and decreased movement of the affected side. The prognosis is excellent; many infants require no treatment or a simple figure of eight bandage to immobilize the bone.

Extremity fractures are less common than fractures of the clavicle and involve the humerus more often than the femur. **Treatment** involves immobilization and a triangular splint bandage for the humerus and traction suspension of the legs for femoral fractures. The prognosis is excellent.

Fractures of the **facial bones** are rare, but dislocation of the cartilaginous part of the nasal septum out of the vomeral groove and columella is common. Clinical manifestations include feeding difficulty, respiratory distress, asymmetrical nares, and a flattened, laterally displaced nose. Treatment reduces the dislocation by elevating the cartilage back into the vomeral groove.

Visceral trauma to the liver, spleen, or adrenal gland occurs in macrosomic infants and in extremely premature infants, with or without breech or vaginal delivery. Rupture of the liver with subcapsular hematoma formation may lead to anemia, hypovolemia, shock, hemoperitoneum, and disseminated intravascular coagulation. Infants with anemia and shock who are suspected to have an intraventricular hemorrhage but with a normal head ultrasound examination should be evaluated for hepatic or splenic rupture. Adrenal hemorrhage may be asymptomatic, detected only by finding calcified adrenal glands in normal infants. Infants with severe adrenal hemorrhage may exhibit a flank mass, jaundice, and hematuria, with or without shock.

Temperature Regulation

After birth, a newborn remains covered by amniotic fluid and situated in a cold environment (20-25°C). An infant's skin temperature may decrease 0.3°C/min, and the core temperature may decrease 0.1°C/min in the delivery room. In the absence of an external heat source, the infant must increase metabolism substantially to maintain body temperature.

Heat loss occurs through four basic mechanisms. In the cold delivery room, the wet infant loses heat predominantly by **evaporation** (cutaneous and respiratory loss when wet or in low humidity), **radiation** (loss to nearby cold, solid surfaces), and **convection** (loss to air current). When the infant is dry, radiation, convection, and **conduction** (loss to object in direct contact with infant) are important causes of heat loss. After birth, all high-risk infants should be dried immediately to eliminate evaporative heat losses. A radiant or convective heat source should be provided for these high-risk infants. Normal term infants should be dried and wrapped in a blanket.

The ideal environmental temperature is the **neutral thermal environment**, the ambient temperature that results in the lowest rate of heat being produced by the infant and maintains normal body temperature. The neutral thermal environmental temperature decreases with increasing gestational and postnatal age. Ambient temperatures less than the neutral thermal environment result in increasing rates of oxygen consumption for heat production, which is designed to maintain normal body temperature. If the ambient temperature decreases further or if oxygen consumption cannot increase sufficiently (due to hypoxia, hypoglycemia, or drugs), the core body temperature decreases.

Heat production by a newborn is created predominantly by nonshivering thermogenesis in specialized areas of tissue containing brown adipose tissue. Brown fat is highly vascular, contains many mitochondria per cell, and is situated around large blood vessels, resulting in rapid heat transfer to the circulation. The vessels of the neck, thorax, and interscapular region are common locations of brown fat. These tissues also are innervated by the sympathetic nervous system, which serves as a primary stimulus for heat production by brown adipose cells. Shivering does not occur in newborns.

Severe **cold injury** in an infant is manifested by acidosis, hypoxia, hypoglycemia, apnea, bradycardia, pulmonary hemorrhage, and a pink skin color. The color is caused by trapping of oxygenated hemoglobin in the cutaneous capillaries. Many of these infants appear dead, but most respond to treatment and recover. Milder degrees of cold injury in the delivery room may contribute to metabolic acidosis and hypoxia after birth. Conversely, hypoxia delays heat generation in cold-stressed infants.

Treatment of severe hypothermia should involve resuscitation and rapid warming of core (e.g., lung and stomach) and external surfaces. Fluid resuscitation also is needed to treat hypovolemia seen in many of these infants. Reduced core temperature (32-35°C) in the immediate newborn period often requires only external warming with a radiant warmer, incubator, or both.

Elevated Temperature

Exposure to ambient temperatures above the neutral thermal environment results in *heat stress* and an elevated core temperature. Sweating is uncommon in newborns and may be noted only on the forehead. In response to moderate heat stress, infants may increase their respiratory rate to dissipate heat. Excessive environmental temperatures may result in heatstroke or in hemorrhagic shock encephalopathy syndrome.

MISCELLANEOUS DISORDERS

Hypocalcemia

Decision-Making Algorithm
Available @ StudentConsult.com

Hypocalcemia

Hypocalcemia is common in sick and premature newborns. Calcium levels are higher in cord blood than in maternal blood because of active placental transfer of calcium to the fetus. Fetal calcium accretion in the third trimester approaches 150 mg/kg/24 hr; fetal bone mineral content doubles between 30 and 40 weeks of gestation. All infants show a slight decline of serum calcium levels after birth, reaching a trough level at 24-48 hours, the point at which hypocalcemia usually occurs. Total serum calcium levels of less than 7 mg/dL and ionized calcium levels of less than 3-3.5 mg/dL are considered hypocalcemia.

The etiology of hypocalcemia varies with the time of onset and the associated illnesses of the child. **Early neonatal hypocalcemia** occurs in the first 3 days of life and is often asymptomatic. Transient hypoparathyroidism and a reduced parathyroid response to the usual postnatal decline of serum calcium levels may be responsible for hypocalcemia in premature infants and infants of diabetic mothers. Congenital absences of the parathyroid gland with DiGeorge syndrome is a cause of hypocalcemia. **Hypomagnesemia** (<1.5 mg/dL) may be seen simultaneously with hypocalcemia, especially in infants of diabetic mothers. Treatment with calcium alone does not relieve symptoms or increase serum calcium levels until hypomagnesemia is also treated. Sodium bicarbonate therapy, phosphate release from cell necrosis, transient hypoparathyroidism, and hypercalcitoninemia may be responsible for early neonatal hypocalcemia associated with asphyxia. Early-onset hypocalcemia associated with asphyxia often occurs with seizures as a result of hypoxic-ischemic encephalopathy.

Late neonatal hypocalcemia, or **neonatal tetany**, often is the result of ingestion of high phosphate–containing milk or the inability to excrete the usual phosphorus in commercial infant formula. Hyperphosphatemia (>8 mg/dL) usually occurs in infants with hypocalcemia after the first week of life. Vitamin D deficiency states and malabsorption also have been associated with late-onset hypocalcemia.

The clinical manifestations of hypocalcemia and hypomagnesemia include apnea, muscle twitching, seizures, laryngospasm, **Chvostek sign** (facial muscle spasm when the side of the face over the seventh nerve is tapped), and **Trousseau sign** (carpopedal spasm induced by partial inflation of a blood pressure cuff). The latter two signs are rare in the immediate newborn period.

Neonatal hypocalcemia may be prevented in high-risk neonates by administration of IV or oral calcium supplementation at a rate of 25-75 mg/kg/24 hr. Early asymptomatic hypocalcemia of preterm infants and infants of diabetic mothers often resolves spontaneously. Symptomatic hypocalcemia should be treated with 2-4 mL/kg of 10% calcium gluconate given intravenously and slowly over 10-15 minutes, followed by a continuous infusion of 75 mg/kg/24 hr of elemental calcium. If hypomagnesemia is associated with hypocalcemia, 50% magnesium sulfate, 0.1 mL/kg, should be given by intramuscular injection and repeated every 8-12 hours.

The **treatment** of late hypocalcemia includes immediate management, as in early hypocalcemia, plus the initiation of feedings with low-phosphate formula. Subcutaneous infiltration of IV calcium salts can cause tissue necrosis; oral supplements are hypertonic and may irritate the intestinal mucosa.

Neonatal Drug Addiction and Withdrawal

Infants may become passively and physiologically addicted to medications or to drugs of abuse (heroin, methadone, barbiturates, tranquilizers, amphetamines) taken chronically by the mother during pregnancy; these infants subsequently may have signs and symptoms of drug withdrawal. Many of these pregnancies are at high risk for other complications related to IV drug abuse, such as hepatitis, acquired immunodeficiency syndrome (AIDS), and syphilis. In addition, the LBW rate and the long-term risk for sudden infant death syndrome are higher in the infants of these high-risk women.

Opiates

Neonatal withdrawal signs and symptoms usually begin at 1-5 days of life with maternal heroin use and at 1-4 weeks with maternal methadone addiction. Clinical manifestations of withdrawal include sneezing, yawning, ravenous appetite, emesis, diarrhea, fever, diaphoresis, tachypnea, high-pitched cry, tremors, jitteriness, poor sleep, poor feeding, and seizures. The illness tends to be more severe during methadone withdrawal. The initial treatment includes swaddling in blankets in a quiet, dark room. When hyperactivity is constant, and irritability interferes with sleeping and feeding, or when diarrhea or seizures are present, pharmacological treatment is indicated. Seizures usually are treated with phenobarbital. The other symptoms may be managed with replacement doses of a narcotic (oral morphine, methadone, buprenorphine) to calm the infant; weaning from narcotics may be prolonged over 1-2 months.

Cocaine

Cocaine use during pregnancy is associated with preterm labor, abruptio placentae, neonatal irritability, and decreased attentiveness. Infants may be small for gestational age and have small head circumferences. Usually no treatment is needed.

CHAPTER 59
Maternal Diseases Affecting the Newborn

Maternal diseases during pregnancy can affect the fetus directly or indirectly (Table 59.1). Autoantibody-mediated diseases can have direct consequences on the fetus and neonate because the antibodies are usually of the immunoglobulin G (IgG) type and can cross the placenta to the fetal circulation.

ANTIPHOSPHOLIPID SYNDROME

Antiphospholipid syndrome is associated with thrombophilia and recurrent pregnancy loss. Antiphospholipid antibodies are found in 2-5% of the general healthy population, but they also may be associated with systemic lupus erythematosus (SLE) and other rheumatic diseases. Obstetric complications arise from the prothrombotic effects of the antiphospholipid antibodies on placental function. Vasculopathy, infarction, and thrombosis have been identified in mothers with antiphospholipid syndrome. Antiphospholipid syndrome can include fetal growth impairment, placental insufficiency, maternal preeclampsia, and premature birth.

IDIOPATHIC (IMMUNE) THROMBOCYTOPENIA

Idiopathic thrombocytopenic purpura (ITP) is seen in approximately 1-2 per 1,000 live births and is an immune process in which antibodies are directed against platelets. Platelet-associated IgG antibodies can cross the placenta and cause thrombocytopenia in the fetus and newborn. The severely thrombocytopenic fetus is at increased risk for intracranial hemorrhage. ITP during pregnancy requires close maternal and fetal management to reduce the risks of life-threatening maternal hemorrhage and trauma to the fetus at delivery. Postnatal management involves observation of the infant's platelet count. For infants

TABLE 59.1 Maternal Disease Affecting the Fetus or Neonate

MATERNAL DISORDER	FETAL/NEONATAL EFFECTS	MECHANISM
Cyanotic heart disease	Intrauterine growth restriction	Low fetal oxygen delivery
Diabetes mellitus		
Mild	Large for gestational age, hypoglycemia	Fetal hyperglycemia—produces hyperinsulinemia promoting growth
Severe	Growth retardation	Vascular disease, placental insufficiency
Drug abuse	Intrauterine growth restriction, neonatal withdrawal	Direct drug effect, plus poor diet
Endemic goiter	Hypothyroidism	Iodine deficiency
Graves disease	Transient thyrotoxicosis	Placental immunoglobulin passage of thyrotropin receptor antibody
Hyperparathyroidism	Hypocalcemia	Maternal calcium crosses to fetus and suppresses fetal parathyroid gland
Hypertension	Intrauterine growth restriction, intrauterine fetal demise	Placental insufficiency, fetal hypoxia
Idiopathic thrombocytopenic purpura	Thrombocytopenia	Nonspecific platelet antibodies cross placenta
Infection	Neonatal sepsis (see Chapter 66)	Transplacental or ascending infection
Isoimmune neutropenia or thrombocytopenia	Neutropenia or thrombocytopenia	Specific antifetal neutrophil or platelet antibody crosses placenta after sensitization of mother
Malignant melanoma	Placental or fetal tumor	Metastasis
Myasthenia gravis	Transient neonatal myasthenia	Immunoglobulin to acetylcholine receptor crosses the placenta
Myotonic dystrophy	Neonatal myotonic dystrophy	Autosomal dominant with genetic anticipation
Phenylketonuria	Microcephaly, retardation, ventricular septal defect	Elevated fetal phenylalanine levels
Rh or other blood group sensitization	Fetal anemia, hypoalbuminemia, hydrops, neonatal jaundice	Antibody crosses placenta directed at fetal cells with antigen
Systemic lupus erythematosus	Congenital heart block, rash, anemia, thrombocytopenia, neutropenia, cardiomyopathy, stillbirth	Antibody directed at fetal heart, red and white blood cells, and platelets; lupus anticoagulant

From Stoll BJ, Kliegman RM. The fetus and neonatal infant. In: Behrman RE, Kliegman RM, Jenson HB, eds. Nelson Textbook of Pediatrics. *16th ed. Philadelphia: Saunders; 2000.*

who have evidence of hemorrhage, single-donor irradiated platelets may be administered to control the bleeding. The infant may benefit from an infusion of intravenous immunoglobulin. Neonatal thrombocytopenia usually resolves within 4-6 weeks.

SYSTEMIC LUPUS ERYTHEMATOSUS

Immune abnormalities in SLE can lead to the production of anti-Ro (SS-A) and anti-La (SS-B) antibodies that can cross the placenta and injure fetal tissue. The most serious complication is damage to the cardiac conducting system, which results in **congenital heart block**. The heart block observed in association with maternal SLE tends to be complete (third degree), although less advanced blocks have been observed. The mortality rate is approximately 20%; most surviving infants require pacing. Neonatal lupus may occur and is characterized by skin lesions (sharply demarcated erythematous plaques or central atrophic macules with peripheral scaling with predilection for the eyes, face, and scalp), thrombocytopenia, autoimmune hemolysis, and hepatic involvement.

NEONATAL HYPERTHYROIDISM

Graves disease is associated with thyroid-stimulating antibodies. The prevalence of clinical hyperthyroidism in pregnancy has been reported to be about 0.1-0.4%; it is the second most common endocrine disorder during pregnancy (after diabetes). Neonatal hyperthyroidism is due to the transplacental passage of thyroid-stimulating antibodies; hyperthyroidism can appear rapidly within the first 12-48 hours. Symptoms may include intrauterine growth restriction, prematurity, goiter (may cause tracheal obstruction), exophthalmos, stare, craniosynostosis (usually coronal), flushing, heart failure, tachycardia, arrhythmias, hypertension, hypoglycemia, thrombocytopenia, and hepatosplenomegaly. Treatment includes propylthiouracil, iodine drops, and propranolol. Autoimmune induced neonatal hyperthyroidism usually resolves in 2-4 months.

TABLE 59.2 Problems of Diabetic Pregnancy

MATERNAL
Ketoacidosis
Hyperglycemia/hypoglycemia
Nephritis
Preeclampsia
Polyhydramnios
Retinopathy
NEONATAL
Birth asphyxia
Birth injury (macrosomia, shoulder dystocia)
Congenital anomalies (lumbosacral dysgenesis—caudal regression)
Congenital heart disease (ventricular and atrial septal defects, transposition of the great arteries, truncus arteriosus, double-outlet right ventricle, coarctation of the aorta)
Hyperbilirubinemia (unconjugated)
Hypocalcemia
Hypoglycemia
Hypomagnesemia
Neurological disorders (neural tube defects, holoprosencephaly)
Organomegaly
Polycythemia (hyperviscosity)
Renal disorders (double ureter, renal vein thrombosis, hydronephrosis, renal agenesis)
Respiratory distress syndrome
Small left colon syndrome
Transient tachypnea of the newborn

TABLE 59.3 Common Teratogenic Drugs

DRUG	RESULTS
Alcohol	Fetal alcohol syndrome, microcephaly, congenital heart disease
Aminopterin	Mesomelia, cranial dysplasia
Coumarin	Hypoplastic nasal bridge, chondrodysplasia punctata
Fluoxetine	Minor malformations, low birth weight, poor neonatal adaptation
Folic acid antagonists*	Neural tube, cardiovascular, renal, and oral cleft defects
Isotretinoin and vitamin A	Facial and ear anomalies, congenital heart disease
Lithium	Ebstein anomaly
Methyl mercury	Microcephaly, blindness, deafness, retardation (Minamata disease)
Misoprostol	Arthrogryposis
Penicillamine	Cutis laxa syndrome
Phenytoin	Hypoplastic nails, intrauterine growth restriction, typical facies
Radioactive iodine	Fetal hypothyroidism
Radiation	Microcephaly
Stilbestrol (DES)	Vaginal adenocarcinoma during adolescence
Streptomycin	Deafness
Testosterone-like drugs	Virilization of female
Tetracycline	Enamel hypoplasia
Thalidomide	Phocomelia
Toluene (solvent abuse)	Fetal alcohol–like syndrome, preterm labor
Trimethadione	Congenital anomalies, typical facies
Valproate	Spina bifida
Vitamin D	Supravalvular aortic stenosis

Trimethoprim, triamterene, phenytoin, primidone, phenobarbital, carbamazepine.

DIABETES MELLITUS

Diabetes mellitus that develops during pregnancy (*gestational diabetes* is noted in about 5% of women) or diabetes that is present before pregnancy adversely influences fetal and neonatal well-being. The effect of diabetes on the fetus depends, in part, on the severity of the diabetic state: age of onset of diabetes, duration of treatment with insulin, and presence of vascular disease. Poorly controlled maternal diabetes leads to maternal and fetal hyperglycemia that stimulates the fetal pancreas, resulting in hyperplasia of the islets of Langerhans. Fetal hyperinsulinemia results in increased fat and protein synthesis, producing a fetus that is large for gestational age. After birth, hyperinsulinemia persists, resulting in fasting neonatal hypoglycemia. Strictly controlling maternal diabetes during pregnancy and preventing hyperglycemia during labor and delivery prevent macrosomic fetal growth and neonatal hypoglycemia. Additional problems of the diabetic mother and her fetus and newborn are summarized in Table 59.2.

OTHER CONDITIONS

Other maternal illnesses, such as severe pulmonary disease (cystic fibrosis), cyanotic heart disease, and sickle cell anemia, may reduce oxygen availability to the fetus. Severe hypertensive or diabetic vasculopathy can result in uteroplacental insufficiency. The fetus and the newborn may also be adversely affected by the medications used to treat maternal illnesses. These effects may appear as teratogenesis (Table 59.3) or as an adverse metabolic, neurological, or cardiopulmonary adaptation to extrauterine life (Table 59.4). Acquired infectious diseases of the mother also may affect the fetus or newborn adversely.

TABLE 59.4 Agents Acting on Pregnant Women That May Adversely Affect the Newborn Infant

AGENT	POTENTIAL CONDITION(S)
Acebutolol	IUGR, hypotension, bradycardia
Acetazolamide	Metabolic acidosis
Adrenal corticosteroids	Adrenocortical failure (rare)
Amiodarone	Bradycardia, hypothyroidism
Anesthetic agents (volatile)	CNS depression
Aspirin	Neonatal bleeding, prolonged gestation
Atenolol	IUGR, hypoglycemia
Blue cohosh herbal tea	Neonatal heart failure
Bromides	Rash, CNS depression, IUGR
Captopril, enalapril	Transient anuric renal failure, oligohydramnios
Caudal-paracervical anesthesia with mepivacaine (accidental introduction of anesthetic into scalp of infant)	Bradypnea, apnea, bradycardia, convulsions
Cholinergic agents (edrophonium, pyridostigmine)	Transient muscle weakness
CNS depressants (narcotics, barbiturates, benzodiazepines) during labor	CNS depression, hypotonia
Cephalothin	Positive direct Coombs test reaction
Fluoxetine	Possible transient neonatal withdrawal, hypertonicity, minor anomalies
Haloperidol	Withdrawal
Hexamethonium bromide	Paralytic ileus
Ibuprofen	Oligohydramnios, PPHN
Imipramine	Withdrawal
Indomethacin	Oliguria, oligohydramnios, intestinal perforation, PPHN
Intravenous fluids during labor (e.g., salt-free solutions)	Electrolyte disturbances, hyponatremia, hypoglycemia
Iodide (radioactive)	Goiter
Iodides	Neonatal goiter
Lead	Reduced intellectual function
Magnesium sulfate	Respiratory depression, meconium plug, hypotonia
Methimazole	Goiter, hypothyroidism
Morphine and its derivatives (addiction)	Withdrawal symptoms (poor feeding, vomiting, diarrhea, restlessness, yawning and stretching, dyspnea and cyanosis, fever and sweating, pallor, tremors, convulsions)
Naphthalene	Hemolytic anemia (in G6PD-deficient infants)
Nitrofurantoin	Hemolytic anemia (in G6PD-deficient infants)
Oxytocin	Hyperbilirubinemia, hyponatremia
Phenobarbital	Bleeding diathesis (vitamin K deficiency), possible long-term reduction in IQ, sedation
Primaquine	Hemolytic anemia (in G6PD-deficient infants)
Propranolol	Hypoglycemia, bradycardia, apnea
Propylthiouracil	Goiter, hypothyroidism
Reserpine	Drowsiness, nasal congestion, poor temperature stability
Sulfonamides	Interfere with protein binding of bilirubin; kernicterus at low levels of serum bilirubin, hemolysis with G6PD deficiency
Sulfonylurea	Refractory hypoglycemia
Sympathomimetic (tocolytic–β agonist) agents	Tachycardia
Thiazides	Neonatal thrombocytopenia (rare)

CNS, Central nervous system; *G6PD*, glucose-6-phosphate dehydrogenase; *IUGR*, intrauterine growth restriction; *PPHN*, persistent pulmonary hypertension of the newborn.

From Stoll BJ, Kliegman RM. The fetus and neonatal infant. In: Behrman RE, Kliegman RM, Jenson HB, eds. Nelson Textbook of Pediatrics. *16th ed. Philadelphia: Saunders; 2000.*

CHAPTER 60

Diseases of the Fetus

The principal determinants of fetal disease include the fetal genotype and the in utero environment. Variation in environmental factors rather than the fetal genetics plays a more significant role in determining overall fetal well-being, although a genetically abnormal fetus may not thrive as well or survive. The ability to assess a fetus genetically, biochemically, and physically is greatly enhanced through the development of amniocentesis, fetoscopy, chorionic villus sampling, fetal blood sampling, genetic testing of circulating fetal DNA in the mother's blood, and real-time ultrasonography.

INTRAUTERINE GROWTH RESTRICTION AND SMALL FOR GESTATIONAL AGE

Fetuses subjected to abnormal maternal, placental, or fetal conditions that restrain growth are a high-risk group and traditionally classified as having intrauterine growth restriction (IUGR). The terms *IUGR* and *small for gestational age (SGA)* are not synonymous. IUGR represents a deviation from expected growth patterns. The decreased fetal growth associated with IUGR is an adaptation to unfavorable intrauterine conditions that result in permanent alterations in metabolism, growth, and development. IUGR most frequently occurs with a variety of maternal conditions that are associated with preterm delivery. SGA describes an infant whose birth weight is statistically less than the 10th percentile or two standard deviations below the mean birth weight for gestational age. The cause of SGA may be pathological, as in an infant with IUGR, or nonpathological, as in an infant who is small but otherwise healthy (Table 60.1).

Only about 50% of IUGR infants are identified before delivery. Measurement and recording of maternal fundal height in conjunction with serial ultrasound assessment of the fetus (growth rate, amniotic fluid volume, malformations, anomalies, and Doppler velocimetry of uterine, placental, and fetal blood flow) can aid detection. When suspected and identified, IUGR and SGA fetuses must be monitored for fetal well-being, and appropriate maternal care needs to be instituted (see Chapter 58).

At birth, infants who are mildly to moderately SGA appear smaller than normal with decreased subcutaneous fat. More severely affected infants may present with a *wasted appearance* with asymmetrical findings, including larger heads for the size of the body (central nervous system sparing), widened anterior fontanelles, small abdomen, thin arms and legs, decreased subcutaneous fat, dry and redundant skin, decreased muscle mass, and thin (often meconium-stained) umbilical cord. Gestational age is often difficult to assess when based on physical appearance and perceived advanced neurological maturity. Physical examination should detail the presence of dysmorphic features, abnormal extremities, or gross anomalies that might suggest underlying congenital malformations, chromosomal defects, or exposure to teratogens. Hepatosplenomegaly, jaundice, and skin rashes in addition to ocular disorders, such as chorioretinitis, cataracts, glaucoma, and cloudy cornea, suggest the presence of a congenital infection or inborn error of metabolism. Infants with severe IUGR or SGA, particularly in conjunction with fetal distress, may have problems at birth that include respiratory acidosis, metabolic acidosis, asphyxia, hypoxemia, hypotension, hypoglycemia, polycythemia, meconium aspiration syndrome, and persistent pulmonary hypertension of the newborn.

TABLE 60.1 Etiologies for Intrauterine Growth Restriction and Small for Gestational Age at Birth

MATERNAL FACTORS
Age (young and advanced)
Cigarette smoking
Genetics (short stature, weight)
Illnesses during pregnancy (preeclampsia, severe diabetes, chronic hypertension, connective tissue disease)
Infections (intrauterine)
Lack of good prenatal care
Oligohydramnios
Poor nutrition
Race (African American)
FETAL FACTORS
Chromosomal abnormality and nonchromosomal syndromes
Congenital infections
Inborn errors of metabolism
Multiple gestations
Insulin resistance or reduced insulin or insulin-like growth factor-1 production
MATERNAL MEDICATIONS
Antimetabolites (methotrexate)
Heavy metals (mercury, lead)
Hydantoin
Narcotics (morphine, methadone)
Steroids (prednisone)
Substance and illicit drug use (alcohol, cocaine)
Warfarin
PLACENTAL AND UTERINE ABNORMALITIES
Abruptio placentae
Abnormal implantation
Abnormal placental vessels
Chorioangioma
Circumvallate placenta
Fetal vessel thrombosis
Ischemic villus necrosis
Multiple gestations
True knots in umbilical cord
Villitis (congenital infection)

Management of IUGR and SGA infants is usually symptomatic and supportive. The diagnostic evaluation at birth should be directed at identifying the cause of the IUGR and SGA, if possible. The consequences of IUGR and SGA depend on the etiology, severity, and duration of growth retardation. The mortality rates of infants who are severely affected are 5-20 times those of infants who are appropriate for gestational age. Postnatal growth and development depend in part on the etiology, the postnatal nutritional intake, and the social environment. Infants who have IUGR and SGA secondary to congenital infection, chromosomal abnormalities, or constitutional syndromes remain small throughout life. Infants who have growth inhibited late in gestation because of uterine constraints, placental insufficiency, or poor nutrition have catch-up growth and, under optimal environmental conditions, approach their inherited growth and development potential.

HYDROPS FETALIS

Decision-Making Algorithm
Available @ StudentConsult.com

Anemia

Hydrops fetalis is caused by immune and nonimmune conditions. Hydrops fetalis is a fetal clinical condition of excessive fluid accumulation in the skin and one or more other body compartments, including the pleural space, peritoneal cavity, pericardial sac, or placenta with resultant high morbidity and mortality. Hydrops initially was described in association with Rhesus blood group isoimmunization. The use of Rho (D) immune globulin has reduced the incidence of isoimmune fetal hydrops. Concurrently the incidence of nonimmune hydrops has increased as a cause of this severe clinical condition.

Fetal hydrops results from an imbalance of interstitial fluid accumulation and decreased removal of fluid by the capillaries and lymphatic system. Fluid accumulation can be secondary to congestive heart failure, obstructed lymphatic flow, or decreased plasma oncotic pressure (hypoproteinemic states). Edema formation is the final common pathway for many disease processes that affect the fetus, including fetal cardiac, genetic, hematological, metabolic, infection, or malformation syndromes.

The diagnostic work-up of the hydropic fetus should focus on discovering the underlying cause. Maternal findings may include hypertension, anemia, multiple gestation, thickened placenta, and polyhydramnios, whereas fetal findings may include tachycardia, ascites, scalp and body wall edema, and pleural and pericardial effusion. Invasive fetal testing may be indicated. Amniocentesis provides amniotic fluid samples for karyotype, culture, alpha-fetoprotein, and metabolic and enzyme analysis. Percutaneous umbilical cord blood sampling can provide fetal blood for chromosomal analysis and hematological and metabolic studies and provide a source for intervention (fetal transfusion for profound anemia).

Management depends on the underlying cause and the gestational age of the fetus. Resuscitative efforts at delivery are often required. It is often necessary to remove ascitic fluid from the abdomen or pleural fluid to improve ventilation. Profound anemia necessitates immediate transfusion with packed red blood cells.

The overall mortality for infants with nonimmune hydrops is approximately 50%. If the diagnosis is made before 24 weeks of gestation with subsequent premature delivery, the survival rate is approximately 4-6%.

CHAPTER 61

Respiratory Diseases of the Newborn

Decision-Making Algorithm
Available @ StudentConsult.com

Acidemia

Respiratory distress that becomes manifested by tachypnea, intercostal retractions, reduced air exchange, cyanosis, expiratory grunting, and nasal flaring is a nonspecific response to serious illness. The differential diagnosis of respiratory distress includes pulmonary, cardiac, hematological, infectious, anatomical, and metabolic disorders that may involve the lungs directly or indirectly. Surfactant deficiency causes **respiratory distress syndrome (RDS)**, resulting in cyanosis and tachypnea; **infection** produces pneumonia, shown by interstitial or lobar infiltrates; **meconium aspiration** results in a chemical pneumonitis with hypoxia and pulmonary hypertension; **hydrops fetalis** causes anemia and hypoalbuminemia with high-output heart failure and pulmonary edema; and congenital or acquired **pulmonary hypoplasia** causes pulmonary hypertension and pulmonary insufficiency. It also is clinically useful to differentiate the common causes of respiratory distress according to gestational age (Table 61.1).

TABLE 61.1 Etiology of Respiratory Distress
PRETERM INFANT
Respiratory distress syndrome (RDS)*
Erythroblastosis fetalis
Nonimmune hydrops
Pulmonary hemorrhage
FULL-TERM INFANT
Primary pulmonary hypertension of the neonate*
Meconium aspiration pneumonia*
Polycythemia
Amniotic fluid aspiration
PRETERM AND FULL-TERM INFANT
Bacterial sepsis (GBS)*
Transient tachypnea*
Spontaneous pneumothorax
Congenital anomalies (e.g., congenital lobar emphysema, cystic adenomatoid malformation, diaphragmatic hernia)
Congenital heart disease
Pulmonary hypoplasia
Viral infection (e.g., herpes simplex, CMV)
Inborn metabolic errors

*Common.
CMV, Cytomegalovirus; *GBS*, group B streptococcus.

In addition to the specific therapy for the individual disorder, supportive care and evaluation of the infant with respiratory distress can be applied to all the problems mentioned earlier (Table 61.2). Blood gas monitoring and interpretation are key components of general respiratory care.

Treatment of hypoxemia requires knowledge of normal values. In term infants, the arterial Pao_2 level is 55-60 mm Hg at 30 minutes of life, 75 mm Hg at 4 hours, and 90 mm Hg at 24 hours. Preterm infants have lower values. $Paco_2$ levels should be 35-40 mm Hg, and the pH should be 7.35-7.40. It is imperative that arterial blood gas analysis be performed in all infants with significant respiratory distress, whether or not cyanosis is perceived. Cyanosis becomes evident when there is 5 g of unsaturated hemoglobin; anemia may interfere with the perception of cyanosis. Jaundice also may interfere with the appearance of cyanosis. Capillary blood gas determinations are useful in determining blood pH and the $Paco_2$ level but may result in falsely low blood Pao_2 readings. Serial blood gas levels may be monitored by an indwelling arterial catheter placed in a peripheral artery or through the umbilical artery. Another method for monitoring blood gas levels is to combine capillary blood gas techniques with noninvasive methods used to monitor oxygen (pulse oximetry or transcutaneous oxygen diffusion).

Metabolic acidosis, defined as a reduced pH (<7.25) and bicarbonate concentration (<18 mEq/L) accompanied by a normal or low $Paco_2$ level, may be caused by hypoxia or by insufficient tissue perfusion. The origin of the disorder may be pulmonary, cardiac, infectious, renal, hematological, nutritional, metabolic, or iatrogenic. The initial approach to metabolic acidosis is to determine the cause and treat the pathophysiological problem. This approach may include, as in the sequence of therapy for hypoxia, increasing the inspired oxygen concentration; applying continuous positive airway pressure (CPAP) nasally; or initiating mechanical ventilation using positive end-expiratory pressure. Patients with hypotension produced by hypovolemia require fluids and may need inotropic or vasoactive drug support. If metabolic acidosis persists despite specific therapy, sodium bicarbonate (1 mEq/kg/dose) may be given by slow intravenous infusion. Near-normal or low Pco_2 levels should be documented before sodium bicarbonate infusion. The buffering effect of sodium bicarbonate results in increased Pco_2 levels, unless adequate ventilation is maintained.

Respiratory acidosis, defined as an elevated Pco_2 level and reduced pH without a reduction in the bicarbonate concentration, may be caused by pulmonary insufficiency or central hypoventilation. Most disorders producing respiratory distress can lead to hypercapnia. Treatment involves assisted ventilation but not sodium bicarbonate. If central nervous system depression of respirations is caused by placental passage of narcotic analgesics, assisted ventilation is instituted first, then the central nervous system depression is reversed by naloxone.

TABLE 61.2 Initial Laboratory Evaluation of Respiratory Distress

TEST	RATIONALE
Chest radiograph	To determine reticular granular pattern of RDS; to determine presence of pneumothorax, cardiomegaly, life-threatening congenital anomalies
Arterial blood gas	To determine severity of respiratory compromise, hypoxemia, and hypercapnia and type of acidosis; severity determines treatment strategy
Complete blood count	Hemoglobin/hematocrit to determine anemia and polycythemia; white blood cell count to determine neutropenia/sepsis; platelet count and smear to determine DIC
Blood culture	To recover potential pathogen
Blood glucose	To determine presence of hypoglycemia, which may produce or occur simultaneously with respiratory distress; to determine stress hyperglycemia
Echocardiogram, ECG	In the presence of a murmur, cardiomegaly, or refractory hypoxia; to determine structural heart disease or PPHN

DIC, Disseminated intravascular coagulation; *ECG*, electrocardiogram; *PPHN*, primary pulmonary hypertension of the newborn; *RDS*, respiratory distress syndrome.

RESPIRATORY DISTRESS SYNDROME (HYALINE MEMBRANE DISEASE)

RDS occurs after the onset of breathing and is associated with an insufficiency of pulmonary surfactant.

Lung Development

The lining of the alveolus consists of 90% type I cells and 10% type II cells. After 20 weeks of gestation, the type II cells contain vacuolated, osmophilic, lamellar inclusion bodies, which are packages of surface-active material (Fig. 61.1). This lipoprotein surfactant is 90% lipid and is composed predominantly of saturated phosphatidylcholine (lecithin), but also contains phosphatidylglycerol, other phospholipids, and neutral lipids. The surfactant proteins, SP-A, SP-B, SP-C, and SP-D, are packaged into the lamellar body and contribute to surface-active properties and recycling of surfactant. Surfactant prevents atelectasis by reducing surface tension at low lung volumes when it is concentrated at end expiration as the alveolar radius decreases; surfactant contributes to lung recoil by increasing surface tension at larger lung volumes when it is diluted during inspiration as the alveolar radius increases. Without surfactant, surface tension forces are not reduced, and atelectasis develops during end expiration as the alveolus collapses.

The timing of surfactant production in quantities sufficient to prevent atelectasis depends on an increase in fetal cortisol levels that begins between 32 and 34 weeks of gestation. By 34-36 weeks, sufficient surface-active material is produced by the type II cells in the lung, is secreted into the alveolar lumen, and is excreted into the amniotic fluid. The concentration of lecithin in amniotic fluid indicates fetal pulmonary maturity. Because the amount of lecithin is difficult to quantify, the ratio of lecithin (which increases with maturity) to sphingomyelin (which remains constant during gestation; L/S ratio) is determined. An L/S ratio of 2 : 1 usually indicates pulmonary maturity. The presence of minor phospholipids, such as phosphatidylglycerol, also is indicative of fetal lung maturity and may be useful in situations in which the L/S ratio is borderline or possibly affected by maternal diabetes, which reduces lung maturity. The absence of phosphatidylglycerol suggests that surfactant might not be mature.

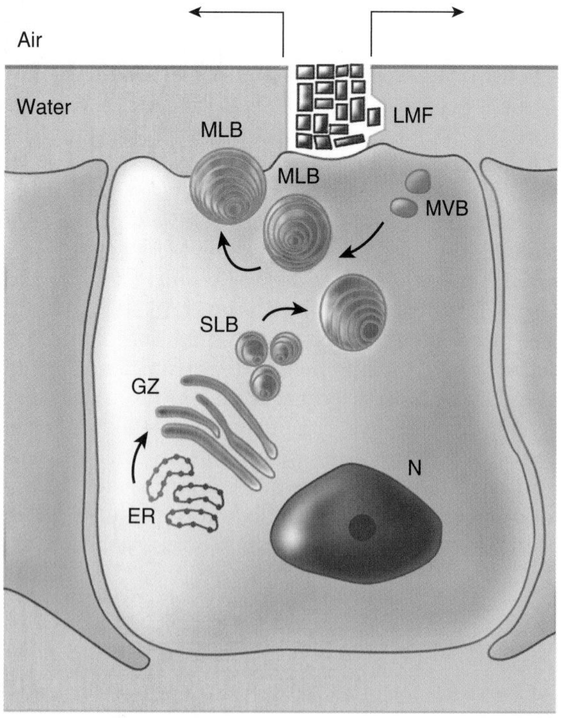

FIGURE 61.1 Proposed pathway of synthesis, transport, secretion, and reuptake of surfactant in the type II alveolar cell. Phospholipids are synthesized in the smooth endoplasmic reticulum (ER). The glucose/glycerol precursor may be derived from lung glycogen or circulating glucose. Phospholipids and surfactant proteins are packaged in the Golgi apparatus (GZ), emerge as small lamellar bodies (SLB), coalesce to mature lamellar bodies (MLB), migrate to the apical membrane, and are released by exocytosis into the liquid hypophase below the air-liquid interface. The tightly coiled lamellar body unravels to form the lattice (tubular) myelin figure (LMF), the immediate precursor to the phospholipid monolayer at the alveolar surface. Reuptake by endocytosis forms multivesicular bodies (MVB) that recycle surfactant. The enzymes, receptors, transporters, and surfactant proteins are controlled by regulatory processes at the transcriptional level in the nucleus (N). Corticosteroid and thyroid hormones are regulatory ligands that may accelerate surfactant synthesis. (From Hansen T, Corbet A. Lung development and function. In: Taeusch HW, Ballard R, Avery ME, eds. *Diseases of the Newborn*. 6th ed. Philadelphia: Saunders; 1991:465.)

Clinical Manifestations

A deficiency of pulmonary surfactant (most often due to prematurity) results in atelectasis, decreased functional residual capacity, arterial hypoxemia, and respiratory distress. Surfactant synthesis may also be reduced as a result of hypovolemia, hypothermia, acidosis, hypoxemia, and rare genetic disorders of surfactant synthesis. These factors also produce pulmonary artery vasospasm, which may contribute to RDS in larger premature infants who have developed sufficient pulmonary arteriole smooth muscle to produce vasoconstriction. Surfactant deficiency–induced atelectasis causes alveoli to be perfused but not ventilated, which results in a pulmonary shunt and hypoxemia. As atelectasis increases, the lungs become increasingly difficult to expand, and lung compliance decreases. Because the chest wall of the premature infant is very compliant, the infant attempts to overcome decreased lung compliance with increasing inspiratory pressures, resulting in retractions of the chest wall. The sequence of decreased lung compliance and chest wall retractions leads to poor air exchange, an increased physiological dead space, alveolar hypoventilation, and hypercapnia. A cycle of hypoxia, hypercapnia, and acidosis acts on type II cells to reduce surfactant synthesis and, in some infants, on the pulmonary arterioles to produce pulmonary hypertension.

Infants at greatest risk for RDS are premature and have an immature L/S ratio. The incidence of RDS increases with decreasing gestational age. RDS develops in 30-60% of infants between 28 and 32 weeks of gestation. Other risk factors include delivery of a previous preterm infant with RDS, maternal diabetes, hypothermia, fetal distress, asphyxia, male sex, white race, being the second-born of twins, and delivery by cesarean section without labor.

RDS may develop immediately in the delivery room in extremely immature infants at 26-30 weeks of gestation. Some more mature infants (34 weeks' gestation) may not show signs of RDS until 3-4 hours after birth, correlating with the initial release of stored surfactant at the onset of breathing accompanied by the ongoing inability to replace the surfactant owing to inadequate stores. **Manifestations** of RDS include cyanosis, tachypnea, nasal flaring, intercostal and sternal retractions, and grunting. Grunting is caused by closure of the glottis during expiration, the effect of which is to maintain lung volume (decreasing atelectasis) and gas exchange during exhalation. Atelectasis is well documented by radiographic examination of the chest, which shows a ground-glass haze in the lung surrounding air-filled bronchi (the air bronchogram; Fig. 61.2). Severe RDS may show an airless lung field *(whiteout)* on a radiograph, even obliterating the distinction between the atelectatic lungs and the heart.

During the first 72 hours, infants with untreated RDS have increasing distress and hypoxemia. In infants with severe RDS, the development of edema, apnea, and respiratory failure necessitates assisted ventilation. Thereafter, uncomplicated cases show a spontaneous improvement that often is heralded by diuresis and a marked resolution of edema. Complications include the development of a pneumothorax, a patent ductus arteriosus (PDA), and bronchopulmonary dysplasia (BPD). The differential diagnosis of RDS includes diseases associated with cyanosis and respiratory distress (see Table 58.10).

Prevention and Treatment

Strategies to prevent preterm birth include maternal cervical cerclage, bed rest, treatment of infections, and administration of tocolytic medications. In addition, prevention of neonatal cold stress, birth asphyxia, and hypovolemia reduces the risk of RDS. If premature delivery is unavoidable, the antenatal administration of corticosteroids (e.g., betamethasone) to the mother (and thus to the fetus) stimulates fetal lung production of surfactant; this approach requires multiple doses for at least 48 hours.

After birth, RDS may be prevented or its severity reduced by intratracheal administration of exogenous surfactant immediately after birth in the delivery room or within a few hours of birth. Exogenous surfactant can be administered repeatedly during the course of RDS in patients receiving endotracheal intubation, mechanical ventilation, and oxygen therapy. Early application of nasal CPAP may also reduce the severity of RDS. Additional management includes the general supportive and ventilation care presented in Table 61.3.

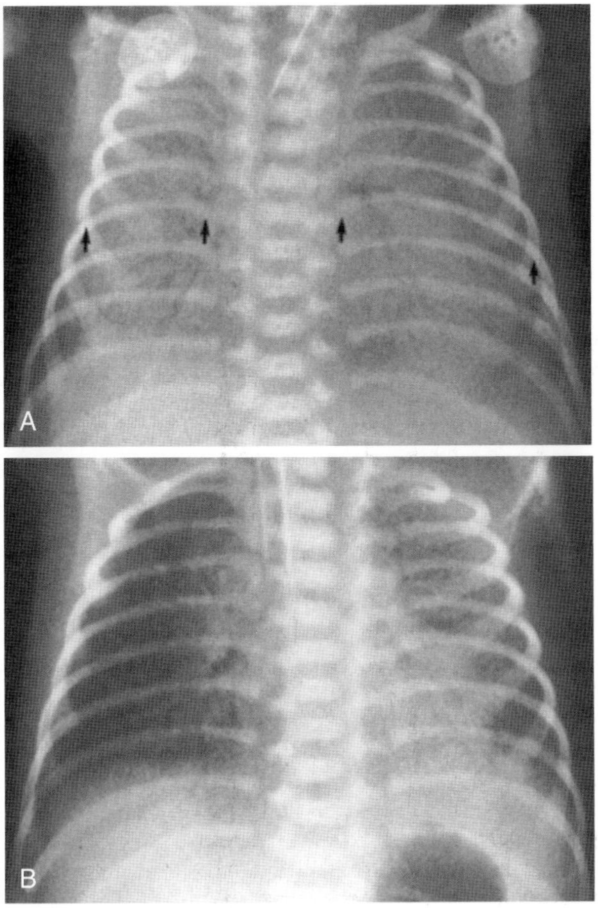

FIGURE 61.2 Respiratory distress syndrome. The infant is intubated, and the lungs show a dense reticulonodular pattern with air bronchograms **(A)**. To evaluate rotation on the frontal chest, the lengths of the posterior ribs are compared from left to right *(arrows)*. Because the infant is supine, the side of the longer ribs indicates to which side the thorax is rotated. In this case, the left ribs are longer, and this radiograph is a left posterior oblique view. Surfactant was administered, resulting in significant improvement in the density of the lung **(B)**. The right lung is slightly better aerated than the left. Uneven distribution of clearing is common. (From Hilton S, Edwards D. *Practical Pediatric Radiology*. 2nd ed. Philadelphia: Saunders; 1994.)

TABLE 61.3 Potential Causes of Neonatal Apnea

Central nervous system	IVH, drugs, seizures, hypoxic injury
Respiratory	Pneumonia, obstructive airway lesions, atelectasis, extreme prematurity (<1,000 g), laryngeal reflex, phrenic nerve paralysis, severe RDS, pneumothorax
Infectious	Sepsis, necrotizing enterocolitis, meningitis (bacterial, fungal, viral)
Gastrointestinal	Oral feeding, bowel movement, gastroesophageal reflux, esophagitis, intestinal perforation
Metabolic	↓ Glucose, ↓ calcium, ↓ Po_2, ↓↑ sodium, ↑ ammonia, ↑ organic acids, ↑ ambient temperature, hypothermia
Cardiovascular	Hypotension, hypertension, heart failure, anemia, hypovolemia, change in vagal tone
Idiopathic	Immaturity of respiratory center, sleep state, upper airway collapse

IVH, Intraventricular hemorrhage; *RDS*, respiratory distress syndrome.

The Pao_2 level should be maintained between 60 and 70 mm Hg (oxygen saturation 90%), and the pH should be maintained above 7.25. An increased concentration of warm and humidified inspired oxygen administered by a nasal cannula or an oxygen hood may be all that is needed for larger premature infants. If hypoxemia (Pao_2 <50 mm Hg) is present, and the needed inspired oxygen concentration is 70-100%, nasal CPAP should be added at a distending pressure of 8-10 cm H_2O. If respiratory failure ensues (Pco_2 >60 mm Hg, pH <7.20, and Pao_2 <50 mm Hg with 100% oxygen), assisted ventilation using a ventilator is indicated. Conventional rate (25-60 breaths/min), high-frequency jet (150-600 breaths/min), and oscillatory (900-3,000 breaths/min) ventilators all have been successful in managing respiratory failure caused by severe RDS. Suggested starting settings on a conventional ventilator are fraction of inspired oxygen, 0.60-1.0; peak inspiratory pressure, 20-25 cm H_2O; positive end-expiratory pressure, 5 cm H_2O; and respiratory rate, 30-50 breaths/min.

In response to persistent hypercapnia, alveolar ventilation (tidal volume − dead space × rate) must be increased. Ventilation can be increased by an increase in the ventilator's rate or an increase in the tidal volume (the gradient between peak inspiratory pressure and positive end-expiratory pressure using a pressure-controlled ventilator). In response to hypoxia, the inspired oxygen content may be increased. Alternatively, the degree of oxygenation depends on the mean airway pressure. Mean airway pressure is directly related to positive end-expiratory pressure, flow, and inspiratory time. Increased mean airway pressure may improve oxygenation by improving lung volume, enhancing ventilation-perfusion matching. Because of the difficulty in distinguishing sepsis and pneumonia from RDS, broad-spectrum parenteral antibiotics (ampicillin and gentamicin) are administered for 48-72 hours, pending the recovery of an organism from a previously obtained blood culture.

COMPLICATIONS OF RESPIRATORY DISTRESS SYNDROME

Patent Ductus Arteriosus

Decision-Making Algorithm
Available @ StudentConsult.com

Heart Murmurs

PDA is a common complication that occurs in many low birth weight infants who have RDS. The incidence of PDA is inversely related to the maturity of the infant. In term newborns, the ductus closes within 24-48 hours after birth. However, in preterm newborns, the ductus frequently fails to close, requiring medical or surgical closure. The ductus arteriosus in a preterm infant is less responsive to vasoconstrictive stimuli, which, when complicated with hypoxemia during RDS, may lead to a persistent PDA that creates a shunt between the pulmonary and systemic circulations.

During the acute phase of RDS, hypoxia, hypercapnia, and acidosis lead to pulmonary arterial vasoconstriction. The pulmonary and systemic pressures may be equal, and flow through the ductus may be small or bidirectional. When RDS improves and pulmonary vascular resistance declines, flow through the ductus arteriosus increases in a left-to-right direction. Significant systemic-to-pulmonary shunting may lead to heart failure and pulmonary edema. Excessive intravenous fluid administration may increase the incidence of symptomatic PDA. The infant's respiratory status deteriorates because of increased lung fluid, hypercapnia, and hypoxemia.

Clinical manifestations of a PDA usually become apparent on day 2-4 of life. Because the left-to-right shunt directs flow to a low-pressure circulation from one of high pressure, the pulse pressure widens; a previously inactive precordium shows an extremely active precordial impulse, and peripheral pulses become easily palpable and bounding. The murmur of a PDA may be continuous in systole and diastole, but usually only the systolic component is auscultated. Heart failure and pulmonary edema result in rales and hepatomegaly. A chest radiograph shows cardiomegaly and pulmonary edema; a two-dimensional echocardiogram shows ductal patency; and Doppler studies show markedly increased left-to-right flow through the ductus.

Treatment of a PDA during RDS involves initial fluid restriction and diuretic administration. If there is no improvement after 24-48 hours, a prostaglandin synthetase inhibitor, indomethacin or ibuprofen, is administered. Contraindications to using indomethacin include thrombocytopenia (platelets <50,000/mm^3), bleeding, serum creatinine measuring more than 1.8 mg/dL, and oliguria. Because 20-30% of infants do not respond initially to indomethacin and because the PDA reopens in 10-20% of infants, a repeat course of indomethacin or surgical ligation is required in some patients.

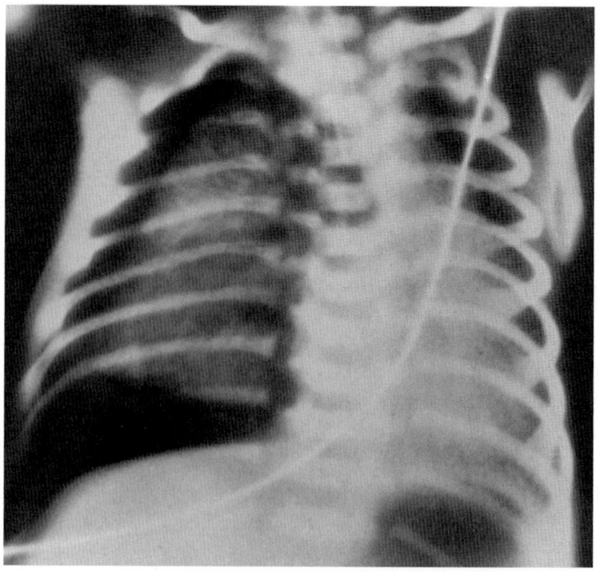

FIGURE 61.3 Pneumothorax. Right-sided hyperlucent pleural air is obvious. The findings of linear interstitial air and the resultant noncompliant but collapsed lung are noted. (From Heller RM, Kirchner SG. *Advanced Exercises in Diagnostic Radiology: the Newborn*. Philadelphia: WB Saunders; 1979.)

Pulmonary Air Leaks

Assisted ventilation with high peak inspiratory pressures and positive end-expiratory pressures may cause overdistention of alveoli in localized areas of the lung. Rupture of the alveolar epithelial lining may produce pulmonary interstitial emphysema as gas dissects along the interstitial space and the peribronchial lymphatics. Extravasation of gas into the parenchyma reduces lung compliance and worsens respiratory failure. Gas dissection into the mediastinal space produces a pneumomediastinum, occasionally dissecting into the subcutaneous tissues around the neck, causing subcutaneous emphysema.

Alveolar rupture adjacent to the pleural space produces a **pneumothorax** (Fig. 61.3). If the gas is under tension, the pneumothorax shifts the mediastinum to the opposite side of the chest, producing hypotension, hypoxia, and hypercapnia. The diagnosis of a pneumothorax may be based on unequal transillumination of the chest and may be confirmed by chest radiograph. Treatment of a symptomatic pneumothorax requires insertion of a pleural chest tube connected to negative pressure or to an underwater drain. Prophylactic or therapeutic use of exogenous surfactant has reduced the incidence of pulmonary air leaks.

Pneumothorax also is observed after vigorous resuscitation, meconium aspiration pneumonia, pulmonary hypoplasia, and diaphragmatic hernia. Spontaneous pneumothorax is seen in fewer than 1% of deliveries and may be associated with renal malformations.

Bronchopulmonary Dysplasia (Chronic Lung Disease)

BPD is a clinical diagnosis defined by oxygen dependence at 36 weeks' postconceptual age and accompanied by characteristic clinical and radiographic findings that correspond to anatomical abnormalities. Oxygen concentrations greater than 40% are toxic to the neonatal lung. Oxygen-mediated lung injury results from the generation of superoxides, hydrogen peroxide, and oxygen free radicals, which disrupt membrane lipids. Assisted ventilation with high peak pressures produces barotrauma, compounding the damaging effects of highly inspired oxygen levels. In most patients, BPD develops after ventilation for RDS that may have been complicated by PDA or pulmonary interstitial emphysema. Inflammation from prolonged assisted ventilation and repeated systemic and pulmonary infections may play a major role. Failure of RDS to improve after 2 weeks, the need for prolonged mechanical ventilation, and oxygen therapy required at 36 weeks' postconceptual age are characteristic of patients with RDS in whom BPD develops. BPD also may develop in infants weighing less than 1,000 g who require mechanical ventilation for poor respiratory drive in the absence of RDS. Fifty percent of infants of 24-26 weeks' gestational age require oxygen at 36 weeks' corrected age.

The **radiographic appearance** of BPD is characterized initially by lung opacification and subsequently by development of cysts accompanied by areas of overdistention and atelectasis, giving the lung a spongelike appearance. The histopathology of BPD reveals interstitial edema, atelectasis, mucosal metaplasia, interstitial fibrosis, necrotizing obliterative bronchiolitis, and overdistended alveoli.

The **clinical manifestations** of BPD are oxygen dependence, hypercapnia with a compensatory metabolic alkalosis, pulmonary hypertension, poor growth, and development of right-sided heart failure. Increased airway resistance with reactive airway bronchoconstriction also is noted and is treated with bronchodilating agents. Severe chest retractions produce negative interstitial pressure that draws fluid into the interstitial space. Together with cor pulmonale, these chest retractions cause fluid retention, necessitating fluid restriction and the administration of diuretics.

Patients with severe BPD may need treatment with mechanical ventilation for many months. To reduce the risk of subglottic stenosis, a tracheotomy may be indicated. To reduce oxygen toxicity and barotrauma, ventilator settings are reduced to maintain blood gases with slightly lower Pa_{O_2} (50 mm Hg) and higher Pa_{CO_2} (50-75 mm Hg) levels than for infants during the acute phase of RDS. Dexamethasone therapy may reduce inflammation, improve pulmonary function, and enhance weaning of patients from assisted ventilation. However, dexamethasone may increase the risk of cerebral palsy or abnormal neuromotor developmental outcome. Older survivors of BPD have hyperinflation, reactive airways, and developmental delay. They are at risk for severe respiratory syncytial virus pneumonia and as infants should receive prophylaxis against respiratory syncytial virus.

Retinopathy of Prematurity (Retrolental Fibroplasia)

Decision-Making Algorithm
Available @ StudentConsult.com

Visual Impairment and Leukocoria

Retinopathy of prematurity (ROP) is caused by the acute and chronic effects of oxygen toxicity on the developing blood vessels of the premature infant's retina. The completely vascularized retina of the term infant is not susceptible to ROP. ROP is a leading cause of blindness in very low birth weight infants (<1,500 g). Excessive arterial oxygen tensions produce vasoconstriction of immature retinal vasculature in the first stage of this disease. Vaso-obliteration follows if the duration and extent of hyperoxia are prolonged beyond the time when vasoconstriction is reversible. Hypercarbia and hypoxia may contribute to ROP. The subsequent proliferative stages are characterized by extraretinal fibrovascular proliferation, forming a ridge between the vascular and avascular portions of the retina, and by the development of neovascular tufts. In mild cases, vasoproliferation is noted at the periphery of the retina. Severe cases may have neovascularization involving the entire retina, retinal detachment resulting from traction on vessels as they leave the optic disc, fibrous proliferation behind the lens producing leukokoria, and synechiae displacing the lens forward, leading to glaucoma. Both eyes usually are involved, but severity may be asymmetrical.

The incidence of ROP may be reduced by careful monitoring of arterial blood gas levels in all patients receiving oxygen. Although there is no absolutely safe Pa_{O_2} level, it is wise to keep the arterial oxygen level between 50 and 70 mm Hg in premature infants. Infants who weigh less than 1,500 g or who are born before 28 weeks' gestational age (some authors say 32 weeks) should be screened when they are 4 weeks of age or more than 34 weeks' corrected gestational age, whichever comes first. Laser therapy or (less often) cryotherapy may be used for vitreous hemorrhage or for severe, progressive vasoproliferation. Surgery is indicated for retinal detachment. Less severe stages of ROP resolve spontaneously and without visual impairment in most patients.

TRANSIENT TACHYPNEA OF THE NEWBORN

Transient tachypnea of the newborn is a self-limited condition characterized by tachypnea, mild retractions, hypoxia, and occasional grunting, usually without signs of severe respiratory distress. Cyanosis, when present, usually requires treatment with supplemental oxygen in the range of 30-40%. Transient tachypnea of the newborn usually is noted in larger premature infants and in term infants born by precipitous delivery or cesarean section without prior labor. Infants of diabetic mothers and infants with poor respiratory drive as a result of placental passage of analgesic drugs are at risk. Transient tachypnea of the newborn may be caused by retained lung fluid or slow resorption of lung fluid. Chest radiographs show prominent central vascular markings, fluid in the lung fissures, overaeration, and occasionally a small pleural effusion. Air bronchograms and a reticulogranular pattern are not seen; their presence suggests another pulmonary process, such as RDS or pneumonia.

MECONIUM ASPIRATION SYNDROME

Meconium-stained amniotic fluid is seen in 15% of predominantly term and post-term deliveries. Although the passage of meconium into amniotic fluid is common in infants born in the breech presentation, meconium-stained fluid should be considered clinically as a sign of fetal distress in all infants. The presence of meconium in the amniotic fluid suggests in utero distress with asphyxia, hypoxia, and acidosis.

Aspiration of amniotic fluid contaminated with particulate meconium may occur in utero in a distressed, gasping fetus; more often, meconium is aspirated into the lung immediately after delivery. Affected infants have abnormal chest radiographs, showing a high incidence of pneumonia and pneumothoraces.

Meconium aspiration pneumonia is characterized by tachypnea, hypoxia, hypercapnia, and small airway obstruction causing a ball-valve effect, leading to air trapping, overdistention, and extra-alveolar air leaks. Complete small-airway obstruction produces atelectasis. Within 24-48 hours, a chemical pneumonitis develops in addition to the mechanical effects of airway obstruction. Abnormal pulmonary function may be caused by the meconium, in part, through inactivation of surfactant. Primary pulmonary hypertension of the newborn (PPHN) frequently accompanies meconium aspiration, with right-to-left shunting caused by increased pulmonary vascular resistance. The chest radiograph reveals patchy infiltrates, overdistention, flattening of the diaphragm, increased anteroposterior diameter, and a high incidence of pneumomediastinum and pneumothoraces. Comorbid diseases include those associated with in utero asphyxia that initiated the passage of meconium.

Treatment of meconium aspiration includes general supportive care and assisted ventilation. Infants with a PPHN-like presentation should be treated for PPHN. If severe hypoxia does not subside with conventional or high-frequency ventilation, surfactant therapy, and inhaled nitric oxide, extracorporeal membrane oxygenation (ECMO) may be beneficial.

Prevention of meconium aspiration syndrome involves careful in utero monitoring to prevent asphyxia. When meconium-stained fluid is observed, the obstetrician should suction the infant's oropharynx before delivering the rest of the infant's body. If the infant is depressed with poor tone, minimal respiratory effort, and cyanosis, the infant's oropharynx should be suctioned, the vocal cords visualized, and the area below the vocal cords suctioned to remove any meconium from the trachea. Saline intrauterine amnioinfusion during labor may reduce the incidence of aspiration and pneumonia.

PRIMARY PULMONARY HYPERTENSION OF THE NEWBORN

PPHN occurs in post-term, term, or near-term infants. PPHN is characterized by severe hypoxemia, without evidence of parenchymal lung or structural heart disease. PPHN is often seen with asphyxia or meconium-stained fluid. The chest radiograph usually reveals normal lung fields rather than the expected infiltrates and hyperinflation that may accompany meconium aspiration. Additional problems that may lead to PPHN are congenital pneumonia, hyperviscosity-polycythemia, congenital diaphragmatic hernia, pulmonary hypoplasia, congenital cyanotic heart disease, hypoglycemia, and hypothermia. Total anomalous venous return associated with obstruction of blood flow may produce a clinical picture that involves severe hypoxia and that is initially indistinguishable from PPHN; however, a chest radiograph reveals severe pulmonary venous engorgement and a small heart. Echocardiography or cardiac catheterization confirms the diagnosis.

Significant right-to-left shunting through a patent foramen ovale, through a PDA, and through intrapulmonary channels is characteristic of PPHN. The pulmonary vasculature often shows hypertrophied arterial wall smooth muscle, suggesting that the process of or predisposition to PPHN began in utero as a result of previous periods of fetal hypoxia. After birth, hypoxia, hypercapnia, and acidosis exacerbate pulmonary artery vasoconstriction, leading to further hypoxia and acidosis. Some infants with PPHN have extrapulmonary manifestations as a result of asphyxia. Myocardial injuries include heart failure, transient mitral insufficiency, and papillary muscle or myocardial infarction. Thrombocytopenia, right atrial thrombi, and pulmonary embolism also may be noted.

The **diagnosis** is confirmed by echocardiographic examination, which shows elevated pulmonary artery pressures and sites of right-to-left shunting. Echocardiography also rules out structural congenital heart disease and transient myocardial dysfunction.

Treatment involves general supportive care; correction of hypotension, anemia, and acidosis; and management of complications associated with asphyxia. If myocardial dysfunction is present, dopamine or dobutamine is needed. The most important therapy for PPHN is assisted ventilation. Reversible mild pulmonary hypertension may respond to conventional assisted ventilation. Patients with severe PPHN do not always respond to conventional therapy. Paralysis with a muscle relaxant may be needed to assist vigorous ventilation. Surfactant replacement seems to have no effect when PPHN is the primary diagnosis. If mechanical ventilation and supportive care are unsuccessful in improving oxygenation, inhaled nitric oxide, a selective pulmonary artery vasodilating agent, should be administered. If hypoxia persists, the patient may be a candidate for ECMO. Infants who require extremely high ventilator settings, marked by an alveolar-to-arterial oxygen gradient greater than 620 mm Hg, have a high mortality rate and benefit from ECMO if they do not respond to nitric oxide. In addition, the oxygenation index (OI) is used to assess the severity of hypoxemia and to guide the timing of interventions such as inhaled nitric oxide and ECMO. The OI is calculated using the equation OI = [(mean airway pressure × fraction of inspired oxygen)/Pao_2] × 100. A high OI indicates severe hypoxemic respiratory failure.

APNEA OF PREMATURITY

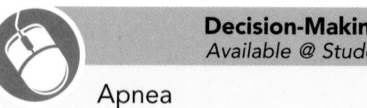

Decision-Making Algorithm
Available @ StudentConsult.com
Apnea

Although apnea typically is associated with immaturity of the respiratory control system, it also may be the presenting sign of other diseases or pathophysiological states that affect preterm infants (see Table 61.3). A thorough consideration of possible causes is always warranted, especially with the onset or unexpected increase in the frequency of episodes of apnea (or bradycardia).

Apnea is defined as the cessation of pulmonary airflow for a specific time interval, usually longer than 10-20 seconds. Bradycardia often accompanies prolonged apnea. **Central apnea** refers to a complete cessation of airflow and respiratory efforts with no chest wall movement. **Obstructive apnea** refers to the absence of noticeable airflow but with the continuation of chest wall movements. **Mixed apnea**, a combination of these two events, is the most frequent type. It may begin as a brief episode of obstruction followed by a central apnea. Alternatively, central apnea may produce upper airway closure (passive pharyngeal hypotonia), resulting in mixed apnea.

A careful evaluation to determine the cause of apnea should be performed immediately in any infant with apnea. The incidence of apnea increases as gestational age decreases. Idiopathic apnea, a disease of premature infants, appears in the absence of any other identifiable disease states during the first week of life and usually resolves by 36-40 weeks of postconceptual age (gestational age at birth + postnatal age). The premature infant's process of regulating respiration is especially vulnerable to apnea. Preterm infants respond paradoxically to hypoxia by developing apnea rather than by increasing respirations as in mature infants. Poor tone of the laryngeal muscles also may lead to collapse of the upper airway, causing obstruction. Isolated obstructive apnea also may occur as a result of flexion or extreme lateral positioning of the premature infant's head, which obstructs the soft trachea.

Treatment of apnea of prematurity involves administration of oxygen to hypoxic infants, transfusion of anemic infants, and physical cutaneous stimulation for infants with mild apnea. Methylxanthines (caffeine or theophylline) are the mainstay of pharmacological treatment of apnea. Xanthine therapy increases minute ventilation, improves the carbon dioxide sensitivity, decreases hypoxic depression of breathing, enhances diaphragmatic activity, and decreases periodic breathing. Treatment usually is initiated with a loading dose followed by maintenance therapy. High-flow nasal cannula therapy and nasal CPAP of 4-6 cm H_2O also are effective and relatively safe methods of treating obstructive or mixed apneas; they may work by stimulating the infant and splinting the upper airway. CPAP also probably increases functional residual capacity, improving oxygenation.

CHAPTER 62

Anemia and Hyperbilirubinemia

ANEMIA

Embryonic hematopoiesis begins by the 20th day of gestation and is evidenced as blood islands in the yolk sac. In midgestation, erythropoiesis occurs in the liver and spleen; the bone marrow becomes the predominant site in the last trimester. Hemoglobin concentration increases from 8-10 g/dL at 12 weeks to 16.5-18 g/dL at 40 weeks. Fetal red blood cell (RBC) production is responsive to erythropoietin; the concentration of this hormone increases with fetal hypoxia and anemia.

After birth, hemoglobin levels increase transiently at 6-12 hours, then decline to 11-12 g/dL at 3-6 months. A premature infant (<32 weeks' gestational age) has a lower hemoglobin concentration and a more rapid postnatal decline of hemoglobin level, which achieves a nadir 1-2 months after birth. Fetal and neonatal RBCs have a shorter life span (70-90 days) and a higher mean corpuscular volume (110-120 fL) than adult cells. In the fetus, hemoglobin synthesis in the last two trimesters of pregnancy produces fetal hemoglobin (hemoglobin F), composed of two alpha chains and two gamma chains. Immediately before term, the infant begins to synthesize beta-hemoglobin chains; the term infant should have some adult hemoglobin (two alpha chains and two beta chains). Fetal hemoglobin represents 60-90% of hemoglobin at term birth. The levels decline to adult levels of less than 5% by 4 months of age.

For a term infant, blood volume is 72-93 mL/kg, and for a preterm infant, blood volume is 90-100 mL/kg. The placenta and umbilical vessels contain approximately 20-30 mL/kg of additional blood that can increase neonatal blood volume and hemoglobin levels transiently for the first 3 days of life if clamping or milking *(stripping)* of the umbilical cord is delayed at birth. Delayed clamping usually has no adverse effects but may increase the risk of polycythemia and jaundice. Early clamping may lead to anemia, a cardiac murmur, poor peripheral perfusion, and less tachypnea. Hydrostatic pressure affects blood transfer between the placenta and the infant at birth. An undesired fetal-to-placental transfusion occurs if the infant is situated above the level of the placenta.

The physiological anemia noted at 2-3 months of age in term infants and at 1-2 months of age in preterm infants is a normal process that does not result in signs of illness and does not require any treatment. It is a physiological condition believed to be related to several factors, including increased tissue oxygenation experienced at birth, shortened RBC life span, and low erythropoietin levels.

Etiology

Decision-Making Algorithms
Available @ StudentConsult.com

Gastrointestinal Bleeding
Anemia
Bleeding
Petechiae/Purpura
Pancytopenia

Symptomatic anemia in the newborn period (Fig. 62.1) may be caused by decreased RBC production, increased RBC destruction, or blood loss.

Decreased Red Blood Cell Production

Anemia caused by decreased production of RBCs appears at birth with pallor, a low reticulocyte count, and absence of erythroid precursors in the bone marrow. Potential causes of neonatal decreased RBC production include bone marrow failure syndromes (congenital RBC aplasia [Blackfan-Diamond anemia]), infection (congenital viral infections [parvovirus, rubella], acquired bacterial or viral sepsis), and congenital leukemia.

Increased Red Blood Cell Destruction

Immunologically mediated hemolysis in utero may lead to **erythroblastosis fetalis**, or the fetus may be spared and **hemolytic disease** may appear in the newborn. Hemolysis of fetal erythrocytes is a result of blood group differences between the sensitized mother and fetus, which causes production of maternal IgG antibodies directed against an antigen on fetal cells.

ABO blood group incompatibility with neonatal hemolysis develops only if the mother has IgG antibodies from a previous exposure to A or B antigens. These IgG antibodies cross the placenta by active transport and affect the fetus or newborn. Sensitization of the mother to fetal antigens may have occurred by previous transfusions or by conditions of pregnancy that result in transfer of fetal erythrocytes into the maternal circulation, such as first-trimester abortion, ectopic pregnancy, amniocentesis, manual extraction of the placenta, version (external or internal) procedures, or normal pregnancy.

ABO incompatibility with sensitization usually does not cause fetal disease other than extremely mild anemia. It may produce **hemolytic disease of the newborn**, which is manifested as significant anemia and hyperbilirubinemia. Because many mothers who have blood group O have IgG antibodies to A and B before pregnancy, the firstborn infant of A or B blood type may be affected. In contrast to Rh disease, ABO hemolytic disease does not become more severe with subsequent pregnancies. Hemolysis with ABO incompatibility is less severe than hemolysis in Rh-sensitized pregnancy, either because the anti-A or anti-B antibody may bind to nonerythrocytic cells that contain A or B antigen or because fetal erythrocytes have fewer A or B antigenic determinants than they have Rh sites. With the declining incidence of Rh hemolytic disease, ABO incompatibility has become the most common cause of neonatal hyperbilirubinemia requiring therapy, currently accounting for approximately 20% of clinically significant jaundice in the newborn.

Erythroblastosis fetalis classically is caused by Rh blood group incompatibility. Most Rh-negative women have no anti-Rh antibodies at the time of their first pregnancy. The Rh antigen system consists of five antigens: C, D, E, c, and e; the d type is not antigenic. In most Rh-sensitized cases, the D antigen of the fetus sensitizes the Rh-negative (d) mother, resulting in IgG antibody production during the first pregnancy. Because most mothers are not sensitized to Rh antigens at the start of pregnancy, Rh erythroblastosis fetalis is usually a disease of the

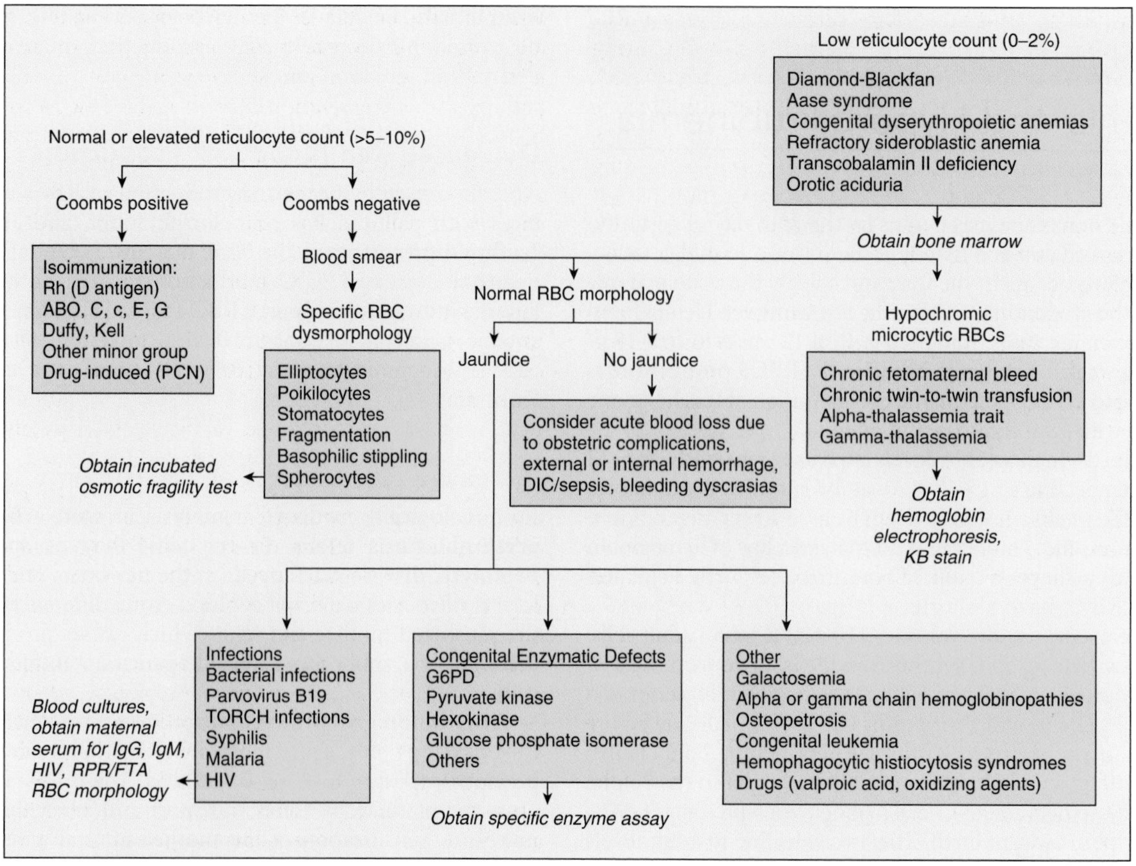

FIGURE 62.1 Differential diagnosis of neonatal anemia. The physician obtains information from the family, maternal and labor and delivery histories, and laboratory tests, including hemoglobin, reticulocyte count, blood type, direct Coombs test, peripheral smear, red blood cell (RBC) indices, and bilirubin concentration. *DIC*, Disseminated intravascular coagulation; *FTA*, fluorescent treponemal antibody test; *G6PD*, glucose-6-phosphate dehydrogenase; *HIV*, human immunodeficiency virus; *KB*, Kleihauer-Betke; *PCN*, penicillin; *RPR*, rapid plasma reagin tests; *TORCH*, toxoplasmosis, other, rubella, cytomegalovirus, herpes simplex. (From Ohls RK. Anemia in the neonate. In: Christensen RD, ed. *Hematologic Problems of the Neonate.* Philadelphia: Saunders; 2000:162.)

second and subsequent pregnancies. The first affected pregnancy results in an antibody response in the mother, which may be detected during antenatal screening with the Coombs test and determined to be anti-D antibody. The first affected newborn may show no serious fetal disease and may manifest hemolytic disease of the newborn only by the development of anemia and hyperbilirubinemia. Subsequent pregnancies result in an increasing severity of response because of an earlier onset of hemolysis in utero. Fetal anemia, heart failure, elevated venous pressure, portal vein obstruction, and hypoalbuminemia result in **fetal hydrops**, which is characterized by ascites, pleural and pericardial effusions, and anasarca (see Chapter 60). The risk of fetal death is high.

The **management** of a pregnancy complicated by Rh sensitization depends on the severity of hemolysis, its effects on the fetus, and the maturity of the fetus at the time it becomes affected. The severity of the hemolysis can be assessed by the quantity of bilirubin transferred from the fetus to the amniotic fluid, quantified by spectrophotometric analysis of the optical density (at 450 nm) of amniotic fluid.

Three zones of optical densities with decreasing slopes toward term gestation have been developed to predict the severity of the illness. The high optical density zone 3 is associated with severe hemolysis. Fetuses in the lower zones probably are not affected. If a fetus's optical density measurement for bilirubin falls into zone 3, and the fetus has pulmonary maturity as determined by the lecithin-to-sphingomyelin ratio, the infant should be delivered and treated in the neonatal intensive care unit. If the lungs are immature and the fetus is between 22 and 33 weeks of gestational age, an ultrasound-guided intrauterine transfusion with O-negative blood into the umbilical vein is indicated and may have to be repeated until pulmonary maturity is reached or fetal distress is detected. Indications for fetal intravascular transfusion in sensitized fetuses between 22 and 32 weeks of gestational age include a fetal hematocrit of less than 25-30%, fetal hydrops, and fetal distress too early in gestation for delivery. Intravascular intrauterine transfusion corrects fetal anemia, improves the outcome of severe hydrops, and reduces the need for postnatal exchange transfusion, but is associated with neonatal anemia as a result of continued hemolysis plus suppressed erythropoiesis.

Prevention of sensitization of the mother carrying an Rh-positive fetus is possible by treating the mother during gestation (>28 weeks' gestational age) and within 72 hours after birth with anti-Rh-positive immune globulin (RhoGAM). The dose of RhoGAM (300 μg) is based on the ability of this amount of anti-Rh-positive antibody to bind all the possible fetal Rh-positive erythrocytes entering the maternal circulation during the fetal-to-maternal transfusion at birth (approximately 30 mL). RhoGAM may bind Rh-positive fetal erythrocytes or interfere with maternal anti-Rh-positive antibody production by another, unknown mechanism. RhoGAM is effective only in preventing sensitization to the D antigen. Other blood group antigens that can cause immune hydrops and erythroblastosis include Rh C, E, Kell, and Duffy. Anti-Kell alloimmunity produces lower amniotic bilirubin levels and a lower reticulocyte count because, in addition to hemolysis, it inhibits erythropoiesis.

Nonimmune causes of hemolysis in the newborn include RBC enzyme deficiencies of the Embden-Meyerhof pathway, such as pyruvate kinase or glucose-6-phosphate dehydrogenase deficiency. RBC membrane disorders are another cause of nonimmune hemolysis. Hereditary spherocytosis is inherited as a severe autosomal recessive form or less severe autosomal dominant form and is the result of a deficiency of spectrin, a protein of the RBC membrane. Hemoglobinopathies, such as thalassemia, are another cause of nonimmunologically mediated hemolysis.

Blood Loss

Decision-Making Algorithms
Available @ StudentConsult.com

Gastrointestinal Bleeding
Bleeding

Anemia from blood loss at birth is manifested by two patterns of presentation, depending on the rapidity of blood loss. **Acute blood loss** after fetal-maternal hemorrhage, rupture of the umbilical cord, placenta previa, or internal hemorrhage (hepatic or splenic hematoma; retroperitoneal) is characterized by pallor, diminished peripheral pulses, and shock. There are no signs of extramedullary hematopoiesis and no hepatosplenomegaly. The hemoglobin content and serum iron levels initially are normal, but the hemoglobin levels decline during the subsequent 24 hours. Newborns with **chronic blood loss** caused by chronic fetal-maternal hemorrhage or a twin-to-twin transfusion present with marked pallor, heart failure, hepatosplenomegaly with or without hydrops, a low hemoglobin level at birth, a hypochromic microcytic blood smear, and decreased serum iron stores. Fetal-maternal bleeding occurs in 50-75% of all pregnancies, with fetal blood losses ranging from 1 to 50 mL; most blood losses are 1 mL or less, 1 in 400 are approximately 30 mL, and 1 in 2,000 are approximately 100 mL.

The diagnosis of fetal-maternal hemorrhage is confirmed by the Kleihauer-Betke acid elution test. Pink fetal RBCs are observed and counted in the mother's peripheral blood smear because fetal hemoglobin is resistant to acid elution; adult hemoglobin is eluted, leaving discolored maternal cells (patients with sickle cell anemia or hereditary persistence of fetal hemoglobin may have a false-positive result, and ABO incompatibility may produce a false-negative result).

Diagnosis and Management

Hemolysis in utero resulting from any cause may produce a spectrum of clinical manifestations at birth. Severe hydrops with anasarca, heart failure, and pulmonary edema may prevent adequate ventilation at birth, resulting in asphyxia. Infants affected with hemolysis in utero have hepatosplenomegaly and pallor and become jaundiced within the first 24 hours after birth. Less severely affected infants manifest pallor and hepatosplenomegaly at birth and become jaundiced subsequently. Patients with ABO incompatibility often are asymptomatic and show no physical signs at birth; mild anemia with jaundice develops during the first 24-72 hours of life.

Because hydrops, anemia, or jaundice is secondary to many diverse causes of hemolysis, a laboratory evaluation is needed in all patients with suspected hemolysis. A complete blood count, blood smear, reticulocyte count, blood type, and direct Coombs test (to determine the presence of antibody-coated RBCs) should be performed in the initial evaluation of all infants with hemolysis. Reduced hemoglobin levels, reticulocytosis, and a blood smear characterized by polychromasia and anisocytosis are expected with isoimmune hemolysis. Spherocytes commonly are observed in ABO incompatibility. The determination of the blood type and the Coombs test identify the responsible antigen and antibody in immunologically mediated hemolysis.

In the absence of a positive Coombs test and blood group differences between the mother and fetus, other causes of nonimmune hemolysis must be considered. RBC enzyme assays, hemoglobin electrophoresis, or RBC membrane tests (osmotic fragility, spectrin assay) should be performed. Internal hemorrhage also may be associated with anemia, reticulocytosis, and jaundice when the hemorrhage reabsorbs; ultrasound evaluation of the brain, liver, spleen, or adrenal gland may be indicated when nonimmune hemolysis is suspected. Shock is more typical in patients with internal hemorrhage, whereas in hemolytic diseases, heart failure may be seen with severe anemia. Evaluation of a possible fetal-maternal hemorrhage should include the Kleihauer-Betke test.

The **treatment** of *symptomatic* neonatal anemia is transfusion of cross-matched packed RBCs. If immune hemolysis is present, the cells to be transfused must be cross-matched against maternal and neonatal plasma. Acute volume loss may necessitate resuscitation with nonblood products, such as saline if blood is not available; packed RBCs can be given subsequently. To correct anemia and any remaining blood volume deficit, 10-15 mL/kg of packed RBCs should be sufficient. Cytomegalovirus-seronegative blood should be given to cytomegalovirus-seronegative infants, and all blood products should be irradiated to reduce the risk of graft-versus-host disease; blood should be screened for HIV, hepatitis B and C, and syphilis. Recombinant erythropoietin may improve the hematocrit in infants with a hyporegenerative anemia after in utero transfusion.

HYPERBILIRUBINEMIA

Hemolytic disease of the newborn is a common cause of neonatal jaundice. Nonetheless, because of the immaturity of the pathways of bilirubin metabolism, many newborn infants without evidence of hemolysis become jaundiced.

Bilirubin is produced by the catabolism of hemoglobin in the reticuloendothelial system. The tetrapyrrole ring of heme is cleaved by heme oxygenase to form equivalent quantities of biliverdin and carbon monoxide. Because no other biologic source of carbon monoxide exists, the excretion of this gas is stoichiometrically identical to the production of bilirubin.

Biliverdin is converted to bilirubin by biliverdin reductase. One gram of hemoglobin produces 35 mg of bilirubin. Sources of bilirubin other than circulating hemoglobin represent 20% of bilirubin production; these sources include inefficient (shunt) hemoglobin production and lysis of precursor cells in bone marrow. Compared with adults, newborns have a twofold to threefold greater rate of bilirubin production (6-10 mg/kg/24 hr vs. 3 mg/kg/24 hr). This increased production is caused, in part, by an increased RBC mass (higher hematocrit) and a shortened erythrocyte life span of 70-90 days compared with the 120-day erythrocyte life span in adults.

Bilirubin produced after hemoglobin catabolism is lipid soluble and unconjugated and reacts as an indirect reagent in the van den Bergh test. Indirect-reacting, unconjugated bilirubin is toxic to the central nervous system and is insoluble in water, limiting its excretion. Unconjugated bilirubin binds to albumin on specific bilirubin binding sites; 1 g of albumin binds 8.5 mg of bilirubin in a newborn. If the binding sites become saturated or if a competitive compound binds at the site, displacing bound bilirubin, free bilirubin becomes available to enter the central nervous system. Organic acids such as free fatty acids and drugs such as sulfisoxazole can displace bilirubin from its binding site on albumin.

Bilirubin dissociates from albumin at the hepatocyte and becomes bound to a cytoplasmic liver protein Y (ligandin). Hepatic conjugation results in the production of bilirubin diglucuronide, which is water soluble and capable of biliary and renal excretion. The enzyme glucuronosyltransferase represents the rate-limiting step of bilirubin conjugation. The concentrations of ligandin and glucuronosyltransferase are lower in newborns, particularly in premature infants, than in older children.

Conjugated bilirubin gives a direct reaction in the van den Bergh test. Most conjugated bilirubin is excreted through the bile into the small intestine and eliminated in the stool. Some bilirubin may undergo hydrolysis back to the unconjugated fraction by intestinal glucuronidase, however, and may be reabsorbed (enterohepatic recirculation). In addition, bacteria in the neonatal intestine convert bilirubin to urobilinogen and stercobilinogen, which are excreted in urine and stool and usually limit bilirubin reabsorption. Delayed passage of meconium, which contains bilirubin, also may contribute to the enterohepatic recirculation of bilirubin.

Bilirubin is produced in utero by the normal fetus and by the fetus affected by erythroblastosis fetalis. Indirect, unconjugated, lipid-soluble fetal bilirubin is transferred across the placenta and becomes conjugated by maternal hepatic enzymes. The placenta is impermeable to conjugated water-soluble bilirubin. Fetal bilirubin levels become only mildly elevated in the presence of severe hemolysis, but may increase when hemolysis produces fetal hepatic inspissated bile stasis and conjugated hyperbilirubinemia. Maternal indirect (but not direct) hyperbilirubinemia also may increase fetal bilirubin levels.

Etiology of Indirect Unconjugated Hyperbilirubinemia

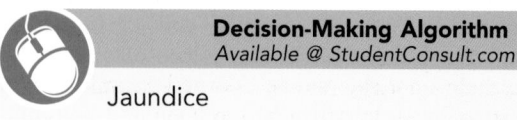

Decision-Making Algorithm
Available @ StudentConsult.com

Jaundice

Physiological jaundice is a common cause of hyperbilirubinemia among newborns. It is a diagnosis of exclusion, made after careful evaluation has ruled out more serious causes of jaundice, such as hemolysis, infection, and metabolic diseases. Physiological jaundice is the result of many factors that are normal physiological characteristics of newborns: increased bilirubin production resulting from an increased RBC mass, shortened RBC life span, and hepatic immaturity of ligandin and glucuronosyltransferase. Physiological jaundice may be exaggerated among infants of Greek and Asian ancestry.

The clinical pattern of physiological jaundice in term infants includes a peak indirect-reacting bilirubin level of no more than 12 mg/dL on day 3 of life. In premature infants, the peak is higher (15 mg/dL) and occurs later (fifth day). The peak level of indirect bilirubin during physiological jaundice may be higher in breast milk–fed infants than in formula-fed infants (15-17 mg/dL versus 12 mg/dL). This higher level may be partly a result of the decreased fluid intake of infants fed breast milk. Jaundice is unphysiological or pathological if it is clinically evident on the first day of life, if the bilirubin level increases more than 0.5 mg/dL/hr, if the peak bilirubin is greater than 13 mg/dL in term infants, if the direct bilirubin fraction is greater than 1.5 mg/dL, or if hepatosplenomegaly and anemia are present.

Crigler-Najjar syndrome is a serious, rare, autosomal recessive, permanent deficiency of glucuronosyltransferase that results in severe indirect hyperbilirubinemia. Type II responds to enzyme induction by phenobarbital, producing an increase in enzyme activity and a reduction of bilirubin levels. Type I does not respond to phenobarbital and manifests as persistent indirect hyperbilirubinemia, often leading to kernicterus. **Gilbert disease** is caused by a mutation of the promoter region of glucuronosyltransferase and results in a mild indirect hyperbilirubinemia. In the presence of another icterogenic factor (hemolysis), more severe jaundice may develop.

Breast milk jaundice may be associated with unconjugated hyperbilirubinemia without evidence of hemolysis during the first to second week of life. Bilirubin levels rarely increase to more than 20 mg/dL. Interruption of breast feeding for 1-2 days results in a rapid decline of bilirubin levels, which do not increase significantly after breast feeding resumes. Breast milk may contain an inhibitor of bilirubin conjugation or may increase enterohepatic recirculation of bilirubin because of breast milk glucuronidase.

Jaundice on the first day of life is always pathological, and immediate attention is needed to establish the cause. Early onset often is a result of hemolysis, internal hemorrhage (cephalhematoma, hepatic or splenic hematoma), or infection (Table 62.1). Infection also is often associated with direct-reacting bilirubin resulting from perinatal congenital infections or from bacterial sepsis.

Physical evidence of jaundice is observed in infants when bilirubin levels reach 5-10 mg/dL (versus 2-3 mg/dL in adults). When jaundice is observed, the laboratory evaluation for hyperbilirubinemia should include a total bilirubin measurement to determine the magnitude of hyperbilirubinemia. Bilirubin levels greater than 5 mg/dL on the first day of life or greater than 13 mg/dL thereafter in term infants should be evaluated further with measurement of indirect and direct bilirubin levels, blood typing, Coombs test, complete blood count, blood smear, and reticulocyte count. These tests must be performed before treatment of hyperbilirubinemia with phototherapy or exchange transfusion. In the absence of hemolysis or evidence

TABLE 62.1 Etiology of Unconjugated Hyperbilirubinemia

	HEMOLYSIS PRESENT	HEMOLYSIS ABSENT
Common	*Blood group incompatibility:* ABO, Rh, Kell, Duffy infection	Physiological jaundice, breast milk jaundice, internal hemorrhage, polycythemia, infant of diabetic mother
Rare	*Red blood cell enzyme defects:* glucose-6-phosphate dehydrogenase, pyruvate kinase *Red blood cell membrane disorders:* spherocytosis, ovalocytosis *Hemoglobinopathy:* thalassemia	Mutations of glucuronyl transferase enzyme (Crigler-Najjar syndrome, Gilbert disease), pyloric stenosis, hypothyroidism, immune thrombocytopenia

for either the common or the rare causes of nonhemolytic indirect hyperbilirubinemia, the diagnosis is either physiological or breast milk jaundice. Jaundice appearing or increasing after 2 weeks of age is pathological and suggests a direct-reacting hyperbilirubinemia.

Etiology of Direct Conjugated Hyperbilirubinemia

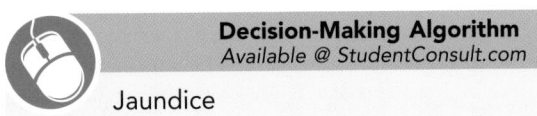

Decision-Making Algorithm
Available @ StudentConsult.com

Jaundice

Direct-reacting hyperbilirubinemia (defined as a direct bilirubin level >2 mg/dL or >20% of the total bilirubin) is never physiological and should always be evaluated thoroughly according to the diagnostic categories (Table 62.2). Direct-reacting bilirubin (composed mostly of conjugated bilirubin) is not neurotoxic to the infant but signifies a serious underlying disorder involving cholestasis or hepatocellular injury. The diagnostic evaluation of patients with direct-reacting hyperbilirubinemia involves the determination of the levels of liver enzymes (aspartate aminotransferase, alkaline phosphatase, alanine aminotransferase, and γ-glutamyl transpeptidase), bacterial and viral cultures, metabolic screening tests, hepatic ultrasound, sweat chloride test, and occasionally liver biopsy. In addition, the presence of dark urine and gray-white (acholic) stools with jaundice after the second week of life strongly suggests biliary atresia. The treatment of disorders manifested by direct bilirubinemia is specific for the diseases that are listed in Table 62.2. These diseases do not respond to phototherapy or exchange transfusion.

TABLE 62.2 Etiology of Conjugated Hyperbilirubinemia

COMMON
Hyperalimentation cholestasis
CMV infection
Other perinatal congenital infections (TORCH)
Inspissated bile from prolonged hemolysis
Neonatal hepatitis
Sepsis
UNCOMMON
Hepatic infarction
Inborn errors of metabolism (galactosemia, tyrosinemia)
Cystic fibrosis
Biliary atresia
Choledochal cyst
α_1-Antitrypsin deficiency
Neonatal iron storage disease (neonatal hemochromatosis)
Alagille syndrome (arteriohepatic dysplasia)
Byler disease, progressive familial intrahepatic cholestasis types 1, 2, 3

CMV, Cytomegalovirus; *TORCH*, toxoplasmosis, other, rubella, cytomegalovirus, herpes simplex.

Kernicterus (Bilirubin Encephalopathy)

Lipid-soluble, unconjugated, indirect bilirubin fraction is toxic to the developing central nervous system, especially when indirect bilirubin concentrations are high and exceed the binding capacity of albumin. Kernicterus results when indirect bilirubin is deposited in brain cells and disrupts neuronal metabolism and function, especially in the basal ganglia. Indirect bilirubin may cross the blood-brain barrier because of its lipid solubility. Other theories propose that a disruption of the blood-brain barrier permits entry of a bilirubin-albumin or free bilirubin–fatty acid complex.

Kernicterus usually is noted when the bilirubin level is excessively high for gestational age. It usually does not develop in term infants when bilirubin levels are less than 20-25 mg/dL, but the incidence increases as serum bilirubin levels exceed 25 mg/dL. Kernicterus may be noted at bilirubin levels less than 20 mg/dL in the presence of sepsis, meningitis, hemolysis, asphyxia, hypoxia, hypothermia, hypoglycemia, bilirubin-displacing drugs (sulfa drugs), and prematurity. Other risks for kernicterus in term infants are hemolysis, jaundice noted within 24 hours of birth, and delayed diagnosis of hyperbilirubinemia. Kernicterus has developed in extremely immature infants weighing less than 1,000 g when bilirubin levels are less than 10 mg/dL because of a more permeable blood-brain barrier associated with prematurity.

The earliest clinical manifestations of kernicterus are lethargy, hypotonia, irritability, poor Moro response, and poor feeding. A high-pitched cry and emesis also may be present. Early signs are noted after day 4 of life. Later signs include bulging fontanelle, opisthotonic posturing, pulmonary hemorrhage, fever, hypertonicity, paralysis of upward gaze, and seizures. Infants with severe cases of kernicterus die in the neonatal period. Spasticity resolves in surviving infants, who may manifest later nerve deafness, choreoathetoid cerebral palsy, mental retardation, enamel dysplasia, and discoloration of teeth as permanent sequelae. Kernicterus may be prevented by avoiding excessively high indirect bilirubin levels and by avoiding conditions or drugs that may displace bilirubin from albumin. Early signs of kernicterus occasionally may be reversed by immediately instituting an exchange transfusion (see later).

Therapy of Indirect Hyperbilirubinemia

Phototherapy is an effective and safe method for reducing indirect bilirubin levels, particularly when initiated before serum bilirubin increases to levels associated with kernicterus. In term infants, phototherapy is begun when indirect bilirubin levels are between 16 and 18 mg/dL. Phototherapy is initiated in premature infants when bilirubin is at lower levels, to prevent bilirubin from reaching the high concentrations necessitating exchange transfusion. Blue lights and white lights are effective in reducing bilirubin levels.

Under the effects of phototherapy light with maximal irradiance in the 425- to 475-nm wavelength band, bilirubin is transformed into isomers that are water soluble and easily excreted. Unconjugated bilirubin (IX) is in the 4Z, 15Z configuration. Phototherapy causes a photochemical reaction producing the reversible, more water-soluble isomer 4Z, 15E bilirubin IX. This isomer can be excreted easily, bypassing the liver's conjugation system. Another photochemical reaction results in the rapid production of lumirubin, a more water-soluble isomer than the aforementioned isomer, which does not spontaneously revert to unconjugated native bilirubin and can be excreted in urine.

Complications of phototherapy include an increased insensible water loss, diarrhea, and dehydration. Additional problems are macular-papular red skin rash, lethargy, masking of cyanosis, nasal obstruction by eye pads, and potential for retinal damage. Skin bronzing may be noted in infants with direct-reacting hyperbilirubinemia. Infants with mild hemolytic disease of the newborn occasionally may be managed successfully with phototherapy for hyperbilirubinemia, but care must be taken to follow these infants for the late occurrence of anemia from continued hemolysis.

Exchange transfusion usually is reserved for infants with dangerously high indirect bilirubin levels who are at risk for kernicterus. As a rule of thumb, a level of 20 mg/dL for indirect-reacting bilirubin is the *exchange number* for infants *with hemolysis* who weigh more than 2,000 g. Asymptomatic infants with physiological or breast milk jaundice may not require exchange transfusion, unless the indirect bilirubin level exceeds 25 mg/dL. The exchangeable level of indirect bilirubin for other infants may be estimated by calculating 10% of the birth weight in grams: the level in an infant weighing 1,500 g would be 15 mg/dL. Infants weighing less than 1,000 g usually do not require an exchange transfusion until the bilirubin level exceeds 10 mg/dL.

The exchange transfusion usually is performed through an umbilical venous catheter placed in the inferior vena cava or, if free flow is obtained, at the confluence of the umbilical vein and the portal system. The level of serum bilirubin immediately after the exchange transfusion declines to levels that are about half of those before the exchange; levels rebound 6-8 hours later as a result of continued hemolysis and redistribution of bilirubin from tissue stores.

Complications of exchange transfusion include problems related to the blood (transfusion reaction, metabolic instability, or infection), the catheter (vessel perforation or hemorrhage), or the procedure (hypotension or necrotizing enterocolitis [NEC]). Unusual complications include thrombocytopenia and graft-versus-host disease. Continuation of phototherapy may reduce the necessity for subsequent exchange transfusions.

Polycythemia (Hyperviscosity Syndrome)

Polycythemia is an excessively high hematocrit (≥65%), which may lead to hyperviscosity that produces symptoms related to vascular stasis, hypoperfusion, and ischemia. As the hematocrit increases from 40% to 60%, there is a small increase in blood viscosity. When the central hematocrit increases to greater than 65%, the blood viscosity begins to increase markedly, and symptoms may appear. Neonatal erythrocytes are less filterable or deformable than adult erythrocytes, which further contributes to hyperviscosity. A central venous hematocrit of 65% or greater is noted in 3-5% of infants. Infants at special risk for polycythemia are term and post-term small for gestational age infants, infants of diabetic mothers, infants with delayed cord clamping, and infants with neonatal hyperthyroidism, adrenogenital syndrome, trisomy 13, trisomy 18, trisomy 21, twin-to-twin transfusion syndrome (recipient), or Beckwith-Wiedemann syndrome. In some infants, polycythemia may reflect a compensation for prolonged periods of fetal hypoxia caused by placental insufficiency; these infants have increased erythropoietin levels at birth.

Polycythemic patients appear plethoric or ruddy and may develop acrocyanosis. Symptoms are a result of the increased RBC mass and of vascular compromise. Seizures, lethargy, and irritability reflect abnormalities of microcirculation of the brain, whereas hyperbilirubinemia may reflect the poor hepatic circulation or the increased amount of hemoglobin that is being broken down into bilirubin. Additional problems include respiratory distress and primary pulmonary hypertension of the newborn (PPHN) that result in part from elevated pulmonary vascular resistance. The chest radiograph often reveals cardiomegaly, increased vascular markings, pleural effusions, and interstitial edema. Other problems are NEC, hypoglycemia, thrombocytopenia, priapism, testicular infarction, hemiplegic stroke, and feeding intolerance. Many of these complications also are related to the primary condition associated with polycythemia (small for gestational age infants are at risk for hypoglycemia and PPHN after periods of hypoxia in utero).

Long-term sequelae of neonatal polycythemia relate to neurodevelopmental abnormalities that may be prevented by treatment of symptomatic infants with partial exchange transfusion after birth. A partial exchange transfusion removes whole blood and replaces it with normal saline.

Coagulation Disorders

Disorders of coagulation are common in the neonatal period. Hemorrhage during this time may be a result of trauma, inherited permanent deficiency of coagulation factors, transient deficiencies of vitamin K–dependent factors, disorders of platelets, and disseminated intravascular coagulation (DIC) seen in sick newborns with shock or hypoxia. Thrombosis also is a potential problem in the newborn because of developmentally lower circulating levels of antithrombin III, protein C (a vitamin K–dependent protein that inhibits factors VIII and V), and the fibrinolytic system.

Coagulation factors do not pass through the placenta to the fetus, and newborn infants have relatively low levels of the vitamin K–dependent factors II, VII, IX, and X. Contact factors XI and XII, prekallikrein, and kininogen also are lower in newborns than in adults. Fibrinogen (factor I); plasma levels of factors V, VIII, and XIII; and platelet counts are within the adult normal range.

Because of the transient, relative deficiencies of the contact and vitamin K–dependent factors, the *partial thromboplastin time* (PTT), which is dependent on factors XII, IX, VIII, X, V, II, and I, is prolonged in the newborn period. Preterm infants have the most marked prolongation of the PTT (50-80 seconds) compared with term infants (35-50 seconds) and older, more mature infants (25-35 seconds). The administration of heparin and the presence of DIC, hemophilia, and severe vitamin K deficiency prolong the PTT.

The *prothrombin time* (PT), which is dependent on factors X, VII, V, II, and I, is a more sensitive test for vitamin K deficiency. The PT is only slightly prolonged in term infants (13-20 seconds) compared with preterm infants (13-21 seconds) and more mature patients (12-14 seconds). Abnormal prolongations of the PT occur with vitamin K deficiency, hepatic injury, and DIC. Levels of *fibrinogen* and *fibrin degradation products* are similar in infants and adults. The *bleeding time,* which reflects platelet function and number, is normal during the newborn period in the absence of maternal salicylate therapy.

Vitamin K is a necessary cofactor for the carboxylation of glutamate on precursor proteins, converting them into the more active coagulation factors II, VII, IX, and X; γ-carboxyglutamic acid binds calcium, which is required for the immediate activation of factors during hemorrhage. There is no congenital deficiency of hepatic synthesis of these precursor proteins, but in the absence of vitamin K, their conversion to the active factor is not possible. Levels of *protein induced by vitamin K absence* increase in vitamin K deficiency and are helpful diagnostic markers; vitamin K administration rapidly corrects the coagulation defects, reducing protein induced by vitamin K absence to undetectable levels.

Although most newborns are born with reduced levels of vitamin K–dependent factors, hemorrhagic complications develop only rarely. Infants at risk for **hemorrhagic disease of the newborn** have the most profound deficiency of vitamin K–dependent factors, and these factors decline further after birth. Because breast milk is a poor source of vitamin K, breast fed infants are at increased risk for hemorrhage that usually occurs between days 3 and 7 of life. Bleeding usually ensues from the umbilical cord, circumcision site, intestines, scalp, mucosa, and skin, but internal hemorrhage places the infant at risk for fatal complications, such as intracranial bleeding.

Hemorrhage on the first day of life resulting from a deficiency of the vitamin K–dependent factors often is associated with administration to the mother of drugs that affect vitamin K metabolism in the infant. This early pattern of hemorrhage has been seen with maternal warfarin or antibiotic (e.g., isoniazid or rifampin) therapy and in infants of mothers receiving phenobarbital and phenytoin. Bleeding also may occur 1-3 months after birth, particularly among breast fed infants. Vitamin K deficiency in breast fed infants also should raise suspicion about the possibility of vitamin K malabsorption resulting from cystic fibrosis, biliary atresia, hepatitis, or antibiotic suppression of the colonic bacteria that produce vitamin K.

Bleeding associated with vitamin K deficiency may be **prevented** by administration of vitamin K to all infants at birth. Before routine administration of vitamin K, 1-2% of all newborns had hemorrhagic disease of the newborn. One intramuscular dose (1 mg) of vitamin K prevents vitamin K–deficiency bleeding. **Treatment** of bleeding resulting from vitamin K deficiency involves intravenous administration of 1 mg of vitamin K. If severe, life-threatening hemorrhage is present, fresh frozen plasma also should be given. Unusually high doses of vitamin K may be needed for hepatic disease and for maternal warfarin or anticonvulsant therapy.

Clinical Manifestations and Differential Diagnoses of Bleeding Disorders

Decision-Making Algorithms
Available @ StudentConsult.com

Bleeding
Petechiae/Purpura

Bleeding disorders in a newborn may be associated with cutaneous bleeding, such as cephalhematoma, subgaleal hemorrhage, ecchymosis, and petechiae. Facial petechiae are common in infants born by vertex presentation, with or without a nuchal cord, and usually are insignificant. Mucosal bleeding may appear as hematemesis, melena, or epistaxis. Internal hemorrhage results in organ-specific dysfunction, such as seizures associated with intracranial hemorrhage. Bleeding from venipuncture or heelstick sites, circumcision sites, or the umbilical cord also is common with bleeding disorders.

The differential diagnosis depends partly on the clinical circumstances associated with the hemorrhage. In a **sick newborn**, the differential diagnosis should include DIC, hepatic failure, and thrombocytopenia. Thrombocytopenia in an ill neonate may be secondary to consumption by trapping of platelets in a hemangioma **(Kasabach-Merritt syndrome)** or may be associated with perinatal, congenital, or bacterial infections; NEC; thrombotic endocarditis; PPHN; organic acidemia; maternal preeclampsia; or asphyxia. Thrombocytopenia also may be due to peripheral washout of platelets after an exchange transfusion. Treatment of a sick infant with thrombocytopenia should be directed at the underlying disorder, supplemented by infusions of platelets, blood, or both.

The etiology of DIC in a newborn includes hypoxia, hypotension, asphyxia, bacterial or viral sepsis, NEC, death of a twin while in utero, cavernous hemangioma, nonimmune hydrops, neonatal cold injury, neonatal neoplasm, and hepatic disease. The treatment of DIC should be focused primarily on therapy for the initiating or underlying disorder. Supportive management of consumptive coagulopathy involves platelet transfusions and factor replacement with fresh frozen plasma. Heparin and factor C concentrate should be reserved for infants with DIC who also have thrombosis.

Disorders of hemostasis in a *well child* are not associated with systemic disease in a newborn, but reflect coagulation factor or platelet deficiency. Hemophilia initially is associated with cutaneous or mucosal bleeding and no systemic illness. If bleeding continues, hypovolemic shock may develop. Bleeding into the brain, liver, or spleen may result in organ-specific signs and shock.

In a *well child,* thrombocytopenia may be part of a syndrome such as Fanconi anemia syndrome (involving hypoplasia and aplasia of the thumb), radial aplasia-thrombocytopenia syndrome (thumbs present), or Wiskott-Aldrich syndrome. Various maternal drugs also may reduce the neonatal platelet count without producing other adverse effects. These drugs include sulfonamides, quinidine, quinine, and thiazide diuretics.

The most common causes of thrombocytopenia in well newborns are transient isoimmune thrombocytopenia and transient neonatal thrombocytopenia. **Isoimmune thrombocytopenia** is caused by antiplatelet antibodies produced by the HPLA1-negative mother after her sensitization to specific paternal platelet antigen (HPA-1a and HPA-5b represent 85% and 10% of cases, respectively) expressed on the fetal platelet. The incidence is 1 in 1,000 to 1 in 2,000 births. This response to maternal-sensitized antibodies that produce isoimmune thrombocytopenia is analogous to the response that produces erythroblastosis fetalis. The maternal antiplatelet antibody does not produce maternal thrombocytopenia, but after crossing the placenta this IgG antibody binds to fetal platelets that are trapped by the reticuloendothelial tissue, resulting in thrombocytopenia. Infants with thrombocytopenia produced in this manner are at risk for development of petechiae, purpura, and intracranial hemorrhage (an incidence of 10-15%) before or after birth. Vaginal delivery may increase the risk of neonatal bleeding; cesarean section may be indicated.

Specific **treatment** for severe thrombocytopenia (<20,000 platelets/mm^3) or significant bleeding is transfusion of ABO-compatible and RhD-compatible, HPA-1a-negative and HPA-5b-negative maternal platelets. Because the antibody in isoimmune thrombocytopenia is directed against the fetal rather than the maternal platelet, thrombocytapheresis of the mother yields sufficient platelets to treat the affected infant. After one platelet transfusion, the infant's platelet count dramatically increases and usually remains in a safe range. Without treatment, thrombocytopenia resolves during the first month of life as the maternal antibody level declines. *Treatment* of the mother with intravenous immunoglobulin or the thrombocytopenic fetus with intravascular platelet transfusion (cordocentesis) is also effective. Cesarean section reduces the risk of intracranial hemorrhage.

Neonatal thrombocytopenia in infants born to women with idiopathic thrombocytopenic purpura (ITP) also is a result of placental transfer of maternal IgG antibodies. In ITP, these autoantibodies are directed against all platelet antigens; mother and newborn may have low platelet counts. The risks of hemorrhage in an infant born to a mother with ITP may be lessened by cesarean section and by treatment of the mother with corticosteroids.

Treatment of an affected infant born to a mother with ITP may involve prednisone and intravenous immunoglobulin. In an emergency, random donor platelets may be used and may produce a transient increase in the infant's platelet count. Thrombocytopenia resolves spontaneously during the first month of life as maternal-derived antibody levels decline. Elevated levels of platelet-associated antibodies also have been noted in thrombocytopenic infants with sepsis and thrombocytopenia of unknown cause who were born to mothers without demonstrable platelet antibodies.

The laboratory evaluation of an infant (well or sick) with bleeding must include a platelet count, blood smear, and evaluation of PTT and PT. Isolated thrombocytopenia in a well infant suggests immune thrombocytopenia. Laboratory evidence of DIC includes a markedly prolonged PTT and PT (minutes rather than seconds), thrombocytopenia, and a blood smear suggesting a microangiopathic hemolytic anemia (burr or fragmented blood cells). Further evaluation reveals low levels of fibrinogen (<100 mg/dL) and elevated levels of fibrin degradation products. Vitamin K deficiency prolongs the PT more than the PTT, whereas hemophilia resulting from factors VIII and IX deficiency prolongs only the PTT. Specific factor levels confirm the diagnosis of hemophilia.

CHAPTER 63

Necrotizing Enterocolitis

Necrotizing enterocolitis (NEC) is a syndrome of intestinal injury and is the most common intestinal emergency occurring in preterm infants admitted to the neonatal intensive care unit. NEC occurs in 1-3 per 1,000 live births and 1-8% of admissions to the neonatal intensive care unit. Prematurity is the most consistent and significant factor associated with neonatal NEC. The disease occurs in 4-13% of infants who weigh less than 1,500 g at birth. NEC is infrequent in term infants (<10% of affected infants).

Most cases of NEC occur in premature infants born before 34 weeks' gestation who have been fed enterally. Prematurity is associated with immaturity of the gastrointestinal tract, including decreased integrity of the intestinal mucosal barrier, depressed mucosal enzymes, suppressed gastrointestinal hormones, suppressed intestinal host defense system, decreased coordination of intestinal motility, and differences in blood flow autoregulation, which is thought to play a significant role in the pathogenesis of NEC. More than 90% of infants diagnosed with NEC have been fed enterally, but NEC has been reported in infants who have never been fed. Feeding with human milk has shown a beneficial role in reducing the incidence of NEC. In addition, probiotics may offer potential benefits for the preterm infant by increasing mucosal barrier function, improving nutrition, upregulating the immune system, and reducing mucosal colonization by potential pathogens. It also is theorized that compromised intestinal blood flow contributes to NEC.

Early clinical signs of NEC include abdominal distention, feeding intolerance/increased gastric residuals, emesis, rectal bleeding, and occasional diarrhea. As the disease progresses, patients may develop marked abdominal distention, bilious emesis, ascites, abdominal wall erythema, lethargy, temperature instability, increased episodes of apnea/bradycardia, disseminated intravascular coagulation, and shock. With abdominal perforation, the abdomen may develop a bluish discoloration.

The white blood cell count can be elevated, but often it is depressed. Thrombocytopenia is common. In addition, infants may develop coagulation abnormalities along with metabolic derangements, including metabolic acidosis, electrolyte imbalance, and hypoglycemia and hyperglycemia. No unique infectious agent has been associated with NEC; bacteriological and fungal cultures may prove helpful but not conclusive.

Radiographic imaging is essential to the diagnosis of NEC. The earliest radiographic finding is intestinal ileus, often associated with thickening of the bowel loops and air-fluid levels. The pathognomonic radiographic finding is **pneumatosis intestinalis** caused by hydrogen gas production from pathogenic bacteria present between the subserosal and muscularis layers of the bowel wall. Radiographic findings also may include a fixed or persistent dilated loop of bowel, intrahepatic venous gas, and *pneumoperitoneum* seen with bowel perforation.

The **differential diagnosis** of NEC includes sepsis with intestinal ileus or a volvulus. Both conditions can present with systemic signs of sepsis and abdominal distention. The absence of pneumatosis on abdominal radiographs does not rule out the diagnosis of NEC; other causes of abdominal distention and perforation (gastric or ileal perforation) should be considered and investigated. Patients diagnosed with Hirschsprung enterocolitis or severe gastroenteritis may present with pneumatosis intestinalis.

The **management** of NEC includes the discontinuation of enteral feedings, gastrointestinal decompression with nasogastric suction, fluid and electrolyte replacement, total parenteral nutrition, and systemic broad-spectrum antibiotics. When the diagnosis of NEC is made, consultation with a pediatric surgeon should be obtained. Even with aggressive and appropriate medical management, 25-50% of infants with NEC require surgical intervention. The decision to perform surgery is obvious when the presence of a pneumoperitoneum is observed on abdominal radiograph. Other, not so obvious indications for surgical intervention include rapid clinical deterioration despite medical therapy, rapid onset and progression of pneumatosis, abdominal mass, and intestinal obstruction. The surgical procedure of choice is laparotomy with removal of the frankly necrotic and nonviable bowel. Many extremely small infants are managed initially with primary peritoneal drainage followed by surgical intervention as needed later, when the infant is stable and a laparotomy can be performed safely. The long-term outcome includes intestinal strictures requiring further surgical intervention, short bowel syndrome with poor absorption of enteral fluids and nutrients, associated cholestasis with resultant cirrhosis and liver failure from prolonged parenteral nutrition, and neurodevelopmental delay from prolonged hospitalization.

CHAPTER 64

Hypoxic-Ischemic Encephalopathy, Intracranial Hemorrhage, and Seizures

The human newborn spends more time asleep (predominantly in rapid eye movement or active sleep) than in a wakeful state and is totally dependent on adults. Primitive reflexes, such as the Moro, grasp, stepping, rooting, sucking, and crossed extensor reflexes, are readily elicited and are normal for this age. In addition, the newborn has a wealth of cortical functions that are less easily shown (e.g., the ability to extinguish repetitive or painful stimuli). The newborn also has the capacity for attentive eye fixation and differential responses to the mother's voice. During the perinatal period, many pathophysiological mechanisms can adversely and permanently affect the developing brain, including prenatal events, such as hypoxia, ischemia, infections, inflammation, malformations, maternal drugs, and coagulation disorders, as well as postnatal events, such as birth trauma, hypoxia-ischemia, inborn errors of metabolism, hypoglycemia, hypothyroidism, hyperthyroidism, polycythemia, hemorrhage, and meningitis.

NEONATAL SEIZURES

Decision-Making Algorithms
Available @ StudentConsult.com

Seizures and Other Paroxysmal Disorders
Hypocalcemia

Seizures during the neonatal period may be the result of multiple causes, with characteristic **historical and clinical manifestations**. Seizures caused by **hypoxic-ischemic encephalopathy** (postasphyxial seizures), a common cause of seizures in the full-term infant, usually occur 12-24 hours after a history of birth asphyxia and often are refractory to conventional doses of anticonvulsant medications. Postasphyxial seizures also may be caused by metabolic disorders associated with neonatal asphyxia, such as hypoglycemia and hypocalcemia. **Intraventricular hemorrhage (IVH)** is a common cause of seizures in premature infants and often occurs between 1 and 3 days of age. Seizures with IVH are associated with a bulging fontanelle, hemorrhagic spinal fluid, anemia, lethargy, and coma. Seizures caused by **hypoglycemia** often occur when blood glucose levels decline to the lowest postnatal value (at 1-2 hours of age or after 24-48 hours of poor nutritional intake). Seizures caused by **hypocalcemia** and **hypomagnesemia** develop in high-risk infants and respond well to therapy with calcium, magnesium, or both.

Seizures noted in the delivery room often are caused by direct *injection of local anesthetic agents* into the fetal scalp (associated with transient bradycardia and fixed dilated pupils), severe *anoxia*, or *congenital brain malformation*. Seizures after the first 5 days of life may be the result of *infection* or *drug withdrawal*. Seizures associated with lethargy, acidosis, and a family history of infant deaths may be the result of an *inborn error of metabolism*. An infant whose parent has a history of a neonatal seizure also is at risk for *benign familial seizures*. In an infant who appears well, a sudden onset on day 1-3 of life of seizures that are of short duration and that do not recur may be the result of a *subarachnoid hemorrhage*. Focal seizures often are the result of local cerebral infarction.

Seizures may be difficult to differentiate from benign jitteriness or from tremulousness in infants of diabetic mothers, in infants with narcotic withdrawal syndrome, and in any infants after an episode of asphyxia. In contrast to seizures, jitteriness and tremors are sensory dependent, elicited by stimuli, and interrupted by holding the extremity. Seizure activity becomes manifested as coarse, fast and slow clonic activity, whereas jitteriness is characterized by fine, rapid movement. Seizures may be associated with abnormal eye movements, such as tonic deviation to one side. The electroencephalogram often shows seizure activity when the clinical diagnosis is uncertain. Identifying seizures in the newborn period is often difficult because the infant, especially the low birth weight infant, usually does not show the tonic-clonic major motor activity typical of the older child (Table 64.1). Subtle seizures are a common manifestation in newborns. The subtle signs of seizure activity include apnea, eye deviation, tongue thrusting, eye blinking, fluctuation of vital

TABLE 64.1 Clinical Characteristics of Neonatal Seizures

DESIGNATION	CHARACTERIZATION
Focal clonic	Repetitive, rhythmic contractions of muscle groups of the limbs, face, or trunk May be unilateral or multifocal May appear synchronously or asynchronously in various body regions Cannot be suppressed by restraint
Focal tonic	Sustained posturing of single limbs Sustained asymmetrical posturing of the trunk Sustained eye deviation Cannot be provoked by stimulation or suppressed by restraint
Myoclonic	Arrhythmic contractions of muscle groups of the limbs, face, or trunk Typically not repetitive or may recur at a slow rate May be generalized, focal, or fragmentary May be provoked by stimulation
Generalized tonic	Sustained symmetrical posturing of limbs, trunk, and neck May be flexor, extensor, or mixed extensor/flexor May be provoked by stimulation May be suppressed by restraint or repositioning
Ocular signs	Random and roving eye movements or nystagmus Distinct from tonic eye deviation
Orobuccolingual movements	Sucking, chewing, tongue protrusions May be provoked by stimulation
Progression movements	Rowing or swimming movements of the arms Pedaling or bicycling movements of the legs May be provoked by stimulation May be suppressed by restraint or repositioning

From Mizrahi EM. Neonatal seizures. In: Shinnar S, Branski D, eds. Pediatric and Adolescent Medicine, *vol 6,* Childhood Seizures. *Basel: S. Karger; 1995.*

signs, and staring. Continuous bedside electroencephalographic monitoring can help identify subtle seizures.

The **diagnostic evaluation** of infants with seizures should involve an immediate determination of capillary blood glucose levels with a Chemstrip. In addition, blood concentrations of sodium, calcium, glucose, and bilirubin should be determined. When infection is suspected, cerebrospinal fluid and blood specimens should be obtained for culture. After the seizure has stopped, a careful examination should be done to identify signs of increased intracranial pressure, congenital malformations, and systemic illness. If signs of elevated intracranial pressure are absent, a lumbar puncture should be performed. If the diagnosis is not apparent at this point, further evaluation should involve magnetic resonance imaging, computed tomography, or cerebral ultrasound and tests to determine the presence of an inborn error of metabolism. Determinations of inborn errors of metabolism are especially important in infants with unexplained lethargy, coma, acidosis, ketonuria, or respiratory alkalosis.

The **treatment** of neonatal seizures may be specific, such as treatment of meningitis or the correction of **hypoglycemia**, **hypocalcemia**, **hypomagnesemia**, **hyponatremia**, or **vitamin B_6 deficiency** or **dependency**. In the absence of an identifiable cause, therapy should involve an anticonvulsant agent, such as 20-40 mg/kg of phenobarbital, 10-20 mg/kg of phenytoin, or 0.1-0.3 mg/kg of diazepam. Treatment of status epilepticus requires repeated doses of phenobarbital and may require diazepam or midazolam, titrated to clinical signs. The long-term outcome for neonatal seizures usually is related to the underlying cause and to the primary pathology, such as hypoxic-ischemic encephalopathy, meningitis, drug withdrawal, stroke, or hemorrhage.

INTRACRANIAL HEMORRHAGE

Intracranial hemorrhage may be confined to one anatomical area of the brain, such as the subdural, subarachnoid, periventricular, intraventricular, intraparenchymal, or cerebellar region. **Subdural hemorrhages** are seen in association with birth trauma, cephalopelvic disproportion, forceps delivery, large for gestational age infants, skull fractures, and postnatal head trauma. The subdural hematoma does not always cause symptoms immediately after birth; with time, however, the red blood cells (RBCs) undergo hemolysis and water is drawn into the hemorrhage because of the high oncotic pressure of protein, resulting in an expanding symptomatic lesion. Anemia, vomiting, seizures, and macrocephaly may occur in an infant who is 1-2 months of age and has a subdural hematoma. **Child abuse** in this situation should be suspected and appropriate diagnostic evaluation undertaken to identify other possible signs of skeletal, ocular, or soft tissue injury. Occasionally, a massive subdural hemorrhage in the neonatal period is caused by rupture of the vein of Galen or by an inherited coagulation disorder, such as hemophilia. Infants with these conditions exhibit shock, seizures, and coma. The **treatment** of all symptomatic subdural hematomas is surgical evacuation.

Subarachnoid hemorrhages may be spontaneous, associated with hypoxia, or caused by bleeding from a cerebral arteriovenous malformation. Seizures are a common presenting manifestation, and the *prognosis* depends on the underlying injury. Treatment is directed at the seizure and the rare occurrence of posthemorrhagic hydrocephalus.

Periventricular hemorrhage and **IVH** are common in very low birth weight infants; the risk decreases with increasing gestational age. Fifty percent of infants weighing less than 1,500 g have evidence of intracranial bleeding. The pathogenesis for these hemorrhages is unknown (they usually are not caused by coagulation disorders), but the initial site of bleeding may be the weak blood vessels in the periventricular germinal matrix. The vessels in this area have poor structural support. These vessels may rupture and hemorrhage because of passive changes in cerebral blood flow occurring with the variations of blood pressure that sick premature infants often exhibit (failure of autoregulation). In some sick infants, these blood pressure variations are the only identifiable etiological factors. In others, the disorders that may cause the elevation or depression of blood pressure or that interfere with venous return from the head (venous stasis) increase the risk of IVH; these disorders include asphyxia, pneumothorax, mechanical ventilation, hypercapnia, hypoxemia, prolonged labor, breech delivery, patent ductus arteriosus, heart failure, and therapy with hypertonic solutions such as sodium bicarbonate.

Most periventricular hemorrhages and IVHs occur in the first 3 days of life. It is unusual for IVH to occur after day 5 of life. The clinical manifestations of IVH include seizures, apnea, bradycardia, lethargy, coma, hypotension, metabolic acidosis, anemia not corrected by blood transfusion, bulging fontanelle, and cutaneous mottling. Many infants with small hemorrhages (grade 1 or 2) are asymptomatic; infants with larger hemorrhages (grade 4) often have a catastrophic event that rapidly progresses to shock and coma.

The diagnosis of IVH is confirmed and the severity graded by ultrasound through the anterior fontanelle or computed tomography examination. Grade 1 IVH is confined to the germinal matrix; grade 2 is an extension of grade 1, with blood noted in the ventricle without ventricular enlargement; grade 3 is an extension of grade 2 with ventricular dilation; and grade 4 has blood in dilated ventricles and in the cerebral cortex, either contiguous with or distant from the ventricle. Grade 4 hemorrhage has a poor prognosis, as does the development of periventricular, small, echolucent cystic lesions, with or without porencephalic cysts and posthemorrhagic hydrocephalus. Periventricular cysts often are noted after the resolution of echodense areas in the periventricular white matter. The cysts may correspond to the development of **periventricular leukomalacia**, which may be a precursor to cerebral palsy. Extensive intraparenchymal echodensities represent hemorrhagic necrosis. They are associated with a high mortality rate and have a poor neurodevelopmental prognosis for survivors.

Treatment of an acute hemorrhage involves standard supportive care, including ventilation for apnea and blood transfusion for hemorrhagic shock. Posthemorrhagic hydrocephalus may be managed with serial daily lumbar punctures, an external ventriculostomy tube, or a permanent ventricular-peritoneal shunt. Implementation of the shunt often is delayed because of the high protein content of the hemorrhagic ventricular fluid.

HYPOXIC-ISCHEMIC ENCEPHALOPATHY

Conditions known to reduce uteroplacental blood flow or to interfere with spontaneous respiration lead to perinatal hypoxia, lactic acidosis, and, if severe enough to reduce cardiac output or cause cardiac arrest, ischemia. The combination of the reduced availability of oxygen for the brain resulting from hypoxia and the diminished or absent blood flow to the brain resulting from ischemia leads to reduced glucose for metabolism and to an accumulation of lactate that produces local tissue acidosis. After reperfusion, hypoxic-ischemic injury also may be complicated by cell necrosis and vascular endothelial edema, reducing blood flow distal to the involved vessel. Typically, hypoxic-ischemic encephalopathy in the term infant is characterized by cerebral edema, cortical necrosis, and involvement of the basal ganglia, whereas in the preterm infant it is characterized by periventricular leukomalacia. Both lesions may result in cortical atrophy, mental retardation, and spastic quadriplegia or diplegia.

The clinical manifestations and characteristic course of hypoxic-ischemic encephalopathy vary according to the severity of the injury (Table 64.2). Infants with severe stage

TABLE 64.2 Hypoxic-Ischemic Encephalopathy in Term Infants

SIGNS	STAGE 1	STAGE 2	STAGE 3
Level of consciousness	Hyperalert	Lethargic	Stuporous
Muscle tone	Normal	Hypotonic	Flaccid
Tendon reflexes/clonus	Hyperactive	Hyperactive	Absent
Moro reflex	Strong	Weak	Absent
Pupils	Mydriasis	Miosis	Unequal, poor light reflex
Seizures	None	Common	Decerebration
Electroencephalography	Normal	Low voltage changing to seizure activity	Burst suppression to isoelectric
Duration	>24 hr if progresses, otherwise may remain normal	24 hr to 14 days	Days to weeks

Modified from Sarnat HB, Sarnat MS. Neonatal encephalopathy following fetal distress. Arch Neurol. *1976;33:696.*

3 hypoxic-ischemic encephalopathy are usually hypotonic, although occasionally they initially appear hypertonic and hyperalert at birth. As cerebral edema develops, brain functions are affected in a descending order; cortical depression produces coma, and brainstem depression results in apnea. As cerebral edema progresses, refractory seizures begin 12-24 hours after birth. Concurrently the infant has no signs of spontaneous respirations, is hypotonic, and has diminished or absent deep tendon reflexes. Hypoxic-ischemic encephalopathy in term infants is often managed with induced hyperthermia.

Survivors of stage 3 hypoxic-ischemic encephalopathy have a high incidence of seizures and serious neurodevelopmental handicaps. The prognosis of severe asphyxia also depends on other organ system injury (see Table 58.6). Another indicator of poor prognosis is time of onset of spontaneous respiration as estimated by Apgar score. Infants with Apgar scores of 0-3 at 10 minutes have a 20% mortality and a 5% incidence of cerebral palsy; if the score remains this low by 20 minutes, the mortality increases to 60%, and the incidence of cerebral palsy increases to 57%.

CHAPTER 65

Sepsis and Meningitis

Systemic and local infections (lung, cutaneous, ocular, umbilical, kidney, bone-joint, and meningeal) are common in the newborn period. Infection may be acquired in utero through the transplacental or transcervical routes and during or after birth. Ascending infection through the cervix, with or without rupture of the amniotic fluid membranes, may result in amnionitis, funisitis (infection of the umbilical cord), congenital pneumonia, and sepsis. The bacteria responsible for ascending infection of the fetus are common bacterial organisms of the maternal genitourinary tract, such as group B streptococci, *Escherichia coli, Haemophilus influenzae*, and *Klebsiella*. Herpes simplex virus (HSV)-1 or, more often, HSV-2 also causes ascending infection that at times may be indistinguishable from bacterial sepsis. Syphilis and *Listeria monocytogenes* are acquired by transplacental infection.

Maternal humoral immunity may protect the fetus against some neonatal pathogens, such as group B streptococci and HSV. Nonetheless, various deficiencies of the neonatal antimicrobial defense mechanism probably are more important than maternal immune status as a contributing factor for neonatal infection, especially in the low birth weight infant. The incidence of sepsis is approximately 1:1,500 in full-term infants and 1:250 in preterm infants. The sixfold-higher rate of sepsis in preterm infants relates to the more immature immunological systems of preterm infants and to their prolonged periods of hospitalization, which increase risk of nosocomially acquired infectious diseases.

Preterm infants before 32 weeks of gestational age have not received the full complement of maternal antibodies (immunoglobulin G [IgG]), which cross the placenta by active transport predominantly in the latter half of the third trimester. In addition, although low birth weight infants may generate IgM antibodies, their own IgG response to infection is reduced. These infants also have deficiencies of the alternate and, to a smaller degree, the classic complement activation pathways, which results in diminished complement-mediated opsonization. Newborn infants also show a deficit in phagocytic migration to the site of infection (to the lung) and in the bone marrow reserve pool of leukocytes. In addition, in the presence of suboptimal activation of complement, neonatal neutrophils ingest and kill bacteria less effectively than adult neutrophils do. Neutrophils from sick infants seem to have an even greater deficit in bacterial killing capacity compared with phagocytic cells from normal neonates.

Defense mechanisms against viral pathogens also may be deficient in a newborn. Neonatal antibody-dependent, cell-mediated immunity by the natural killer lymphocytes is deficient in the absence of maternal antibodies and in the presence of reduced interferon production; reduced antibody levels occur in premature infants and in infants born during a primary viral infection of the mother, such as with enteroviruses, HSV-2, or cytomegalovirus. In addition, antibody-independent cytotoxicity may be reduced in lymphocytes of newborns.

Bacterial sepsis and meningitis often are linked closely in neonates. Despite this association, the incidence of meningitis relative to neonatal sepsis has been on a steady decline. The incidence of meningitis is approximately 1 in 20 cases of sepsis. The causative organisms isolated most frequently are the same as for neonatal sepsis: group B streptococci, *E. coli*, and *L. monocytogenes*. Gram-negative organisms, such as *Klebsiella*, *Salmonella*, and *Serratia marcescens*, are more common in less developed countries, and coagulase-negative staphylococcus needs to be considered in very low birth weight infants. Male infants seem to be more susceptible to neonatal infection than female infants. Severely premature infants are at even greater risk secondary to less effective defense mechanisms and deficient transfer of antibodies from the mother to the fetus (which occurs mostly after 32 weeks' gestation). Neonates in the neonatal intensive care unit live in a hostile environment, with exposure to endotracheal tubes, central arterial and venous catheters, and blood draws, all predisposing to bacteremia and meningitis. Genetic factors have been implicated in the ability of bacteria to cross the blood-brain barrier. This penetration has been noted for group B streptococci, *E. coli*, *Listeria*, *Citrobacter*, and *Streptococcus pneumoniae*.

Neonatal sepsis presents during three periods. **Early-onset sepsis** often begins in utero and usually is a result of infection caused by the bacteria in the mother's genitourinary tract. Organisms related to this sepsis include group B streptococci, *E. coli*, *Klebsiella*, *L. monocytogenes*, and nontypeable *H. influenzae*. Most infected infants are premature and show nonspecific cardiorespiratory signs, such as grunting, tachypnea, and cyanosis at birth. Risk factors for early-onset sepsis include vaginal colonization with group B streptococci, prolonged rupture of the membranes (>24 hours), amnionitis, maternal fever or leukocytosis, fetal tachycardia, and preterm birth. African American race and male sex are unexplained additional risk factors for neonatal sepsis.

Early-onset sepsis (birth to 7 days) is an overwhelming multiorgan system disease frequently manifested as respiratory failure, shock, meningitis (in 30% of cases), disseminated intravascular coagulation, acute tubular necrosis, and symmetrical peripheral gangrene. Early manifestations—grunting, poor feeding, pallor, apnea, lethargy, hypothermia, or an abnormal cry—may be nonspecific. Profound neutropenia, hypoxia, and hypotension may be refractory to treatment with broad-spectrum antibiotics, mechanical ventilation, and vasopressors such as dopamine. In the initial stages of early-onset septicemia in a preterm infant, it is often difficult to differentiate sepsis from respiratory distress syndrome. Because of this difficulty, premature infants with respiratory distress syndrome receive broad-spectrum antibiotics.

The clinical manifestations of sepsis are difficult to separate from the manifestations of meningitis in the neonate. Infants with early-onset sepsis should be evaluated by blood and cerebrospinal fluid (CSF) cultures, CSF Gram stain, cell count, and protein and glucose levels. Normal newborns generally have an elevated CSF protein content (100-150 mg/dL) and may have 25-30/mm^3 white blood cells (mean, 9/mm^3), which are 75% lymphocytes in the absence of infection. Some infants with neonatal meningitis caused by group B streptococci do not have an elevated CSF leukocyte count but are seen to have microorganisms in the CSF on Gram stain. In addition to culture, other methods of identifying the pathogenic bacteria are the determination of bacterial DNA in samples of CSF. In cases of neonatal meningitis, the ratio of CSF glucose to blood glucose usually is less than 50%. The polymerase chain reaction test primarily is used to identify viral infections. Serial complete blood counts should be performed to identify neutropenia, an increased number of immature neutrophils (bands), and thrombocytopenia. C-reactive protein levels are often elevated in neonatal patients with bacterial sepsis.

A chest radiograph also should be obtained to determine the presence of pneumonia. In addition to the traditional neonatal pathogens, pneumonia in very low birth weight infants may be the result of acquisition of maternal genital mycoplasmal agent (e.g., *Ureaplasma urealyticum* or *Mycoplasma hominis*). Arterial blood gases should be monitored to detect hypoxemia and metabolic acidosis that may be caused by hypoxia, shock, or both. Blood pressure, urine output, and peripheral perfusion should be monitored to determine the need to treat septic shock with fluids and vasopressor agents.

The mainstay of treatment for sepsis and meningitis is antibiotic therapy. Antibiotics are used to suppress bacterial growth, allowing the infant's defense mechanisms time to respond. In addition, support measures, such as assisted ventilation and cardiovascular support, are equally important to the management of the infant. A combination of ampicillin and an aminoglycoside (usually gentamicin) for 10-14 days is effective treatment against most organisms responsible for early-onset sepsis. The combination of ampicillin and cefotaxime also is proposed as an alternative method of treatment. If meningitis is present, the treatment should be extended to 21 days or 14 days after a negative result from a CSF culture. Persistently positive results from CSF cultures are common with neonatal meningitis caused by gram-negative organisms, even with appropriate antibiotic treatment, and may be present for 2-3 days after antibiotic therapy. If gram-negative meningitis is present, some authorities continue to treat with an effective penicillin derivative combined with an aminoglycoside, whereas most change to a third-generation cephalosporin. High-dose penicillin (250,000-450,000 U/kg/24 hr) is appropriate for group B streptococcal meningitis. Inhaled nitric oxide, extracorporeal membrane oxygenation (in term infants), or both may improve the outcome of sepsis-related pulmonary hypertension. Intratracheal surfactant may reverse respiratory failure. Intrapartum penicillin empirical prophylaxis for group B streptococcal colonized mothers or mothers with risk factors (fever, preterm labor, previous infant with group B streptococci, and amnionitis) has reduced the rate of early-onset infection.

Late-onset sepsis (8-28 days) usually occurs in a healthy full-term infant who was discharged in good health from the normal newborn nursery. Clinical manifestations may include lethargy, poor feeding, hypotonia, apathy, seizures, bulging fontanelle, fever, and direct-reacting hyperbilirubinemia. In addition to bacteremia, hematogenous seeding may result in focal infections, such as meningitis (in 75% of cases), osteomyelitis (group B streptococci, *Staphylococcus aureus*), arthritis (gonococcus, *S. aureus*, *Candida albicans*, gram-negative bacteria), and urinary tract infection (gram-negative bacteria).

The evaluation of infants with late-onset sepsis is similar to that for infants with early-onset sepsis, with special attention given to a careful physical examination of the bones (infants with osteomyelitis may exhibit pseudoparalysis) and to the laboratory examination and culture of urine obtained by sterile suprapubic aspiration or urethral catheterization. Late-onset sepsis may be caused by the same pathogens as early-onset sepsis, but infants exhibiting sepsis late in the neonatal period also may have infections caused by the pathogens usually found in older infants (*H. influenzae*, *S. pneumoniae*, and *Neisseria meningitidis*). In addition, viral agents (HSV, cytomegalovirus, or enteroviruses) may manifest with a late-onset, sepsis-like picture.

Because of the increased rate of resistance of *H. influenzae* and pneumococcus to ampicillin, some centers begin treatment with ampicillin and a third-generation cephalosporin (and vancomycin if meningitis is present) when sepsis occurs in the last week of the first month of life. The treatment of late-onset neonatal sepsis and meningitis is the same as that for early-onset sepsis.

CHAPTER 66

Congenital Infections

An infection acquired transplacentally during gestation is a congenital infection. Numerous pathogens that produce mild or subclinical disease in older infants and children can cause severe disease in neonates who acquire such infections prenatally or perinatally. Sepsis, meningitis, pneumonia, and other infections caused by numerous perinatally acquired pathogens are the cause of significant neonatal morbidity and mortality. Congenital infections include a well-known group of fungal, bacterial, and viral pathogens: toxoplasmosis, rubella, cytomegalovirus (CMV), herpes simplex virus (HSV), varicella-zoster virus, congenital syphilis, parvovirus, human immunodeficiency virus (HIV), hepatitis B, Zika virus, *Neisseria gonorrhoeae*, *Chlamydia*, and *Mycobacterium tuberculosis*.

Many of the clinical manifestations of congenital infections are similar, including intrauterine growth restriction, nonimmune hydrops, anemia, thrombocytopenia, jaundice, hepatosplenomegaly, chorioretinitis, and congenital malformations. Some unique manifestations and epidemiological characteristics of these infections are listed in Table 66.1. Evaluation of patients thought to have a congenital infection should include attempts to isolate the organism by culture (for rubella, CMV, HSV, gonorrhea, and *M. tuberculosis*), to identify

TABLE 66.1 Perinatal Congenital Infections (TORCH)

AGENT	MATERNAL EPIDEMIOLOGY	NEONATAL FEATURES
Toxoplasma gondii	Heterophil-negative mononucleosis Exposure to cats or raw meat or immunosuppression High-risk exposure at 10-24-wk gestation	Hydrocephalus, abnormal spinal fluid, intracranial calcifications, chorioretinitis, jaundice, hepatosplenomegaly, fever Many infants asymptomatic at birth Treatment: pyrimethamine plus sulfadiazine
Rubella virus	Unimmunized seronegative mother; fever ± rash Detectable defects with infection: by 8 wk, 85% 9-12 wk, 50% 13-20 wk, 16% Virus may be present in infant's throat for 1 yr Prevention: vaccine	Intrauterine growth restriction, microcephaly, microphthalmia, cataracts, glaucoma, "salt and pepper" chorioretinitis, hepatosplenomegaly, jaundice, PDA, deafness, blueberry muffin rash, anemia, thrombocytopenia, leukopenia, metaphyseal lucencies, B-cell and T-cell deficiency Infant may be asymptomatic at birth
CMV	Sexually transmitted disease: primary genital infection may be asymptomatic Heterophil-negative mononucleosis; infant may have viruria for 1-6 yr	Sepsis, intrauterine growth restriction, chorioretinitis, microcephaly, periventricular calcifications, blueberry muffin rash, anemia, thrombocytopenia, neutropenia, hepatosplenomegaly, jaundice, deafness, pneumonia Many asymptomatic at birth Prevention: CMV-negative blood products Possible treatment: ganciclovir
Herpes simplex type 2 or 1 virus	Sexually transmitted disease: primary genital infection may be asymptomatic; intrauterine infection rare, acquisition at time of birth more common	Intrauterine infection: chorioretinitis, skin lesions, microcephaly Postnatal: encephalitis, localized or disseminated disease, skin vesicles, keratoconjunctivitis Treatment: acyclovir
Varicella-zoster virus	Intrauterine infection with chickenpox Infant develops severe neonatal varicella with maternal illness 5 days before or 2 days after delivery	Microphthalmia, cataracts, chorioretinitis, cutaneous and bony aplasia/hypoplasia/atrophy, cutaneous scars Zoster as in older child Prevention of neonatal condition with VZIG Treatment of ill neonate: acyclovir
Treponema pallidum (syphilis)	Sexually transmitted infection Maternal primary asymptomatic: painless "hidden" chancre Penicillin, not erythromycin, prevents fetal infection	Presentation at birth as nonimmune hydrops, prematurity, anemia, neutropenia, thrombocytopenia, pneumonia, hepatosplenomegaly Late neonatal as snuffles (rhinitis), rash, hepatosplenomegaly, condylomata lata, metaphysitis, cerebrospinal fluid pleocytosis, keratitis, periosteal new bone, lymphocytosis, hepatitis Late onset: teeth, eye, bone, skin, central nervous system, ear Treatment: penicillin
Parvovirus	Etiology of fifth disease; fever, rash, arthralgia in adults	Nonimmune hydrops, fetal anemia Treatment: in utero transfusion
HIV	AIDS; most mothers are asymptomatic and HIV positive; high-risk history; prostitute, drug abuse, married to bisexual, or hemophiliac	AIDS symptoms develop between 3 and 6 mo of age in 10-25%; failure to thrive, recurrent infection, hepatosplenomegaly, neurological abnormalities Management: trimethoprim/sulfamethoxazole, AZT, other antiretroviral agents Prevention: prenatal, intrapartum, postpartum AZT; avoid breast feeding
Hepatitis B virus	Vertical transmission common; may result in cirrhosis, hepatocellular carcinoma	Acute neonatal hepatitis; many become asymptomatic carriers Prevention: HBIG, vaccine
Neisseria gonorrhoeae	Sexually transmitted infection, infant acquires at birth Treatment: cefotaxime, ceftriaxone	Gonococcal ophthalmia, sepsis, meningitis Prevention: silver nitrate, erythromycin eye drops Treatment: ceftriaxone
Chlamydia trachomatis	Sexually transmitted infection, infant acquires at birth Treatment: oral erythromycin	Conjunctivitis, pneumonia Prevention: erythromycin eye drops Treatment: oral erythromycin
Mycobacterium tuberculosis	Positive PPD skin test, recent converter, positive chest radiograph, positive family member Treatment: INH and rifampin ± ethambutol	Congenital rare septic pneumonia; acquired primary pulmonary TB; asymptomatic, follow PPD Prevention: INH, BCG, separation Treatment: INH, rifampin, pyrazinamide
Trypanosoma cruzi (Chagas disease)	Central South American native, immigrant, travel Chronic disease in mother	Failure to thrive, heart failure, achalasia Treatment: nifurtimox
Zika virus	see text	see text

AZT, Zidovudine (azidothymidine); *BCG*, bacille Calmette-Guerin; *CMV*, cytomegalovirus; *HBIG*, hepatitis B immune globulin; *INH*, isoniazid; *PDA*, patent ductus arteriosus; *PPD*, purified protein derivative; *TB*, tuberculosis; *VZIG*, varicella-zoster immune globulin.

the antigen of the pathogen (for hepatitis B and *Chlamydia trachomatis*), to identify the pathogen's genome with polymerase chain reaction (PCR), and to identify specific fetal production of antibodies (immunoglobulin M [IgM] or increasing titer of IgG for *Toxoplasma*, syphilis, parvovirus, HIV, or *Borrelia*).

Treatment is not always available, specific, or effective. Nonetheless, some encouraging results have been reported for preventing the disease and for specifically treating the infant when the correct diagnosis is made (see Table 66.1).

TOXOPLASMOSIS

Decision-Making Algorithms
Available @ StudentConsult.com

Abnormal Head Size, Shape, and Fontanels
Visual Impairment and Leukocoria
Petechiae/Purpura

Vertical transmission of *Toxoplasma gondii* occurs by transplacental transfer of the organism from the mother to the fetus after an acute maternal infection. Fetal infection rarely can occur after reactivation of disease in an immunocompromised pregnant mother. Transmission from an acutely infected mother to her fetus occurs in about 30-40% of cases, but the rate varies directly with gestational age. Transmission rates and the timing of fetal infection correlate directly with placental blood flow; the risk of infection increases throughout gestation to 90% or greater near term, and the time interval between maternal and fetal infection decreases.

The severity of fetal disease varies inversely with the gestational age at which maternal infection occurs. Most infants have subclinical infection with no overt disease at birth; however, specific ophthalmologic and central nervous system (CNS) evaluations may reveal abnormalities. The classic findings of hydrocephalus, chorioretinitis, and intracerebral calcifications suggest the diagnosis of congenital toxoplasmosis. Affected infants tend to be small for gestational age, develop early-onset jaundice, have hepatosplenomegaly, and present with a generalized maculopapular rash. Seizures are common, and skull films may reveal diffuse cortical calcifications in contrast to the periventricular pattern observed with CMV. These infants are at increased risk for long-term neurological and neurodevelopmental complications.

Serological tests are the primary means of diagnosis. IgG-specific antibodies achieve a peak concentration 1-2 months after infection and remain positive indefinitely. For infants with seroconversion or a fourfold increase in IgG titers, specific IgM antibody determinations should be performed to confirm disease. Especially for congenital infections, measurement of IgA and IgE antibodies can be useful to confirm the disease. Thorough ophthalmologic, auditory, and neurological evaluations (head computed tomography and cerebrospinal fluid [CSF] examination) are indicated.

For symptomatic and asymptomatic congenital infections, initial therapy should include pyrimethamine (supplemented with folic acid) combined with sulfadiazine. Duration of therapy is often prolonged, even up to 1 year. Optimal dosages of medications and duration of therapy should be determined in consultation with appropriate specialists.

RUBELLA

Decision-Making Algorithms
Available @ StudentConsult.com

Abnormal Head Size, Shape, and Fontanelles
Visual Impairment and Leukocoria
Heart Murmurs
Hearing Loss

With the widespread use of vaccination, congenital rubella is rare in developed countries. Acquired in utero during early gestation, rubella can cause severe neonatal consequences. The occurrence of congenital defects approaches 85% if infection is acquired during the first 4 weeks of gestation; close to 40% spontaneously abort or are stillborn. If infection occurs during weeks 13-16, 35% of infants can have abnormalities. Infection after 4 months' gestation does not seem to cause disease.

The most common characteristic abnormalities associated with congenital rubella include ophthalmologic (cataracts, retinopathy, and glaucoma), cardiac (patent ductus arteriosus and peripheral pulmonary artery stenosis), auditory (sensorineural hearing loss), and neurological (behavioral disorders, meningoencephalitis, and developmental delay) conditions. In addition, infants can present with growth retardation, hepatosplenomegaly, early-onset jaundice, thrombocytopenia, radiolucent bone disease, and purpuric skin lesions ("blueberry muffin" appearance from dermal erythropoiesis).

Detection of rubella-specific IgM antibody usually indicates recent infection. Measurement of rubella-specific IgG over several months can be confirmatory. Rubella virus can be isolated from blood, urine, CSF, and throat swab specimens. Infants with congenital rubella are chronically and persistently infected and tend to shed live virus in urine, stools, and respiratory secretions for 1 year. Infants should be isolated while in the hospital and kept away from susceptible pregnant women when sent home.

CYTOMEGALOVIRUS

Decision-Making Algorithms
Available @ StudentConsult.com

Visual Impairment and Leukocoria
Hepatomegaly
Hearing Loss
Petechiae/Purpura

CMV is the most common congenital infection and the leading cause of sensorineural hearing loss, mental retardation, retinal disease, and cerebral palsy. Congenital CMV occurs in about 0.5-1.5% of births. When primary infection occurs in mothers during a pregnancy, the virus is transmitted to the fetus in approximately 35% of cases. Rates of CMV infection are three to seven times greater in infants born to adolescent mothers compared to others. The risk of transmission of CMV to the fetus is independent of gestational age at the time of maternal infection. The earlier in gestation that the primary maternal infection occurs, the more symptomatic the infant will be at birth. The most common sources of CMV for primary infections occurring in mothers during pregnancy are sexual contacts and contact with young children. It is well known that CMV can be transmitted to the fetus even when maternal infection occurred long before conception. This transmission can occur as the result of virus reactivation, chronic infection, or reinfection with a new strain.

More than 90% of infants who have congenital CMV infection exhibit no clinical evidence of disease at birth. Approximately 10% of infected infants are small for gestational age and have symptoms at birth. Findings include microcephaly, thrombocytopenia, hepatosplenomegaly, hepatitis, intracranial calcifications, chorioretinitis, and hearing abnormalities. Some infants can present with a blueberry muffin appearance as the result of dermal erythropoiesis. Skull films may reveal periventricular calcifications. An additional 10% of infected infants may not present until later in infancy or early childhood, when they are found to have sensorineural hearing loss and developmental delays. Mortality is 10-15% in symptomatic newborns. Perinatal CMV infection acquired during birth or from mother's milk is not associated with newborn illness or CNS sequelae.

Congenital CMV infection is diagnosed by detection of virus in the urine or saliva. Detection is often accomplished by traditional virus culture methods but can take several weeks to obtain a result. Rapid culture methods using centrifugation to enhance infectivity and monoclonal antibody to detect early antigens in infected tissue culture can give results in 24 hours. PCR also can be used to detect small amounts of CMV DNA in the urine. Detection of CMV within the first 3 weeks after birth is considered proof of congenital CMV infection.

Trial studies in severely symptomatic newborns of the antiviral agent ganciclovir have shown a lack of progression of hearing loss.

HERPES SIMPLEX VIRUS

HSV-2 accounts for 90% of primary genital herpes. About 70-85% of neonatal herpes simplex infections are caused by HSV-2. Most commonly, neonatal infections are acquired from the mother shortly before (ascending infection) or during passage through the birth canal at delivery. The incidence of neonatal HSV is estimated to range from 1 in 3,000 to 1 in 20,000 live births. Infants with HSV infections are more likely to be born prematurely (40% of affected infants are <36 weeks' gestation). The risk of infection at delivery in an infant born vaginally to a mother with primary genital herpes is about 33-50%. The risk to an infant born to a mother with a reactivated infection is less than 5%. More than 75% of infants who acquire HSV infection are born to mothers who have no previous history or clinical findings consistent with HSV infection.

Most infants are normal at birth, and symptoms of infection develop at 5-10 days of life. Symptoms of neonatal HSV infection include disseminated disease involving multiple organ systems, most notably the liver and lungs; localized infection to the CNS; or localized infection to the skin, eyes, and mouth. Symptoms may overlap, and in many cases of disseminated disease, skin lesions are a late finding. Disseminated infection should be considered in any infant with symptoms of sepsis, liver dysfunction, and negative bacteriological cultures. HSV infection also should be suspected in any neonate who presents with fever, irritability, abnormal CSF findings, and seizures. Initial symptoms can occur anytime between birth and 4 weeks of age, although disseminated disease usually occurs during the first week of life. HSV infections are often severe, and a delay in treatment can result in significant morbidity and mortality.

For the diagnosis of neonatal HSV infection, specimens for culture should be obtained from any skin vesicle, nasopharynx, eyes, urine, blood, CSF, stool, or rectum. Positive cultures obtained from these sites more than 48 hours after birth indicate intrapartum exposure. PCR is a sensitive method for detecting HSV DNA in blood, skin lesions, and CSF.

Parenteral acyclovir is the treatment of choice for neonatal HSV infections. Acyclovir should be administered to all infants suspected to have infection or diagnosed with HSV. The most benign outcome with regard to morbidity and mortality is observed in infants with disease limited to the skin, eyes, and mouth.

CONGENITAL SYPHILIS

Decision-Making Algorithms
Available @ StudentConsult.com

Rhinorrhea
Abnormal Head Size, Shape, and Fontanels
Red Eye
Hoarseness
Hepatomegaly
Hearing Loss
Lymphadenopathy

Congenital syphilis most commonly results from transplacental infection of the fetus, although the fetus can acquire infection by contact with a chancre at birth. In addition, hematogenous infection can occur throughout pregnancy. The longer the time elapsed between the mother's infection and pregnancy, the less likely she is to transmit the disease to the fetus.

Intrauterine infection can result in stillbirth, hydrops fetalis, or prematurity. Clinical symptoms vary but include hepatosplenomegaly, snuffles, lymphadenopathy, mucocutaneous lesions, osteochondritis, rash, hemolytic anemia, and thrombocytopenia. Untreated infants, regardless of whether they manifest symptoms at birth, may develop late symptoms, which usually appear after 2 years of age and involve the CNS, bones, joints, teeth, eyes, and skin. Some manifestations of disease may not become apparent until many years after birth, such as interstitial keratitis, eighth cranial nerve deafness, Hutchinson teeth, bowing of the shins, frontal bossing, mulberry molars, saddle nose, rhagades, and Clutton joints. The combination of interstitial keratitis, eighth cranial nerve deafness, and Hutchinson teeth is commonly referred to as the *Hutchinson triad* (see Table 66.1).

Many infants are asymptomatic at the time of diagnosis. If untreated, most infants develop symptoms within the first 5 weeks of life. The most striking lesions affect the mucocutaneous tissues and bones. Early signs of infection may be poor feeding and snuffles (syphilitic rhinitis). Snuffles are more severe and persistent than the common cold and are often bloody. A maculopapular desquamative rash develops over the palms and soles and around the mouth and anus. The rash may progress to become vesicular with bullae. Severely ill infants may be born with hydrops and have profound anemia. Severe consolidated pneumonia may be present at birth, and there may be laboratory findings consistent with a glomerulonephritis. CSF evaluation may reveal a pleocytosis and elevated protein. More than 90% of symptomatic infants exhibit radiographic abnormalities of the long bones consistent with osteochondritis and perichondritis.

No newborn should be discharged from the hospital without knowledge or determination of the mother's serological status for syphilis. All infants born to seropositive mothers require a careful examination and a quantitative nontreponemal syphilis test. Dark-field examination of direct fluorescent antibody staining of organisms obtained by scraping a skin or mucous membrane lesion is the quickest and most direct method of diagnosis. More commonly, serological testing is used. The nontreponemal reaginic antibody assays—the Venereal Disease Research Laboratory (VDRL) and the rapid plasma reagin—are helpful as indicators of disease. The test performed on the infant should be the same as that performed on the mother to enable comparison of results. An infant should be evaluated further if the maternal titer has increased fourfold, if the infant's titer is fourfold greater than the mother's titer, if the infant is symptomatic, or if the mother has inadequately treated syphilis. A mother infected later in pregnancy may deliver an infant who is incubating active disease. The mother and infant may have negative serological testing at birth. When clinical or serological tests suggest congenital syphilis, CSF should be examined microscopically, and a CSF VDRL test should be performed. An increased CSF white blood cell count and protein concentration suggests neurosyphilis; a positive CSF VDRL is diagnostic.

Parenteral penicillin is the preferred drug of choice for treatment of syphilis. Penicillin G for 10-14 days is the only documented effective therapy for infants who have congenital syphilis and neurosyphilis. Infants should have repeat nontreponemal antibody titers repeated at 3, 6, and 12 months to document falling titers. Infants with neurosyphilis must be followed carefully with serological testing and CSF determinations every 6 months for at least 3 years or until CSF findings are normal.

HUMAN IMMUNODEFICIENCY VIRUS

See Chapter 125.

HEPATITIS B

See Chapter 113.

NEISSERIA GONORRHOEAE

Decision-Making Algorithm
Available @ StudentConsult.com

Hepatomegaly

N. gonorrhoeae infection in a newborn usually involves the eyes (ophthalmia neonatorum). Other sites of infection include scalp abscesses (often associated with fetal monitoring with scalp electrodes), vaginitis, and disseminated disease with bacteremia, arthritis, or meningitis. Transmission to the infant usually occurs during passage through the birth canal when mucous membranes come in contact with infected secretions.

Infection usually is present within the first 5 days of life and is characterized initially by a clear, watery discharge, which rapidly becomes purulent. There is marked conjunctival hyperemia and chemosis. Infection tends to be bilateral; however, one eye may be clinically worse than the other. Untreated infections can spread to the cornea (keratitis) and anterior chamber of the eye. This extension can result in corneal perforation and blindness.

Recommended treatment for isolated infection, such as ophthalmia neonatorum, is one intramuscular dose of ceftriaxone. Infants with gonococcal ophthalmia should receive eye irrigations with saline solution at frequent intervals before discharge. Topical antibiotic therapy alone is inadequate and is unnecessary when recommended systemic antimicrobial therapy is given. Infants with gonococcal ophthalmia should be hospitalized and evaluated for disseminated disease (sepsis, arthritis, meningitis). Disseminated disease should be treated with antimicrobial therapy (ceftriaxone or cefotaxime) for 7 days. Cefotaxime can be used in infants with hyperbilirubinemia. If documented, infants with meningitis should be treated for 10-14 days.

Tests for concomitant infection with *C. trachomatis*, congenital syphilis, and HIV should be performed. Results of the maternal test for hepatitis B surface antigen should be confirmed. Topical prophylaxis with silver nitrate, erythromycin, or tetracycline is recommended for all newborns for the prevention of gonococcal ophthalmia.

CHLAMYDIA

Decision-Making Algorithm
Available @ StudentConsult.com

Hepatomegaly

C. trachomatis is the most common reportable sexually transmitted infection, with a high rate of infection among sexually active adolescents and young adults. Prevalence of the organism in pregnant women ranges from 6% to 12% and can be 40% in adolescents. *Chlamydia* can be transmitted from the genital tract of an infected mother to her newborn. Acquisition occurs in about 50% of infants born vaginally to infected mothers. Transmission also has been reported in some infants delivered by cesarean section with intact membranes. In infected infants, the risk of conjunctivitis is 25-50%, and the risk of pneumonia is 5-20%. The nasopharynx is the most commonly infected anatomical site.

Neonatal chlamydial conjunctivitis is characterized by ocular congestion, edema, and discharge developing 5-14 days to several weeks after birth and lasting for 1-2 weeks. Clinical manifestations vary from mild conjunctivitis to intense inflammation and swelling. Both eyes are almost always involved; however, one eye may appear to be more swollen and infected than the other. The cornea is rarely involved, and preauricular adenopathy is rare.

Pneumonia in a young infant can occur between 2 and 19 weeks of age and is characterized by an afebrile illness with a repetitive staccato cough, tachypnea, and rales. Wheezing is uncommon. Hyperinflation with diffuse infiltrates can be seen on chest radiograph. Nasal stuffiness and otitis media can occur.

Diagnosis can be made by scraping the conjunctiva and culturing the material. Giemsa staining of the conjunctival scrapings revealing the presence of blue-stained intracytoplasmic inclusions within the epithelial cells is diagnostic. PCR is also available. Infants with conjunctivitis and pneumonia are treated with oral erythromycin for 14 days. Topical treatment of conjunctivitis is ineffective and unnecessary. The recommended topical prophylaxis with silver nitrate, erythromycin, or tetracycline for all newborns for the prevention of gonococcal ophthalmia does not prevent neonatal chlamydial conjunctivitis.

MYCOBACTERIUM TUBERCULOSIS

See Chapter 124.

ZIKA VIRUS

Zika virus is an arthropod-borne flavivirus carried and transmitted by mosquitoes, and is associated with severe congenital anomalies. Zika virus is a neurotropic virus that particularly targets progenitor cells. Zika virus causes a maternal infection leading to a placental infection and injury to the fetus. The infection is transmitted to the fetal brain where it kills neuronal progenitor cells disrupting neuronal proliferation, migration, and differentiation. In utero infections can be transmitted to the fetus at any time during the pregnancy and result in severe brain abnormalities (i.e., microcephaly, cerebellar hypoplasia, ventriculomegaly, lissencephaly) and craniofacial malformations. Additionally, the virus can result in pulmonary hypoplasia and multiple congenital contractures.

Suggested Readings

Engle WE. Infants born late preterm: definition, physiologic and metabolic immaturity, and outcomes. *NeoReviews*. 2009;10:e280.
Frankovich J, Sandborg C, Barnes P, et al. Neonatal lupus and related autoimmune disorders of infants. *NeoReviews*. 2008;9:e207–e217.
HAPO Study Cooperative Research Group. Hyperglycemia and adverse pregnancy outcomes. *N Engl J Med*. 2008;358(19):1991–2002.
Jesse N, Neu J. Necrotizing enterocolitis: relationship to innate immunity, clinical features and strategies for prevention. *NeoReviews*. 2006;7:e143.
Kates EH, Kates JS. Anemia and polycythemia in the newborn. *Pediatr Rev*. 2007;28:33–34.
Kattwinkel J, Perlman J. The neonatal resuscitation program: the evidence evaluation process and anticipating edition 6. *NeoReviews*. 2010;11:e673.
Shankaran S. Neonatal encephalopathy: treatment with hypothermia. *NeoReviews*. 2010;11:e85.
Silva RA, Moshfeghi DM. Interventions in retinopathy of prematurity. *NeoReviews*. 2012;13:e476.
Steinhorn RH, Farrow KN. Pulmonary hypertension in the neonate. *NeoReviews*. 2007;8:e14–e21.
Wong RJ, Stevenson DK, Ahlfors CE, et al. Neonatal jaundice: bilirubin physiology and clinical chemistry. *NeoReviews*. 2007;8:e58–e67.

PEARLS FOR PRACTITIONERS

CHAPTER 58

Assessment of the Mother, Fetus, and Newborn

- High-risk pregnancies include those with intrauterine growth restriction (IUGR), maternal hypertension or diabetes, autoimmune diseases (systemic lupus erythematosus [SLE]), and those with prior intrauterine fetal demise or neonatal deaths.
- Additional high-risk pregnancies include those with oligo- or polyhydramnios, multiple gestation, or macrosomic fetuses.
- Polyhydramnios is associated with fetal central nervous system (CNS) anomalies as well as high gastrointestinal obstruction.
- Low birthweight is defined by birthweight <2,500 g.
- Vitamin K must be given to all newborns to prevent hemorrhagic disease of the newborn.
- The Apgar examination performed at 1 and 5 minutes assesses fetal to neonatal transition and identifies infants in need of resuscitation.
- Hair tufts over the lumbosacral area suggest a neural tube anomaly.
- Leukokoria may be due to cataracts, ocular tumor, chorioretinitis, retinopathy of prematurity, or persistent hyperplastic primary vitreous.
- Shock in the delivery room is often due to blood loss such as fetal to maternal hemorrhage or internal bleeding (liver, spleen).
- Erb-Duchenne palsy involves the 5th and 6th cervical nerves.
- Early neonatal hypocalcemia may be due to maternal hyperparathyroidism, or neonatal DiGeorge syndrome; it is also seen in infants of diabetic mothers, preterm infants, or following birth asphyxia.
- About 10% of neonates will require some form of intervention and/or resuscitation in the delivery room.
- Since most medical centers now use Erythromycin eye ointment following delivery, any eye redness or purulent discharge needs immediate attention and potential treatment.
- The biophysical profile, which includes fetal movement, fetal breathing, fetal tone, amniotic fluid volume, and fetal heart rate reactivity, is often used to assess fetal well-being. A score of <6 out of 10 indicates possible fetal compromise and may necessitate delivery of the infant.
- Pulse oximetry screening (preductal and postductal) should be performed on all infants before discharge from the hospital. A difference of >3% is suggestive of cyanotic heart disease.
- Hearing loss is a most common congenital condition in the United States; each infant should be screened for hearing loss prior to being discharged from the hospital.
- Failure of a term infant to pass urine in the first 24 hours or meconium in the first 48 hours warrant further evaluation.
- Rule of 2s and congenital heart failure: Heart failure at 2 days is most likely caused by transposition of the great arteries (as the patent ductus arteriosus [PDA] closes), at 2 weeks, coarctation of the aorta, and at 2 months, ventricular septal defect.

- Transposition of the great arteries is the most common cyanotic heart disease to present in the neonatal period, whereas tetralogy of Fallot will most commonly present outside the neonatal period.
- Tetralogy of Fallot is the most common congenital cyanotic heart disease to present in the pediatric population.

CHAPTER 59
Maternal Diseases Affecting the Newborn

- Maternal diabetes mellitus represents a high risk for teratogenic changes in the fetus (i.e., congenital heart disease, caudal regression).
- For the fetus, insulin is the primary growth hormone; in situations where fetal insulin levels are increased, the fetus can be overgrown (macrosomic, large for gestational age).
- Infants of diabetic mothers are at risk for birth trauma, hypoglycemia, hypocalcemia, hyperbilirubinemia (increased red cell mass), cardiac disease, and caudal regression.
- All pregnant mothers should be screened for HIV. In addition, serologies for the following should be known at the time of birth: complete blood type; immunity for rubella, syphilis, and chlamydia status; gonorrhea and group B streptococcus cultures (usually obtained at ~35 weeks' gestation); and hepatitis B titers.
- Autoimmune diseases of the mother may affect the fetus by placental transfer of IgG autoantibodies such as seen in maternal immune thrombocytopenia, SLE, hyperthyroidism, or myasthenia gravis.

CHAPTER 60
Diseases of the Fetus

- Causes of IUGR include poor maternal nutrition, maternal hypertension, fetal anomalies or infection, and twin-twin transfusion syndrome.
- The quadruple test and testing fetal DNA in the maternal circulation screen for chromosomal disorders.
- Hepatosplenomegaly, jaundice, dermatitis, chorioretinitis, and micro- or hydrocephaly in an infant with IUGR suggests an intrauterine infection.
- Organ anomalies such as congenital heart disease, oral clefts, and limb anomalies suggest a congenital malformation syndrome.
- Hydrops fetalis is often due to fetal anemia secondary to immune hemolysis or decreased red cell production.
- Nonimmune hydrops has many etiologies including infection, malignancy, autoinflammatory diseases, and complex congenital anomalies.

CHAPTER 61
Respiratory Diseases of the Newborn

- Respiratory distress may manifest by cyanosis, sternal and intercostal retractions, nasal flaring, and expiratory grunting.
- Common causes of respiratory distress include infection, respiratory distress syndrome (RDS; hyaline membrane disease), and congenital anomalies of the airway, lung, or diaphragm.
- Maternal betamethasone therapy reduces the risk of RDS in at-risk premature infants.
- A patent ductus arteriosus may present with a widened pulse pressure, worsening hypoxia and hypercarbia, and signs of heart failure with a new cardiac murmur.
- Bronchopulmonary dysplasia may develop in infants with severe ventilator treated RDS and manifests as persistent ventilator and oxygen requirements and chronic changes on chest x-ray.
- Primary pulmonary hypertension of the newborn (PPHN) often accompanies birth asphyxia, meconium aspiration syndrome, pulmonary hypoplasia, and a congenital diaphragmatic hernia.
- PPHN is managed by oxygen and ventilation therapy; if these are unsuccessful, patients may be treated with inhaled nitric oxide and then extracorporeal membrane oxygenation (ECMO).

CHAPTER 62
Anemia and Hyperbilirubinemia

- Neonatal anemia is often due to immune mediated hemolysis, red cell membrane defects, or red cell enzyme deficiencies. Rarely is it due to decrease production as seen in Blackfan-Diamond syndrome.
- Prevention of hemolytic disease of the newborn due to Rh factor incompatibility is possible by administering RhoGAM to the Rh-negative mother during gestation and within 3 days after the delivery of the Rh-positive infant.
- Fetal to maternal hemorrhage may produce fetal anemia and may be detected by the Kleihauer-Betke test.
- Physiological jaundice is an indirect hyperbilirubinemia peaking on day 3 of life in term babies; the peak may be later in premature infants.
- Breast milk jaundice is an indirect hyperbilirubinemia that occurs 1-2 weeks after birth; its cause is unknown.
- Visible jaundice in the first day of life and any direct hyperbilirubinemia are due to potentially serious pathological processes and require immediate evaluation.

CHAPTER 63
Necrotizing Enterocolitis

- Necrotizing enterocolitis (NEC) manifests with a sepsis-like presentation and with abdominal distention and tenderness.
- Abdominal x-rays in NEC demonstrate pneumatosis intestinalis, portal-hepatic gas, pneumoperitoneum, or intestinal distention.
- Significant bilious emesis is considered a neonatal emergency and deserves further evaluation with an upper gastrointestinal tract series to rule out malrotation and midgut volvulus.

CHAPTER 64

Hypoxic-Ischemic Encephalopathy, Intracranial Hemorrhage, and Seizures

- Seizures in a neonate within the first 24 hours of birth are most likely secondary to birth asphyxia or hypoxia during labor and delivery.
- Therapeutic hypothermia has been shown to reduce the risk of neurodevelopmental disability following moderate to severe in utero hypoxia or ischemia; the outcome is best if hypothermia can be started before 6 hours of age.

CHAPTER 65

Sepsis and Meningitis

- Maternal chorioamnionitis puts the fetus at the greatest risk for a poor pregnancy and delivery outcome.
- Fever in the neonatal period should be considered as caused by significant bacterial infections and herpes virus infection.
- The most common organisms causing early onset neonatal sepsis include group B streptococcus and *Escherichia coli*; a synergistic combination of ampicillin and an aminoglycoside (usually gentamicin) is appropriate initial therapy for early-onset sepsis.
- Antimicrobial stewardship is a coordinated program that promotes the appropriate use of antimicrobials (including antibiotics), improves patient outcomes, reduces microbial resistance, and decreases the spread of infections caused by multi-resistant organisms. This program is of utmost importance in the NICU where the results of antibiotic resistance can be followed and treatment protocols can be modified as needed based on resistance patterns.

CHAPTER 66

Congenital Infections

- "Blueberry muffin" appearance is most commonly seen in neonates with congenital rubella or cytomegalovirus infection. A biopsy of a blueberry muffin lesion will reveal dermal hematopoiesis. The "skin" is the first organ system to produce red cells.

ADOLESCENT MEDICINE

Kim Blake | Lisa M. Allen

CHAPTER 67

Overview and Assessment of Adolescents

The leading causes of mortality (Table 67.1) and morbidity (Table 67.2) in adolescents in the United States are behaviorally mediated. Motor vehicle injuries and other injuries account for more than 75% of all deaths. Unhealthy dietary behaviors and inadequate physical activity result in adolescent obesity, with associated health complications (e.g., diabetes, hypertension).

It is the physician's responsibility to use every opportunity to inquire about risk-taking behaviors (Fig. 67.1), regardless of the presenting issue. Physical symptoms in adolescents are often related to psychosocial problems.

INTERVIEWING ADOLESCENTS

The adolescent interview shifts from information gathering from the parent to the adolescent. Interviewing an adolescent alone and discussing confidentiality are the cornerstones of obtaining information regarding risk-taking behaviors, anticipatory guidance, and protective factors (see Chapters 7 and 9).

The interview should take into account the developmental age of the adolescent (Table 67.3). Conversations about sports, friends, movies, and activities outside of school can be useful for all ages and help build rapport (Fig. 67.2).

Confidentiality is a key element in interviewing an adolescent (Table 67.4). A vital, open discussion about risk-taking behavior is more likely to happen when the adolescent is alone (Table 67.5). Some issues cannot be kept confidential, such as suicidal intent and disclosure of sexual or physical abuse. If there is an ambiguous situation, it is wise to obtain legal, ethical, or social work consultation. In caring for a young adolescent, the health care provider should encourage open discussions with a parent, guardian, or other adult.

The law confers certain rights on adolescents, depending on their health condition and personal characteristics; this allows them to receive health services without parental permission (Table 67.6). Usually adolescents can seek health care without parental consent for reproductive, mental, and emergency health services. Emancipated adolescents and *mature minors* may be treated without parental consent; this status should be documented in the record. The key characteristics of mature minors are their competence and capacity to understand, not their chronological age. There must be a reasonable judgment that the health intervention is in the best interests of the minor.

TABLE 67.1 Leading Causes of Death in Adolescents

RANK	CAUSE	RATE (PER 100,000)
1	Unintentional injuries	26.9
2	Suicide	11.5
3	Assault (homicide)	9.4
4	Malignant neoplasms (cancer)	3.6
5	Diseases of the heart	2.2

From the Centers for Disease Control and Prevention, National Center for Health Statistics: National Vital Statistics *2014.*

TABLE 67.2 Prevalence of Common Chronic Illnesses in Children and Adolescents

ILLNESS	PREVALENCE
PULMONARY	
• Asthma	8-12%
• Cystic fibrosis	1:2,500 white, 1:17,000 black
NEUROMUSCULAR	
• Cerebral palsy	2-3:1,000
• Mental retardation	1-2%
• Seizure disorder	3.5:1,000
• Any seizure	3-5%
• Auditory/visual defects	2-3%
• Traumatic paralysis	2:1,000
• Scoliosis	3% males, 5% females
• Migraine	6-27% (↑ with increasing age)
ENDOCRINE/NUTRITION	
• Diabetes mellitus	1.8:1,000
• Obesity	25-30%
• Anorexia nervosa	0.5-1%
• Bulimia	1% (early adolescence), 5-10% (19-20 years)
• Dysmenorrhea	20%
• Acne	65%

Structured Communication Adolescent Guide (SCAG)

Instructions for scoring this form

After your check-up, please score your doctor (or medical student) using this form.

Examples:

0 = Did Not	**1 = Did**	**2 = Did Well**
Dr. didn't ask at all.	Dr. asked as if reading a list. Dr. asked as if embarrassed. I felt judged. I felt a bit uncomfortable.	Dr. established a relationship. Dr. comfortable with questions. Dr. did not judge. I felt comfortable.

General Rating: Give a general impression of each section.
A = Excellent, B = Good, C = Average, D = Poor, F = Fail

	Did Not 0	Did 1	Did Well 2	Give examples of things that stood out in your interview, one positive and one negative.
A. GETTING STARTED				*Example: I liked that you talked to me and not just my mom.*
1. Greeted me.	0	1	2	
2. Introduced self.	0	1	2	
3. Discussed confidentiality.	0	1	2	
GENERAL RATING A B C D F				

	Did Not 0	Did 1	Did Well 2	Give examples of things that stood out in your interview, one positive and one negative.
B. GATHERING INFORMATION				*Example: I felt bad when you asked about smoking with my mom in the room.*
4. Good body language.	0	1	2	
5. Encouraged me to speak by asking questions other than ones with a yes/no answer.	0	1	2	
6. Encouraged parent to speak *(leave out if no parent present).*	0	1	2	
7. Listened and did not judge me.	0	1	2	
8. Established relationship with me by appropriate choice of words.	0	1	2	
GENERAL RATING A B C D F				

FIGURE 67.1 The Structured Communication Adolescent Guide (SCAG). The SCAG is an interviewing tool developed for learners to use with real or standardized adolescent patients. It incorporates the four major interview components: confidentiality, separation of the adolescent from the adult, psychosocial data gathering (using the HEADDSS mnemonic), and a nonjudgmental approach. The SCAG is at a grade 5 reading level and has demonstrated reliability and validity. A printable version is available through MedEdPORTAL. (From Blake K, Mann K, Kutcher M. The structured communication adolescent guide [SCAG]. *MedEdPORTAL Publ.* 2008;4:798. http://doi.org/10.15766/mep_2374-8265.798.)

	Did Not 0	Did 1	Did Well 2	Give examples of things that stood out in your interview, one positive and one negative.
C. TEEN ALONE				*Example: I was glad you talked about confidentially. I need lots of reassurance that you won't tell my mom.*
9. Separated me and parent. *(Leave out if no parent present.)*	0	1	2	
10. Discussed confidentiality.	0	1	2	
11. Gave me a chance to talk about things other than what I came in to discuss.	0	1	2	
12. Reflected on my feelings or concerns (example: You seem...).	0	1	2	
LIFESTYLES: Physician asks or talks about the following:				
13. **Home:** Family	0	1	2	
14. **Education:** School	0	1	2	
15. **Activities** Friends/social media	0	1	2	
16.	0	1	2	
17. **Alcohol:** Beer and hard liquor	0	1	2	
18. **Drugs:** Cigarettes	0	1	2	
19. Marijuana	0	1	2	
20. Street drugs	0	1	2	
21. **Diet:** Weight/diet/eating habits	0	1	2	
22. **Sex:** Boyfriend/girlfriend	0	1	2	
23. Sexual activity	0	1	2	
24. Safe sex/contraception	0	1	2	
25. **Self:** Body image, self-esteem	0	1	2	*Example: You weren't embarrassed to talk about sex. OR You seemed embarrassed to talk about sex.*
26. Moods/depression/suicide	0	1	2	
GENERAL RATING A	B	C	D	F

	Did Not 0	Did 1	Did Well 2	Comments: Please give examples of things that stood out in your interview.
D. WRAP UP				*Example: I wasn't sure what the next step would be.*
27. Summary, recapped issues	0	1	2	
28. Kept the confidentiality	0	1	2	
29. Asked if there were any questions	0	1	2	
30. Talked about what to do next (plan and follow-up)	0	1	2	
GENERAL RATING A	B	C	D	F

FIGURE 67.1, cont'd

TABLE 67.3 Adolescent Psychological Development

STAGE	AGE	THINKING	CHARACTERISTICS
Early teens	10-14	Concrete ↓	Appearance–"Am I normal?"
			Invincible
			Peer group
			No tomorrow
Middle teens	15-17		Risk-taking increased
			Limit testing
			"Who am I?"
			Experiments with ideas
Late teens	18-21	Formal operational	Future
			Planning
			Partner
			Separation

TABLE 67.4 Guidelines for Confidentiality

Prepare the preadolescent and parent for confidentiality and being interviewed alone.
Discuss confidentiality at the start of the interview.
Conversations with parents/guardians/adolescent are confidential (with exceptions*).
Reaffirm confidentiality when you are alone with your adolescent patient.

**Exceptions to confidentiality include major or impending harm to any person (i.e., abuse, suicide, homicide).*

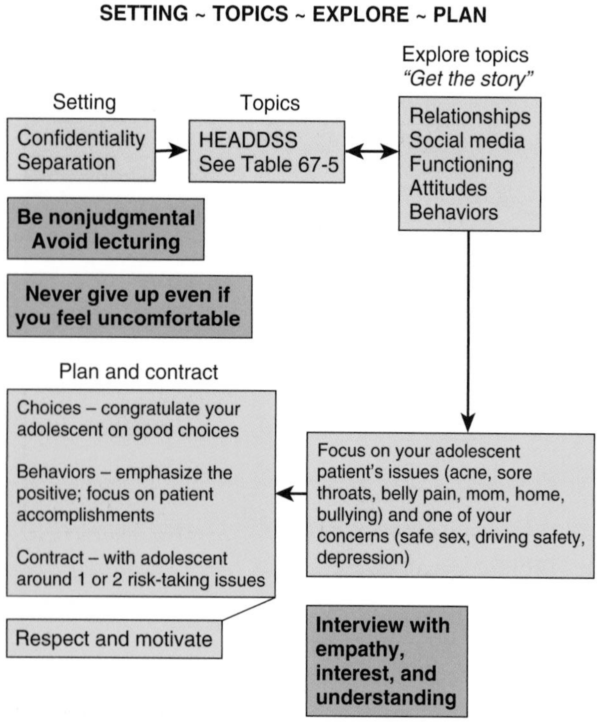

FIGURE 67.2 STEP guide for adolescent interviewing.

TABLE 67.5 Interviewing the Adolescent Alone: Discussion of HEADDSS Topics*

HOME/friends	Family, relationships, and activities. "What do you do for fun?" "What social media do you use?" "How much screen time in a day?"
EDUCATION	"What do you like best at school?" "How's school going?" "Any bullying?"
ALCOHOL	"Are any of your friends drinking?" "Are you drinking?"
DRUGS	Cigarettes, marijuana, street drugs. "Have you ever smoked or tried e-cigarettes?" "Many adolescents experiment with different drugs and substances. . . . Have you tried anything?"
DIET*	Weight, diet/eating habits. "Many adolescents worry about their weight and try dieting. Have you ever done this?"
SEX	Sexual activity, contraception. "Are you going out with anybody?" "Have you dated in the past?"
SUICIDE/ DEPRESSION	Mood swings, depression, suicide attempts or thoughts, self-image. "Feeling down or depressed is common for everyone. Have you ever felt so bad that you wanted to harm yourself?"

**The acronym HEADDSS can represent other terms, that is, A, Activities; D, Depression. Also see Fig. 67.1.*

TABLE 67.6 Legal Rights of Minors

Age of majority (≥18 years of age in most states)
Exceptions in which health care services can be provided to a minor*
Emergency care (e.g., life-threatening condition or condition in which a delay in treatment would increase significantly the likelihood of morbidity)
Diagnosis and treatment of sexuality-related health care
Diagnosis and treatment of drug-related health care
Emancipated minors (physically and financially independent of family; Armed Forces, married, childbirth)
Mature minors (able to comprehend the risks and benefits of evaluation and treatment)
All exceptions ***should be documented clearly in the patient's health record.***

**Determined by individual state laws.*

During the physical examination, the adolescent must be offered a choice between having a parent or a chaperone present.

PHYSICAL GROWTH AND DEVELOPMENT OF ADOLESCENTS

Girls

Breast budding under the areola (**thelarche**) and fine straight pubic hair over the mons pubis (**adrenarche** or **pubarche**) are early pubertal changes occurring at around 11 years of age (range, 8-13 years; see Chapter 174). These changes mark Tanner stage II (the sexual maturity rating) of pubertal development (Figs. 67.3 and 67.4). Completion of the Tanner stages should take 4-5 years. The peak growth spurt usually occurs

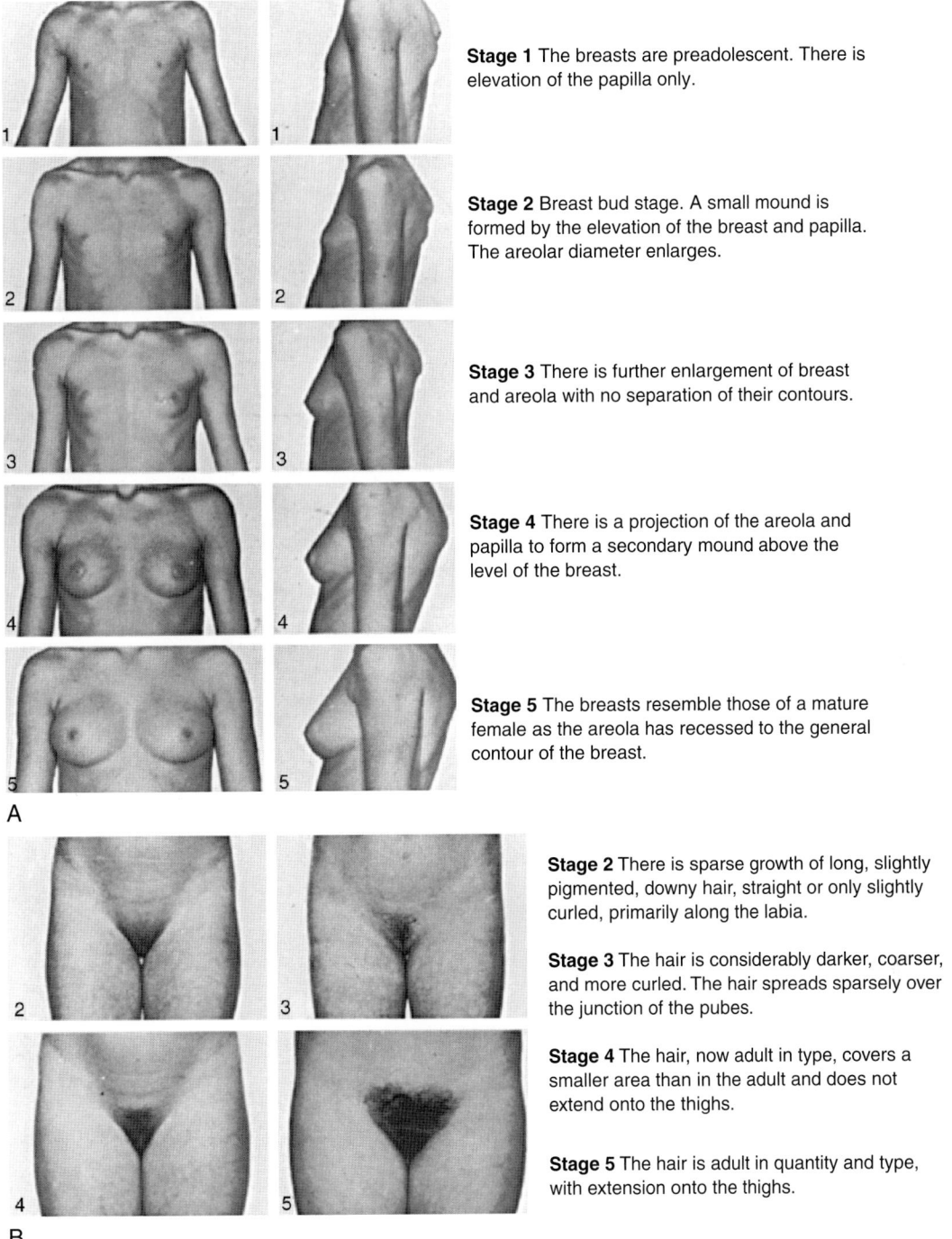

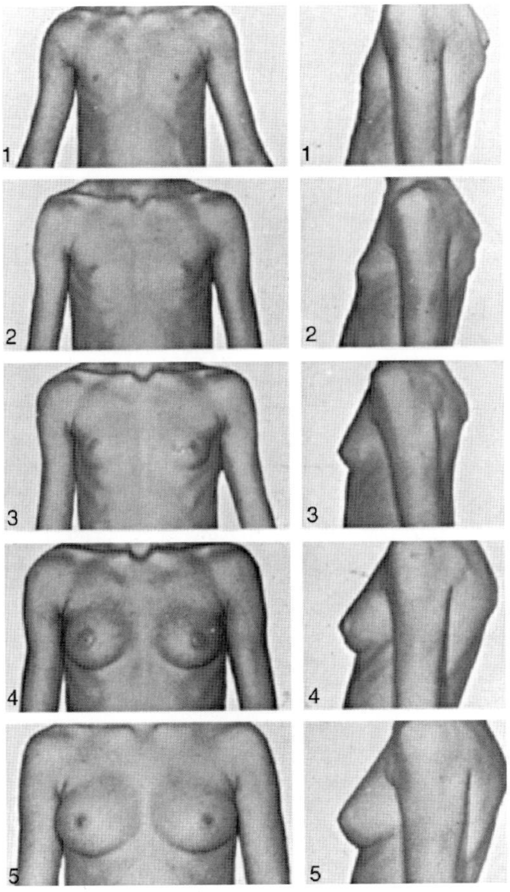

Stage 1 The breasts are preadolescent. There is elevation of the papilla only.

Stage 2 Breast bud stage. A small mound is formed by the elevation of the breast and papilla. The areolar diameter enlarges.

Stage 3 There is further enlargement of breast and areola with no separation of their contours.

Stage 4 There is a projection of the areola and papilla to form a secondary mound above the level of the breast.

Stage 5 The breasts resemble those of a mature female as the areola has recessed to the general contour of the breast.

A

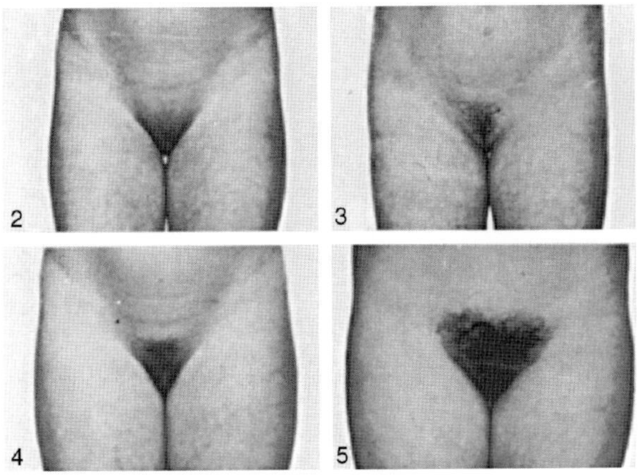

Stage 2 There is sparse growth of long, slightly pigmented, downy hair, straight or only slightly curled, primarily along the labia.

Stage 3 The hair is considerably darker, coarser, and more curled. The hair spreads sparsely over the junction of the pubes.

Stage 4 The hair, now adult in type, covers a smaller area than in the adult and does not extend onto the thighs.

Stage 5 The hair is adult in quantity and type, with extension onto the thighs.

B

FIGURE 67.3 Typical progression of female pubertal development, stages 1-5. **A,** Pubertal development in the size of female breasts. **B,** Pubertal development of female pubic hair. Note that at stage I (not shown) there is no pubic hair. (Courtesy J.M. Tanner, MD, Institute of Child Health, Department of Growth and Development, University of London, London, England.)

approximately 1 year after thelarche, at Tanner stages III to IV of breast development and before the onset of menstruation **(menarche).** Menarche is a relatively late pubertal event. Females grow only 2-5 cm in height after menarche (see Chapter 174).

The mean ages of thelarche and adrenarche are approximately 9 and 10 years for African American and white girls, respectively. The mean ages of menarche are 12.2 and 12.9 years for African American and white girls, respectively. The interval from the initiation of thelarche to the onset of menses (menarche) is 2.3 years plus or minus 1 year. Pubertal changes before 6 years of age in African American girls and 7 years of age in white girls are considered precocious.

Boys

Testicular enlargement (≥2.5 cm) corresponds to Tanner stages I to II for boys (Figs. 67.5 and 67.6). Testicular enlargement is followed by pubic hair development at the base of the penis

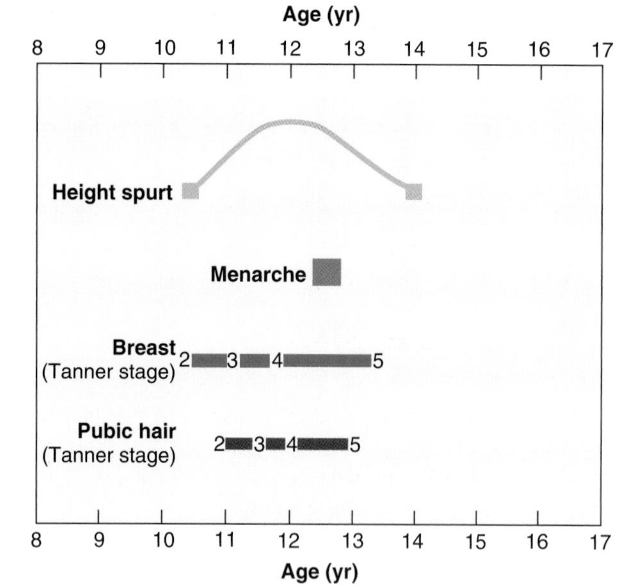

FIGURE 67.4 Sequence of pubertal events in the average American female. More recent studies suggest that breast development may begin at 9 years of age for African American girls and 10 years of age for white girls. (From Brookman RR, Rauh JL, Morrison JA, et al. The Princeton maturation study, 1976, unpublished data for adolescents in Cincinnati, Ohio. Reprinted from *Assessment of Pubertal Development,* Columbus, Ohio, 1986, Ross Laboratories.)

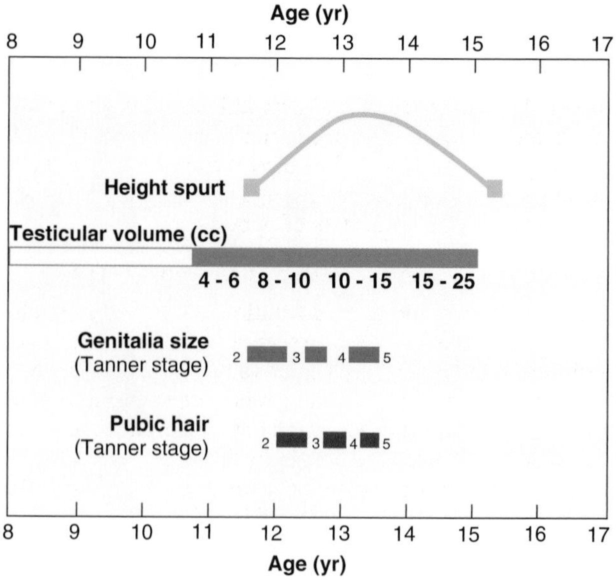

FIGURE 67.6 Sequence of pubertal events in the average American male. Testicular volume less than 4 mL using an orchidometer (Prader Beads) represents a prepubertal stage. (From Brookman RR, Rauh JL, Morrison JA, et al. The Princeton maturation study, 1976, unpublished data for adolescents in Cincinnati, Ohio. Reprinted from *Assessment of Pubertal Development,* Columbus, Ohio, 1986, Ross Laboratories.)

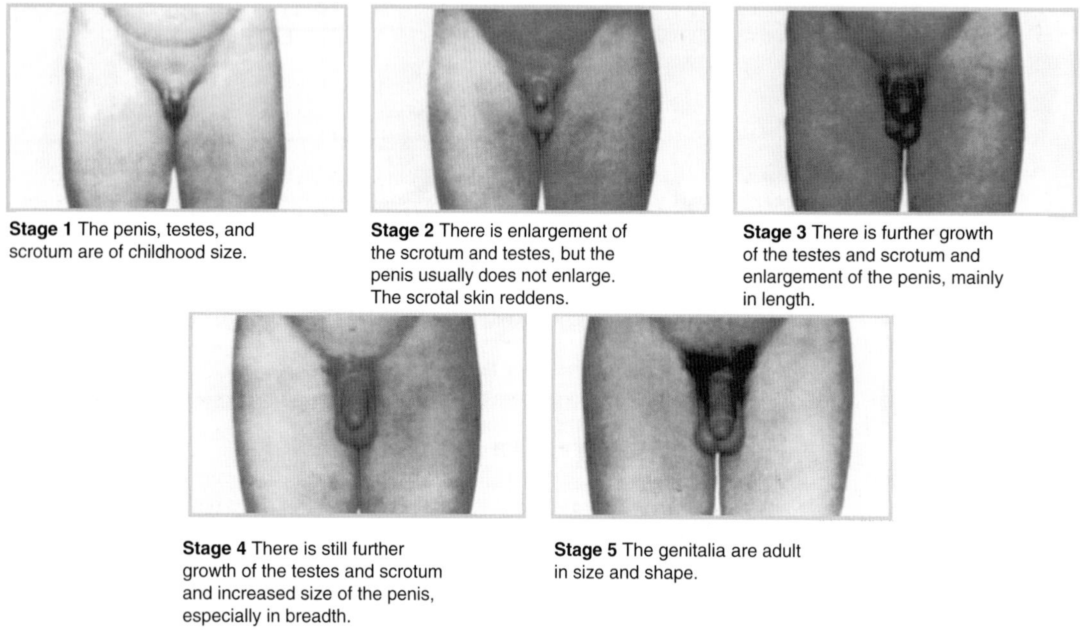

Stage 1 The penis, testes, and scrotum are of childhood size.
Stage 2 There is enlargement of the scrotum and testes, but the penis usually does not enlarge. The scrotal skin reddens.
Stage 3 There is further growth of the testes and scrotum and enlargement of the penis, mainly in length.
Stage 4 There is still further growth of the testes and scrotum and increased size of the penis, especially in breadth.
Stage 5 The genitalia are adult in size and shape.

A

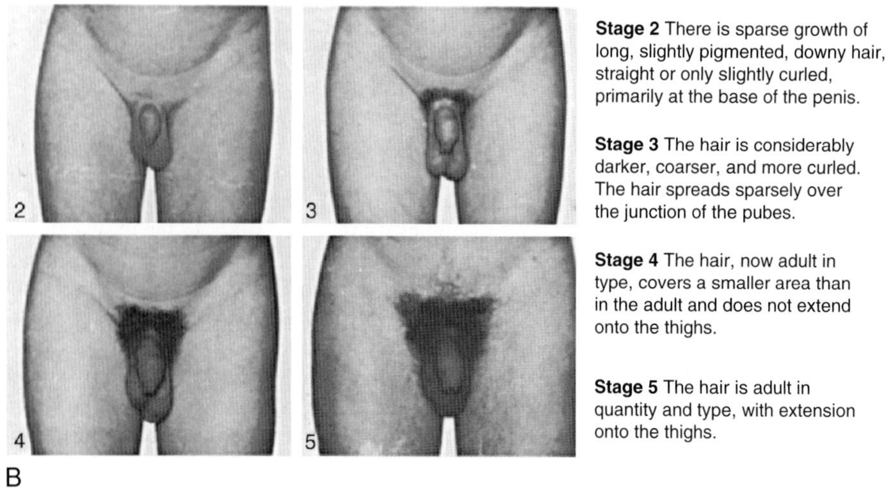

B

FIGURE 67.5 Typical progression of male pubertal development. **A,** Pubertal development in the size of male genitalia. **B,** Pubertal development of male pubic hair. Note that at stage I there is no pubic hair. (Courtesy J.M. Tanner, MD, Institute of Child Health, Department of Growth and Development, University of London, London, England.)

(adrenarche) and then axillary hair within the year. The growth spurt is a relatively late event; it can occur from 10½ to 16 years of age. Deepening of the voice, the appearance of facial hair, and acne indicate the early stages of puberty. See Chapter 174 for discussion of disorders of puberty.

Changes Associated With Physical Maturation

Tanner stages mark biologic maturation, which can be related to specific changes in laboratory values and certain physical conditions. The higher hematocrit values in adolescent boys than in adolescent girls are the result of greater androgenic stimulation of the bone marrow and not loss through menstruation. Alkaline phosphatase levels in boys and girls increase during puberty because of rapid bone turnover, especially during the growth spurt. Worsening of mild scoliosis is common in adolescents during the growth spurt.

PSYCHOLOGICAL GROWTH AND DEVELOPMENT OF ADOLESCENTS

See Table 67.3 and Chapters 7 and 9.

CHAPTER 68
Well-Adolescent Care

When interviewing an adolescent, use a nonjudgmental approach and find some common ground to get the adolescent talking about himself or herself. Try to focus on the positive actions that these adolescents are taking to ensure their physical and mental well-being (protective factors). The HEADDSS (home, education, alcohol, drugs, diet, sex, suicide/depression) mnemonic addresses important risk-taking elements of the history (see Table 67.5). Adolescents who experiment in one area of risk-taking often have contemplated or tried multiple other risk-taking behaviors. When all of the risk-taking information has been gathered, choose one or two health care issues to discuss, making it clear that the information is confidential and that you are there to help the adolescent in a partnership way. Although the focus in adolescent care is on psychosocial issues, a general examination must also be performed (Table 68.1). Pediatric issues, such as immunization (see Chapter 94) and health screening, should be included (see Table 9.5).

TABLE 68.1 Examination of the Adolescent

PHYSICAL EXAMINATION—CHECKLIST
Explain to your patient what you are going to do.
Explain how you are going to do it.
Ask whether your adolescent wants his or her parent in the room.*
Be sensitive to the adolescent's needs.
Always use a sheet or blanket to provide privacy.
Let the adolescent remain dressed and work around the clothing.
Ask some questions as you go through the physical to keep the adolescent at ease. Give reassurance that elements of the physical are normal for this age.
ASSESSMENT
Examination can be used to offer reassurance about normalcy†
Assess the following:
Height/weight/body mass index and plot on percentile charts
Skin for acne
Mouth for periodontal disease
Tanner staging
Breasts and testicles
Thyroid (palpation)
Skeletal: scoliosis, Osgood-Schlatter disease, slipped capital femoral epiphysis
Mental status for depression; use screening tools
Signs of substance abuse, risk-taking behaviors, and trauma

**If not, you will need a chaperone.*
†For example, 70% of boys can have breast enlargement (gynecomastia), and girls often have one breast larger than the other.

EARLY ADOLESCENCE (AGES 10-14 YEARS)

Rapid changes in physical appearance and behavior are the major characteristics of early adolescence, leading to a great deal of self-consciousness and need for privacy. The history focuses on the early adolescent's physical and psychosocial health.

MIDDLE ADOLESCENCE (AGES 15-17 YEARS)

Autonomy and a global sense of identity are the major characteristics of middle adolescence. The history focuses on the middle adolescent's interactions with family, school, and peers. High-risk behaviors as a result of experimentation are common.

LATE ADOLESCENCE (AGES 18-21 YEARS)

Individuality and planning for the future are the major characteristics of late adolescence. Greater emphasis is placed on the late adolescent's responsibility for his or her health.

PELVIC EXAMINATION

A full pelvic examination is rarely required in a virginal adolescent girl. A bimanual rectal-abdominal examination (all midline internal genitalia are immediately anterior to the rectal wall) is as efficient as a vaginal-abdominal examination. In some girls, anesthesia may be required for a full pelvic examination.

Before a pelvic examination, the patient should be informed about the importance of the assessment and what maneuvers will take place; she should be encouraged to ask questions before, during, or after the examination. A chaperone should be offered when a family caregiver is not present. Assuring the patient that she has complete control over the examination and allowing participation by using a mirror or guiding the examiner is important. The examiner should maintain eye contact during the examination. Before all maneuvers, the patient must be informed of what to expect and the sensations that may be experienced.

A padded examination table with the patient in a frog-leg position maximizes comfort during a pelvic examination. Stirrups can be used but are less comfortable. The examination room, lubricants, and instruments should be warm. The examination should be unhurried but efficient.

Inspection of the genitalia includes evaluation of the pubic hair, labia majora and minora, clitoris, urethra, and hymenal ring. When a **speculum examination** is required, it must be performed before bimanual palpation of internal genitalia because lubricants interfere with the evaluation of microscopic and microbiologic samples. The speculum allows visualization of the vaginal walls and cervical os for collection of appropriate specimens, such as cultures or Papanicolaou (Pap) smears. A Pap smear is not needed until the adolescent is sexually active unless there is a history of sexual abuse or vulvar infection with human papillomavirus. In the rare circumstance that a vaginal examination is necessary in a virginal girl, a Huffman (0.5 by 4.5 in.) or Pederson (0.9 by 4.5 in.) speculum should be used. A nonvirginal introitus frequently admits a small to medium-sized adult speculum.

NORMAL VARIANTS OF PUBERTY

Breast Asymmetry and Masses

It is not unusual for one breast to begin growth before (or to grow more rapidly than) the other, with resulting asymmetry. Reassurance that after full maturation the asymmetry will be less obvious and that all women have some degree of asymmetry is needed by some. The breast bud is a pea-sized mass below the nipple that is often tender. Occasionally young women present with a breast mass; usually these are **benign fibroadenomas** or cysts (Table 68.2). Breast cancer is extremely rare in this age group. An ultrasound evaluation is better for the evaluation of young, dense breasts and avoids the radiation exposure of mammography.

Physiological Leukorrhea

Peripubertal girls (sexual maturity rating stage III) often complain of vaginal discharge. If the discharge is clear without symptoms of pruritus or odor, it is most likely physiological leukorrhea, due to ovarian estrogen stimulation of the uterus and vagina. A physical examination should reveal evidence of an estrogenized vulva and hymen without erythema or excoriation. The physician should always be alert for signs of abuse. If there are symptoms, cultures should be obtained. In these circumstances, vaginal cultures can be obtained without a speculum because **sexually transmitted infections** are vaginal until menarche, when cervical infections are the rule. Inspection of physiological leukorrhea shows few white blood cells, estrogen maturation of vaginal epithelial cells, and no pathogens on culture.

TABLE 68.2 Etiology of Breast Masses in Adolescents
Classic or juvenile fibroadenoma (70%)
Fibrocystic disease
Breast cyst
Abscess/mastitis
Intraductal papilloma
Fat necrosis/lipoma
Cystosarcoma phyllodes (low-grade malignancy)
Adenomatous hyperplasia
Hemangioma, lymphangioma, lymphoma (rare)
Carcinoma (<1%)

Irregular Menses

Menarche typically occurs approximately 2 years after thelarche, at the average age of 12.6 years. The initial menses are anovulatory and tend to be irregular in duration. This irregularity may persist for 2-5 years, so reassurance may be required. During this phase, estrogen feedback on the hypothalamus decreases gonadotropin secretion, which reduces estrogen production and induces an estrogen withdrawal bleed that can be prolonged and heavy. Anovulatory bleeding is usually painless. As the hypothalamic-pituitary-gonadal axis matures, the cycle becomes ovulatory and menses are secondary to progesterone withdrawal. When ovulation is established, the average cycle length is 21-45 days. Some adolescents ovulate with their first cycle, as indicated by pregnancy before menarche.

Gynecomastia

Decision-Making Algorithm
Available @ StudentConsult.com
Gynecomastia

Breast enlargement in boys is usually a benign, self-limited condition. Gynecomastia is noted in 50-60% of boys during early adolescence. It is often idiopathic, but it may be noted in various conditions (Table 68.3). Typical findings include the

TABLE 68.3 Etiology of Gynecomastia
Idiopathic
Hypogonadism (primary or secondary)
Liver disease
Renal disease
Hyperthyroidism
Neoplasms
Adrenal
Ectopic human chorionic gonadotropin secretion
Testicular
Drugs
Antiandrogens
Antibiotics (isoniazid, ketoconazole, metronidazole)
Antacids (H_2 blockers)
Cancer chemotherapy (especially alkylating agents)
Cardiovascular drugs
Drugs of abuse
Alcohol
Amphetamines
Heroin
Marijuana
Hormones (for female sex)
Psychoactive agents (e.g., diazepam, phenothiazines, tricyclics)

appearance of a 1-3 cm round, freely mobile, often tender, and firm mass immediately beneath the areola during sexual maturity rating stage III. Large, hard, or fixed enlargements and masses associated with any nipple discharge warrant further investigation. Reassurance is usually the only treatment required. If the condition worsens and is associated with psychological morbidity, it may be treated with bromocriptine. Surgical treatment with reduction mammoplasty can be helpful with massive hypertrophy.

CHAPTER 69

Adolescent Gynecology

MENSTRUAL DISORDERS

Irregular menses is the most common complaint of early adolescent girls. As regular ovulatory cycles become established, pain with menstruation **(dysmenorrhea)** is a frequent complaint.

Amenorrhea

Decision-Making Algorithm
Available @ StudentConsult.com
Amenorrhea

Primary amenorrhea has been classically defined as the complete absence of menstruation by 16 years of age in the presence of secondary sexual characteristics or by 14 years of age in the absence of growth or breast development. Ninety-eight percent of adolescents have onset of menarche by age 15; therefore investigations should begin at that age in young women without menses. Other indications for evaluation include the absence of menses by age of 14 with signs of hirsutism or a history of excessive exercise or an eating disorder, absence of menses at any age with symptoms suggestive of an outflow tract obstruction, or no onset of menses within 3 years of thelarche. **Secondary amenorrhea** refers to the cessation of menses for more than 3 consecutive months any time after menarche.

Primary amenorrhea may be a result of functional or anatomical abnormalities of the hypothalamus, pituitary gland, ovaries, uterus, or vagina. The most common etiologies are premature ovarian insufficiency and müllerian agenesis.

The **history** and **physical examination** should guide the investigation. An outflow tract obstruction should be ruled out in adolescents with primary amenorrhea, cyclic abdominal pain, and normal secondary sexual characteristics. An abdominal mass resulting from accumulated blood may be present. Low outflow tract obstructions, such as an imperforate hymen, are visible on examination. An imperforate hymen is characteristic in appearance, with a blue, bulging membrane. All other obstructed outflow tract anomalies require imaging to confirm the diagnosis. A rectoabdominal examination may allow palpation of a hematocolpos or hematometria. An endocrine evaluation is indicated for girls with primary amenorrhea without secondary sexual characteristics and an unremarkable history and physical examination. An elevated follicle-stimulating hormone (FSH) over 25 IU/L on two occasions 4 weeks apart indicates premature ovarian insufficiency, which may reflect ovarian dysgenesis or ovarian agenesis and warrants a karyotype. **Turner syndrome** is a common cause, but other chromosomal anomalies, fragile X premutation carriers, and autoimmune etiologies should be ruled out. Low levels of FSH and luteinizing hormone (LH) suggest hypothalamic dysfunction, which may be due to constitutional delay (often familial), isolated gonadotropin deficiency, central nervous system (CNS) lesions, or reversible hypogonadotropic hypogonadism (chronic illness, low body weight, stressful life events). Additional hormone evaluation may include thyroid-stimulating hormone and prolactin. Hypothyroidism is a common cause of menstrual dysfunction. A prolactinoma, although rare, must be ruled out.

The most common causes of secondary amenorrhea are pregnancy, anorexia/stress (low LH, FSH, and estradiol), and **polycystic ovary syndrome (PCOS).** In PCOS, there may be symptoms of androgen excess, such as acne and hirsutism, weight gain, and, with insulin resistance, acanthosis. If hirsutism or virilization is present, free and total testosterone, androstenedione, and dihydroepiandrosterone sulfate should be measured to rule out ovarian or adrenal tumors. A normal 17-hydroxyprogesterone level rules out late-onset **congenital adrenal hyperplasia.** The diagnosis of PCOS may be difficult in adolescence as there is considerable overlap between normal pubertal development and PCOS. After excluding other etiologies of irregular menses and hyperandrogenism, current recommendations are that PCOS may be diagnosed with infrequent menstrual bleeding (or amenorrhea) that has persisted for more than 2 years after menarche in conjunction with clinical or biochemical evidence of hyperandrogenism. Hyperandrogenism in adolescents is defined as moderate or severe hirsutism, persistent acne/poorly responsive to treatment, or persistent elevation of total and/or free testosterone. There are no compelling criteria for polycystic ovarian morphology on imaging in adolescents; therefore, at present, ovarian ultrasound imaging can be deferred during the evaluation of PCOS in this age group. Patients may have impaired glucose tolerance or hypercholesterolemia even in adolescence; hence they should be screened for these issues.

In a patient with amenorrhea (primary or secondary), normal secondary sex characteristics, a negative pregnancy test, normal prolactin and thyroid-stimulating hormone, and no evidence of outflow tract obstruction, the total effect of estrogen on the uterus (rather than a single point estradiol level) can be determined by a **progesterone withdrawal test.** To achieve this, 5-10 mg of medroxyprogesterone (depending on body weight) is given daily for 5-10 days. If the uterus is normal and primed by estrogen (an intact hypothalamic-pituitary-gonadal [HPO] axis) with no outflow tract obstruction, there should be bleeding within 1 week after the last progesterone tablet. If there is bleeding, the amenorrhea is secondary to anovulation. If there is no progesterone withdrawal bleeding, the uterus has been insufficiently exposed to estrogen, and there is systemic estrogen deficiency.

Therapy for the amenorrhea should be directed at the cause. Anovulation can be managed with either cyclic progesterone withdrawal or combined hormonal contraceptives (CHCs). In irreversible hypothalamic amenorrhea ovarian failure, there is an associated hypoestrogenism. Therapy is directed at replacing estrogen and progesterone, either with a combined hormone replacement regimen or a CHC. With reversible etiologies of hypothalamic amenorrhea, therapy is directed at changing the underlying state: reducing stress, reducing excess exercise, or changing disordered eating to allow reversal of the amenorrheic state. PCOS usually can be treated effectively with weight loss, exercise, progesterone withdrawal, or CHC. If there is evidence of androgen excess, CHCs reduce androgen production from the ovaries and increase sex hormone–binding globulin to reduce the amount of available androgen. Spironolactone helps treat hirsutism, and when there is evidence of insulin insensitivity, metformin can restore ovulatory cycles. Contraception should be prescribed if applicable.

Abnormal Uterine Bleeding

Decision-Making Algorithm
Available @ StudentConsult.com

Abnormal Vaginal Bleeding

Normal ovulatory menses occur between 21 and 45 days apart, measuring from the first day of menstruation to the first day of the next menstruation. The average duration of flow is 3-7 days; more than 7 days is considered prolonged. More than 8 well-soaked pads or 12 tampons per day may be considered excessive, although classically blood loss is difficult to estimate. Table 69.1 defines menstrual disorders according to the new International Federation of Gynecology and Obstetrics nomenclature and classification of **abnormal uterine bleeding (AUB).** If the menstrual problem is unclear and nonacute, observation and charting on a menstrual calendar are warranted. Excessively heavy, prolonged, or infrequent bleeding in the first year after menarche is often physiological anovulation but should be investigated, especially if it causes iron-deficiency anemia or is associated with other symptoms such as hyperandrogenism, galactorrhea, etc.

The differential diagnosis of AUB using the polyp, adenomyosis, leiomyoma, and malignancy (PALM) COEIN classification system is found in Table 69.2. This classification system has been adopted in multiple guidelines. The PALM categories include extremely rare causes of AUB in this age group. Far more common are the categories of AUB-C (coagulopathy) and AUB-O (ovulatory). **Anovulation** is the most common etiology of AUB in adolescents. Ovulation is a later event in puberty. Without progesterone from the corpus luteum, unopposed estrogen causes endometrial hyperplasia and irregular endometrial shedding, which can be prolonged and heavy, sometimes life threatening. Progesterone induces a secretory endometrium. When progesterone is withdrawn, the endometrium sheds in a synchronous fashion with myometrial and vascular contractions (causing dysmenorrhea but limiting blood loss). For the first 1-2 years after menarche, the majority of adolescent cycles are anovulatory. After 1 year of regular cycles, irregular bleeding usually indicates an organic abnormality. The differential diagnosis of anovulatory bleeding at that time would include thyroid dysfunction, PCOS, and adrenal and pituitary disorders. Approximately 20% of adolescents with heavy or prolonged menses have a coagulation disorder (even higher if presenting in early menarche) and 10% have other pathology. Clues on history to suspect a coagulopathy are onset of heavy menses with menarche, severity requiring admission or blood transfusion, failure of initial medical therapy and a family history of a bleeding disorder, or a personal history of bleeding. If an underlying pathology is discovered, treatment should be directed at the primary disorder and the secondary menstrual dysfunction. It is important to remember that AUB in adolescents can be the result of complications of sexual activity, including pregnancy, sexually transmitted infections (STIs), or as a side effect of contraception (AUB-I (iatrogenic).

A thorough history with a menstrual calendar indicating the amount of flow and associated symptoms is followed by physical examination, including a pelvic examination in a sexually active adolescent. Physical examination should also assess for signs of anemia, bruising, or petechiae, and signs of hyperandrogenism or thyroid disease. A complete blood count, pregnancy test, thyroid-stimulating hormone (TSH), and coagulation screen should be performed if appropriate. With a suspicion of PCOS or in the setting of clinical hyperandrogenism, free or total testosterone and DHEAS may be included. In sexually active adolescents, **STIs** should be ruled out. Due to the infrequency of structural etiologies of AUB at this age, pelvic ultrasound has no role in the initial investigations of AUB.

TABLE 69.1 Definition of Menstrual Disorders

CLINICAL DIMENSION	DESCRIPTIVE TERM	DEFINITION
Frequency	Frequent menstrual bleeding	<21 days/cycle
	Infrequent menstrual bleeding	>35 days/cycle
Regularity	Amenorrhea	Absent for 6 mo or more
	Irregular menstrual bleeding	>20-day variation in cycle length
Duration	Prolonged menstrual bleeding	>8 days of flow
	Shortened menstrual bleeding	<2 days of flow
Flow	Heavy menstrual bleeding	>80 mL loss
	Light menstrual bleeding	<5 mL loss
Intermenstrual bleeding		Bleeding between normally timed periods

TABLE 69.2 Differential Diagnosis of Abnormal Uterine Bleeding—PALM COEIN Classification

P—Polyps
A—Adenomyosis
L—Leiomyoma
M—Malignancy
C—Coagulopathies
O—Ovulatory disorder
E—Endometrial
I—Iatrogenic
N—Not otherwise specified

Unpredictable, heavy, and prolonged menses may impair school attendance and social functioning; iron-deficiency anemia is associated with lower academic scores. **Treatment** is indicated for AUB that affects the quality of life. Chronic and acute bleeding can be managed with CHCs; multiple daily doses may be initially required until blood loss is controlled. Occasionally uncontrollable bleeding requires hospitalization for intravenous fluids, consideration of blood transfusion, and high-dose estrogen. Iron therapy is also important. If the etiology of bleeding is related to an immature HPO axis, use of CHCs to regulate menstruation and allow the HPO axis to mature is appropriate; 6-12 months of therapy may be sufficient. CHCs are prescribed either cyclically or in an extended fashion (avoiding frequent hormone free intervals) and can manage heavy menstrual bleeding in individuals with **bleeding disorders** (von Willebrand disease, platelet function defects, idiopathic thrombocytopenic purpura, etc.). Tranexamic acid, an antifibrinolytic, is an additional therapeutic option for decreasing flow in heavy menstrual bleeding; it does not provide cycle regulation or contraceptive benefits. For young women with a contraindication to estrogen, progestin-only methods can also be prescribed. The levonorgestrel-releasing intrauterine system, a long-acting contraceptive, can provide over 70% reduction in blood loss in AUB as well as effective contraception for sexually active adolescents. Parents are often concerned that CHC use will cause their daughter to become sexually active, but literature and experience do not support this.

Dysmenorrhea

Decision-Making Algorithm
Available @ StudentConsult.com
Dysmenorrhea

The most common gynecological complaint of young women is painful menstruation, or dysmenorrhea, during the first 1-3 days of bleeding. **Primary dysmenorrhea** is defined as pelvic pain during menstruation in the absence of pelvic pathology and is a feature of ovulation. It typically develops 1-3 years after menarche, with an increasing incidence to age 24 as ovulatory cycles are established. The release of prostaglandins and leukotrienes from the degenerating endometrium after progesterone levels decline causes increased uterine tone and increased frequency and dysrhythmia of uterine contractions. This creates excessive uterine pressures and ischemia, which heightens the sensitivity of pain fibers to bradykinin and other physical stimuli.

Secondary dysmenorrhea is menstrual pain associated with pelvic pathology; it represents 10% of dysmenorrhea in this age group and is caused most frequently by **endometriosis** or **pelvic inflammatory disease.** Adolescents with endometriosis usually have mild to moderate disease on laparoscopy. Severe dysmenorrhea with onset immediately following menarche should raise the consideration of an asymmetrically obstructed outflow tract (e.g., obstructed hemivagina and ipsilateral renal anomaly or functional noncommunicating uterine horn). The types of dysmenorrhea usually can be distinguished by history and physical examination. Secondary dysmenorrhea often is more severe, fails initial medical therapy, and is more commonly associated with atypical features (chronic pain, dyschezia, dyspareunia). Severe dysmenorrhea in a patient with a known renal anomaly should raise the suspicion of a müllerian anomaly. Ultrasound is preferred as the initial screen for obstructing genital tract lesions. Magnetic resonance imaging is the gold standard for diagnosing complex reproductive tract anomalies in this age group. Laparoscopy is required to diagnose endometriosis and pelvic inflammatory disease with certainty, although it is usually reserved for patients who fail medical therapy.

Treatment of primary dysmenorrhea should be considered with symptoms causing significant distress. First-line therapy is nonsteroidal antiinflammatory drugs (NSAIDs; Table 69.3). To maximize pain relief, NSAIDs should be taken before or as soon as menstruation begins, closely following the dosing schedule. Typically NSAIDs are needed for 2-3 days. If NSAIDs fail to provide adequate relief, CHCs or long-acting reversible contraceptives (LARCs) may be added. These contraceptives may be first-line therapy, depending on need for pregnancy prevention. If dysmenorrhea persists despite an adequate trial of CHCs (>4 months), an alternative diagnosis, such as endometriosis, should be considered. When CHCs fail, a laparoscopy may be performed before advancing therapy to confirm the diagnosis and excise endometriotic lesions. More commonly, additional medical options are pursued for symptom relief. Extended CHC therapy (84 days of active CHC followed by a 5- to 7-day hormone-free interval) may control symptoms. Alternatives are dienogest 2 mg daily, depot medroxyprogesterone acetate (150 mg) every 3 months, or insertion of a levonorgestrel-releasing intrauterine system. Endometriosis may be treated with gonadotropin-releasing hormone agonists (nafarelin or leuprolide), adding norethindrone in older adolescents (>16 years of age) when symptom relief is required.

PREGNANCY

The median age of first intercourse in the United States is 17 years for girls and 16 years for boys; this is similar to the ages in other developed countries. Although the age of coital initiation

TABLE 69.3 Treatment of Dysmenorrhea
NSAIDs
Over-the-counter medications
Ibuprofen or naproxen sodium taken every 4 hr
Prescription
Ibuprofen 400 mg PO qid
Naproxen 500 mg PO stat then 250-500 mg PO bid
Mefenamic acid 500 mg PO stat then 250 mg qid or 500 mg PO tid
Diclofenac 100 mg PO stat then 50 mg tid
Combined hormonal contraceptives—cyclic or continuous
Progestogen-only pill
Depo-medroxyprogesterone acetate—150 mg IM every 12-14 wk or 104 mg sq
LNG intrauterine system (52 mg)

IM, Intramuscularly; *LNG*, levonorgestrel; *NSAIDs*, nonsteroidal antiinflammatory drugs.

is similar among different socioeconomic groups, the prevalence of adolescent childbearing is greatest in the lower socioeconomic strata. Annually, 14 million births occur globally to women aged 14-19 years. Risk factors for adolescent pregnancy include lower socioeconomic status, lower educational attainment, low self-esteem, lack of access to contraception, alcohol and drug use, and adverse early life experiences in the home. Approximately 553,000 U.S. females 15-19 years of age become pregnant each year. Sixty percent of those pregnancies result in births, 26% in abortions, and the remainder are pregnancy losses. Primarily due to the increased use of contraceptives, the teen birth rate in the United States was reduced to a record low in 2013, with an overall decrease of 57% since 1991. Adolescents who continue their pregnancies have an increased incidence of preterm and very preterm births, low birth weight infants, infant neonatal admission, postneonatal mortality, child abuse, subsequent maternal unemployment, and poor maternal educational achievement. Children of adolescent parents compared with their peers are more likely to have lower educational achievements, be involved with drugs and alcohol, and become adolescent parents.

Pregnancy risks are influenced by behavior and socioeconomic status as well as inherent biologic risks within adolescents. Within adolescence, pregnancies to women <15 years of age pose higher risks than those in women ≥16 years of age. Prenatal care should be adapted to the adolescent to improve pregnancy outcome. Multidisciplinary care, a comprehensive nutrition program, and social support improve pregnancy outcomes.

Diagnosis

Pregnancy should be considered and ruled out in any adolescent presenting with secondary amenorrhea. Frequently pregnant adolescents delay seeking a diagnosis until several periods have been missed and initially may not disclose having had intercourse. Young adolescents may present with other symptoms, such as vomiting, vague pains, or deteriorating behavior and may report normal periods. Because of the varied presentations of adolescent pregnancy, a thorough menstrual history should be obtained from all menstruating adolescents. Urine pregnancy tests are sensitive approximately 7-10 days after conception. Sexual assault or coercion should be screened for in all cases of adolescent pregnancy. It is important to recognize that adolescents' pregnancies are not all unwanted or unplanned. Sensitivity to that awareness and to culture is important in the approach to the pregnant adolescent.

When pregnancy is confirmed, immediate gestational dating is important to assist in planning. An ultrasound examination for dating is recommended. Options are to continue the pregnancy or abortion (if not beyond 20-24 weeks' gestation). With the former, the adolescent may choose to parent the child or have the child adopted. Pregnant adolescents should be encouraged to involve their families in decision making.

Continuation of the Pregnancy

Adolescents who continue their pregnancies need pregnancy care that is adapted for their developmental needs. Multidisciplinary adolescent-specific antenatal care has been documented to decrease risks of adolescent pregnancy such as preterm birth, low birth weight, and neonatal admissions to intensive care settings. Care must be easily accessible to the adolescent. Their socioeconomic situation should be evaluated in an effort to optimize the infant's health and development. Pregnant adolescents should be screened frequently for mood disorders, alcohol and/or drug use, STIs, and interpersonal violence, as reported rates are higher in this age group than in adults. Pregnancy is the most common cause for young women to drop out of school, so special attention should be given to keeping the adolescent in school during and after pregnancy. Contraceptive planning should be initiated in the antenatal care period with continued focus postpartum, including education about contraceptives to decrease repeat pregnancy rates.

Termination

If a pregnant adolescent chooses to terminate her pregnancy, she should be referred immediately to a nonjudgmental abortion service. The options for pregnancy termination depend on the gestational age. Surgical procedures include manual vacuum aspiration (<8 weeks' gestational age), suction curettage (<12-14 weeks' gestational age, depending on the provider), and dilation and evacuation (14-20 weeks' gestational age). Early pregnancy (<8 weeks' gestational age) can be terminated medically with oral mifepristone (RU-486) in combination with misoprostol, methotrexate with misoprostol, or misoprostol alone. Adolescents may not present early enough to explore this option. Psychosocial support and subsequent contraceptive counseling and implementation should be available to adolescents who choose abortion.

CONTRACEPTION

Adolescents may begin intercourse without reliable or consistent use of birth control. While the proportion of adolescents using contraception the first time they have sex has increased, 20% still initiate intercourse with no contraception, with higher rates in younger adolescents. All methods of contraception significantly reduce the risk of pregnancy when used in a consistent and correct fashion. The best form of contraception is the one an individual will use; thus counseling adolescents about all methods and supporting their choice is important. Contraceptives can be divided into user-based methods and LARCs. Although LARCs are recommended as first-line contraceptives to decrease pregnancy, birth, and abortion rates, only the minority of adolescent women currently use these methods. However, studies have shown that if accurate information is provided and barriers such as cost and access are removed, the majority of adolescents choose a LARC method. It is important to remind young women that steroidal contraception or LARCs do not provide any protection from STIs, and condoms should be used to reduce the risk of infection.

Steroidal Contraception

Long-Acting Reversible Contraceptives

Implants

The subdermal progestin etonogestrel implant is a single rod inserted subcutaneously in the upper inner arm. Effective for 3 years, it has the lowest failure rate of any contraceptive method (0.05% out of 100 women during the first year of typical use).

The primary mechanism of action is suppression of ovulation; there may be additional efficacy from the effects of the progestin on cervical mucus and the endometrium. Quick starts are possible, with insertion on the day of presentation once pregnancy has been excluded. The implant does not need to be inserted at any particular time in the menstrual cycle. The most common side effect is the irregular and unpredictable bleeding pattern that is most common in the first 3 months of use. Adolescents should be counseled regarding the expected change in bleeding. Continuation rates of use among adolescents of this method at 1 year have been reported at over 80%.

Intrauterine Devices

Intrauterine devices (IUDs) are inserted into the uterus, where they release either copper ions or levonorgestrel. Either IUD method is safe for adolescents. A sterile foreign-body reaction in the uterine cavity is a common mechanism of action of both IUD methods. In addition, the copper IUD impairs sperm function and fertilization, while the levonorgestrel IUDs induce an atrophic endometrium as well as thickening cervical mucus. The copper IUD has the longest approval for duration of use at 10 years; however, it may increase the amount and duration of bleeding as well as dysmenorrhea. The levonorgestrel-releasing intrauterine systems contain differing amounts of levonorgestrel (13.5 mg or 52 mg), with durations of use of 3 years and 5 years respectively. All levonorgestrel IUDs affect bleeding patterns. The 52-mg products decrease menstrual flow, resulting in amenorrhea in approximately 20% of users at 1 year. They are used therapeutically for heavy menstrual bleeding and dysmenorrhea. The 13.5-mg product decreases menstrual flow but with less achievement of amenorrhea. All IUDs are highly effective (failure rates of <1%), with even lower failure rates of levonorgestrel IUDs. Although a small increased risk of pelvic inflammatory disease exists for 21 days after insertion of an IUD, the risk following that transient period lowers to the level of an adolescent without an IUD for the remainder of use. Adolescents should be screened for STIs at the time of IUD insertion, with treatment provided as soon as possible for positive results or if there is a concern for compliance at the time of IUD insertion. Insertion in nulliparous women can be aided by the use of a paracervical block. The use of condoms should be encouraged to reduce the risk of STIs.

Hormonal Injections

Depo-medroxyprogesterone acetate (DMPA) is available in two formulations: intramuscular injection of 150 mg every 12-14 weeks or 104 mg/0.65 mL for subcutaneous use every 12-14 weeks. The primary mechanism of action is suppression of ovulation with a secondary effect of progestin on cervical mucus. Progestin-only contraception is associated with menstrual irregularities (70% amenorrhea and 30% frequent menstrual bleeding). Weight gain on DMPA is unpredictable. The average weight gain is 5 pounds in the first year. Individuals who gain more than 5% of weight early on are at greater risk of excess weight gain overall. Current information on the concerns of possible effect on bone mineral density suggests reversibility of effect. The potential impact on bone density should not prevent health care providers from prescribing DMPA methods to adolescents after appropriate counseling. Continuation of DMPA in adolescents at 1 year is less than with other LARCs.

Combined Hormonal Contraceptives

CHCs are available in oral, transdermal, and vaginal routes of administration. All contain a synthetic estrogen and progesterone that suppress gonadotropin secretion and ovarian follicle development and ovulation. CHCs also produce an atrophic endometrium (inhospitable for blastocyst implantation) and thicken cervical mucus to inhibit sperm penetration. Contraindications and relative contraindications to CHCs are listed in Tables 69.4 and 69.5. CHCs are 99% effective if taken regularly and have numerous noncontraceptive benefits (decreased acne, less dysmenorrhea, and lighter menstrual flow). Unfortunately typical use among adolescents often result in much higher failure rates and continuations rate at 1 year are low. There are many formulations of combined oral contraceptives available that vary in the amount of estrogen, progestin, and packing (with or without placebo week, duration of active pills, duration of hormone-free intervals). Unless the adolescent shows the ability to take a pill daily, contraception with oral combined contraceptive pills should be avoided. The contraceptive patch is a 25-cm^2 pink patch containing ethinyl estradiol and norelgestromin that is applied to the skin of the torso, buttocks, or arm for 1 week followed by removal and application of a new patch for a total of 3 weeks of patch use. A patch-free week then follows for a withdrawal bleed. The 4-week cycle is repeated. In women weighing 90 kg or more, the contraceptive patch is less efficacious. The contraceptive vaginal ring is a flexible, Silastic ring. The ring releases a constant rate of 15 mg of ethinyl estradiol and 0.120 mg of etonogestrel per day. Each ring is used continuously for 3 weeks and then removed. A new ring

TABLE 69.4 Absolute Contraindications to Combined Hormonal Contraceptives

Smoking and age >35 yr and >15 cigarettes/day
Hypertension (systolic ≥160 mm Hg or diastolic ≥100 mm Hg) or associated with vascular disease
Current venous thromboembolic disease (not on therapy or on therapy for >3 mo with high risk of recurrence)
History of venous thromboembolic disease at high risk of recurrence
Major surgery with prolonged immobilization
Ischemic heart disease
Peripartum cardiomyopathy with moderately or severely impaired cardiac function or within 6 mo of pregnancy
Complicated solid organ transplantation
Complicated valvular heart disease (pulmonary hypertension, atrial fibrillation, history of subacute bacterial endocarditis)
Migraine with focal neurological symptoms any age
Breast cancer (current)
Diabetes with retinopathy/nephropathy/neuropathy or duration of diabetes of >20 yr duration
Severe cirrhosis
Liver tumor (adenoma or hepatoma)
Acute hepatitis
Systemic lupus with positive antiphospholipid antibody levels (or unknown levels)
Thrombogenic mutations

TABLE 69.5 Relative Contraindications to Combined Hormonal Contraceptives
<1 mo postpartum and breast feeding or <21 days postpartum not breast feeding
Adequately controlled hypertension
Hypertension adequately controlled or systolic 140-159 mm Hg, diastolic 90-99 mm Hg
Migraine without aura and age >35 yr
Currently symptomatic gallbladder disease medically treated
Peripartum cardiomyopathy, normal or mildly impaired cardiac function >6 mo from pregnancy
History of combined oral contraceptive–related cholestasis
History of malabsorptive bariatric surgery procedure
Past breast cancer with no evidence of current disease for 5 yr
History of venous thromboembolic disease at low risk for recurrence
Acute venous thromboembolic event on treatment for at least 3 mo at low risk of recurrence
Smoking > age 35 and <15 cigarettes per day
Drug interactions (ritonavir-boosted protease inhibitors, certain anticonvulsants (phenytoin, carbamazepine, primidone, lamotrigine, topiramate, barbiturates), rifampicin, rifabutin therapy)

is inserted 7 days later. Any CHC can be used in an extended fashion by missing hormone-free days to induce long intervals between withdrawal bleeding.

After a history and physical examination, CHCs can be started on the first day of the next menstrual period or as a "Quick Start." The Quick Start method refers to starting on any day of the cycle, usually on the day of the visit to the health care provider, as long as pregnancy has been ruled out. Blood pressure measurement to rule out preexisting hypertension should be obtained before prescribing a CHC. Initially the adolescent should be seen monthly to reinforce good contraceptive use and safer sex.

Initial **side effects,** such as nausea, breast tenderness, and breakthrough bleeding, are common and usually transient. CHCs do not generally cause weight gain. Usually 3-4 months on one CHC are needed to determine acceptability. If there is breakthrough bleeding, the physician should determine compliance with the method (especially with oral pills) before changing methods. Adolescents should be taught the appropriate response to missed doses. Health care providers usually suggest the use of additional contraception in the first month.

Progestogen-Only Pill

Although not as widely used as CHCs, the progestin-only pill, *norethindrone*, is a safe and effective form of contraception when used consistently. It is supplied in packages of 28 tablets, each containing norethindrone with no hormone-free interval. It prevents pregnancy through reduced volume, increased viscosity, and altered molecular structure of cervical mucus, resulting in little or no sperm penetration. In addition, endometrial changes reduce the potential for implantation, and ovulation is partially or completely suppressed. Approximately 40% of women using progestogen-only contraceptives continue to ovulate. Progestogen-only contraception is indicated for women who have a contraindication to estrogen-based contraceptives (see Table 69.4) or have estrogen-related side effects.

Barrier Methods

Condoms

Latex condoms will provide protection not only against pregnancy but will also reduce the risk of STIs, including human immunodeficiency virus (HIV), when used correctly. Polyurethane and other nonlatex male condoms have an increased risk of breakage and slippage. Condoms may be chosen by individuals who have infrequent intercourse. Latex and polyurethane condoms are available over the counter without the need for a physician visit or prescription. The female condom is an additional barrier method made of polyurethane that affords females more control, but adolescents usually do not consider it aesthetically pleasing. Condoms are commonly recommended in the context of "dual" protection for adolescents. Any adolescent using barrier methods should be counseled regarding emergency contraceptive (EC) options.

Sponge, Caps, and Diaphragm

The vaginal sponge is a spermicide-impregnated synthetic sponge that is effective for 24 hours of intercourse. The sponge has higher rates of failure compared with other methods of contraception. Nonoxynol-9 (the spermicide) increases the risk of vaginal and cervical irritation or abrasion and therefore also the risk of transmission of HIV. The cervical cap, made of silicone, is available in several sizes; the choice of size depends on the user's pregnancy history. The cap is placed on the cervix by the user before intercourse. This method is technically difficult, especially for an adolescent. The *diaphragm* is an intravaginal barrier method used in conjunction with a gel. The user must be fitted for a diaphragm by a health care provider, but it is technically simpler to use than the cap because the edges go into the vaginal fornices. The efficacy of the diaphragm and the cap was studied with use of a spermicidal gel, which is no longer available. Thus the efficacy of these methods with use of an acid-buffering lubricant to inhibit sperm motility is not known. All of these methods need to be left in place for 6 hours after the last act of intercourse for optimal efficacy.

Emergency Postcoital Contraception

Emergency postcoital contraception should be discussed at every visit. A prescription should be given in advance of need when no over-the-counter access is available. Emergency contraception (EC) reduces the risk of pregnancy after unprotected intercourse. Indications and contraindications to emergency postcoital contraception are listed in Table 69.6. There are several forms of EC. The copper IUD can be inserted up to 7 days from the act of unprotected intercourse; it is the most effective EC method with an efficacy of greater than 99%. Levonorgestrel 0.75 mg, two tablets given once (total dose of 1.5 mg), is approved for use up to 72 hours after unprotected intercourse with efficacy up to 5 days. Effectiveness is higher the earlier the method is used after unprotected intercourse. Women with a BMI >25 kg/m^2 may experience reduced efficacy, but regardless of BMI, hormonal EC methods may retain effectiveness and should not be withheld if a copper IUD EC is not available or acceptable. Any CHC pill may be prescribed to deliver two doses of the equivalent of 100 mg of ethinyl estradiol and 500 µg of levonorgestrel 12 hours apart. The CHC method is associated with significantly more nausea and

TABLE 69.6 Emergency Contraception
INDICATIONS
• No method of contraception being used
• Condom breaks, slips, or leaks
• Diaphragm or cervical cap dislodged/removed <6 hr
• Missed hormonal contraceptive
• Error in using withdrawal (ejaculation on external genitalia or in vagina)
• Sexual assault on no reliable contraceptive
CONTRAINDICATIONS
• Known pregnancy
• If strong contraindications to estrogens, use progestin
• If uterine anomaly—contraindication to intrauterine device

vomiting than the progestin-only regimen and is less effective. The antiprogestin mifepristone is an effective postcoital contraceptive in a 30 mg dose; however, it is not approved for this use in the United States. When women are prescribed or use emergency contraception, a pregnancy test should be completed if normal menstrual bleeding does not occur within 21 days with Progestin or IUD methods or by 28 days with CHC method. Young women who use EC should be counseled on alternative contraceptive methods.

Coitus Interruptus

Withdrawal is a common method of birth control used by sexually active adolescents. It is ineffective because sperm are released into the vagina before ejaculation, and withdrawal may occur after ejaculation has begun.

Rhythm Method (Periodic Coital Abstinence)

The rhythm method is the practice of periodic abstinence just before, during, and after ovulation. This method requires the user to have an accurate knowledge of her cycle, awareness of clues indicating ovulation, and discipline. Adolescents tend to have unpredictable cycles and, consequently, less predictable ovulation, so it is difficult to determine with any accuracy a time of the month that can be considered completely safe.

Oral and Anal Sex

Some adolescents engage in oral or anal sex because they believe that it eliminates the need for contraception. Many do not consider this activity as "having sex." Condoms generally are not used during oral or anal sex, but the risk of acquiring an STI is still present. Adolescents should be asked specifically about nonvaginal forms of sexual activity. Adolescents who engage in oral and anal sex require STI and HIV counseling and screening.

RAPE

Rape is a legal term for nonconsensual intercourse. Almost half of rape victims are adolescents, and the perpetrator is known in 50% of cases. Although gathering historical and physical evidence for a criminal investigation is important, the physician's primary responsibility is to perform these functions in a supportive, nonjudgmental manner. The history should include details of the sexual assault, time from the assault until presentation, whether the victim cleaned herself, date of last menstrual period, and previous sexual activity if any.

For optimal results, forensic material should be collected within 72 hours of the assault. Clothes, especially undergarments, need to be placed in a paper bag for drying (plastic holds humidity, which allows organisms to grow, destroying forensic evidence). The patient should be inspected for bruising and bites as well as oral, genital, and anal trauma. Photographs are the best record to document injuries. Specimens should be obtained from the fingernails, mouth, vagina, pubic hair, and anus. The sexual assault kit provides materials to obtain DNA from semen, saliva, blood, fingernail scrapings, and pubic hair. A wet mount of vaginal fluids shows the presence or absence of sperm under the microscope. Cultures for STIs should be taken but are often negative (unless the patient was previously infected) because 72 hours are needed for the bacterial load to be sufficient for a culture. Blood should be drawn for baseline HIV and syphilis (Venereal Disease Research Laboratories [VDRL] test). All materials must be maintained in a "chain of evidence" that cannot be called into question in court.

Therapy after a rape includes prophylaxis for EC and STI and, if indicated, hepatitis immune globulin and hepatitis vaccine. A single oral dose of cefixime, 400 mg, and azithromycin, 1 g, treats *Chlamydia,* gonorrhea, and syphilis. An alternative regimen is a single intramuscular dose of ceftriaxone, 125 mg, with a single oral dose of azithromycin, 1 g. For prophylaxis against bacterial vaginosis and *Trichomonas,* a single oral dose of metronidazole, 2 g, is recommended. If the HIV status of the perpetrator is known and is positive, exposure to blood, genital secretions, or other potentially infective fluids occurred, and the individual is seeking assistance within 72 hours, a 28-day course of highly active antiretroviral therapy should be considered and initiated as soon as possible. If the assailant's HIV status is unknown, an individualized approach should be taken in deciding on postexposure prophylaxis, assessing for risk of infection (trauma at time of assault, prevalence of HIV in the region, nature of exposure) and the patient's wishes. Consider consulting an HIV specialist for advice. Repeat cultures, wet mounts, and a pregnancy test should be performed 3 weeks after the assault, followed by serology for syphilis, hepatitis, and HIV at 12 weeks. Long-term sequelae are common; patients should be offered immediate and ongoing psychological support, such as that offered by local rape crisis services.

CHAPTER 70
Eating Disorders

Eating disorders are common chronic diseases in adolescents, especially in females. The *Diagnostic and Statistical Manual of Mental Disorders,* fifth edition (DSM-V), classifies these as psychiatric illnesses. The diagnosis in young adolescents (pre-growth spurt, premenstrual) may not follow the typical diagnostic criteria (Table 70.1).

ANOREXIA NERVOSA

The prevalence of anorexia nervosa is 1.5% in teenage girls. The female-to-male ratio is approximately 20:1, and the condition shows a familial pattern. The cause of anorexia nervosa is unknown but involves a complex interaction between social, environmental, psychological, and biologic events (Fig. 70.1), with risk factors having been identified (Fig. 70.2).

Clinical Manifestations and Diagnosis

Screening for eating disorders is important and is best done as part of the larger psychosocial screen for risk-taking factors (see Fig. 67.1). Although it is recommended that the adolescent be interviewed alone, he or she may minimize the problem; thus it is also important to interview the parent(s) alone. The first event usually described by an affected patient is a behavioral change in eating or exercise (i.e., food obsession, food-related ruminations, mood changes). The patient has an unrealistic body image and feels too fat, despite appearing excessively thin. The parents' response to this situation can be anger, self-blame, focusing attention on the child, ignoring the disorder, or approving the behavior.

The physician should be nonjudgmental, collect information, and assess the differential diagnosis. The **differential diagnosis** of weight loss includes gastroesophageal reflux, peptic ulcer, malignancy, chronic diarrhea, malabsorption, inflammatory

TABLE 70.1 Normal Adolescent Milestones

PSYCHOLOGICAL STAGES	ISSUES THAT CAN TRIGGER EATING DISORDERS
Early adolescence—increased body awareness	Fear of growing up
Middle adolescence—increased self-awareness	Rebelliousness
	Social media, especially attention to models and celebrities
	Competition and achievement
Late adolescence—identity	Anxiety and worry for the future
	Need for control

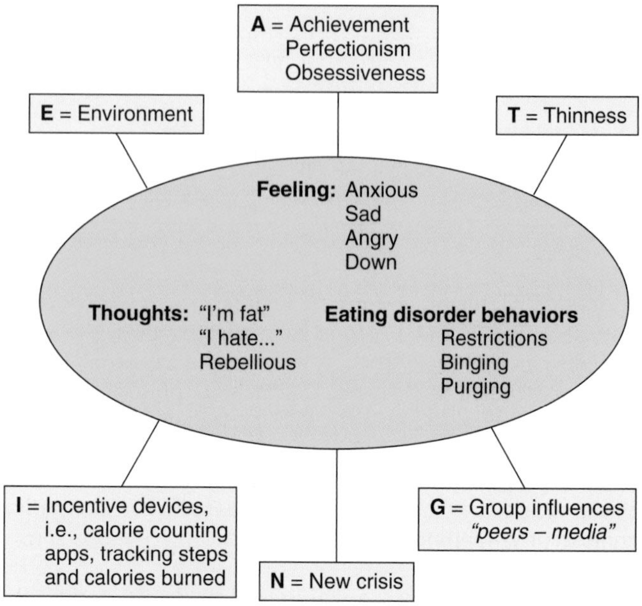

FIGURE 70.1 The eating disorder cycle.

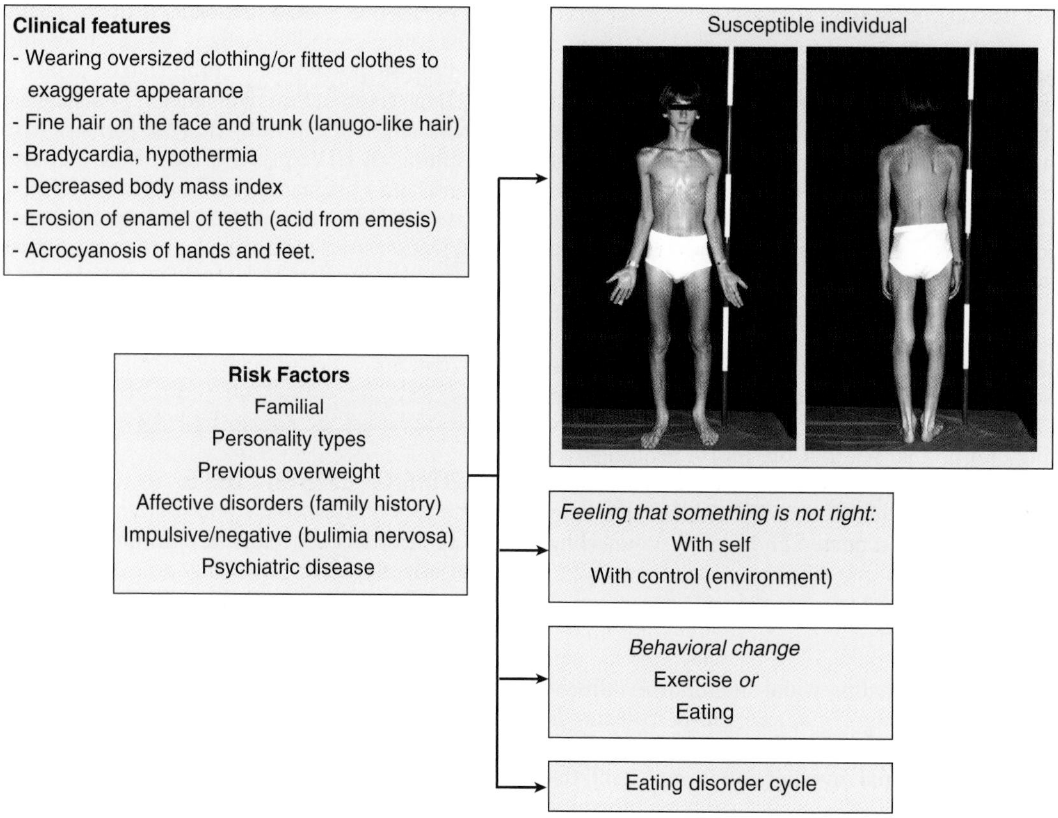

Clinical features
- Wearing oversized clothing/or fitted clothes to exaggerate appearance
- Fine hair on the face and trunk (lanugo-like hair)
- Bradycardia, hypothermia
- Decreased body mass index
- Erosion of enamel of teeth (acid from emesis)
- Acrocyanosis of hands and feet.
Susceptible individual
Risk Factors
Familial
Personality types
Previous overweight
Affective disorders (family history)
Impulsive/negative (bulimia nervosa)
Psychiatric disease
Feeling that something is not right:
With self
With control (environment)
Behavioral change
Exercise or
Eating
Eating disorder cycle

FIGURE 70.2 The slippery slope to eating disorders.

TABLE 70.2 Diagnostic Criteria for Anorexia Nervosa
Refusal to maintain body weight at or above a minimally normal weight for age and height (e.g., weight loss leading to body weight <85% of ideal)*
Intense fear of gaining weight or becoming fat, even though underweight
Denial of the seriousness of the low body weight—a disturbance in the way in which one's body weight or shape is experienced
Amenorrhea in postmenarche females*

The diagnostic criteria may be difficult to meet in a young adolescent. Allow for a wide spectrum of clinical features.

TABLE 70.3 When to Hospitalize an Anorexic Patient
Weight loss >25% ideal body weight*
Risk of suicide
Bradycardia, hypothermia
Dehydration, hypokalemia, dysrhythmias
Outpatient treatment fails

Less weight loss may trigger hospitalization in a young adolescent.

bowel disease, increased energy demands, hypothalamic lesions, hyperthyroidism, diabetes mellitus, and Addison disease. Psychiatric disorders must also be considered (e.g., drug abuse, depression, obsessive-compulsive disorder).

The **clinical features** of anorexia can include wearing oversized, layered clothing to hide appearance or, conversely, tight-fitting clothing to exaggerate appearance. Other signs include fine hair on the face and trunk (lanugo-like hair), rough and scaly skin, bradycardia, hypothermia, decreased body mass index, erosion of tooth enamel (due to acid from emesis), and acrocyanosis of the hands and feet. Signs of hyperthyroidism should not be present (see Chapter 175). The diagnostic criteria for anorexia nervosa are listed in Table 70.2.

Treatment and Prognosis

Treatment requires a multidisciplinary approach, including a feeding program as well as individual and family therapy. Feeding is accomplished through voluntary intake of regular foods, nutritional formula orally, or by nasogastric tube. When vital signs are stable, discussion and negotiation of a detailed treatment contract with the patient and the parents are essential. The first step is to restore body weight. Hospitalization may be necessary (Table 70.3). When 80% of normal weight is achieved, the patient is given freedom to gain weight at a personal pace. The *prognosis* includes a 3-5% mortality (suicide, malnutrition) rate, the development of bulimic symptoms (30% of individuals), and persistent anorexia nervosa syndrome (20% of individuals).

BULIMIA NERVOSA

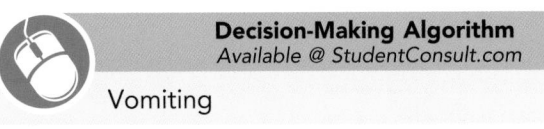

Decision-Making Algorithm
Available @ StudentConsult.com

Vomiting

TABLE 70.4 Diagnostic Criteria for Bulimia Nervosa
Recurrent episodes of binge eating, at least twice a week for 3 mo, characterized by the following:
Eating an amount of food that is definitely larger than most people would eat during a discrete period
A sense of lack of control over eating during the episode (e.g., a feeling that one cannot stop eating or control what/how much one is eating)
Compensatory behavior to prevent weight gain (i.e., self-induced vomiting, misuse of laxatives or diuretics, excessive exercise)
Self-evaluation unduly influenced by body shape and weight
Disturbance does not occur exclusively during episodes of anorexia nervosa

Table 70.4 presents the diagnostic criteria for bulimia nervosa. The prevalence of bulimia nervosa is 5% in female college students. The female-to-male ratio is 10 : 1. Binge-eating episodes consist of large quantities of what the adolescent perceives as forbidden foods or leftovers, consumed rapidly, followed by vomiting. Metabolic abnormalities can result from the excessive vomiting or laxative and diuretic intake. Binge-eating episodes and the loss of control over eating often occur in young women who are slightly overweight with a history of dieting.

Nutritional, educational, and self-monitoring techniques are used to increase awareness of the maladaptive behavior, following which efforts are made to change the eating behavior. Patients with bulimia nervosa may respond to antidepressant therapy, which may help impulse control and/or depression. There may be family histories of affective disorders. Patients feel embarrassed, guilty, and ashamed of their actions. Attempted suicide and completed suicide (5%) are important concerns.

CHAPTER 71

Substance Abuse

The age at which street drugs are first used is decreasing (now <12 years), and females are overtaking males in terms of substance use. Ninety percent of adult smokers begin their habit during the adolescent years. Marijuana and stimulant drug use is increasing. Inhalant use (glue solvents, aerosol products) is prevalent among younger adolescents and in Native Americans. The use of *club drugs* by adolescents from upper-income groups at rave parties (3,4-methylenedioxymethamphetamine ["ecstasy"]) and so-called date-rape drugs (gamma-hydroxybutyrate or flunitrazepam [Rohypnol]) has risen sharply. Anabolic steroid use has increased among adolescent boys seeking enhanced athletic performance.

A history of drug use should be taken in a nonjudgmental and supportive manner and should include the types of substances as well as the frequency, timing, circumstances, and outcomes of substance use. Table 71.1 is a helpful screening tool. There are few physical findings even with chronic adolescent substance use. An adolescent may present in an overdose or in an intoxicated state, or in a psychosis triggered by a hallucinogen, such as phencyclidine ("angel dust"). Club drugs have direct (coma and seizures) and indirect (sexual assault and dehydration) adverse effects. Anabolic steroids also have direct (gynecomastia and testicular atrophy) and indirect (mood swings and violence) adverse effects.

ACUTE OVERDOSE

Decision-Making Algorithms
Available @ StudentConsult.com

Seizures and other paroxysmal disorders
Ataxia
Altered mental status

TABLE 71.1 CRAFFT: A Screening Tool for Adolescent Substance Abuse

C	Car	Driving under the influence of drugs
R	Relax	Using drugs to relax, fit in, feel better
A	Alone	Drugs/alcohol consumption while alone
F	Forgetting	Forgetting things as a result of drugs/alcohol
F	Family/friends	Family and friends tell teen to stop/cut down
T	Trouble	Getting into trouble because of drugs/alcohol

Many drugs (most commonly alcohol, amphetamines, opiates, and cocaine) can result in a toxicological emergency, often with first-time use (Table 71.2). Initial management should be directed at appropriate supportive medical treatment, with follow-up counseling after the toxic effects have diminished.

ACUTE AND CHRONIC EFFECTS

Heavy alcohol use can cause acute gastritis and acute pancreatitis. Intravenous drug use can result in hepatitis B, bacterial endocarditis, osteomyelitis, septic pulmonary embolism, infection, and acquired immunodeficiency syndrome (AIDS). Chronic marijuana or tobacco use is associated with bronchoconstriction and bronchitis. Compulsive drug or alcohol use results in an adolescent being unable to navigate out of the psychosocial sequelae that attend such habituation (e.g., stealing, prostitution, drug dealing, unemployment, school failure, social isolation).

TREATMENT

Specific management of substance use by adolescents depends on many individual patient factors. Because of the highly addictive (physical and psychological) nature of many substances, residential drug treatment facilities are suggested, especially for younger adolescents.

TABLE 71.2 Substances Abused by Adolescents: Names and Acute Effects

SUBSTANCE (STREET/ALTERNATIVE NAME)	EFFECTS AND FACTS	ROUTE OF ADMINISTRATION (TIME OF ACTION)	DETECTION
Alcohol/Liquor	Disinhibition, ataxia, slurred speech, respiratory and CNS depression	Oral (depends on amount and tolerance)	Urine and blood
Nicotine	Relaxation, CNS dependence, ↑ blood pressure, ↑ heart rate, ↓ temperature	Inhaled (minutes); snuffed, dipped, chewed	Urine up to 1 mo
Marijuana (cannabis, weed, joints)	Euphoria, relaxation, ↑ appetite, ↓ reaction time	Inhaled (minutes) Oral (30 min+)	Urine up to 1 mo
STIMULANTS			
Cocaine (coke, crack)	Alertness, euphoria Insomnia, ↓ appetite, irritability, paranoia	Inhaled and snorted (quick high); Oral (longer effect)	Urine up to 48 hr
Amphetamines (bennies, black beauties, ice)	Insomnia, ↓ appetite, irregular heartbeat, hypertension	Inhaled, oral, injection	
HALLUCINOGENS			
Mescaline (buttons, cactus, mesc)	Psychosis, dilated pupils	Injected, sniffed, ingested (onset: 20-90 min; duration 6-12 hr)	Immunoassay
Psilocybin (magic mushrooms, shrooms)	Dysphoria	Ingested (dry, raw mushrooms; tea) (onset: 20-90 min; duration 6-12 hr)	
LSD (acid)	"Artistic high" "Lucy in the sky with diamonds"	Oral: Tablets, liquid, absorbed through mouth using drug-soaked paper (onset: 20-90 min; duration 6-12 hr)	
Phencyclidine (PCP, angel dust)	Microdots in many colors Can induce suicide attempts	Ingested, inhaled, injected (onset: 20-90 min; duration 6-12 hr)	
MDMA (ecstasy, molly) (both stimulant and hallucinogen)	Euphoria, drowsiness, memory impairment	Oral: tablet or liquid (duration: 3-6 hr)	Ecstasy not detected by urine screen

TABLE 71.2 Substances Abused by Adolescents: Names and Acute Effects—cont'd

SUBSTANCE (STREET/ ALTERNATIVE NAME)	EFFECTS AND FACTS	ROUTE OF ADMINISTRATION (TIME OF ACTION)	DETECTION
OPIATES	Euphoria, ataxia, miosis, slurred speech	Oral, IV, smoked, snorted, and sniffed	Urine or blood
Heroin (H, horse, smack)	Euphoria, alternating wakefulness and drowsiness	Injected, smoked, snorted	
Opium and heroin (free base)	A common adolescent mix	Injected, smoked	
Oxycodone (cotton, hillbilly)	Pain relief, sedation	Oral, IV, inhaled	
TRANQUILIZERS			
Flunitrazepam (Rohypnol, roofies, date rape drugs)		Often mixed in alcohol	Urine 1-24 hr
Sedatives (barbs, downers)	Sedation	Oral	Urine or blood
INHALANTS (SOLVENTS, GASOLINE)	Like alcohol	Inhaled	
ANABOLIC STEROIDS	To enhance athletic performance	Oral	Urine

Common side effects (with suggested treatment) of substance abuse drugs are paranoia (haloperidol), seizures (diazepam), hyperthermia (slow cooling), hypertension (β-blockers), and opiate overdose (naloxone).
CNS, Central nervous system; EDMA, 3,4-ethylenedioxy-N-methylamphetamine; LSD, lysergic acid diethylamide; PCP, phencyclidine.
Data from U.S. Department of Health and Human Services. Reducing Tobacco Use: A Report of the Surgeon General. Atlanta, Georgia: U.S. Department of Health and Human Services, Centers for Disease Control and Prevention, National Center for Chronic Disease Prevention and Health Promotion, Office on Smoking and Health. https://www.cdc.gov/tobacco/data_statistics/sgr/2000/complete_report/index.htm; 2000.

Suggested Readings

ACOG Committee Opinion No 651. Menstruation in girls and adolescents: using the menstrual cycle as a vital sign. *Obstet Gynecol.* 2015;126(6):e143–e146.

Blake K, Mann K, Kutcher M. The structured communication adolescent guide (SCAG). *MedEdPORTAL.* https://www.mededportal.org/publication/798; 2008. Accessed November 8, 2016.

Brodie N, Silberholz EA, Spector ND, et al. Important considerations in adolescent health maintenance: long acting reversible contraception, human papillomavirus vaccination and heavy menstrual bleeding. *Curr Opin Pediatr.* 2016;28(6):778–785.

Das JK, Salam RA, Arshad A, et al. Interventions for adolescent substance abuse: an overview of systematic reviews. *J Adolesc Health.* 2016;59(4S):S 61–S75.

Fleming N, O'Driscoll T, Becker G, et al; CANPAGO COMMITTEE. Adolescent pregnancy guidelines. *J Obstet Gynaecol Can.* 2015;37(8):740–759.

Hartman L, Monasterio E, Hwang L. Adolescent contraception: review and guidance for pediatric clinicians. *Curr Probl Pediatr Adolesc Health Care.* 2012;24:221–263.

Keel PK, Brown TA. Update on course and outcome in eating disorders. *Int J Eat Disord.* 2010;43(3):195–204.

Klein D, Goldenring J, Adelman W. HEEADSSS 3.0 the psychosocial interview for adolescents updated for a new century fueled by media. *Contemp Pediatr.* 2014;31:16–28.

Lauterstein D, Hoshino R, Gordon T, et al. The changing face of tobacco use among United States youth. *Curr Drug Abuse Rev.* 2014;7(1): 29–43.

Norris ML, Spettigue WJ, Katzman DK. Update on eating disorders: current perspectives on avoidant/restrictive food intake disorder in children and youth. *Neuropsychiatr Dis Treat.* 2016;12:213–218.

The Emergency Contraception Website. Office of Population Research, Princeton, NJ. http://ec.princeton.edu/; 2016 Accessed November 8, 2016.

Williams C, Creighton S. Menstrual disorders in adolescents: review of current practice. *Horm Res Paediatr.* 2012;78(30):135–143.

PEARLS FOR PRACTITIONERS

CHAPTER 67

Overview and Assessment of Adolescents

General Adolescent

- Leading causes of adolescent deaths in the United States are:
  - Unintentional injuries (i.e., motor vehicle), suicide, homicide
- Physical symptoms in an adolescent are often related to psychosocial problems.
- A psychosocial history including protective and risk-taking behaviors is important.

Key elements for interviewing an adolescent alone:

- Discussing confidentiality
- Separating the caregiver and adolescent
- Being nonjudgmental—build rapport by discussing activities (social media), movies, etc.

- Use HEADDSS approach (**H**ome, **E**ducation [friends/bullies], **A**ctivities/**A**lcohol, **D**rugs [include e-cigarettes], **D**iet, **D**epression/**S**uicide, **S**exual activity, **S**elf).
- Explain which issues cannot be kept confidential: suicidal intent; serious harm to someone else; or experiencing or planning physical or sexual abuse/neglect.

Mature Minor

- Has competence and capacity to understand (is not age-specific)
- Can be treated without parental consent
- Any intervention should be in the best interest of the minor (and documented)

CHAPTER 68

Well-Adolescent Care

Laboratory and Physical Changes

- High hematocrit values (boys > girls) because of androgenic stimulation of the bone marrow
- Alkaline phosphatase levels increase during puberty because of rapid bone turnover
- Worsening of mild scoliosis during growth spurt

Physical growth and development of adolescents (can start earlier in African Americans)

- Females: onset 8-13 years (Tanner stages I to II) with thelarche (breast budding); pubarche (axillary hair, body odor, mild acne)
  - Growth spurt occurs 1 year after thelarche (Tanner stages III to V)
  - Menarche, mean age 12.5 yrs
- Boys: onset 9-14 yrs (Tanner stages I to II) with testicular enlargement; pubarche (axillary and facial hair, body odor, mild acne)
  - Penile enlargement, then growth spurt

STAGE	AGE	CHARACTERISTICS
Early teens	10-14	Focus on appearance; invincible; peer group is everything; no tomorrow; concrete thinking
Middle teens	15-17	Risk taking; experimentation; questioning who am i? no tomorrow; concrete thinking
Late teens	18-21	Future planning; separate from family; partner; formal operational thinking

CHAPTER 69

Adolescent Gynecology

- Evaluation for primary amenorrhea should be initiated by age 15 or earlier in the presence of cyclic pelvic pain, suspicion of an eating disorder, or hyperandrogenism.
- Pregnancy should be excluded in any adolescent presenting with amenorrhea.
- Treatment in reversible causes of hypothalamic amenorrhea (disordered eating/eating disorder, stress) are directed at changing the underlying state to allow resumption of menses.
- Physiological anovulation is the most common etiology of abnormal uterine bleeding (AUB) in adolescents; treatment may still be required if the associated symptoms affect quality of life.
- A coagulopathy should be considered in adolescents with heavy menstrual bleeding that begins at menarche, especially with anemia or a family/personal history of bleeding.
- Polycystic ovary syndrome (PCOS) is difficult to diagnose in adolescence as it overlaps with many physiological changes in puberty; the diagnosis should be considered with the persistence of both infrequent menstrual bleeding and clinical or biochemical hyperandrogenism.
- First-line therapies for primary dysmenorrhea should consider the need for contraception for an adolescent and include combined hormonal contraceptives, progestin-only contraception, and levonorgestrel intrauterine device (IUD).
- Failure of nonsteroidal antiinflammatory drugs (NSAIDs) and hormonal contraceptives for dysmenorrhea should prompt investigation for secondary etiologies such as endometriosis, pelvic inflammatory disease (PID), or müllerian anomalies.
- Multidisciplinary adolescent-specific antenatal care can decrease risks associated with teen pregnancy, such as preterm birth, low birth weight infants, and neonatal admissions to intensive care settings.
- Long-acting reversible contraceptives are an acceptable method for adolescents with high continuation rates and should be offered as first-line methods.
- Users of barrier methods of contraception should be counseled on emergency contraception (EC).

CHAPTER 70

Eating Disorders

Anorexia nervosa (1-2% of teenage girls, female-to-male ratio 20:1)

- Initial signs are behavioral changes in eating, exercise, and mood
- Unrealistic body image "feels too fat" despite appearing excessively thin
- Amenorrhea in postmenarche females
- Diagnostic criteria may be difficult to meet in a younger adolescent
- Physical signs: oversized clothing, fine hair on face and trunk (lanugo-like hair), bradycardia, hypothermia, decreased body mass index, erosion of enamel of teeth

Bulimia (5% in females, female-to-male ratio 10:1)

- Binge eating at least twice a week for 3 months
- Eating excessive food within a set period of time
- Sense of lack of control
- Behavior to prevent gaining weight (vomiting, laxatives, diuretics, and exercise)

When to hospitalize an anorexic patient

- Weight loss >25% of ideal body weight (less weight loss accepted in young adolescent)
- Risk of suicide; outpatient treatment fails
- Bradycardia, hypothermia; dehydration, hypokalemia, dysrhythmias

CHAPTER 71

Substance Abuse

- Use the screening tool CRAFFT (**C**ar, **R**elax, **A**lone, **F**orgetting, **F**amily/Friends, **T**rouble) to screen for risk-taking behaviors.

Substances abused by adolescents

- Depressants, barbiturates, tranquilizers (Rohypnol, "roofies," "date rape" drugs), opioids (heroin, oxycontin, gamma hydroxybutyrate [GHB]), stimulants (amphetamines ["ice"], cocaine ["crack"], methylphenidate [Ritalin]), hallucinogens (D-lysergic acid diethylamide [LSD], phencyclidine [PCP, "angel dust"], psilocybin ["magic mushrooms"]), marijuana (cannabis, "weed"), "ecstasy" (club drugs: combinations [i.e., of hallucinogens and amphetamines]), Anabolic steroids
- Common side effects (with suggested **treatment**) of substance-abuse drugs are paranoia **(haloperidol)**, seizures **(diazepam)**, hyperthermia **(slow cooling)**, hypertension **(β-blockers)**, and opiate overdose **(naloxone)**

IMMUNOLOGY

James W. Verbsky

CHAPTER 72

Immunological Assessment

The major components of host defense include anatomical barriers, and the innate and adaptive immune systems. Integrity of the **anatomical** and **mucociliary barrier** (i.e., skin and mucous membranes) is essential for protection against infection, and defects in this barrier function can lead to infections (Table 72.1). The **innate immune system** acts as the first line of defense against pathogens, responding rapidly but nonspecifically before the development of the more versatile **adaptive immune system**. The **innate immune system** includes soluble factors, including acute-phase proteins, cytokines, chemokines, and complement, as well as cellular components, including neutrophils, monocytes/macrophages, innate lymphoid cells, and natural killer (NK) cells. The **adaptive immune system** is made up of T and B lymphocytes and their effector molecules (Table 72.2).

Recognition of pathogens by the innate immune system is facilitated by receptors on macrophages, NK cells, and neutrophils that recognize conserved pathogen motifs called **pathogen-associated molecular patterns (PAMPs)**, including lipopolysaccharide of gram-negative bacteria, lipoteichoic acid of gram-positive bacteria, mannans of yeast, and specific nucleotide sequences of bacterial and viral DNA. Recognition of PAMPs by the innate immune system leads to the production of cytokines that initiate inflammation and induce an acute phase response (e.g., C-reactive protein, mannose-binding lectin, complement) and chemokines that recruit inflammatory cells, ultimately resulting in the activation of the adaptive immune system. Complement protein activation on pathogens facilitates their uptake by phagocytic cells or results in lysis of pathogens. Polymorphonuclear neutrophils ingest pyogenic bacteria and some fungi. Macrophages are effective in killing facultative intracellular organisms such as *Mycobacterium, Toxoplasma, Salmonella*, and *Legionella*. NK lymphocytes mediate cytotoxic activity against virus-infected cells and cancer cells.

The key features of the **adaptive immune system** are antigen specificity and the development of immunological memory, produced by expansion and maturation of antigen-specific T cells and B cells. Antibodies (immunoglobulin) produced by **B cells** neutralize toxins released by pathogens, opsonize pathogens to facilitate uptake by phagocytic cells, activate complement causing cytolysis of the pathogen, and direct NK cells to kill infected cells through antibody-mediated cytotoxicity. **T cells** kill virus-infected cells and cancer cells, activate macrophage to kill intracellular pathogens, and deliver the necessary signals for B-cell antibody synthesis and memory B-cell formation. Immunodeficiency can result from defects in one or more components of innate or adaptive immunity, leading to recurrent, opportunistic, or life-threatening infections. Primary

TABLE 72.1 Anatomical and Mucociliary Defects that Result in Recurrent or Opportunistic Infections

ANATOMICAL DEFECTS IN UPPER AIRWAYS
Aspiration syndromes (gastroesophageal reflux, ineffective cough, foreign body)
Cleft palate, eustachian tube dysfunction
Adenoidal hypertrophy
Nasal polyps
Obstruction of paranasal sinus drainage (osteomeatal complex disease), encephaloceles
Post-traumatic or congenital sinus tracts (CSF rhinorrhea)
ANATOMICAL DEFECTS IN THE TRACHEOBRONCHIAL TREE
Tracheoesophageal fistula, bronchobiliary fistula
Pulmonary sequestration, bronchogenic cysts
Vascular ring
Tumor, foreign body, or enlarged lymph nodes
PHYSIOLOGICAL DEFECTS IN UPPER AND LOWER AIRWAYS
Primary ciliary dyskinesia syndromes
Cystic fibrosis
Bronchopulmonary dysplasia
Bronchiectasis
Allergic disease (allergic rhinitis, asthma)
Chronic cigarette smoke exposure
OTHER DEFECTS
Burns
Chronic atopic dermatitis
Ureteral obstruction, vesicoureteral reflux
IV drug use
Central venous line, artificial heart value, CSF shunt, peritoneal dialysis catheter, urinary catheter
Dermal sinus tract

CSF, Cerebrospinal fluid; *IV*, intravenous.

TABLE 72.2 Cytokines and Chemotactic Cytokines and Their Functions

FACTOR	SOURCE	FUNCTION
IL-1	Macrophages	Co-stimulatory effect on T cells, enhances antigen presentation, acute phase response, fever
IL-2	T cells	Primary T-cell growth factor; B-cell and NK cell growth factors; required for T-regulatory cell function and survival
IL-3	T cells	Mast cell growth factor; multicolony-stimulating factor
IL-4	T cells	T-cell growth factor; enhances IgE synthesis; enhances B-cell differentiation; mast cell growth
IL-5	T cells	Enhances eosinophil differentiation; enhances immunoglobulin synthesis; enhances IgA synthesis
IL-6	T cells, macrophages, fibroblasts, endothelium	Enhances immunoglobulin synthesis, antiviral activity, induces acute phase response, fever, hematopoietic effects
IL-7	Stromal cells	Enhances growth of pre-T cells
IL-8	T cells, macrophages, epithelium	Neutrophil-activating protein; T-lymphocyte and neutrophil chemotactic factor
IL-9	T cells	Acts in synergy with IL-4 to induce IgE production, mast cell growth
IL-10	T cells, including regulatory T cells, macrophages	Cytokine synthesis inhibitory factor; suppresses macrophage function; enhances B-cell growth; inhibits IL-12 production; suppresses inflammation at mucosal surfaces
IL-12	Macrophages, neutrophils	NK cell stimulatory factor; cytotoxic lymphocyte maturation factor; enhances IFN-γ synthesis; inhibits IL-4 synthesis
IL-13	T cells	Enhances IgE synthesis; enhances B-cell growth; inhibits macrophage activation; causes airway hyperreactivity
IL-17	T cells	Induces IL-1β and IL-6 synthesis, important in fungal infections
IL-18	Macrophages	Enhances IFN-γ synthesis
IFN-γ	T cells	Macrophage activation; inhibits IgE synthesis; antiviral activity
TGF-β	T cells, including regulatory T cells, many other cells	Inhibits T-cell and B-cell proliferation and activation, induces T-regulatory cells
RANTES	T cells, endothelium	Chemokine for monocytes, T cells, eosinophils
MIP-1α	Mononuclear cells, endothelium	Chemokine for T cells; enhances differentiation of $CD4^+$ T cells
Eotaxin 1, 2, and 3	Epithelium, endothelium, eosinophils, fibroblasts, macrophages	Chemokine for eosinophils, basophils, and Th2 cells
IP-10	Monocytes, macrophages, endothelium	Chemokine for activated T cells, monocytes, and NK cells

IFN, Interferon; *Ig*, immunoglobulin; *IL*, interleukin; *NK*, natural killer; *RANTES*, regulated on activation, normal T expressed and secreted; *TGF-β*, transforming growth factor β; *Th2*, T-helper 2.

immunodeficiency diseases are relatively rare individually, but together they cause significant chronic disease, morbidity, and mortality (Table 72.3).

HISTORY

The frequency, severity, and location of infections and the pathogens involved can help differentiate infections in a normal host from infections in an immunodeficient patient (see Table 72.3). Although otitis media and sinopulmonary infections are common in children, recurrent infections, invasive or deep seeded infections, infections that require multiple rounds of oral or intravenous antibiotics, or infections with opportunistic infections suggest a primary immunodeficiency. Recurrent sinopulmonary infections with encapsulated bacteria suggest a defect in antibody-mediated immunity because these pathogens evade phagocytosis. Failure to thrive, diarrhea, malabsorption, and infections with opportunistic infections (i.e., fungi, *Candida* sp, *Pneumocystis jiroveci [carinii]*) suggest T-cell immunodeficiency. Recurrent viral infections can result from T-cell or NK-cell deficiency. Deep-seated abscesses and infections with *Staphylococcus aureus, Serratia marcescens,* and *Aspergillus* suggest a disorder of neutrophil function, such as chronic granulomatous disease (CGD). Delayed separation of the umbilical cord, especially in the presence of omphalitis and later onset periodontal disease, in addition to poorly formed abscesses, indicates leukocyte adhesion deficiency. Neisserial infections or early onset autoimmunity may suggest a complement defect.

Age of onset of symptoms can be helpful in defining an immune deficiency, although significant variability does occur. Neutrophil defects (e.g., congenital neutropenia, leukocyte adhesion deficiency) typically present in the first several months of life. Antibody defects (e.g., agammaglobulinemia) and T-cell defects (e.g., severe combined immunodeficiency [SCID]) typically present after 3 months of life after maternal antibody levels have waned. Presentation with symptoms of an antibody deficiency in adolescence or young adulthood suggests common variable immunodeficiency (CVID) rather than congenital agammaglobulinemia, although milder phenotypes of primary

TABLE 72.3 Clinical Characteristics of Primary Immunodeficiencies

B-CELL DEFECTS
Recurrent pyogenic infections with extracellular encapsulated organisms, such as *Streptococcus pneumoniae, Haemophilus influenzae* type b, and group A streptococcus
Otitis, sinusitis, recurrent pneumonia, bronchiectasis, and conjunctivitis
Few problems with fungal or viral infections (except enterovirus and poliomyelitis)
Diarrhea common, especially secondary to infection with *Giardia lamblia*
Minimal growth retardation
Compatible with survival to adulthood or for several years after onset unless complications occur
COMPLEMENT DEFECTS
Recurrent bacterial infections with extracellular encapsulated organisms, such as *S. pneumoniae* and *H. influenzae*
Susceptibility to recurrent infections with *Neisseria meningitides*
Increased incidence of autoimmune disease
Severe or recurrent skin and respiratory tract infection
T-CELL DEFECTS
Recurrent infections with less virulent or opportunistic organisms, such as fungi, *Candida* sp, mycobacteria, viruses, and protozoa as well as bacteria
Growth retardation, malabsorption, diarrhea, and failure to thrive common
Anergy
Susceptible to graft versus host disease from nonirradiated blood or from maternal engraftment
Fatal reactions may occur from live virus or bacille Calmette-Guérin vaccination
Increased incidence of malignancy
Poor survival beyond infancy or early childhood
NEUTROPHIL DEFECTS
Recurrent dermatological infections with bacteria such as *Staphylococcus, Pseudomonas,* and *Escherichia coli,* and fungi such as *Aspergillus*
Subcutaneous, lymph node, lung, and liver abscesses
Pulmonary infections common, including abscess and pneumatocele formation, contributing to chronic disease
Bone and joint infection common
Delayed separation of umbilical cord
Absence of pus at site(s) of infection
Poor wound healing

immunodeficiency disease may not present until later in life. The presence of associated problems, such as congenital heart disease and hypocalcemia (DiGeorge syndrome), abnormal gait and telangiectasia (ataxia-telangiectasia), atopic dermatitis (hyper-IgE syndrome, Omenn syndrome), and easy bruising or a bleeding disorder (Wiskott-Aldrich syndrome), can be informative in guiding an immune work-up. A **family history** of a primary immune deficiency or death of a young child due to infections should prompt an immune evaluation, particularly in the setting of recurrent infections.

TABLE 72.4 Causes of Secondary Immunodeficiency

VIRAL INFECTIONS
HIV (destroys CD4 T cells)
Measles
Rubella
Influenza
METABOLIC DISORDERS
Diabetes mellitus
Malnutrition
Uremia
Sickle cell disease
Zinc and vitamin deficiency
Multiple carboxylase deficiency
Burns
PROTEIN-LOSING STATES
Nephrotic syndrome
Protein-losing enteropathy
OTHER CAUSES
Prematurity
Immunosuppressive agents (e.g., corticosteroids, radiation, and antimetabolites)
Malignancy (leukemia, Hodgkin disease, nonlymphoid cancer)
Acquired asplenia
Acquired neutropenia (autoimmune, viral, or drug-induced)
Stem cell transplantation/graft versus host disease
Systemic lupus erythematosus and other autoimmune diseases
Sarcoidosis

PHYSICAL EXAMINATION

Recurrent infection in immune deficient children is associated with pathology at sites of infection resulting in substantial morbidity, such as scarring of tympanic membranes leading to hearing loss, chronic lung disease due to recurrent pneumonia, or failure to thrive due to gastrointestinal involvement. Height and weight percentiles, nutritional status, and presence of subcutaneous fat should be assessed. Oral thrush, purulent nasal or otic discharge, and chronic rales may be evidence of repeated or persistent infections. Absence of lymphoid tissue (e.g., tonsils) suggests agammaglobulinemia or SCID, whereas increased size of lymphoid tissue suggests CVID, CGD, or human immunodeficiency virus (HIV) infection. Cerebellar ataxia and telangiectasia indicate ataxia-telangiectasia. Severe eczema and inflammatory bowel disease are seen in the immune regulation with polyendocrinopathy and enteropathy that is X-linked (IPEX) syndrome, whereas eczema and petechiae or bruises suggest Wiskott-Aldrich syndrome.

DIFFERENTIAL DIAGNOSIS

There are many secondary causes of immunodeficiency that should be considered, particularly if the immunological testing is nonrevealing (Table 72.4). In patients with primary immunodeficiencies, infections develop at multiple sites (e.g., ears, sinuses, lungs, skin), whereas in individuals with anatomical problems (e.g., sequestered pulmonary lobe, ureteral reflux), infections are confined to a single anatomical site. Asplenia is associated with recurrent and severe infections, even in the presence of protective antibody titers. Infection with HIV should be considered in any patient presenting with a history suggesting a T-cell immunodeficiency.

DIAGNOSTIC EVALUATION

The diagnosis of patients with primary immunodeficiency diseases depends on early recognition of signs and symptoms of primary immunodeficiency, followed by laboratory tests to evaluate immune function (see Table 72.3; Fig. 72.1).

Laboratory Tests

A diagnosis of primary immunodeficiency disease cannot be established without the use of laboratory tests based on the clinical history (Table 72.5). A **complete blood count with differential** should always be obtained to identify patients with neutropenia or lymphopenia (SCID) as well as the presence of eosinophils (allergic disease) and anemia (chronic disease). **Serum immunoglobulin levels** are essential to the work-up of suspected primary immunodeficiency. Antibody levels vary with age, with normal adult values of immunoglobulin G (IgG) at full-term birth from transplacental transfer of maternal IgG, a physiological nadir occurring between 3 and 6 months of age, and a gradual increase to adult values over several years. IgA and IgM are low at birth, and levels increase gradually over several years, with IgA taking the longest to reach normal adult values. Low albumin levels with low immunoglobulin levels suggest low synthetic rates for all proteins or increased loss of proteins, as in protein-losing enteropathy. High immunoglobulin levels suggest intact B-cell immunity and can be found in diseases with recurrent infections, such as CGD, immotile cilia syndrome, cystic fibrosis, HIV infection, and autoimmune diseases. Elevated IgE levels can be found in a number of immune deficiencies such as hyper-IgE syndrome, as well as in atopic individuals.

Specific antibody titers after childhood vaccination (tetanus, diphtheria, *Haemophilus influenzae* type b, or *Streptococcus pneumoniae* vaccines) reflect the capacity of the immune system to synthesize specific antibodies and to develop memory B cells. If titers are low, immunization with a specific vaccine and titers obtained 4-6 weeks later confirm response to the immunization. Poor response to bacterial polysaccharide antigens is normal before 24 months of age but is also associated with IgG subclass deficiency or specific antibody deficiency. The development of protein-conjugate polysaccharide vaccines has prevented infections with encapsulated organisms in early childhood. Antibody responses to the *S. pneumoniae* serotypes found in the 23-valent

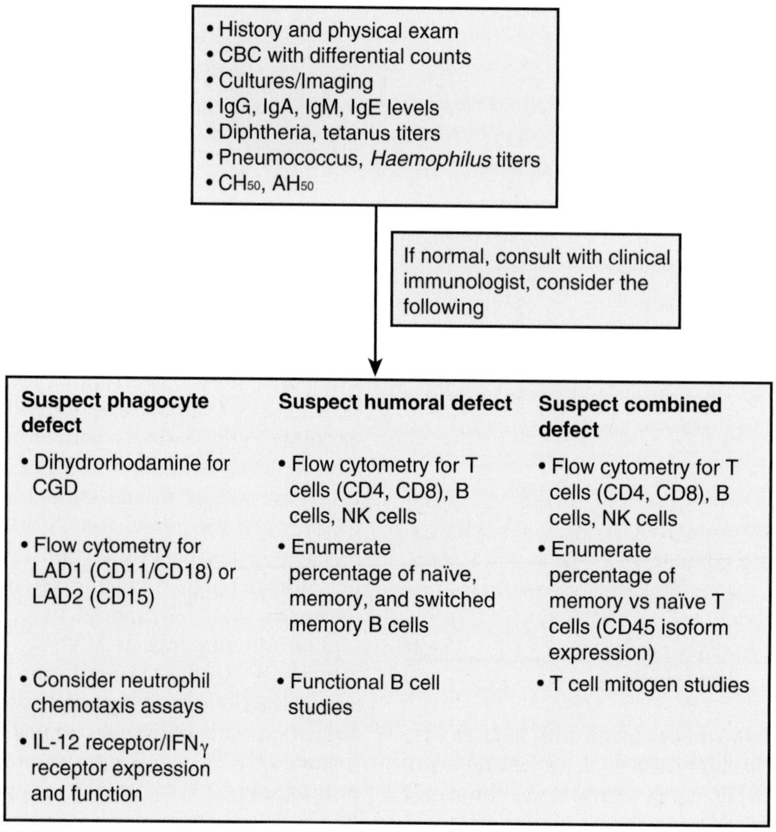

FIGURE 72.1 Initial work-up and follow-up studies of patients with suspected immune deficiency. Consultation with a clinical immunologist is recommended to guide advanced testing and interpret results. *CBC*, Complete blood count; *CGD*, chronic granulomatous disease; *IFN*, interferon; *Ig*, immunoglobulin; *IL*, interleukin; *LAD*, leukocyte adhesion defect; *NK*, natural killer cell. (From Kliegman RM, Lye PS, Bordini BJ, Toth H, Basel D, eds. *Nelson Pediatric Symptom-Based Diagnosis*. Philadelphia: Elsevier; 2018, Fig. 41.1.)

TABLE 72.5 Tests for Suspected Immune Deficiency

GENERAL
Complete blood count, including hemoglobin, differential white blood cell count and morphology, and platelet count
Radiographs to document infection in chest, sinus, mastoids, and long bones, if indicated by clinical history
Cultures, if appropriate
ANTIBODY-MEDIATED IMMUNITY
Quantitative immunoglobulin levels: IgG, IgA, IgM, IgE, isohemagglutinin titers (anti-A, anti-B, measures IgM function)
Specific antibody levels:
Protein antigens: diphtheria, tetanus
Protein-conjugated antigens: *Haemophilus influenzae, Streptococcus pneumoniae* (conjugate vaccine)
Polysaccharide antigens: *S. pneumoniae* (unconjugated vaccine)
B-cell numbers and subsets by flow cytometry
CELL-MEDIATED IMMUNITY
Lymphocyte count and morphology
Delayed hypersensitivity skin tests (*Candida*, tetanus toxoid, mumps): measure T-cell and macrophage function
T-cell and NK cell numbers and subsets by flow cytometry
T-lymphocyte functional analyses (mitogen responses, cytokines)
NK cell cytotoxicity assays
PHAGOCYTE FUNCTION
Neutrophil cell count and morphology
Nitroblue tetrazolium dye test/dihydrorhodamine 123 using flow cytometry
Staphylococcal killing, chemotaxis assay
Myeloperoxidase stain
COMPLEMENT
Total hemolytic complement CH_{50}: measures classic and common pathway activity
AH_{50}: measures alternative and common pathway activity
Levels of individual complement components
C1-inhibitor level and function

Ig, Immunoglobulin; *NK*, natural killer.

polysaccharide vaccine, but not in the conjugate vaccine, can be used to test antibody responses to polysaccharide antigens.

Delayed-type hypersensitivity skin tests to protein antigens such as tetanus, diphtheria, *Candida*, or mumps demonstrate the presence of antigen-specific T cells and functional antigen-presenting cells. If delayed-type hypersensitivity skin test results are negative, patients should receive a booster vaccination and be retested 4 weeks later.

Lymphocyte phenotyping by flow cytometry enumerates the percentage and absolute numbers of T-cell, B-cell, and NK-cell subsets. Flow cytometry can also test for the presence of proteins that are necessary for normal immunity, such as major histocompatibility complex molecules or adhesion molecules, as well as intracellular analysis of signaling proteins and cytokines. **T-cell proliferation** assays to mitogens (phytohemagglutinin, concanavalin A, pokeweed mitogen, or CD3) or antigens (tetanus toxoid or *Candida*) are in vitro assays that confirm the capacity of T cells to proliferate in response to a nonspecific stimulus (mitogens) or the presence of antigen-specific memory T cells (antigens). **Tests for cytokine synthesis, intracellular signaling pathways, or expression of activation markers** may be performed in specialized research laboratories.

Complement assays include the CH_{50} test, which measures the presence of proteins in the classic pathway of complement (C1, C2, C3, C4), and the AH_{50} test, which tests the proteins of the alternative pathway of complement (C3, factor B, properdin). If both the CH_{50} and AH_{50} levels are abnormal, a defect in the common pathway is likely (C5-C9). Specialized laboratories can measure the presence or function of specific complement proteins. Tests for C1-inhibitor antigen levels and function are used to diagnose hereditary or acquired angioneurotic edema.

Tests for neutrophil function include the nitroblue tetrazolium (NBT) or dihydrorhodamine 123 (DHR) test for CGD, in which oxygen radicals generated by activated neutrophils reduce NBT to an insoluble blue dye and DHR to a fluorescent molecule. Patients with CGD have no blue-staining neutrophils with NBT and little fluorescence when DHR is used. In vitro tests for evaluation of neutrophil phagocytosis, chemotaxis, and bacterial killing are available in some laboratories. Tests for the expression of adhesion molecules such as CD18 (leukocyte function–associated antigen type 1, LFA-1) and CD15 (LFA-2) can be performed by flow cytometry.

Genetic testing to confirm the diagnosis of a primary immunodeficiency can be performed in specialized laboratories and may be helpful for deciding on a course of treatment, determining the natural history and prognosis of the disease, genetic counseling, and prenatal diagnosis. In patients in whom DiGeorge syndrome is suspected, fluorescent in situ hybridization or chromosomal microarray studies for deletions of chromosome 22 can be helpful. In patients in whom ataxia-telangiectasia is suspected, chromosomal studies for breakage in chromosomes 7 and 14 are useful.

Diagnostic Imaging

The absence of a thymus on chest x-ray suggests DiGeorge syndrome or other defects in T-cell development. Abnormalities in the cerebellum are found in patients with ataxia-telangiectasia. Otherwise the use of diagnostic imaging in the evaluation of immunodeficiency diseases is essentially limited to the diagnosis of infectious diseases.

CHAPTER 73

Lymphocyte Disorders

Disorders that affect lymphocyte development or function result in significant immunodeficiency because lymphocytes provide antigen specificity and memory responses. Hematopoietic stem cells give rise to lymphoid precursors that develop into T lymphocytes in the thymus or B lymphocytes in the bone marrow (Fig. 73.1). Isolated B-cell disorders result in **antibody deficiency diseases,** whereas T-cell disorders usually cause **combined immunodeficiency** because they are necessary for cell-mediated immunity to clear intracellular pathogens and for antibody synthesis by B cells. Natural killer (NK) cells are an important

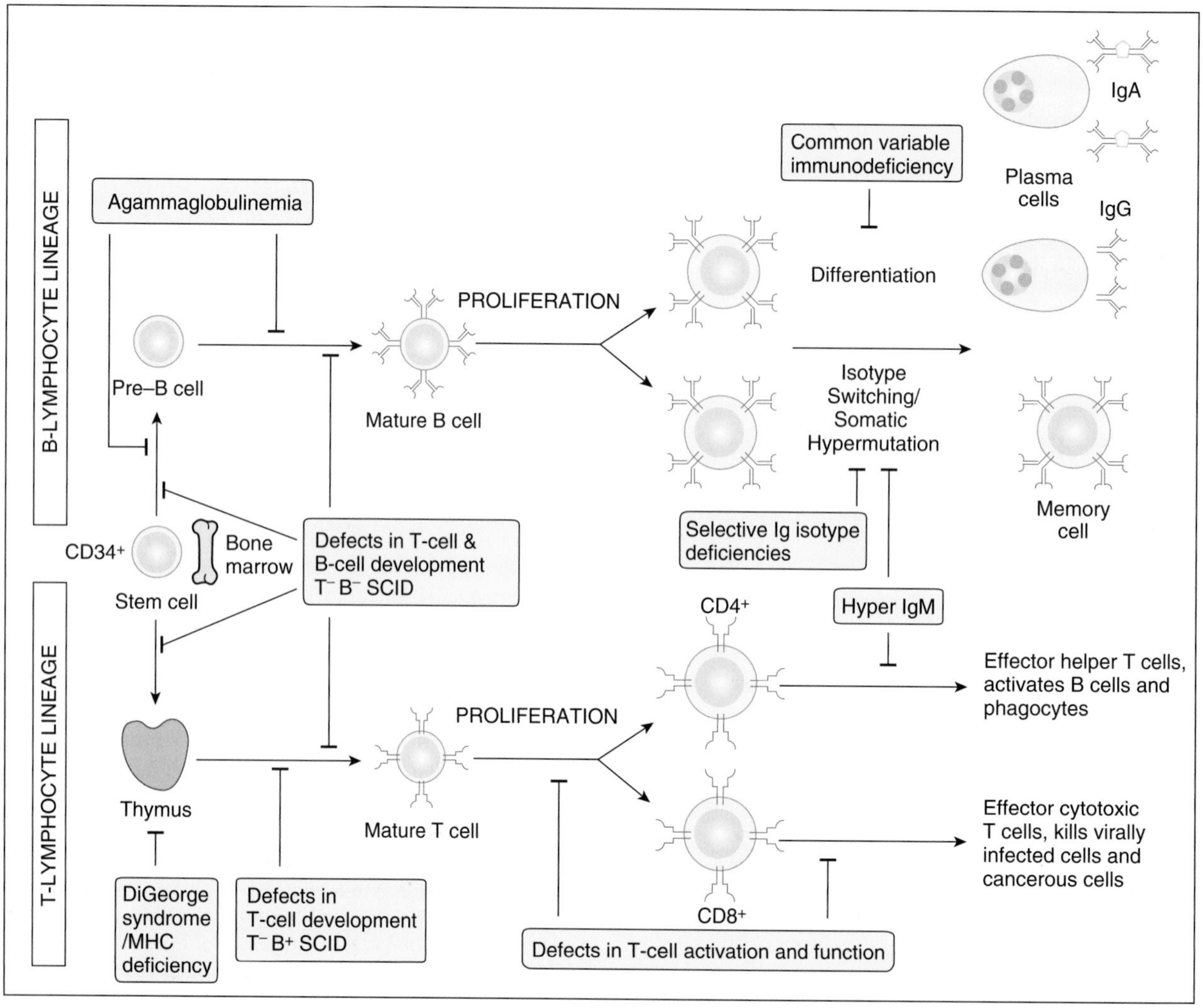

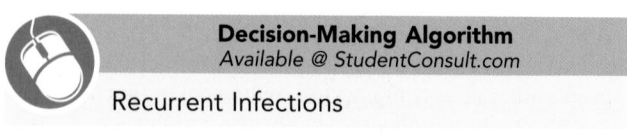

FIGURE 73.1 Sites of cellular abnormalities in congenital immunodeficiencies. In primary immunodeficiency diseases, the maturation or activation of B or T lymphocytes may be blocked at different stages. *B*, B lymphocyte; *Ig*, immunoglobulin; *MHC*, major histocompatibility complex; *SCID*, severe combined immunodeficiency; *T*, T lymphocyte. (Modified from Abbas AK, Lichtman AH, Pober JS. *Cellular and Molecular Immunology*. 3rd ed. Philadelphia: Saunders; 1997.)

component of the **innate immune response**, develop from lymphoid precursors, and can kill virus-infected cells and tumor cells. Antibodies can enhance NK cell function by antibody-mediated cellular cytotoxicity.

ETIOLOGY AND CLINICAL MANIFESTATIONS

Antibody Deficiency Diseases

Decision-Making Algorithm
Available @ StudentConsult.com

Recurrent Infections

Disorders of B cells result in an increased susceptibility to infections by encapsulated bacteria and certain viruses.

Agammaglobulinemia results from the absence or defective function of B cells with subsequent severe decrease in immunoglobulin (Ig) levels and an absence of specific antibody. **X-linked agammaglobulinemia** affects males and is characterized by a profound deficiency of B cells, severe hypogammaglobulinemia, and absence of lymphoid tissue (Table 73.1; see Fig. 73.1). The defect is caused by mutations in a gene encoding the tyrosine kinase *Btk* on chromosome Xq22 that is involved in signaling of the pre–B-cell receptor and the B-cell antigen receptor. **Autosomal recessive agammaglobulinemia** results from defects in components of the pre–B-cell and B-cell antigen receptor complexes and includes mutations in the μ heavy chain gene, γ5, Igα, Igβ, and BLNK. X-linked agammaglobulinemia is more common than the autosomal recessive forms.

Patients with agammaglobulinemia usually present during the first 6-12 months of life as maternally derived antibodies wane, although patients can present years later. These patients develop infections with *Streptococcus pneumoniae, Haemophilus influenzae* type b, *Staphylococcus aureus,* and *Pseudomonas,* organisms for which antibody is an important opsonin. They also have increased susceptibility to giardiasis and enteroviral infections, leading to chronic enteroviral meningoencephalitis and vaccine-associated poliomyelitis (if immunized with oral live, attenuated poliovirus vaccine).

Common variable immunodeficiency (CVID) is a heterogeneous disorder characterized by hypogammaglobulinemia

TABLE 73.1 Antibody Deficiency Diseases

DISORDER	GENETICS	ONSET	MANIFESTATIONS	PATHOGENESIS	ASSOCIATED FEATURES
Agammaglobulinemia	X-linked, AR	Infancy (6-9 mo)	Recurrent infections, sinusitis, pneumonia, meningitis (encapsulated bacteria, enteroviruses)	Arrest in B-cell differentiation (pre-B level); mutations in: *Btk* gene (X-linked); μ chain, BLNK, Igα, Igβ, γ5, BLNK (AR)	Lymphoid hypoplasia
Common variable immunodeficiency	AR; AD; sporadic	2nd to 3rd decade	Sinusitis, bronchitis, pneumonia, chronic diarrhea	Arrest in plasma cell differentiation, mutations in ICOS, TACI, CD19, CD81, CD20, CD21	Autoimmune disease, RA, SLE, Graves disease, ITP, malignancy, granulomatous disease
Transient hypogammaglobulinemia of infancy		Infancy (3-7 mo)	Recurrent viral and pyogenic infections	Unknown; delayed plasma cell maturation	Frequently in families with other immunodeficiencies
IgA deficiency	Variable	Variable	Sinopulmonary infections; can be normal	Failure of IgA expression	IgG subclass deficiency common, autoimmune diseases
IgG subclass deficiency	Variable	Variable	Sinopulmonary infections; can be normal	Defect in IgG isotype production	IgA deficiency, ataxia telangiectasia, polysaccharide antibody deficiency
Specific antibody deficiency	Variable	After 2 years of age	Sinopulmonary infections	Unknown	IgG subclass deficiency
Hyper-IgM syndrome	AR	Variable	Sinopulmonary infections	Defect in AID, UNG	Autoimmunity

AD, Autosomal dominant; *AID,* activation-induced cytidine deaminase; *AR,* autosomal recessive; *Ig,* immunoglobulin; *ITP,* idiopathic thrombocytopenic purpura; *RA,* rheumatoid arthritis; *SLE,* systemic lupus erythematosus; *UNG,* uracil-DNA glycosylase.

developing after an initial period of normal immune function, most commonly in the second and third decades of life (see Table 73.1). Serum immunoglobulin G (IgG) levels are less than 500 mg/dL (usually <300 mg/dL) with IgA levels less than 10 mg/dL and/or low IgM levels. Antibody titers to protein antigens, such as tetanus and diphtheria, and to polysaccharide antigens, such as pneumococcus, are low or absent. T-cell numbers and function are highly variable, and B-cell numbers can be normal or low. Patients exhibit normal-sized or enlarged tonsils and lymph nodes and may have splenomegaly. They are susceptible to frequent respiratory tract infections due to *S. pneumoniae, H. influenzae* type b, and *Mycoplasma*. Gastrointestinal infections with *Giardia*, *Campylobacter*, *Salmonella*, *Helicobacter,* and enteroviruses are common. Autoimmune hemolytic anemia and thrombocytopenia occur frequently, and granulomatous disease affecting the gastrointestinal tract, liver, and lungs leads to significant morbidity. Cancer, especially lymphoma, is a major cause of mortality.

The gene defects leading to the majority of cases of CVID are unknown. Some patients have a defect in inducible co-stimulator (ICOS) on activated T cells, transmembrane activator and calcium-modulating cyclophilin ligand interactor (TACI), CD19, CD21, CD81, or BAFF-R. It is important to exclude X-linked agammaglobulinemia, X-linked lymphoproliferative disease, or hyper-IgM syndrome as well as other causes of hypogammaglobulinemia, such as hypogammaglobulinemia associated with thymoma, protein losing enteropathy, or medications, before making the diagnosis of CVID.

Selective **IgA deficiency** is defined as serum IgA levels less than 10 mg/dL with normal levels of other Igs. The diagnosis cannot be confirmed until the patient is at least 4 years of age when IgA levels should reach adult levels. Selective IgA deficiency occurs in approximately 1 in 500 individuals. Most patients with selective IgA deficiency are asymptomatic. In others it is associated with recurrent sinopulmonary infections, IgG_2 subclass deficiency, specific antibody deficiency, food allergy, autoimmune disease, or celiac disease. IgA deficiency occurs in families, suggesting autosomal inheritance.

IgG subclass deficiency occurs when the level of antibodies in one or more of the four IgG subclasses is selectively decreased while total IgG levels are normal. Normal individuals can express low levels of one or more subclasses, so a history of recurrent infections is important. An inability to synthesize specific antibody titers to protein or polysaccharide antigens is the best marker of IgG subclass deficiency associated with recurrent infections requiring therapy.

Transient hypogammaglobulinemia of infancy is a temporary condition characterized by a prolongation of the physiological hypogammaglobulinemia of infancy. The Ig nadir at 6 months of age is accentuated, with Ig levels less than 200 mg/dL. Ig levels remain diminished throughout the first year of life and usually increase to normal, age-appropriate levels, generally by 2-4 years of age. The incidence of sinopulmonary infection is increased in some patients. The diagnosis is supported by normal levels of both B and T cells and by normal antibody responses to protein antigens such as diphtheria and tetanus toxoids. The transient nature of this disorder cannot be confirmed, however, until Ig levels return to normal ranges.

Specific antibody deficiency syndrome is characterized by recurrent infections with normal Ig levels and normal lymphocyte numbers and subsets, but an inability to synthesize specific antibody to polysaccharide antigens, such as to the 23-valent pneumococcal vaccine. The pathogenesis of this disorder is unknown. Lack of specific antibody titers explains the recurrent infections and justifies therapy.

Combined Immunodeficiency Diseases

Decision-Making Algorithms
Available @ StudentConsult.com

Petechiae/Purpura
Recurrent Infections

Disorders that affect T-cell development or function usually result in combined immunodeficiency because T cells provide necessary signals for B-cell differentiation. **X-linked hyper-IgM syndrome**, the most common form of hyper-IgM syndrome, is a combined immunodeficiency with deficient T-cell function due to defects in CD40 ligand. Defects in CD40 cause **autosomal recessive hyper-IgM syndrome** and present similarly to X-linked hyper-IgM syndrome (Fig. 73.2 and Table 73.2). Hyper-IgM syndrome is characterized by a failure of Ig isotype switching from IgM and IgD to IgG, IgA, or IgE, and a lack of memory responses. Affected patients have normal or elevated serum levels of IgM with low or absent levels of IgG, IgA, and IgE. Ig isotype switching allows a B cell to maintain antigen specificity while altering Ig function, and is directed by cytokines and interaction between CD40 ligand on CD4 T cells and CD40 on B cells (see Fig. 73.2). Signal transduction via CD40 activates several signaling molecules and transcription factors, including nuclear factor κB (NF-κB) and two enzymes, activation-induced cytidine deaminase (AID) and uracil-DNA glycosylase (UNG), which are required for class switching. Deficiency of AID or UNG presents with a failure of Ig isotype switching without any abnormality in T-cell function. These forms of hyper IgM are antibody deficiency diseases and not combined immunodeficiencies and do not exhibit susceptibility to opportunistic infections (see Table 73.1).

All patients with hyper-IgM syndrome have increased susceptibility to sinopulmonary infections, whereas patients with defects in CD40 ligand or CD40 are susceptible to opportunistic infections, such as *P. jiroveci (carinii)* and *Cryptosporidium parvum*. Signaling via CD40 on B cells and other antigen-presenting cells leads to upregulation of co-stimulatory molecules important for promoting T-cell differentiation and for activating cell-mediated immune responses. The hyper-IgM phenotype is also found in an X-linked disorder associated with ectodermal dysplasia, resulting from defects in the gene encoding the NF-κB essential modulator (NEMO). Patients with defects in NEMO are susceptible to a wider spectrum of infectious organisms, especially meningitis and infection with atypical mycobacteria, because NF-κB signaling is important for the function of both innate and adaptive immune systems.

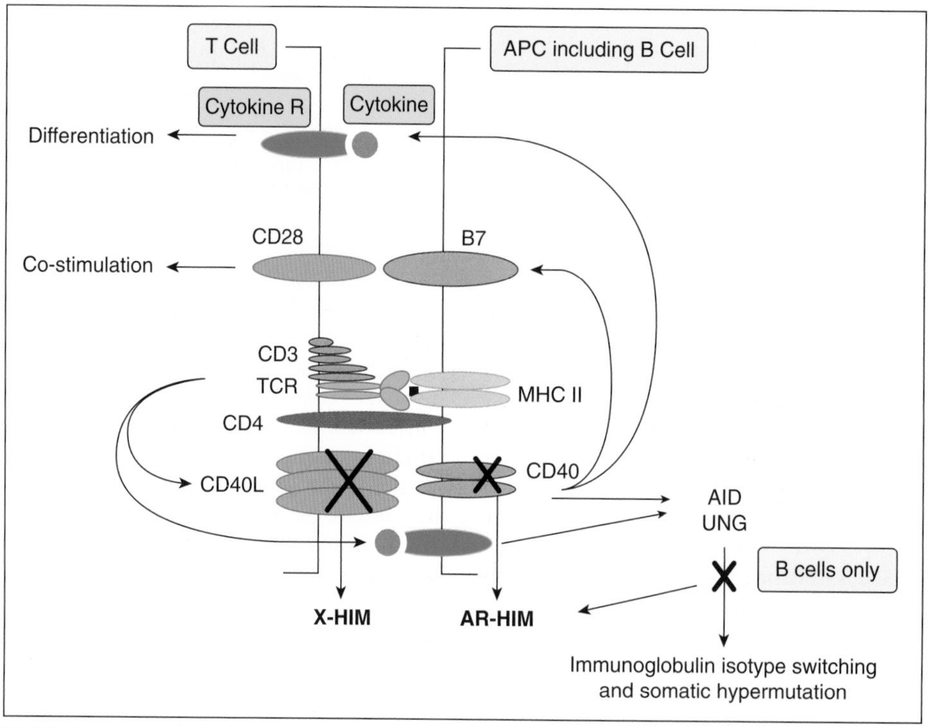

FIGURE 73.2 Schematic representation of the interaction between a CD4 T cell and a B cell. T-cell activation follows T-cell receptor (TCR) recognition of peptide antigen presented via major histocompatibility complex (MHC) class II molecules resulting in CD40 ligand (CD40L) expression and cytokine synthesis. CD40L stimulates the B cell via CD40, resulting in expression of co-stimulatory molecules (B7) that are important in T-cell priming and cytokine synthesis that drives T-cell differentiation. CD40 and cytokine signaling in B cells activate activation-induced cytidine deaminase (AID) and uracil-DNA glycosylase (UNG) to promote Ig isotype switching and somatic hypermutation. Defects in CD40L cause X-linked hyper IgM (X-HIM), and defects in CD40, AID, or UNG cause autosomal recessive hyper IgM (AR-HIM). Defects in either CD40L or CD40 affect T-cell co-stimulation and priming, leading to T-cell defects and susceptibility to opportunistic infections, whereas defects in AID and UNG maintain normal T-cell co-stimulation and function.

TABLE 73.2 Combined Immunodeficiency Diseases

DISORDER	GENETICS	ONSET	MANIFESTATIONS	PATHOGENESIS	ASSOCIATED FEATURES
Hyper-IgM syndrome (see Table 73.1)	X-linked, AR	First year	Sinopulmonary infections, opportunistic infections, *Pneumocystis jiroveci*	Defect in CD40 ligand (X-linked) or CD40 (AR)	Neutropenia, liver disease, cancer
DiGeorge anomaly	22q11.2 (or 10p) deletion	Newborn, early infancy	Hypocalcemic tetany, pyogenic infections, partial or complete T-cell deficiency	Hypoplasia of third and fourth pharyngeal pouch	Congenital heart disease (aortic arch anomalies), hypoparathyroidism, micrognathia, hypertelorism
Severe combined immunodeficiency (T– B+ SCID)	X-linked; AR	1-3 mo	Candidiasis, all types of infections, failure to thrive, chronic diarrhea	Mutation in IL-2Rγ chain, Jak3 kinase, ZAP-70, IL-7Ra, CD3 subunits	GVHD from maternal-fetal transfusions, severe GVHD from nonirradiated blood transfusion
Severe combined immunodeficiency (T– B– SCID)	AR	1-3 mo	Same as T– B+ SCID	Mutation in RAG1/2, Artemis, ADA/PNP deficiency	Same as T– B+ SCID ADA deficiency: chondro-osseous dysplasia PNP deficiency: neurological disorders
Omenn syndrome	AR	1-3 mo	Same as T– B– SCID, exfoliative erythroderma, lymphadenopathy, hepatosplenomegaly	Hypomorphic mutations in SCID-causing genes (RAG1/2, Artemis)	Restricted T-cell receptor heterogeneity, eosinophilia, elevated IgE
Reticular dysgenesis (T– B– SCID)	AR	1-3 mo	Same as T– B– SCID	Defective maturation of common stem cells due to *AK2* mutations	Agammaglobulinemia, alymphocytosis, agranulocytosis
Bare lymphocyte syndrome (MHC class I deficiency)	AR	First decade	Sinopulmonary infections	Mutation in TAP1 or TAP2 (transporter associated with antigen processing)	Decreased CD8 T cells, chronic lung inflammation
Bare lymphocyte syndrome (MHC class II deficiency)	AR	Early infancy	Respiratory tract infections, chronic diarrhea, viral infections	Mutations in CIITA, RFX5, RFXAP, and RFX-B (DNA binding factors)	Decreased CD4 T cells, autoimmune disease

ADA, Adenosine deaminase; *AR,* autosomal recessive; *GVHD,* graft versus host disease; *IL,* interleukin; *IL-2Rγ,* interleukin-2 receptor gamma chain; *MHC,* major histocompatibility complex; *PNP,* purine nucleoside phosphorylase; *SCID,* severe combined immunodeficiency; *T– B+,* T– cells absent and B cells present; *T– B–,* T cells absent and B cells absent.

Severe combined immunodeficiency (SCID) is characterized by a profound lack of T-cell numbers or function, and B-cell dysfunction resulting from the absence of B cells from the gene defect itself, or secondary to lack of T-cell function (see Table 73.2). T cells develop from bone marrow–derived precursors in the thymus (see Fig. 73.2), where they undergo several stages of development characterized by DNA recombination of the variable region of T-cell antigen receptor genes to generate a diverse T-cell receptor repertoire. A process of positive selection occurs in the thymus to select thymocytes with antigen receptors that can interact with major histocompatibility complex (MHC) molecules to ensure their survival (see Fig. 73.2). Thymocytes differentiate into CD4 or CD8 T cells if they interact with MHC class II or class I molecules, respectively. Some of the positively selected thymocytes, however, have antigen receptors that recognize self-antigens presented by MHC molecules in the thymus. These cells are deleted in the thymus by a process of negative selection. Positive selection and negative selection in the thymus ensure that the mature T cells that leave the thymus can function with the individual's MHC molecules and recognize a multitude of foreign antigens without mounting autoimmune responses. SCID can result from any specific genetic mutation that interferes with T-cell development in the thymus or T-cell function in the periphery.

Clinical manifestations of SCID include failure to thrive, severe bacterial infections, chronic candidiasis and other fungal infections, chronic viral infections, infection with *P. jiroveci (carinii)* and other opportunistic organisms, and intractable diarrhea. Patients often have skin disease similar to eczema, possibly related to graft versus host disease (GVHD) from engraftment of maternal lymphocytes, which usually is not fatal. Patients with SCID are extremely susceptible to fatal GVHD from lymphocytes in blood transfusions and can be infected by cytomegalovirus-positive blood products. *Patients with T-cell disorders should always receive irradiated, leukopoor, CMV negative blood products.*

X-linked SCID, the most common form, is caused by mutations in the gene on chromosome Xq13.1 coding for the common gamma chain of the interleukin-2 (IL-2), IL-4, IL-7, IL-9, IL-15, and IL-21 receptors. Affected patients have no T cells or NK cells in the peripheral blood but have normal numbers of B cells. Ig levels are low or undetectable because there are no CD4 T cells to stimulate B cells. The defect in T-cell development results from a failure of signaling via the IL-7 receptor, and IL-15 is required for NK-cell development. There are many causes of **autosomal recessive SCID.** Defects in Janus kinase 3 (Jak3), which binds to the common gamma chain, results in a similar phenotype as X-linked SCID. Defects in the IL-7 receptor, ZAP-70, and subunits of the CD3 molecule result in a deficiency of T cells with normal B-cell and NK-cell numbers. In addition there is a variety of defects that affect DNA recombination in T and B cells, including two genes called *recombinase activating gene (RAG)1* and *RAG2* as well as other genes important in DNA excision and repair such as *Artemis.* Defects in any of the genes that abolish DNA recombination or DNA repair result in autosomal recessive SCID with no T cells or B cells present. Mutations in *RAG1, RAG2,* or *Artemis* that preserve limited function result in **Omenn syndrome,** a variant form of SCID that is characterized by exfoliative erythroderma, lymphadenopathy, hepatosplenomegaly, marked eosinophilia, elevated serum IgE, and impaired T-cell function. Patients with Omenn syndrome have T cells in the periphery, but these T cells have a limited repertoire.

Deficiencies in **adenosine deaminase (ADA)** and **purine nucleoside phosphorylase,** two enzymes involved in the purine salvage pathway, also result in SCID. Accumulation of nucleoside substrates or their metabolic products in the plasma and urine is toxic to lymphocytes, including T, B, and NK cells. Most patients exhibit severe infection early in life, although the diagnosis in patients with partial enzyme function may not be established until after 5 years of age or, occasionally, in adulthood. Patients with late-onset diagnosis are generally lymphopenic; they may have B cells and normal total Ig levels but little functional antibody.

Bare lymphocyte syndrome results from defects in transcription factors that regulate expression of MHC class II molecules or genes that affect transport of antigen peptides, which leads to the absence of either MHC class I or MHC class II molecules. Lymphoid tissue and B cells may be present in normal amounts, but CD4 T cells are decreased or absent in class II deficiency, whereas CD8 cells are decreased or absent in class I deficiency. Some patients may have normal numbers of CD4 or CD8 T cells, but none of the T cells are functional because peptide antigens cannot be presented to T cells.

DiGeorge syndrome, also known as **velocardiofacial syndrome** or **CATCH 22 syndrome (c**ardiac anomalies, **a**bnormal facies, **t**hymic hypoplasia, **c**left palate, and **h**ypocalcemia), is the result of dysmorphogenesis of the third and fourth pharyngeal pouches, resulting in hypoplasia of the thymus required for T-cell maturation. Most, but not all, patients with DiGeorge syndrome have a deletion on chromosome 22q11.2. DiGeorge syndrome is classically characterized by hypocalcemic tetany, conotruncal and aortic arch anomalies, and increased infections. The diagnosis is established by fluorescent in situ hybridization or a polymerase chain reaction with a DNA probe to detect deletions in chromosome 22q11.2. Most patients have partial immune defects with low T-cell numbers and function that generally improve with age. Severe T-cell deficiency is rare, but when it occurs, it presents similarly to SCID due to a complete lack of T cells. Most important, DiGeorge syndrome and bare lymphocyte syndrome do not respond well to bone marrow transplantation as do other forms of SCID because the defects are in the thymus, although transfer of mature T cells during transplant may confer some immune function. Thymic transplants have been utilized in cases of severe T-cell lymphopenia in DiGeorge syndrome.

Wiskott-Aldrich syndrome is an X-linked disorder characterized by thrombocytopenia, eczema, defects in cell-mediated and humoral immunity, and a predisposition to lymphoproliferative disease (Table 73.3). It is caused by mutations of the gene on chromosome Xp11.22 coding for the Wiskott-Aldrich syndrome protein (WASP), expressed in lymphocytes, platelets, and monocytes. Deficiency of this protein results in elevated levels of IgE and IgA, decreased IgM, poor responses to polysaccharide antigens, waning T-cell function, and profound thrombocytopenia. Opportunistic infections and autoimmune cytopenias become problematic in older children. **Isolated X-linked thrombocytopenia** also results from mutations of the identical gene. One third of patients with Wiskott-Aldrich syndrome die as a result of hemorrhage, and two thirds die as a result of recurrent infection caused by bacteria, cytomegalovirus, *P. jiroveci (carinii),* or herpes simplex virus. Stem cell transplantation has corrected the immunological and hematological problems in some patients.

Ataxia-telangiectasia is a syndrome caused by the ataxia-telangiectasia, mutated *(ATM)* gene on chromosome 11q22.3 (see Table 73.3). Patients have cutaneous and conjunctival telangiectasias and progressive cerebellar ataxia with degeneration of Purkinje cells. IgA deficiency, IgG_2 subclass deficiency of variable severity, low IgE levels, and variably depressed T-cell function may be seen. The normal function of the *ATM* gene appears to be involved in detecting DNA damage and blocking cell growth division until the damage is repaired. Ataxia-telangiectasia cells are exquisitely sensitive to irradiation, and malignancies including leukemia or lymphoma can occur. Diabetes also may be present, and sexual maturation is delayed. There is no uniformly effective therapy, but antimicrobial therapy and intravenous immunoglobulin (IVIG) replacement therapy may be helpful.

Decision-Making Algorithms
Available @ StudentConsult.com

Involuntary Movements
Ataxia
Recurrent Infections

Chronic mucocutaneous candidiasis (autoimmune-polyendocrinopathy-candidiasis-ectodermal dystrophy [APECED]) is characterized by chronic or recurrent candidal infections of the mucous membranes, skin, and nails (see Table 73.3). There is normal antibody production but significantly decreased or absent lymphocyte proliferation and delayed skin reactivity to *Candida.* Patients usually do not respond to topical antifungal therapy and must be treated with oral antifungal agents. In most patients, an autoimmune endocrine disorder, such as hypoparathyroidism and Addison disease, develops by early adulthood. Other autoimmune disorders have been reported. The insidious onset requires the need for frequent evaluation for autoimmune endocrine disorders. This disease results from a defect in the gene for the transcription factor autoimmune regulator *(AIRE),* which is necessary for expression of peripheral tissue antigens in the thymus, resulting in a negative selection in the thymus and in tolerance to these tissues in normal individuals. Although originally thought to be a T-cell defect, patients with APECED produce neutralizing antibodies to cytokines important in the control of fungal infection, including IL-17.

Patients with **X-linked lymphoproliferative disease** (see Table 73.3) exhibit dysregulated immune responses to Epstein-Barr virus (EBV). Boys with this disease are normal until infected with EBV, which is acutely fatal in 80% of patients. X-linked

TABLE 73.3 Other Immunodeficiency Diseases

DISORDER	GENETICS	ONSET	MANIFESTATIONS	PATHOGENESIS	ASSOCIATED FEATURES
Wiskott-Aldrich syndrome	X-linked, (Xp11.22)	Early infancy	Thrombocytopenia and bleeding, atopic dermatitis, recurrent infections	53-kDa protein (WASP) defect	Polysaccharide antibody deficiency, small platelets, decreased cell-mediated immunity, lymphoproliferation
Ataxia-telangiectasia	AR (11q22.3)	2-5 yr	Recurrent otitis media, pneumonia, meningitis with encapsulated organisms	*ATM* gene mutation Disorder of DNA double-strand break repair	Neurological and endocrine dysfunction, malignancy, telangiectasis; sensitivity to radiation
Nijmegen breakage syndrome	AR (8q21)	Infancy	Sinopulmonary infections, bronchiectasis, urinary tract infections	Defect in chromosomal repair mechanisms; hypomorphic mutation in *NBS1* (Nibrin)	Sensitivity to ionizing radiation; microcephaly with mild neurological impairment; malignancy
Cartilage-hair hypoplasia (short-limbed dwarf)	AR (9p13–21)	Birth	Variable susceptibility to infections	Mutation in *RMRP*	Metaphyseal dysplasia, short extremities
Chronic mucocutaneous candidiasis (APECED)	AR	3-5 yr	Candidal infections of mucous membranes, skin, and nails	Mutations in *AIRE* gene	Autoimmune endocrinopathies
X-linked lymphoproliferative syndromes	X-linked	Variable	Variable decrease in T, B, and NK cell function, hypogammaglobulinemia	Mutation in *SH2D1A* (SAP: SLAM-associated protein) or *XIAP*	Life-threatening Epstein-Barr virus infection, lymphoma or Hodgkin disease, aplastic anemia, lymphohistiocytic disorder
Hyper-IgE syndrome	AD, AR	Variable	Skin and pulmonary abscesses, fungal infections, eczema, elevated IgE	Mutation in STAT3 (AD), TYK2 (AR), and DOCK8 (AR)	Coarse facial features, failure to shed primary teeth, frequent fractures (STAT3), viral and other infections (TYK2 and DOCK8)

AD, Autosomal dominant; *APECED,* autoimmune-polyendocrinopathy-candidiasis-ectodermal dystrophy; *AR,* autosomal recessive; *NK,* natural killer.

lymphoproliferative type 1 (XLP-1) is caused by a mutation in the gene called *SH2D1A* at chromosome Xq25, which codes for an adapter protein involved in signal transduction of lymphocytes. With EBV infection, affected boys exhibit a clinical phenotype similar to hemophagocytic lymphohistiocytosis with extensive expansion of CD8 T cells, hepatic necrosis, and death. Boys who survive initial EBV infection have significant hypogammaglobulinemia and are at high risk for developing aplastic anemia and lymphoma. A similar disorder is seen in boys with mutations in *XIAP*, which results in X-linked lymphoproliferative disorder type 2. The patients can also present with early onset colitis, and do not exhibit a susceptibility to lymphoma.

Hyper-IgE syndrome is characterized by markedly elevated serum IgE levels, a rash that resembles atopic dermatitis, eosinophilia, and staphylococcal abscesses of the skin, lungs, joints, and viscera (see Table 73.3). Infections with *H. influenzae* type b, *Candida,* and *Aspergillus* also may occur. These patients have coarse facial features, joint laxity, osteopenia with fractures, and may have giant pneumatoceles in the lungs after staphylococcal pneumonias. Although serum IgG, IgA, and IgM levels are normal, humoral immune responses to specific antigens are reduced, as is cell-mediated immunity. Long-term treatment with antistaphylococcal medications is indicated, and Ig replacement therapy may be helpful. Most patients have an autosomal dominant form of inheritance, whereas some patients have an autosomal recessive inheritance. Defects in the *TYK2* and *DOCK8* genes have been found in patients with autosomal recessive hyper-IgE syndrome, and defects in the *STAT3* gene were identified in autosomal dominant hyper-IgE syndrome.

TREATMENT

The approach to therapy of lymphocyte disorders depends on the diagnosis, clinical findings, and laboratory findings (Table 73.4). When immunodeficiency is suspected and while the evaluation is in process, all blood products need to be irradiated and negative for cytomegalovirus. Lymphocytes present in blood products can cause fatal **GVHD** in patients with SCID. Cytomegalovirus infection can be fatal in an immunodeficiency patient undergoing stem cell transplantation. Live-virus vaccines should be withheld from patients *and* household members until a diagnosis is established.

Infections should be treated with appropriate antibiotics; **antibiotic prophylaxis** can be used to prevent recurrent infections, provide a better quality of life, and decrease possible consequences. Patients with severe T-cell deficiencies should receive prophylaxis against *Pneumocystis* and fungi until treated with stem cell transplantation. Patients with milder forms of antibody deficiency diseases may benefit from **vaccination** with protein-conjugate vaccines to *H. influenzae* type b and *S. pneumonia.*

Ig replacement therapy, intravenously or subcutaneously, is a lifesaving therapy for patients with severe antibody deficiency diseases and SCID. It provides passive immunity against common microorganisms and reduces the frequency and

TABLE 73.4 General Management of Patients with Immunodeficiency
Avoid transfusions with blood products unless they are irradiated and cytomegalovirus-negative.
Avoid live-virus vaccines, especially in patients with severe T-cell deficiencies or agammaglobulinemia, and in household members.
Use prophylaxis to *Pneumocystis jiroveci (carinii)* in T-cell immunodeficiency, and in X-linked hyper IgM, consider antifungal prophylaxis in T-cell immunodeficiency.
Follow pulmonary function in patients with recurrent pneumonia.
Use chest physiotherapy and postural drainage in patients with recurrent pneumonia.
Consider using prophylactic antibiotics because minor infections can quickly disseminate.
Examine diarrheal stools for *Giardia lamblia* and *Clostridium difficile*.
Avoid unnecessary exposure to individuals with infection.
Boil water for T-cell defects and hyper-IgM syndrome (*Cryptosporidium* risk).
Use Ig for severe antibody deficiency states (400-600 mg/kg monthly IV or SC).

severity of infection in most patients. Ig replacement therapy is usually administered at a total monthly dose of 400-600 mg/kg of body weight administered intravenously every 3-4 weeks or subcutaneously by infusion pump every 1-2 weeks. IVIG therapy should be monitored by regularly measuring trough Ig levels and, more important, the patient's clinical course. Patients who continue to have recurrent infections, especially in the last week before the administration of IVIG, may require higher doses or more frequent administration. A combination of prophylactic antibiotics and Ig replacement therapy may be indicated in patients who continue to have recurrent infections. **Complications of IVIG** therapy include transfusion reactions with chills, fever, and myalgias. They usually can be prevented in subsequent infusions by pretreatment with an antihistamine, an antipyretic, and by a slower rate of infusion. Headache from aseptic meningitis can develop after IVIG therapy, usually in the first 24 hours. It most often responds to treatment with ibuprofen. Allergic reactions to IVIG can occur in patients with absent IgA, although these reactions are rare. Subcutaneous administration of Ig has fewer adverse effects but may be complicated by local reactions at the site(s) of infusion. The risk of transmission of infectious agents, despite preparation from large numbers of selected donors, is extremely low.

Therapy for severe T-cell disorders is stem cell transplantation, preferably from a human leukocyte antigen–matched sibling (see Chapter 76). Ig replacement provides passive antibody-mediated immunity. Some patients continue to have poor B-cell function after stem cell transplantation and require lifelong Ig replacement therapy. **GVHD,** in which the transplanted cells initiate an immune response against the host tissues, is the main complication of stem cell transplantation. Patients with the ADA deficiency form of SCID who lack matched sibling donors can receive repeated intramuscular replacement doses of ADA, stabilized by coupling to polyethylene glycol. Gene therapy has been performed in patients with common gamma chain deficiency and ADA deficiency by transfer of a normal gene into bone marrow stem cells, which are infused into the patient. Gene therapy for common gamma chain deficiency was successful in most of the treated patients; however, it was complicated by the development of leukemia in some patients. Newer viral vectors have been developed without the risk of leukemia, making gene therapy a likely option in the future for patients with SCID.

PREVENTION AND NEWBORN SCREENING

Population-based screening programs for SCID are underway because early identification of SCID prior to infectious complications improves outcomes. Polymerase chain reaction amplification of T-cell receptor excision circles (TRECs) formed during T-cell receptor recombination can be performed on newborn screening blood spots to detect severe T-cell lymphopenia. Newborn screening for TRECs has been shown to detect SCID at birth, and this test has been recommended for universal screening.

CHAPTER 74

Neutrophil Disorders

Neutrophils play important roles in immunity and wound healing; their primary function is ingesting and killing pathogens. Neutrophil disorders can result from deficient cell numbers or defective function (Table 74.1). Patients with neutrophil disorders are susceptible to a variety of bacterial infections and certain fungi. Suggestive signs include mucous membrane infections (gingivitis), abscesses in the skin and viscera, lymphadenitis, poor wound healing, delayed umbilical cord separation, or absence of pus. Neutrophils develop in the bone marrow from hematopoietic stem cells by the action of several colony-stimulating factors, including stem cell factor, granulocyte-monocyte colony-stimulating factor, granulocyte colony-stimulating factor (G-CSF), and interleukin-3. On leaving the bone marrow, mature neutrophils are found in the circulation or reside in the marginating pool. Adhesion molecules are necessary for neutrophils to roll and adhere to vascular endothelium and extravasate from the blood into sites of infection, where they phagocytose and kill pathogens, especially those coated by complement or antibodies. Chemotactic factors, including the complement fragment C5a, interleukin-8, and bacterial formulated peptides, mobilize neutrophils to enter tissues and sites of infections. Neutrophils kill ingested pathogens using granular enzymes or by activation of oxygen radicals.

ETIOLOGY AND CLINICAL MANIFESTATIONS

Disorders of Neutrophil Numbers

Decision-Making Algorithms
Available @ StudentConsult.com

Diarrhea
Neutropenia
Failure to Thrive

TABLE 74.1 Phagocytic Disorders

NAME	GENETICS	DEFECT	COMMENT
Congenital neutropenia, cyclic neutropenia	AR (*HAX1, GFI1*, others) AD (*GFI1, ELANE*)	Severe neutropenia	Cellulitis, pharyngitis, gingivitis, lymphadenitis, abscesses, typhlitis, and pneumonia
Chronic granulomatous disease	X-linked (gp91^{phox}), AR (p22^{phox}, p47^{phox}, and p67^{phox})	Bactericidal	X-linked recessive (66%), autosomal recessive (33%); eczema, osteomyelitis, granulomas, abscesses caused by *Staphylococcus aureus, Burkholderia cepacia, Aspergillus fumigatus*, colitis
Chédiak-Higashi syndrome (1q42l-44)	AR (*LYST*)	Bactericidal plus chemotaxis; poor natural killer function	Autosomal recessive; oculocutaneous albinism, neuropathy, giant neutrophilic cytoplasmic inclusions; malignancy, neutropenia
Myeloperoxidase deficiency	AR (*MPO*)	Bactericidal, fungicidal	Reduced chemiluminescence; autosomal recessive (1 : 4,000); persistent candidiasis in diabetic patients
Glucose-6-phosphate dehydrogenase deficiency	AR (*G6PD*)	Bactericidal	Phenotypically similar to chronic granulomatous disease
Leukocyte adhesion deficiency	AR (*ITGB2, FUCT1*)	Adherence, chemotaxis, phagocytosis; reduced lymphocyte cytotoxicity	Delayed separation or infection of umbilical cord; lethal bacterial infections without pus; autosomal recessive; neutrophilia
Shwachman-Diamond syndrome	AR (*SBDS*)	Chemotaxis, neutropenia	Pancreatic insufficiency, metaphyseal chondrodysplasia; autosomal recessive

AR, Autosomal recessive; *AD*, autosomal dominant.

The normal neutrophil count varies with age. **Neutropenia** is defined as an absolute neutrophil count (ANC) less than 1,500/mm^3 for white children 1 year of age or older. African American children normally have lower total white blood cell and neutrophil counts. The effect of neutropenia depends on its severity. The susceptibility to infection is minimally increased until the ANC is less than 1,000/mm^3. Most patients do well with an ANC greater than 500/mm^3. At these levels, localized infections are more common than generalized bacteremia. Serious bacterial infections are more common with an ANC less than 200/mm^3. The major types of infections associated with neutropenia are cellulitis, pharyngitis, gingivitis, lymphadenitis, abscesses (cutaneous or perianal), enteritis (typhlitis), and pneumonia. The sites of the infection usually are colonized heavily with normal bacterial flora that becomes invasive in the presence of neutropenia. Neutropenia may be congenital or acquired (Table 74.2) and may be associated with specific diseases, especially infections (Table 74.3), or result from drug reactions (Table 74.4).

There are several forms of congenital neutropenia. **Severe congenital neutropenia (Kostmann syndrome)** is an autosomal recessive disorder in which myeloid cells fail to mature beyond the early stages of the promyelocyte due to mutations in the *HAX-1* gene. The peripheral blood may show an impressive monocytosis. Although endogenous G-CSF levels are increased, exogenous G-CSF produces a rise in the neutrophil count, improving the care of these children. Acute myeloid leukemia has developed in a few patients who have survived into adolescence. Stem cell transplantation may be curative. Defects in *G6PC3, GFI1*, and other genes have also been shown to cause severe congenital neutropenia. **Cyclic neutropenia** is a stem cell disorder in which all marrow elements cycle resulting in transient neutropenia. It may be transmitted as an autosomal dominant, recessive, or sporadic disorder. Because of the short half-life of neutrophils in the blood (6-7 hours) compared to platelets (10 days) and red blood cells (120 days), neutropenia is the only clinically significant abnormality. The usual cycle is 21 days, with neutropenia lasting 4-6 days, accompanied by monocytosis and often by eosinophilia. Severe, debilitating bone pain is common when the neutrophil count is low. G-CSF results in increasing neutrophil numbers and a shorter duration of neutropenia. Defects in *ELANE*, the gene encoding for neutrophil elastase, has been found in patients with cyclic neutropenia. Further analysis has demonstrated *ELANE* mutations in some cases of severe congenital neutropenia.

Severe congenital neutropenia that may be either persistent or cyclic also is a component of **Shwachman-Diamond syndrome**, an autosomal recessive syndrome of pancreatic insufficiency accompanying bone marrow dysfunction. This is a panmyeloid disorder in which neutropenia is the most prominent manifestation. Metaphyseal dysostosis and dwarfism may occur. Patients usually respond to G-CSF. A gain of function mutation in the Wiskott-Aldrich syndrome protein has also been associated with an X-linked form of severe congenital neutropenia. **Benign congenital neutropenia** is a functional diagnosis for patients with significant neutropenia in whom major infectious complications do not develop. Many patients whose ANC ranges from 100-500/mm^3 have an increased frequency of infections, particularly respiratory infections, but the major problem is the slow resolution of infections that develop. These disorders may be sporadic or familial and, in some instances, are transmitted as an autosomal dominant disorder. Severe congenital neutropenia may be associated with severe combined immunodeficiency in **reticular dysgenesis**, a disorder of hematopoietic stem cells affecting all bone marrow lineages due to mutations in the *AK2* gene.

Isoimmune neutropenia occurs in neonates as the result of transplacental transfer of maternal antibodies to fetal neutrophil antigens. The mother is sensitized to specific neutrophil antigens on fetal leukocytes that are inherited from the father and are not present on maternal cells. Isoimmune neonatal neutropenia, similar to isoimmune anemia and thrombocytopenia,

TABLE 74.2 Mechanisms of Neutropenia
ABNORMAL BONE MARROW
Marrow Injury
Drugs: idiosyncratic, cytotoxic (myelosuppressive)
Radiation
Chemicals: DDT, benzene
Immune-mediated: T and B cell and immunoglobulin
Infections (viruses, rickettsia)
Infiltrative processes: tumor, storage disease
Myelodysplasia
Aplastic anemia
Maturation Defects
Folic acid deficiency
Vitamin B_{12}
Copper
Congenital Disorders
Severe congenital neutropenia (HAX-1, G6PC3, ELANE, GFI-1)
Cyclic neutropenia (ELANE)
Cartilage hair hypoplasia
Shwachman-Diamond syndrome
Diamond-Blackfan syndrome
Griscelli syndrome
Chédiak-Higashi syndrome
WHIM syndrome (warts, hypogammaglobulinemia, infections, myelokathexis)
Glycogen storage disease type Ib
Methylmalonic acidemia
PERIPHERAL CIRCULATION
Pseudoneutropenia: Shift to Bone Marrow/Spleen
Splenomegaly
Severe infection
Intravascular
Destruction: neonatal isoimmune, autoimmune, hypersplenism
Autoimmune diseases (systemic lupus erythematosus, rheumatoid arthritis, Sjögren syndrome)

ELA-2, Elastase 2; *G6PC3*, glucose-6-phosphatase catalytic subunit 3; *GFI-1*, growth factor independent 1; *HAX-1*, HS1-associated protein X-1.

is a transient process (see Chapters 62 and 151). Cutaneous infections are common, and sepsis is rare. Early treatment of infection while the infant is neutropenic is the major goal of therapy. Intravenous immune globulin may decrease the duration of neutropenia.

Autoimmune neutropenia usually develops in children 5-24 months of age and often persists for prolonged periods. Neutrophil autoantibodies may be IgG, IgM, IgA, or a combination of these. Usually the condition resolves in 6 months to 4 years. Although intravenous immune globulin and corticosteroids have been used, most patients respond to G-CSF. Autoimmune neutropenia may rarely be an early manifestation of systemic lupus erythematosus, rheumatoid arthritis, or autoimmune lymphoproliferative disease.

TABLE 74.3 Infection-Associated Neutropenia
BACTERIAL
Typhoid-paratyphoid
Brucellosis
Neonatal sepsis
Meningococcemia
Overwhelming sepsis
Congenital syphilis
Tuberculosis
VIRAL
Measles
Hepatitis B
HIV
Rubella
Cytomegalovirus
Influenza
Epstein-Barr virus
RICKETTSIAL
Rocky Mountain spotted fever
Typhus
Ehrlichiosis
Rickettsialpox

HIV, Human immunodeficiency virus.

TABLE 74.4 Drug-Associated Neutropenia
CYTOTOXIC
Myelosuppressive, chemotherapeutic agents
Immunosuppressive agents
IDIOSYNCRATIC
Indomethacin
Para-aminophenol derivatives
Pyrazolone derivatives (aminopyrine, dipyrone, oxyphenbutazone)
Chloramphenicol
Sulfonamides
Antithyroid drugs (propylthiouracil, methimazole, carbimazole)
Phenothiazines (chlorpromazine, phenothiazines)
Penicillins and semisynthetic penicillins

Modified from Dale DC. Neutropenia. In: Lichtman MA, Kipps TJ, Seligsohn U, et al., eds. Williams Hematology. *8th ed. New York: McGraw-Hill; 2010.*

Disorders of Neutrophil Migration

Neutrophils normally adhere to endothelium and migrate to areas of inflammation by the interaction of membrane proteins, called *integrins* and *selectins,* with endothelial cell adhesion molecules. A hallmark of defects in neutrophil migration is the absence of pus at sites of infection. In **leukocyte adhesion deficiency type I (LAD-I)**, infants lacking the β_2 integrin CD18 exhibit the condition early in infancy with failure of separation of the umbilical cord (often 2 months after birth) with attendant omphalitis and sepsis (see Table 74.1). The neutrophil count usually is greater than $20,000/mm^3$ because of failure of the neutrophils to adhere normally to vascular endothelium and to migrate out of blood to the tissues (Fig. 74.1). Cutaneous, respiratory, and mucosal infections occur. Children with this condition often have severe gingivitis. Sepsis can lead to death in early childhood. This disorder is transmitted as an autosomal recessive trait. Stem cell transplantation can be lifesaving.

LAD-II results from impairment of neutrophil rolling along the vascular wall, which is the first step in neutrophil migration into tissues and sites of infection. Rolling is mediated by sialylated and fucosylated tetrasaccharides related to the sialylated Lewis X (S-LeX) blood group found on the surface of neutrophils, monocytes, and activated lymphocytes binding to selectin molecules on vascular endothelium (see Fig. 74.1). LAD-II results from a defect in the FUCT1 protein resulting in abnormal fucose metabolism leading to the absence of S-LeX blood group on the surface of neutrophils and other leukocytes. LAD-III is a rare disorder caused by defects in the KINDLIN-3 protein resulting in defective neutrophil adhesion as well as platelet defects. Defective migration of neutrophils has also been described in **Hyper-IgE syndrome** and with mutations in the *RAC2* gene (see Chapter 73 and Table 74.1).

Disorders of Neutrophil Function

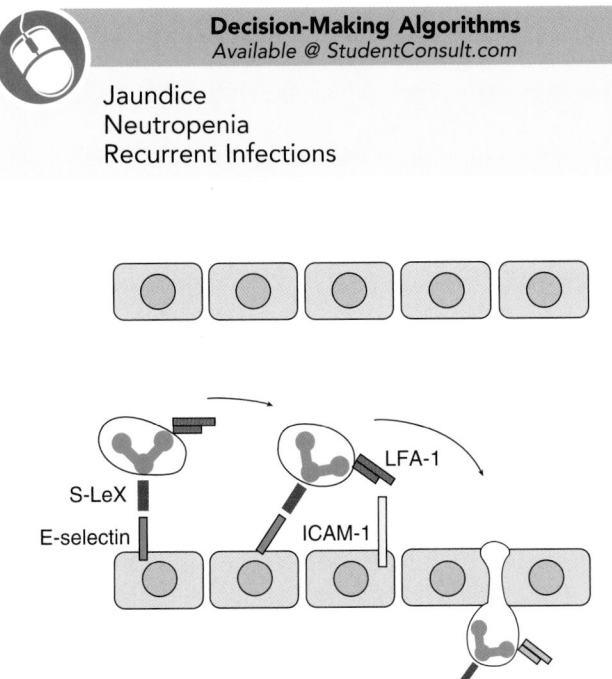

Decision-Making Algorithms
Available @ StudentConsult.com

Jaundice
Neutropenia
Recurrent Infections

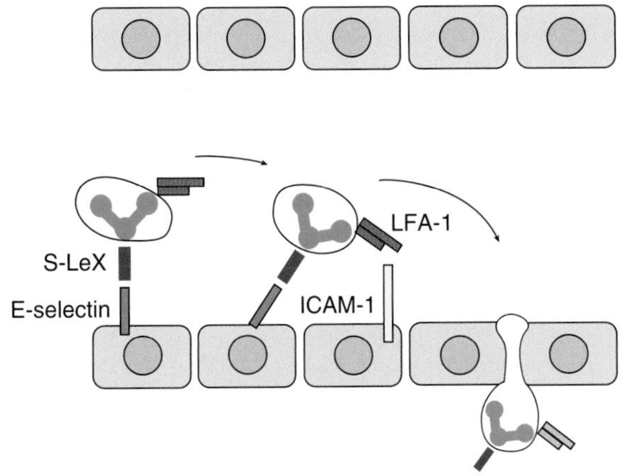

FIGURE 74.1 Schematic representation of neutrophil migration from the vascular space across the vascular endothelium into tissues. Neutrophils bind to selectin (E- or P-selectin) molecules on the surface of vascular endothelium via sialylated and fucosylated tetrasaccharides related to the S-LeX blood group found on the surface of neutrophils. The bound neutrophils roll along the endothelium and become tightly bound by the interaction of the adhesion molecule leukocyte function-associated antigen type 1 (LFA-1) on the neutrophil and intercellular adhesion molecule type 1 (ICAM-1) on vascular endothelium, allowing neutrophils to move through the endothelium and into the tissue spaces. (Modified from Janeway CA, Travers P, Walport M, et al. *Immunobiology: The Immune System in Health and Disease*. 4th ed. New York: Elsevier; 1999.)

Defects in neutrophil function are relatively rare inherited disorders and tend to be associated with a marked susceptibility to bacterial and fungal infection. **Chronic granulomatous disease (CGD)** is a disorder of white blood cells that results from defective intracellular killing of bacteria and intracellular pathogens by neutrophils and macrophages because of an inability to activate the "respiratory burst," the catalytic conversion of molecular oxygen to superoxide (O_2^-). Reduced nicotinamide adenine dinucleotide phosphate oxidase, the enzyme that catalyzes the respiratory burst, consists of four subunits: $gp91^{phox}$, $p22^{phox}$, $p47^{phox}$, and $p67^{phox}$. Defects in any of these enzymes lead to an inability to kill catalase-positive pathogens such as *Staphylococcus aureus* and enteric gram-negative bacteria *(Burkholderia)* and fungi *(Aspergillus fumigatus, Candida albicans)*. The $gp91^{phox}$ gene is located on chromosome Xp21.1 and is responsible for the most common form of the disease. The other gene defects are inherited in an autosomal recessive manner. The chromosome locations for these genes are 16q24 for $p22^{phox}$, 7q11.23 for $p47^{phox}$, and 1q25 for $p67^{phox}$. Glucose-6-phosphate dehydrogenase also is involved in the production of superoxide, and severe forms of glucose-6-phosphate dehydrogenase deficiency also result in CGD. Patients characteristically have lymphadenopathy, hypergammaglobulinemia, hepatosplenomegaly, dermatitis, failure to thrive, anemia, chronic diarrhea, and abscesses. Infections occur in the lungs, the middle ear, gastrointestinal tract, skin, urinary tract, lymph nodes, liver, and bones. Granulomas are prominent and may obstruct the pylorus or ureters.

Chédiak-Higashi syndrome, an abnormality of secondary granules, is an autosomal recessive disorder caused by a mutation in a cytoplasmic protein *(LYST)* thought to be involved in organellar protein trafficking, resulting in a fusion of the primary and secondary granules in neutrophils. Giant granules are present in many cells, including lymphocytes, platelets, and melanocytes. Patients usually have partial oculocutaneous albinism. The defect in Chédiak-Higashi syndrome results in defective neutrophil and natural killer cell function, leading to recurrent and sometimes fatal infections with streptococci and staphylococci. Most patients progress to an accelerated phase associated with Epstein-Barr virus infection and characterized by a **lymphoproliferative syndrome** with generalized lymphohistiocytic infiltrates, fever, jaundice, hepatomegaly, lymphadenopathy, and pancytopenia. The condition resembles hemophagocytic lymphohistiocytosis.

LABORATORY DIAGNOSIS

The evaluation of a neutropenic child depends on clinical signs of infection, family and medication history, age of the patient, cyclic or persistent nature of the condition, signs of bone marrow infiltration (malignancy or storage disease), and evidence of involvement of other cell lines. Neutropenia is confirmed by a complete blood count and differential. A bone marrow aspirate and biopsy may be necessary to determine whether the neutropenia is due to a failure of production in the bone marrow, infiltration of the bone marrow, or loss of neutrophils in the periphery. Antineutrophil antibodies help diagnose autoimmune neutropenia.

Neutrophil chemotactic defects can be excluded by the presence of neutrophils at the site of infection. The **Rebuck skin window** is a 4-hour in vivo test for neutrophil chemotaxis that is not performed routinely by most laboratories. In vitro studies of neutrophil migration are available in specialized laboratories. Flow cytometry for the presence of adhesion molecules, such as CD18 or CD15, can help diagnose leukocyte adhesion defects. Point mutations that affect the function of the adhesion molecule but do not alter antibody binding are missed using flow cytometry. CGD can be diagnosed by the flow cytometry-based test using **dihydrorhodamine 123** or the nitroblue tetrazolium test (see Chapter 72). Light microscopy of neutrophils for the presence of giant granules can help diagnose Chédiak-Higashi syndrome.

TREATMENT

Therapy for neutropenia depends on the underlying cause. Patients with severe bacterial infections require broad-spectrum antibiotics; the resolution of neutropenia is the most important prognostic factor. Most patients with severe congenital neutropenia or autoimmune neutropenia respond to therapy with G-CSF. Granulocyte transfusion should be reserved for life-threatening infection. Chronic mild neutropenia not associated with immunosuppression can be managed expectantly with prompt antimicrobial treatment of soft tissue infections, which usually are caused by *S. aureus* or group A streptococcus.

Frequent courses of antibiotics, including trimethoprim-sulfamethoxazole prophylaxis, and surgical débridement of infections are required in **CGD.** Because *A. fumigatus* can cause serious infection in patients with CGD, moldy hay, decomposing compost, and other nests of fungi must be avoided, and prophylactic antifungals can be helpful. The frequency of infection in CGD is lessened by treatment with **recombinant interferon-γ** administered subcutaneously three times a week. Stem cell transplantation (see Chapter 76) may be lifesaving in CGD, LAD-1, and Chédiak-Higashi syndrome.

PROGNOSIS AND PREVENTION

The prognosis depends on the particular defect. Milder and transient defects in neutrophil numbers have a better prognosis. Prolonged absence of neutrophils or their function has a poor prognosis, especially with the risk of bacterial and fungal sepsis. Treatment with prophylactic antibiotics and interferon-γ has improved the prognosis of patients with CGD. Stem cell transplantation is the only currently available mode of therapy that can reverse the poor prognosis of severe neutrophil defects. As in other genetic defects, prenatal diagnosis and genetic counseling are possible for all known gene mutations.

CHAPTER 75

Complement System

The **complement system** consists of plasma and membrane proteins that function in the innate immune response as well as facilitate adaptive immunity. **Complement proteins** can kill pathogens with or without antibodies, opsonize pathogens to facilitate their uptake by phagocytes, or mediate inflammation. The complement system can be activated through three pathways—classic, alternative, or lectin—that involve a cascade-like, sequential activation of complement factors resulting in an amplified response (Fig. 75.1). Disorders of the complement system predispose to recurrent infection, autoimmunity, and angioedema (Table 75.1).

TABLE 75.1 Deficiency of Complement and Associated Disease

DEFICIENT PROTEIN	ASSOCIATED DISEASE
C1q, C1r	SLE, glomerulonephritis; encapsulated bacterial infections
C2	SLE, glomerulonephritis; encapsulated bacterial infections
C3	Recurrent bacterial infections, rare glomerulonephritis, or SLE
C4	SLE, glomerulonephritis; encapsulated bacterial infections
C5	Recurrent meningococcal infections
C6	Recurrent meningococcal infections
C7	Recurrent meningococcal infections
C8	Recurrent meningococcal infections
C9	Occasional meningococcal infection
Properdin	Recurrent infections, severe meningococcal infection
MBL	Increased susceptibility to infections
Factor H	Glomerulonephritis, atypical HUS
Factor I	Recurrent infections, glomerulonephritis
MCP	Glomerulonephritis, atypical HUS
C1 inhibitor	Hereditary angioedema

HUS, Hemolytic uremic syndrome; *MBL*, mannose-binding lectin; *MCP*, membrane cofactor protein; *SLE*, systemic lupus erythematosus.

ETIOLOGY

The three pathways for complement activation are initiated by different mechanisms. The **classic pathway** is activated by antigen-antibody complexes or by C-reactive protein. The **alternative pathway** may be activated by C3b generated through classic complement activation or by spontaneous hydrolysis of C3 on microbial surfaces. The **lectin pathway** is initiated by the interaction of mannose-binding lectin with microbial carbohydrate. Activation of the classic pathway by an antigen-antibody complex is initiated by the binding of C1q to the Fc portion of an antibody molecule in the immune complex. C1r auto-activates and cleaves C1s, which cleaves C4 and then C2, forming the C3 convertase, C4b2a. C4b2a is activated by the lectin pathway when mannose-binding protein binds to sugar residues on the surface of pathogens, and mannose-binding protein–associated proteases (MASP) cleave C4 and C2. The alternative pathway is always active at a low level and is amplified when active C3 binds to a surface that lacks regulatory proteins. C3b generated from C3 binds to factor B, which is cleaved by factor D to form the alternative pathway C3 convertase, C3bBb. Properdin binds to and stabilizes the C3 convertase (see Fig. 75.1). The C3 convertase can cleave C3 resulting in further C3b deposition and activation of the alternative pathway that acts as an amplification loop by generating more C3b, or it can form the C5 convertase, which initiates the formation of a

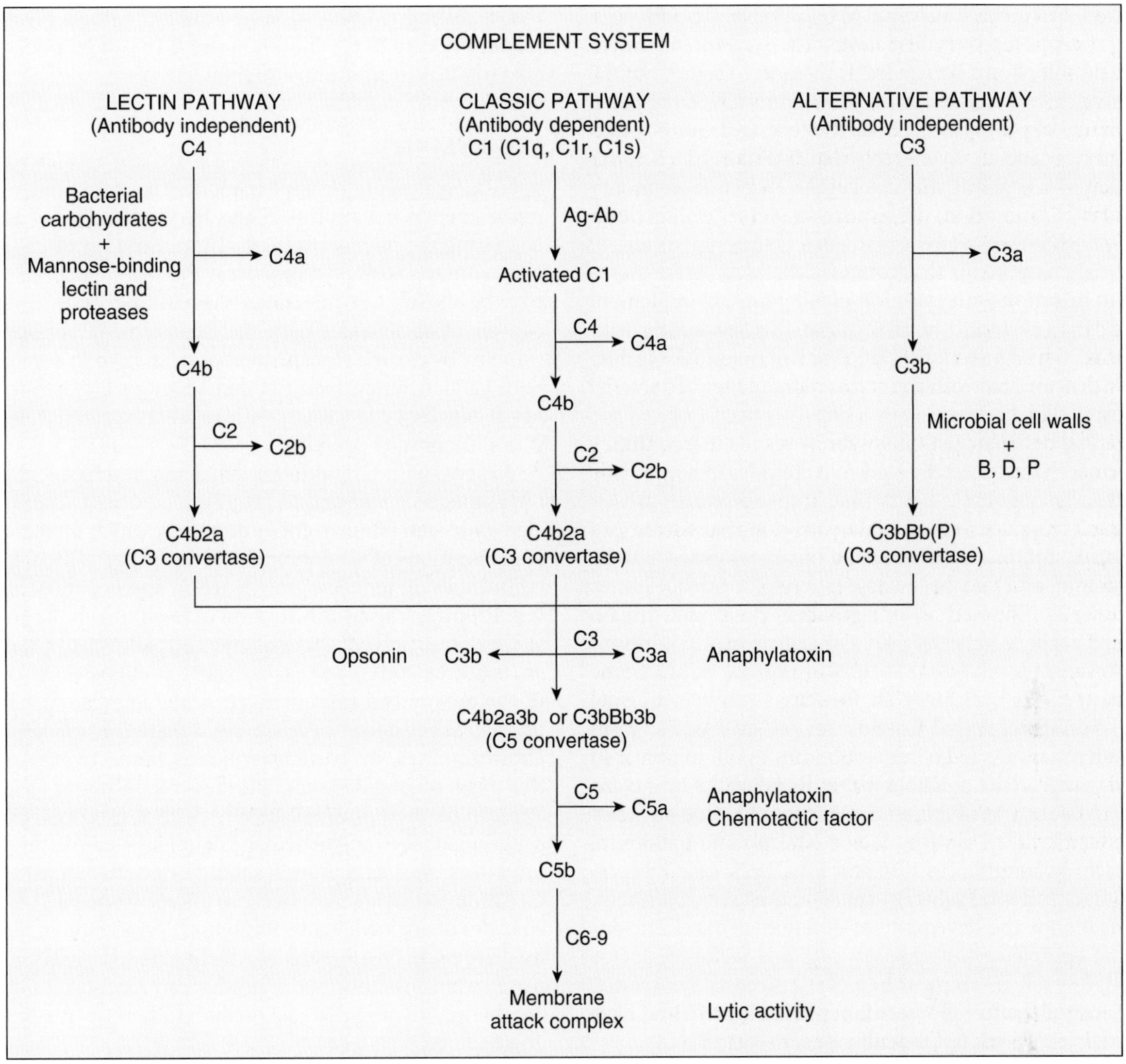

FIGURE 75.1 Complement component cascade involving the classic, alternative, and lectin pathways. The initiating events for the pathways differ, but they result in the production of C3 cleaving enzyme activity, which is the pivotal step as the three pathways converge to the terminal activation sequences. *Ag-Ab*, Antigen-antibody complex; *B*, factor B; *D*, factor D (factor B clearing enzyme); *P*, properdin.

membrane attack complex (MAC). The MAC is a complex of C5b, C6, C7, C8, and several C9 molecules that is common to all three pathways (see Fig. 75.1). The MAC generates pores in the cell membrane, leading to lysis of the cells. C3a and C5a, produced by cleavage of C3 and C5, respectively, can release histamine from mast cells and basophils, leading to increased vascular permeability and smooth muscle contraction. In addition, C5a has chemotactic activity, attracting phagocytes to the site of complement activation, and it can cause degranulation of phagocytic cells. C3b acts as an opsonin when attached to the surface of a pathogen by binding to phagocytes via complement receptor 1 (CR1). Its degradation product, iC3b, can bind to CR3 on the surface of phagocytes leading to the ingestion of the C3b-coated or iC3b-coated pathogen. iC3b and its breakdown product C3dg can bind complement receptor 2 (CR2) on B cells leading to activation and differentiation.

The complement system is under tight regulation because it has potent inflammatory activity and the potential to cause significant damage to host cells. The complement cascade is inherently regulated by the short half-life C4b and C3b and by instability of the C3 convertases, C4b2a, and C3bBb. C1-inhibitor regulates the cascade by blocking active sites on C1r, C1s, and the MASP. Factor I destabilizes C3 convertase complexes and degrades the active fragments. Other inhibitors include membrane proteins, such as decay accelerating factor, CR1, membrane cofactor protein (MCP), and plasma proteins such as C4b-binding protein and factor H. Formation of the MAC can be blocked by cell surface CD59, protein S, and other plasma proteins. Deficiency of any of these regulatory proteins can result in an inflammatory response, tissue damage, or excessive complement consumption.

Disorders of complement proteins can result from inherited deficiency or can be secondary to increased consumption. The consequences of decreased complement depend on the affected factor (see Table 75.1). **Deficiencies of early components** of the classic pathway (C1, C2, or C4) are not usually associated with severe infections, although patients with C2 deficiency may present with milder recurrent infections. Patients with C1,

C2, or C4 deficiency are susceptible to autoimmune diseases, especially systemic lupus erythematosus. The exact mechanism of this susceptibility is not known but is thought to arise from the role of these early components in clearing immune complexes.

Deficiency of properdin, C3, or the terminal components predisposes patients to severe recurrent infections. Deficiency of C3, the major opsonin, due to a genetic defect or secondary to excessive consumption, predisposes patients to infections, especially with encapsulated organisms. Deficiency of one of the terminal components that compose the MAC predisposes patients to infection with *Neisseria meningitidis*. Complement deficiency may be found in 40% of patients presenting with recurrent neisserial infections. Deficiency of mannose-binding lectin also is associated with an increased frequency of bacterial infections, including sepsis.

Congenital deficiency of C1-inhibitor results in **hereditary angioedema**, characterized by recurrent episodes of nonpruritic angioedema lasting 48-72 hours that occur spontaneously or after minor trauma, stress, or anxiety. Abdominal edema can cause acute abdominal pain; edema of the upper airway can be life threatening and may necessitate emergency tracheostomy. The disorder is inherited as an autosomal dominant disease and results from a heterozygous deficiency of C1-inhibitor leading to serum levels less than 30% of normal values. Some mutations (type II hereditary angioedema) result in normal levels of C1-inhibitor with defective function. An acquired form of angioedema results from autoantibodies to C1-inhibitor in lymphoid malignancies or autoimmune disorders but is uncommon in childhood. C1-inhibitor is a regulator of Hageman factor (clotting factor XIIa), clotting factor XIa, plasma kallikrein, and plasmin in addition to C1r and C1s. Lack of inhibition of the contact system, Hageman factor and plasma kallikrein, is responsible for the development of angioedema. Deficiencies in the complement regulatory proteins factor H, factor I, and MCP result in **atypical hemolytic uremic syndrome, membranoproliferative glomerulonephritis type II**, and have been linked to **age-related macular degeneration**.

LABORATORY STUDIES

The **CH_{50} test** is a widely available test of classic complement pathway function, based on an antibody-dependent hemolytic assay, which measures the serum dilution that results in lysis of 50% of sheep red blood cells. The CH_{50} test depends on the function of all nine complement proteins, C1 through C9. The **AH_{50} test**, which measures complement activation using red blood cells from different species (e.g., rabbit) that can activate the alternative pathway without antibody, is less widely available than the CH_{50} test and requires the alternative pathway components and C5 to C9. Abnormal results of both tests indicate a deficiency in a terminal component common to both pathways, whereas an abnormal result of one or the other test indicates a deficiency of an early component of the respective pathway. If the CH_{50} or AH_{50} levels are abnormal, individual components can be analyzed in specialized laboratories.

Determination of C1-inhibitor levels and function is needed to diagnose hereditary angioedema. Some functional tests miss rare mutations that allow C1-inhibitor to bind C1s, but not one or more of the other enzymes with which it interacts. Low C1-inhibitor levels or function results in chronically decreased C4 levels and decreased C2 levels during acute attacks. Low C1q levels are found in acquired C1-inhibitor deficiency, which distinguishes it from hereditary angioedema. Tests for autoantibodies to C1-inhibitor and C1q can be performed by enzyme-linked immunosorbent assay.

TREATMENT

Specific treatment of complement deficiencies with component replacement is not available. Long, frequent courses of antibiotics constitute the primary therapy. Immunization of patients and close contacts with pneumococcal and meningococcal vaccines may be useful, but infections may still occur in immunized complement-deficient patients. Replacement of complement proteins by plasma transfusion has been used in some patients with C2 deficiency, factor H deficiency, or factor I deficiency. MCP deficiency is treated with renal transplantation because it is a membrane protein.

Patients with C1-inhibitor deficiency and frequent episodes of angioedema respond to prophylactic use of an oral attenuated androgen (**stanozolol** or **danazol**), which increases serum concentrations of C1-inhibitor. Adverse effects, including masculinization in females, growth arrest, and hepatitis, limit their use. Prophylactic administration of fresh frozen plasma before surgery can prevent angioedema, but administration during an acute episode may exacerbate the episode. Angioedema of the airway can present as an acute emergency, necessitating a tracheostomy because administration of epinephrine, antihistamines, or corticosteroids is ineffective in reversing this type of angioedema. Purified C1-inhibitor is available and can be used prophylactically (before surgery) and during acute episodes of angioedema. Angiotensin-converting enzyme inhibitors, such as captopril, should be avoided in patients with C1-inhibitor deficiency because these drugs can precipitate episodes of angioedema by inhibiting degradation of kinins that mediate edema formation. Novel therapeutic agents, including a kallikrein inhibitor and a bradykinin receptor 2 antagonist, are being investigated as potential therapy for hereditary angioedema.

CHAPTER 76

Hematopoietic Stem Cell Transplantation

Hematopoietic stem cell transplantation (HSCT) can cure some patients with primary immunodeficiency disease (Table 76.1). Use of HSCT is limited to immunodeficiency diseases, some metabolic storage diseases (see Chapters 55 and 56), malignancies (see Chapter 154), aplastic anemia (see Chapter 150), hemoglobinopathies (see Chapter 150), and a few other disorders.

The principle of HSCT is to replace a patient's defective bone marrow stem cells with normal stem cells. Hematopoietic stem cells reside in the bone marrow but can also be obtained from peripheral blood or cord blood. Peripheral blood does not contain a significant proportion of stem cells unless the donor's bone marrow is actively stimulated to generate stem cells. Cord blood is a good source of stem cells and is used for sibling and unrelated HSCT.

TABLE 76.1 Immunodeficiency Diseases Curable by Stem Cell Transplantation

Severe combined immunodeficiency (SCID)
X-linked SCID (γ_c deficiency)
Jak3 kinase deficiency
ZAP 70 deficiency and other T-cell activation defects
RAG1/RAG2 deficiency and other $T^- B^-$ SCID
Omenn syndrome
Adenosine deaminase deficiency
Purine nucleoside phosphorylase deficiency
Reticular dysgenesis
Bare lymphocyte syndrome
Wiskott-Aldrich syndrome
X-linked hyper IgM
X-linked lymphoproliferative syndromes
Chronic granulomatous disease
Autoimmune lymphoproliferative syndrome (Fas defect)
Severe congenital neutropenia
Shwachman-Diamond syndrome
Immune dysregulation, polyendocrinopathy, enteropathy, X-linked (IPEX)
Cyclic neutropenia
Chédiak-Higashi syndrome
Leukocyte adhesion deficiency type I
Familial hemophagocytic lymphohistiocytosis

Major histocompatibility complex (MHC) compatibility is crucial in the choice of a stem cell donor to avoid rejection of the donor cells by the host immune system and to prevent graft versus host disease (GVHD) caused by contaminating mature T cells. The donor stem cells give rise to T cells that develop in the host thymus and need to interact with donor and host antigen-presenting cells. In cases with MHC mismatched donors, mature T cells need to be removed from the donor to reduce the risk of **GVHD**; this complication outweighs the disadvantage of a prolonged time of 90-120 days before T-cell development. Patients are at risk for developing **B-cell lymphoproliferative disease**, usually associated with Epstein-Barr virus, when T-cell–depletion techniques are used, likely due to the delay in T-cell engraftment.

The most important factor affecting outcomes in HSCT is the similarity of the donor MHC. The best outcomes are obtained using MHC-identical siblings (25% chance of a matched sibling) as donors, followed by matched unrelated donors. Unlike transplantation for other disorders, MHC haploidentical bone marrow from a parent (preferred) or a sibling can be used to treat severe combined immunodeficiency (SCID), likely the result of these patients lacking functioning T cells. Stem cells from a partially mismatched donor, such as a parent, can give rise to a functioning immune system because the patient shares at least half of the MHC molecules with the donor stem cells.

MHC molecules are highly polymorphic, and typing is currently performed on DNA rather than by serology. Bone marrow and cord blood registries are available worldwide. Searching and identifying a donor can be a lengthy process, especially for some underrepresented ethnic backgrounds. Finding a suitable cord blood donor is faster because the cord blood already has been obtained and stored, whereas bone marrow donors have to be identified, located, and tested. A matched sibling, if available, is the preferred source of hematopoietic stem cells.

Patients with SCID are ideal candidates for HSCT, which is the main option for treatment of SCID, although research is ongoing with gene therapy. Patients are unlikely to survive beyond 1-2 years of age without transplantation, and they have no T-cell function to reject donor cells. Thus they may not need to undergo conditioning with chemotherapy or irradiation before transplantation. The development of transplantation using T-cell–depleted, haploidentical bone marrow from a parent for SCID has provided almost every patient with SCID a potential donor. The mother is the preferred source for haploidentical bone marrow, if she is able to donate, because some transfer of maternal T cells can occur during pregnancy, and these maternal T cells can reject cells obtained from the father. The survival rate after HSCT for SCID is approximately 90% with MHC-identical and 60% with haploidentical bone marrow transplantation. Early transplant before the acquisition of infection improves outcomes. Because newborn screening for SCID is now possible, stem cell transplantation can occur as early as possible when the infants are healthy, providing the best opportunity for a cure.

The decision to treat other primary immunodeficiency diseases with HSCT is more difficult because it is difficult to predict the prognosis of a particular patient because of the variability in clinical course of most primary immunodeficiency diseases. This must be weighed with the risks of transplantation. In addition, HSCT for other primary immunodeficiencies is less successful than for SCID because patients typically have some T-cell function and require conditioning with the risks that it entails. The availability of a matched related sibling favors the decision to perform HSCT. Disorders of B cells have not been treated with HSCT because, in many cases, donor B cells do not engraft, and patients usually do well with intravenous immunoglobulin. Regardless, a variety of primary immunodeficiencies have been treated with HSCT (see Table 76.1).

COMPLICATIONS

Rejection of the grafted cells is the first potential complication of HSCT and depends on the immunocompetence of the patient, the degree of MHC incompatibility, and the number of cells administered. Preconditioning with myeloablative drugs, such as busulfan and cyclophosphamide, can prevent graft rejection but may be complicated by pulmonary toxicity and by venoocclusive disease of the liver, which results from damage to the hepatic vascular endothelium and can be fatal. Myeloablation results in anemia, leukopenia, and thrombocytopenia, making patients susceptible to infection and bleeding disorders. Neutropenic precautions should be maintained and patients supported with red blood cell and platelet transfusions until the red blood cell, platelet, and neutrophil lineages engraft. Reduced intensity preconditioning has been used recently to prevent graft rejection and decrease the adverse effects of myeloablation. **B-cell lymphoproliferative** disorder can develop after T-cell depleted bone marrow transplantation. **GVHD** can arise from an MHC-mismatched transplantation or from mismatch in minor histocompatibility antigens that are not tested for before transplantation. T-cell depletion of haploidentical bone marrow reduces the risk of GVHD. Patients with SCID transplanted with T-cell–depleted haploidentical bone marrow do not usually develop severe GVHD. **Acute GVHD** begins 6 or more days after transplantation and can result from transfusion of nonirradiated blood products in patients with no T-cell function. Acute GVHD presents with fever, skin rash, and severe diarrhea. Patients develop a high, unrelenting fever; a morbilliform maculopapular erythematous rash that is painful and pruritic; hepatosplenomegaly and abnormal liver function tests; and nausea, vomiting, abdominal pain, and watery diarrhea. Acute GVHD is staged from grades 1-4, depending on the degree of skin, fever, gastrointestinal, and liver involvement. **Chronic GVHD** results from acute GVHD lasting longer than 100 days and can develop without acute GVHD or after acute GVHD has resolved. Chronic GVHD is characterized by skin lesions (hyperkeratosis, reticular hyperpigmentation, fibrosis, and atrophy with ulceration), limitation of joint movement, interstitial pneumonitis, and immune dysregulation with autoantibody and immune complex formation.

Suggested Readings

Bousfiha A, Jeddane L, Al-Herz W, et al. The 2015 IUIS Phenotypic Classification for Primary Immunodeficiencies. *J Clin Immunol.* 2015;35(8):727–738.

Frank MM. Complement disorders and hereditary angioedema. *J Allergy Clin Immunol.* 2010;125(2 suppl 2):S262–S271.

Kang EM, Marciano BE, DeRavin S, et al. Chronic granulomatous disease: overview and hematopoietic stem cell transplantation. *J Allergy Clin Immunol.* 2011;127(6):1319–1326.

Klein C. Genetic defects in severe congenital neutropenia: emerging insights into life and death of human neutrophil granulocytes. *Annu Rev Immunol.* 2011;29:399–413.

Picard C, Al-Herz W, Bousfiha A, et al. Primary immunodeficiency diseases: an update on the classification from the international union of immunological societies expert committee for primary immunodeficiency 2015. *J Clin Immunol.* 2015;35(8):696–726.

Ricklin D, Hajishengallis G, Yang K, et al. Complement: a key system for immune surveillance and homeostasis. *Nat Immunol.* 2010;11:785–797.

Szabolcs P, Cavazzana-Calvo M, Fischer A, et al. Bone marrow transplantation for primary immunodeficiency diseases. *Pediatr Clin North Am.* 2010;57:207–237.

PEARLS FOR PRACTITIONERS

CHAPTER 72

Immunological Assessment

- Primary immune deficiency disorders (PIDDs) result in severe, recurrent, or unusual (opportunistic) infections.
- Secondary causes of immune deficiency (e.g., protein losing enteropathy, drug effects, impaired barrier function such as eczema or burns, anatomical defects, malignancies) should be considered.
- PIDDs typically present in childhood, but can occur at any age, and the age of onset can give clues to the diagnosis.
  - Congenital neutropenia and other phagocyte defects typically present with infections in the first several months of life.
  - Severe combined immunodeficiency (SCID) and other serious combined immunodeficiencies present within the first year of life.
  - Antibody deficiencies typically present after 6 months of age but can present after several years of life.
  - Common variable immunodeficiency (CVID) typically presents in young adulthood.
- The type and location of infections can help to narrow the diagnosis.
  - Gingivitis, poor wound healing, omphalitis, granulomas, or abscesses without pus point to a neutrophil/phagocyte defect.
  - Recurrent sinopulmonary infections suggest a humoral or B-cell defect.
  - Infections with opportunistic infections or severe viral infections suggests a T-cell or combined immunodeficiency.
  - Neiserria infections or early onset autoimmunity may represent a complement defect.
- The initial work-up of a suspected PIDDs is guided by the differential.
  - Suspected neutrophil/phagocyte defects: complete blood count with differential, examination of peripheral smear, dihydrorhodamine 123 (DHR) or nitroblue tetrazolium (NBT) test of the NADPH oxidase pathway, antineutrophil antibody
  - Suspected humoral or B-cell disorder: immunoglobulin G (IgG), IgA, IgM levels, specific titers to diphtheria, tetanus, and pneumococcus
  - Suspected T-cell or combined defect: IgG, IgA, IgM levels, specific titers to diphtheria, tetanus, and pneumococcus, flow cytometry for lymphocyte subsets
  - Suspected complement defects: CH_{50}, AH_{50}
- Genetic testing can confirm a PIDD and may have implications as to treatment and long-term monitoring.
- Treatment of PIDDs is tailored to the diagnosis.
  - Humoral/B-cell defects are treated with immunoglobulin replacement.
  - Neutrophil/phagocyte defects are treated with granulocyte colony-stimulating factor (G-CSF) or hematopoietic stem cell transplant (HSCT).
  - T cells/combined defects are treated with intravenous immunoglobulin (IVIG) replacement until HSCT can be performed.
  - Complement defects are treated with frequent vaccinations and in some cases antibiotic prophylaxis.
- Practical aspects of patients with PIDDs
  - No live-virus vaccines. If patient has SCID, family members should not receive live viral vaccines as well
  - Clean water sources, which may involve boiling water
  - All blood products given to patients with PIDDs should be cytomegalovirus (CMV) negative and irradiated
  - Limit sick contacts

CHAPTER 73

Lymphocyte Disorders

- Agammaglobulinemia may be inherited as either an X-linked or autosomal recessive disorder.
- Patients with agammaglobulinemia have an increased risk of infection with bacteria as well as enteroviruses and giardia.
- CVID has low IgG levels with low IgA or IgM levels.
- Patients with CVID are at risk for infection, autoimmunity, and lymphoma.
- Hyper-IgM syndrome may be inherited as an X-linked or autosomal recessive disorder.
- SCID diseases present with failure to thrive, severe bacterial or virus infections, diarrhea, eczema-like skin rash, and graft versus host disease from transfused lymphocytes.
- DiGeorge syndrome is characterized by hypocalcemia, congenital heart disease, T-cell immunodeficiency, and deletions on chromosome 22q11.2.

CHAPTER 74

Neutrophil Disorders

- Neutrophil disorders may manifest with abscesses, lymphadenitis, gingivitis, poor wound healing, delayed separation of the umbilical cord, or poor pus formation.
- Neutropenia is defined as an absolute neutrophil count of <1,500/mm^3 in white children >1 year of age. It is somewhat lower in black children.
- Cyclic neutropenia has ~21-day cycles of low neutrophil counts that then recover.
- Autoimmune neutropenia develops in children between 5 and 24 months of age and may persist; it responds to G-CSF.
- Chronic granulomatous disease results from defective intracellular neutrophil killing of bacteria that produce catalase.

CHAPTER 75

Complement System

- Deficiencies of early components of the classic compliment pathway are associated with severe infections.
- Patients with C1, C2, or C4 deficiency are at risk for autoimmune diseases (systemic lupus erythematosus).
- Deficiency of C3, properdin, or terminal complement components results in severe infection.
- Deficiency of C1 inhibitor produces hereditary angioedema.

CHAPTER 76

Hematopoietic Stem Cell Transplantation

- Hematopoietic stem cell transplantation has been used to treat malignancies, some metabolic disorders, aplastic anemia, immunodeficiency or immune dysregulation syndromes, and hemoglobinopathies.

ALLERGY

Kristen K. Volkman | Asriani M. Chiu

CHAPTER 77

Allergy Assessment

Atopy is a result of a complex interaction between multiple genes and environmental factors. It implies specific immunoglobulin (Ig)E-mediated diseases, including allergic rhinitis, asthma, and food allergy. An **allergen** is an antigen that triggers an IgE response in genetically predisposed individuals.

Hypersensitivity disorders of the immune system are classified into four groups, based on the mechanism of tissue inflammation (Table 77.1). **Type I reactions** result from the binding of antigen to cell surface-bound IgE on high-affinity IgE receptors on tissue mast cells, circulating basophils, or both, causing the release of preformed chemical mediators, such as histamine and tryptase, and newly generated mediators, such as leukotrienes, prostaglandins, and platelet-activating factor. These mediators contribute to the development of allergic symptoms, with anaphylaxis as the most profound syndrome. Several hours after the initial response, a **late-phase reaction** may develop with an influx of other inflammatory cells such as basophils, eosinophils, monocytes, lymphocytes, and neutrophils, and their inflammatory mediators. Recruitment of these cells leads to more persistent and chronic symptoms.

Type II (cytotoxic antibody) reactions involve IgM, IgG, or IgA antibodies binding to cell surface antigens and activating the entire complement pathway resulting in lysis of the cell or release of anaphylatoxins, such as C3a, C4a, and C5a (see Chapter 75). These anaphylatoxins trigger mast cell degranulation, resulting in inflammatory mediator release. The target can be cell surface membrane antigens, such as red blood cells causing hemolytic anemia, platelet cell surface molecules, glomerular basement membrane molecules, acetylcholine receptor α chain at the neuromuscular junction, and thyroid-stimulating hormone receptor on thyroid cells causing Graves disease.

Type III (immune complex) reactions involve the formation of antigen-antibody or immune complexes that enter into the circulation and are deposited in tissues such as blood vessels and filtering organs (i.e., liver, spleen, and kidney). These complexes initiate tissue injury by activating the complement cascade and recruiting neutrophils that release their toxic mediators. Local reactions caused by the injection of antigen into tissue are called **Arthus reactions.** The administration of large amounts of antigen leads to **serum sickness**. Other type III reactions include hypersensitivity pneumonitis and some vasculitic syndromes.

Type IV (cellular immune–mediated or delayed-hypersensitivity) reactions involve recognition of antigen by sensitized T cells. Antigen-presenting cells present peptides on the cell surface in association with major histocompatibility complex class II (MHC-II) molecules. Memory T cells recognize the peptide/MHC-II complex resulting in cytokine release (e.g., interferon-γ, tumor necrosis factor-α, and granulocyte-macrophage colony-stimulating factor), which activates and

TABLE 77.1 Gell and Coombs Classification of Hypersensitivity Disorders

TYPE	INTERVAL BETWEEN EXPOSURE AND REACTION	EFFECTOR MOLECULE	TARGET OR ANTIGEN	EXAMPLES OF MEDIATORS	EXAMPLES
I Immediate Late phase	<30 min 2-12 hr	IgE	Pollens, food, venom, drugs	Histamine, tryptase, leukotrienes, prostaglandins, platelet-activating factor	Anaphylaxis, urticaria, allergic rhinitis, allergic asthma
II Cytotoxic antibody	Variable (minutes to hours)	IgM, IgG, IgA	Red blood cells, platelets	Complement	Hemolytic anemia, thrombocytopenia, Goodpasture syndrome
III Immune complex	1-3 wk after drug exposure	Antigen-antibody complexes	Blood vessels, liver, spleen, kidney, lung	Complement, anaphylatoxin	Serum sickness, hypersensitivity pneumonitis
IV Delayed type	2-7 days after drug exposure	Lymphocytes	*Mycobacterium tuberculosis*, chemicals	Cytokines (IFN-γ, TNFα, GM-CSF)	TB skin test reactions, contact dermatitis, graft-versus-host disease

CSF, Cerebrospinal fluid; *GM-CSF*, granulocyte-macrophage colony-stimulating factor; *IFN-γ*, interferon-γ; *TB*, tuberculosis; *TNFα*, tumor necrosis factor-α.

attracts tissue macrophages. **Contact allergies** (e.g., nickel dermatitis and poison ivy) and immunity to tuberculosis are examples of type IV reactions.

HISTORY

Decision-Making Algorithm
Available @ StudentConsult.com
Recurrent Infections

The history may reveal allergic symptoms after exposure to a potential trigger that usually has occurred upon previous exposures.

A family history of allergic disease is often present in affected patients. Multiple genes predispose to atopy. If one parent has allergies, the risk that a child will develop an allergic disease is 25%. If both parents have allergies, the risk increases to 50-70%. Similar atopic diseases tend to occur in families.

PHYSICAL EXAMINATION

Decision-Making Algorithm
Available @ StudentConsult.com
Recurrent Infections

Allergic disease may involve the skin, nose, eyes, lungs, or gastrointestinal tract alone or in combination. Many patients have more than one organ system involved.

Children with allergic rhinitis exhibit frequent nasal itching and rubbing of the nose with the palm of the hand, called the **allergic salute**, which leads to a transverse nasal crease across the nose. Pale nasal mucosa and edematous turbinates are common examination findings. **Allergic shiners**, blue-gray to purple discoloration below the lower eyelids attributed to venous congestion, along with swollen eyelids or conjunctival injection are often present in children. Dermatologic findings of atopy include pruritic, erythematous plaques of atopic dermatitis, prominent creases under the lower eyelids **(Dennie–Morgan folds** or **Dennie lines)**, urticaria, and **keratosis pilaris** (asymptomatic horny follicular papules on the extensor surfaces of the arms). Wheezing may be noted on auscultation of the lower respiratory tract.

INITIAL DIAGNOSTIC EVALUATION

Screening Tests

Decision-Making Algorithms
Available @ StudentConsult.com
Eosinophilia
Recurrent Infections

Atopy is characterized by elevated levels of IgE (Table 77.2) and **eosinophilia** (3-10% of white blood cells or an absolute eosinophil count of >250 eosinophils/mm^3) with a predominance of T helper (Th)2 cytokines, including interleukin (IL)-4, IL-5, and IL-13. Extreme eosinophilia suggests a nonallergic disorder such as infection, hypereosinophilic syndrome, drug reaction, or malignancy (Table 77.3).

TABLE 77.2 Disorders Associated With Elevated Serum Immunoglobulin E
Allergic disease
Atopic dermatitis (eczema)
Tissue-invasive helminthic infections
Hyperimmunoglobulin-E syndrome
Allergic bronchopulmonary aspergillosis
Wiskott-Aldrich syndrome
Bone marrow transplantation
Hodgkin disease
Bullous pemphigoid
Idiopathic nephrotic syndrome

TABLE 77.3 Disorders Associated With Eosinophilia
ALLERGIC DISEASE
Allergic rhinitis
Atopic dermatitis
Asthma
GASTROINTESTINAL
Eosinophilic esophagitis and gastroenteritis
Allergic colitis
Inflammatory bowel disease
INFECTIOUS
Tissue-invasive helminthic infections
NEOPLASTIC
Eosinophilic leukemia
Hodgkin disease
RESPIRATORY
Eosinophilic pneumonia
Allergic bronchopulmonary aspergillosis
SYSTEMIC
Idiopathic hypereosinophilic syndrome
Adrenal insufficiency
Mastocytosis
IATROGENIC
Drug-induced

There are two methods for identifying allergen-specific IgE: in vivo skin testing and in vitro serum testing (Table 77.4). **In vivo skin testing** introduces allergen into the skin via a prick/puncture or intradermal injection. The allergen diffuses through the skin to interact with IgE that is bound to mast cells. Cross-linking of IgE causes mast cell degranulation, which results in histamine release and the development of a **central wheal and erythematous flare**. The wheal and flare are measured 15-20 minutes after the allergen has been applied.

TABLE 77.4 Comparison of In Vivo Skin Tests and In Vitro Serum IgE Antibody Immunoassay in Allergic Diagnosis

IN VIVO SKIN TEST	IN VITRO SERUM IMMUNOASSAY
Less expensive	Patient/physician convenience
Greater sensitivity	Not suppressed by antihistamines
Wide allergen selection	Preferable to skin testing for dermatographism, widespread dermatitis, or uncooperative children
Results available immediately	

From Skoner DP. Allergic rhinitis: definition, epidemiology, pathophysiology, detection, and diagnosis. J Allergy Clin Immunol. *2001;108:S2–S8.*

Properly performed skin tests are the most sensitive method for detecting the presence of allergen-specific IgE.

In vitro serum testing, such as immunoassays like the enzyme-linked immunosorbent assay **(ELISA)**, measures levels of antigen-specific IgE. Many allergists and laboratories regard the ImmunoCAP System (ThermoFisher Scientific, Waltham, Massachusetts) as the method of choice. This method uses a solid phase and shows higher sensitivity, specificity, and reproducibility. The assay uses a quantitative fluorescent immunoassay (FEIA) that is more sensitive than other methods. Serum-based tests are indicated for patients who have dermatographism or extensive dermatitis; who cannot discontinue medications, such as antihistamines that interfere with skin test results; or who are noncompliant for skin testing. The presence of specific IgE antibodies suggests sensitization but is not sufficient for the diagnosis of allergic disease. Diagnosis must be based on the physician's assessment of the entire clinical picture, including the history and physical examination, the presence of specific IgE antibodies, and the correlation with IgE-mediated symptoms.

DIAGNOSTIC IMAGING

Diagnostic imaging has a limited role in the evaluation of allergic disease. Chest radiography is helpful with the differential diagnosis of asthma. Sinus radiography and computed tomography may be useful, but when these images are abnormal, they do not distinguish allergic disease from nonallergic disease.

CHAPTER 78

Asthma

ETIOLOGY

Inflammatory cells (mast cells, eosinophils, T lymphocytes, neutrophils), chemical mediators (histamine, leukotrienes, platelet-activating factor, bradykinin), and chemotactic factors (cytokines, eotaxin) mediate the underlying inflammation found in asthmatic airways. Inflammation contributes to **airway hyperresponsiveness** (airways constricting in response to allergens, irritants, viral infections, and exercise). It also results in edema, increased mucus production in the lungs, influx of inflammatory cells into the airway tissue, and epithelial cell denudation. Chronic inflammation can lead to **airway remodeling**, which results from a proliferation of extracellular matrix proteins and vascular hyperplasia and may lead to irreversible structural changes and progressive loss of pulmonary function.

EPIDEMIOLOGY

Asthma is the most common chronic disease of childhood in industrialized countries, affecting nearly 7 million children younger than 18 years of age in the United States. From 2001 to 2010, individuals with asthma increased by 2.9% per year. In adults, females are more likely than males to have asthma, but in children the reverse is true. Among children less than 18 years of age, asthma prevalence increased by 1.4% per year. In 2010, pediatric hospitalizations for asthma numbered close to 140,000. Mortality from asthma occurs; in 2014, 187 deaths were attributed to asthma. For children, the death rate is 2.5 per million.

CLINICAL MANIFESTATIONS

Decision-Making Algorithms
Available @ StudentConsult.com

Rhinorrhea
Cough
Wheezing
Chest Pain

Children with asthma have symptoms of coughing, wheezing, shortness of breath, exercise intolerance, or chest tightness. The history should elicit the frequency, severity, and precipitating factors as well as a family history of asthma and allergy. Common exacerbating factors include viral infections, exposure to allergens and irritants (e.g., smoke, air pollution, strong odors, fumes), exercise, emotions, and change in weather/humidity. Nocturnal symptoms are common. Rhinosinusitis, gastroesophageal reflux, and aspirin can aggravate asthma. Treatment of these conditions may lessen the frequency and severity of asthma.

During acute episodes, tachypnea, tachycardia, cough, wheezing, and a prolonged expiratory phase may be present. Physical findings may be subtle. Wheezing may not be prominent if there is poor aeration from airway obstruction. As the attack progresses, cyanosis, diminished air movement, retractions, agitation, inability to speak, tripod sitting position, diaphoresis, and pulsus paradoxus (decrease in blood pressure of >15 mm Hg with inspiration) may be observed. Physical examination may show evidence of other atopic diseases such as eczema or allergic rhinitis.

LABORATORY AND IMAGING STUDIES

While no single test or study can confirm the diagnosis of asthma, many elements contribute to establishing the diagnosis.

Objective measurements of pulmonary function **(spirometry)** aid in the diagnosis and direct the treatment of asthma. Spirometry is used to monitor response to treatment, assess degree of reversibility to therapeutic intervention, and measure

TABLE 78.1 Differential Diagnosis of Cough and Wheeze in Infants and Children

UPPER AIRWAY DISEASES	OBSTRUCTION INVOLVING LARGE AIRWAYS	OBSTRUCTION INVOLVING SMALL AIRWAYS	OTHER
Allergic rhinitis Sinusitis	Tracheal or bronchial foreign body Paradoxical vocal fold motion Vascular rings or laryngeal webs Enlarged lymph nodes or tumor	Viral bronchiolitis or obliterative bronchiolitis Cystic fibrosis Bronchopulmonary dysplasia (chronic lung disease of prematurity)	Recurrent cough not caused by asthma (infection, habit cough, postnasal drip) Aspiration from swallowing mechanism dysfunction or gastroesophageal reflux disease

From Guilbert TW, Lemanske RF, Jackson DJ. Diagnosis of asthma in infants and children. In: Adkinson NF Jr, Bochner BS, Burks AW, et al., eds. Middleton's Allergy: Principles and Practice. *8th ed. Philadelphia: Saunders; 2014:870.*

TABLE 78.2 Mnemonic of Causes of Cough in the First Months of Life

C—Cystic fibrosis
R—Respiratory tract infections
A—Aspiration (swallowing dysfunction, gastroesophageal reflux, tracheoesophageal fistula, foreign body)
D—Dyskinetic cilia
L—Lung and airway malformations (laryngeal webs, laryngotracheomalacia, tracheal stenosis, vascular rings and slings)
E—Edema (heart failure, congenital heart disease)

From Schidlow DV. Cough. In: Schidlow DV, Smith DS, eds. A Practical Guide to Pediatric Disease. *Philadelphia: Hanley & Belfus; 1994.*

the severity of an asthma exacerbation. Children older than 5 years of age can usually perform spirometry maneuvers. Variability in predicted peak flow reference values make spirometry preferred over peak flow measures in the diagnosis of asthma. For younger children who cannot perform spirometry maneuvers or peak flow, a therapeutic trial of controller medications aids in the diagnosis of asthma.

Allergy skin testing should be included in the evaluation of all children with persistent asthma but not during an exacerbation of symptoms. Positive skin test results, identifying sensitization to **aeroallergens** (e.g., pollens, mold, dust mite, pet dander), correlate strongly with bronchial allergen provocative challenges. In vitro serum tests, such as enzyme-linked immunosorbent assay (ELISA), are generally less sensitive in defining clinically pertinent allergens, are more expensive, and require several days for results, compared to several minutes for skin testing (see Table 77.4).

An **x-ray** should be performed with the first episode of asthma or with recurrent episodes of undiagnosed cough or wheeze to exclude anatomic abnormalities. Repeat chest x-rays are not needed with new episodes unless there is fever (suggesting pneumonia) or localized findings on physical examination.

Two novel forms of monitoring asthma and airway inflammation directly include **exhaled nitric oxide analysis** and quantitative analysis of expectorated sputum for eosinophilia.

DIFFERENTIAL DIAGNOSIS

Many childhood conditions can cause wheezing and coughing like asthma (Table 78.1), but not all cough and wheeze is asthma. Misdiagnosis delays correcting the underlying cause and exposes children to inappropriate therapy (Table 78.2).

Allergic bronchopulmonary aspergillosis is a hypersensitivity reaction to antigens of the mold *Aspergillus fumigatus.* It occurs primarily in patients with steroid-dependent asthma and in patients with cystic fibrosis.

TREATMENT

Optimal medical treatment of asthma includes several key components: environmental control, pharmacologic therapy, and patient education, including attainment of self-management skills. Because many children with asthma have coexisting allergies, steps to minimize allergen exposure should be taken (Table 78.3). For all children with asthma, exposures to tobacco and wood smoke and to persons with viral infections should be minimized. Influenza immunization is indicated. Asthma medications can be divided into long-term control medications and quick-relief medications.

Long-Term Control Medications

Inhaled Corticosteroids

Inhaled corticosteroids are the most effective antiinflammatory medications for the treatment of chronic, persistent asthma and are the preferred therapy when initiating long-term control therapy. Early intervention with inhaled corticosteroids reduces morbidity but does not alter the natural history of asthma. Regular use reduces airway hyperreactivity, the need for rescue bronchodilator therapy, risk of hospitalization, and risk of death from asthma. Inhaled corticosteroids are available as inhalation aerosols, dry powder inhalers, and a nebulizer solution.

The potential risks of inhaled corticosteroids are favorably balanced with their benefits. A reduction in growth velocity may occur with poorly controlled asthma or inhaled corticosteroid use. Low-to-medium dose inhaled corticosteroids may decrease growth velocity, although these effects are small (approximately 1 cm in the first year of treatment), generally not progressive, and may be reversible. Height measurements should be monitored. Inhaled corticosteroids do not have clinically significant adverse effects on hypothalamic-pituitary-adrenal axis function, glucose metabolism, subcapsular cataracts, or glaucoma when used at low-to-medium doses in children. Rinsing the mouth after inhalation and using large volume spacers help lessen the local adverse effects of dysphonia and candidiasis and decrease systemic absorption from the gastrointestinal tract. Inhaled corticosteroids should be titrated to the lowest dose needed to

TABLE 78.3 Controlling Factors Contributing to Asthma Severity

MAJOR INDOOR TRIGGERS FOR ASTHMA	SUGGESTIONS FOR REDUCING EXPOSURE
Viral upper respiratory tract (RSV, influenza virus)	Limit exposure to viral infections (day care with fewer children)
	Annual influenza immunization for children with persistent asthma
Tobacco smoke, wood smoke	No smoking around the child or in child's home
	Help parents and caregivers quit smoking
	Eliminate use of wood stoves and fireplaces
Dust mites	ESSENTIAL ACTIONS
	Encase pillow, mattress, and box spring in allergen-impermeable encasements
	Wash bedding in hot water weekly
	DESIRABLE ACTIONS
	Avoid sleeping or lying on upholstered furniture
	Minimize number of stuffed toys in child's bedroom
	Reduce indoor humidity to <50%
	If possible, remove carpets from bedroom and play areas; if not possible, vacuum weekly
Animal dander	Remove the pet from the home or keep outdoors (if removal is not acceptable)
	Keep pet out of bedroom/no sleeping with pet
	Use a filter on air ducts in child's room
	Wash pet weekly (the evidence to support this has not been firmly established)
Cockroach allergens	Do not leave food or garbage exposed
	Pesticides
	Sealing cracks and holes
Indoor mold	Avoid vaporizers
	Reduce indoor humidity to <50%
	Use of mold inhibiting cleaner
	Use of dehumidifier
	Fix leaky faucets, pipes

RSV, Respiratory syncytial virus.
From American Academy of Allergy Asthma & Immunology. Pediatric Asthma: Promoting Best Practice. *Milwaukee, WI: American Academy of Allergy Asthma & Immunology; 1999:50.*

maintain control of a child's asthma. For children with severe asthma, high dose inhaled corticosteroids may be needed to minimize oral corticosteroid use, but other "add-on" therapy should be considered (see the following sections).

Leukotriene Modifiers

Leukotrienes, synthesized via the arachidonic acid metabolism cascade, are potent mediators of inflammation and smooth muscle bronchoconstriction. Leukotriene modifiers are oral, daily-use medications that inhibit these biologic effects in the airway. Two classes of leukotriene modifiers include cysteinyl leukotriene receptor antagonists (zafirlukast and montelukast) and leukotriene synthesis inhibitors (zileuton). The leukotriene receptor antagonists have much wider appeal than zileuton. Zafirlukast is approved for children older than 5 years of age and is given twice daily. Montelukast is dosed once daily at night as 4-mg granules or chewable tablets (for children 6 months to 5 years of age), 5-mg chewable tablets (6-14 years of age), and 10-mg tablets (≥15 years of age). Pediatric studies show the usefulness of leukotriene modifiers in mild asthma and the attenuation of exercise-induced bronchoconstriction. These agents may be helpful as steroid-sparing agents in patients with asthma that is more difficult to control.

Long-Acting β_2-Agonists

Long-acting β_2-agonists, formoterol and salmeterol, have twice-daily dosing and relax airway smooth muscle for 12 hours but do not have any significant antiinflammatory effects. Adding a long-acting bronchodilator to inhaled corticosteroid therapy is more beneficial than doubling the dose of inhaled corticosteroids. Multiple formulations are available. Formoterol is approved for use in children older than 5 years of age for maintenance asthma therapy and for prevention of exercise-induced asthma. It has a rapid onset of action similar to albuterol (15 minutes). Salmeterol is approved for children 4 years of age or older and has an onset of 30 minutes. Because combination inhalers administer two medications simultaneously, compliance is generally improved.

Theophylline

Theophylline was more widely used previously, but because current management is aimed at inflammatory control, its popularity has declined. It is mildly to moderately effective as a bronchodilator and is considered an alternative, add-on treatment to low- and medium-dose inhaled corticosteroids. However, its therapeutic window is narrow necessitating monitoring of blood levels.

Biologics

Omalizumab is a humanized anti-IgE monoclonal antibody that prevents binding of free IgE to high-affinity receptors on basophils and mast cells. It is approved for moderate to severe allergic asthma in children 6 years of age and older. Omalizumab is delivered by subcutaneous injection every 2-4 weeks, depending on body weight and pretreatment serum IgE level.

Mepolizumab is an add-on maintenance therapy for severe asthma with an eosinophilic phenotype in patients aged 12 years and older. It is an anti-interleukin-5 monoclonal antibody injected subcutaneously every 4 weeks. Mepolizumab decreases the production and survival of eosinophils, a major inflammatory cell involved in asthma pathogenesis.

Quick-Relief Medications

Short-Acting β_2-Agonists

Short-acting β_2-agonists such as albuterol and levalbuterol are effective bronchodilators that exert their effect by relaxing bronchial smooth muscle within 5-10 minutes of administration. These effects last 4-6 hours. Generally, a short-acting β_2-agonist is prescribed for acute symptoms and as prophylaxis before allergen exposure and exercise. The inhaled route is preferred because adverse effects—tremor, prolonged tachycardia, and irritability—are less. **Overuse** of β_2-agonists implies inadequate control, and a change in medications may be warranted. The definition of bronchodilator *overuse* depends on the severity of the child's asthma; use of more than one metered dose inhaler canister per month or daily use suggests poor control.

Anticholinergic Agents

Ipratropium bromide is a short-acting anticholinergic bronchodilator that relieves bronchoconstriction, decreases mucus hypersecretion, and counteracts cough-receptor irritability by binding acetylcholine at the muscarinic receptors found in bronchial smooth muscle. It seems to have an additive effect with β_2-agonists when used for acute asthma exacerbations.

A long-acting anticholinergic agent (tiotropium) is approved for use in moderate to severe persistent asthma in children 12 years or older. It inhibits muscarinic receptors on bronchial smooth muscle to induce bronchodilation.

Oral Corticosteroids

Short bursts of oral corticosteroids (3-10 days) are administered to children with acute exacerbations. The usual dose is 1-2 mg/kg/day of prednisone for 5 days. Oral corticosteroids are available in liquid or tablet formulations. Prolonged use of oral corticosteroids can result in systemic adverse effects such as hypothalamic-pituitary-adrenal suppression, cushingoid features, weight gain, hypertension, diabetes, cataracts, glaucoma, impaired immunity, osteoporosis, and growth suppression. Children with severe asthma may require oral corticosteroids over extended periods. The dose should be tapered as soon as possible to the minimum effective dose, preferably administered on alternate days.

Administration of two doses of dexamethasone for the treatment of acute asthma exacerbations has been used, usually in an emergency room setting for intermittent, mild persistent, or moderate persistent asthma. This oral corticosteroid has properties that may increase compliance with therapy, decrease missed school days, and decrease readmission rates. Results are mixed and have not been translated to outpatient settings.

Approach to Therapy

Therapy is based on the concept that chronic airway inflammation is a fundamental feature of asthma, which can vary in intensity over time, requiring treatment to be adjusted accordingly. Classification of asthma severity is emphasized for initiation of therapy in patients not currently receiving controller medications. Assessing control is emphasized for monitoring and adjusting therapy. A stepwise approach is used for management of infants and young children 0-4 years of age, children 5-11 years of age (Fig. 78.1), and youths 12 years or older, and adults (Fig. 78.2). Medication type, dose, and dosing intervals are determined by the level of asthma severity or asthma control. Therapy is then increased **(stepped up)** as necessary and decreased **(stepped down)** when possible. A short-acting bronchodilator should be available for all children with asthma. A child with intermittent asthma has asthma symptoms less than two times per week. To determine whether a child is having more persistent asthma, using the **Rules of Two** is helpful: daytime symptoms occurring two or more times per week or nocturnal awakenings two or more times per month implies a need for daily antiinflammatory medication.

Inhaled corticosteroids are the preferred initial long-term control therapy for children of all ages (Fig. 78.3). Daily long-term control therapy is recommended for infants and young children 0-4 years of age who had four or more episodes of wheezing in the previous year that lasted more than 1 day, affected sleep, and who have a positive asthma predictive index. For children over 5 years of age with moderate persistent asthma, combining long-acting bronchodilators with low-to-medium doses of inhaled corticosteroids improves lung function and reduces rescue medication use. For children with severe persistent asthma, a high-dose inhaled corticosteroid combined with a long-acting bronchodilator is the preferred therapy. The guidelines also recommend that treatment be reevaluated within 4-6 weeks of initiating therapy. Once asthma is under control, control should be assessed on an ongoing basis every 1-6 months. The asthma should be well controlled for at least 3 months before stepping down therapy.

COMPLICATIONS

Most asthma exacerbations can be successfully managed at home. **Status asthmaticus** is an acute exacerbation of asthma that does not respond adequately to therapeutic measures and may require hospitalization. Exacerbations may progress over several days or occur suddenly and can range in severity from mild to life threatening. Significant respiratory distress, dyspnea, wheezing, cough, and a decrease in **spirometry** or **peak expiratory flow rate (PEFR)** characterize deterioration in asthma control. During a severe episode, pulse oximetry is helpful in monitoring oxygenation. In status asthmaticus, arterial blood gases may be necessary for measurement of ventilation. As airway obstruction worsens and chest compliance decreases, carbon dioxide retention can occur. In the face of tachypnea, a *normal* P_{CO_2} (35-45 mm Hg) indicates impending respiratory arrest.

First-line management of asthma exacerbations includes supplemental oxygen if needed and repetitive or continuous administration of short-acting bronchodilators. Early administration of oral or intravenous corticosteroids (Fig. 78.4) is important in treating the underlying inflammation. Administration of anticholinergic agents (ipratropium) with bronchodilators decreases rates of hospitalization and duration of time in the emergency department. Intravenous magnesium sulfate is administered in the emergency department if there is clinical deterioration despite treatment with β_2-agonists, ipratropium, and systemic corticosteroids. The typical dose of magnesium sulfate is 25-75 mg/kg (maximum 2.0 g) intravenously administered over 20 minutes. Intramuscular epinephrine or subcutaneous terbutaline are rarely used except when severe asthma is associated with anaphylaxis or unresponsive to continuous administration of short-acting bronchodilators.

PROGNOSIS

For some children, symptoms of wheezing with respiratory infections subside in the preschool years, whereas others have more persistent asthma symptoms. Prognostic indicators for children younger than 3 years of age who are at risk for persistent asthma are known as the Modified Asthma Predictive Index for children (Table 78.4). Atopy is the strongest

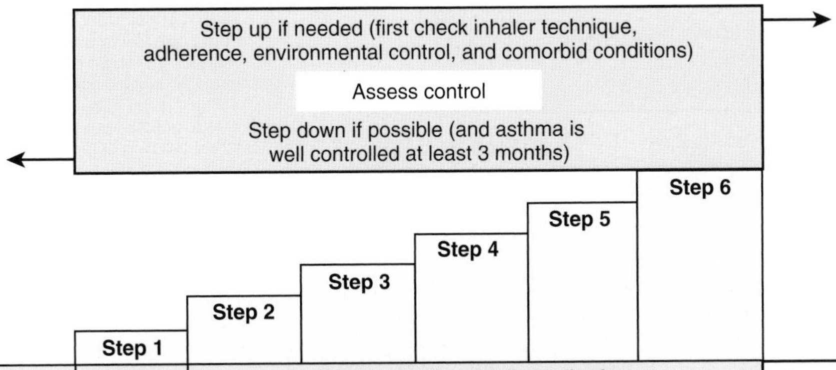

Children 0–4 years of age

	Step 1	Step 2	Step 3	Step 4	Step 5	Step 6
	Intermittent asthma	**Persistent asthma: Daily medication** Consult with asthma specialist if Step 3 care or higher is required. Consider consultation at Step 2.				
Preferred	SABA PRN	Low-dose ICS	Medium-dose ICS	Medium-dose ICS + LABA *or* Montelukast	High-dose ICS + LABA *or* Montelukast	High-dose ICS + **LABA or Montelukast** + **Oral corticosteroids ICS**
Alternative		Cromolyn *or* Montelukast				
	Each Step: Patient Education and Environmental Control					
Quick-Relief Medication	• SABA as needed for symptoms. Intensity of treatment depends on severity of symptoms. • With viral respiratory symptoms: SABA q 4–6 hours up to 24 hours (longer with physician consult). Consider short course of oral systemic corticosteroids if exacerbation is severe or patient has history of previous severe exacerbations. Caution: Frequent use of SABA may indicate the need to step up treatment. See text for recommendations on initiating daily long-term-control therapy.					

Notes

- The stepwise approach is meant to assist, not replace, the clinical decision making required to meet individual patient needs.
- If an alternative treatment is used and response is inadequate, discontinue it and use the preferred treatment before stepping up.
- If clear benefit is not observed within 4–6 weeks, and patient's/family's medication technique and adherence are satisfactory, consider adjusting therapy or an alternative diagnosis.
- Studies on children 0–4 years of age are limited. Step 2 preferred therapy is based on Evidence A. All other recommendations are based on expert opinion and extrapolation from studies in older children.
- Clinicians who administer immunotherapy should be prepared and equipped to identify and treat anaphylaxis that may occur.

Key: Alphabetical listing is used when more than one treatment option is listed within either preferred or alternative therapy. *ICS*, Inhaled corticosteroid; *LABA*, inhaled long-acting $beta_2$-agonist; *LTRA*, leukotriene receptor antagonist, oral corticosteroids, oral systemic corticosteroids; *SABA*, inhaled short-acting $beta_2$-agonist

Children 5–11 Years of Age

	Step 1	Step 2	Step 3	Step 4	Step 5	Step 6
	Intermittent Asthma	**Persistent Asthma: Daily Medication** Consult with asthma specialist if Step 4 care or higher is required. Consider consultation at Step 3.				
Preferred	SABA PRN	Low-dose ICS	Low-dose ICS + LABA, LTRA, *or* Theophylline *OR*	Medium-dose ICS + LABA	High-dose ICS + LABA	High-dose ICS + LABA + Oral corticosteroids
Alternative		Cromolyn LTRA Nedocromil, *or* Theophylline	Medium-dose ICS	Medium-dose ICS + LTRA *or* Theophylline	High-dose ICS + LTRA *or* Theophylline	High-dose ICS + LTRA *or* Theophylline + Oral corticosteroids
	Each Step: Patient Education and Environmental Control, and Management of Comorbidities Steps 2–4: Consider subcutaneous allergen immunotherapy for patients who have persistent, allergic asthma.					
Quick-Relief Medication	• SABA as needed for symptoms. Intensity of treatment depends on severity of symptoms: up to 3 treatments at 20-minute intervals as needed. Short course of oral systemic corticosteroids may be needed. Caution: Increasing use of SABA or use >2 days a week for symptom relief (not prevention of EIB) generally indicates inadequate control and the need to step up treatment.					

- The stepwise approach is meant to assist, not replace, the clinical decision making required to meet individual patient needs.
- If an alternative treatment is used and response is inadequate, discontinue it and use the preferred treatment before stepping up.
- Theophylline is a less desirable alternative due to the need to monitor serum concentration levels.
- Steps 1 and 2 medications are based on Evidence A. Step 3 ICS and ICS plus adjunctive therapy are based on Evidence B for efficacy of each treatment and extrapolation from comparator trials in older children and adults–comparator trials are not available for this age group; Steps 4–6 are based on expert opinion and extrapolation from studies in older children and adults.
- Immunotherapy for Steps 2–4 is based on Evidence B for house-dust mites, animal danders, and pollens; evidence is weak or lacking for molds and cockroaches. Evidence is strongest for immunotherapy with single allergens. The role of allergy in asthma is greater in children than adults.
- Clinicians who administer immunotherapy should be prepared and equipped to identify and treat anaphylaxis that may occur.

Key: Alphabetical listing is used when more than one treatment option is listed within either preferred or alternative therapy. *ICS*, Inhaled corticosteroid; *LABA*, inhaled long-acting $beta_2$-agonist; *LTRA*, leukotriene receptor antagonist; *SABA*, inhaled short-acting $beta_2$-agonist

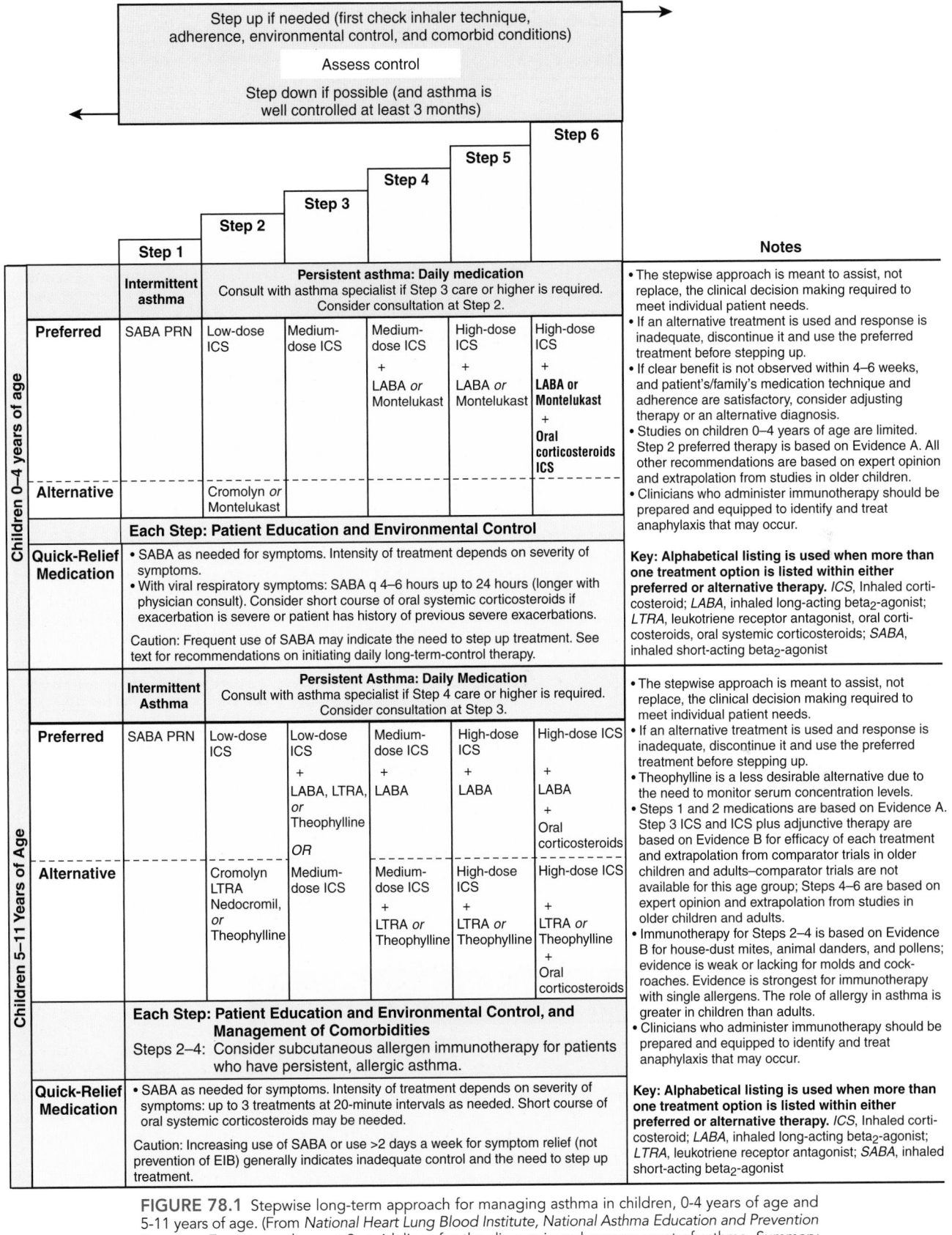

FIGURE 78.1 Stepwise long-term approach for managing asthma in children, 0-4 years of age and 5-11 years of age. (From *National Heart Lung Blood Institute, National Asthma Education and Prevention Program.* Expert panel report 3: guidelines for the diagnosis and management of asthma. Summary report 2007, NIH Publication No. 08-5846, Bethesda, MD, 2007, U.S. Department of Health and Human Services, 42, <http://www.nhlbi.nih.gov/guidelines/asthma/asthsumm.pdf>.)

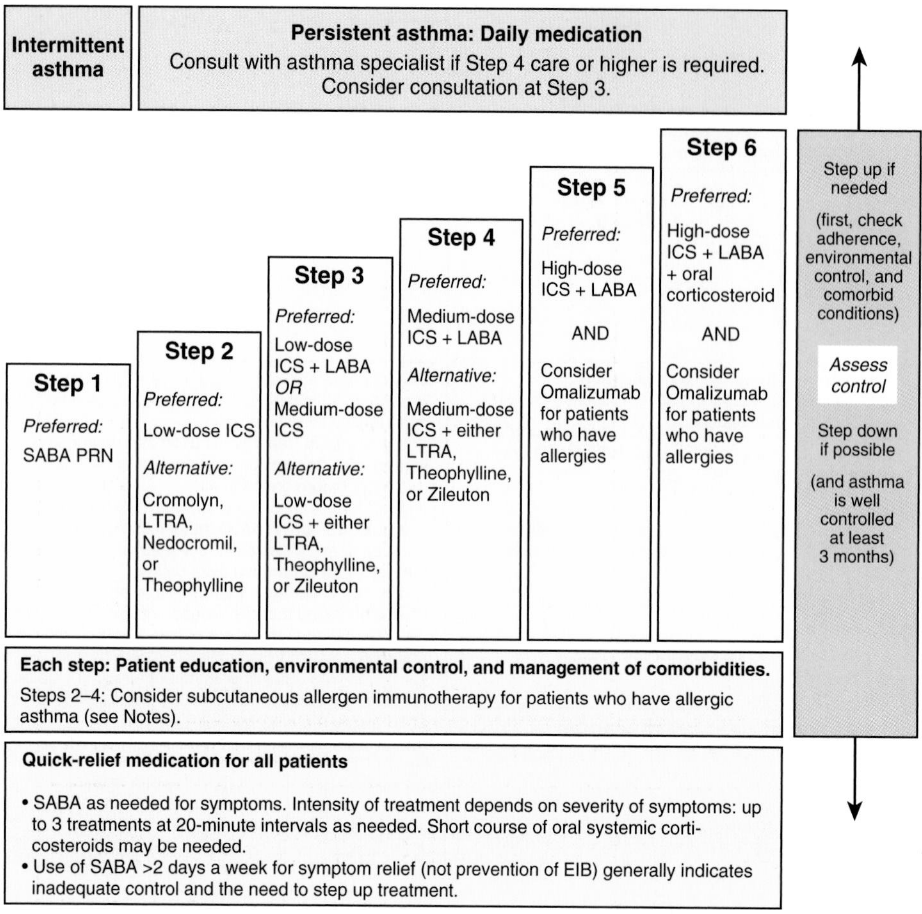

Key: **Alphabetical order is used when more than one treatment option is listed within either preferred or alternative therapy.** *ICS*, Inhaled corticosteroid; *LABA*, long-acting inhaled beta$_2$-agonist; *LTRA*, leukotriene receptor antagonist; *SABA*, inhaled short-acting beta$_2$-agonist

Notes:

- The stepwise approach is meant to assist, not replace, the clinical decision making required to meet individual patient needs.
- If alternative treatment is used and response is inadequate, discontinue it and use the preferred treatment before stepping up.
- Zileuton is a less desirable alternative due to limited studies as adjunctive therapy and the need to monitor liver function. Theophylline requires monitoring of serum concentration levels.
- In Step 6, before oral corticosteroids are introduced, a trial of high-dose ICS + LABA + either LTRA, Theophylline, or Zileuton may be considered, although this approach has not been studied in clinical trials.
- Step 1, 2, and 3 preferred therapies are based on Evidence A; Step 3 alternative therapy is based on Evidence A for LTRA, Evidence B for Theophylline, and Evidence D for Zileuton. Step 4 preferred therapy is based on Evidence B, and alternative therapy is based on Evidence B for LTRA and Theophylline and Evidence D Zileuton. Step 5 preferred therapy is based on Evidence B. Step 6 preferred therapy is based on (EPR–2 1997) and Evidence B for Omalizumab.
- Immunotherapy for Steps 2–4 is based on Evidence B for house-dust mites, animal danders, and pollens; evidence is weak or lacking for molds and cockroaches. Evidence is strongest for immunotherapy with single allergens. The role of allergy in asthma is greater in children than in adults.
- Clinicians who administer immunotherapy or Omalizumab should be prepared and equipped to identify and treat anaphylaxis that may occur.

FIGURE 78.2 Stepwise approach for managing asthma in youths 12 years of age or older and adults. (From *National Heart Lung Blood Institute, National Asthma Education and Prevention Program.* Expert panel report 3: guidelines for the diagnosis and management of asthma. Summary report 2007, NIH Publication No. 08-5846, Bethesda, MD, 2007, U.S. Department of Health and Human Services, 45, <http://www.nhlbi.nih.gov/guidelines/asthma/asthsumm.pdf>.)

TABLE 78.4 Modified Asthma Predictive Index for Children

At least four wheezing episodes *plus*:	
1 Major criteria	Or 2 Minor criteria
Parental asthma	Allergic rhinitis
Eczema	Wheezing apart from colds
Inhalant allergen sensitization	Eosinophils ≥ 4%
	Food allergen sensitization

From Liu AH, Martinez FD. Natural history of allergic diseases and asthma. In: Leung DYM, Szefler SJ, Bonilla FA, et al., eds. Pediatric Allergy: Principles and Practice. *3rd ed. Philadelphia: Elsevier; 2016. Fig. 2.4.*

Drug	Low Daily Dose: Child 0–4 Years of Age	Low Daily Dose: Child 5–11 Years of Age	Low Daily Dose: ≥12 Years of Age and Adults	Medium Daily Dose: Child 0–4 Years of Age	Medium Daily Dose: Child 5–11 Years of Age	Medium Daily Dose: ≥12 Years of Age and Adults	High Daily Dose: Child 0–4 Years of Age	High Daily Dose: Child 5–11 Years of Age	High Daily Dose: ≥12 Years of Age and Adults
Beclomethasone HFA 40 or 80 μg/puff	NA	80–160 μg	80–240 μg	NA	>160–320 μg	>240–480 μg	NA	>320 μg	>480 μg
Budesonide DPI 90, 180, or 200 μg/inhalation	NA	180–400 μg	180–600 μg	NA	>400–800 μg	>600–1,200 μg	NA	>800 μg	>1,200 μg
Budesonide Inhaled Inhalation suspension for nebulization	0.25–0.5 mg	0.5 mg	NA	>0.5–1.0 mg	1.0 mg	NA	>1.0 mg	2.0 mg	NA
Flunisolide 250 μg/puff	NA	500–750 μg	500–1,000 μg	NA	1,000–1,250 μg	>1,000–2,000 μg	NA	>1,250 μg	>2,000 μg
Flunisolide HFA 80 μg/puff	NA	160 μg	320 μg	NA	320 μg	>320–640 μg	NA	≥640 μg	>640 μg
Fluticasone **HFA/MDI:** 44, 110, or 220 μg/puff	176 μg	88–176 μg	88–264 μg	>176–352 μg	>176–352 μg	>264–440 μg	>352 μg	>352 μg	>440 μg
DPI: 50, 100, or 250 μg/inhalation	NA	100–200 μg	100–300 μg	NA	>200–400 μg	>300–500 μg	NA	>400 μg	>500 μg
Mometasone DPI 200 μg/inhalation	NA	NA	200 μg	NA	NA	400 μg	NA	NA	>400 μg
Triamcinolone acetonide 75 μg/puff	NA	300–600 μg	300–750 μg	NA	>600–900 μg	>750–1,500 μg	NA	>900 μg	>1,500 μg

Key: *DPI*, Dry power inhaler; *HFA*, hydrofluoroalkane; *MDI*, metered-dose inhaler; *NA*, not available (either not approved, no data available, or safety and efficacy not established for this age group)

Therapeutic Issues:

- The most important determinant of appropriate dosing is the clinician's judgment of the patient's response to therapy. The clinician must monitor the patient's response on several clinical parameters and adjust the dose accordingly. Once control of asthma is achieved, the dose should be carefully titrated to the minimum dose required to maintain control.
- Preparations are not interchangeable on a μg or per puff basis. This figure presents estimated comparable daily doses. See EPR–3 Full Report 2007 for full discussion.
- Some doses may be outside package labeling, especially in the high-dose range. Budesonide nebulizer suspension is the only inhaler corticosteroid (ICS) with FDA-approved labeling for children <4 years of age.
- For children <4 years of age: The safety and efficacy of ICSs in children <1 year has not been established. Children <4 years of age generally require delivery of ICS (budesonide and fluticasone HFA) through a face mask that should fit snugly over nose and mouth and avoid nebulizing in the eyes. Wash face after each treatment to prevent local corticosteroid side effects. For budesonide, the dose may be administered 1–3 times daily. Budesonide suspension is compatible with Albuterol, Ipratropium, and Levalbuterol nebulizer solutions in the same nebulizer. Use only jet nebulizers, as ultrasonic nebulizers are ineffective for suspensions. For Fluticasone HFA, the dose should be divided 2 times daily; the low dose for children <4 years of age is higher than for children 5–11 years of age due to lower dose delivered with face mask and data on efficacy in young children.

Potential Adverse Effects of Inhaled Corticosteroids:

- Cough, dysphonia, oral thrush (candidiasis).
- Spacer or valved holding chamber with non-breath-actuated MDIs and mouthwashing and spitting after inhalation decrease local side effects.
- A number of the ICSs, including Fluticasone, Budesonide, and Mometasone, are metabolized in the gastrointestinal tract and liver by CYP 3A4 isoenzymes. Potent inhibitors of CYP 3A4, such as Ritonavir and Ketoconazole, have the potential for increasing systemic concentrations of these ICSs by increasing oral availability and decreasing systemic clearance. Some cases of clinically significant Cushing syndrome and secondary adrenal insufficiency have been reported.
- In high doses, systemic effects may occur, although studies are not conclusive, and clinical significance of these effects has not been established (e.g., adrenal suppression, osteoporosis, skin thinning, and easy bruising). In low-to-medium doses, suppression of growth velocity has been observed in children, but this effect may be transient, and the clinical significance has not been established.

FIGURE 78.3 Estimated comparative daily dosages for inhaled corticosteroids. (From *National Heart Lung Blood Institute, National Asthma Education and Prevention Program*. Expert panel report 3: guidelines for the diagnosis and management of asthma. Summary report 2007, NIH Publication No. 08-5846, Bethesda, MD, 2007, U.S. Department of Health and Human Services, 49, <http://www.nhlbi.nih.gov/guidelines/asthma/asthsumm.pdf>.)

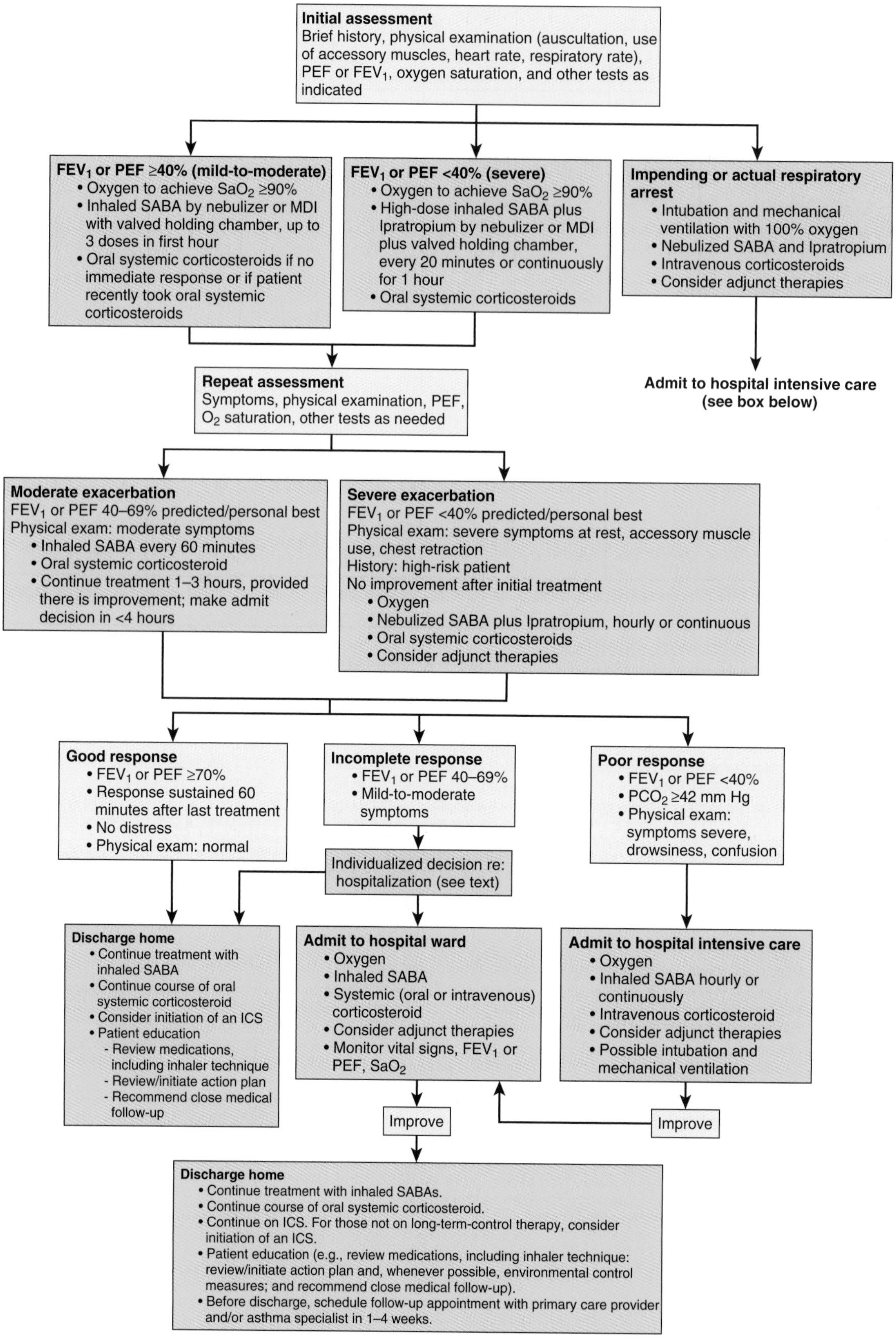

Key: *FEV_1*, Forced expiratory volume in 1 second; *ICS*, inhaled corticosteroid; *MDI*, metered-dose inhaler; *PCO_2*, partial pressure carbon dioxide; *PEF*, peak expiratory flow; *SABA*, short-acting beta$_2$-agonist; *SaO_2*, oxygen saturation

FIGURE 78.4 Management of asthma exacerbations: emergency department and hospital-based care. (From *National Heart Lung Blood Institute, National Asthma Education and Prevention Program*. Expert panel report 3: guidelines for the diagnosis and management of asthma. Summary report 2007, NIH Publication No. 08-5846, Bethesda, MD, 2007, U.S. Department of Health and Human Services, 55, <http://www.nhlbi.nih.gov/guidelines/asthma/asthsumm.pdf>.)

predictor for wheezing continuing into persistent asthma (Table 78.5).

PREVENTION

Education plays an important role in helping patients and their families adhere to the prescribed therapy and needs to begin at the time of diagnosis. Successful education involves teaching basic asthma facts, explaining the role of medications, teaching environmental control measures, and improving patient skills in the use of spacer devices for metered dose inhalers and peak flow monitoring. Families should have an asthma management plan (Fig. 78.5) for daily care and for exacerbations.

Peak flow monitoring is a self-assessment tool that may be helpful for children with asthma over 5 years of age who are poor perceivers of airway obstruction, have moderate to severe asthma, or have a history of severe exacerbations. Peak flow monitoring also can be useful in children who are still learning to recognize asthma symptoms. It must be emphasized that peak flow monitoring is not for the diagnosis of asthma but for monitoring.

A child's personal best peak flow (PEFR) is the highest value achieved over a 2-week period when asthma is controlled. Percentages based on the best PEFR reading may then be incorporated into a written asthma management plan as a means of providing an objective indication of airway obstruction in order to guide home-based asthma care. Limitations exist, however, to PEFR: they are effort and technique dependent, peak flow meters may lose accuracy with time, and appropriate range meters (low versus high) must be provided.

In addition, the medical literature has not shown consistently that monitoring PEFR is valuable for home-based asthma care. Likewise, written asthma management plans have not been shown consistently to be useful in asthma care at home. However, utilizing both of these two tools simultaneously trend toward a significant impact on asthma monitoring and management. Perhaps the most significant factor to positively impact asthma outcomes is simply having a plan in place to manage changes in asthma symptomatology.

TABLE 78.5 Risk Factors for Persistent Asthma

Allergy	Atopic dermatitis
	Allergic rhinitis
	Elevated total serum IgE levels (first year of life)
	Peripheral blood eosinophilia >4% (2-3 yr of age)
	Inhalant and food allergen sensitization
Gender	Males
	• Transient wheezing
	• Persistent allergy-associated asthma
	Females
	• Asthma associated with obesity and early-onset puberty
	• "Triad" asthma (adulthood)
Parental asthma	
Lower respiratory tract infections	Rhinovirus, respiratory syncytial virus
	Severe bronchiolitis (i.e., requiring hospitalization)
	Pneumonia
Environmental tobacco smoke exposure (including prenatal)	

Triad asthma—Nasal polyps, aspirin sensitivity, asthma.
From Liu AH, Martinez FD. Natural history of allergic diseases and asthma. In: Leung DYM, Szefler SJ, Bonilla FA, et al., eds. Pediatric Allergy: Principles and Practice. *3rd ed. Philadelphia: Elsevier; 2016:10.*

Children with asthma should be seen not only when they are ill but also when they are healthy. Regular office visits allow the health care team to review **adherence** to medication and control measures and to determine whether doses of medications need adjustment.

Asthma Action Plan

For: ______ Doctor: ______ Date: ______

Doctor's Phone Number ______ Hospital/Emergency Department Phone Number ______

GREEN ZONE

Doing Well

- No cough, wheeze, chest tightness, or shortness of breath during the day or night
- Can do usual activities

And, if a peak flow meter is used,

Peak flow: more than ______ (80 percent or more of my best peak flow)

My best peak flow is: ______

Take these long-term-control medicines each day (include an anti-inflammatory).

Medicine	How much to take	When to take it

Identify and avoid and control the things that make your asthma worse, like (list here):

______ ______ ______

Before exercise, if prescribed, take: ☐ 2 or ☐ 4 puffs ______ 5 to 60 minutes before exercise

YELLOW ZONE

Asthma Is Getting Worse

- Cough, wheeze, chest tightness, or shortness of breath, or
- Waking at night due to asthma, or
- Can do some, but not all, usual activities

-Or-

Peak flow: ______ to ______ (50 to 79 percent of my best peak flow)

First: **Add: quick-relief medicine–and keep taking your GREEN ZONE medicine.**

______ (short-acting $beta_2$-agonist) ☐ 2 or ☐ 4 puffs, every 20 minutes for up to 1 hour ☐ Nebulizer, once

Second: If applicable, remove yourself from the thing that made your asthma worse.

If your symptoms (and peak flow, if used) return to GREEN ZONE after 1 hour of above treatment:

☐ Continue monitoring to be sure you stay in the green zone.

-Or-

If your symptoms (and peak flow, if used) do not return to GREEN ZONE after 1 hour of above treatment:

☐ Take: ______ (short-acting $beta_2$-agonist) ☐ 2 or ☐ 4 puffs or ☐ Nebulizer

☐ Add: ______ (oral corticosteroid) mg per day. For ______ (3–10) days

☐ Call the doctor ______ (phone) ☐ before/ ☐ within ______ hours after taking the oral corticosteroid.

RED ZONE

Medical Alert!

- Very short of breath, or
- Quick-relief medicines have not helped, or
- Cannot do usual activities, or
- Symptoms are same or get worse after 24 hours in Yellow Zone.

-Or-

Peak flow: less than ______ (50 percent of my best peak flow)

Take this medicine:

☐ ______ (short-acting $beta_2$-agonist) ☐ 4 or ☐ 6 puffs or ☐ Nebulizer

☐ ______ (oral corticosteroid) mg

Then call your doctor NOW. Go to the hospital or call an ambulance if

- You are still in the red zone after 15 minutes AND
- You have not reached your doctor.

DANGER SIGNS

- Trouble walking and talking due to shortness of breath
- Lips or fingernails are blue

- Take ☐ 4 or ☐ 6 puffs of your quick-relief medicine **AND**
- Go to the hospital or call for an ambulance ______ (phone) **NOW!**

FIGURE 78.5 Asthma self-management guideline. (From *National Heart Lung Blood Institute, National Asthma Education and Prevention Program*. Expert panel report 3: guidelines for the diagnosis and management of asthma. Summary report 2007, NIH Publication No. 05-5251, Bethesda, MD, 2007, U.S. Department of Health and Human Services, 119, <http://www.nhlbi.nih.gov/guidelines/asthma/asthgdln.pdf>.)

CHAPTER 79

Allergic Rhinitis

ETIOLOGY

Rhinitis describes diseases that involve inflammation of the nasal epithelium and is characterized by sneezing, pruritus, rhinorrhea, and congestion. There are many different causes of rhinitis in children, but approximately half of all cases are caused by allergies.

Allergic rhinitis, commonly known as **hay fever,** is caused by an IgE-mediated allergic response. During the early allergic phase, mast cells degranulate and release preformed chemical mediators, such as histamine and tryptase, and newly generated mediators such as leukotrienes, prostaglandins, and platelet-activating factor. After a quiescent phase in which other cells are recruited, a late phase occurs approximately 4-8 hours later. Eosinophils, basophils, CD4 T cells, monocytes, and neutrophils release their chemical mediators, which leads to the development of chronic nasal inflammation.

Allergic rhinitis can be seasonal, perennial, or episodic depending on the particular causative allergen and exposure. Some children experience perennial symptoms with seasonal exacerbations. **Seasonal allergic rhinitis** is caused by airborne pollens, which have seasonal patterns. Typically trees pollinate in the spring, grasses in late spring to summer, and weeds in the summer and fall. The pollen, microscopic in size, can travel airborne hundreds of miles and be inhaled easily into the respiratory tract. **Perennial allergic rhinitis** is primarily caused by indoor allergens, such as house dust mites, animal dander, mold, and cockroaches. **Episodic rhinitis** occurs with intermittent exposure to allergens, such as visiting a friend's home where a pet dwells.

EPIDEMIOLOGY

Chronic rhinitis is one of the most common disorders encountered in infants and children. Overall allergic rhinitis is observed in 10-25% of the general population, with children and adolescents more commonly affected than adults. The prevalence of physician-diagnosed allergic rhinitis has been estimated at 40%.

CLINICAL MANIFESTATIONS

Decision-Making Algorithms
Available @ StudentConsult.com

Rhinorrhea
Red Eye
Cough
Hoarseness

The hallmark symptoms of allergic rhinitis are clear thin rhinorrhea, nasal congestion, sneezing paroxysms, and pruritus of the eyes, nose, ears, and palate. Postnasal drip may result in frequent attempts to clear the throat, nocturnal cough, and hoarseness. It is important to correlate the onset, duration, and severity of symptoms with seasonal or perennial exposures, changes in the home or school environment, and exposure to nonspecific irritants such as tobacco smoke.

The physical examination includes a thorough nasal examination and an evaluation of the eyes, ears, throat, chest, and skin. Physical findings may be subtle. Classic physical findings include pale or bluish, boggy and edematous nasal turbinates with clear, watery secretions. Frequent nasal itching and rubbing of the nose superiorly with the palm of the hand, the **allergic salute,** can lead to a transverse nasal crease found across the nose. Children may produce clucking sounds by rubbing the soft palate with their tongue. Oropharyngeal examination may reveal lymphoid hyperplasia of the posterior oropharynx or visible mucus or both. Orthodontic abnormalities may be seen in children with chronic mouth breathing. **Allergic shiners,** dark, edematous infraorbital areas caused by venous congestion, along with eyelid edema or conjunctival injection, are often present in children. Retracted tympanic membranes from eustachian tube dysfunction or serous otitis media also may be present. Evidence of other atopic diseases, such as asthma or eczema, may be present, which helps lead the clinician to the correct diagnosis.

LABORATORY AND IMAGING STUDIES

Allergy testing can be performed by in vivo skin tests or by in vitro serum tests (enzyme linked immunosorbent assay [ELISA]) to pertinent allergens found in the patient's environment (see Table 77.4). Skin tests (prick/puncture) provide immediate and accurate results. Positive tests correlate strongly with nasal and bronchial allergen provocative challenges. In vitro serum tests are useful for patients with diffuse dermatitis, dermatographism, poor tolerance to skin testing, or for those taking medications that interfere with skin testing. Disadvantages of serum tests include increased cost, inability to obtain immediate results, and reduced sensitivity compared with skin tests. Testing should include relevant allergens in the home and regional flora. Broad screening testing without regard to symptoms is not recommended. Measurement of total serum IgE or blood eosinophils generally is not helpful. The presence of eosinophils on the nasal smear suggests a diagnosis of allergy, but eosinophils also can be found in patients with **nonallergic rhinitis with eosinophilia**. Nasal smear eosinophilia is often predictive of a good clinical response to nasal corticosteroid sprays, but is not commonly performed in clinical practice.

DIFFERENTIAL DIAGNOSIS

Rhinitis can be divided into allergic and nonallergic rhinitis (Table 79.1). Nonallergic rhinitis describes a group of nasal diseases in which there is no evidence of allergic etiology. It can be divided further into nonanatomic and anatomic etiologies. The most common form of nonallergic rhinitis in children is infectious rhinitis, which may be acute or chronic. Acute infectious rhinitis **(the common cold)** is caused by viruses, including rhinoviruses and coronaviruses, and typically resolves within 7-10 days (see Chapter 102). An average child has three to six common colds per year, with the most affected being younger children and children attending day care. Infection is suggested by the presence of sore throat, fever, and poor appetite, especially with a history of exposure to others with colds. Chronic infectious **rhinosinusitis**, or sinusitis, should be suspected if there is mucopurulent nasal discharge with

TABLE 79.1 Classification of the Etiology of Rhinitis in Children

	NONALLERGIC	
ALLERGIC	**Nonanatomic**	**Anatomic**
Seasonal	Nonallergic, noninfectious (vasomotor) rhinitis	Adenoidal hypertrophy
Perennial	Infectious rhinosinusitis	CSF rhinorrhea
Episodic	Nonallergic rhinitis with eosinophilia	Choanal atresia
	Rhinitis medicamentosa	Congenital anomalies
		Foreign body
		Nasal polyps
		Septal deviation
		Tumors
		Turbinate hypertrophy

CSF, Cerebrospinal fluid.

symptoms that persist beyond 10 days (see Chapter 104). Classic signs of acute sinusitis in older children include facial tenderness, tooth pain, headache, and fever. Classic signs are usually not present in young children who may present with postnasal drainage with cough, throat clearing, halitosis, and rhinorrhea. The character of the nasal secretions with infectious rhinitis varies from purulent to minimal or absent. Coexistence of middle ear disease, such as otitis media or eustachian tube dysfunction, may be additional clues of infection.

Nonallergic, noninfectious rhinitis (formerly known as *vasomotor rhinitis*) can manifest as rhinorrhea and sneezing in children with profuse clear nasal discharge. Exposure to irritants, such as cigarette smoke and dust, and strong fumes and odors, such as perfumes and chlorine in swimming pools, can trigger these nasal symptoms. Nonallergic rhinitis with eosinophilia syndrome is associated with clear nasal discharge and eosinophils on nasal smear and is seen infrequently in children. Cold air **(skier's nose),** hot/spicy food ingestion **(gustatory rhinitis),** and exposure to bright light **(reflex rhinitis)** are examples of nonallergic, noninfectious rhinitis. Treatment with topical ipratropium before exposure may be helpful.

Rhinitis medicamentosa is due primarily to overuse of topical nasal decongestants, such as oxymetazoline, or phenylephrine, resulting in rebound nasal congestion. This condition is not common in younger children. Adolescents or young adults may become dependent on these over-the-counter medications. Treatment requires discontinuation of the offending decongestant spray, topical corticosteroids, and frequently, a short course of oral corticosteroids.

The most common anatomic problem seen in young children is obstruction secondary to adenoidal hypertrophy, which can be suspected from symptoms such as mouth breathing, snoring, hyponasal speech, sleep disordered breathing, and persistent rhinitis with or without chronic otitis media. Infection of the nasopharynx may be secondary to infected hypertrophied adenoid tissue.

Choanal atresia is the most common congenital anomaly of the nose and consists of either bony or membranous septum between the nose and pharynx, either unilateral or bilateral. Bilateral choanal atresia classically presents in neonates as cyclic cyanosis because neonates are obligate nose breathers. Airway obstruction and cyanosis are relieved when the mouth is opened to cry and recurs when the calm infant reattempts to breathe through the nose. Some newborns show respiratory difficulty while feeding only. Nearly half of infants with choanal atresia have other congenital anomalies as a part of the **CHARGE association** (**c**oloboma, congenital **h**eart disease, choanal **a**tresia, **r**etardation, **g**enitourinary defects, **e**ar anomalies). Unilateral choanal atresia may go undiagnosed until later in life and presents with symptoms of unilateral nasal obstruction and discharge.

Nasal polyps typically appear as bilateral, gray, glistening tissue originating from the sinus ostia and may be associated with anosmia, nasal obstruction, and clear or purulent nasal discharge. Nasal polyps are rare in children younger than 10 years of age but if present, warrant evaluation for an underlying disease process, such as cystic fibrosis or primary ciliary dyskinesia. **Aspirin exacerbated respiratory disease** consists of asthma, aspirin sensitivity, and nasal polyps with chronic or recurrent sinusitis.

Foreign bodies are seen more commonly in young children who place food, small toys, stones, or other objects in their nose. The index of suspicion should be raised by a history of unilateral, purulent nasal discharge or foul odor. The foreign body can often be seen on anterior nasal examination.

TREATMENT

Management of allergic rhinitis is based on disease severity, impact of the disease on the patient, and the ability of the patient to comply with recommendations. Treatment modalities include allergen avoidance, pharmacologic therapy, and immunotherapy. Environmental control and steps to minimize allergen exposure, similar to preventive steps for asthma, should be implemented whenever possible (see Table 78.3).

Pharmacotherapy

Intranasal corticosteroids are the most effective pharmacologic therapy for treatment of allergic and nonallergic rhinitis. These include beclomethasone, budesonide, ciclesonide, flunisolide, fluticasone, mometasone, and triamcinolone. These topical agents work to reduce inflammation, edema, and mucus production. They are effective for symptoms of nasal congestion, rhinorrhea, pruritus, and sneezing but less helpful for ocular symptoms. Daily administration is necessary for maximum effectiveness. Nasal corticosteroid sprays have been used safely in long-term therapy. Deleterious effects on adrenal function or nasal membranes have not been reported when these agents are used appropriately. The most common adverse effects include local irritation, burning, and sneezing, which occur in 10% of patients. Nasal bleeding from improper technique (spraying the nasal septum) can occur. Rare cases of nasal septal perforation have been reported.

Antihistamines are the medications used most frequently to treat allergic rhinitis. They are useful in treating rhinorrhea, sneezing, nasal itching, and ocular itching but are less helpful in treating nasal congestion. **First-generation antihistamines,** such as diphenhydramine and hydroxyzine, easily cross the blood-brain barrier with sedation as the most common reported adverse effect. Use of first-generation antihistamines in children has an adverse effect on cognitive and academic function. In very young children, a paradoxical stimulatory central nervous system effect resulting in irritability and restlessness has been noted. Other adverse effects of first-generation antihistamines include anticholinergic effects, such as blurred vision, urinary retention, dry mouth, tachycardia, and constipation. **Second-generation antihistamines**, such as cetirizine, desloratadine, fexofenadine, levocetirizine, and loratadine, are less likely to cross the blood-brain barrier resulting in less sedation. Cetirizine, fexofenadine, levocetirizine, and loratadine are available without prescription. Azelastine and olopatadine, topical nasal antihistamine sprays, are approved for children older than 5 years and 6 years, respectively.

Decongestants, taken orally or intranasally, may be used to relieve nasal congestion. Oral medications, such as pseudoephedrine and phenylephrine, are available either alone or in combination with antihistamines. Adverse effects of oral decongestants include insomnia, nervousness, irritability, tachycardia, tremors, and palpitations; oral decongestants are not recommended for children less than 4 years old. For older children participating in sports, oral decongestant use may be restricted. Topical nasal decongestant sprays are effective for immediate relief of nasal obstruction but should not be used more than 3 consecutive days to prevent rhinitis medicamentosa.

Topical ipratropium bromide, an anticholinergic nasal spray, is used primarily for nonallergic rhinitis and rhinitis associated with viral upper respiratory infection. Leukotriene modifiers have been studied in the treatment of allergic rhinitis. Montelukast is approved for use in seasonal allergic rhinitis.

Immunotherapy

If environmental control measures and medication intervention are only partially effective or produce unacceptable adverse effects, immunotherapy may be recommended. The mechanism of action for allergen immunotherapy is complex but includes increased production of an IgG-blocking antibody, decreased production of specific IgE, and alteration of cytokine expression produced in response to an allergen challenge. Immunotherapy is effective for desensitization to pollens, dust mites, and cat and dog proteins. Use in young children may be limited by the need for frequent injections. Immunotherapy must be administered in a physician's office with 30 minutes of observation after the allergen injection. Anaphylaxis may occur, and the physician must be experienced in the treatment of these severe adverse allergic reactions.

COMPLICATIONS

Approximately 60% of children with allergic rhinitis have symptoms of bronchial hyperresponsiveness (see Chapter 78). Chronic allergic inflammation leads to chronic cough from postnasal drip, eustachian tube dysfunction and otitis media, sinusitis, and tonsillar and adenoid hypertrophy, which may lead to obstructive sleep apnea. Children with allergic rhinitis may experience sleep disturbances, limitations of activity, irritability, and mood and cognitive disorders that adversely affect their performance at school and their sense of well-being.

PROGNOSIS AND PREVENTION

Seasonal allergic rhinitis is a common and prominent condition that may not improve as children grow older. Patients become more adept at self-management. Perennial allergic rhinitis improves with allergen control of indoor allergens.

Removal or avoidance of the offending allergen is advised. The only effective measure for minimizing pet allergen exposure is removal of the pet from the home. Avoidance of pollen and outdoor molds can be accomplished by staying indoors in a controlled environment. Air conditioning and keeping windows and doors closed lower exposure to pollen. High-efficiency particle air filters reduce exposure to allergens (e.g., pet dander). Sealing the mattress and pillow in allergen-proof encasings is the most effective strategy for reduction of dust mite allergen. Bedding should be washed in hot water (>130°F) every week.

CHAPTER 80

Atopic Dermatitis

ETIOLOGY

Atopic dermatitis is a chronic, pruritic, relapsing inflammatory skin condition. The pathogenesis is multifactorial and involves a complex interplay of genetics, immunologic abnormalities, impaired skin barrier function, environmental interactions, and infectious triggers. A diverse set of genes encoding epidermal structural proteins (filaggrin) and elements of the immune system play a major role in atopic dermatitis.

Several immunoregulatory abnormalities have been described in patients with atopic dermatitis. There is an exaggerated cutaneous inflammatory response to environmental triggers, including irritants and allergens. Activated Langerhans cells in the dermis expressing surface-bound immunoglobulin (Ig)E stimulate T cells. In acute lesions, activated Th2 lymphocytes infiltrate the dermis. They initiate and maintain local tissue inflammation primarily through interleukin-4 (IL-4), IL-13, and IL-5, promoting IgE production and eosinophil differentiation, respectively. As the disease progresses from an acute to chronic phase, the Th2 response switches to Th1/Th0 response. Chronic lesions are characterized by increased IL-12 and IL-18.

Patients with atopic dermatitis have **hyperirritable skin**, and many factors can cause the disease to worsen or relapse. Known triggers include anxiety and stress, climate (extremes of temperature and humidity), irritants, allergens, and infections. Approximately 30% of infants and young children with severe atopic dermatitis have coexisting food allergies. The more severe the atopic dermatitis and the younger the patient, the more likely a food allergy will be identified as a contributing factor. Egg allergy is the most common cause of food-induced eczematous reactions.

EPIDEMIOLOGY

The prevalence of atopic dermatitis increased two- to threefold over the past 30 years. Approximately 15-20% of children and 2-10% of adults are affected. Atopic dermatitis often starts in early infancy. Approximately 50% of affected children show symptoms in the first year of life, and 80% experience disease onset before 5 years of age. Atopic dermatitis is often the first manifestation of the atopic march. Approximately 80% of children with atopic dermatitis develop other allergic diseases, such as asthma or allergic rhinitis. Symptoms of dermatitis often disappear at the onset of respiratory allergy.

CLINICAL MANIFESTATIONS

The clinical manifestations of atopic dermatitis vary with age. In infants, atopic dermatitis involves the face, scalp, cheeks, and extensor surfaces of the extremities (Fig. 80.1). The diaper area is spared. In older children, the rash localizes to the antecubital and popliteal fossae, head and neck. In adolescents and adults, lichenified plaques are seen in flexural areas (Fig. 80.2) and head and neck regions. Pruritus has a significant impact on the child and family's quality of life since it is often worse at night, disturbing sleep. Physical examination may also show hyperlinearity of the palms and soles, dermatographism, pityriasis alba, creases under the lower eyelids (**Dennie–Morgan folds or Dennie lines**), and **keratosis pilaris** (asymptomatic horny follicular papules on the extensor surfaces of the arms).

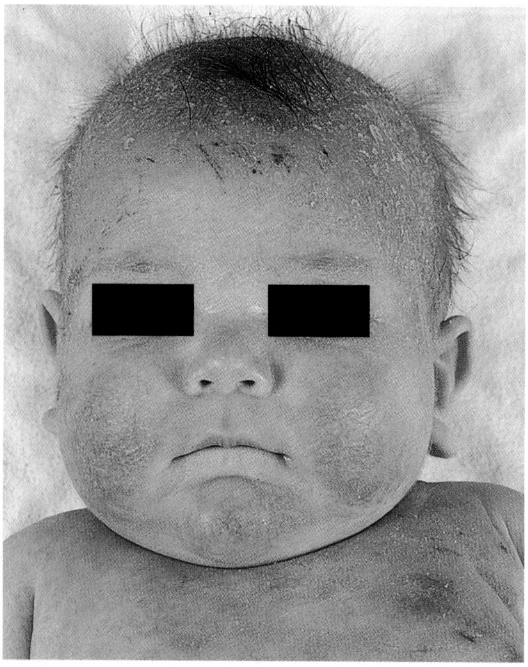

FIGURE 80.1 Atopic dermatitis typical cheek involvement. (From Eichenfield LF, Frieden IJ, Esterly NB. *Textbook of Neonatal Dermatology*. Philadelphia: Saunders; 2001:242.)

LABORATORY AND IMAGING STUDIES

The diagnosis of atopic dermatitis is based on clinical features rather than laboratory tests (Table 80.1). Skin biopsy is of little value, but it may be performed to exclude other skin diseases that mimic atopic dermatitis. Skin testing or serum specific IgE testing may be helpful in assessing the contribution of food or environmental allergies to disease expression if history is suggestive.

DIFFERENTIAL DIAGNOSIS

Many conditions share signs and symptoms of atopic dermatitis (Table 80.2). Infants presenting in the first year of life with failure to thrive, recurrent skin or systemic infections, and scaling, erythematous rash should be evaluated for immunodeficiency disorders. Wiskott-Aldrich syndrome is an X-linked recessive syndrome characterized by atopic dermatitis, thrombocytopenia, small-sized platelets, and recurrent infections. Langerhans cell histiocytosis is characterized by hemorrhagic or petechial lesions. Scabies is an intensely pruritic skin condition caused by the human scabies mite. The presence of burrows in interdigital spaces and flexor surfaces of the wrists, elbows, axilla, or genitals is pathognomonic. Burrows may be few in number or absent, however.

TREATMENT

The goals of eczema therapy are to reduce the number and severity of flares and to increase the number of disease-free

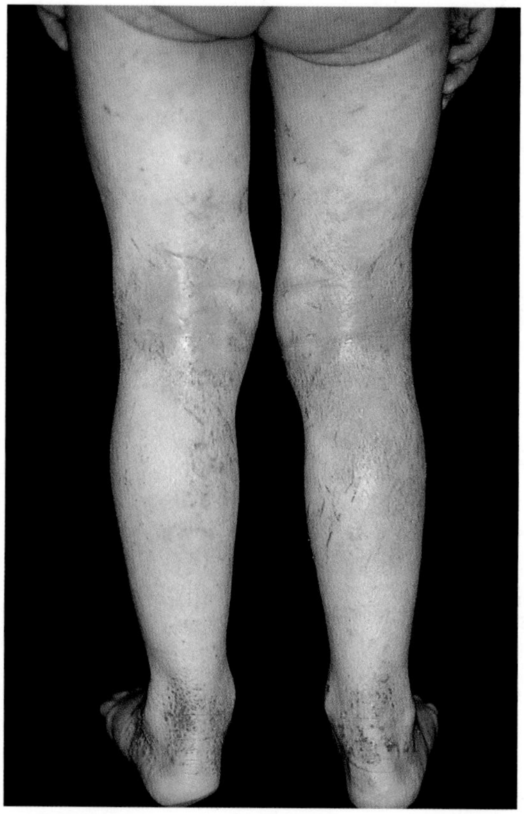

FIGURE 80.2 Rubbing and scratching the inflamed flexural areas cause thickened (lichenified) skin. (From Habif T. *Clinical Dermatology*. 4th ed. Philadelphia: Elsevier; 2004. Fig. 5.13.)

TABLE 80.1 Clinical Features of Atopic Dermatitis

ESSENTIAL FEATURES
• Pruritus • Facial and extensor eczema in infants and children • Flexural eczema in adults • Chronic or relapsing dermatitis
FREQUENTLY ASSOCIATED FEATURES
• Personal or family history of atopic disease • Xerosis • Cutaneous infections • Nonspecific dermatitis of the hands or feet • Elevated serum IgE levels • Positive immediate-type allergy skin tests • Early age of onset
OTHER FEATURES
• Ichthyosis, palmar hyperlinearity, keratosis pilaris • Pityriasis alba • Nipple eczema • Dermatographism and delayed blanch response • Anterior subcapsular cataracts, keratoconus • Dennie-Morgan infraorbital folds, orbital darkening • Facial erythema or pallor • Perifollicular accentuation

From Noovak N, Leung DYM. Role of barrier dysfunction and immune response in atopic dermatitis. In: Leung DYM, Szefler SJ, Bonilla FA, et al., eds. Pediatric Allergy: Principles and Practice. *3rd ed. Philadelphia: Elsevier; 2016:438.*

TABLE 80.2 Differential Diagnosis of Atopic Dermatitis

CONGENITAL DISORDERS
Netherton syndrome
Familial keratosis pilaris
CHRONIC DERMATOSES
Seborrheic dermatitis
Contact dermatitis (allergic or irritant)
Nummular eczema
Psoriasis
Ichthyoses
INFECTIONS AND INFESTATIONS
Scabies
HIV-associated dermatitis
Dermatophytosis
MALIGNANCIES
Cutaneous T-cell lymphoma (mycosis fungoides/Sezary syndrome)
Langerhan cell histiocytosis
AUTOIMMUNE DISORDERS
Dermatitis herpetiformis
Pemphigus foliaceus
Graft-versus-host disease
Dermatomyositis
IMMUNODEFICIENCIES
Wiskott-Aldrich syndrome
Severe combined immunodeficiency
Hyper IgE syndrome
DOCK8 associated immunodeficiency
IPEX
METABOLIC DISORDERS
Zinc deficiency
Pyridoxine (vitamin B_6) and niacin deficiency
Multiple carboxylase deficiency
Phenylkenonuria

DOCK 8, Dedicator of cytokinesis 8; *HIV,* human immunodeficiency virus; *IPEX,* immunodeficiency polyendocrinopathy X-linked.
From Boguniewicz M, Leung DYM. Management of atopic dermatitis. In: Leung DYM, Szefler SJ, Bonilla FA, et al., eds. Pediatric Allergy: Principles and Practice. *3rd ed. Philadelphia: Elsevier; 2016:449.*

periods. Successful management involves skin hydration with emollients, pharmacologic therapy to reduce pruritus and inflammation, and identification and avoidance of triggers. Patients with atopic dermatitis have impaired skin barrier function and enhanced transepidermal water loss. Daily, lukewarm baths for 15-20 minutes followed immediately by the application of fragrance-free emollients to retain moisture are a major component of therapy. Prevention of xerosis is important for pruritus control and for maintaining the integrity of the epithelial barrier. Emollients should be ointments or creams. Lotions are not as effective because they contain water or alcohol and may have a drying effect owing to evaporation. A mild nonsoap cleanser also is recommended.

Topical antiinflammatory agents, including corticosteroids and immunomodulators, are the cornerstone of therapy for acute flares and prevention of relapses. Topical corticosteroids are used for reducing inflammation and pruritus. They are effective for the acute and chronic phases of the disease. Ointments generally are preferred over creams and lotions because of enhanced potency due to easier skin penetration. Corticosteroids are ranked by potency into seven classes. The least potent corticosteroid that is effective should be used. Higher potency corticosteroids may be necessary to diminish the dermatitis flare but should be used for limited periods. Low-potency, nonfluorinated corticosteroids should be used on the face, intertriginous areas (groin, axilla), and large areas to reduce the risk of adverse effects. Reduced efficacy of topical corticosteroids may be related to disease severity rather than glucocorticoid resistance. Local adverse effects (skin atrophy and striae) and systemic adverse effects (hypothalamic-pituitary-adrenal axis suppression and hyperglycemia) are related to the potency, length of use, and applied surface area. In infants and younger children, the possibility of corticosteroid-induced adverse effects may be greater. When control of inflammatory lesions is achieved, most patients can be managed with emollients and low-potency topical corticosteroids.

The topical immunomodulating drugs tacrolimus and pimecrolimus are approved as second-line agents for short-term and intermittent treatment of atopic dermatitis in patients unresponsive to or intolerant of other therapies. They are approved for use in children older than 2 years of age. These agents may be used on all body locations and are especially useful on delicate skin sites, such as the face, neck, and axilla, without the adverse effect of cutaneous atrophy seen with topical corticosteroids. These medications have a potential increased cancer risk, and their long-term safety has not been established.

Other less serious adverse effects include local burning sensation and the need for sun protection.

COMPLICATIONS

Defective cell-mediated immunity leads to increased susceptibility to many bacterial, viral, and fungal infections of the skin. More than 90% of patients with atopic dermatitis have colonization of lesional skin with *Staphylococcus aureus (S. aureus)*, and more than 75% of patients have colonization of uninvolved skin. Colonization and infection by *S. aureus* are associated with disease severity. *S. aureus* secretes exotoxins that act as superantigens, stimulating T cells and increasing IgE production. Secondarily infected atopic dermatitis often presents as impetiginous, pustular lesions with crusting and honey-colored exudate. Topical antibiotics, such as mupirocin or retapamulin, can be used to treat local areas of infection. Oral antibiotics such as cephalexin, dicloxacillin, or amoxicillin-clavulanate can be used for multifocal disease or for infection around the eyes and mouth that is difficult to treat topically. Bacterial cultures may be helpful in patients who do not respond to oral antibiotics or who have infection after multiple antibiotic courses. The incidence of community-acquired methicillin-resistant *S. aureus* is increasing.

Herpes simplex superinfection of affected skin, or **Kaposi varicelliform eruption** or **eczema herpeticum,** results in vesiculopustular lesions that appear in clusters and can become hemorrhagic. Herpes simplex virus infection can be misdiagnosed as bacterial infection and should be considered if skin lesions fail to respond to antibiotics.

In individuals with atopic dermatitis, smallpox vaccination or exposure to a vaccinated individual may lead to **eczema vaccinatum,** a localized vaccinial superinfection of affected skin. Eczema vaccinatum may progress to generalized vaccinia with vaccinial lesions appearing at sites distant from the inoculation. In patients with underlying immunodeficiencies, this complication may be life threatening.

Widespread infections with human papillomavirus (warts) and molluscum contagiosum are also common in children with atopic dermatitis.

PROGNOSIS

Atopic dermatitis is a chronic, relapsing skin disorder that tends to be more severe and prominent in young children. Symptoms become less severe in two thirds of children, with complete remission for approximately 20%. Early onset disease that is more widespread with concomitant asthma and allergic rhinitis, family history of atopic dermatitis, and elevated serum IgE levels may predict a more persistent course. Patients and families should be taught that a single cause and cure for atopic dermatitis is unlikely but that good control is possible for the majority of affected patients.

PREVENTION

An important step in the management of atopic dermatitis is to identify and avoid allergens and irritants. Common irritants include soaps, detergents, fragrances, chemicals, smoke, and extremes of temperature and humidity. Since wool and synthetic fabrics can be irritating to the skin, 100% cotton fabric is preferred. Sweating is a recognized trigger. Fingernails should be trimmed frequently to minimize excoriations from scratching.

In infants and younger children who do not respond to the usual therapies, identifying and removing a food allergen from the diet may lead to clinical improvement. Food allergy is not a common trigger for older patients. Other environmental exposures, such as dust mites, can also contribute to the disease state.

CHAPTER 81

Urticaria, Angioedema, and Anaphylaxis

ETIOLOGY

Urticaria, commonly referred to as **hives**, is swelling of the dermis and one of the most common skin conditions seen in clinical practice. **Angioedema** results from a process similar to urticaria, but the reaction extends below the dermis. Urticaria and angioedema occur in response to the release of inflammatory mediators including histamine, leukotrienes, platelet-activating factor, prostaglandins, and cytokines from mast cells residing in the skin. A variety of stimuli can trigger mast cells to release their chemical mediators. Typically mast cells degranulate when antigen cross links cell surface immunoglobulin (Ig)E. Release of mediators results in vasodilation, increased vascular leak, and pruritus. In addition, basophils from the peripheral blood can localize to tissue and release mediators. Patients with urticaria have elevated histamine content in the skin that is more easily released.

Anaphylaxis is mediated by IgE, whereas **anaphylactoid reactions** result from mechanisms that are due to nonimmunologic mechanisms. Both reactions are acute, severe, and can be life threatening due to massive release of inflammatory mediators. Urticaria, angioedema, and anaphylaxis are best considered as symptoms because they have a variety of causes.

Not all mast cell activation is IgE-mediated. Immunologic, nonimmunologic, physical, and chemical stimuli can produce degranulation of mast cells and basophils. **Anaphylatoxins**, C3a and C5a, can cause histamine release in a non–IgE-mediated reaction. Anaphylatoxins are generated in serum sickness (see Chapter 82) and in infectious, neoplastic, and rheumatic diseases. In addition, mast cell degranulation can occur from direct pharmacologic effect or physical or mechanical activation, such as urticaria after exposure to opiate medications or dermatographism (see below).

Urticaria and angioedema can be classified into three subcategories: acute, chronic, and physical. By definition **acute urticaria** and **angioedema** are hives and diffuse swelling that last less than 6 weeks. Often the history is quite helpful in eliciting the cause of the acute reaction (Table 81.1). An IgE mechanism is more commonly found in acute urticaria than in chronic urticaria. In the pediatric population, viral illnesses are responsible for the majority of acute urticaria.

Chronic urticaria and **angioedema** are characterized by persistence of symptoms beyond 6 weeks (Table 81.1). Some have daily symptoms of hives and swelling, whereas others have intermittent or recurrent episodes. Chronic urticaria can be

TABLE 81.1 Etiologies of Acute and Chronic Urticaria

ACUTE URTICARIA	CHRONIC URTICARIA
Food	Physical
Medication	Chronic spontaneous (formerly idiopathic)
Insect sting or bite	Autoantibody associated
Infection	
Contact allergy	
Transfusion reaction	
Idiopathic	

idiopathic with unknown causal factors. Thirty five to 40% of chronic urticaria cases have an autoimmune process due to IgG autoantibodies binding directly to IgE or the high-affinity IgE receptor. **Physical urticaria** and **angioedema** are characterized by known eliciting external factors that may include pressure, cold, heat, exercise, vibration, or exposure to sun.

The most common physical urticaria is dermatographism, affecting 2-5% of persons. **Dermatographism** means "writing on the skin" and is easily diagnosed by firmly scratching the skin with a blunt point, such as the wooden tip of a cotton swab or tongue depressor. It is characterized by an urticarial reaction localized to the site of skin trauma. It has been suggested that trauma induces an IgE-mediated reaction causing histamine to be released from the mast cells.

Cholinergic urticaria, characterized by the appearance of 1-3 mm wheals surrounded by large erythematous flares after an increase in core body temperature, occurs commonly in young adults. Lesions may develop during strenuous exercise, after a hot bath, or with emotional stress. The lack of airway symptoms differentiates it from exercise-induced anaphylaxis.

Cold urticaria occurs with exposure to cold and may develop within minutes on areas directly exposed to cold or on rewarming of the affected areas. Ingestion of cold drinks may precipitate lip swelling. Cold urticaria syndromes can be categorized into acquired and familial disorders. Severe reactions resulting in death can occur with swimming or diving into cold water. Patients must never swim alone, should avoid total body exposure to cold, and should have auto-injectable epinephrine available.

Hereditary angioedema (HAE) is an autosomal dominant disease due to a deficiency of C1-esterase inhibitor. The genetic defect may be caused by spontaneous mutation since approximately 25% of cases occur in patients without any family history. The disease is estimated to affect approximately 10,000 persons in the United States. It is characterized by unpredictable, recurrent attacks of episodic swelling that involves the face, peripheral extremities, genitalia, abdomen, oropharynx, and pharynx. Episodes are often triggered by trauma. Asphyxiation from laryngeal attacks is a significant cause of mortality. Patients with HAE rarely have urticaria associated with angioedema, and the swelling is not relieved with antihistamines or oral corticosteroids. The majority of patients (85%) have **type I** disease, which is due to decreased production of C1-esterase inhibitor. A minority of patients (15%) have **type II** disease, which is due to production of dysfunctional C1-esterase inhibitor. A low C4 level serves as an initial screening test. Patients with reduced C4 should have quantitative and functional levels of C1-esterase inhibitor measured. C2 levels are low during an

TABLE 81.2 Hereditary Angioedema Treatment

DRUG CLASS AND NAME	INDICATION	APPROVED AGE
C1INH concentrate	Acute attacks	
Berinert		Children and adults
Ruconest		≥12 yr of age
Plasma kallikrein inhibitor	Acute attacks	
Ecallantide		≥16 yr of age
Bradykinin B_2 receptor antagonist	Acute attacks	
Icatibant		≥18 yr of age
17α-Alkylated androgens	Long-term prophylaxis	
Danazol		Adults
Stanozolol		Children and adults
C1INH concentrate	Long-term prophylaxis	
Cinryze		≥12 yr of age

From BL Zuraw. Urticaria and angioedema. In: Leung DYM, Szefler SJ, Bonilla FA, et al., eds. Pediatric Allergy: Principles and Practice. *3rd ed. Philadelphia: Elsevier; 2016:465–466.*

TABLE 81.3 Common Causes of Anaphylaxis in Children

IgE-MEDIATED ANAPHYLAXIS	NONIMMUNOLOGIC
Food	Exercise
Drug	Direct mast cell degranulation
Insect sting or bite	
Latex	
Allergen immunotherapy	
Biologic agent	
Allergen challenge	
Blood products	

Modified from FER Simons. Anaphylaxis: assessment and management. In: Leung DYM, Szefler SJ, Bonilla FA, et al., eds. Pediatric Allergy: Principles and Practice. *3rd ed. Philadelphia: Elsevier; 2016:526.*

acute attack. **HAE with normal C1 inhibitor** (formerly known as type III HAE) patients have normal laboratory evaluation of C1-esterase inhibitor. These patients are more typically females. Treatment for HAE is divided into on-demand treatment for acute attacks and prophylaxis (Table 81.2). Prophylactic C1INH concentrate has advantage over other prophylactic therapies in terms of availability, effectiveness, and side effects. Bradykinin is an important mediator in the pathophysiology of HAE, and newer treatments are aimed at blocking this mediator.

Anaphylactic reactions are type I IgE-mediated reactions and result from many causes (Table 81.3). Cross linking of cell surface IgE by allergen leads to high-affinity IgE receptor activation on the mast cell and basophil resulting in release of mediators, including histamine, tryptase, tumor necrosis factor, platelet-activating factor, leukotrienes, prostaglandins, and cytokines. Other cell types involved in the reactions include monocytes, macrophages, eosinophils, neutrophils, and platelets. The mediator release results in the clinical picture of anaphylaxis.

Anaphylactoid reactions are due to nonimmunologic mechanisms. Mast cells and basophils can be activated by direct, nonspecific stimulation, although the exact underlying mechanism is unknown. Reactions to opiates and radiocontrast material are classic examples. Complement system activation also can result in mast cell and basophil activation. **Anaphylatoxins,** C3a and C5a, are named because of their ability to trigger mediator release and are generated in serum sickness. There are other causes of anaphylactoid reactions for which the mechanism has not been clarified.

EPIDEMIOLOGY

Urticaria and angioedema are common skin conditions affecting 15-25% of individuals at some point in their lives. Most cases of urticaria are self-limited, but for some patients, they are chronic. In approximately 50% of patients, urticaria and angioedema occur together. In the remaining 50%, 40% have urticaria alone and 10% have angioedema alone. The incidence of anaphylaxis in children is unknown.

CLINICAL MANIFESTATIONS

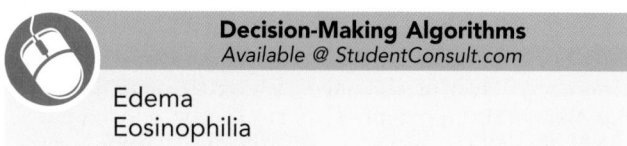

Decision-Making Algorithms
Available @ StudentConsult.com

Edema
Eosinophilia

Raised, erythematous lesions with pale centers that are intensely pruritic characterize **urticaria** (Fig. 81.1). The lesions vary in size and can occur anywhere on the body. Typically, urticaria arises suddenly and may resolve within 1-2 hours or may persist for up to 24 hours. **Angioedema** is a similar process that involves the deeper dermis or subcutaneous tissue, with swelling as the principal symptom. Generally, angioedema is not pruritic, may be mildly painful, and persists for longer than 24 hours. In rare cases it may become life threatening if swelling affects the upper airway.

The clinical manifestations of **anaphylaxis** and **anaphylactoid** reactions are the same for children and adults. The signs and symptoms vary and can range from mild skin findings to a fatal reaction. Ninety percent of patients present with cutaneous symptoms, including urticaria, angioedema, flushing, and warmth, but the absence of dermal symptoms does not exclude the diagnosis of anaphylaxis. Other affected organ systems include the respiratory tract (rhinorrhea, oropharyngeal edema, laryngeal edema, hoarseness, stridor, wheezing, dyspnea, and asphyxiation), cardiovascular system (tachycardia, hypotension, shock, syncope, and arrhythmias), gastrointestinal tract (nausea, abdominal pain, diarrhea, and vomiting) and neurological system (syncope, seizure, dizziness, and a sense of impending doom). The severity of an anaphylactic reaction is often proportionate to the speed of symptom onset.

LABORATORY AND IMAGING STUDIES

The laboratory evaluation of patients with urticaria and angioedema must be tailored to the clinical situation. Acute urticaria and angioedema do not require specific laboratory evaluation except to document the suspected cause. For patients with chronic urticaria and angioedema, current recommendations advise against routine lab testing unless history suggests a potential etiology. Patients with recurrent angioedema *without* urticaria should be evaluated for HAE (Table 81.4).

Measurement of the mast cell mediators, histamine and tryptase, may be helpful when the diagnosis of anaphylaxis is in question. A tryptase level is a more useful test because histamine is released quickly, has a very short half-life, and is often difficult to detect in the serum. Serum tryptase levels peak 1-1.5 hours after anaphylaxis. Elevated levels may be helpful in establishing the diagnosis, but normal tryptase levels do not rule out the diagnosis. It is best to measure a serum tryptase level

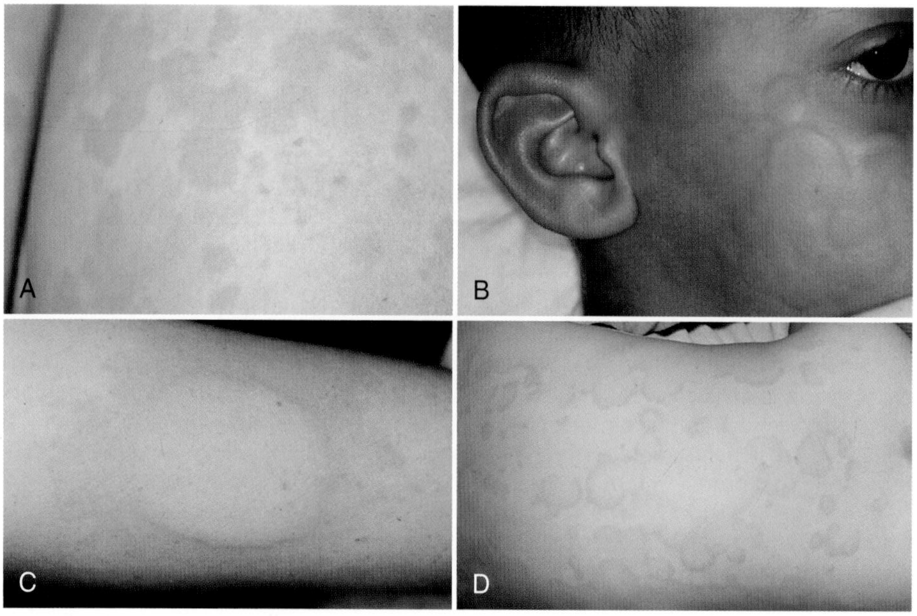

FIGURE 81.1 Examples of urticaria. (From Zitelli BJ, Davis HW, eds. *Pediatric Physical Diagnosis Electronic Atlas*. Philadelphia: Mosby; 2004.)

TABLE 81.4 Complement Evaluation of Patients With Recurrent Angioedema

ASSAY	IDIOPATHIC ANGIOEDEMA	TYPE I HEREDITARY ANGIOEDEMA	TYPE II HEREDITARY ANGIOEDEMA	HEREDITARY ANGIOEDEMA WITH NORMAL C1 INHIBITOR	ACQUIRED C1-ESTERASE INHIBITOR DEFICIENCY	VASCULITIS
C4	Normal	Low	Low	Normal	Low	Low or normal
C1-esterase inhibitor level	Normal	Low	Normal	Normal	Low	Normal
C1-esterase inhibitor function	Normal	Low	Low	Normal	Low	Normal
C1q	Normal	Normal	Normal	Normal	Low	Low or normal

From Zuraw BL. Urticaria and angioedema. In: Leung DYM, Szefler SJ, Bonilla FA, et al., eds. Pediatric Allergy: Principles and Practice. *3rd ed. Philadelphia: Elsevier; 2016:463.*

1-2 hours after the onset of symptoms. It also can be measured retrospectively on stored serum that is less than 2 days old.

DIFFERENTIAL DIAGNOSIS

The diagnosis of urticaria and angioedema is straightforward; finding the etiology may be more difficult. Other dermatologic conditions can mimic urticaria. **Erythema multiforme** has target-shaped, erythematous, macular, or papular lesions that may look similar to urticaria, but the lesions are fixed and last for several days. Other dermatologic diseases such as dermatitis herpetiformis and bullous pemphigoid are quite pruritic, and early on, the lesions may resemble urticaria. Mastocytosis is characterized by mast cell infiltration of various organs, including the skin. Some patients have skin lesions similar in appearance to urticaria rather than the classic urticaria pigmentosa. Urticaria pigmentosa appears as hyperpigmented, red-brown macules that may coalesce. When these lesions are stroked, they urticate, which is called the **Darier sign**. A rare disorder that should be included in the differential diagnosis of urticaria is **Muckle-Wells syndrome**. It is an autosomal dominant autoinflammatory disorder characterized by episodic urticaria presenting in infancy with sensorineural deafness, amyloidosis, arthralgias, and skeletal abnormalities. Another rare syndrome is **Schnitzler syndrome**, which is characterized by chronic urticaria, macroglobulinemia, bone pain, anemia, fever, fatigue, and weight loss. **Urticarial vasculitis** is a small vessel vasculitis with histological features of a leukocytoclastic response. The main distinguishing feature is that the lesions last longer than 24 hours, may be tender, and leave behind skin pigmentation. Skin biopsy is required for definitive diagnosis.

The diagnosis of anaphylaxis is usually apparent from the acute and often dramatic onset of multisystem involvement of the skin, respiratory tract, and cardiovascular system. Sudden cardiovascular collapse in the absence of cutaneous symptoms suggests vasovagal collapse, seizure disorder, aspiration, pulmonary embolism, or myocardial infarction. Laryngeal edema, especially with abdominal pain, suggests HAE. Many patients with anaphylaxis are initially thought to have septic shock (see Chapter 40).

TREATMENT

Avoidance of triggering agents is important in the management of acute urticaria and angioedema. Most cases resolve spontaneously. However, use of pharmacologic agents will provide symptom relief and include H_1 antihistamines. If acute urticaria and angioedema do not respond to this therapy, a short course of oral steroids may be considered.

Chronic urticaria treatment employs H_1 antihistamines. Second-generation H_1 antihistamines, such as cetirizine, desloratadine, fexofenadine, levocetirizine, and loratadine, are preferred because they have fewer adverse effects. If second-generation H_1 antihistamine monotherapy does not provide adequate relief, increasing the dose of antihistamines is indicated as is the addition of a sedating H_1 antihistamine at bedtime or H_2 antihistamines, such as cimetidine or ranitidine. While results on the effectiveness of antileukotriene medications as mono and add-on therapy is mixed, a trial of this medication can be considered. Omalizumab, a monoclonal anti-IgE antibody, was approved for the treatment of chronic urticaria and has proven to be effective. Other immunomodulating agents, such as cyclosporine, hydroxychloroquine, methotrexate, cyclophosphamide, and intravenous immunoglobulin, have been used. However, data supporting their use are limited, and they require laboratory monitoring due to potential adverse effects. Corticosteroids are effective in treating chronic urticaria, although adverse effects from long-term use mandate using the lowest dose for a brief time and not for chronic use.

Anaphylaxis is a medical emergency. Prompt recognition and immediate treatment are crucial (Fig. 81.2). Early administration of intramuscular epinephrine is the mainstay of therapy and should be given at the same time that basic measures of cardiopulmonary resuscitation are being performed. If the child is not in a medical setting, emergency medical services should be activated. Supplemental oxygen and intravenous fluid should be administered with the child lying in Trendelenburg. An airway must be secured as intubation or tracheotomy may be required. Additional pharmacologic therapies, such as corticosteroids, antihistamines, H_2-receptor antagonists, and bronchodilators, may be given to improve symptoms. Up to 30% of people with anaphylaxis have **biphasic** or **protracted** anaphylaxis.

A person with **biphasic anaphylaxis** has both early- and late-phase reactions. The biphasic reaction is a recurrence of anaphylactic symptoms after an initial remission, occurring within 8-72 hours after the initial reaction. A person with **protracted anaphylaxis** has signs and symptoms that persist for hours or even days despite treatment, although this is rare.

PREVENTION

Prevention of urticaria, angioedema, and anaphylaxis focuses on avoidance of known triggers. A referral to an allergy specialist for a thorough history, diagnostic testing if indicated, and

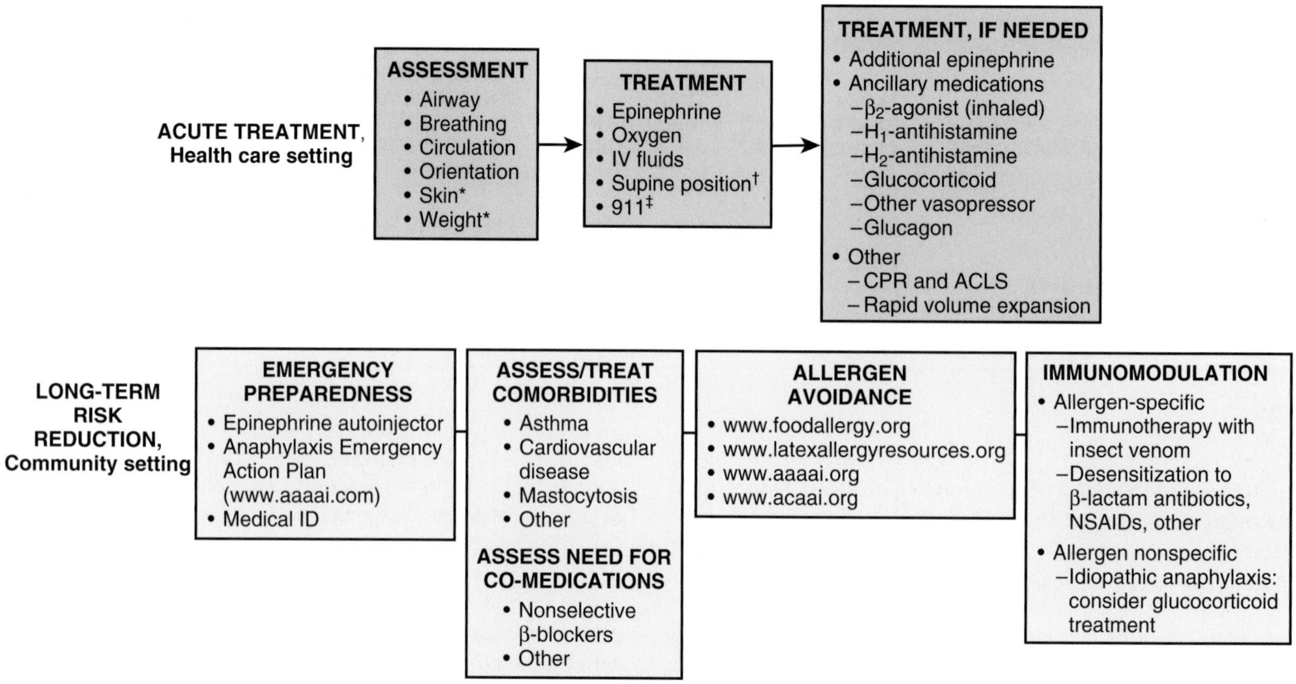

FIGURE 81.2 Summary of anaphylaxis management. Acute treatment is the same regardless of the mechanism or trigger involved in anaphylaxis. In contrast, for long-term risk reduction, avoidance measures, and immunomodulation are trigger-specific; currently immunomodulation is available only for a minority of individuals with anaphylaxis. All at-risk individuals need to have comorbidities and current medications assessed, be taught the importance of emergency preparedness, and be instructed in the use of auto-injectable epinephrine. *ACLS*, Advanced cardiac life support; *CPR*, cardiopulmonary resuscitation; *CVS*, cardiovascular; *GI*, gastrointestinal; *ID*, identification (e.g., bracelet, wallet card); *IV*, intravenous; *NSAIDs*, nonsteroidal antiinflammatory drugs. *The skin should be inspected, and weight estimation is important, especially in infants and children, and also in overweight and obese teens and adults, in order to calculate an optimal dose of epinephrine and other medications needed in treatment and resuscitation. †Supine position, as tolerated, to prevent empty ventricle syndrome. ‡Call 911/emergency medical services for anaphylaxis occurring in community health care facilities such as medical, dental, or infusion clinics, where optimal backup might not be available for resuscitation. (From Simon FER. Anaphylaxis. *J Allergy Clin Immunol.* 2008;121:S405.)

recommendations for avoidance is suggested for patients following severe reactions or anaphylaxis. Skin testing and serum IgE-specific testing are available for foods, inhalants, insect venoms, drugs (penicillin), vaccines, and latex. Educating the patient and family members about the signs and symptoms of anaphylaxis and using auto-injectable epinephrine early result in better outcomes. Fatal anaphylaxis has occurred despite timely and appropriate treatment. Medical informational jewelry with appropriate information should be worn. Medications such as β-blockers, angiotensin-converting enzyme inhibitors, and monoamine oxidase inhibitors should be discontinued because they may exacerbate anaphylaxis or interfere with its treatment.

CHAPTER 82

Serum Sickness

ETIOLOGY

Serum sickness is a type III hypersensitivity reaction (see Table 77.1). The patient's immune system recognizes the proteins in a drug or antiserum as foreign and produces antibodies against them. The newly formed antibodies bind with the foreign protein to form antigen-antibody or immune complexes, which may enter the circulation and be deposited in blood vessels and filtering organs. These complexes cause tissue injury by activating the complement cascade and recruiting neutrophils, resulting in increased capillary permeability, toxic mediator release, and tissue damage.

EPIDEMIOLOGY

Immune complexes were first described after administration of heterologous serum, such as horse serum for diphtheria treatment. The availability of human-derived biologics, bioengineered antibodies, and alternative pharmacotherapies has greatly reduced the incidence of serum sickness. Common inciting agents include blood products and foreign proteins, such as antithymocyte globulin and antivenoms. Medications frequently implicated include penicillin, sulfonamides, minocycline, cefaclor, hydantoins, and thiazides.

CLINICAL MANIFESTATIONS

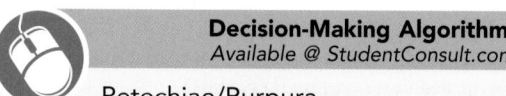

Decision-Making Algorithm
Available @ StudentConsult.com

Petechiae/Purpura

The symptoms of serum sickness typically occur 7-21 days after the administration of drugs, foreign proteins, or infections. Symptom onset may be more rapid (within 1-4 days) in previously sensitized individuals. The classic clinical manifestations consist of fever, polyarticular arthralgias, lymphadenopathy, and cutaneous symptoms. Cutaneous lesions vary and may include urticaria, angioedema, erythema multiforme, morbilliform rash, and palpable purpura or serpiginous rash at the interface of the dorsal and palmar or plantar aspects of the hands and feet. Carditis, glomerulonephritis, Guillain-Barre syndrome, encephalomyelitis, and peripheral neuritis are rare complications.

LABORATORY AND IMAGING STUDIES

Laboratory tests may show an elevated erythrocyte sedimentation rate, presence of circulating immune complexes, and depressed complement (C3 and C4) levels. Skin biopsy specimens show immune deposits of IgM, IgA, IgE, or C3. Hematuria or proteinuria or both may be present. The diagnosis is established by history of exposure to an inciting cause, characteristic clinical manifestations, and laboratory testing showing circulating immune complexes and depressed complement levels.

TREATMENT AND PREVENTION

Serum sickness is self-limited and resolves within 1-2 weeks. Therefore treatment is symptomatic relief. Antihistamines may be administered to relieve pruritus. Nonsteroidal anti-inflammatory drugs reduce fever and joint pain, and if necessary, prednisone (1-2 mg/kg orally daily) is administered with a tapering dose. Allergy skin testing does not predict the likelihood of serum sickness development and is not indicated.

The primary means of prevention is to avoid exposure to the implicated cause.

CHAPTER 83

Insect Allergies

ETIOLOGY

Systemic allergic reactions usually result from stinging insects of the order **Hymenoptera**, which include **apids** (honeybee and bumblebee), **vespids** (yellow jacket, wasp, yellow-face and white-face hornets), and **formicids** (fire and harvester ants). Honeybees have a barbed stinger that remains embedded after a sting. Yellow jackets are responsible for most allergic reactions in most parts of the United States, whereas wasps are the most frequent cause of sting reactions in Texas. Fire ants are found in southeastern and south central United States.

Biting insects rarely cause anaphylaxis. Anaphylaxis has been described, however, after the bites from the kissing bug *Triatoma*, bed bugs, blackflies, and deerflies. Large local reactions from biting insects, such as mosquitoes, fleas, and flies, are a more common occurrence. The reaction appears urticarial and is caused by the salivary secretions deposited by the biting insect and does not represent an allergic response.

EPIDEMIOLOGY

Insect sting allergy may develop at any age and typically manifests after several uneventful stings. Although children are stung more frequently than adults, systemic allergic reactions occur in only about 1% of children and 3% of adults. Reactions in adults are generally more severe than in children and can result in death. Large local reactions to insect stings are more common in children, with an estimated incidence of 20% for children and 10% for adults.

CLINICAL MANIFESTATIONS

The diagnosis of insect sting allergy is dependent on the history of the reaction and the presence of venom-specific IgE. Normal reactions to insect stings, which are observed in 90% of children, include localized pain, swelling, and erythema at the sting site that usually subside within 24 hours. Large local reactions occur in approximately 10% of patients. They are usually late-phase, IgE-mediated reactions, with large swelling, contiguous to the sting site that develops over 24-48 hours and resolves within 2-7 days. Virtually all individuals with large local reactions have similar reactions with subsequent stings. Systemic reactions are IgE mediated and occur in 1% of children. They can be mild and nonlife-threatening with cutaneous symptoms only or life-threatening with respiratory, cardiovascular, or neurologic symptoms of anaphylaxis (see Chapter 81). Toxic reactions may result if a person receives a large number of simultaneous stings (50-100). Symptoms include malaise, nausea, and emesis resulting from the toxic effects of the venom. Unusual reactions, such as vasculitis, nephrosis, neuritis, serum sickness, and encephalitis, rarely are associated with insect stings (Table 83.1).

TABLE 83.1 Classification of Insect Sting Reactions

REACTION TYPE	CHARACTERISTICS
Normal	<2 inches in diameter
	Transient pain and erythema
	Duration <24 hr
Large local reaction	>2 inches in diameter
	Swelling contiguous to the site
	Duration 2-7 days
Systemic	
Nonlife-threatening	Immediate generalized reaction confined to the skin (erythema, urticaria, angioedema)
Life-threatening	Immediate generalized reaction not confined to the skin with respiratory (laryngeal edema, bronchospasm) or cardiovascular (hypotension, shock) symptoms
Toxic	Follows multiple simultaneous stings, produced by exogenous vasoactive amines in venom
Unusual	Serum sickness, vasculitis, nephrosis, neuritis, encephalitis
	Symptoms start several days to weeks after the insect sting.

LABORATORY AND IMAGING STUDIES

A positive skin test to Hymenoptera venom extract demonstrates the presence of venom-specific IgE and in the context of a positive sting reaction history helps identify specific insects to which an individual is allergic. Venom-specific IgE antibodies also may be measured by in vitro serum tests. Both testing methods should be considered complementary because neither test alone detects all patients with insect sting allergy. Future reactions correlate more with past individual patterns than the level of sensitivity of venom skin testing or serum specific IgE testing.

Pediatric patients presenting with history of anaphylaxis to stinging insect venoms require evaluation of a baseline tryptase level to screen for an underlying mast cell disorder in addition to assessment of specific IgE. Patients with mast cell disorders are at higher risk for severe reactions to stings. Likewise, they are more likely to have no skin manifestations during their reaction, systemic reactions to vespid stings, hypotensive anaphylaxis, and negative evaluation of specific IgE despite a highly suggestive history. Mast cell disorders have further implications for venom immunotherapy. During immunotherapy, these patients have higher risk of side effects, higher risk of systemic sting reactions, and higher risk of relapse after discontinuing therapy. They should receive venom immunotherapy indefinitely.

DIFFERENTIAL DIAGNOSIS

A history of an immediate systemic reaction is necessary before venom testing and consideration of immunotherapy. Testing for venom-specific IgE without a history of a systemic reaction to a sting is not recommended. Identification of the offending insect is often unreliable. Honeybee stings may be identified by the stinger that remains in place. Vespid stings are usually unprovoked and occur at summer's end when the insects are more aggressive.

TREATMENT

Local reactions should be treated by cleaning the site, applying cold compresses, and administering oral antihistamines and analgesics. Occasionally, large local reactions may be mistaken for cellulitis. Infection is unlikely if reaction occurs within 24-48 hours after a sting. Treatment is with an oral corticosteroid for 4-5 days rather than oral antibiotics.

Treatment of systemic reactions is guided by the severity of the reaction, but epinephrine is the cornerstone of therapy and should be administered without delay. Antihistamines may be administered concurrently with epinephrine. Corticosteroids should be given to prevent recurrent or prolonged symptoms. For severe reactions, intravenous fluids and epinephrine, oxygen, and respiratory support in an intensive care unit may be needed. After acute care of a systemic sting reaction, patients should be provided an epinephrine auto-injector, referral to an allergist, and instructions on prevention of insect stings.

COMPLICATIONS

At least 50-100 fatalities per year in the United States are attributed to insect sting reactions. Most deaths (80%) occur in adults older than 40 years of age, but only 2% occur in individuals younger than 20 years of age. Approximately one half of deaths occur in persons without a previous history of a sting reaction.

PROGNOSIS

Successfully avoiding the stinging insect is the most important prognostic factor. More than 85% of adults who complete 5 years of immunotherapy tolerate sting challenges without systemic reactions for 5-10 years after completion.

PREVENTION

Measures to reduce the chance of accidental sting include exterminating infested areas, avoid eating or drinking outdoors, wearing long pants and shoes, and avoiding brightly colored clothing, fragrances, or hairspray when outdoors. Common insect repellents are not effective against Hymenoptera.

Current recommendations are to administer **venom immunotherapy** to individuals who have had a systemic life-threatening reaction from an insect sting and have positive venom skin tests or elevated venom-specific IgE. All persons with a history of systemic reactions to stinging insects should be instructed in the use of an epinephrine auto-injector and encouraged to wear medical information jewelry. Children younger than 16 years of age who have had only a cutaneous reaction generally do not require immunotherapy because their risk of life-threatening reaction is low.

CHAPTER 84

Adverse Reactions to Foods

ETIOLOGY AND EPIDEMIOLOGY

An **adverse reaction to food** is a generic description of any untoward reaction after food ingestion, including toxic reactions such as food poisoning and nontoxic reactions, which can be subdivided further into nonimmune and immune reactions. Lactose intolerance represents a nonimmune reaction. Food allergy or hypersensitivity reactions encompass immune reactions to food and can be divided further into immunoglobulin (Ig)E-mediated reactions, which are typically rapid in onset, and non-IgE-mediated reactions.

Oral tolerance is the suppression of the immune response to the array of dietary elements ingested daily. **Food allergy** or **hypersensitivity reactions** are the result of immune reactions to glycoproteins and develop in genetically predisposed individuals. In children, cow's milk, eggs, peanuts, soybean, wheat, tree nuts, fish, and shellfish cause 90% of IgE-mediated reactions. In older children and adults, peanuts, tree nuts, fish, and shellfish account for most reactions. Exposure to the allergenic food protein results in cross linking of cell surface specific IgE molecules found on mast cells and basophils resulting in activation and degranulation. Numerous potent mediators and cytokines are released. Non-IgE-mediated reactions typically occur hours to days after the allergen ingestion and manifest as gastrointestinal symptoms. A cell-mediated immune mechanism may be responsible.

Approximately 6-8% of children are affected with food allergy. In adults this declines to 1-2%.

CLINICAL MANIFESTATIONS

Symptoms of hypersensitivity reactions vary from involvement of the skin, gastrointestinal tract, and respiratory tract to anaphylaxis. Non-IgE-mediated food allergy typically presents during infancy as proctitis/proctocolitis, enteropathy, or enterocolitis (Table 84.1).

LABORATORY AND IMAGING STUDIES

In suspected IgE-mediated food reactions, skin prick allergy testing and serum specific IgE testing to foods help confirm the suspected food allergy. Despite the availability of two methods to evaluate food allergy, neither test can predict the severity of the reaction nor the quantity of food ingested to elicit symptoms. Positive skin tests or serum specific tests to foods in the context of a positive history can only indicate risk of an allergic reaction when exposed to that allergen.

DIAGNOSIS

A careful history focuses on symptoms, the time interval from ingestion to onset of symptoms, the quantity of food necessary to evoke the reaction, the most recent reaction, patterns of reactivity, and associated factors such as exercise and medication use. Skin prick testing can be performed to confirm suspected IgE-mediated food allergies. The history dictates what food allergens should be evaluated. Testing to a wide variety of food allergens as a screening tool has little clinical value and is strongly

TABLE 84.1 Food Allergic Disorders

DISORDER	AGE GROUP	CHARACTERISTICS	DIAGNOSIS	PROGNOSIS/COURSE
IgE-MEDIATED				
Acute gastrointestinal hypersensitivity	Any	Onset: minutes to 2 hr Nausea, abdominal pain, emesis, diarrhea Typically in conjunction with cutaneous and/or respiratory symptoms	History, positive PST, and/or serum food-IgE Confirmatory OFC	Variable, food-dependent Milk, soy, egg, and wheat typically outgrown Peanut, tree nuts, seeds, and shellfish typically persist
Pollen-food allergy syndrome (oral allergy syndrome)	Any, most common in young adults (50% of birch pollen allergic adults)	Immediate symptoms on contact of raw fruit or vegetables with oral mucosa Pruritus, tingling, erythema, or angioedema of the lips, tongue, oropharynx, throat pruritus/tightness	History	Severity of symptoms may vary with pollen season Symptoms may improve with pollen immunotherapy in subset of patients
Acute urticarial and angioedema	Any	Pruritic, evanescent skin rash (hives) and swelling within minutes to 2 hr after food ingestion; food identified as etiology in 20%	History, positive PST and/or serum food-IgE level; confirmed by OFC if necessary	Varies, food-dependent; milk, soy, egg, and wheat typically outgrown; peanut, tree nuts, seeds, and shellfish typically persistent
Allergic rhinoconjunctivitis	Any	Ocular pruritus, conjunctival injection and watery discharge, nasal pruritus, congestion, rhinorrhea, sneezing within minutes to 2 hr after food ingestion or inhalation; cutaneous and gastrointestinal manifestations typical	History, PST and/or serum food-IgE level; OFC	Varies
Acute bronchospasm	Any	Cough, wheezing, dyspnea on food ingestion or inhalation; possible risk factor for severe anaphylaxis; cutaneous and gastrointestinal manifestations typical	History, PST and/or serum food-IgE level; OFC	Varies
IgE- AND/OR NON-IgE-MEDIATED				
Allergic eosinophilic esophagitis	Any, but especially infants, children, adolescents	Children: chronic/intermittent symptoms of gastroesophageal reflux, emesis, dysphagia, abdominal pain, irritability Adults: abdominal pain, dysphagia, food impaction	History, positive PST, and/or food-IgE in 50%, but poor correlation with clinical symptoms. Elimination diet and OFC Endoscopy, biopsy provides conclusive diagnosis and response to treatment information	Variable, not well established, improvement with elimination diet within 6-8 wk Elemental diet may be required Often responds to swallowed topical steroids

Continued

TABLE 84.1 Food Allergic Disorders—cont'd

DISORDER	AGE GROUP	CHARACTERISTICS	DIAGNOSIS	PROGNOSIS/COURSE
Allergic eosinophilic gastroenteritis	Any	Chronic/intermittent abdominal pain, emesis, irritability, poor appetite, failure to thrive, weight loss, anemia, protein-losing gastroenteropathy	History, positive PST, and/or food-IgE in 50%, but poor correlation with clinical symptoms, elimination diet, and OFC Endoscopy, biopsy provides conclusive diagnosis and response to treatment information	Variable, not well established, improvement with elimination diet within 6-8 wk Elemental diet may be required
Atopic dermatitis	Infant and child; 90% start <5 yr	Relapsing pruritic vesiculopapular rash; generalized in infants, localized to flexor areas in older children; food allergy in about 30% of children with severe atopic dermatitis	History, PST and/or serum food-IgE level; elimination diet and OFC	60-80% improve significantly or allergy resolves by adolescence
Asthma	Any	Chronic cough, wheezing, dyspnea; food allergy is risk factor for intubation in children who have asthma	History, PST and/or serum food-IgE level; OFC	Varies
NON-IgE-MEDIATED				
Allergic proctocolitis	Young infants (<6 mo), frequently breastfed	Blood-streaked or heme-positive stools, otherwise healthy-appearing	History, prompt response (resolution of gross blood in 48 hr) to allergen elimination Biopsy conclusive but not necessary in vast majority	Majority able to tolerate milk or soy by 1-2 yr of age
Food protein-induced enterocolitis syndrome	Young infants	Chronic: emesis, diarrhea, failure to thrive on chronic exposure Subacute: repetitive emesis, dehydration (15% shock), diarrhea on repeat exposure after elimination period Breast feeding protective	History, response to dietary restriction PST is negative; OFC	Most resolve in 1-3 yr; rarely persists into late teenage years
Dietary protein-induced enteropathy	Young infants; incidence has decreased	Protracted diarrhea, (steatorrhea), emesis, failure to thrive, anemia in 40%	History, endoscopy, and biopsy Response to dietary restriction	Most resolve in 1-2 yr
Celiac disease (gluten-sensitive enteropathy)	Any	Chronic diarrhea, malabsorption, abdominal distention, flatulence, failure to thrive, or weight loss May be associated with oral ulcers and/or dermatitis herpetiformis	Biopsy diagnostic: villus atrophy Screening with serum IgA antitissue transglutaminase and antigliadin Resolution of symptoms with gluten elimination and relapse on oral challenge	Lifelong
Contact dermatitis	Any; more common in adults	Relapsing, pruritic eczematous rash, often on hands or face; often occurs in occupational contact with food stuff	History, patch testing	Varies
Dermatitis herpetiformis	Any	Intensely pruritic vesicular rash on extensor surfaces and buttocks	Biopsy diagnostic, shows IgA granule deposits at the dermal-epidermal junction; resolves with dietary gluten avoidance	Lifelong
Pulmonary hemosiderosis (Heiner syndrome)	Infants, children (rare)	Chronic cough, hemoptysis, lung infiltrates, wheezing, anemia; described in cow's milk– and buckwheat-allergic infants	History, PST and serum food-IgE negative but milk and buckwheat IgG precipitins positive; lung biopsy with deposits of IgG and IgA	

OFC, Oral food challenge; *PST*, prick skin test.
Modified from Nowak-Węgrzyn A, Burks AW, Sampson HA. Reactions to foods. In: Adkinson NF Jr, Bochner BS, Burks AW, et al., eds. Middleton's Allergy: Principles and Practice. *8th ed. Philadelphia: Elsevier; 2013:1323–1328.*

discouraged. A negative skin test virtually excludes an IgE-mediated mechanism. A positive skin test indicates sensitization but does not prove clinical reactivity and must be interpreted in the context of the history.

An in vitro serum-specific IgE assay can be used to help confirm clinical allergy as well. Many allergists and laboratories regard the ImmunoCAP system as the method of choice. This method uses a quantitative fluorescent immunoassay, which is more sensitive and has improved specificity and reproducibility compared to other assays. These tests provide supplementary information to skin tests. Researchers have tried to determine levels of food-specific IgE at which clinical reactions are highly likely to occur (Table 84.2). Patients with allergen-specific IgE levels greater than 95% of the predictive value will likely be symptomatic upon ingestion, so an oral food challenge is not necessary. Monitoring the allergen-specific IgE level and/or wheal size on skin prick testing may be helpful in predicting whether a child has outgrown the food allergy. Oral food challenges remain the standard of diagnosis and can be performed to determine whether a child has developed oral tolerance to the food allergen.

Component resolved diagnostics (CRD) have gained attention in the area of food allergy testing. CRD refers to a testing method employing allergens purified from natural sources or recombinant DNA technology. Hence, an individual allergen is being evaluated versus whole allergens in hopes of improved information about risk, tolerance, and prognosis. CRD is helpful in peanut and hazelnut allergy, but not for cow's milk, egg, or soy allergies.

TREATMENT

Currently, the only treatment modality of IgE-mediated food allergy is avoidance. This requires the education of the patient and family on how to avoid ingestion of the responsible allergen and when to initiate therapy if ingestion occurs. If the food allergen is ingested and symptoms of an IgE-mediated reaction ensue, auto-injectable epinephrine should be administered intramuscularly followed by emergent evaluation by medical personnel. There is no role for antihistamines in this setting because the severity of the reaction is unpredictable. There are approximately 100 deaths per year due to food allergies, and most cases are secondary to a delay or no administration of epinephrine.

Novel therapies for IgE-mediated food allergy are currently being investigated to either desensitize patients to food allergens or induce tolerance. Oral immunotherapy entails ingesting increasing amounts of the food allergen to achieve desensitization. Sublingual immunotherapy requires placing increasing doses of food allergen under the tongue. This treatment has been shown to be effective for desensitization, but compliance is poor. In epicutaneous therapy, food allergens are embedded in a patch that is applied to the skin. While still in clinical trials, these therapies may become common clinical practice within this century.

TABLE 84.2 Interpretation of Serum IgE Antibody Concentrations

FOOD		FOOD-SPECIFIC IgE ANTIBODY CONCENTRATIONS AT OR ABOVE WHICH CLINICAL REACTIONS ARE HIGHLY LIKELY (KUa/L)	POSITIVE PREDICTIVE VALUE (%)
Egg	>2 yr of age	7	98
	≤2 yr of age	2	95
Milk	>2 yr of age	15	95
	≤2 yr of age	5	95
Peanut		14	95-100
Fish		20	100
Soybean		30	73
Wheat		26	74
Tree nuts		~15	≈5

Modified from Sampson HA. Food allergy. J Allergy Clin Immunol. 2003;111:S544.

COMPLICATIONS

Anaphylaxis is the most serious complication of allergic food reactions and can result in death (see Chapter 81). Patients also need to be monitored for alterations in growth and potential nutritional deficiencies from food avoidance. This is especially important for children avoiding multiple foods or if one of their food allergens is cow's milk.

PROGNOSIS AND PREVENTION

The natural history of food allergies or "is my child going to outgrow this?" is a common concern of parents. With new data, counseling parents on the future likelihood of developing oral tolerance to a food allergen has changed over the last several years and for some foods is multifactorial. For cow's milk allergic patients who have multiple food allergies, asthma, and allergic rhinitis, 21% of patients will have persistent milk allergy at age 16 years. But 85% of children who do not have additional atopic disease develop cow's milk tolerance by 3 years of age. Similarly, 66% of children with egg allergy but no other atopic disease develop tolerance by 5 years of age, but 32% of those with additional atopic disease will still be sensitive to egg by age 16 years. The natural histories of soy and wheat allergy are similar: oral tolerance in 25-29% by age 4 years, 45-56% by age 6 or 8 years, and 65-69% by age 10 or 12 years. Previously, most children with peanut allergy were thought to nearly never develop oral tolerance. However, 20% of children with peanut allergy outgrow their allergy. Nine percent of tree nut allergic patients will develop oral tolerance. Food allergies to seafood continue to be a lifelong affliction.

Avoidance of the suspect food is crucial. Careful reading of food labels is a priority. Medical information jewelry with appropriate information should be worn. The Food Allergy Research & Education organization (www.foodallergy.org) is a useful educational resource for families and physicians.

Recommendations for prevention of allergic diseases aimed at the *high-risk* newborn who has not manifested atopic disease include (1) exclusive breast feeding for the first 4-6 months or (2) using an extensively hydrolyzed formula for the first 4-6 months and introducing solid foods between 4 and 6 months of age. Other approaches, such as maternal avoidance diets during pregnancy and during lactation, as well as avoidance of allergenic foods for infants beyond 6 months of age, are unproven.

In 2015, the Learning Early About Peanut Allergy (LEAP) study showed that early introduction of peanut in high-risk infants significantly decreased the development of peanut allergy. Likewise, the Persistence of Oral Tolerance to Peanut (LEAP-On) trial revealed that this effect is durable.

CHAPTER 85

Adverse Reactions to Drugs

ETIOLOGY

An **adverse drug reaction** is defined as an unwanted, negative consequence associated with the use of a drug or biologic agent. Drug reactions can be classified as immunologic or nonimmunologic reactions (Table 85.1). Nearly 75-80% of adverse drug reactions are caused by a predictable, nonimmunologic mechanism, and between 5 and 10% of all drug reactions are explained by an immune-mediated mechanism (Table 77.1). The remaining drug reactions are caused by an unpredictable mechanism, which may or may not be immune-mediated. Many drug reactions cannot be classified because the exact immune mechanism has not been defined. Most drugs cannot elicit an immune response because of their small size; rather, the drug or a metabolite acts as a hapten and binds to larger molecules, such as tissue or serum proteins, a process called **haptenation**. The multivalent hapten-protein complex forms a new immunogenic epitope that stimulates T and B lymphocyte responses.

EPIDEMIOLOGY

Drug reactions to penicillins and cephalosporins are the most common allergic drug reactions encountered in the pediatric population. Approximately 6-10% of children are labeled as *penicillin allergic.* Risk factors for drug reactions include previous drug exposure, increasing age (>20 years of age), parenteral or topical administration, higher dose, intermittent repeated exposure, and a genetic predisposition of slow drug metabolism. An atopic background does not predispose an individual to the development of drug reactions but may indicate a greater risk of serious reaction.

CLINICAL MANIFESTATIONS

Allergic reactions can be classified as **immediate (anaphylactic) reactions**, which occur within 60 minutes of drug administration; **accelerated reactions**, which begin 1-72 hours after drug administration; and **late reactions**, which occur after 72 hours. The most common form of adverse drug reaction is cutaneous. Accelerated reactions are usually dermatologic or serum sickness reactions. Late reactions include desquamating dermatitis, Stevens-Johnson syndrome, toxic epidermal necrolysis, and serum sickness.

LABORATORY AND IMAGING STUDIES

Skin testing protocols are standardized for penicillin and are well described for other agents, such as local anesthetics, muscle relaxants, vaccines, and insulin. Positive skin testing to such

TABLE 85.1 Classification of Adverse Drug Reactions

TYPE	EXAMPLE
IMMUNOLOGIC	
Type I reaction (IgE-mediated)	Anaphylaxis from β-lactam antibiotic
Type II reaction (cytotoxic)	Hemolytic anemia from cephalosporins
Type III reaction (immune complex)	Serum sickness from antithymocyte globulin
Type IV reaction (delayed, cell-mediated)	Contact dermatitis from topical antihistamine
Specific T-cell activation	Morbilliform rash from sulfonamides
Fas/Fas ligand-induced apoptosis	Stevens-Johnson syndrome; toxic epidermal necrolysis
Other	Drug-induced lupus-like syndrome; anticonvulsant hypersensitivity syndrome
NONIMMUNOLOGIC	
Predictable	
Pharmacologic adverse effect	Dry mouth from antihistamines; tremor from albuterol
Secondary pharmacologic adverse effect	Thrush while taking antibiotics; *Clostridium difficile*-associated colitis (pseudomembranous colitis) from clindamycin (and other antibiotics)
Drug toxicity	Hepatotoxicity from methotrexate
Drug-drug interactions	Increased carbamazepine levels with clarithromycin
Drug overdose	Hepatic necrosis from acetaminophen
Unpredictable	
Pseudoallergic	Anaphylactoid reaction after radiocontrast media
Idiosyncratic	Hemolytic anemia in a patient with G6PD deficiency after primaquine therapy
Intolerance	Tinnitus after a single, small dose of aspirin

G6PD, Glucose-6-phosphate dehydrogenase.
Modified from Riedl MA, Casillas AM. Adverse drug reactions: types and treatment options. Am Fam Physician. *2003;68(9):1781–1790.*

reagents confirms the presence of antigen-specific IgE and supports the diagnosis of a type I hypersensitivity reaction in the appropriate clinical setting.

DIFFERENTIAL DIAGNOSIS

The broadest experience with managing adverse drug reactions is with penicillin. Penicillin allergy should be evaluated when the individual is well and not in acute need of treatment. Penicillin skin testing is helpful for IgE-mediated reactions because of its negative predictive value; only 1-3% of patients with negative skin tests have a reaction, which is mild, when re-exposed to penicillin. Skin testing for penicillin should be performed using the **major determinant, penicilloyl polylysine** (available as Pre-Pen [ALK-Abelló, Inc, Hørsholm, Denmark]), and **minor determinants**, which include penicillin G, penicilloate, and penilloate. Skin testing to penicillin does not predict non-IgE-mediated reactions. For patients with a history consistent with serum sickness or desquamative-type reactions, skin testing should not be performed and penicillin should be avoided indefinitely.

The risk of having an allergic reaction to a cephalosporin in a child who has reacted positively to penicillin skin testing is less than 2%. It is believed that the first-generation cephalosporins are more likely than second-generation or third-generation cephalosporins to be cross-reactive. This is due to the chemical similarity of side chains of the β-lactam ring between penicillin and first-generation cephalosporins.

TREATMENT

If penicillin skin testing is positive, penicillin should be avoided, and an alternative antibiotic should be used. If there is a definite need for penicillin, **desensitization** can be accomplished by administration of increasing amounts of drug over a short time in a hospital setting. The exact mechanism of desensitization is unclear; however, it is thought to render mast cells unresponsive to the drug. To maintain desensitization, the drug must be given at least twice daily. If the drug is stopped for longer than 48 hours, the patient is no longer *desensitized* and the same protocol must be repeated before continuing antibiotic use.

For other antibiotics, the relevant allergenic determinants produced by metabolism or degradation are not well defined. Skin testing to the native antibiotic in nonirritating concentrations can be performed. However, a negative response does not exclude allergy while a positive response suggests the presence of IgE-mediated allergy. In the case of a negative skin test response, a graded challenge or test dose may be administered, depending on the clinical history of the reaction. Patients who have experienced Stevens-Johnson syndrome, toxic epidermal necrolysis, or serum sickness should not be challenged.

COMPLICATIONS

Anaphylaxis is the most serious complication of IgE-mediated drug reactions and can result in death (see Chapter 81).

PROGNOSIS

Most drug reactions do not seem to be allergic in nature. Repeated, intermittent exposure during childhood or early adulthood contributes to an increased incidence of adverse drug reactions in adults.

PREVENTION

Avoidance of the suspect drug is paramount. Medical information jewelry with appropriate information should be worn. In the medical community, responsible antibiotic use has been emphasized to improve patient outcomes, decrease selection for resistant organisms, and minimize spread of multidrug resistant organisms. Ideally, sensitive and specific testing to any drug for allergy evaluation is highly desirable. However, standardized testing reagents do not exist except for penicillin. The penicillin family of antimicrobials are very effective to treat a multitude of pediatric infections. So limiting their use due to suspected drug allergy may result in undesirable outcomes. Approximately 10% of patients report they have a drug allergy to penicillin, but after evaluation 90% of these patients are proven to tolerate the medication.

One of the most common concerns in regard to allergic drug reactions is cross-reactivity between penicillin and cephalosporins. In children with a history of penicillin allergy, it is important to determine whether they are truly allergic by skin testing to penicillin using the major and minor determinants. If penicillin skin testing is negative, there is a very low risk of an allergic reaction to cephalosporins. A positive penicillin skin test leads to use of an alternate non-cross-reacting antibiotic, a graded challenge to the required cephalosporin under appropriate monitoring or desensitization to the required cephalosporin.

For children with a history of a cephalosporin allergy who require another cephalosporin, consider using a graded challenge with a cephalosporin with a different side chain.

Suggested Readings

Du Toit G, Roberts G, Sayre PH, et al. Randomized trial of peanut consumption in infants at risk for peanut allergy. *NEJM.* 2015;372(9):803–813.

Du Toit G, Sayre PH, Roberts G, et al. Effect of avoidance on peanut allergy after early peanut consumption. *NEJM.* 2016;374:1435–1443.

Greenberger P, Grammer L. Northwestern University allergy-immunology syllabus 2012: residents and students. *Allergy Asthma Proc.* 2012;33(3):Suppl 1.

Keeney GE, Gray MP, Morrison AK, et al. Dexamethasone for acute asthma exacerbations in children: a meta-analysis. *Pediatrics.* 2014;133(3): 493–499.

Leung DYM, Szefler SJ, Bonilla FA, et al. *Pediatric Allergy: Principles and Practice.* 3rd ed. Elsevier; 2015.

National Heart, Lung, and Blood Institute and National Asthma Education and Prevention Program. Expert panel report 3: guidelines for the diagnosis and management of asthma. Full report 2007. *NTH Publication No. 08-4051.* U.S. Department of Health and Human Services: Bethesda, MD. http://www.nhlbi.nih.gov/guidelines/asthma/asthgdln.htm.

National Heart, Lung, and Blood Institute and National Asthma Education and Prevention Program. Expert panel report 3: guidelines for the diagnosis and management of asthma. Summary report 2007. *NTH Publication No. 08–5846.* U.S. Department of Health and Human Services: Bethesda, MD. http://www.nhlbi.nih.gov/guidelines/asthma/asthsumm.pdf.

Pesek RD, Jones SM. Current and emerging therapies for IgE-mediated food allergy. *Curr Allergy Asthma Rep.* 2016;16(4):28.

Schussler E, Kattan J. Allergen component testing in the diagnosis of food allergy. *Curr Allergy Asthma Rep.* 2015;15(9):55.

Shearer WT, Leung DYM. 2010 primer on allergic and immunologic diseases. *J Allergy Clin Immunol.* 2010;125:S1–S2.

Summary of the New Food Allergy Guidelines for Primary Care Physicians. American Academy of Allergy, Asthma & Immunology. January 2012.

Williams HC. Atopic dermatitis. *NEJM.* 2005;352:2314–2324.

Zuraw BL. Hereditary angioedema. *NEJM.* 2008;359:1027–1036.

PEARLS FOR PRACTITIONERS

CHAPTER 77

Allergy Assessment

- Type I immediate hypersensitivity reactions involve immunoglobulin E (IgE) antibodies bound to mast cell and basophil cell surfaces. Upon binding of antigen to these antibodies, chemical mediators such as histamine, tryptase, leukotrienes, and prostaglandins are released, resulting in allergic symptoms, the most serious syndrome being anaphylaxis.
- Type II cytotoxic antibody reactions occur when antibodies (IgM, IgG, or IgA) bind to cell surface antigens causing complement activation and ultimately, cell lysis, or release of anaphylatoxins. Examples of Type II disease are hemolytic anemia and Goodpasture syndrome.
- Type III immune complex reactions result when antigen-antibody complexes are formed causing injury to vasculature and organs such as liver, spleen, and kidney. The classic Type III reaction is serum sickness.
- Type IV delayed type hypersensitivity reactions result when T cells recognize antigens in the context of major histocompatibility complex class II, which activates cytokine release. Contact dermatitis to poison ivy represents an example of Type IV delayed type hypersensitivity reactions.
- The history, family history, and physical examination may indicate existing atopic disease in patients.
- Allergic rhinitis, allergic asthma, and food allergies are examples of atopic disease involving IgE antibodies.
- Of the two methods for assessing antigen-specific IgE antibodies, in vivo skin testing (via prick or intradermal testing) is the most sensitive method. Serum-based testing with quantitative fluorescent immunoassay proves to be useful in those patients unable to have skin testing performed such as dermatographism or extensive dermatitis.
- The presence of specific IgE antibodies does not equate to diagnosis of allergic disease. Rather, positive results must be correlated with the history. Therefore obtaining screening tests of multiple allergens is not recommended.

CHAPTER 78

Asthma

- Asthma involves many different cells, chemical mediators, and chemotactic factors resulting in airway inflammation and airway hyperresponsiveness. Typical symptoms included cough, wheeze, shortness of breath, and chest tightness.
- Evaluation of patients with asthma should include history, response to treatment, spirometry (>5 years of age), allergy testing, and chest radiograph, if warranted.
- Treatment of asthma involves numerous interventions: environmental control of potential allergens, patient and care giver education, reduction of exposure to nonspecific irritants such as secondhand tobacco smoke, pharmacologic therapy, and yearly influenza vaccination.
- To relieve smooth muscle airway bronchoconstriction, short-acting β_2 agonists should be employed on an as-needed basis and/or prior to physical activity.
- The most effective antiinflammatory pharmacologic therapy for persistent asthma is inhaled corticosteroids, emphasizing finding the minimum dose that is able to achieve control and minimize risk and impairment from the disease.
- All metered-dose inhalers need to be administered with the use of an aerochamber to maximize lung deposition of the medication.
- For some patients with more severe asthma, additional therapies may be required to achieve treatment goals: combination therapy with long-acting β_2 agonists, leukotriene modifiers, theophylline, omalizumab and other biologic agents, anticholinergic agents, allergen immunotherapy, and oral corticosteroids.
- Use of peak flow monitoring and written asthma action plans may assist patients and their parents with at-home monitoring and adherence to medical therapy.
- Asthma exacerbations may be treated with frequent administration of short acting bronchodilators and a course of systemic corticosteroids. Despite these interventions, status asthmaticus may ensue, requiring supplemental oxygen, continuous bronchodilation, intravenous corticosteroids, blood gas monitoring, magnesium sulfate, and hospitalization.

CHAPTER 79

Allergic Rhinitis

- Allergic rhinitis and conjunctivitis are IgE-mediated atopic diseases in response to relevant aeroallergens in a perennial and/or seasonal fashion. Common symptoms include nasal pruritus, sneezing, clear rhinorrhea, nasal obstruction, lacrimation, ocular pruritus, and conjunctival injection.
- Like asthma, treatment for allergic rhinitis and conjunctivitis employs numerous modalities: education, avoidance of triggers, pharmacologic therapy, and immunotherapy.
- The most effective pharmacologic class of medications for the treatment of allergic rhinitis is intranasal corticosteroids. When used properly, these sprays are efficacious and have no effects on the hypothalamic-pituitary-adrenal axis. Other treatments include oral and nasal antihistamines, oral decongestants, and leukotriene modifiers.

CHAPTER 80

Atopic Dermatitis

- Atopic dermatitis is a chronic relapsing skin condition characterized by pruritus and skin inflammation. The pathogenesis is complex and multifactorial.

- Restoring the skin barrier is an important treatment modality as is control of pruritus, reduction of inflammation, and minimizing exposure to known triggers.
- In severe atopic dermatitis, 30% of patients may have a food allergy trigger; for moderate eczema, 15%; for mild, less than 10%.

CHAPTER 81

Urticaria, Angioedema, and Anaphylaxis

- The pathophysiology of urticaria involves swelling of the dermis due to inflammatory mediators released from skin mast cells.
- Angioedema is swelling below the dermis.
- Acute urticaria refers to urticaria occurring less than 6 weeks duration and chronic urticaria occurs 6 weeks or more. A causal agent is more likely to be found in acute urticaria such as a food, medication, insect sting, infection, blood transfusion, or contact agent. But with chronic urticaria, an etiology is less likely to be found and most cases are idiopathic.
- Physical urticaria refers to lesions due to physical stimuli like dermatographia, cold, heat, and/or exercise and pressure.
- There are two types of hereditary angioedema, and both are inherited in an autosomal dominant fashion. Type I accounts for the majority of cases and is due to decreased production of C1-esterase inhibitor. Patients with type II have normal levels of C1-esterase inhibitor, but function is reduced.
- Patients with hereditary angioedema with normal C1 inhibitor experience angioedema like Type I and II hereditary angioedema but have normal levels and function of C1-esterase inhibitor.
- Anaphylaxis refers to a syndrome of symptoms (usually involving two or more organ systems) due to type I immediate hypersensitivity. Causative agents are numerous.
- Anaphylactoid reactions result from direct, nonspecific mast cell and basophil activation but are not immune mediated. Examples include reactions to radiocontrast media and opiates.

CHAPTER 82

Serum Sickness

- Serum sickness is the prototypical type III reaction where antibody binds to antigen forming immune complexes that can cause vascular injury or end-organ damage. Symptoms classically are fever, arthralgias, lymphadenopathy, and rash.

CHAPTER 83

Insect Allergies

- Stinging insect hypersensitivity refers to allergic reactions to Hymenoptera, which include bees, yellow jackets, wasps, hornets, and fire ants. Biting insects such as the kissing bug, bed bugs, blackflies, and deerflies have also caused cases of anaphylaxis.
- Patients of any age who suffer from anaphylaxis due to Hymenoptera stings with positive specific IgE testing benefit from immunotherapy and should have an auto-injector of epinephrine. However, patients less than 16 years of age who experience only cutaneous symptoms do not require testing, immunotherapy, or epinephrine since their risk of life-threatening reaction is low.

CHAPTER 84

Adverse Reactions to Foods

- Cow's milk, egg, soy, wheat, peanut, tree nut, finned fish, and shellfish account for 90% of IgE-mediated food allergies in children.
- Positive food skin and/or serum specific IgE testing alone does not equate to clinical reactivity and must be interpreted in the context of the history. In fact, the clinical history should dictate what food allergens should be tested; testing to many different foods as a screening tool has very little clinical value and is strongly discouraged.
- Neither skin nor serum testing for food allergies can predict severity of allergy nor the amount required to elicit a reaction. Only risk for an allergic reaction can be inferred from a positive allergy test to a food.
- Currently, treatment of food allergies is avoidance and the use of auto-injectable epinephrine in the case of accidental ingestion resulting in symptoms. There are other novel treatment modalities in clinical trials.
- Studies indicate that even for high-risk infants, early introduction of peanut into the diet decreased the development of peanut allergy.

CHAPTER 85

Adverse Reaction to Drugs

- Predictable adverse drug reactions are classified as either immunologic or nonimmunologic with the former being less common.
- Standardized allergy skin testing for reactions due to IgE is available for penicillin determinants but unavailable for most other medications. Drug challenges and drug desensitizations may be an appropriate approach in this setting.

RHEUMATIC DISEASES OF CHILDHOOD

Hilary M. Haftel

CHAPTER 86

Rheumatic Assessment

The **rheumatic diseases (collagen vascular** or **connective tissue diseases)** of childhood are characterized by autoimmunity and inflammation, which may be localized or generalized. The classic rheumatic diseases of children include juvenile idiopathic arthritis (JIA), formerly called *juvenile rheumatoid arthritis*, systemic lupus erythematosus (SLE), and juvenile dermatomyositis (JDM). Vasculitis is a component of many rheumatic diseases. **Musculoskeletal pain syndromes** are a set of overlapping conditions characterized by poorly localized pain involving the extremities. Scleroderma, Behçet syndrome, and Sjögren syndrome are rare in childhood. The differential diagnosis of rheumatological disorders typically includes infections, postinfectious processes, and malignancies (Table 86.1).

HISTORY

The history can identify symptoms that reflect the source of the inflammation, including whether it is localized or systemic. Symptoms of systemic inflammation tend to be nonspecific. **Fever**, caused by cytokine release, can take many patterns. A hectic fever, without periodicity or pattern, is commonly found in vasculitides such as Kawasaki disease but also occurs in children with underlying infection. Certain illnesses, such as systemic JIA, produce a patterned fever with regular temperature spikes once or twice a day. Other rheumatic illnesses cause low-grade fevers. Charting the child's fever pattern, particularly in the absence of antipyretics, is useful. Rashes occur in many forms, from evanescent to fixed and scarring (see Table 86.1). Other systemic symptoms (malaise, anorexia, weight loss, and fatigue) can vary from mild to debilitating.

Symptoms of localized inflammation vary depending on the involved site. **Arthritis**, or inflammation of the synovium **(synovitis)**, leads to joint pain, swelling, and impaired ability to use the affected joint. Morning stiffness or gelling is commonly described. The child may be slow to arise in the morning or after long periods of inactivity and may have a limp. Children may refrain from usual activities and athletics. **Enthesitis** is inflammation at the insertion of a ligament to a bone. **Serositis**, inflammation of serosal lining such as pleuritis, pericarditis, or peritonitis, gives rise to chest pain, shortness of breath, or abdominal pain. **Myositis**, inflammation of the muscle, may lead to symptoms of muscle pain, weakness, or difficulty performing tasks of daily living. **Vasculitis**, inflammation of the blood vessels, leads to nonspecific symptoms of rash (petechiae, purpura) and edema when small vessels deep in the papillary dermis are involved; involvement of medium-sized vessels results in a circumscribed tender nodule.

PHYSICAL EXAMINATION

A thorough history and physical examination is frequently sufficient to narrow the differential diagnosis and elicit the diagnosis. The child's overall appearance, evidence of growth failure, or failure to thrive may point to a significant underlying inflammatory disorder. The head and neck examination may show evidence of mucosal ulceration, seen in diseases such as SLE. The eye examination may show pupillary irregularity and synechiae from uveitis or the nonpurulent conjunctivitis of Kawasaki disease. Diffuse lymphadenopathy may be found and is nonspecific. The respiratory and cardiac examinations may show pericardial or pleural friction rubs, indicating serositis. Splenomegaly or hepatomegaly raises suspicion of activation of the reticuloendothelial system that occurs in systemic JIA or SLE.

The joint examination is crucial for the diagnosis of arthritis and may identify evidence of inflammation, such as joint swelling, effusion, tenderness, and erythema from increased blood flow. Joint contractures may be seen if the process is chronic. The joint lining, or synovium, may be thickened from chronic inflammation. Activation of epiphyseal growth plates in an area of arthritis can lead to localized bony proliferation and limb length discrepancies. Conversely, inflammation at sites of immature growth centers may lead to maldevelopment of bones, such as the carpals or tarsals, resulting in crowding, or the temporomandibular joints, resulting in micrognathia. A rash or evidence of underlying skin disorders, such as skin thickening from scleroderma or sclerodactyly, may be noted. Chronic Raynaud phenomenon may result in nail fold capillary changes, ulceration, or digital tuft wasting.

COMMON MANIFESTATIONS

The rheumatic diseases of childhood encompass a heterogeneous group of diseases with a shared underlying pathogenesis: disordered functioning of the immune system leading to inflammation directed against native proteins, with secondary increases in numbers of activated lymphocytes, inflammatory cytokines, and circulating antibodies. This antibody production can be nonspecific, or it can be targeted against specific native

TABLE 86.1 Differential Diagnosis of Pediatric Arthritis Syndromes

CHARACTERISTIC	SYSTEMIC LUPUS ERYTHEMATOSUS	JUVENILE IDIOPATHIC ARTHRITIS	RHEUMATIC FEVER	LYME DISEASE	LEUKEMIA	GONOCOCCEMIA	KAWASAKI DISEASE
Sex	F > M	Type-dependent	M = F	M = F	M = F	F > M	M = F
Age	10–20 yr	1–16 yr	5–15 yr	>5–20 yr	2–10 yr	>12 yr	<5 yr
Arthralgia	Yes	Yes	Yes	Yes	Yes	Yes	Yes
Morning stiffness	Yes	Yes	No	No	No	No	No
Rash	Butterfly; discoid	Salmon-pink macules (systemic)	Erythema marginatum	Erythema migrans	No	Palms/soles, papulopustules	Diffuse maculopapular (nonspecific), desquamation
Monarticular, oligoarticular	Yes	50%	No	Yes	Yes	Yes	—
Polyarticular	Yes	Yes	Yes	No	Yes	No	Yes
Small joints	Yes	Yes	No	Rare	Yes	No	Yes
Temporomandibular joint	No	Rare	No	Rare	No	No	No
Eye disease	Uveitis/retinitis	Iridocyclitis (rare in systemic)	No	Conjunctivitis, keratitis	No	No	Conjunctivitis, uveitis
Total WBC count	Decreased	Increased (decreased in macrophage activation syndrome)	Normal to increased	Normal	Increased or neutropenia ± blasts	Increased	Increased
ANA*	Positive (>99%)	Positive (50%)	Negative	Negative	Negative	Negative	Negative
Rheumatoid factor*	Positive or negative	Positive (10%) (polyarticular)	Negative	Negative	Negative	Negative	Negative
Other laboratory results	↓ Complement, ↑antibodies to double-stranded DNA	Anti-CCP antibody + in adult type RA	↑ASO anti-DNase B	↑Cryoglobulin, ↑immune complexes	+ Bone marrow	+ Culture for *Neisseria gonorrhoeae*	Thrombocytosis, ↑ immune complexes
Erosive arthritis	Rare	Yes	Rare	Rare	No	Yes	No
Other clinical manifestations	Proteinuria, serositis	Fever, serositis (systemic)	Carditis, nodules, chorea	Carditis, neuropathy, meningitis	Thrombocytopenia	Sexual activity, menses	Fever, lymphadenopathy, swollen hands/feet, mouth lesions
Pathogenesis	Autoimmune	Autoimmune	Group A streptococcus	*Borrelia burgdorferi*	Acute lymphoblastic leukemia	*N. gonorrhoeae*	Unknown
Treatment	NSAIDs, corticosteroids, hydroxychloroquine, immunosuppressive agents	NSAIDs, methotrexate, hydroxychloroquine, sulfasalazine, biologic agents	Penicillin prophylaxis, aspirin, corticosteroids	Amoxicillin, doxycycline, ceftriaxone	Corticosteroids, chemotherapy	Ceftriaxone	Intravenous immunoglobulin, aspirin

**Up to 20% of normal children will have a false-positive ANA or RF, most likely due to infection.*
ANA, Antinuclear antibody; *ASO,* antistreptolysin-O titer; *CCP,* cyclic citrullinated protein; *NSAID,* nonsteroidal antiinflammatory drug; *TNF,* tumor necrosis factor; *WBC,* white blood cell.

TABLE 86.2 Manifestations of Autoantibodies
Coombs-positive hemolytic anemia
Immune neutropenia
Immune thrombocytopenia
Thrombosis (anticardiolipin, antiphospholipid, lupus anticoagulant)
Immune lymphopenia
Antimitochondrial (primary biliary cirrhosis, SLE)
Antimicrosomal (chronic active hepatitis, SLE)
Antithyroid (thyroiditis, SLE)
ANCA-cytoplasmic (granulomatosis with polyangiitis)
ANCA-perinuclear (microscopic polyangiitis or other vasculitides)
Anti-CCP (rheumatoid positive JIA)
ANTINUCLEAR ANTIBODIES TO SPECIFIC NUCLEAR ANTIGENS AND ASSOCIATED MANIFESTATIONS
Single-stranded DNA (nonspecific, indicates inflammation)
Double-stranded DNA (SLE, renal disease)
DNA-histone (drug-induced SLE)
Sm (Smith) (SLE, renal, CNS)
RNP (ribonucleoprotein) (SLE, Sjögren syndrome, scleroderma, polymyositis, MCTD)
Ro (Robert: SSA) (SLE, neonatal lupus-congenital heart block, Sjögren syndrome)
La (Lane: SSB) (SLE, neonatal lupus [congenital heart block], Sjögren syndrome)
Jo-1 (polymyositis, dermatomyositis)
Scl-70 (systemic sclerosis)
Centromere (CREST; limited scleroderma)
PM-Scl (scleroderma, UCTD)

ANCA, Antineutrophil cytoplasmic antibody; *CCP,* cyclic citrullinated protein; *CNS,* central nervous system; *CREST syndrome,* calcinosis, Raynaud phenomenon, esophageal dysfunction, sclerodactyly, telangiectasia; *JIA,* juvenile idiopathic arthritis; *MCTD,* mixed connective tissue disease; *SLE,* systemic lupus erythematosus; *SSA,* Sjögren syndrome antigen A; *SSB,* Sjögren syndrome antigen B; *UCTD,* undifferentiated connective tissue disease.
Modified from Condemi J. The autoimmune disease. JAMA. *1992;268:2882–2892.*

proteins, leading to subsequent disease manifestations (Table 86.2). Although immune system hyperactivity may be self-limited, the hallmark of most rheumatic diseases of childhood is chronicity, or the perpetuation of the inflammatory process, which can lead to long-term disability.

INITIAL DIAGNOSTIC EVALUATION

Although rheumatic diseases sometimes present with nonspecific symptoms, especially early in the course, over time a characteristic set of symptoms and physical findings can be elicited. In conjunction with carefully chosen confirmatory laboratory tests, an appropriate differential diagnosis is made, and eventually the correct diagnosis and treatment plan is developed.

Most rheumatological diagnoses are established by clinical findings and fulfillment of classification criteria. Laboratory testing should be judicious and based on a differential diagnosis rather than random screening in search of a diagnosis. Laboratory tests confirm clinical diagnoses rather than develop them.

LABORATORY TESTING

Evidence of an underlying systemic inflammation may be indicated by elevated acute phase reactants, especially the erythrocyte sedimentation rate, but also the white blood cell count, platelet count, and C-reactive protein. The complete blood count may demonstrate a normochromic, normocytic anemia of chronic disease. These laboratory findings are nonspecific for any particular rheumatological diagnosis. Certain laboratory tests may help confirm a diagnosis, such as autoantibody production in SLE or muscle enzyme elevation in JDM, or identify increased risk for complications, such as uveitis in a patient with JIA with a positive antinuclear antibody.

DIAGNOSTIC IMAGING

Radiological studies should focus on areas of concern identified by history or physical examination. Radiography of joints in patients with arthritis on examination may be beneficial, but radiographic abnormalities may lag far behind the clinical examination. Tests with greater sensitivity, such as magnetic resonance imaging (MRI), may be useful when trying to differentiate between synovitis and traumatic soft tissue injury. MRI may also be useful to identify evidence of central nervous system involvement with SLE or evidence of myositis with JDM.

CHAPTER 87

Henoch-Schönlein Purpura

ETIOLOGY

Henoch-Schönlein purpura (HSP) is a vasculitis of unknown etiology characterized by inflammation of small blood vessels with leukocytic infiltration of tissue, hemorrhage, and ischemia. The immune complexes associated with HSP are predominantly composed of immunoglobulin A (IgA), suggesting a hypersensitivity process.

EPIDEMIOLOGY

HSP is the most common systemic vasculitis of childhood and cause of *nonthrombocytopenic* purpura, with an incidence of 13 per 100,000 children. It occurs primarily in children 3-15 years of age, although it has been described in adults. HSP is slightly more common in boys than girls and occurs more frequently in the winter than in the summer months.

CLINICAL MANIFESTATIONS

Decision-Making Algorithms
Available @ StudentConsult.com

Red Urine and Hematuria
Proteinuria
Scrotal Pain
Fever and Rash
Petechiae/Purpura

HSP is characterized by rash, arthritis, and less frequently gastrointestinal or renal vasculitis. The hallmark of HSP is **palpable purpura**, caused by small vessel inflammation in the skin, leading to extravasation of blood into the surrounding tissues, frequently with IgA deposition. The rash is classically found in dependent areas: below the waist, on the buttocks, and lower extremities (Fig. 87.1). The rash can begin as small macules or urticarial lesions but rapidly progresses to purpura with areas of ecchymosis. The rash also can be accompanied by edema, particularly of the calves and dorsum of the feet, scalp, and scrotum or labia. HSP occasionally is associated with encephalopathy, pancreatitis, and orchitis.

Arthritis occurs in 80% of patients with HSP and is most common in the lower extremities, particularly the ankles and knees. The arthritis is acute and very painful, with refusal to bear weight. Joint swelling can be confused with peripheral edema seen with the rash of HSP.

Gastrointestinal involvement occurs in about one half of affected children and most typically presents as mild to moderate crampy abdominal pain, thought to be due to small vessel involvement of the gastrointestinal tract leading to ischemia. Less commonly, significant abdominal distention, bloody diarrhea, intussusception, or abdominal perforation occurs and requires emergent intervention. Gastrointestinal involvement is typically seen during the acute phase of the illness. It may precede the onset of rash.

One third of children with HSP develop renal involvement, which can be acute or chronic. Although renal involvement is mild in most cases, acute glomerulonephritis manifested by hematuria, hypertension, or acute renal failure can occur. Most cases of glomerulonephritis occur within the first few months of presentation, but rarely patients develop late renal disease, which ultimately can lead to chronic renal disease, including renal failure.

LABORATORY AND IMAGING STUDIES

Erythrocyte sedimentation rate, C-reactive protein, and white blood cell count are elevated in patients with HSP. The platelet count is the most important test, because HSP is characterized by nonthrombocytopenic purpura with a normal, or even high, platelet count, differentiating HSP from other causes of purpura that are associated with thrombocytopenia such as autoimmune thrombocytopenia, systemic lupus erythematosus, or leukemia. A urinalysis screens for evidence of hematuria. A serum blood urea nitrogen and creatinine should be obtained to evaluate renal function. Testing the stool for blood may identify evidence of gut ischemia. Any question of gut perforation requires radiological investigation.

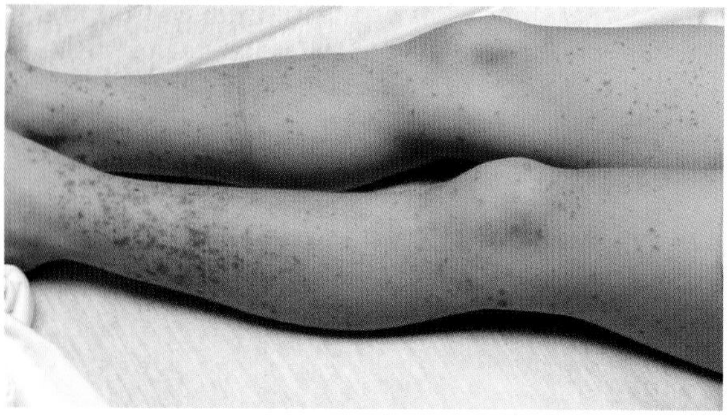

FIGURE 87.1 Rash of Henoch-Schönlein purpura on the lower extremities of a child. Note evidence of both purpura and petechiae.

DIFFERENTIAL DIAGNOSIS

The diagnosis of HSP is based on the presence of two of four criteria (Table 87.1), which provides 87.1% sensitivity and 87.7% specificity for the disease. The differential diagnosis includes other systemic vasculitides (Table 87.2) and diseases associated with thrombocytopenic purpura, such as idiopathic thrombocytopenic purpura and leukemia.

TABLE 87.1 Criteria for Diagnosis of Henoch-Schönlein Purpura*

CRITERIA	DEFINITION
Palpable purpura	Raised, palpable hemorrhagic skin lesions in the absence of thrombocytopenia
Bowel angina	Diffuse abdominal pain or the diagnosis of bowel ischemia
Diagnostic biopsy	Histological changes showing granulocytes in the walls of arterioles or venules; IgA deposits in vessel wall
Pediatric age group	Age <20 yr at onset of symptoms

**The diagnosis of Henoch-Schönlein purpura is based on the presence of two of four criteria.*

TABLE 87.2 Classification of Vasculitides

ANTINEUTROPHIL CYTOPLASMIC ANTIBODY-ASSOCIATED VASCULITIS
Granulomatosis with polyangiitis (GPA) (formerly known as Wegener granulomatosis)
Polyarteritis nodosa
Eosinophilic granulomatosis with polyangiitis (formerly known as Churg-Strauss syndrome)
Microscopic polyangiitis (MPA)
HYPERSENSITIVITY SYNDROMES
Henoch-Schönlein purpura
Serum sickness (e.g., drug-related)
Vasculitis associated with infections
CONNECTIVE TISSUE DISEASES
Systemic lupus erythematosus
Dermatomyositis
Juvenile idiopathic arthritis
GIANT CELL ARTERITIS
Temporal arteritis
Takayasu arteritis
OTHERS
Behçet syndrome
Kawasaki disease
Hypocomplementemic urticarial vasculitis

TREATMENT

Therapy for HSP is supportive. A short-term course of nonsteroidal antiinflammatory drugs can be administered for the acute arthritis. Systemic corticosteroids usually are reserved for children with gastrointestinal disease and provide significant relief of abdominal pain. A typical dosing regimen is prednisone, 1 mg/kg/day for 1-2 weeks, followed by a taper schedule. Recurrence of abdominal pain as corticosteroids are weaned may necessitate a longer course of treatment. Acute nephritis typically is treated with corticosteroids but may require more aggressive immunosuppressive therapy.

COMPLICATIONS

Most cases of HSP are monophasic, lasting 3-4 weeks and resolving completely. The rash can wax and wane, however, for 1 year after the initial episode of HSP. Parents should be warned regarding possible recurrences. The arthritis of HSP does not leave any permanent joint damage; it does not typically recur. Gastrointestinal involvement can lead to temporary abnormal peristalsis that poses a risk of intussusception, which may be followed by complete obstruction or infarction with bowel perforation. Any child with a recent history of HSP who presents with acute abdominal pain, obstipation, or diarrhea should be evaluated for intussusception. Renal involvement rarely may lead to renal failure.

PROGNOSIS

The prognosis of HSP is excellent. Most children have complete resolution of the illness without any significant sequelae. HSP patients with renal disease (elevated blood urea nitrogen, persistent high-grade proteinuria) are at highest risk for long-term complications such as hypertension or renal insufficiency, particularly if the initial course was marked by significant nephritis. There is a long-term risk of progression to end-stage renal disease in less than 1% of children with HSP. The rare patients who develop end-stage renal disease may require renal transplantation. HSP may recur in the transplanted kidney.

CHAPTER 88

Kawasaki Disease

ETIOLOGY

Kawasaki disease (KD) is a vasculitis of unknown etiology that is characterized by multisystem involvement and inflammation of small- to medium-sized arteries with resulting aneurysm formation.

EPIDEMIOLOGY

KD is the second most common vasculitis of childhood. It is more common in children of Asian descent. It has been described in variable frequency in all parts of the world; the highest frequency is in Japan. KD most commonly occurs in children younger than 5 years of age, with a peak between 2 and 3 years, and is rare in children older than 7 years. The incidence in the United States is approximately 6 per 100,000 children who are younger than 5 years of age. A seasonal variability has been described with a peak between February and May, but the disease occurs throughout the year.

CLINICAL MANIFESTATIONS

The clinical course of KD can be divided into three phases, each with its own unique manifestations. Aneurysmal involvement of the coronary arteries is the most important manifestation of KD.

Acute Phase

Decision-Making Algorithms
Available @ StudentConsult.com

Lymphadenopathy
Fever Without a Source
Fever of Unknown Origin

The acute phase of KD, which lasts 1-2 weeks, is marked by sudden onset of a high, hectic **fever** without an apparent source. The onset of fever is followed by **conjunctival erythema**; mucosal changes, including dry, **cracked lips** and a **strawberry tongue; cervical lymphadenopathy**; and swelling of the hands and feet (Fig. 88.1). Conjunctivitis is bilateral, bulbar, and nonsuppurative. Cervical lymphadenopathy is found in 70% of children and should be greater than 1.5 cm in diameter for the purposes of diagnosis. A rash, which can vary in appearance, occurs in 80% of children with KD and may be particularly accentuated in the inguinal area and on the chest. Extreme irritability is prominent, especially in infants. Abdominal pain and hydrops of the gallbladder, cerebrospinal fluid pleocytosis, sterile pyuria, and arthritis, particularly of medium-sized to large joints, may occur. Carditis in the acute phase may be manifested by tachycardia, shortness of breath, or overt heart failure. **Giant coronary artery aneurysms**, which are rare but occur most commonly in very young children, can appear during this phase.

Subacute Phase

The subacute phase, which lasts until about the 4th week, is characterized by gradual resolution of fever (if untreated) and other symptoms. **Desquamation** of the skin, particularly of the fingers and toes, appears at this point. The platelet count, previously normal or slightly depressed, increases to a significant degree (often >1 million/mm^3). This phase heralds the onset of **coronary artery aneurysms**, which may also appear in the convalescent phase and pose the highest risk of morbidity and mortality. Risk factors for development of coronary artery aneurysms include prolonged fever, prolonged elevation of inflammatory parameters such as the erythrocyte sedimentation rate (ESR), age younger than 1 year or older than 6 years, poor response to therapy, and male gender.

Convalescent Phase

The convalescent phase begins with the disappearance of clinical symptoms and continues until the ESR returns to normal, usually

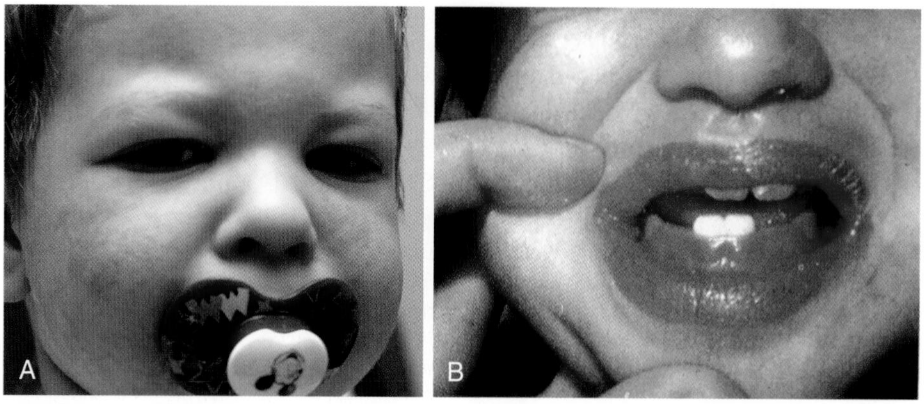

FIGURE 88.1 Facial features of Kawasaki disease with **(A)** morbilliform rash and nonsuppurative conjunctivitis and **(B)** red, chapped lips.

6-8 weeks after the onset of illness. Beau lines of the fingernails may appear during this phase.

LABORATORY AND IMAGING STUDIES

It is particularly important to exclude other causes of fever, notably infection. It is appropriate to obtain blood and urine cultures and to perform a chest x-ray. In the acute phase, inflammatory parameters are elevated, including white blood cell count, C-reactive protein, and the ESR, which can be profoundly elevated (often >80 mm/hr). Platelet counts may be inappropriately low or normal. A lumbar puncture, if performed to exclude infection, may reveal pleocytosis. Tests of hepatobiliary function may be abnormal. Greatly elevated platelet counts develop during the subacute phase. The development of coronary artery aneurysms is monitored by performing two-dimensional echocardiograms, usually during the acute phase, at 2-3 weeks, and again at 6-8 weeks. More frequent echocardiograms and, potentially, coronary angiography are indicated for patients who develop coronary artery abnormalities.

TABLE 88.1 Criteria for Diagnosis of Kawasaki Disease
Fever of >5 days' duration associated with at least four* of the following five changes:
Bilateral nonsuppurative conjunctivitis
One or more changes of the mucous membranes of the upper respiratory tract, including pharyngeal injection, dry fissured lips, injected lips, and "strawberry" tongue
One or more changes of the extremities, including peripheral erythema, peripheral edema, periungual desquamation, and generalized desquamation
Polymorphous rash, primarily truncal
Posterior cervical lymphadenopathy >1.5 cm in diameter
Disease cannot be explained by some other known disease process

**A diagnosis of Kawasaki disease can be made if fever and only three changes are present in conjunction with coronary artery disease documented by two-dimensional echocardiography or coronary angiography.*

DIFFERENTIAL DIAGNOSIS

The diagnosis of KD is based on the presence of fever for more than 5 days without an identifiable source and the presence of four of five other clinical criteria (Table 88.1).

The diagnosis of **incomplete (atypical) KD**, which occurs more commonly in infants, is made when fever is present for at least 5 days, even if only two or three clinical criteria are present, particularly in the presence of coronary artery aneurysms. The diagnosis of KD should be considered in infants younger than 6 months of age with fever for at least 7 days even if no other criteria are present. Because many of the manifestations of KD are found in other illnesses, many diagnoses must be considered and excluded before the diagnosis of KD can be established (Table 88.2).

TREATMENT

Intravenous immunoglobulin (IVIG) is the mainstay of therapy for KD, although the mechanism of action is unknown. A single dose of IVIG (2 g/kg over 12 hours) usually results in rapid defervescence and resolution of clinical illness in most patients and, more important, reduces the incidence of coronary artery aneurysms. Aspirin is initially given in **antiinflammatory doses** (80-100 mg/kg/day divided every 6 hours) in the acute phase. Once the fever resolves, aspirin is reduced to **antithrombotic doses** (3-5 mg/kg/day as a single dose) and given through the subacute and convalescent phases, usually for 6-8 weeks, until follow-up echocardiography documents the absence or resolution of coronary artery aneurysms.

Up to 10% of children with KD initially fail to respond satisfactorily to IVIG therapy. Most of these patients respond to retreatment with IVIG, but an alternative preparation of IVIG may be required. Corticosteroids or infliximab are used less frequently in KD, as opposed to other vasculitides, but may have a role during the acute phase if active carditis is apparent or for children with persistent fever after two doses of IVIG.

COMPLICATIONS

Most cases resolve without sequelae. Myocardial infarction has been documented, most likely caused by stenosis of a coronary artery at the site of an aneurysm. Coronary artery aneurysms found on autopsy in older children following sudden cardiac death may have been due to past KD. Other complications are listed in Table 88.3.

TABLE 88.2 Differential Diagnosis of Kawasaki Disease
INFECTIOUS
Scarlet fever
Epstein-Barr virus
Adenovirus
Meningococcemia
Measles
Rubella
Roseola infantum
Staphylococcal toxic shock syndrome
Scalded skin syndrome
Toxoplasmosis
Leptospirosis
Rocky Mountain spotted fever
INFLAMMATORY
Juvenile idiopathic arthritis (systemic)
Polyarteritis nodosa
Behçet syndrome
HYPERSENSITIVITY
Drug reaction
Stevens-Johnson syndrome

TABLE 88.3 Complications of Kawasaki Disease
Coronary artery thrombosis
Peripheral artery aneurysm
Coronary artery aneurysms
Myocardial infarction
Myopericarditis
Heart failure
Hydrops of gallbladder
Aseptic meningitis
Irritability
Arthritis
Sterile pyuria (urethritis)
Thrombocytosis (late)
Diarrhea
Pancreatitis
Peripheral gangrene

PROGNOSIS

IVIG reduces the prevalence of coronary artery disease from 20% to 25% in children treated with aspirin alone to 2-4% in children treated with IVIG and aspirin. Prolonged inflammation (greater than 10 days) puts the patient at greater risk for developing coronary artery aneurysms. Other than the risk of persistent coronary artery aneurysms, KD has an excellent prognosis.

CHAPTER 89

Juvenile Idiopathic Arthritis

ETIOLOGY

The chronic arthritides of childhood include several types, the most common of which is juvenile idiopathic arthritis (JIA), formerly called *juvenile rheumatoid arthritis (JRA)*. The classification of JIA includes several other types of juvenile arthritis, such as enthesitis-related arthritis, spondyloarthropathies, and psoriatic arthritis. The etiology of this autoimmune disease is unknown. The common underlying manifestation of this group of illnesses is the presence of chronic **synovitis**, or inflammation of the synovial lining of the joint. The synovium becomes thickened and hypervascular with infiltration by lymphocytes, which also can be found in the synovial fluid along with inflammatory cytokines. The inflammation leads to production and release of tissue proteases and collagenases. If left untreated, the inflammation can lead to tissue destruction, particularly of the articular cartilage and, eventually, the underlying bony structures.

EPIDEMIOLOGY

JIA is the most common chronic rheumatological disease of childhood, with a prevalence of 1 : 1,000 children. The disease has two peaks, one at 1-3 years and one at 8-12 years, but it can occur at any age. Girls are affected more commonly than boys, particularly with the oligoarticular form of the illness.

CLINICAL PRESENTATION

Decision-Making Algorithms
Available @ StudentConsult.com

Red Eye
Limp
Arthritis
Knee Pain
Extremity Pain

JIA can be divided into several subtypes, depending on the number of joints involved (<5 versus 5 or more), the presence of sacroiliac involvement, and the presence of systemic features, each with particular disease characteristics (Table 89.1). Although the onset of the arthritis is slow, the actual joint swelling is often noticed acutely by the child or parent, such as after an accident or fall, and can be confused with trauma (even though traumatic effusions are rare in children). The child may develop pain and stiffness in the joint that limit use, but refusing to bear weight on the joint is rare. Morning stiffness and gelling also can occur in the joint and, if present, can be followed in response to therapy.

On physical examination, signs of inflammation are present, including joint tenderness, erythema, and effusion (Fig. 89.1). Joint range of motion may be limited because of pain, swelling, or contractures from lack of use. In children, because of the presence of an active growth plate, it may be possible to find bony abnormalities of the surrounding bone, causing bony

TABLE 89.1 Features of Juvenile Idiopathic Arthritis Subgroups

FEATURE	OLIGOARTICULAR	POLYARTICULAR	SYSTEMIC	SPONDYLOARTHROPATHIES
No. joints	<5	≥5	Varies, usually ≥5	Varies
Types of joints	Medium to large (also small in extended oligoarthritis)	Small to medium	Small to medium	Medium to large, including sacroiliac joints
Gender predominance	F > M (especially in younger children)	F > M	F = M	M > F
Systemic features	None	Some constitutional	Prominent	Some constitutional
Eye disease	+++ (uveitis)	++ (uveitis)	+ (uveitis)	++ (iritis)
Extraarticular manifestations	None	None	Systemic features	Enthesopathy, psoriasis, bowel disease
ANA positivity	++	+	—	—
RF or anti-CCP positivity		+ (in older children with early-onset RA)		
Outcomes	Excellent, >90% complete remission	Good, >50% complete remission, some risk of disability	Variable, depends on extent of arthritis	Variable

ANA, Antinuclear antibody; *CCP*, cyclic citrullinated peptide; *RA*, rheumatoid arthritis; *RF*, rheumatoid factor.

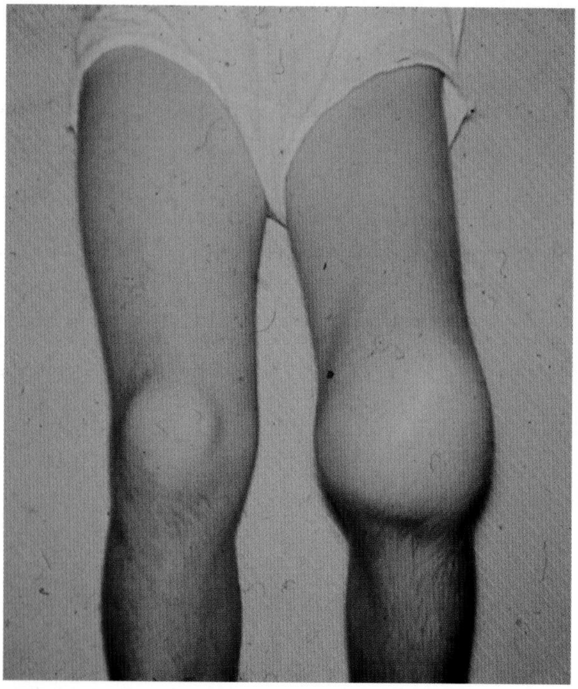

FIGURE 89.1 An affected knee in a patient with oligoarticular juvenile idiopathic arthritis. Note sizeable effusion, bony proliferation, and flexion contracture.

proliferation and localized growth disturbance. In a lower extremity joint, a leg length discrepancy may be appreciable if the arthritis is asymmetric.

All children with chronic arthritis are at risk for chronic **iridocyclitis** or **uveitis.** There is an association between human leukocyte antigens (HLAs; HLA-DR5, HLA-DR6, and HLA-DR8) and uveitis. The presence of a positive **antinuclear antibody** identifies children with arthritis who are at higher risk for chronic uveitis. Although all children with JIA are at increased risk, the subgroup of children, particularly young girls, with oligoarticular (<5 affected joints) JIA and a positive antinuclear antibody are at highest risk, with an incidence of uveitis of 80%. The uveitis associated with JIA can be asymptomatic until the point of visual loss, making it the primary treatable cause of blindness in children. It is crucial for children with JIA to undergo regular ophthalmological screening with a slit-lamp examination to identify anterior chamber inflammation and to initiate prompt treatment of any active disease.

Oligoarticular Juvenile Idiopathic Arthritis

Oligoarticular JIA is defined as the presence of arthritis in fewer than five joints within 6 months of diagnosis. This is the most common form of JIA, accounting for approximately 50% of cases.

Oligoarticular JIA presents in young children, with a peak at 1-3 years and another peak at 8-12 years. The arthritis is found in medium-sized to large joints; the knee is the most common joint involved, followed by the ankle and the wrist. It is unusual for small joints, such as the fingers or toes, to be involved, although this may occur. Neck, jaw, and hip involvement are also uncommon. Children with oligoarticular JIA may be otherwise well without any evidence of systemic inflammation (fever, weight loss, or failure to thrive) or any laboratory evidence of systemic inflammation (elevated white blood cell count or erythrocyte sedimentation rate). A subset of these children later develops polyarticular disease (called *extended oligoarthritis*).

Polyarticular Juvenile Idiopathic Arthritis

Polyarticular JIA describes children with arthritis in five or more joints within the first 6 months of diagnosis and accounts for about 40% of cases. Children with polyarticular JIA tend to have symmetric arthritis, which can affect any joint but typically involves the small joints of the hands, feet, ankles, wrists, and knees. The cervical spine can be involved, leading to fusion of the spine over time. In contrast to oligoarticular JIA, children with polyarticular disease can present with evidence

TABLE 89.2 Comparison of Juvenile Idiopathic Arthritis and Spondyloarthropathies

CLINICAL MANIFESTATIONS	JIA	JAS	PSA	IBD
Gender predominance	F	M	Equal	Equal
Peripheral arthritis	+++	+	++	+
Back symptoms	–	+++	+	++
Family history	–	++	++	+
ANA positivity	++	–	–	–
HLA-B27 positivity	–	++	–	
RF or anti-CCP antibody positivity	+ (in late-onset JIA)	–	–	–
Extraarticular manifestations	Systemic symptoms (systemic JIA)	Enthesopathy	Psoriasis, nail changes	Bowel symptoms
Eye disease	Anterior uveitis iritis	Iritis	Posterior uveitis	Anterior uveitis

ANA, Antinuclear antibody; *CCP*, cyclic citrullinated peptide; *HLA*, human leukocyte antigen; *IBD*, inflammatory bowel disease; *JAS*, juvenile ankylosing spondylitis; *JIA*, juvenile idiopathic arthritis; *PSA*, psoriatic arthritis; *RF*, rheumatoid factor.

of systemic inflammation, including malaise, low-grade fever, growth retardation, anemia of chronic disease, and elevated markers of inflammation. Polyarticular JIA can present at any age, although there is a peak in early childhood. There is a second peak in adolescence, but these children differ by the presence of a positive **rheumatoid factor** or **anti-CCP antibody** and most likely represent a subgroup with true adult rheumatoid arthritis; the clinical course and prognosis are similar to the adult entity.

Systemic Juvenile Idiopathic Arthritis

A small subgroup of patients (approximately 10%) with juvenile arthritis does not present with onset of arthritis but rather with preceding **systemic inflammation**. This form of JIA, thought to be an autoinflammatory disease, manifests with a typical recurring, spiking fever, usually once or twice per day, which can occur for several weeks to months. This is accompanied by a rash, typically **morbilliform** and **salmon-colored**. The rash may be evanescent and occur at times of high fever only. Rarely the rash can be urticarial in nature. Internal organ involvement also occurs. Serositis, such as pleuritis and pericarditis, occurs in 50% of children. Pericardial tamponade may rarely occur. Hepatosplenomegaly occurs in 70% of children. Children with systemic JIA appear sick; they have significant constitutional symptoms, including malaise and failure to thrive. Laboratory findings show the inflammation, with elevated erythrocyte sedimentation rate, C-reactive protein, white blood cell count, and platelet counts and anemia. The arthritis of JIA follows the systemic inflammation by 6 weeks to 6 months. The arthritis is typically polyarticular in nature and can be extensive and resistant to treatment, placing these children at highest risk for long-term disability.

Spondyloarthropathies

The spondyloarthropathies describe a group of arthritides that include inflammation of the axial skeleton and sacroiliac joints and enthesitis, or inflammation of tendinous insertions. These include juvenile ankylosing spondylitis, psoriatic arthritis, and the arthritis of inflammatory bowel disease. This group of diseases can also present with peripheral arthritis and can be initially classified in other subgroups. It is only later, when the patient develops evidence of sacroiliac arthritis, psoriasis, or gastrointestinal disease, that the diagnosis becomes clear (Table 89.2). Other important features of this group include the frequent presence of HLA-B27 and the need for earlier treatment with tumor necrosis factor (TNF) blockers.

LABORATORY AND IMAGING STUDIES

Most children with oligoarticular JIA have no laboratory abnormalities. Children with polyarticular and systemic disease commonly show elevated acute phase reactants and anemia of chronic disease. In all pediatric patients with joint or bone pain, a complete blood count should be performed to exclude leukemia, which also can present with limb pain (see Chapter 155). All patients with oligoarticular JIA should have an antinuclear antibody test to help identify those at higher risk for uveitis. Older children and adolescents with polyarticular disease should have a rheumatoid factor and anti-CCP antibody performed to identify children with early onset adult rheumatoid arthritis.

Diagnostic arthrocentesis may be necessary to exclude suppurative arthritis in children who present with acute onset of monarticular symptoms. The synovial fluid white blood cell count is typically less than 50,000 to 100,000/mm^3 and should be predominantly lymphocytes, rather than neutrophils seen with suppurative arthritis. Gram stain, PCR, and culture should be negative (see Chapter 118).

The most common radiological finding in the early stages of JIA is a normal bone x-ray. Over time, periarticular osteopenia, resulting from decreased mineralization, is most commonly found. Growth centers may be slow to develop, whereas there may be accelerated maturation of growth plates or evidence of bony proliferation. Erosions of bony articular surfaces may be a late finding. If the cervical spine is involved, fusion of C1-4 may occur, and atlantoaxial subluxation may be demonstrable.

DIFFERENTIAL DIAGNOSIS

The diagnosis of JIA is established by the presence of arthritis, the duration of the disease for at least 6 weeks, and exclusion of other possible diagnoses. Although a presumptive diagnosis of systemic JIA can be established for a child during the systemic

TABLE 89.3 Differential Diagnosis of Juvenile Arthritis
CONNECTIVE TISSUE DISEASES
Juvenile idiopathic arthritis
Systemic lupus erythematosus
Juvenile dermatomyositis
Scleroderma with arthritis
INFECTIOUS ARTHRITIS
Bacterial arthritis
Viral arthritis
Fungal arthritis
Lyme disease
REACTIVE ARTHRITIS
Poststreptococcal arthritis
Rheumatic fever
Toxic synovitis
Henoch-Schönlein purpura
Reiter syndrome
ORTHOPEDIC DISORDERS
Traumatic arthritis
Legg-Calve-Perthes disease
Slipped capital femoral epiphysis
Osteochondritis dissecans
Chondromalacia patellae
MUSCULOSKELETAL PAIN SYNDROMES
Growing pains
Hypermobility syndromes
Myofascial pain syndromes/fibromyalgia
Complex regional pain syndrome
HEMATOLOGICAL/ONCOLOGICAL DISORDERS
Leukemia
Lymphoma
Sickle cell disease
Thalassemia
Malignant and benign tumors of bone, cartilage, or synovium
Metastatic bone disease
Hemophilia
MISCELLANEOUS
Rickets/metabolic bone disease
Lysosomal storage diseases
Heritable disorders of collagen

phase, a definitive diagnosis is not possible until arthritis develops. Children must be younger than 16 years of age at the time of onset of the disease; the diagnosis of JIA does not change when the child becomes an adult. Because there are so many other causes of arthritis, these disorders need to be excluded before providing a definitive diagnosis of JIA (Table 89.3). The acute arthritides can affect the same joints as JIA but have a shorter time course.

TREATMENT

The treatment of JIA focuses on suppressing inflammation, preserving and maximizing function, preventing deformity, and preventing blindness. Nonsteroidal antiinflammatory drugs (NSAIDs) are the first choice in the treatment of JIA. Naproxen, sulindac, ibuprofen, indomethacin, and others have been used successfully. Systemic corticosteroid medications, such as prednisone and prednisolone, should be avoided in all but the most extreme circumstances, such as for severe systemic JIA with internal organ involvement or for significant active arthritis leading to the inability to ambulate. In this circumstance, the corticosteroids are used as **bridging therapy** until other medications take effect. For patients with a few isolated inflamed joints, intraarticular corticosteroids may be helpful.

Second-line medications, such as hydroxychloroquine and sulfasalazine, have been used in patients whose arthritis is not completely controlled with NSAIDs alone. **Methotrexate**, given either orally or subcutaneously, has become the drug of choice for polyarticular and systemic JIA, which may not respond to baseline agents alone. Methotrexate can cause bone marrow suppression and hepatotoxicity; regular monitoring can minimize these risks. Leflunomide, with a similar adverse effect profile to methotrexate, has also been used. Biologic agents that inhibit TNFα and block the inflammatory cascade, including **etanercept, infliximab**, and **adalimumab**, are effective in the treatment of JIA and may be superior to methotrexate in the spondyloarthropathy group. The risks of these agents are greater, however, and include serious infection and, possibly, increased risk of malignancy. **Anakinra**, an interleukin-1 receptor antagonist, is very beneficial in the treatment of the systemic features of systemic JIA.

COMPLICATIONS

Complications with JIA result primarily from the loss of function of an involved joint secondary to contractures, bony fusion, or loss of joint space. Physical and occupational therapies, professionally and through home programs, are crucial to preserve and maximize function. More serious complications stem from associated uveitis; if left untreated, it can lead to serious visual loss or blindness.

A very serious complication of sJIA, **macrophage activation syndrome** (MAS), has received increasing recognition. Occurring in more than 10% of sJIA patients, MAS can be seen in the context of overwhelming inflammation, which leads to activation of proliferation of T lymphocytes and macrophages, resulting in overwhelming release of proinflammatory cytokines. The patient develops high fevers, hepatosplenomegaly, neurological abnormalities, and bleeding diathesis. Laboratory studies reveal pancytopenia, profoundly elevated ferritin, transaminases, and triglycerides, as well as elevated soluble CD25. There is evidence of disseminated intravascular coagulation with low fibrinogen, increased D-dimer, and abnormal blood smear. Bone marrow sampling may identify mature macrophages displaying **hemophagocytic** activity. MAS can lead to multisystem organ failure. Even with early detection and aggressive treatment, mortality rates for MAS approximate 8%.

PROGNOSIS

The prognosis of JIA is excellent, with an overall 85% complete remission rate. Children with oligoarticular JIA uniformly tend to do well, whereas children with polyarticular disease and systemic disease constitute most children with functional disability. Systemic disease, a positive rheumatoid factor or anti-CCP antibody, poor response to therapy, and the presence of erosions on x-ray all connote a poorer prognosis. The importance of physical and occupational therapy cannot be overstated because when the disease remits, the physical limitations remain with the patient into adulthood.

CHAPTER 90

Systemic Lupus Erythematosus

ETIOLOGY

Systemic lupus erythematosus (SLE) is a multisystem disorder of unknown etiology characterized by a production of large amounts of **circulating autoantibodies**. This antibody production may be due to loss of T-lymphocyte control on B-lymphocyte activity, leading to hyperactivity of B lymphocytes, which leads to nonspecific and specific antibody and autoantibody production. These antibodies form immune complexes that become trapped in the microvasculature, leading to inflammation and ischemia.

EPIDEMIOLOGY

Although SLE affects primarily women ages 20-40, approximately 5% of cases present in childhood, mainly around puberty. SLE is rare in children younger than 9 years of age. Although there is a female predominance of this disease in adolescence and adulthood, there is an equal gender distribution in children. The overall prevalence of SLE in the pediatric population is 10-25 cases per 100,000 children.

CLINICAL MANIFESTATIONS

Patients with SLE can present either in an abrupt fashion with fulminant disease or in an indolent manner (Tables 90.1 and 90.2). Nonspecific symptoms are common but can be quite profound and may include significant fatigue and malaise, low-grade fever, and weight loss.

Skin disease can be a prominent finding, occurring in up to 95% of patients. A raised, erythematous rash on the cheeks, called a *malar butterfly rash*, is common (Fig. 90.1). This rash can also occur across the bridge of the nose, on the forehead, and on the chin. **Photosensitivity** can be problematic, particularly during the summer months. Both of these rashes improve with appropriate therapy. The rash of **discoid lupus**, by contrast, is an inflammatory process that leads to disruption of the dermal-epidermal junction, resulting in permanent scarring and loss of pigmentation in the affected area. If discoid lupus occurs in the scalp, permanent alopecia ensues because of loss of hair follicles. **Alopecia** and **Raynaud phenomenon** occurs, although not specific for SLE, and livedo reticularis also can occur.

Mouth and nasal sores resulting from mucosal ulceration are a common complaint in patients with SLE and can lead to ulceration and perforation of the nasal septum. Because of reticuloendothelial system stimulation, lymphadenopathy and splenomegaly are common findings in SLE. In particular, axillary lymphadenopathy can be a sensitive indicator of disease activity. Serositis can be seen, with chest pain and pleural or pericardial friction rubs or frank effusion.

Renal involvement is one of the most serious manifestations of SLE and is common in pediatric SLE, occurring in 50-70% of children. Renal disease may range from microscopic proteinuria or hematuria to gross hematuria, nephrotic syndrome, and renal failure. Hypertension or the presence of edema suggests lupus renal disease.

Arthralgias and arthritis are common. The arthritis is rarely deforming and typically involves the small joints of the hands; any joint may be involved. Myalgias or frank myositis, with muscle weakness and muscle fatigability, may occur. SLE can affect the central nervous system (CNS), leading to a myriad of symptoms ranging from poor school performance and difficulty concentrating, to seizures, psychosis, and stroke.

TABLE 90.1 American College of Rheumatology Criteria for Diagnosis of Systemic Lupus Erythematosus*

PHYSICAL SIGNS
Malar butterfly rash
Discoid lupus
Photosensitivity
Oral and nasopharyngeal ulcers
Nonerosive arthritis (more than two joints with effusion and tenderness)
Pleuritis or pericarditis (serositis)
Seizures or psychosis in absence of metabolic toxins or drugs
LABORATORY DATA
Renal disease (nephritis):
Proteinuria (>500 mg/24 hr) or
Cellular casts (RBC, granular, or tubular)
Hematological disease:
Hemolytic anemia with reticulocytosis or
Leukopenia (<4,000 on two occasions) or
Lymphopenia (<1,500 on two occasions) or
Thrombocytopenia (<100,000/mm^3)
SEROLOGICAL DATA
Positive anti-dsDNA or
Positive anti-Sm or
Evidence of presence of antiphospholipid antibodies
IgG or IgM anticardiolipin antibodies or
Lupus anticoagulant or
False-positive VDRL for >6 mo
Positive ANA in absence of drugs known to induce lupus

**These are the 1997 revised criteria for diagnosing systemic lupus erythematosus (SLE). A patient must have 4 of the 11 criteria to establish the diagnosis of SLE. These criteria may be present at the same or at different times during the patient's illness. Additional, less specific diagnostic manifestations are noted in Table 90.2.*

ANA, Antinuclear antibody; *RBC*, red blood cell; *VDRL*, Venereal Disease Research Laboratory.

TABLE 90.2 Additional Manifestations of Systemic Lupus Erythematosus
SYSTEMIC
Fever
Malaise
Weight loss
Fatigue
MUSCULOSKELETAL
Myositis, myalgia
Arthralgia
CUTANEOUS
Raynaud phenomenon
Alopecia
Urticaria-angioedema
Panniculitis
Livedo reticularis
NEUROPSYCHIATRIC
Personality disorders
Stroke
Peripheral neuropathy
Chorea
Transverse myelitis
Migraine headaches
Depression
CARDIOPULMONARY
Endocarditis
Myocarditis
Pneumonitis
OCULAR
Episcleritis
Sicca syndrome
Retinal cytoid bodies
GASTROINTESTINAL
Pancreatitis
Mesenteric arteritis
Serositis
Hepatomegaly
Hepatitis (chronic lupoid)
Splenomegaly
RENAL
Nephritis
Nephrosis
Uremia
Hypertension
REPRODUCTIVE
Repeat spontaneous abortions
Neonatal lupus erythematosus
Congenital heart block in fetus

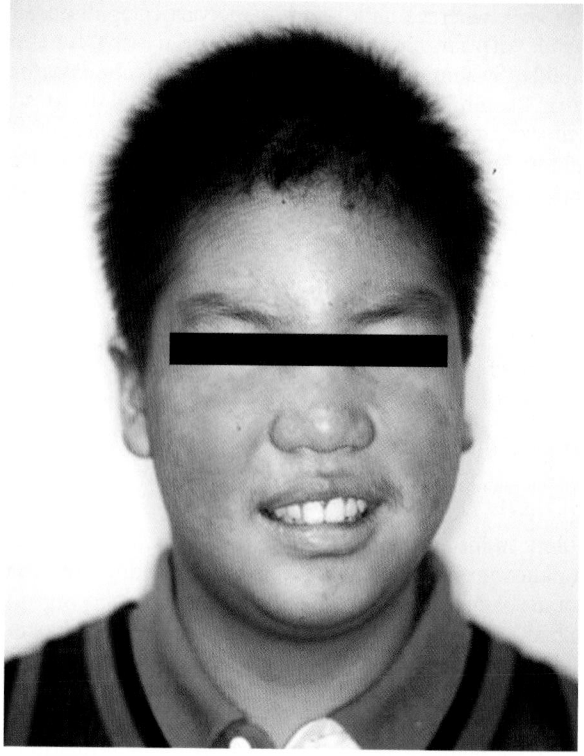

FIGURE 90.1 Malar butterfly rash on teenage boy with systemic lupus erythematosus. Note erythema on cheeks and chin, sparing the nasolabial folds.

LABORATORY AND IMAGING STUDIES

Testing for SLE is performed to establish the diagnosis, determine prognosis, and monitor response to therapy. Although nonspecific, a positive **antinuclear antibody** is found in more than 97% of patients with SLE, usually at high titers. Because of its high sensitivity, a negative antinuclear antibody has a high negative predictive value for SLE. The presence of **antibodies to double-stranded DNA** should raise suspicion for SLE because these antibodies are present in most patients with SLE and are found almost exclusively in the disease. Titers of anti-double-stranded DNA antibodies are quantifiable and vary with disease activity. Antibodies directed against Sm (Smith) are specific to SLE but are found in only approximately 30% of persons with SLE, limiting its clinical utility. Antibodies to Ro (SSA) and La (SSB) can also be found in patients with SLE, but they also occur in patients with Sjögren syndrome.

Likewise, patients with SLE can have antibodies directed against phospholipids, which also can be seen in other rheumatological diseases and in primary antiphospholipid syndrome. These antibodies lead to an increased risk of arterial and venous thrombosis and can be detected by the presence of anticardiolipin antibodies, a false-positive Venereal Disease Research Laboratory (VDRL) test, or a prolonged activated partial thromboplastin time.

Hematological abnormalities also are prevalent in patients with SLE. Leukopenia, primarily manifest as lymphopenia, is common. Thrombocytopenia and anemia of chronic disease may be found. Patients with SLE can develop a Coombs-positive autoimmune hemolytic anemia. Excessive antibody production can lead to polyclonal hypergammopathy, with an elevated globulin fraction in the serum. Excessive circulating antibodies and immune complexes also lead to the consumption of complement proteins, with low levels of C3 and C4 and decreased complement function as measured by CH50. Effective therapy returns the low complement levels to normal. This is one way to monitor therapy, except in patients with familial deficiency in complement components, which itself predisposes to SLE.

Urinalysis may show hematuria and proteinuria, identifying patients with lupus nephritis. Serum blood urea nitrogen and creatinine evaluate renal function. Hypoalbuminemia and hypoproteinemia may be present due to leakage at the glomerular level. Elevation of muscle enzymes may be a clue for the presence of myositis. Elevated cerebrospinal fluid (CSF) protein and an elevated IgG-to-albumin ratio when comparing CSF with serum (IgG index) can indicate antibody production in the CSF and help diagnose SLE affecting the CNS. CNS lupus has a specific pattern on gadolinium-enhanced magnetic resonance imaging.

DIFFERENTIAL DIAGNOSIS

Because SLE is a multisystem disease, it can be difficult to diagnose early in the disease course. Suspicion must be high in patients who present with diffuse symptoms, particularly adolescent girls. Many of the clinical manifestations of SLE are found in other inflammatory illnesses and during acute or chronic infection. Criteria have been developed for the diagnosis of SLE (see Table 90.1). The presence of 4 of 11 of these criteria has 98% sensitivity and 97% specificity for SLE.

TREATMENT

Corticosteroids have been the mainstay of treatment for SLE for decades. Initial use of pulse methylprednisolone and high-dose oral prednisone (up to 2 mg/kg) frequently is required, followed by cautious tapering to minimize recurrence of symptoms. Nonsteroidal antiinflammatory drugs have been used to treat the arthralgias and arthritis associated with SLE. Hydroxychloroquine is used not only for the treatment of lupus skin disease, such as discoid lupus, but as maintenance therapy. Hydroxychloroquine treatment results in longer periods of wellness between flares of disease as well as decreased numbers of flares.

Corticosteroids and hydroxychloroquine frequently are not sufficient therapies for lupus nephritis or cerebritis. Cyclophosphamide is effective for the worst forms of lupus nephritis, with significant improvements in outcome and decreased rates of progression to renal failure. Mycophenolate mofetil may also have a role in the treatment of lupus nephritis. CNS lupus responds to cyclophosphamide. For patients who are not able to tolerate the tapering of corticosteroids, the use of steroid-sparing agents, such as azathioprine, methotrexate, or mycophenolate mofetil, may be indicated.

Patients with SLE should be counseled to wear sun block and avoid sun exposure because exposure to the sun precipitates flares of the disease. Because of this prohibition, patients benefit from calcium and vitamin D supplementation to reduce the risk of osteoporosis that may result from prolonged corticosteroid use. Early treatment of hyperlipidemia to decrease long-term cardiovascular complications is also indicated.

COMPLICATIONS

Long-term complications include avascular bone necrosis secondary to corticosteroid use, infections, and myocardial infarction. Adult patients with SLE develop accelerated atherosclerosis, not only because of prolonged corticosteroid use but also due to the underlying disease. All patients with SLE should be counseled regarding their weight and maintaining an active lifestyle to reduce other cardiac risk factors.

PROGNOSIS

Outcomes for SLE have improved significantly over the past several decades and depend largely on the organ systems that are involved. Worse prognoses are seen in patients with severe lupus nephritis or cerebritis, with risk of chronic disability or progression to renal failure. With current therapy for the disease and the success of renal transplantation, however, most patients live well into adulthood.

CHAPTER 91

Juvenile Dermatomyositis

ETIOLOGY

The etiology of juvenile dermatomyositis (JDM) is unknown. It is characterized by the activation of T and B lymphocytes, leading to vasculitis affecting small vessels of skeletal muscle, with immune complex deposition and subsequent inflammation of blood vessels and muscle and inflammation of the skin. JDM may follow infections, allergic reactions, or sun exposure, but no causal relationship has been shown.

EPIDEMIOLOGY

JDM is a rare disease, with an incidence of less than 0.1 : 100,000 children. JDM can occur in all age groups with a peak incidence between 4 and 10 years. The disease is slightly more common in girls than boys.

CLINICAL MANIFESTATIONS

Dermatomyositis tends to present in a slow, progressive fashion, with insidious onset of fatigue, malaise, and progressive muscle weakness, accompanied by low-grade fevers and rash. Some children present in an acute fashion, however, with rapid onset of severe disease.

The muscle disease of JDM primarily affects the proximal muscles, particularly the hip and shoulder girdles, and the abdominal and neck muscles. Children have difficulty climbing steps, getting out of chairs, and getting off the floor. The patient may have a positive **Gower sign**. In severe cases, the patient is not able to sit up from a supine position or even lift the head off the examination table (see Chapter 182). If muscles of the upper airway and pharynx are involved, the patient's voice will sound nasal and the patient may have difficulty swallowing.

A classic **JDM rash** occurs on the face and across the cheeks but also can be found on the shoulders and back **(shawl sign)**. Patients may have **heliotrope discoloration** of the eyelids. Scaly, red plaques **(Gottron papules)** classically are found across the knuckles but can be found on the extensor surfaces of any joint. Patients may have periungual erythema and **dilated nailfold capillaries**. Less commonly, patients develop cutaneous vasculitis, with inflammation, erythema, and skin breakdown.

At some point, approximately 15% of patients with JDM develop arthritis that commonly affects small joints but may involve any joint. Raynaud phenomenon, hepatomegaly, and splenomegaly may also occur.

LABORATORY AND IMAGING STUDIES

Many patients with JDM have no evidence of systemic inflammation (normal blood count and erythrocyte sedimentation rate). Evidence of myositis can be identified in 98% of children with active JDM by elevated serum muscle enzymes, including aspartate aminotransferase, alanine aminotransferase, creatine phosphokinase, aldolase, and lactate dehydrogenase. Electromyography and muscle biopsy can document the myositis. Magnetic resonance imaging is a noninvasive means of showing muscle inflammation.

DIFFERENTIAL DIAGNOSIS

Diagnosis of JDM is based on the presence of documented muscle inflammation in the setting of classic rash (Table 91.1). A small percentage of children have muscle disease without skin manifestations, but polymyositis is sufficiently rare in children that they should have a muscle biopsy to exclude other causes of muscle weakness, such as muscular dystrophy (particularly in boys). The differential diagnosis also includes postinfectious myositis and other myopathies (see Chapter 182).

TREATMENT

Methotrexate, supplemented by short-term use of systemic corticosteroids, is the cornerstone of therapy for JDM. Initial treatment with pulse intravenous methylprednisolone is followed by several months of tapering doses of oral prednisone. Early institution of methotrexate significantly decreases the duration of corticosteroid use and its associated toxicities. Intravenous immunoglobulin is useful as adjunctive therapy. In severe or refractory cases, it may be necessary to use cyclosporine or cyclophosphamide. Hydroxychloroquine or dapsone has been used for the skin manifestations. These drugs do not significantly affect the muscle disease. Exposure to the sun worsens the cutaneous manifestations and exacerbates the muscle disease; sunlight may lead to flare. Patients should be advised to wear sun block and refrain from prolonged sun exposure. Accordingly supplementation with calcium and active forms of vitamin D is also indicated.

TABLE 91.1 Criteria for Diagnosis of Juvenile Dermatomyositis*
Rash typical of dermatomyositis
Symmetric proximal muscle weakness
Elevated muscle enzymes (ALT, AST, LDH, CPK, and aldolase)
EMG abnormalities typical of dermatomyositis (fasciculations, needle insertion irritability, and high-frequency discharges)
Positive muscle biopsy specimen with chronic inflammation

**To make a definitive diagnosis of dermatomyositis, four of five criteria are required.*

ALT, Alanine aminotransferase; *AST*, aspartate aminotransferase; *CPK*, creatine phosphokinase; *EMG*, electromyography; *LDH*, lactate dehydrogenase.

COMPLICATIONS

The most serious complication of JDM is the development of **calcinosis**. Dystrophic calcification can occur in the skin and soft tissues in any area of the body; it ranges from mild to extensive **(calcinosis universalis)**. Although it is difficult to predict who will develop calcinosis, it occurs more commonly in children with cutaneous vasculitis, prolonged disease activity, or delays in onset of therapy. Patients with JDM who develop vasculitis also are at risk for gastrointestinal perforation and gastrointestinal bleeding. JDM has been associated with lipoatrophy and insulin resistance, which can progress to type 2 diabetes. Control of insulin resistance frequently leads to improvement in muscle disease in these patients.

PROGNOSIS

The outcome of JDM depends greatly on the extent of muscle disease and the time between disease onset and initiation of therapy. JDM follows one of three clinical courses: a monophasic course, in which patients are treated and improve without significant sequelae; a chronic recurrent course; and a chronic progressive course marked by poor response to therapy and resulting loss of function. Patients who ultimately develop calcinosis are at risk for chronic loss of mobility, depending on the extent of calcium deposition. The association of dermatomyositis with malignancy seen in adults does not occur in children.

CHAPTER 92

Musculoskeletal Pain Syndromes

GROWING PAINS

Growing pains, or benign musculoskeletal pain syndrome, occur in 10-20% of school-age children. The peak age range is 3-7 years; the syndrome seems to be more common in boys than girls. There is no known etiology, although there seems to be a familial predisposition.

Children with growing pains complain of deep, crampy pain in the calves and thighs. It most typically occurs in the evening or as nocturnal pain that occasionally can awaken the child from sleep. Growing pains tend to be more common in children who are extremely active; bouts are exacerbated by increased physical activity. The physical examination is unremarkable, with no evidence of arthritis or muscular tenderness or weakness. Laboratory studies or x-rays, if performed, are normal.

The **diagnosis** of growing pains is based on a typical history and a normal physical examination. **Hypermobility** excludes the diagnosis. It is important to consider leukemia as a cause of nocturnal leg pain in children of this age group, so it is prudent to document a normal complete blood count.

The **treatment** of growing pains consists of reassurance and a regular bedtime ritual of stretching and relaxation. The pain can be relieved by massage. Some patients may benefit from a nighttime dose of acetaminophen or an analgesic dose of a nonsteroidal antiinflammatory drug (NSAID). Occasionally nocturnal awakening has been of long duration, leading to disruptive behavior patterns. In these cases, intervention must be aimed at decreasing the secondary gain associated with nighttime parental attention and should focus on sleep hygiene. Other than the negative behavioral patterns that can occur, there are no significant complications. Growing pains are not associated with other illnesses and resolve over time.

BENIGN HYPERMOBILITY

Hypermobility syndromes are disorders of unknown etiology that cause musculoskeletal pain secondary to excessive mobility of joints. These disorders most commonly present in children 3-10 years of age. Girls are more commonly affected than boys. There is a familial predisposition to hypermobility syndromes. Specific diseases causing hypermobility include Marfan syndrome, homocystinuria, Stickler syndrome, Ehlers-Danlos syndromes, osteogenesis imperfecta, Williams syndrome, and trisomy 21. Most children with hypermobility do not have an identifiable associated syndrome or disease.

Hypermobility can be isolated to a specific joint group or can present as a generalized disorder. Symptoms vary depending on the joints involved. The most consistent symptom is pain, which may occur during the day or night. The discomfort may increase after exertion but rarely interferes with regular physical activity. Children with hypermobility of the ankles or feet may complain of chronic leg or back pain.

Joint hypermobility may be quite marked. Range of motion may be exaggerated with excessive flexion or extension at the metacarpophalangeal joints, wrists, elbows, or knees (genu recurvatum; Fig. 92.1). There may be excessive pronation of the ankles. Hypermobility of the foot (flat foot; *pes planus*) is shown by the presence of a longitudinal arch of the foot that disappears with weight bearing and may be associated with a shortened Achilles tendon (see Chapter 200). These findings are rarely associated with tenderness on examination. No laboratory test abnormalities are apparent, and radiographs of affected joints are normal.

The diagnosis of isolated hypermobility is made on the basis of physical examination with demonstration of exaggerated mobility of a joint. Generalized hypermobility is diagnosed by the presence of sufficient criteria (Table 92.1) and the absence of evidence of other underlying disorders. Excessive skin elasticity, easy bruisability, or mitral valve prolapse suggests **Ehlers-Danlos syndrome** or **Marfan syndrome** rather than benign hypermobility.

The **treatment** of hypermobility consists of reassurance and regular stretching, similar to treatment for other benign musculoskeletal disorders. NSAIDs can be administered as needed but do not need to be prescribed on a regular basis. Arch supports can be helpful in children with symptomatic pes planus but are not indicated in the absence of symptoms. Benign hypermobility tends to improve with increasing age and is not associated with long-term complications.

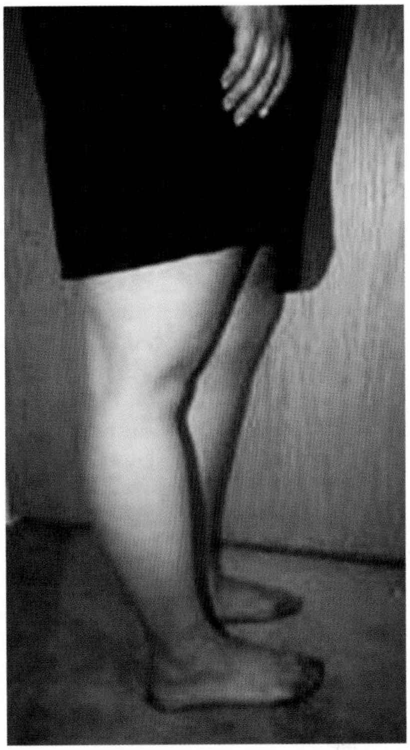

FIGURE 92.1 Hyperextension of the knees—an example of hypermobility.

TABLE 92.1 Criteria for Hypermobility

MODIFIED CRITERIA OF CARTER AND WILKINSON
Three of Five Are Required to Establish a Diagnosis of Hypermobility:
• Touch thumb to volar forearm • Hyperextend metacarpophalangeal joints so fingers parallel forearm • >10° hyperextension of elbows • >10° hyperextension of knees • Touch palms to floor with knees straight
Beighton Scale
• ≥6 points defines hypermobility: touch thumb to volar forearm (one point each for right and left) • Extend fifth metacarpophalangeal joint to 90° (one point each for right and left) • >10° hyperextension of elbow (one point each for right and left) • >10° hyperextension of knee (one point each for right and left) • Touch palms to floor with knees straight (one point)
Other Noncriteria Features of Many Children With Hypermobility:
• Put heel behind head • Excessive internal rotation to hip • Excessive ankle dorsiflexion • Excessive eversion of the foot • Passively touch elbows behind the back

Data from Carter C, Wilkins J. Persistent joint laxity and congenital dislocation of the hip. J Bone Joint Surg Br. *1964;46:40-45.*

MYOFASCIAL PAIN SYNDROMES AND FIBROMYALGIA

The myofascial pain syndromes are a group of noninflammatory disorders characterized by diffuse musculoskeletal pain, the presence of multiple **tender points**, fatigue, malaise, and poor sleep patterns. The etiology of these disorders is unknown, although there seems to be a familial predisposition. Although these disorders sometimes follow viral infection or trauma, no causal relationship has been shown. The myofascial pain syndromes are most common in adults but can occur in children (particularly >12 years of age). The syndromes are more common in girls than in boys. The prevalence of fibromyalgia in children has been reported to be 6%.

Patients with myofascial pain syndromes complain of long-standing diffuse pain in muscles and in the soft tissues around joints that can occur at any time of day, awaken the patient from sleep, and interfere with regular activities. There is frequently a high degree of school absenteeism, despite maintaining adequate school performance. A significant percentage of patients with myofascial pain syndromes exhibit symptoms consistent with depression. An increased incidence of sexual abuse has been reported in children presenting with fibromyalgia.

Physical examination is typically unremarkable with the exception of the presence of specific points that are painful—not just tender—to digital palpation. These points often are located on the neck, back, lateral epicondyles, greater trochanter, and knees. There is no evidence of arthritis or muscular weakness.

Patients with myofascial pain syndromes frequently undergo extensive medical testing because of the concern for underlying inflammatory disease. These tests are invariably normal. Children may have a false-positive antinuclear antibody, which is found in 20% of the normal pediatric population.

The **diagnosis** of myofascial pain syndrome is based on the presence of multiple tender points in the absence of other illness. To fulfill strict criteria for a diagnosis of fibromyalgia, the patient must have a history of diffuse pain for at least 3 months and the presence of multiple pain sites and an elevated symptom profile as measured by formal instruments. It is important to exclude underlying inflammatory diseases, such as systemic lupus erythematosus, or the postinfectious fatigue that characteristically follows Epstein-Barr virus and influenza virus infection. Mood and conversion disorders also should be considered.

Treatment consists of pain control, usually using NSAIDs, physical therapy, relaxation techniques, and education regarding sleep hygiene. Patients may require medications, such as amitriptyline to regulate sleep or gabapentin to reduce pain sensitivity. Education and reassurance are crucial. Because of the disability associated with myofascial pain syndromes, patients and parents frequently believe that the child has a serious underlying condition and may be resistant to reassurance. It should be emphasized that there is no simple cure, and time and perseverance are required.

The long-term outcomes in the myofascial pain syndromes vary. Patients and families who focus on therapy and are positive in their approach tend to have better outcomes. Patients who demand prolonged evaluations, especially from multiple health care providers, may do more poorly. Overall children with fibromyalgia and myofascial pain syndromes have better prognoses than their adult counterparts.

Suggested Readings

Barut K, Sahin S, Kasapcopur O. Pediatric vasculitis. *Curr Opin Rheumatol.* 2016;28(1):29–38.

Cattalini M, Khubchandani R, Cimaz R. When flexibility is not necessarily a virtue: a review of hypermobility syndromes and chronic or recurrent musculoskeletal pain in children. *Pediatr Rheumatol Online J.* 2015;13(1):40.

Couture J, Silverman ED. Update on the pathogenesis and treatment of childhood-onset systemic lupus erythematosus. *Curr Opin Rheumatol.* 2016;28(5):488–496.

Giancane G, Consolaro A, Lanni S, et al. Juvenile idiopathic arthritis: diagnosis and treatment. *Rheumatol Ther.* 2016;3(2):187–207.

Rider LG, Nistala K. The juvenile idiopathic inflammatory myopathies: pathogenesis, clinical and autoantibody phenotypes, and outcomes. *J Intern Med.* 2016;280(1):24–28.

Thakral A, Klein-Gitelman MS. An update of treatment and management of pediatric systemic lupus erythematosus. *Rheumatol Ther.* 2016;3(2):209–219.

Zhu FH, Ang JY. The clinical diagnosis and management of kawasaki disease: a review and update. *Curr Infect Dis Rep.* 2016;18(10):32.

PEARLS FOR PRACTITIONERS

CHAPTER 86

Rheumatic Assessment

- The hallmarks of rheumatic diseases of childhood are inflammation and autoimmunity, which may be localized or generalized.
- The differential diagnosis of rheumatological disease typically includes infections, postinfectious processes, and malignancy.
- The diagnosis of most rheumatological diseases can be made from the history and physical exam, in conjunction with carefully chosen confirmatory laboratory or radiological tests.
- Enthesitis is inflammation at the insertion of a ligament to a bone such as at the heel.
- Vasculitis often results in a petechial or purpuric rash.
- Morning stiffness may be seen in rheumatological disorders.
- Certain laboratory tests will reveal generalized inflammation, such as an elevated white blood cell or platelet count or an elevated ESR or CRP; they may also reveal the presence of an anemia of chronic disease. Other laboratory tests, such as those that measure autoantibodies, are used to detect only specific disorders.

CHAPTER 87

Henoch-Schönlein Purpura

- Henoch-Schönlein purpura (HSP) is a vasculitis of unknown etiology, which may be hypersensitivity in nature. The hallmark of HSP is nonthrombocytopenic palpable purpura, which predominantly occurs on the buttocks and lower extremities. Other features of HSP include arthritis, gastrointestinal, and renal involvement.
- The differential diagnosis includes other vasculitis syndromes, leukemia, and immune thrombocytopenic purpura.
- Treatment of HSP is largely supportive; nonsteroidal anti-inflammatory drugs (NSAIDs) are used for arthritis. In rare cases, such as gastrointestinal (GI) involvement or active nephritis, steroids are used.
- The prognosis of HSP is excellent. Most cases of HSP are uniphasic and resolve within 3-4 weeks, but the GI symptoms can recur as steroids are weaned, and the rash of HSP can recur for 12-15 months. In rare cases, patients can develop chronic renal disease.
- Immunoglobulin (Ig)A is often present in skin and renal lesions.

CHAPTER 88

Kawasaki Disease

- Kawasaki disease is a vasculitis that typically affects children under the age of seven and runs a triphasic course: acute, subacute, and convalescent. The acute phase, which lasts 1-2 weeks, is characterized by a high, hectic fever, followed by conjunctival erythema, mucosal changes, cervical lymphadenopathy, swelling of the hands and feet, and elevated inflammatory parameters. The subacute phase is noted by desquamation of the skin, reactive thrombocytosis, and development of coronary artery aneurysms. The convalescent phase, which occurs 6-8 weeks into the illness, is characterized by the resolution of symptoms and development of dystrophic nail changes.
- The diagnosis of Kawasaki disease is made based on the presence of fever for more than 5 days without an identifiable source and the presence of four of five other clinical criteria: bilateral nonsuppurative conjunctivitis, mucosal changes, extremity changes, polymorphous rash, and posterior cervical lymphadenopathy greater than 1.5 cm in diameter.
- The most serious complication of Kawasaki disease is coronary artery aneurysms. The main treatment of Kawasaki disease is intravenous Ig, which has been shown to reduce the incidence of coronary artery aneurysms from 20-25% to <5%.

CHAPTER 89

Juvenile Idiopathic Arthritis

- Juvenile idiopathic arthritis (JIA) is the most common rheumatological disease of childhood and is classified into subtypes including oligoarticular, polyarticular, systemic, juvenile psoriatic arthritis, and spondyloarthropathies.
- Chronic arthritis is characterized by gradual onset, morning stiffness and joint pain, swelling, erythema, and limitation of range of motion, either from pain or contracture. Due to the presence of active growth plates, patients also develop localized growth disturbance, which causes the ends of the surrounding bones to be longer and wider.
- Systemic JIA differs from the other subtypes of arthritis, as the presence of arthritis is preceded by a systemic inflammatory process characterized by high diurnal fever, rash, hepatosplenomegaly, and elevated inflammatory parameters.
- The treatment of JIA consists in controlling the inflammation and preserving joint function. Nonsteroidal antiinflammatory medications are considered first line of therapy, followed by methotrexate and then biologic agents. Steroids are used sparingly as bridge therapy and are not used for maintenance therapy. Prognosis of JIA overall is excellent with an overall 85% complete remission rate. Higher rates of remission are seen in the oligoarticular group and are lowest in the systemic and polyarticular groups.
- The most common complication of JIA is uveitis. The uveitis is frequently asymptomatic until the point of visual loss and therefore requires regular screening with a slit-lamp exam. All children with JIA are at increased risk for uveitis, but those with a positive antinuclear antibody are at even higher risk and need to be screened more often.
- The most severe complication of JIA is macrophage activation syndrome (MAS), which can occur in systemic JIA. MAS is caused by massive release of cytokines in the context of overwhelming inflammation leading to pancytopenia, liver dysfunction, disseminated intravascular coagulation, and multiorgan failure. Even with appropriate treatment, mortality rates from MAS are approximately 8%.

CHAPTER 90

Systemic Lupus Erythematosus

- Systemic lupus erythematosus is a multisystem disease characterized by large amounts of circulating antibodies, both nonspecific and specific autoantibodies, which form an immune complex that becomes trapped in the microvasculature, leading to inflammation and ischemia.
- The most serious features of systemic lupus erythematosus (SLE) are nephritis and central nervous system (CNS) involvement, which can lead to long-term morbidity. Other features include malar rash, discoid rash, photosensitivity, mucosal ulceration, arthritis, myositis, and hemolytic anemia. Because the features are nonspecific, diagnosis is made based on specific criteria, including the presence of specific autoantibodies such as antinuclear antibody and anti-double-stranded DNA antibody.
- Corticosteroids have been the mainstay of treatment for SLE. For more aggressive disease, such as renal or CNS disease, medications like cyclophosphamide may be used. In patients for which steroids cannot be reduced, steroid-sparing agents such as methotrexate, mycophenolate mofetil, or azathioprine may be used.
- Long-term outcomes in SLE have improved significantly and are determined primarily by the presence or absence of nephritis or neurological involvement, with most patients living well into adulthood.

CHAPTER 91

Juvenile Dermatomyositis

- Juvenile dermatomyositis (JDM) is a rare disease characterized by inflammation of muscles and skin, leading to stereotypical rashes. Patients have muscle weakness, particularly in proximal muscle groups, which can develop slowly or in a fulminant fashion. Involvement of muscles of the upper airway can lead to difficulty phonating or swallowing. The skin disease is characterized by a facial rash, heliotrope discoloration of the eyelids, and scaly red patches on extensor surfaces (Gottron papules). Patients can also develop arthritis.
- Diagnosis of JDM is made by the presence of classic rash and myositis, as evidenced by elevated muscle enzymes, muscle biopsy, or abnormal electromyography (EMG) or magnetic resonance imaging (MRI).
- Treatment of JDM consists of an initial course of corticosteroids and a longer course of a steroid-sparing agent—most commonly methotrexate.
- Prognosis in JDM depends greatly on the extent of muscle disease and the time between disease onset and initiation of therapy. Most patients have excellent outcomes, although a small percentage will have a chronic, progressive disease course.
- The most common complication of JDM is calcinosis. Dystrophic calcification can occur in the skin and soft tissues and can range from mild to extensive. Treatments for calcinosis have been largely ineffective.

CHAPTER 92

Musculoskeletal Pain Syndromes

- Growing pains are very common in the pediatric age group, affecting 10-20% of school-age children. Children complain of deep achy pain in their legs, particularly at night, but have no evidence of underlying disease. Treatment is symptomatic, but other causes of nocturnal leg pain, particularly leukemia, must be excluded first.
- Hypermobility syndromes can be either generalized, as seen in benign hypermobility or Ehlers-Danlos syndrome, or localized, such as in pes planus (flat feet). Beighton criteria are used to diagnose generalized hypermobility. Treatment is symptomatic and focused on stretching, joint protection, arch supports when appropriate, and NSAID therapy as needed.
- Myofascial pain syndromes, such as fibromyalgia, are characterized by diffuse musculoskeletal pain, tender points, and generalized malaise, fatigue, and poor sleep patterns. These syndromes are noninflammatory, and an underlying cause for the pain cannot be found. Comorbid depression is not uncommon.
- The treatment of myofascial pain syndrome consists of pain control (usually using NSAIDs), physical therapy, relaxation techniques, and education regarding sleep hygiene. Long-term outcomes vary.

SECTION **16**

INFECTIOUS DISEASES

Matthew P. Kronman | Claudia S. Crowell | Surabhi B. Vora

CHAPTER **93**

Infectious Disease Assessment

Overlapping clinical symptoms caused by infectious and noninfectious illnesses make the diagnosis of some diseases difficult. Clinicians are concerned that an untreated minor infection may progress to a life-threatening illness, if appropriate treatment is not given. However, unnecessary treatment with antimicrobial agents may lead to emergence of antimicrobial-resistant organisms, in addition to antibiotic-associated diarrhea or allergic reactions. Therefore accurate diagnosis of infectious and noninfectious diseases is critical to ensure the provision of specific treatment only as indicated, and thereby reduce the unnecessary use of antibiotics.

A thorough patient assessment, including a detailed history, complete physical examination, and appropriate diagnostic testing, is the cornerstone of optimal care.

INITIAL DIAGNOSTIC EVALUATION

The ability to diagnose specific infections accurately begins with an understanding of the epidemiology; risk factors, including exposures to sick contacts or environmental risks (e.g., travel, zoonoses); and infection susceptibility related either to age (reflecting the maturity of the immune system) or to primary or secondary immunodeficiencies. Obtaining a thorough history and physical examination identifies most of these elements (Tables 93.1 and 93.2) and guides the appropriate use of other diagnostic tests.

Unique questions that help identify whether an infection is causing the patient's symptoms include a detailed environmental history (including sick contacts, travel, food, water, and animal exposure; see Table 93.1). Certain infections are more common in specific geographic areas. For instance, parasitic infections are more common in tropical climates. Certain fungal infections have specific geographic distribution (coccidioidomycosis in the southwestern United States, blastomycosis in the upper Midwest, and histoplasmosis in central United States). In other areas, fungal pneumonias are rare except in immunocompromised persons.

An immunization history is critical for determining susceptibility to vaccine preventable diseases. Family history, especially that of unexpected deaths of male infants, may suggest familial immunodeficiency (see Chapters 73 through 76). Localization of symptoms to a specific body site may narrow diagnostic possibilities (see Table 93.2).

A complete physical examination is essential to identify signs of infection, which may be systemic (e.g., fever and shock) or focal (e.g., swelling, erythema, tenderness, and limitation of function). Many infectious diseases are associated with characteristic cutaneous signs (see Table 97.1). Accurate otolaryngological examination is critical for diagnosing upper respiratory tract infections and otitis media, the most common childhood infectious diseases in the United States.

DIFFERENTIAL DIAGNOSIS

Decision-Making Algorithms
Available @ StudentConsult.com

Fever and Rash
Fever Without a Source
Fever of Unknown Origin

Fever does not always represent infection. Rheumatological diseases, inflammatory bowel disease, Kawasaki disease, poisoning, periodic fever syndromes, and malignancy also may present with fever. Particularly, children with overwhelming infection may be afebrile or hypothermic. Common symptoms, such as bone pain or lymphadenopathy that suggest infection, may also be due to leukemia, lymphoma, juvenile idiopathic arthritis, or Kawasaki disease (see Chapters 88, 89, and 153). Acute mental status changes or focal neurological impairment could be manifestations of infections (encephalitis, meningitis, or brain abscess) or noninfectious causes (brain or spinal tumors, inflammatory conditions, postinfectious sequelae, or impairment from toxic ingestions or inhalants). Many manifestations of mucosal allergy (rhinitis, diarrhea) may mimic common infectious diseases (see Chapter 77).

Some infections are prone to recurrence, especially if treatment is suboptimal (inadequate antimicrobial or insufficient duration). Recurrent, severe, or unusual (opportunistic) infections suggest the possibility of immunodeficiency (see Chapters 72 and 125).

SCREENING TESTS

Laboratory diagnosis of infection includes examination of bacterial morphology using Gram stain, various culture techniques, molecular microbiologic methods (e.g., polymerase chain reaction or matrix-assisted laser desorption/ionization time of flight), and assessment of the immune response with

TABLE 93.1 Clues From the History for Risk of Infection
Season of year
Age
General health
Weight change
Fever—presence, duration, and pattern
Previous similar symptoms
Previous infections and other illnesses
Previous surgeries, dental procedures
Preceding trauma
Presence of outbreaks or epidemics in the community
Exposures to infected individuals
Exposures to farm or feral animals and pets
Exposures to ticks and mosquitoes
Sexual history, including possibility of sexual abuse
Illicit drug use
Transfusion of blood or blood products
Travel history
Daycare or school attendance
Sources of water and food (e.g., undercooked meat, unpasteurized dairy products)
Home sanitary facilities and hygiene
Pica
Exposure to soil-borne and waterborne organisms (e.g., swimming in brackish water)
Presence of foreign bodies (e.g., indwelling catheters, shunt, grafts)
Immunization history
Immunodeficiency (chemotherapy, acquired, congenital)
Current medications

antibody titers or skin testing. The **acute phase response** is a nonspecific metabolic and inflammatory response to infection, trauma, autoimmune disease, and some malignancies. **Acute phase reactants**, such as erythrocyte sedimentation rate, C-reactive protein, and procalcitonin, are commonly elevated during an infection but are not specific for infection and do not identify any specific infection. These tests can be used to monitor response to therapy.

A **complete blood count** is frequently obtained for evidence of infection. The initial response to infection, especially in children, is usually a **leukocytosis** (increased number of circulating leukocytes) with an initial neutrophilic response to both bacterial and viral infections. With most viral infections, this response is transient and is followed quickly by a characteristic mononuclear response. In general, bacterial infections are associated with greater neutrophil counts than viral infections (Table 93.3). A **left-shift** is an increase in the numbers of circulating immature cells of the neutrophil series, including band forms, metamyelocytes, and myelocytes. It indicates the rapid release of cells from the bone marrow and is characteristic of both the early stages of infection and, if sustained, bacterial infections. Transient lymphopenia at the beginning of illness and lasting 24-48 hours has been described with many viral infections. **Atypical lymphocytes** are mature T lymphocytes with larger, eccentrically placed, and indented nuclei classically seen with infectious mononucleosis caused by Epstein-Barr virus. Other infections associated with atypical lymphocytosis include cytomegalovirus infection, toxoplasmosis, viral hepatitis, rubella, roseola, mumps, and some drug reactions. **Eosinophilia** is characteristic of allergic diseases but may be seen with tissue-invasive multicellular parasites, such as the migration of the larval stages of parasites through skin, connective tissue, and viscera. High-grade eosinophilia (>30% eosinophils, or a total eosinophil count >3,000/μL) frequently occurs during the muscle invasion phase of trichinellosis, the pulmonary phases of ascariasis and hookworm infection (eosinophilic pneumonia), and the hepatic and central nervous system phases of visceral larva migrans.

Other common screening tests include **urinalysis** for urinary tract infections, transaminases for liver inflammation, and **lumbar puncture** for evaluation of the cerebrospinal fluid if there is concern for meningitis or encephalitis (see Chapters 100 and 101). Various tests may help distinguish viral versus bacterial infection, but definitive diagnosis requires identifying the agent by culture or molecular means.

Cultures are the mainstay of diagnosis of many infections. **Blood cultures** are sensitive and specific for bacteremia, which may be primary or secondary to a focal infection (osteomyelitis, gastroenteritis, pyelonephritis, and endocarditis). Urine cultures are important to confirm urinary tract infection, which may be occult in young infants. Cultures should be obtained with every lumbar puncture, aspiration, or biopsy of other fluid collections or masses. Specific types of cultures (bacterial, fungal, viral, or mycobacterial) are guided by the clinical problem. Tissue culture techniques are used to identify viruses and intracellular bacterial pathogens.

Antibiotics often are begun before a definitive diagnosis is established, complicating the ability to rely on subsequent cultures for microbiologic diagnosis (see Chapter 95). Although persistent or progressive symptoms, despite antibiotic treatment, may indicate the need to change the regimen, more frequently this indicates the need to stop all antibiotics to facilitate definitive diagnosis by obtaining appropriate cultures. Antibiotics should not be given before obtaining appropriate cultures unless there is a life-threatening situation (e.g., septic shock).

Rapid tests, such as antigen tests, are useful for preliminary diagnosis and are available for numerous bacterial, viral, fungal, and parasitic infections. **Serological tests,** using enzyme-linked immunosorbent assay or Western blotting, showing an immunoglobulin (Ig)M response, high IgG titer, or seroconversion between acute and convalescent sera, also can be used for diagnosis. **Molecular tests,** such as **polymerase chain reaction** (nucleic acid amplification tests) for DNA or RNA, offer the specificity of culture, high sensitivity, and rapid results. When an unusual infection is suspected, a microbiologist should be consulted before samples are obtained.

DIAGNOSTIC IMAGING

The choice of diagnostic imaging modality should be based on the location of the findings and the differential diagnosis. In the absence of localizing signs, and during an acute infection, imaging of the entire body is less productive. **Plain x-rays** are useful initial tests for respiratory tract infections.

TABLE 93.2 Localizing Manifestations of Infection

SITE	LOCALIZING SYMPTOMS	LOCALIZING SIGNS*
Eye	Eye pain, double vision, photophobia, conjunctival discharge	Periorbital erythema, periorbital edema, drainage, chemosis, limitation of extraocular movements
Ear	Ear pain, drainage	Red, bulging tympanic membrane, drainage from ear canal
Upper respiratory tract	Rhinorrhea, sore throat, cough, drooling, stridor, trismus, sinus pain, tooth pain, hoarse voice	Nasal congestion, pharyngeal erythema, enlarged tonsils with exudate, swollen red epiglottis, regional lymphadenopathy
Lower respiratory tract	Cough, chest pain, dyspnea, sputum production, cyanosis	Tachypnea, crackles, wheezing, localized diminished breath sounds, intercostal retractions
Gastrointestinal tract	Nausea, vomiting, diarrhea, abdominal pain (focal or diffuse), anorexia, weight loss	Hypoactive or hyperactive bowel sounds, abdominal tenderness (focal or generalized), hematochezia
Liver	Anorexia, vomiting, dark urine, light stools	Jaundice, hepatomegaly, hepatic tenderness, bleeding diatheses, coma
Genitourinary tract	Dysuria, frequency, urgency, flank or suprapubic pain, vaginal discharge	Costovertebral angle or suprapubic tenderness, cervical motion and adnexal tenderness
Central nervous system	Lethargy, irritability, headache, neck stiffness, seizures	Nuchal rigidity, Kernig sign, Brudzinski sign, bulging fontanelle, focal neurological deficits, altered mental status, coma
Cardiovascular	Dyspnea, palpitations, fatigue, exercise intolerance, chest pain	Tachycardia, hypotension, cardiomegaly, hepatomegaly, splenomegaly, crackles, petechiae, Osler nodes, Janeway lesions, Roth spots, new or change in murmur, distended neck veins, pericardial friction rub, muffled heart sounds
Musculoskeletal	Limp, bone pain, limited function (pseudoparalysis)	Local swelling, erythema, warmth, limited range of motion, point bone tenderness, joint line tenderness

**Fever usually accompanies infection as a systemic manifestation.*

TABLE 93.3 Differentiating Viral From Bacterial Infections

VARIABLE	VIRAL	BACTERIAL
Petechiae	Present	Present
Purpura	Rare	If severe
Leukocytosis	Uncommon*	Common
Left-shift (↑ bands)	Uncommon	Common
Neutropenia	Possible	Suggests overwhelming infection
↑ ESR	Unusual*	Common
↑ CRP	Unusual	Common
↑ TNF, IL-1, PAF	Uncommon	Common
Meningitis (pleocytosis)	Lymphocytic†	Neutrophilic
Meningeal signs positive‡	Present	Present

**Adenovirus and herpes simplex may cause leukocytosis and increased ESR; Epstein-Barr virus may cause petechiae and increased ESR.*
†Early viral (enterovirus, arbovirus) meningitis initially may have a neutrophilic pleocytosis.
‡Nuchal rigidity, bulging fontanelle, Kernig sign, Brudzinski sign.
CRP, C-reactive protein; *ESR*, erythrocyte sedimentation rate; *IL*, interleukin; *PAF*, platelet-activating factor; *TNF*, tumor necrosis factor.

Ultrasonography is a noninvasive, nonirradiating technique well suited to infants and children for imaging solid organs. It also is useful to identify soft tissue abscesses with lymphadenitis and to diagnose suppurative arthritis of the hip. **Computed tomography (CT; with contrast enhancement)** and **magnetic resonance imaging (MRI; with gadolinium enhancement)** allow characterization of lesions and precise anatomical localization and are the modalities of choice for the brain. CT shows greater bone detail, and MRI shows greater tissue detail. MRI is especially useful for diagnosis of osteomyelitis, myositis, and necrotizing fasciitis. High-resolution CT is useful for complicated chest infections. Judicious use of CT scans is important because of the long-term effects of radiation on children's health. Contrast studies (upper gastrointestinal series, barium enema) are used to identify mucosal lesions of the gastrointestinal tract, whereas CT or MRI is preferred for evaluation of appendicitis and intraabdominal masses. A voiding cystourethrogram may be used to evaluate for vesicoureteral reflux, a predisposing factor for upper urinary tract infections. **Radionuclide scans,** such as technetium-99m for osteomyelitis and dimercaptosuccinic acid for acute pyelonephritis, are often informative.

CHAPTER 94

Immunization and Prophylaxis

IMMUNIZATION

Childhood immunization has markedly reduced the impact of major infectious diseases. **Active immunization** induces immunity through the administration of all or part of a microorganism or a modified product of a microorganism (e.g., toxoid). **Passive immunization** involves administration of protective antibodies and includes transplacental transfer of maternal antibodies and the administration of preformed antibody, either as immunoglobulin or as monoclonal antibody.

Vaccinations may be with live-attenuated viruses (measles, mumps, rubella [MMR], varicella, nasal influenza, oral polio), inactivated or killed viruses (intramuscular polio, hepatitis A, intramuscular influenza), recombinant products (hepatitis B, human papillomavirus), live reassortants (rotavirus), or immunogenic components of bacteria (pertussis, *Haemophilus influenzae* type b, *Neisseria meningitidis*, and *Streptococcus pneumoniae*), including toxoids (diphtheria, tetanus). Many purified polysaccharides are T-cell independent antigens that initiate B-cell proliferation without involvement of CD4 T lymphocytes and are poor immunogens in children younger than 2 years of age. Conjugation of a polysaccharide to a **protein carrier** induces a T-cell dependent response in infants and creates immunogenic vaccines for *H. influenzae* type b, *S. pneumoniae*, and *N. meningitidis*.

Childhood immunization standards and recommendations in the United States (Figs. 94.1 and 94.2) are formulated by the Advisory Committee on Immunization Practices of the Centers for Disease Control and Prevention (ACIP), the American Academy of Pediatrics, and the American Academy of Family Physicians. In the United States, due to state laws requiring immunization for school entry, approximately 95% of children entering kindergarten are vaccinated for the common infectious diseases. The ACIP recommends that children in the United States routinely receive vaccines against 16 diseases (see Fig. 94.1). This schedule includes up to 23 injections in four to five visits by 18 months of age. Children who are at increased risk for pneumococcal infections should receive the pneumococcal polysaccharide vaccine as well. Infants and children who are at increased risk for meningococcal infections should receive the two- or four-dose meningococcal series depending on age. Children who are behind in immunization should receive catch-up immunizations as rapidly as feasible. Infants born prematurely, regardless of birth weight, should be vaccinated at the same chronological age and according to the same schedule as full-term infants and children (see Fig. 94.2). The single exception to this practice is providing hepatitis B vaccine at 1 month of age instead of at birth for infants weighing less than 2,000 g if the mother is hepatitis B virus surface antigen (HB_sAg)-negative. Vaccines for adolescents should be given at

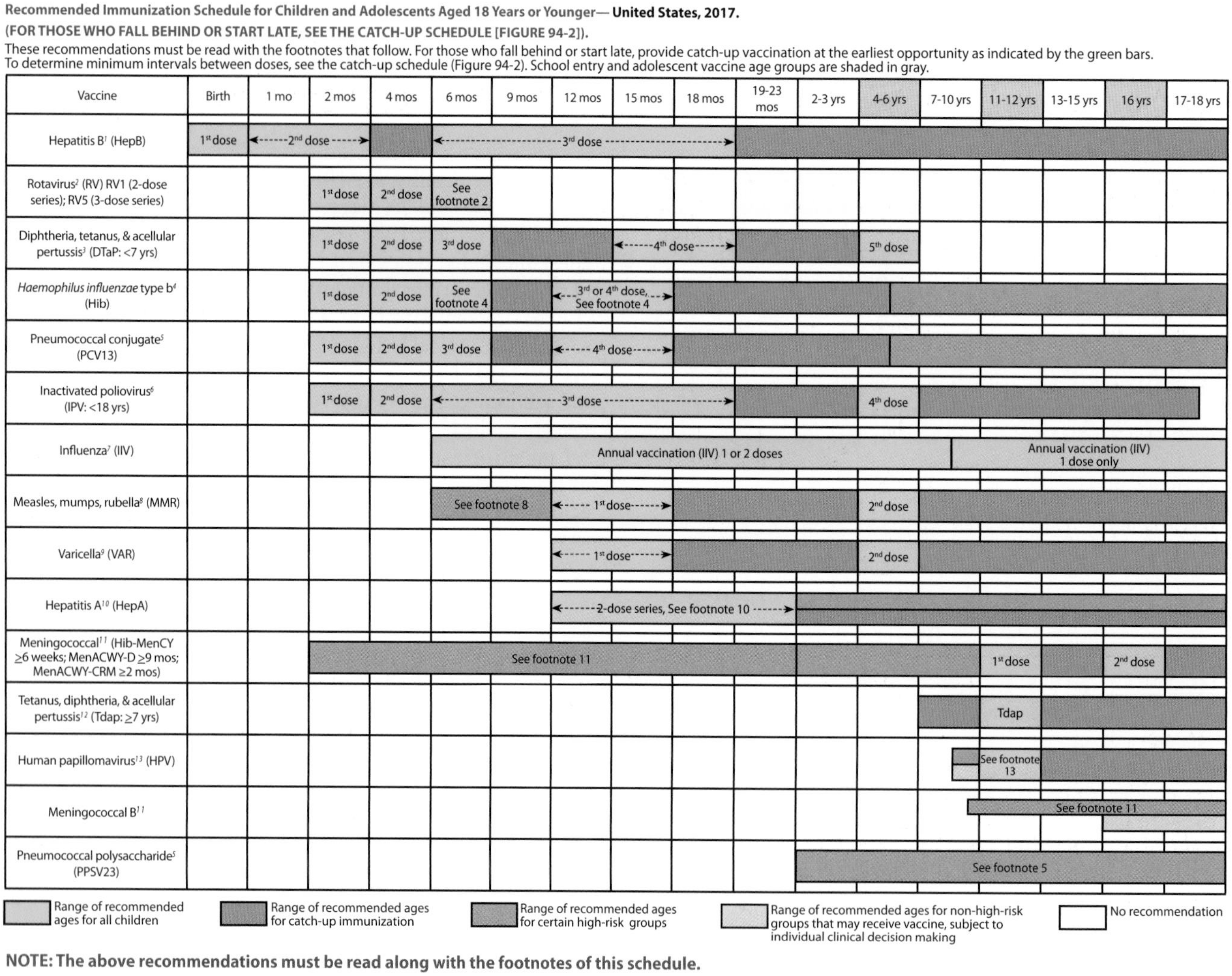

FIGURE 94.1 Recommended immunization schedules for persons aged 0 through 18 years—United States, 2017. (Approved by the Advisory Committee on Immunization Practices; American Academy of Pediatrics; American Academy of Family Physicians; and American College of Obstetricians and Gynecologists; Courtesy of the U.S. Department of Health and Human Services, Centers for Disease Control and Prevention, http://www.cdc.gov/vaccines/schedules/hcp/child-adolescent.html.)

Catch-up immunization schedule for persons aged 4 months through 18 years who start late or who are more than 1 month behind—United States, 2017.
The figure below provides catch-up schedules and minimum intervals between doses for children whose vaccinations have been delayed. A vaccine series does not need to be restarted, regardless of the time that has elapsed between doses. Use the section appropriate for the child's age. Always use this table in conjunction with Figure 94-1 and the footnotes that follow Figure 94-1.

Vaccine	Minimum Age for Dose 1	Minimum Interval Between Doses			
		Dose 1 to Dose 2	Dose 2 to Dose 3	Dose 3 to Dose 4	Dose 4 to Dose 5
Children age 4 months through 6 years					
Hepatitis B[1]	Birth	4 weeks	8 weeks *and* at least 16 weeks after first dose. Minimum age for the final dose is 24 weeks.		
Rotavirus[2]	6 weeks	4 weeks	4 weeks[2]		
Diphtheria, tetanus, and acellular pertussis[3]	6 weeks	4 weeks	4 weeks	6 months	6 months[3]
Haemophilus influenzae type b[4]	6 weeks	4 weeks if first dose was administered before the 1st birthday. 8 weeks (as final dose) if first dose was administered at age 12 through 14 months. No further doses needed if first dose was administered at age 15 months or older.	4 weeks[4] if current age is younger than 12 months **and** first dose was administered at younger than age 7 months, **and** at least 1 previous dose was PRP-T (ActHib, Pentacel, Hiberix) or unknown. 8 weeks *and* age 12 through 59 months (as final dose)[4] • if current age is younger than 12 months **and** first dose was administered at age 7 through 11 months; OR • if current age is 12 through 59 months **and** first dose was administered before the 1st birthday, **and** second dose administered at younger than 15 months; OR • if both doses were PRP-OMP (PedvaxHIB; Comvax) **and** were administered before the 1st birthday. No further doses needed if previous dose was administered at age 15 months or older.	8 weeks (as final dose) This dose only necessary for children age 12 through 59 months who received 3 doses before the 1st birthday.	
Pneumococcal[5]	6 weeks	4 weeks if first dose administered before the 1st birthday. 8 weeks (as final dose for healthy children) if first dose was administered at the 1st birthday or after. No further doses needed for healthy children if first dose was administered at age 24 months or older.	4 weeks if current age is younger than 12 months and previous dose given at <7 months old. 8 weeks (as final dose for healthy children) if previous dose given between 7-11 months (wait until at least 12 months old); OR if current age is 12 months or older and at least 1 dose was given before age 12 months. No further doses needed for healthy children if previous dose administered at age 24 months or older.	8 weeks (as final dose) This dose only necessary for children aged 12 through 59 months who received 3 doses before age 12 months or for children at high risk who received 3 doses at any age.	
Inactivated poliovirus[6]	6 weeks	4 weeks[6]	4 weeks[6]	6 months[6] (minimum age 4 years for final dose).	
Measles, mumps, rubella[8]	12 months	4 weeks			
Varicella[9]	12 months	3 months			
Hepatitis A[10]	12 months	6 months			
Meningococcal[11] (Hib-MenCY ≥6 weeks; MenACWY-D ≥9 mos; MenACWY-CRM ≥2 mos)	6 weeks	8 weeks[11]	See footnote 11	See footnote 11	
Children and adolescents age 7 through 18 years					
Meningococcal[11] (MenACWY-D ≥9 mos; MenACWY-CRM ≥2 mos)	Not Applicable (N/A)	8 weeks[11]			
Tetanus, diphtheria; tetanus, diphtheria, and acellular pertussis[12]	7 years[12]	4 weeks	4 weeks if first dose of DTaP/DT was administered before the 1st birthday. 6 months (as final dose) if first dose of DTaP/DT or Tdap/Td was administered at or after the 1st birthday.	6 months if first dose of DTaP/DT was administered before the 1st birthday.	
Human papillomavirus[13]	9 years	Routine dosing intervals are recommended.[13]			
Hepatitis A[10]	N/A	6 months			
Hepatitis B[1]	N/A	4 weeks	8 weeks **and** at least 16 weeks after first dose.		
Inactivated poliovirus[6]	N/A	4 weeks	4 weeks[6]	6 months[6]	
Measles, mumps, rubella[8]	N/A	4 weeks			
Varicella[9]	N/A	3 months if younger than age 13 years. 4 weeks if age 13 years or older.			

NOTE: The above recommendations must be read along with the footnotes of this schedule that follow Figure 94-1.

FIGURE 94.2 Catch-up immunization schedule for persons aged 4 months through 18 years who start late or who are more than 1 month behind—United States, 2017. This figure provides catch-up schedules and minimum intervals between doses for children whose vaccinations have been delayed. A vaccine series does not need to be restarted, regardless of the time that has elapsed between doses. Use the section appropriate for the child's age. Always use this table in conjunction with the Recommended Immunization Schedule for 2016 and the footnotes that follow. (Approved by the Advisory Committee on Immunization Practices; American Academy of Pediatrics; American Academy of Family Physicians; and American College of Obstetricians and Gynecologists; Courtesy of the U.S. Department of Health and Human Services, Centers for Disease Control and Prevention, http://www.cdc.gov/vaccines/schedules/hcp/child-adolescent.html.)

11-12 years of age (see Fig. 94.1), with completion of any vaccine series at 13-18 years of age and a booster for *N. meningitidis* at 16 years of age.

Vaccines should be administered after obtaining informed consent. The **National Childhood Vaccine Injury Act** requires that all health care providers provide parents or patients with copies of **Vaccine Information Statements** prepared by the Centers for Disease Control and Prevention (http://www.cdc.gov/vaccines/hcp/vis/index.html) before administering each vaccine dose.

Most vaccines are administered by intramuscular or subcutaneous injection. The preferred sites for administration are the anterolateral aspect of the thigh in infants and the deltoid region in children and adults. Multiple vaccines can be administered simultaneously at anatomically separate sites (different limbs, or separated by >1 in) without diminishing the immune response. MMR and varicella vaccines should be administered simultaneously or more than 28 days apart. The conjugate and polysaccharide pneumococcal vaccines should be spaced at least 8 weeks apart when both are indicated, and the conjugate vaccine should be administered first, if possible. Tuberculosis testing, either with a skin test or gamma interferon release blood test, can be performed at the time of vaccination. If tuberculosis testing is not performed at the same visit as MMR vaccination, then testing should be delayed for 6 weeks as MMR vaccination can temporarily suppress response to tuberculin antigens. Administration of blood products and immunoglobulin can diminish response to live-virus vaccines administered before the recommended interval.

General contraindications to vaccination include serious allergic reaction (anaphylaxis) after a previous vaccine dose or to a vaccine component, immunocompromised states, or pregnancy (live-virus vaccines), and moderate or severe acute illness with or without fever. History of *anaphylactic-like* reactions to eggs has historically been a contraindication to influenza and yellow fever vaccines, which are produced in embryonated chicken eggs; however, in 2016 the ACIP recommended that even persons with severe egg allergy could receive any licensed influenza vaccine. Current preparations of measles and mumps vaccines, which are produced in chick embryo fibroblast tissue culture, do not contain significant amounts of egg proteins and may be administered without testing children with history of egg allergy. Mild acute illness with or without fever, convalescent phase of illness, recent exposure to infectious diseases, current antimicrobial therapy, breast feeding, mild to moderate local reaction or low-grade to moderate fever after previous vaccination, and a history of penicillin or other nonvaccine allergy or receiving allergen extract immunotherapy are **not contraindications** to immunization.

Severe immunosuppression resulting from congenital immunodeficiency, human immunodeficiency virus (HIV) infection, leukemia, lymphoma, cancer therapy, or a prolonged course of high-dose corticosteroids (≥2 mg/kg/day for >2 weeks) predisposes to complications and is a contraindication for live-virus vaccines. For HIV-infected children who do not have evidence of severe immunosuppression, MMR vaccination is recommended at 12 months and 4-6 years of age. Varicella vaccine is contraindicated for persons with cellular immunodeficiency but is recommended for persons with impaired humoral immunity (hypogammaglobulinemia or dysgammaglobulinemia) and at 12 months of age for HIV-infected children without evidence of severe immunosuppression, given as two doses 3 months apart.

The National Childhood Vaccine Injury Act requires that clinically significant adverse events after vaccination be reported to the **Vaccine Adverse Event Reporting System (VAERS)** (http://www.vaers.hhs.gov or (800) 822-7967). Suspected cases of vaccine-preventable diseases should be reported to state or local health departments. The act also established the **National Vaccine Injury Compensation Program,** a no-fault system in which persons thought to have suffered an injury or death as a result of administration of a covered vaccine can seek compensation.

PROPHYLAXIS

Prophylaxis may include antibiotics, immunoglobulin or monoclonal antibody, and vaccine, alone or in combination. They may be used preexposure, for perinatal exposure, and postexposure for persons at increased risk for infection. **Primary prophylaxis** is used to prevent infection before a first occurrence. **Secondary prophylaxis** is used to prevent recurrence after a first episode.

Meningococcus

Primary prophylaxis to all close contacts of index cases of *N. meningitidis* infection should be administered as soon as possible (see Chapter 100). Prophylaxis is recommended for all household contacts, especially young children; child care or preschool contacts in the 7 days before illness onset; contacts with direct exposure to the index patient's secretions through kissing, sharing of toothbrushes or eating utensils in the 7 days before illness onset; and for mouth-to-mouth resuscitation or unprotected contact during endotracheal intubation within 7 days before illness onset. Prophylaxis is also recommended for contacts who frequently sleep or eat in the same dwelling as the index patient or passengers seated directly next to the index case during airline flights lasting longer than 8 hours. Chemoprophylaxis is not recommended for casual contacts with no history of direct exposure to the patient's oral secretions (school or work), indirect contact with the index patient, or medical personnel without direct exposure to the patient's oral secretions. Rifampin twice daily for 2 days, ceftriaxone once, and ciprofloxacin once (≥1 month of age) are the recommended regimens. Azithromycin may be used in the case of resistant organisms.

Tetanus

All postexposure wound treatment begins with immediate, thorough cleansing using soap and water, removal of foreign bodies, and debridement of devitalized tissue. Tetanus prophylaxis after wounds and injuries includes vaccination of persons with incomplete immunization and tetanus immunoglobulin for contaminated wounds (soil, feces, saliva), puncture wounds, avulsions, and wounds resulting from missiles, crushing, burns, and frostbite (Table 94.1).

Rabies

Rabies immune globulin (RIG) and rabies vaccine are extremely effective for prophylaxis after exposure to rabies, but are of no known benefit after symptoms appear. Because rabies is one of the deadliest infections, recognition of potential exposure and prophylaxis are crucial. Any healthy-appearing domestic animal (dog, cat) responsible for an apparently unprovoked bite should be observed for 10 days for signs of rabies, without immediate treatment of the victim. Prophylaxis should be administered if the animal is rabid or suspected to be rabid, or if the animal develops signs of rabies while under observation. A captured wild animal should be euthanized (by animal control officials) without a period of observation and its brain examined for evidence of rabies. If the biting animal is not captured, particularly if it is a wild animal of a species known to harbor the virus in the region, rabies should be presumed and prophylaxis administered to the victim. Bats, raccoons, skunks, foxes, coyotes, and bobcats are the most important wild animal potential sources of rabies infection. Prophylaxis also should be provided following exposure to a bat for persons who might be unaware or unable to relate that a bite or direct contact has occurred, such as a mentally disabled person, a sleeping child, or an unattended infant. Local public health departments are important resources for determining rabies risk based on local epidemiology.

All rabies postexposure management begins with immediate thorough cleansing of the bite using soap and water. RIG at a dose of 20 IU/kg should be administered, with the full dose of RIG infiltrated subcutaneously into the area around the wound, if possible. Any remaining RIG that cannot be infiltrated into the wound should be administered as an intramuscular injection. Inactivated rabies vaccine should be administered simultaneously as soon as possible, at a site away from where RIG was administered, with additional vaccine doses at 3, 7, and 14 days.

TABLE 94.1 Guide to Tetanus Prophylaxis in Routine Wound Management

PREVIOUS TETANUS IMMUNIZATION (DOSES)	CLEAN, MINOR WOUNDS: DTap, Tdap, OR Td[†]	CLEAN, MINOR WOUNDS: TIG[‡]	ALL OTHER WOUNDS*: DTap, Tdap, OR Td[†]	ALL OTHER WOUNDS*: TIG[‡]
Uncertain or <3 doses	Yes	No	Yes	Yes
≥3 doses	No if <10 yr since last tetanus-containing vaccine dose	No	No if <5 yr since last tetanus-containing vaccine dose	No
	Yes if ≥10 yr since the last tetanus toxoid-containing vaccine dose	No	Yes if ≥5 yr since the last tetanus toxoid-containing vaccine dose	No

*Such as, but not limited to, wounds contaminated with dirt, feces, soil, or saliva; puncture wounds; avulsions; and wounds resulting from missiles, crushing, burns, and frostbite.
[†]Tdap is preferred for children ≥7 years of age who have never received Tdap.
[‡]Immune globulin intravenous should be used if TIG is not available.
Tdap, Tetanus and diphtheria toxoids, acelluar pertussis vaccine; *Td*, tetanus-diphtheria toxoid; *TIG*, tetanus immunoglobulin.
From Pickering LK, ed. Red Book: 2015 Report of the Committee on Infectious Diseases. *30th ed. Elk Grove Village, IL. Copyright 2015 American Academy of Pediatrics. Reproduced with permission.*

CHAPTER 95

Antiinfective Therapy

The selection of antiinfective therapy depends on a number of factors: the site of infection and clinical syndrome, host immunity, probable causative agents, the pathogen's susceptibility to antimicrobial agents and the local epidemiology of resistance, the pharmacokinetics of the selected agents, and their pharmacodynamics in specific patient populations.

Empirical or presumptive antiinfective therapy is based on a clinical diagnosis combined with published evidence and experience of the probable causative pathogens. **Definitive therapy** relies on microbiologic diagnosis by isolation or other direct evidence of a pathogen. Microbiological diagnosis through culture permits characterization of the pathogen's antiinfective drug **susceptibilities** and delivery of the appropriate antiinfective agent to the site of infection in concentrations sufficient to kill or alter the pathogen and facilitate an effective immune response. Antiviral therapy must include consideration of the intracellular nature of viral replication and, to avoid toxicity to host cells, must be targeted to viral-specific proteins, such as the thymidine kinase of herpesviruses or the reverse transcriptase of HIV.

Empirical antimicrobial therapy is best initiated after obtaining appropriate cultures of fluids or tissues. In high-risk circumstances, such as neonatal sepsis or bacteremia in immunocompromised persons, empirical therapy includes broad-spectrum antimicrobials (see Chapters 96 and 120). Empirical antimicrobial therapy may be tailored to specific pathogens based on the clinical diagnosis (e.g., streptococcal pharyngitis) or defined risks (e.g., close exposure to tuberculosis). Definitive therapy can additionally minimize drug toxicity, development of resistant microorganisms, and cost.

Antimicrobial agents are an adjunct to the normal host immune response. Infections associated with foreign bodies, such as an intravascular catheter, are difficult to eradicate with antimicrobials alone because of organism-produced biofilms that impair phagocytosis. Similarly it is difficult for phagocytic cells to eradicate bacteria amid vegetations of fibrin and platelets on infected heart valves. Prolonged bactericidal therapy is required with these infections, and outcomes are not always satisfactory. Foreign body devices may have to be removed if sterilization does not occur promptly. Infections in closed spaces with limited perfusion (e.g., abscesses or chronic osteomyelitis with poorly perfused bone) are difficult to cure without surgical drainage, debridement of the infected tissue, and re-establishment of a good vascular supply.

Optimal antimicrobial therapy requires an understanding of both the **pharmacokinetics** (e.g., bioavailability and tissue penetration) of the administered drugs and their **pharmacodynamics** (e.g., metabolism and excretion by the body) in specific patient populations. The bioavailability of orally administered antibiotics varies depending on the acid stability of the drug, degree of gastric acidity, and whether it is taken with food, antacids, H_2 blockers, or other medications. An ileus, underlying intestinal disease, or profuse diarrhea may alter intestinal transit time and result in unpredictable absorption.

The **site and nature** of the infection may affect the choice of antimicrobials. Aminoglycosides, active against aerobic organisms only, have significantly reduced activity in abscesses with low pH and oxygen tension. Infections of the central nervous system or the eye necessitate treatment with antimicrobials that penetrate and achieve therapeutic levels in these sites.

Limited renal function (as in premature infants or those with renal failure) requires lengthening dosing intervals to allow time for excretion of certain drugs. The larger volume of distribution of certain hydrophilic antimicrobials and increased renal clearance (e.g., in cystic fibrosis) requires higher doses to achieve therapeutic levels. Weight-based dosage regimens may result in overdoses in obese children due to significantly smaller volumes of distribution for hydrophilic drugs. Determining serum drug levels for antibiotics with narrow safety margins (e.g., aminoglycosides and vancomycin) minimizes adverse effects of treatment.

Drug-drug interactions must be considered when multiple antimicrobial agents are used to treat infection, or for patients on other medications (e.g., chemotherapy or immunosuppressants). Use of two or more antimicrobial agents may be justified before organism identification or for the benefit of different mechanisms of action. Several antimicrobials are administered routinely in combination (e.g., trimethoprim-sulfamethoxazole, amoxicillin-clavulanate) because of **synergism** (significantly greater bacterial killing or spectrum of activity than when either is used alone). The use of a bacteriostatic drug, such as a tetracycline, along with a β-lactam agent, effective against growing organisms only, may result in antibiotic **antagonism,** or less bacterial killing in the presence of both drugs, than if either is used alone.

CHAPTER 96

Fever Without a Focus

Decision-Making Algorithms
Available @ StudentConsult.com

Fever Without a Source
Fever of Unknown Origin

Core body temperature is normally maintained within 1-1.5°C in a range of 37-38°C. Normal body temperature is generally considered to be 37°C (98.6°F; range, 97-99.6°F). Normal diurnal variation exists, with maximum temperature in the late afternoon. Rectal temperatures higher than 38°C (>100.4°F) generally are considered abnormal, especially if associated with symptoms.

Normal body temperature is maintained by a complex regulatory system in the anterior hypothalamus. The development of fever begins with the release of endogenous pyrogens into the circulation as the result of infection, inflammatory processes, or malignancy. Microbes and microbial toxins act as **exogenous pyrogens** by stimulating release of **endogenous pyrogens,** including cytokines such as interleukin-1, interleukin-6, tumor necrosis factor, and interferons. These cytokines reach the anterior hypothalamus, liberating arachidonic acid, which is metabolized to prostaglandin E_2. Elevation of the hypothalamic thermostat occurs via a complex interaction of complement and prostaglandin E_2 production. Antipyretics (acetaminophen, ibuprofen, aspirin) inhibit hypothalamic cyclooxygenase, decreasing production of prostaglandin E_2. Aspirin is associated with Reye syndrome in children and is not recommended as an antipyretic. The response to antipyretics does not distinguish bacterial from viral infections.

The **pattern of fever** in children may vary, depending on age and the nature of the illness. Neonates may not have a febrile response and may be instead be hypothermic, despite significant infection, whereas older infants and children younger than 5 years of age may have an exaggerated febrile response with temperatures of up to 105°F (40.6°C) in response to either a serious bacterial infection or an otherwise benign viral infection. Fever to this degree is unusual in older children and adolescents and suggests a serious process. The fever pattern does not reliably distinguish fever caused by infectious microorganisms from that resulting from malignancy, autoimmune diseases, or drugs.

Children with fever without a focus present a diagnostic challenge that includes identifying bacteremia and sepsis. **Bacteremia,** the presence of bacteria in the bloodstream, may be primary or secondary to a focal infection. **Sepsis** is the systemic response to infection that is manifested by hyperthermia or hypothermia, tachycardia, tachypnea, and shock (see Chapter 40). Children with septicemia and signs of central nervous system dysfunction (irritability, lethargy), cardiovascular impairment (cyanosis, poor perfusion), and disseminated intravascular coagulation (petechiae, ecchymosis) are readily recognized as **toxic appearing** or **septic.** Most febrile illnesses in children may be categorized as follows:

- **Fever of short duration** accompanied by localizing signs and symptoms, in which a diagnosis can often be established by clinical history and physical examination
- **Fever without localizing signs (fever without a focus),** frequently occurring in children younger than 3 years of age, in which a history and physical examination fail to establish a cause
- **Fever of unknown origin (FUO),** defined as fever for >14 days without an identified etiology despite history, physical examination, and routine laboratory tests, or after 1 week of intense evaluation

FEVER IN INFANTS YOUNGER THAN 3 MONTHS OF AGE

Fever or **temperature instability** in infants younger than 3 months of age is associated with a higher risk of **serious bacterial infections** than in older infants. These younger infants usually exhibit only fever and poor feeding, without localizing signs of infection. Most febrile illnesses in this age group are caused by common viral pathogens, but serious bacterial infections include **bacteremia** (caused by group B streptococcus [GBS], *Escherichia coli,* and *Listeria monocytogenes* in neonates; and *Streptococcus pneumoniae, Haemophilus influenzae* type b [Hib], nontyphoidal *Salmonella,* and *Neisseria meningitidis* in 1- to 3-month-old infants), **urinary tract infection (UTI)** *(E. coli),* **pneumonia** *(S. pneumoniae,* GBS, or *Staphylococcus aureus),* **meningitis** (GBS, *E. coli, L. monocytogenes, S. pneumoniae, N. meningitidis,* Hib, herpes simplex virus [HSV], enteroviruses), **bacterial diarrhea** *(Salmonella, Shigella, E. coli),* and **osteomyelitis** or **septic arthritis** *(S. aureus* or GBS).

Differentiating between viral and bacterial infections in young infants is difficult, but emerging studies demonstrate that doing so may be possible with the examination of inflammatory markers and gene expression profiles. Febrile infants <3 months of age who appear ill, especially if follow-up is uncertain, and all febrile infants <4 weeks of age should be admitted to the hospital for empirical antibiotics pending culture results. After blood, urine, and cerebrospinal fluid cultures are obtained, broad-spectrum parenteral antibiotics (typically ampicillin with cefotaxime or gentamicin) are administered. The choice of antibiotics depends on the pathogens suggested by localizing findings. The possibility of neonatal HSV should also be considered in febrile children <4 weeks old, and empirical acyclovir begun in those in whom neonatal HSV is a concern. Well-appearing febrile infants ≥4 weeks of age without an identifiable focus and with certainty of follow-up are at a low risk of developing a serious bacterial infection (0.8% develop bacteremia, and 2% develop a serious localized bacterial infection). Specific criteria identifying these low-risk infants include age older than 1 month, well-appearing without a focus of infection, no history of prematurity or prior antimicrobial therapy, a white blood cell (WBC) count of 5,000 to 15,000/µL, urine with <10 WBCs/high-power field, and spinal fluid, if obtained, with less than 5-10 WBC per microliter. Fecal leukocyte testing and chest radiograph can be considered in infants with diarrhea or respiratory signs. Low-risk infants may be followed as outpatients without empirical antibiotic treatment, or, alternatively, may be treated with intramuscular ceftriaxone. Regardless of antibiotic treatment, close follow-up for at least 72 hours, including re-evaluation in 24 hours or immediately with any clinical change, is essential.

FEVER IN CHILDREN 3 MONTHS TO 3 YEARS OF AGE

A common problem is the evaluation of a febrile but well-appearing child 3 months to 3 years of age without localizing signs of infection. Although most of these children have self-limited viral infections, some have **occult bacteremia** (bacteremia without identifiable focus) or UTIs, and a few have severe and potentially life-threatening illnesses. It is difficult, even for experienced clinicians, to differentiate patients with occult bacteremia from those with benign illnesses.

Observational assessment is a key part of the evaluation. Descriptions of normal appearance and **alertness** include *child looking at the observer* and *looking around the room,* with eyes that are *shiny* or *bright.* Descriptions that indicate severe impairment include *glassy eyes* and *stares vacantly into space.* Observations, such as *sitting, moving arms and legs on table or lap,* and *sits without support* reflect normal motor ability, whereas *no movement in mother's arms* and *lies limply on table* indicate severe impairment. Normal behaviors, such as *vocalizing spontaneously, playing with objects, reaching for objects, smiling,* and *crying with noxious stimuli,* reflect **playfulness;** abnormal behaviors reflect **irritability.** Normally, crying children are **consolable** and *stop crying when held by the parent,* whereas severe impairment is indicated by *continual cry despite being held and comforted.*

Children between 3 months and 3 years of age are at increased risk for infection with organisms with polysaccharide capsules, including *S. pneumoniae,* Hib, *N. meningitidis,* and nontyphoidal *Salmonella.* Effective phagocytosis of these organisms requires opsonic antibody. Transplacentally acquired maternal immunoglobulin (Ig)G initially provides immunity to these organisms, but as the IgG gradually dissipates, the risk of infection increases. In the United States, use of conjugate Hib and *S. pneumoniae* vaccines has dramatically reduced the incidence of these infections, and determining the child's immunization status is essential to evaluate the risk of these infections. An approach to evaluating these children is outlined in Fig. 96.1.

Most episodes of fever in children younger than 3 years of age have a demonstrable source of infection elicited by history, physical examination, or a simple laboratory test. In this age group, the most commonly identified serious bacterial infection is a UTI. A blood culture to evaluate for occult bacteremia, and urinalysis and urine culture to evaluate for a UTI, should be considered for all children younger than 3 years of age with ongoing fever without localizing signs. Stool culture should be obtained in those with diarrhea marked by blood or mucous. Ill-appearing children should be admitted to the hospital and treated with empirical antibiotics.

Approximately 0.2% of well-appearing febrile children 3-36 months of age vaccinated against *S. pneumoniae* and Hib and without localizing signs have occult bacteremia. Risk factors for occult bacteremia include temperature of 102.2°F (39°C) or greater, WBC count of 15,000/mm^3 or more, and elevated absolute neutrophil count, band count, erythrocyte sedimentation rate, or C-reactive protein. No combination of demographic factors (socioeconomic status, race, gender, and age), clinical parameters, or laboratory tests in these children reliably predicts occult bacteremia. Occult bacteremia in otherwise

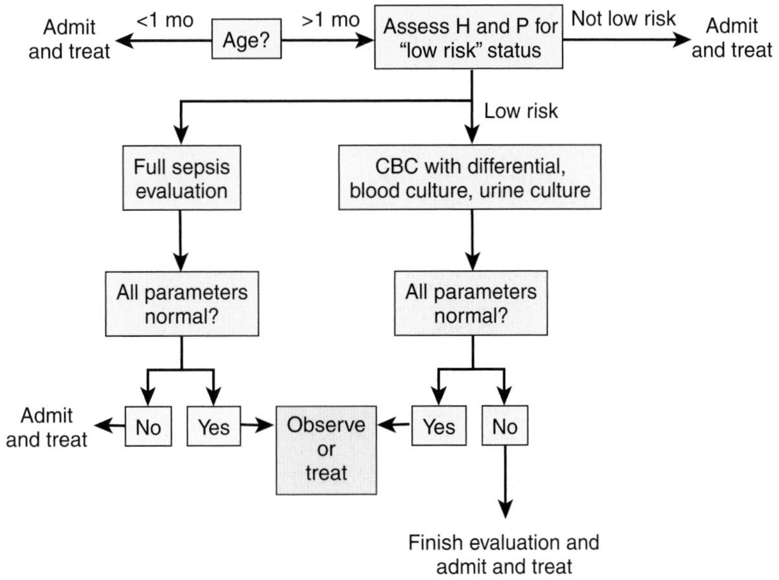

FIGURE 96.1 Approach to a child younger than 36 months of age with fever without localizing signs. The specific management varies, depending on the age and clinical status of the child. *CBC,* Complete blood count; *H and P,* history and physical.

healthy children is usually transient and self-limited but may progress to serious localizing infections. Well-appearing children usually are followed as outpatients without empirical antibiotic treatment. Regardless of antibiotic treatment, close follow-up for at least 72 hours, including re-evaluation in 24 hours or immediately with any clinical change, is essential. Children with a positive blood culture require immediate re-evaluation, repeat blood culture, consideration for lumbar puncture, and empirical antibiotic treatment.

Children with **sickle cell disease** have both impaired splenic function and properdin-dependent opsonization that places them at increased risk for bacteremia due to encapsulated organisms, especially during the first 5 years of life. Children with sickle cell disease and fever who appear seriously ill, have a temperature of ≥104°F (40°C), or WBC count <5,000/mm^3 or >30,000/mm^3 should be hospitalized and treated empirically with antibiotics. Other children with sickle cell disease and fever should have blood culture, empirical treatment with ceftriaxone, and close outpatient follow-up. Osteomyelitis resulting from *Salmonella* or *S. aureus* is more common in children with sickle cell disease; blood culture is not always positive in the presence of osteomyelitis.

FEVER OF UNKNOWN ORIGIN

Decision-Making Algorithm
Available @ StudentConsult.com
Fever of Unknown Origin

FUO is defined as temperature >100.4°F (38°C) lasting for >14 days without an obvious cause despite a complete history, physical examination, and routine screening laboratory evaluation. It is important to distinguish persistent fever from recurrent or periodic fevers, which usually represent serial acute illnesses.

The initial FUO evaluation requires a thorough history and physical examination supplemented with a few screening laboratory tests (Fig. 96.2). Additional laboratory and imaging tests are guided by abnormalities on initial evaluation. Important historical elements include the impact the fever has on the child's health and activity; weight loss; the use of drugs, medications, or immunosuppressive therapy; a history of unusual, severe, or

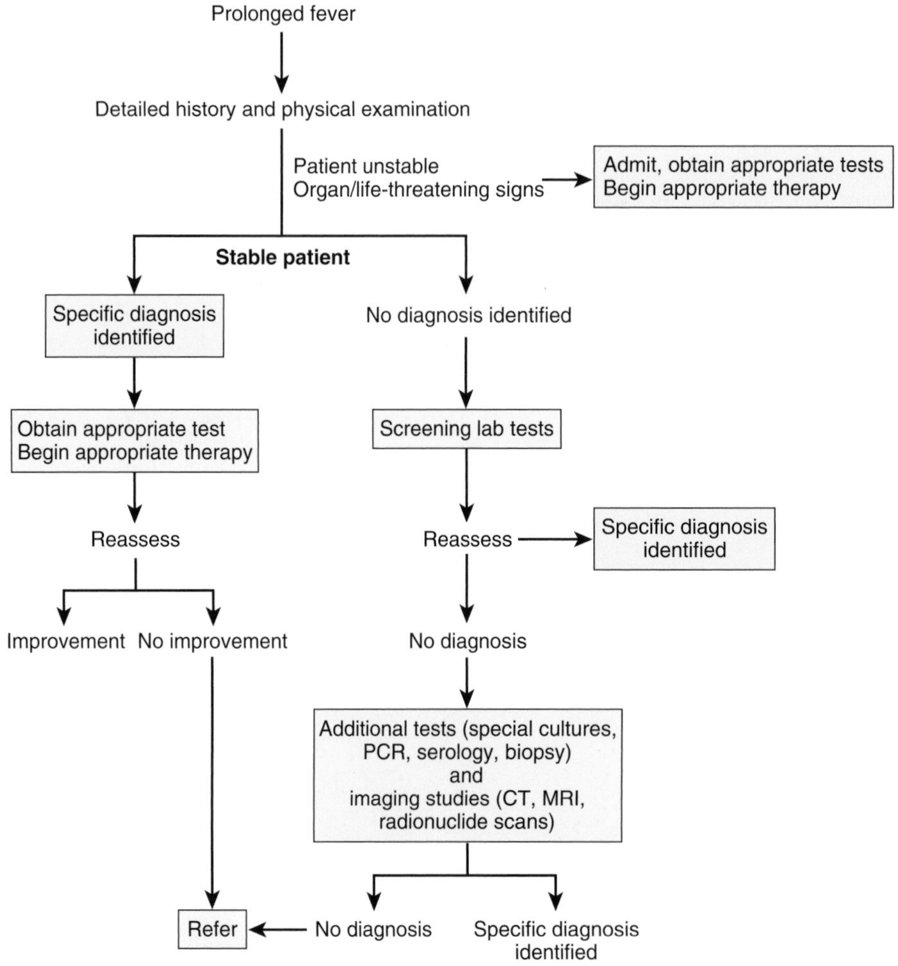

FIGURE 96.2 Approach to the evaluation of fever of unknown origin in children. Screening laboratory tests include complete blood count with and differential, erythrocyte sedimentation rate, C-reactive protein, basic metabolic panel, hepatic transaminase levels, urinalysis, and cultures of urine and blood. Chest radiograph should be included for patients with pulmonary symptoms. *CT*, Computed tomography; *MRI*, magnetic resonance imaging; *PCR*, polymerase chain reaction; *WBC*, white blood cells.

chronic infection suggesting immunodeficiency (see Chapter 72); immunizations; exposure to unprocessed or raw foods; a history of pica and exposure to soil-borne or waterborne organisms; exposure to industrial or hobby-related chemicals; blood transfusions; domestic or foreign travel; exposure to animals; exposure to ticks or mosquitoes; ethnic background; recent surgical procedures or dental work; tattooing and body piercing; and sexual activity.

The etiology of most occult infections causing FUO is an unusual presentation of a common disease. Sinusitis, endocarditis, intraabdominal abscesses (perinephric, intrahepatic, subdiaphragmatic), and central nervous system lesions (tuberculoma, cysticercosis, abscess, toxoplasmosis) may be relatively asymptomatic. **Infections** are the most common cause of FUO in children, accounting for approximately 40-50% of FUO episodes, followed by **inflammatory diseases** (about 20% of all episodes), **malignancy** (about 10% of all episodes), and other etiologies (Table 96.1). Approximately 15% of children with FUO have no diagnosis. Fever eventually resolves in many of these cases, usually without sequelae, although some may develop definable signs of rheumatic disease over time. Common infections causing FUO in patients with known or newly diagnosed **immunodeficiency** include viral hepatitis, Epstein-Barr virus, cytomegalovirus, *Bartonella henselae,* ehrlichiosis, *Salmonella,* and tuberculosis.

Factitious fever or fever produced or feigned intentionally by the patient **(Munchausen syndrome)** or the parent of a child **(Munchausen syndrome by proxy)** is an important consideration, particularly if family members are familiar with health care practices (see Chapter 22). Fever should be recorded in the hospital by a reliable individual who remains with the patient when the temperature is taken. Continuous observation over a long period and repetitive evaluation are essential.

Screening tests for FUO include complete blood count with WBC and differential, erythrocyte sedimentation rate, C-reactive protein, procalcitonin, basic metabolic panel, hepatic transaminase levels, urinalysis, and cultures of urine and blood. Chest radiograph should be included for patients with pulmonary symptoms. Additional tests for FUO may include throat culture, stool culture, tuberculin skin test or interferon-gamma release assay, HIV, Epstein-Barr virus, cytomegalovirus, and *B. henselae* antibodies. Consultation with infectious disease, immunology, rheumatic disease, or oncology specialists should be considered. Further tests may include lumbar puncture for cerebrospinal fluid analysis and culture; evaluation for rheumatic disease with antinuclear antibody, rheumatoid factor, ferritin, and serum complement (C3, C4, CH_{50}); uric acid and lactate dehydrogenase; computed tomography or magnetic resonance imaging of the chest, abdomen, and head; radionuclide scans; and bone marrow biopsy for cytology and culture.

TABLE 96.1 Causes of Fever of Unknown Origin in Children

INFECTIONS	Lymphogranuloma venereum
Localized Infections	Meningococcemia (chronic)
Abscesses: abdominal, brain, dental, hepatic, pelvic, perinephric, rectal, subphrenic, splenic, periappendiceal, psoas, pyomyositis	*Mycoplasma pneumoniae*
Cholangitis	Psittacosis
Diskitis	Relapsing fever (*Borrelia recurrentis,* other *Borrelia*)
Infective endocarditis	Salmonellosis
Mastoiditis	*Spirillum minus* (rat-bite fever)
Osteomyelitis	*Streptobacillus moniliformis* (rat-bite fever)
Pneumonia	Syphilis
Pyelonephritis	Tuberculosis
Septic arthritis	Whipple disease
Sinusitis	Yersiniosis
Bacterial Diseases	**Viral Diseases**
Actinomycosis	Cytomegalovirus
Bartonella henselae (cat-scratch disease)	Hepatitis viruses
Brucellosis	HIV (and associated opportunistic infections)
Campylobacter	Infectious mononucleosis (Epstein-Barr virus)
Chlamydia	**Rickettsial Diseases**
Francisella tularensis (tularemia)	Ehrlichiosis
Gonococcemia (chronic)	Q fever (*Coxiella burnetii*)
Leptospirosis	Rocky Mountain spotted fever
Listeria monocytogenes (listeriosis)	Tick-borne typhus
Lyme disease (*Borrelia burgdorferi*)	

Continued

TABLE 96.1 Causes of Fever of Unknown Origin in Children—cont'd

INFECTIONS	Hepatoma
Fungal Diseases	Hodgkin disease
Blastomycosis (extrapulmonary)	Inflammatory pseudotumor
Coccidioidomycosis (disseminated)	Leukemia
Histoplasmosis (disseminated)	Lymphoma
Parasitic Diseases	Neuroblastoma
Extraintestinal amebiasis	Pheochromocytoma
Baylisascaris	Wilms tumor
Babesiosis	MISCELLANEOUS
Malaria	Addison disease
Toxoplasmosis	Anhidrotic ectodermal dysplasia
Trichinosis	Autonomic neuropathies
Trypanosomiasis	Castleman disease
Visceral larva migrans (*Toxocara*)	Chronic active hepatitis
INFLAMMATORY DISEASES	Cyclic neutropenia
Autoimmune lymphoproliferative syndrome	Diabetes insipidus (central and nephrogenic)
Behçet syndrome	Fabry disease
Chronic recurrent multifocal osteomyelitis	Factitious fever
Drug fever	Familial dysautonomia
Granulomatosis with polyangiitis	Familial Mediterranean fever
Hypersensitivity pneumonitis	Granulomatous hepatitis
Juvenile dermatomyositis	Hemophagocytic syndromes
Juvenile idiopathic arthritis (systemic onset, Still disease)	Hypertriglyceridemia
Inflammatory bowel disease (Crohn disease, ulcerative colitis)	Hypothalamic-central fever
Kawasaki disease	Ichthyosis
Polyarteritis nodosa	Infantile cortical hyperostosis
Rheumatic fever	Kikuchi-Fujimoto disease
Sarcoidosis	Metal fume fever
Serum sickness	Pancreatitis
Systemic lupus erythematosus	Periodic fever syndromes
Weber-Christian disease	Poisoning
MALIGNANCIES	Postoperative (pericardiotomy, craniectomy)
Atrial myxoma	Pulmonary embolism
Cholesterol granuloma	Thrombophlebitis
Ewing sarcoma	Thyrotoxicosis

Modified from Nield LS, Kamat D: Fever without a focus. In: Kliegman RM, Stanton BF, St. Geme III JW, Schor NF, eds. Nelson Textbook of Pediatrics, *ed 20, Philadelphia, 2016, Elsevier.*

CHAPTER 97

Infections Characterized by Fever and Rash

Decision-Making Algorithm
Available @ StudentConsult.com

Fever and Rash

Rashes are a common manifestation of many infections; this chapter describes five common childhood viral exanthems characterized by fever and rash. Rash distribution and appearance provide important clues to the differential diagnosis, including other infectious agents (Table 97.1).

MEASLES (RUBEOLA)

Etiology

Measles (rubeola) is highly contagious and is caused by a single-stranded RNA paramyxovirus with one antigenic type. Humans are the only natural host. The measles virus infects the upper respiratory tract and regional lymph nodes and is spread systemically during a brief, low-titer primary viremia. A secondary viremia occurs within 5-7 days as virus-infected monocytes spread the virus to the respiratory tract, skin, and other organs. The virus is present in respiratory secretions, blood, and the urine of infected individuals. It is transmitted by droplets or via the airborne route and is extremely contagious. Infected persons are contagious from 1-2 days before onset of symptoms—from about 5 days before to 4 days after the appearance of rash—and immunocompromised persons can have prolonged excretion of contagious virus.

Epidemiology

Measles remains endemic in regions of the world where measles vaccination is not readily available and is responsible for about 20 million infections and 150,000 deaths annually. There have typically been fewer than 100 cases of measles reported annually in the United States; however, outbreaks have occurred resulting from imported virus after international travel, and in 2014 there were over 650 measles cases in the United States. Infections of nonimmigrant children may occur during outbreaks among those too young to be vaccinated or in communities with low immunization rates. Most young infants are protected by transplacentally acquired maternal antibody until the end of their first year.

Clinical Manifestations

Measles infection is divided into four phases: incubation, prodromal (catarrhal), exanthematous (rash), and recovery. The incubation period is 8-12 days from exposure to symptom onset and a mean of 14 days (range: 7-21) from exposure to rash onset. The manifestations of the 3-day prodromal period are cough, coryza, conjunctivitis, and the pathognomonic **Koplik**

TABLE 97.1 Differential Diagnosis of Fever and Rash

LESION	PATHOGEN OR DISEASE
Macular or Maculopapular Rash	
Viruses	Adenovirus
	Measles
	Rubella
	Roseola (HHV-6 or HHV-7)
	Erythema infectiosum (5th disease, parvovirus B19)
	Epstein-Barr virus
	Enteroviruses
	Parechoviruses
	HBV (papular acrodermatitis or Gianotti-Crosti syndrome)
	HIV
Bacteria	Erythema marginatum (rheumatic fever)
	Scarlet fever (group A streptococcus)
	Erysipelas (group A streptococcus)
	Arcanobacterium haemolyticum
	Secondary syphilis
	Leptospirosis
	Pseudomonas aeruginosa
	Meningococcal infection (early)
	Salmonella typhi (typhoid fever, "rose spots")
	Lyme disease (erythema migrans)
	Mycoplasma pneumoniae
Rickettsiae	Rocky Mountain spotted fever (early)
	Typhus (scrub, endemic)
	Ehrlichiosis
Other	Kawasaki disease
	Rheumatoid arthritis
	Drug reaction
Diffuse Erythroderma	
Bacteria	Scarlet fever (group A streptococcus)
	Staphylococcal scalded skin syndrome
	Toxic shock syndrome *(Staphylococcus aureus,* group A streptococcus)
Fungi	*Candida albicans*
Other	Kawasaki disease
Urticarial Rash	
Viruses	Epstein-Barr virus
	HBV
	HIV
Bacteria	*M. pneumoniae*
	Group A streptococcus
Other	Drug reaction
	Serum sickness
Vesicular, Bullous, Pustular	
Viruses	Herpes simplex viruses
	Varicella-zoster virus
	Coxsackievirus

Continued

TABLE 97.1 Differential Diagnosis of Fever and Rash—cont'd

LESION	PATHOGEN OR DISEASE
Vesicular, Bullous, Pustular—cont'd	
Bacteria	Staphylococcal scalded skin syndrome
	Staphylococcal bullous impetigo
	Group A streptococcal crusted impetigo
Rickettsiae	Rickettsialpox
Other	Toxic epidermal necrolysis
	Erythema multiforme
	Stevens-Johnson syndrome
Petechial-Purpuric	
Viruses	Adenovirus
	Atypical measles
	Congenital rubella
	Congenital cytomegalovirus
	Enterovirus
	Papular-purpuric gloves and socks (parvovirus B19)
	HIV
	Hemorrhagic fever viruses
Bacteria	Sepsis (meningococcal, gonococcal, pneumococcal, *Haemophilus influenzae* type b)
	Infective endocarditis
	Ecthyma gangrenosum *(P. aeruginosa)*
	Vibrio vulnificus
Rickettsiae	Rocky Mountain spotted fever
	Epidemic typhus
	Ehrlichiosis
Other	Vasculitis
	Thrombocytopenia
	Henoch-Schönlein purpura
	Acute hemorrhagic edema of infancy
	Malaria
Necrotic Eschar	
Bacteria	*Bacillus anthracis*
	Francisella tularensis
Fungi	*Aspergillus, Mucor*
Erythema Nodosum	
Viruses	Epstein-Barr virus
	HBV
Bacteria	Group A streptococcus
	Mycobacterium tuberculosis
	Yersinia
	Cat-scratch disease *(Bartonella henselae)*
Fungi	Coccidioidomycosis
	Histoplasmosis
Other	Sarcoidosis
	Inflammatory bowel disease
	Estrogen-containing oral contraceptives
	Systemic lupus erythematosus
	Behçet disease

HBV, Hepatitis B virus; *HHV*, human herpesvirus.

spots (gray-white, sand-grain-sized dots on the buccal mucosa opposite the lower molars) that last 12-24 hours. The conjunctiva may reveal a characteristic transverse line of inflammation along the eyelid margin **(Stimson line)**. The classic symptoms of cough, coryza, and conjunctivitis occur during the secondary viremia of the exanthematous phase, which often is accompanied by high fever (40-40.5°C [104-105°F]). The macular rash begins on the head (often above the hairline) and spreads over most of the body in a cephalad to caudal pattern over 24 hours. Areas of the rash are often confluent. The rash fades in the same pattern, and illness severity is related to the extent of the rash. It may be petechial or hemorrhagic **(black measles).** As the rash fades, it undergoes brownish discoloration and desquamation.

Cervical lymphadenitis, splenomegaly, and mesenteric lymphadenopathy with abdominal pain may be noted with the rash. Otitis media, pneumonia, and diarrhea are more common in infants. Liver involvement is more common in adults.

The term **modified measles** describes mild cases of measles occurring in persons with partial protection against measles. Modified measles occurs in persons vaccinated before 12 months of age or with co-administration of immune serum globulin, in infants with disease modified by transplacentally acquired antibody, or in persons receiving immunoglobulin.

Laboratory and Imaging Studies

Routine laboratory findings are nonspecific and do not aid in diagnosis. Leukopenia is characteristic. In patients with acute encephalitis, the cerebrospinal fluid reveals an increased protein, a lymphocytic pleocytosis, and normal glucose levels. Measles virus culture is not generally available, though identification of measles RNA via reverse transcriptase-polymerase chain reaction (PCR) may be available through state public health departments or the Centers for Disease Control and Prevention (CDC). Serological testing for immunoglobulin (Ig)M antibodies that appear within 1-2 days of the rash and persist for 1-2 months in unimmunized persons confirms the clinical diagnosis, though IgM antibodies may be present only transiently in immunized people. Suspected cases should be **reported immediately** to the local or state health department.

Differential Diagnosis

The constellation of fever, rash, cough, and conjunctivitis is highly suggestive of measles. Koplik spots are pathognomonic but not always present at the time the rash is most pronounced. Confirmation is by diagnostic antibody increases in acute and convalescent sera. Measles must be differentiated from rubella, roseola, enteroviral or adenoviral infection, infectious mononucleosis, toxoplasmosis, meningococcemia, scarlet fever, rickettsial disease, Kawasaki disease, serum sickness, and drug rash.

Treatment

Routine supportive care includes maintaining adequate hydration and antipyretics. High-dose vitamin A supplementation improves the outcome of infants with measles in developing countries. The World Health Organization recommends routine administration of vitamin A for 2 days to all children with acute measles, regardless of country of residence.

Complications and Prognosis

Otitis media is the most common complication of measles infection. Interstitial (measles) pneumonia can occur, or pneumonia may result from secondary bacterial infection with *Streptococcus pneumoniae, Staphylococcus aureus,* or group A streptococcus. Persons with impaired cell-mediated immunity may develop **giant cell (Hecht) pneumonia,** which is usually fatal. Myocarditis and mesenteric lymphadenitis are infrequent complications.

Encephalomyelitis occurs in 1-2 per 1,000 cases and usually occurs 2-5 days after the onset of the rash. Early encephalitis probably is caused by direct viral infection of brain tissue, whereas later onset encephalitis is a demyelinating, and probably an immunopathological, phenomenon. **Subacute sclerosing panencephalitis (SSPE)** is a late neurological complication of slow measles infection that is characterized by progressive behavioral and intellectual deterioration and eventual death. It occurs in approximately 1 in every 1 million cases of measles, an average of 8-10 years after measles. There is no effective treatment.

Deaths most frequently result from bronchopneumonia or encephalitis, with much higher risk in persons with malignancy, severe malnutrition, age under 5 years, or immunocompromise (such as HIV infection). Late deaths in adolescents and adults usually result from SSPE. Other forms of measles encephalitis in immunocompetent persons are associated with a mortality rate of approximately 15%, with 20-30% of survivors having serious neurological sequelae.

Prevention

Live measles vaccine prevents infection and is recommended as measles, mumps, and rubella (MMR) for children at 12-15 months and 4-6 years of age. The MMRV (MMR combined with varicella vaccine) is an alternative vaccine for children 12 months to 12 years of age, provided there are no contraindications, but is associated with a higher rate of febrile seizures following administration. The second dose of MMR is not a booster dose but significantly reduces the primary vaccine failure rate, from <5% to <1%. Contraindications to measles vaccine include immunocompromised states or an immunosuppressive course of corticosteroids (>2 mg/kg/day or >20 mg/day for those weighing >10 kg, for >14 days); pregnancy; or recent administration of immunoglobulin (within 3-11 months, depending on dose). MMR vaccination is recommended for all HIV-infected persons without evidence of severe immunosuppression (low age-specific CD4 T lymphocytes), children with cancer in remission who have not received chemotherapy in the previous 3 months, and children who have not received immunosuppressive corticosteroids in the previous month. Susceptible household contacts with a chronic disease or who are immunocompromised should receive **postexposure prophylaxis** with measles vaccine within 72 hours of measles exposure or immunoglobulin within 6 days of exposure.

RUBELLA (GERMAN OR 3-DAY MEASLES)

Etiology

Rubella, also known as **German measles** or **3-day measles,** is caused by a single-stranded RNA virus with a glycolipid envelope and is a member of the togavirus family. Humans are the only natural host. Rubella virus invades the respiratory epithelium and disseminates via a primary viremia. After replication in the reticuloendothelial system, a secondary viremia ensues, and the virus can be isolated from peripheral blood monocytes, cerebrospinal fluid, and urine. Rubella virus is most contagious through direct or droplet contact with nasopharyngeal secretions from 2 days before until 5-7 days after rash onset, although the virus may be present in nasopharyngeal secretions from 7 days before until 14 days after the rash.

Infection **in utero** results in significant morbidity from **congenital rubella syndrome (CRS)** with associated ophthalmological, cardiac, and neurological manifestations (see Chapter 66). Maternal infection during the first trimester results in fetal infection with generalized vasculitis in more than 90% of cases. Infants with CRS may shed the virus in nasopharyngeal secretions and urine for >12 months after birth and transmit it to susceptible contacts.

Epidemiology

In unvaccinated populations, rubella usually occurs in the spring, with epidemics occurring in cycles of every 6-9 years. Approximately 25-50% of cases are subclinical. Fewer than 20 cases of rubella now occur annually in the United States. Outbreaks occasionally occur in nonvaccinated groups from internationally imported cases. Transplacentally acquired antibody is protective during the first 6 months of life.

Clinical Manifestations

Decision-Making Algorithm
Available @ StudentConsult.com
Fever and Rash

The incubation period for postnatal rubella is typically 16-18 days (range: 14-21 days). The mild catarrhal symptoms of the prodromal phase of rubella may go unnoticed. The characteristic signs of rubella are retroauricular, posterior cervical, and posterior occipital lymphadenopathy accompanied by an erythematous, maculopapular, discrete rash. The rash begins on the face and spreads to the body, lasting for 3 days, and is less prominent than that of measles. Rose-colored spots on the soft palate, known as **Forchheimer spots,** develop in 20% of patients and may appear before the rash. Other manifestations of rubella include mild pharyngitis, conjunctivitis, anorexia, headache, malaise, and low-grade fever. Polyarthritis, usually of the hands, may occur, especially among adult females, but usually resolves without sequelae. Paresthesias and tendinitis may occur.

Laboratory and Imaging Studies

Routine laboratory findings are nonspecific and generally do not aid in diagnosis. The white blood cell count usually is normal or low, and thrombocytopenia rarely occurs. Diagnosis is confirmed by serological testing for IgM antibodies (typically positive 5 days after symptom onset) or by a fourfold or greater increase in specific IgG antibodies in paired acute and convalescent sera. **CRS** cases can have detectable IgM until 3 months of age and stable or rising IgG titers over the first 7-11 months of age. False-positive IgM results can occur. Cases of suspected CRS and postnatal rubella infection should be reported to the local and state health department.

Differential Diagnosis

The rash must be differentiated from measles, roseola, enteroviral or adenoviral infection, infectious mononucleosis, toxoplasmosis, scarlet fever, rickettsial disease, Kawasaki disease, serum sickness, and drug rash.

Treatment

There is no specific therapy for rubella, and treatment is supportive.

Complications and Prognosis

Other than **CRS** (see Chapter 66) arising from rubella infection during pregnancy, complications are rare. Deaths rarely occur with rubella encephalitis.

Prevention

Live rubella vaccine prevents infection and is recommended as MMR for children at 12-15 months and at 4-6 years of age. After vaccination, rubella virus is shed from the nasopharynx for several weeks, but it is not communicable. In children, rubella vaccine rarely is associated with adverse effects, but in postpubertal females, it causes arthralgias in 25% of vaccinated individuals and acute arthritis-like symptoms in 10% of vaccinated individuals. These symptoms typically develop 1-3 weeks after vaccination and last 1-3 days.

Contraindications to rubella vaccine include immunocompromised states or an immunosuppressive course of corticosteroids (>2 mg/kg/day or >20 mg/day for those weighing >10 kg, for >14 days); pregnancy; or recent administration of immunoglobulin (within 3-11 months, depending on dose). Vaccine virus has been recovered from fetal tissues, although no cases of **CRS** have been identified among infants born to women inadvertently vaccinated against rubella during pregnancy. Nevertheless, women are cautioned to avoid pregnancy for 28 days after receiving the rubella-containing vaccine. All pregnant women should have prenatal serological testing to determine their immune status to rubella, and susceptible mothers should be vaccinated after delivery and before hospital discharge.

Susceptible, nonpregnant persons exposed to rubella should receive rubella vaccination. Immunoglobulin is not recommended for postexposure prophylaxis of susceptible, pregnant women exposed to rubella.

ROSEOLA INFANTUM (EXANTHEM SUBITUM)

Etiology

Roseola infantum (exanthem subitum, sixth disease) is caused primarily by human herpesvirus type 6 (HHV-6), and by HHV-7 in 10-30% of cases. HHV-6 and HHV-7 are large, enveloped double-stranded DNA viruses that are members of the herpesvirus family. Two species of HHV-6—HHV-6A and HHV-6B—exist, with almost all postnatal infections caused by HHV-6B. These viruses infect mature mononuclear cells and cause a relatively prolonged (3-5 days) viremia during primary infection. They can be detected in the saliva of healthy adults, which suggests, as with other herpesviruses, the development of lifelong latent infection and intermittent viral shedding.

Epidemiology

Transplacentally acquired antibody protects most infants until 6 months of age. The incidence of infection increases as maternally derived antibody levels decline. By 12 months of age, approximately 60-90% of children have antibodies to HHV-6, and essentially all children are seropositive by 2-3 years of age. The virus is likely acquired from asymptomatic adults who periodically shed these viruses. HHV-6 is a major cause of acute febrile illnesses in infants and may be responsible for up to 20% of visits to the emergency department for children 6-18 months of age.

Clinical Manifestations

Roseola is characterized by high fever (often >40°C) with an abrupt onset that lasts 3-5 days. A maculopapular, rose-colored rash erupts coincident with defervescence, although it may be present earlier. The rash usually lasts 1-3 days but may fade rapidly and is not present in all infants with HHV-6 infection. Upper respiratory symptoms, nasal congestion, erythematous tympanic membranes, and cough may occur. Gastrointestinal symptoms are described. Roseola is associated with approximately one third of febrile seizures. Roseola caused by HHV-6 and HHV-7 are clinically indistinguishable, although HHV-6-associated roseola typically occurs in younger infants. Reactivation of HHV-6 following bone marrow transplantation may result in bone marrow suppression, hepatitis, rash, and encephalitis.

Laboratory and Imaging Studies

Routine laboratory findings are nonspecific and do not aid in diagnosis. Encephalitis with roseola is characterized by pleocytosis (30-200 cells/mm^3) with mononuclear cell predominance, elevated protein concentration, and normal glucose concentration. Serological testing showing a fourfold rise in acute and convalescent sera or documentation of HHV-6 DNA by PCR in the cerebrospinal fluid is diagnostic. PCR has also been used to detect HHV-6 in blood but may not be sensitive in primary infection.

Differential Diagnosis

The pattern of high fever for 3-5 days without significant physical findings followed by onset of rash with subsequent defervescence is characteristic. Many febrile illnesses may be easily confused with roseola during the preeruptive stage. Serious infections must be excluded, although most children are alert, behave normally, and continue with their usual daily activities.

Treatment

There is no specific therapy for roseola. Routine supportive care includes maintaining adequate hydration and antipyretics. In immunocompromised hosts, use of ganciclovir or foscarnet can be considered.

Complications and Prognosis

The prognosis for roseola is excellent. A few deaths have been attributed to HHV-6, usually in cases complicated by encephalitis or virus-associated **hemophagocytosis syndrome.**

Prevention

No preventative measures are available.

ERYTHEMA INFECTIOSUM (FIFTH DISEASE)

Etiology

Erythema infectiosum (fifth disease) is caused by the human parvovirus B19, a single-stranded DNA virus producing a benign viral exanthem in healthy children. The viral affinity for red blood cell progenitor cells makes it an important cause of aplastic crisis in patients with hemolytic anemias, including sickle cell disease, spherocytosis, and thalassemia. Parvovirus B19 also causes fetal anemia and hydrops fetalis after primary infection during pregnancy. The cell receptor for parvovirus B19 is the **erythrocyte P antigen,** a glycolipid present on erythroid cells. The virus replicates in actively dividing erythroid stem cells, leading to cell death that results in erythroid aplasia and anemia.

Epidemiology

Erythema infectiosum is common. Parvovirus B19 seroprevalence is only 2-9% in children younger than 5 years of age but increases to 15-35% in children 5-18 years and 30-60% in adults. Community epidemics usually occur in the spring. The virus is transmitted by respiratory secretions and by blood product transfusions.

Clinical Manifestations

The incubation period is typically 4-14 days and, rarely, may last 21 days. Parvovirus B19 infections usually begin with a mild, nonspecific illness characterized by fever, malaise, myalgias, and headache. In some cases, the characteristic rash appears 7-10 days later. Erythema infectiosum is manifested by rash, low-grade or no fever, and occasionally pharyngitis and mild conjunctivitis. The rash appears in three stages. The initial stage is typically a **"slapped cheek" rash** with circumoral pallor. An erythematous symmetric, maculopapular, truncal rash appears 1-4 days later, then fades as central clearing takes place, giving a distinctive **lacy, reticulated rash** that lasts 2-40 days (mean: 11 days). This rash may be pruritic, does not desquamate, and may recur with exercise, bathing, rubbing, or stress. Adolescents and adults may experience myalgia, significant arthralgias or arthritis, headache, pharyngitis, coryza, and gastrointestinal upset.

Children with shortened erythrocyte life span (e.g., sickle cell disease) may develop a **transient aplastic crisis,** which is characterized by ineffective erythroid production typically lasting 7-10 days (see Chapter 150). Most children with parvovirus B19-induced transient aplastic crisis have multiple symptoms, including fever, lethargy, malaise, pallor, headache, gastrointestinal symptoms, and respiratory symptoms. The reticulocyte count is extremely low, and the hemoglobin level is lower than usual for the patient. Transient neutropenia and thrombocytopenia also commonly occur.

Persistent parvovirus B19 infection may develop in children with immunodeficiency, causing severe anemia resulting from pure red blood cell aplasia. These children do not display the typical manifestations of erythema infectiosum.

Laboratory and Imaging Studies

Hematological abnormalities occur with parvovirus infection, including reticulocytopenia lasting 7-10 days, mild anemia, thrombocytopenia, lymphopenia, and neutropenia. Parvovirus B19 can be detected by PCR and by electron microscopy of erythroid precursors in the bone marrow. Serological tests showing specific IgM antibody to parvovirus are diagnostic, demonstrating an infection that probably occurred in the prior 2-4 months. Parvovirus PCR of blood and cerebrospinal fluid is also available, primarily for use in severe illness or immunocompromised patients.

Differential Diagnosis

The diagnosis of erythema infectiosum in children is established on the basis of the clinical findings of typical facial rash with absent or mild prodromal symptoms, followed by a reticulated rash over the body that waxes and wanes. The differential diagnosis includes measles, rubella, scarlet fever, enteroviral or adenoviral infection, infectious mononucleosis, Kawasaki disease, systemic lupus erythematosus, serum sickness, and drug reaction.

Treatment

There is no specific therapy other than routine supportive care. Transfusions may be required for transient aplastic crisis. Intrauterine transfusion has been performed for hydrops fetalis associated with fetal parvovirus B19 infection. Intravenous immunoglobulin may be used for immunocompromised persons with severe anemia or chronic infection.

Complications and Prognosis

The prognosis for erythema infectiosum is excellent. Fatalities associated with transient aplastic crisis are rare. Parvovirus B19 is not teratogenic, but in utero infection of fetal erythroid cells may result in fetal heart failure, hydrops fetalis, and fetal death. Of the approximately 50% of women of childbearing age susceptible to parvovirus B19 infection, 30% of exposed women develop infection, with 25% of exposed fetuses becoming infected and 10% of these culminating in fetal death.

Prevention

The greatest risk is to pregnant women. Effective control measures are limited. The exclusion of affected children from school is not recommended because children generally are not infectious by the time the rash is present. Good handwashing and hygiene are practical measures that should help reduce transmission.

VARICELLA-ZOSTER VIRUS INFECTION (CHICKENPOX AND ZOSTER)

Etiology

Chickenpox and zoster are caused by varicella-zoster virus (VZV), an enveloped, icosahedral, double-stranded DNA virus that is a member of the herpesvirus family. Humans are the only natural host. **Chickenpox (varicella)** is the manifestation of primary infection. VZV infects susceptible individuals via the conjunctivae or respiratory tract and replicates in the nasopharynx and upper respiratory tract. It disseminates by a primary viremia and infects regional lymph nodes, the liver, the spleen, and other organs. A secondary viremia follows, resulting in a cutaneous infection with the typical vesicular rash. After resolution of chickenpox, the virus persists in latent infection in the dorsal root ganglia cells. **Zoster (shingles)** is the manifestation of reactivated latent infection of endogenous VZV. Chickenpox is highly communicable in susceptible individuals, with a secondary attack rate of more than 90%. The period of communicability ranges from 2 days before to 7 days after the onset of the rash, when all lesions are crusted.

Epidemiology

In the prevaccine era, the peak age of occurrence was 5-10 years, with peak seasonal infection in late winter and spring. In the postvaccine era, the incidence of varicella has declined in all age groups, with the peak incidence now in 10-14-year-olds. Transmission is by direct contact, droplet, and air. **Zoster**, however, is contagious by direct contact. Only 5% of cases of zoster occur in children younger than 15 years of age. The overall incidence of zoster (215 cases per 100,000 person-years) results in a cumulative lifetime incidence of approximately 10-20%, with 75% of cases occurring after 45 years of age. The incidence of zoster is increased in immunocompromised persons.

Clinical Manifestations

Decision-Making Algorithms
Available @ StudentConsult.com

Ataxia
Alopecia
Vesicles and Bullae
Fever and Rash
Petechiae/Purpura

The incubation period of varicella is generally 14-16 days, with a range of 10-21 days after exposure. Prodromal symptoms of fever, malaise, and anorexia may precede the rash by 1 day. The characteristic rash appears initially as small red papules that rapidly progress to nonumbilicated, oval, "teardrop" vesicles on an erythematous base. The fluid progresses from clear to cloudy, and the vesicles ulcerate, crust, and heal. New crops appear for 3-4 days, usually beginning on the trunk followed by the head, the face, and, less commonly, the extremities. There may be a total of 100-500 lesions, with all forms of lesions being present at the same time. Pruritus is universal and marked. Lesions may be present on mucous membranes. Lymphadenopathy may be generalized. The severity of the rash varies, as do systemic signs and fever, which generally abate after 3-4 days.

The preeruption phase of **zoster** includes intense localized and burning pain and tenderness **(acute neuritis)** along a dermatome, accompanied by malaise and fever. In several days, the eruption of papules, which quickly vesiculate, occurs in the dermatome or in two adjacent dermatomes. Groups of lesions occur for 1-7 days and then progress to crusting and healing. Thoracic and lumbar regions are typically involved. Lesions generally are unilateral and are accompanied by regional lymphadenopathy. In one third of patients, a few vesicles occur outside the primary dermatome. Any branch of cranial nerve V may be involved, which also may cause corneal and intraoral lesions. Involvement of cranial nerve VII may result in facial paralysis and ear canal vesicles **(Ramsay Hunt syndrome).** Ophthalmic zoster may be associated with ipsilateral cerebral angiitis and stroke. Immunocompromised persons may have unusually severe, painful herpes zoster that involves cutaneous and, rarely, visceral dissemination (to liver, lungs, and central nervous system). **Postherpetic neuralgia,** defined as pain persisting longer than 1 month, is uncommon in children.

Laboratory and Imaging Studies

Laboratory testing confirmation for diagnosis is usually unnecessary. PCR is the current diagnostic method of choice, and genotyping to distinguish vaccine and wild-type strains is available through the CDC. Detection of varicella-specific antigen in vesicular fluid by immunofluorescence using monoclonal antibodies or demonstration of a fourfold antibody increase of acute and convalescent sera is also diagnostic but not as sensitive as PCR.

Differential Diagnosis

The diagnosis of varicella and zoster is based on the distinctive characteristics of the rash. **Eczema herpeticum,** or **Kaposi**

varicelliform eruption, is a localized, vesicular eruption caused by herpes simplex virus (HSV) that develops on skin affected by underlying eczema or trauma. The differentiation between zoster and HSV infection may be difficult because HSV may cause eruption that appears to be in a dermatomal distribution. Coxsackievirus A infection has a vesiculopustular appearance, but lesions are usually localized to the extremities and oropharynx. A previously healthy patient with more than one recurrence probably has the HSV infection, which can be confirmed by viral culture or PCR.

Treatment

Symptomatic therapy of varicella includes nonaspirin antipyretics, cool baths, and careful hygiene. Routine oral administration of acyclovir is not recommended in otherwise healthy children with varicella. The decision to use antiviral medications, the route, and the duration of treatment depend on host factors and the risk for severe infection or complications. Early therapy with antivirals (especially within 24 hours of rash onset) in immunocompromised persons is effective in preventing severe complications, including pneumonia, encephalitis, and death from varicella. Acyclovir or valacyclovir may be considered in those at risk of severe varicella, such as unvaccinated persons older than 12 years; those with chronic cutaneous or pulmonary disease; receiving short-course, intermittent, or aerosolized corticosteroids; or receiving long-term salicylate therapy. The dose of acyclovir used for VZV infections is much higher than that for HSV.

Antiviral treatment of zoster accelerates cutaneous healing, hastens the resolution of acute neuritis, and reduces the risk of postherpetic neuralgia. Oral famciclovir and valacyclovir have much greater oral bioavailability than acyclovir and are recommended for treatment of zoster in adults. Acyclovir is recommended for children and is an alternative therapy for adults.

Complications and Prognosis

Secondary infection of skin lesions by streptococci or staphylococci is the most common complication. These infections may be mild, resembling impetigo, or life-threatening with toxic shock syndrome or necrotizing fasciitis. Pneumonia is uncommon in healthy children but occurs in 15-20% of healthy adults and immunocompromised persons. Myocarditis, pericarditis, orchitis, hepatitis, ulcerative gastritis, glomerulonephritis, and arthritis may complicate varicella. Reye syndrome may follow varicella; thus salicylate use is contraindicated during varicella infection.

Neurological complications frequently include postinfectious encephalitis, cerebellar ataxia, nystagmus, and tremor. Less common neurological complications include Guillain-Barré syndrome, transverse myelitis, cranial nerve palsies, optic neuritis, and hypothalamic syndrome.

Primary varicella can be a fatal disease in immunocompromised persons as a result of visceral dissemination, encephalitis, hepatitis, and pneumonitis. The mortality rate approaches 15% in children with leukemia who do not receive prophylaxis or therapy for varicella (see Chapter 72).

A severe form of neonatal varicella may develop in newborns of mothers with primary varicella (but not shingles) occurring 5 days before to 2 days after delivery. The fetus is exposed to a large inoculum of virus, but is born before the maternal antibody response develops and can cross the placenta. These infants should be treated as soon as possible with varicella-zoster immunoglobulin (VZIG) or intravenous immunoglobulin if VZIG is unavailable, to attempt to prevent or ameliorate the infection.

Primary varicella usually resolves spontaneously. The mortality rate is much higher for persons older than 20 years of age and for immunocompromised persons. Zoster usually is self-limited, especially in children. Advanced age and severity of pain at presentation and at 1 month are predictors of prolonged pain. Scarring is more common with zoster because of the involvement of the deeper layers of the skin.

Prevention

Children with chickenpox should not return to school until all vesicles have crusted. A hospitalized child with chickenpox and immunocompromised patients with zoster should be isolated in a negative-pressure room to prevent transmission. Zoster transmission can be minimized by covering the affected area.

A live, two-dose attenuated varicella vaccine is recommended for all children. The first dose should be administered at age 12-15 months and the second dose at 4-6 years. The varicella vaccine is 85% effective in preventing any disease and 97% effective in preventing moderately severe and severe disease. Transmission of vaccine virus from a healthy vaccinated individual is rare but possible.

Passive immunity can be provided by VZIG, which is indicated within 96 hours of exposure for susceptible individuals at increased risk for severe illness, such as immunocompromised children and some hospitalized preterm infants. Administration of VZIG does not eliminate the possibility of disease in recipients and prolongs the incubation period up to 28 days.

CHAPTER 98

Cutaneous Infections

SUPERFICIAL BACTERIAL INFECTIONS

Impetigo

Decision-Making Algorithms
Available @ StudentConsult.com

Vesicles and Bullae
Fever and Rash

Nonbullous or crusted impetigo is caused most often by *Staphylococcus aureus* and occasionally by group A streptococcus. It begins as a single erythematous papulovesicle that progresses to one or many **honey-colored, crusted lesions** weeping serous drainage. **Bullous impetigo** accounts for approximately 10% of all impetigo. The skin lesions are thin-walled (0.5-3 cm) bullae with erythematous margins resembling second-degree burns, and are associated with *S. aureus* phage type 71. Impetigo most frequently occurs on the face, around the nares and mouth, and on the extremities. Fever is uncommon. The diagnosis usually is established by the clinical appearance alone.

Recommended treatment for nonbullous impetigo is topical 2% mupirocin or oral antistaphylococcal antibiotics. Extensive or disseminated lesions, bullous impetigo, lesions around the eyes, or lesions otherwise not amenable to topical therapy are best treated with oral antibiotics. Streptococcal impetigo is associated with increased risk of postinfectious glomerulonephritis, but not acute rheumatic fever (see Chapter 163). Antibiotic treatment does not decrease the risk of postinfectious glomerulonephritis, but it does decrease the possible spread of nephritogenic strains to close contacts. Children with impetigo should remain out of school or day care until 24 hours of antibiotic therapy have been completed.

Cellulitis

Decision-Making Algorithms
Available @ StudentConsult.com

Red Eye
Extremity Pain

Cellulitis is infection involving the subcutaneous tissues and the dermis and is usually caused by *S. aureus* or group A streptococci. Cellulitis typically presents with indurated, warm, and erythematous macules with indistinct borders that can expand rapidly. Additional manifestations commonly include fever, lymphangitis, and regional lymphadenitis. **Erysipelas** is a superficial variant of cellulitis usually caused by group A streptococcus that involves the dermis only. The rapidly advancing lesions are tender, bright red in appearance, and have sharp margins. The patients may appear toxic. Blood cultures are recommended for erysipelas. Empirical antibiotic treatment for cellulitis is recommended with a first-generation cephalosporin unless the local *S. aureus* methicillin-resistance rate is high, in which case alternatives include clindamycin or trimethoprim-sulfamethoxazole. Many patients may be managed with oral antibiotics and close follow-up; hospitalization and intravenous antibiotics are recommended for erysipelas and cellulitis of the face, hands, feet, or perineum; those with lymphangitis; and those not responding to outpatient therapy.

Ecthyma usually is caused by group A streptococcus and may complicate impetigo. Initially it is characterized by a lesion with a rim of erythematous induration surrounding an eschar, which, if removed, reveals a shallow ulcer. **Ecthyma gangrenosum** is a serious skin infection occurring in immunocompromised persons due to hematogenous spread of septic emboli to the skin, classically caused by *Pseudomonas aeruginosa,* other gram-negative organisms, or occasionally *Aspergillus.* The lesions begin as purple macules that undergo central necrosis to become exquisitely tender, deep, punched-out ulcers 2-3 cm in diameter with a dark necrotic base, raised red edges, and sometimes a yellowish-green exudate. Fever usually is present.

Necrotizing fasciitis is the most extensive form of cellulitis and involves deeper subcutaneous tissues and fascial planes. It may progress to **myonecrosis** of the underlying muscle. Common causes include *S. aureus* and group A streptococcus alone or in combination with anaerobic organisms, such as *Clostridium perfringens.* Risk factors include underlying immunodeficiency, recent surgery or trauma, and varicella infection. Lesions progress rapidly with raised or sharply demarcated margins, although disease typically extends on a deeper plane beyond superficially evident lesions. Warning signs of necrotizing fasciitis include pain out of proportion to evident skin lesions, shock or toxic appearance, or crepitus due to subcutaneous gas formation by anaerobes. Necrotizing fasciitis is a surgical emergency, and early consultation with an experienced surgeon is recommended. Adjunctive tests such as magnetic resonance imaging can confirm the presence of gas in tissues, but obtaining imaging should not delay surgical consultation. Treatment includes rapid surgical debridement of all necrotic tissues and broad-spectrum intravenous antibiotics, such as clindamycin plus cefotaxime or ceftriaxone, with or without an aminoglycoside or vancomycin.

Folliculitis

Folliculitis refers to small, dome-shaped pustules or erythematous papules predominantly caused by *S. aureus* and is located in hair follicles, with superficial, limited inflammatory reaction in the surrounding tissue. **Furuncles (boils)** are deeper hair follicle infections that manifest as nodules with intense surrounding inflammatory reaction. These occur most frequently on the neck, trunk, axillae, and buttocks. A **carbuncle** represents the deepest of hair follicle infections and is characterized by multiseptate, loculated abscesses. Boils and carbuncles frequently require incisional drainage. Superficial folliculitis can be treated with topical therapy, such as an antibacterial chlorhexidine wash or an antibacterial lotion or solution such as clindamycin 1%, applied twice a day for 7-10 days. Oral antibiotics are necessary for unresponsive cases, or for furuncles and carbuncles.

P. aeruginosa folliculitis **(hot tub folliculitis)** presents as pruritic papules; pustules; or deeper, purple-red nodules predominantly on skin areas covered by a swimsuit after bathing in hot tubs. Folliculitis develops 8-48 hours after exposure, usually without associated systemic symptoms, and resolves in 1-2 weeks without treatment.

Perianal Dermatitis

Perianal dermatitis (perianal streptococcal disease) is caused by group A streptococcus and is characterized by well-demarcated, very tender, marked perianal erythema extending 2 cm from the anus. Manifestations include anal pruritus and painful defecation, sometimes with blood-streaked stools. The differential diagnosis includes diaper dermatitis, candidiasis, pinworm infection, and anal fissures. Optimal treatment is oral penicillin or amoxicillin.

SUPERFICIAL FUNGAL INFECTIONS

Decision-Making Algorithms
Available @ StudentConsult.com

Alopecia
Lymphadenopathy

TABLE 98.1 Superficial Fungal Infections

NAME	ETIOLOGY	MANIFESTATIONS	DIAGNOSIS	THERAPY
Dermatophytes				
Tinea capitis (ringworm)	*Microsporum audouinii, Trichophyton tonsurans, Microsporum canis*	Prepubertal infection of scalp, hair-shafts; *black dot* alopecia; *T. tonsurans* common in African Americans	*M. audouinii* fluorescence: blue-green with Wood lamp*; +KOH, culture	Griseofulvin; terbinafine, itraconazole
Kerion	Inflammatory reaction to tinea capitis	Swollen, boggy, crusted, purulent, tender mass with lymphadenopathy; secondary distal *id* reaction common	As above	As above, plus steroids for *id* reactions
Tinea corporis (ringworm)	*M. canis, Trichophyton rubrum,* others	Slightly pruritic ringlike, erythematous papules, plaques with scaling and slow outward expansion of the border; check cat or dog for *M. canis*	+KOH, culture; *M. canis* fluorescence: blue-green with Wood lamp; differential diagnosis: granuloma annulare, pityriasis rosea, nummular eczema, psoriasis	Topical miconazole, clotrimazole, terbinafine, tolnaftate, ciclopirox, oxiconazole, or butenafine
Tinea cruris (jock itch)	*Epidermophyton floccosum, Trichophyton mentagrophytes, T. rubrum*	Symmetric, pruritic, scrotal sparing, scaling plaques	+KOH, culture; differential diagnosis: erythrasma *(Corynebacterium minutissimum)*	See Tinea corporis, Therapy; wear loose cotton underwear
Tinea pedis (athlete's foot)	*T. rubrum, T. mentagrophytes*	Moccasin or interdigital distribution, dry scales, interdigital maceration with secondary bacterial infection	+KOH, culture; differential diagnosis: *C. minutissimum* erythrasma	Medications as above; wear cotton socks
Tinea unguium (onychomycosis)	*T. mentagrophytes, T. rubrum, Candida albicans*	Uncommon before puberty; peeling of distal nail plate; thickening, splitting of nails	+KOH, culture	Oral terbinafine or itraconazole
Tinea versicolor	*Malassezia furfur*	Tropical climates, steroids or immunosuppressive drugs; uncommon before puberty; chest, back, arms; oval hypopigmented or hyperpigmented in African Americans, red-brown in Caucasians; scaling patches	+KOH; orange-gold fluorescence with Wood lamp; differential diagnosis: pityriasis alba	Topical selenium sulfide, oral ketoconazole
Yeast				
Candidiasis	*C. albicans*	Diaper area, intense erythematous plaques or pustules, isolated or confluent	+KOH, culture	Topical nystatin; oral nystatin treats concomitant oral thrush

**Wood lamp examination uses an ultraviolet source in a completely darkened room.* Trichophyton *usually has no fluorescence.*
KOH, Potassium hydroxide.

Cutaneous fungal infections are common in children (Table 98.1). The estimated lifetime risk of developing a **dermatophytosis** is 10-20%. Diagnosis is usually established by visual inspection and may be confirmed by potassium hydroxide (KOH) examination or fungal culture of skin scrapings from the margins of the lesion. **Recommended tinea treatment** is usually for 4-6 weeks and 2 weeks after resolution; topical antifungal creams (e.g., miconazole, clotrimazole, ketoconazole, tolnaftate) are appropriate for tinea corporis, tinea pedis, and tinea cruris, whereas tinea capitis requires oral treatment. The diagnosis of **onychomycosis** should be confirmed by KOH examination and fungal culture. Recommended treatment is terbinafine or itraconazole for at least 12 weeks.

SUPERFICIAL VIRAL INFECTIONS

Herpes Simplex Virus

Decision-Making Algorithms
Available @ StudentConsult.com

Sore Throat
Vaginal Discharge
Seizures and Other Paroxysmal Disorders
Vesicles and Bullae
Fever and Rash
Lymphadenopathy

Primary herpetic infections can occur after inoculation of the virus at any mucocutaneous site. Herpes simplex virus type 1 (HSV-1) is common in children and classically causes gingivostomatitis, whereas HSV-2 classically infects the genitalia as a sexually transmitted infection (see Chapter 116), though HSV-1 may cause approximately 30% of genital herpes, and HSV-2 can cause gingivostomatitis. For the cutaneous manifestations of neonatal HSV infection, see Chapter 65.

Herpes gingivostomatitis involves the gingivae and the vermilion border of the lips. Herpes labialis **(cold sores or fever blisters)** is limited to the vermilion border involving skin and mucous membranes. Clinical manifestations of primary HSV gingivostomatitis include typical oropharyngeal vesicular lesions with high fever, malaise, stinging mouth pain, drooling, fetid breath, and cervical lymphadenopathy.

Herpetic skin lesions are quite painful and characteristically begin as erythematous papules that quickly progress to the characteristically grouped, 2-4 mm, fluid-filled vesicles on an erythematous base. Removal of the vesicle roof reveals a small, sharply demarcated ulcer with a punched-out appearance. The characteristic grouped vesicles distinguish HSV from chickenpox (see Chapter 97). Within several days, the vesicles become pustular, rupture, and encrust. Diagnosis is made clinically, or with viral culture, fluorescent antibody staining, or most often polymerase chain reaction. Scarring is uncommon, but there may be residual hyperpigmentation. After primary infection, the virus remains latent in nerve dorsal root ganglia. About 20-40% of adults experience recurrent oral episodes of HSV labialis throughout life. Recurrences occur in roughly the same location and may be preceded by prodromal symptoms of tingling or burning without fever or lymphadenopathy.

Viral paronychia **(herpetic whitlow)** is a painful, localized infection of a digit, usually of the distal pulp space, with erythematous and occasionally vesiculopustular eruption. It occurs in children who suck their thumbs, bite their nails, and those with herpetic gingivostomatitis. **Herpes gladiatorum** occurs in wrestlers and rugby players who acquire cutaneous herpes from close body contact with other players' cutaneous infections. Cutaneous HSV infection in persons with an underlying skin disorder (e.g., atopic dermatitis) can result in **eczema herpeticum (Kaposi varicelliform eruption),** a disseminated cutaneous infection. There may be hundreds of herpetic vesicles over the body, usually concentrated in the areas of skin affected by the underlying disorder.

Treatment with oral valacyclovir or famciclovir may shorten duration of disease for primary and recurrent infection. Prophylactic antiviral therapy may be warranted in those with frequent recurrences. Neonates, persons with eczema, and persons with immunodeficiency are at increased risk for disseminated and severe HSV disease and should receive intravenous acyclovir therapy.

Human Papillomaviruses (Warts)

Decision-Making Algorithms
Available @ StudentConsult.com

Hoarseness
Vaginal Discharge

Warts are caused by the human papillomaviruses (HPVs), nonenveloped, double-stranded DNA viruses that infect skin and mucous membrane keratinocytes. More than 100 HPV serotypes have been identified, with different serotypes accounting for the variation in location and clinical presentations. There are 15-20 **oncogenic (high-risk)** types, including 16, 18, 31, 33, 35, 39, 45, 51, 52, and 58. HPV types 16 and 18 are associated with 70% of cases of cervical cancer as well as vulvar and vaginal cancers. Common **nononcogenic (low-risk)** types include 1, 2, 3, 6, 10, 11, 40, 42, 43, 44, and 54. Regardless of the infecting serotype, all warts are associated with hyperplasia of the epidermal cells.

Warts occur at all ages. **Common warts (verruca vulgaris),** associated with HPV types 1 and 2, are the most frequent form (71%). They occur in school-age children, with a prevalence of 4-20%. They are transmitted by direct contact or by fomites and have an incubation period of approximately 1 month before clinical presentation. The common wart is a painless, well-circumscribed, small (2-5 mm) papule with a papillated or verrucous surface typically distributed on the fingers, toes, elbows, and knees. They also may be found on the nose, ears, and lips. **Filiform warts** are verrucous, exophytic, 2-mm papules that have a narrow or pedunculated base. **Flat warts (verruca plana)** are associated with HPV types 3 and 10 and are multiple, flat-topped 2-4-mm papules clustered on the dorsal surface of the hands, on the soles of the feet **(plantar warts),** or on the face. Plantar warts may be painful because of the effect of pressure and friction on the lesions. **Genital warts (condylomata acuminata)** are associated with the HPV types 6 and 11 (90%). They are flesh-colored, hyperpigmented, or erythematous lesions that are filiform, fungating, or plaque-like in appearance and involve multiple sites on the vulva, vagina, penis, or perineum. Genital warts are the most common sexually transmitted infection, with 1 million new cases annually.

Warts typically are self-limited and resolve spontaneously over years without specific treatment. Treatment options are available for common and flat warts as well as condylomata acuminata. Topical preparations for common and flat warts disrupt infected epithelium (using salicylic acid, liquid nitrogen, or laser therapy) and result in the cure of approximately 75% of patients. Treatment of anogenital warts requires assessment of size, number, patient preference, cost, convenience, and adverse effects. Medications may include topical podophyllotoxin or imiquimod. Additional treatment methods include laser ablation and immunotherapy with intralesional interferon; immunotherapy may result in significant toxicities.

The most serious consequence of HPV infection is **cervical cancer** (more than 12,000 new cases annually) as well as vulvar, vaginal, penile, anal, and head and neck cancers. Three main recombinant HPV vaccines are available. A quadrivalent vaccine against serotypes 6, 11, 31, and 33 was licensed in 2006 for use in all children and adults between 9 and 26 years of age. A 9-valent vaccine protecting against serotypes 6, 11, 16, 18, 31, 33, 45, 52, and 58 was licensed in 2014 for use in females 9 through 26 years and males 9 through 15 years. A bivalent vaccine against serotypes 16 and 18 is also available for females only. The three-dose regimen of these vaccines has >98% efficacy in preventing the precancerous dysplasia that precedes cervical cancer.

Molluscum Contagiosum

Molluscum contagiosum virus, a poxvirus that replicates in host epithelial cells, produces discrete, small (2-4 mm), pearly flesh-colored or pink, nontender, dome-shaped papules with central umbilication. Papules occur most commonly in intertriginous regions, such as the axillae, groin, and neck. They rarely occur on the face or in the periocular region. The infection typically affects toddlers and young children and is acquired through direct contact with infected individuals. Spread occurs by autoinoculation. Infection with molluscum contagiosum may be complicated by a surrounding dermatitis. Severely immunocompromised persons or persons with extensive atopic dermatitis often have widespread lesions.

Diagnosis is clinical. Lesions are self-limited, resolving over months to years, and usually no specific treatment is recommended. Available treatment options are limited to destructive modalities, such as cryotherapy with topical liquid nitrogen, vesicant therapy with topical 0.9% cantharidin, or removal by curettage, and should be reserved for extensive disease.

CHAPTER 99

Lymphadenopathy

ETIOLOGY

Decision-Making Algorithm
Available @ StudentConsult.com

Lymphadenopathy

TABLE 99.1 Infectious Causes of Generalized Lymphadenopathy

VIRAL
Epstein-Barr virus (infectious mononucleosis)
Cytomegalovirus (infectious mononucleosis-like syndrome)
HIV (acute retroviral syndrome)
Hepatitis B virus
Hepatitis C virus
Varicella
Adenoviruses
Rubeola (measles)
Rubella
BACTERIAL
Endocarditis
Brucella (brucellosis)
Leptospira interrogans (leptospirosis)
Streptobacillus moniliformis (bacillary rat-bite fever)
Mycobacterium tuberculosis (tuberculosis)
Treponema pallidum (secondary syphilis)
FUNGAL
Coccidioides immitis (coccidioidomycosis)
Histoplasma capsulatum (histoplasmosis)
PROTOZOAL
Toxoplasma gondii (toxoplasmosis)
Trypanosoma cruzi (Chagas disease)

Lymphoid tissue steadily enlarges until puberty and subsequently undergoes progressive atrophy. Lymph nodes are most prominent in children 4-8 years of age. Normal lymph node size is 10 mm in diameter, with the exceptions of 15 mm for inguinal nodes, 5 mm for epitrochlear nodes, and 2 mm for supraclavicular nodes, which are usually not palpable. **Lymphadenopathy** is enlargement of lymph nodes and occurs in response to a wide variety of infectious, inflammatory, and malignant processes. **Generalized lymphadenopathy** is enlargement of two or more noncontiguous lymph node groups, whereas **regional lymphadenopathy** involves one lymph node group only.

Lymphadenitis is acute or chronic inflammation of lymph nodes. Acute lymphadenitis usually results when bacteria and toxins from a site of acute inflammation are carried via lymph to regional nodes. Numerous infections cause lymphadenopathy and lymphadenitis (Tables 99.1 and 99.2). Causes of inguinal regional lymphadenopathy also include sexually transmitted infections (see Chapter 116). Regional lymphadenitis associated with a characteristic skin lesion at the site of inoculation defines various **lymphocutaneous syndromes**. **Lymphangitis** is an inflammation of subcutaneous lymphatic channels that presents as an acute bacterial infection, usually caused by *Staphylococcus aureus* and group A streptococci.

Cervical lymphadenitis is the most common regional lymphadenitis among children and is associated most commonly with pharyngitis caused by group A streptococcus (see Chapter 103), respiratory viruses, and Epstein-Barr virus (EBV). Other common infectious causes of cervical lymphadenitis include *Bartonella henselae* (cat-scratch disease) and nontuberculous mycobacteria; tularemia, endemic mycoses, *Nocardia*, and *Actinomyces* are less common causes.

EPIDEMIOLOGY

Acute cervical lymphadenitis as a complication of group A streptococcal infection parallels the incidence of streptococcal pharyngitis (see Chapter 103). Many cases are caused by *S. aureus*. EBV and cytomegalovirus (CMV) are ubiquitous, with most infections occurring in young children, who may often be asymptomatic or only mildly symptomatic. Risk factors for other specific causes of lymphadenopathy may be indicated by past medical and surgical history; preceding trauma; exposure to animals; contact with persons infected with tuberculosis; sexual history; travel history; food and ingestion history, especially of undercooked meat or unpasteurized dairy products; and current medications.

CLINICAL MANIFESTATIONS

The exact location and detailed measurement of the size, shape, characteristics, and number of involved nodes should be noted, including their consistency, mobility, tenderness, warmth, fluctuance, firmness, and adherence to adjacent tissues.

TABLE 99.2 Infectious Causes of Regional Lymphadenopathy
NONVENEREAL ORIGIN
Staphylococcus aureus
Group A streptococcus
Group B streptococcus (in infants)
Bartonella henselae (cat-scratch disease)
Yersinia pestis (plague)
Francisella tularensis (glandular tularemia)
Mycobacterium tuberculosis
Nontuberculous mycobacteria
Sporothrix schenckii (sporotrichosis)
Epstein-Barr virus
Toxoplasma gondii
SEXUALLY TRANSMITTED INFECTIONS (PRIMARILY INGUINAL LYMPHADENOPATHY)
Neisseria gonorrhoeae (gonorrhea)
Treponema pallidum (syphilis)
Herpes simplex virus
Haemophilus ducreyi (chancroid)
Chlamydia trachomatis serovars L_{1-3} (lymphogranuloma venereum)
LYMPHOCUTANEOUS SYNDROMES
Bacillus anthracis (anthrax)
F. tularensis (ulceroglandular tularemia)
B. henselae (cat-scratch disease)
Pasteurella multocida (dog or cat bite)
Rickettsialpox
Spirillum minus (spirillary rat-bite fever)
Y. pestis (plague)
Nocardia (nocardiosis)
Cutaneous diphtheria (*Corynebacterium diphtheriae*)
Cutaneous coccidioidomycosis (*Coccidioides immitis*)
Cutaneous histoplasmosis (*Histoplasma capsulatum*)
Cutaneous leishmaniasis
Cutaneous sporotrichosis (*S. schenckii*)
Tinea capitis

Important findings include presence or absence of dental disease, oropharyngeal or skin lesions, ocular disease, other nodal enlargement, and any other signs of systemic illness, including hepatosplenomegaly and skin lesions.

Acute cervical lymphadenopathy associated with pharyngitis is characterized by small and rubbery lymph nodes in the anterior cervical chain with minimal to moderate tenderness. **Suppurative cervical lymphadenitis**, frequently caused by *S. aureus* or group A streptococcus, shows erythema and warmth of the overlying skin with moderate to exquisite tenderness.

EBV is the primary cause of **infectious mononucleosis,** a clinical syndrome characterized by fever, fatigue and malaise, cervical or generalized lymphadenopathy, tonsillitis, and pharyngitis. The pharynx shows enlarged tonsils and exudate and, sometimes, an enanthem with pharyngeal petechiae. Lymphadenopathy is most prominent in the anterior and posterior cervical and submandibular lymph nodes and less commonly involves axillary and inguinal lymph nodes. Other findings include splenomegaly in 50% of cases, hepatomegaly in 10-20%, and maculopapular or urticarial rash in 5-15%. A diffuse, erythematous rash develops in approximately 80% of mononucleosis patients treated with amoxicillin. EBV, a member of the herpesvirus family, infects B lymphocytes and is spread by salivary secretions. After primary infection, EBV is maintained latently in multiple episomes in the cell nucleus of resting B lymphocytes and establishes a lifelong infection that remains clinically inapparent. Most persons shed EBV intermittently, with approximately 20% of healthy individuals shedding EBV at any given time.

CMV, *Toxoplasma gondii,* adenoviruses, hepatitis B virus, hepatitis C virus, and acute HIV infection, also known as **acute retroviral syndrome,** can cause an infectious mononucleosis-like syndrome with lymphadenopathy. Compared with EBV infection, infectious mononucleosis-like illness caused by CMV has minimal pharyngitis and often more prominent splenomegaly; it often presents with fever only. The most common manifestation of toxoplasmosis is asymptomatic cervical lymphadenopathy, but approximately 10% of cases of acquired toxoplasmosis develop chronic posterior cervical lymphadenopathy and fatigue, usually without significant fever.

The cause of **cat-scratch disease** is *B. henselae,* a small, pleomorphic, gram-negative bacillus that stains with Warthin-Starry silver stain. *B. henselae* causes apparently asymptomatic bacteremia in cats; kittens under 1 year of age are more likely to harbor the organism. *B. henselae* is transmitted to humans by bites and scratches, which may be minor. *B. henselae* also causes bacillary angiomatosis and peliosis hepatis in persons with HIV infection (see Chapter 125). Cat-scratch disease typically presents with a cutaneous papule or conjunctival granuloma at the site of bacterial inoculation, followed by lymphadenopathy of the draining regional nodes. The nodes are tender with suppuration in approximately 10% of cases. Lymphadenopathy may persist 1-4 months. Less common features of cat-scratch disease include erythema nodosum, osteolytic lesions, encephalitis, oculoglandular (Parinaud) syndrome, hepatic or splenic granulomas, endocarditis, polyneuritis, and transverse myelitis.

Lymphadenitis caused by **nontuberculous mycobacteria** usually is unilateral in the cervical, submandibular, or preauricular nodes and is more common in toddlers. The nodes are relatively painless and firm initially, but gradually soften, rupture, and drain over time. The local reaction is circumscribed, and overlying skin may develop a violaceous discoloration without warmth. Fever and systemic symptoms are minimal or absent. Nontuberculous mycobacteria are ubiquitous in soil, vegetation, dust, and water. *Mycobacterium* species commonly causing lymphadenitis in children includes *M. avium* complex, *M. scrofulaceum,* and *M. kansasii. M. tuberculosis* uncommonly causes cervical lymphadenitis.

LABORATORY AND IMAGING STUDIES

Initial laboratory tests of regional lymphadenopathy include a complete blood count and inflammatory markers. Infectious mononucleosis is characterized by lymphocytosis with **atypical lymphocytes**; thrombocytopenia and elevated hepatic enzymes are common.

Cultures of infected skin lesions and tonsillar exudates should be obtained. Isolation of group A streptococci from the oropharynx suggests, but does not confirm, streptococcal cervical lymphadenitis. A blood culture should be obtained from children with systemic signs and symptoms of bacteremia.

Serological testing (or polymerase chain reaction) for EBV and for *B. henselae* should be obtained if there are appropriate findings. The most reliable test for diagnosis of acute EBV infection is the IgM antiviral capsid antigen (Fig. 99.1). Heterophil antibody is also diagnostic but is not reliably positive in children younger than 4 years with infectious mononucleosis.

Extended diagnostic work-up for lymphadenopathy is guided by the specific risk factors in the history and physical examination findings. Chest radiograph, throat culture, antistreptolysin O titer, and serological tests for CMV, HIV, toxoplasmosis, syphilis, tularemia, *Brucella,* histoplasmosis, and coccidioidomycosis may be indicated. Genital tract evaluation and specimens should be obtained with regional inguinal lymphadenopathy (see Chapter 116). Screening for tuberculosis can be performed using the standard tuberculin skin test or an interferon-gamma release assay; both may be positive with atypical mycobacterial infection.

Aspiration is indicated for acutely inflamed, fluctuant cervical lymph nodes, especially those larger than 3 cm in diameter or not responding to antibiotic treatment. Ultrasound or computed tomography may help in establishing the extent of lymphadenopathy and defining whether the mass is solid, cystic, or suppurative with abscess formation. Pus from fluctuant lesions should be examined by Gram and acid-fast stains and cultured for aerobic and anaerobic bacteria and mycobacteria. Biopsy should be performed if **lymphoma** is suspected because of firm, matted, nontender nodes and other systemic findings.

If the diagnosis remains uncertain and lymphadenopathy persists despite empirical antibiotic therapy for presumed *S. aureus* and group A streptococcus, excisional biopsy of the entire node should be performed, if possible. This is curative for nontuberculous mycobacterial lymphadenitis. Biopsy material should be submitted for histopathology as well as Gram, acid-fast, Giemsa, periodic acid-Schiff, Warthin-Starry silver (*B. henselae*), and methenamine silver stains. Cultures for aerobic and anaerobic bacteria, mycobacteria, and fungi should be performed.

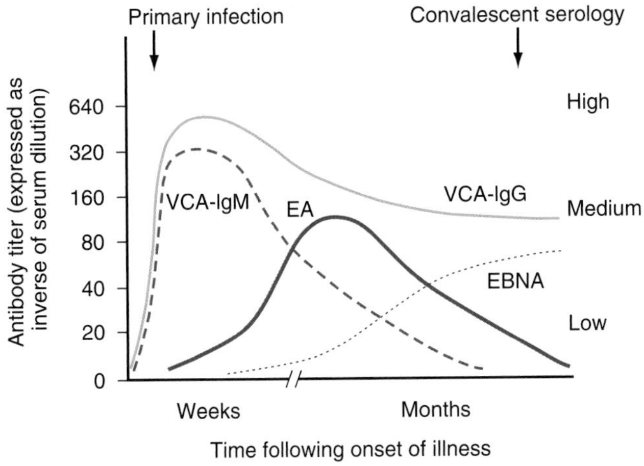

FIGURE 99.1 Idealized time course for the development of antibody to different Epstein-Barr virus antigens after primary infection with the virus. *IgM*, Immunoglobulin M; *VCA*, viral capsid antigen. (From Katz BZ. Epstein-Barr Virus [Mononucleosis and Lymphoproliferative Disorders]. In: Long SS, Pickering LK, Prober CG, eds. *Principles and Practice of Pediatric Infectious* Diseases. 4th ed. Philadelphia: Elsevier; 2012. Fig. 208-3.)

DIFFERENTIAL DIAGNOSIS

Noninfectious causes of cervical swelling and/or lymphadenopathy include congenital and acquired cysts, Kawasaki disease, autoimmune diseases (e.g., sarcoidosis or Kikuchi-Fujimoto disease), benign neoplasms, and malignancies. The differential diagnosis for generalized lymphadenopathy includes juvenile idiopathic arthritis; systemic lupus erythematosus; and serum sickness and other adverse drug reactions, especially with phenytoin and other antiepileptic medications, allopurinol, isoniazid, antithyroid medications, and pyrimethamine. Leukemia, lymphoma, and occasionally neuroblastoma may have lymph nodes that are usually painless, uninflamed, matted, and firm (see Chapters 155 and 156). A syndrome of **periodic fever, aphthous stomatitis, pharyngitis, and adenitis** is an occasional cause of recurrent fever and cervical lymphadenitis (see Chapter 103).

TREATMENT

Management of *lymphadenopathy* and *lymphadenitis* depends on patient age, associated findings, node size and location, and severity of the acute systemic symptoms. In children, most cases of cervical lymphadenopathy, without other signs of acute inflammation, require no specific therapy and usually regress within 2-3 weeks. Progression to lymphadenitis or development of generalized lymphadenopathy requires further evaluation.

The specific treatment of cervical lymphadenitis depends on the underlying etiology. Empirical treatment targeting *S. aureus* and group A streptococcus includes a penicillinase-resistant penicillin (e.g., oxacillin) or first-generation cephalosporin (e.g., cefazolin). For patients with hypersensitivity to β-lactam antibiotics, or if community-acquired methicillin-resistant *S. aureus* is suspected, clindamycin is appropriate. Response to empirical antibiotic therapy for suppurative cervical lymphadenitis obviates the need for further evaluation. Absence of a clinical response within 48-72 hours is an indication for further laboratory evaluation and possible excisional biopsy and culture.

There is no specific treatment for infectious mononucleosis. Cat-scratch disease usually does not require treatment because the lymphadenopathy resolves in 2-4 months without sequelae. Azithromycin may hasten resolution and reduces node size at 30 days, but no benefit is evident at 90 days. Aspiration and drainage are indicated for suppurative nodes. The recommended treatment of cervical lymphadenitis caused by nontuberculous mycobacteria is complete surgical excision. Antimycobacterial drugs are necessary only if there is recurrence or inability to excise infected nodes completely, or if *M. tuberculosis* is identified, which requires 6 months of antituberculous chemotherapy (see Chapter 124).

COMPLICATIONS AND PROGNOSIS

Most acute infections caused by *S. aureus* and group A streptococcus respond to treatment and have an excellent prognosis. Complications such as abscess formation, cellulitis, and bacteremia may occur. Abscess formation is treated with incision and drainage in conjunction with appropriate antibiotic therapy.

Infectious mononucleosis usually resolves in 2-4 weeks, but fatigue and malaise may wax and wane for several weeks to months. EBV also is associated with numerous complications during the acute illness. Neurological complications include seizures, aseptic meningitis syndrome, Bell palsy, transverse myelitis, encephalitis, and Guillain-Barré syndrome. Hematological complications include Coombs-positive hemolytic anemia, antibody-mediated thrombocytopenia, hemophagocytic syndrome, and, rarely, aplastic anemia. Corticosteroids have been used for respiratory compromise resulting from tonsillar hypertrophy, which responds rapidly, and for thrombocytopenia, hemolytic anemia, and neurological complications. Splenic rupture is very rare. **X-linked lymphoproliferative disease,** which results from a mutation of the *SH2D1A* gene located in the Xq25 region, manifests as fulminant infectious mononucleosis with primary EBV infection, and progresses to malignant lymphoproliferative disease or dysgammaglobulinemia.

EBV infection, as with other herpesviruses, persists for life, but no symptoms are attributed to intermittent reactivation in immunocompetent hosts. EBV is causally associated with nasopharyngeal carcinoma; Burkitt lymphoma; Hodgkin disease; leiomyosarcoma in immunocompromised persons; and EBV lymphoproliferative disease, especially in posttransplant patients and in those with acquired immunodeficiency syndrome (AIDS).

Lymphadenitis caused by nontuberculous mycobacteria has an excellent prognosis. Surgical excision of cervical lymphadenitis caused by nontuberculous mycobacteria is curative in >97% of cases.

PREVENTION

The incidence of suppurative regional lymphadenitis reflects the incidence of predisposing conditions, such as dental disease, streptococcal pharyngitis, otitis media, impetigo, and other infections involving the face and scalp. There are no guidelines to prevent lymphadenitis caused by nontuberculous mycobacteria.

CHAPTER 100

Meningitis

ETIOLOGY

Meningitis, inflammation of the leptomeninges, can be caused by bacteria, viruses, or—rarely—fungi. The term **aseptic meningitis** principally refers to viral meningitis, but meningitis with negative cerebrospinal fluid (CSF) bacterial cultures may be seen with other infectious organisms (Lyme disease, syphilis, tuberculosis), parameningeal infections (brain abscess, epidural abscess, venous sinus empyema), chemical exposure (nonsteroidal antiinflammatory drugs, intravenous immunoglobulin), autoimmune disorders, and other diseases, including Kawasaki disease.

The organisms commonly causing bacterial meningitis (Table 100.1) before the availability of current conjugate vaccines were *Haemophilus influenzae, Streptococcus pneumoniae,* and *Neisseria meningitidis.* In the United States, the rates of *H. influenzae* type b and *S. pneumoniae* meningitis have declined substantially after the introduction of targeted vaccines. The bacteria causing neonatal meningitis are the same as those causing neonatal sepsis (see Chapter 65). In older children, *S. pneumoniae* and *N. meningitidis* remain the most common causes of bacterial meningitis. Staphylococcal meningitis primarily occurs after neurosurgery or penetrating head trauma.

TABLE 100.1 Bacterial Causes of Meningitis

AGE	MOST COMMON	LESS COMMON
Neonatal	Group B streptococcus *Escherichia coli* Other enteric gram-negative bacilli	*Listeria monocytogenes* *Enterococcus faecalis* *Neisseria meningitidis* *Streptococcus pneumoniae* Other Streptococci *Citrobacter species* *Salmonella* *Pseudomonas aeruginosa* *Haemophilus influenzae* *Staphylococcus aureus* (NICU only)
>1-3 months	*S. pneumoniae* Gram-negative bacilli Group B streptococcus	*N. meningitidis*
>3 months	*S. pneumoniae* *Neisseria meningitidis*	Gram-negative bacilli Group B streptococcus

NICU, Neonatal intensive care unit.

Partially treated meningitis refers to bacterial meningitis complicated by antibiotic treatment before the lumbar puncture (LP), which may result in negative CSF cultures, although other CSF findings suggestive of bacterial infection persist. In this case, the etiology can sometimes be confirmed by polymerase chain reaction (PCR) of the CSF.

The most common viruses causing meningitis are enteroviruses and parechoviruses. Other viruses that can cause meningitis include herpes simplex virus (HSV), Epstein-Barr virus (EBV), cytomegalovirus (CMV), lymphocytic choriomeningitis virus (LCMV), many arboviruses (see Chapter 101), and human immunodeficiency virus (HIV). The mumps virus can cause meningitis in unvaccinated children. Less frequent infectious causes of meningitis include *Borrelia burgdorferi* (Lyme disease), *Bartonella henselae* (cat-scratch disease), *Mycobacterium tuberculosis, Toxoplasma,* fungi *(Cryptococcus, Histoplasma, Blastomycosis,* and *Coccidioides),* and parasites *(Angiostrongylus cantonensis, Naegleria fowleri,* and *Acanthamoeba).*

EPIDEMIOLOGY

The incidence of bacterial meningitis is highest among children under 1 year of age, especially infants <2 months. Extremely high rates are found in Native Americans, Alaskan Natives, and Australian aboriginals, suggesting that genetic factors play a role in susceptibility. Other risk factors include acquired or congenital immunodeficiencies, functional or anatomical asplenia, cochlear implantation, penetrating head trauma, recent neurosurgical procedure, and crowding, such as that which occurs in some daycare centers or college and military dormitories. A CSF leak (fistula), resulting from congenital anomaly or following a basilar skull fracture, increases the risk of meningitis, especially that caused by *S. pneumoniae.*

Enteroviruses and parechoviruses cause meningitis with peaks during summer and fall in temperate climates. These infections are more prevalent among infants and school-age children and immunocompromised persons. The prevalence of arboviral meningitis or encephalitis is determined by geographic distribution and seasonal activity of the arthropod (mosquito) vectors. In the United States, most arboviral infections occur during the summer and fall.

CLINICAL MANIFESTATIONS

Decision-Making Algorithms
Available @ StudentConsult.com

Apnea
Stiff or Painful Neck
Headaches
Hearing Loss
Fever Without a Source
Irritable Infant

Preceding upper respiratory tract symptoms may occur; however, rapid onset is typical of infections with *S. pneumoniae* and *N. meningitidis.* Indications of meningeal inflammation include headache, irritability, nausea, nuchal rigidity, lethargy, photophobia, and vomiting. Fever is usually present. Kernig and Brudzinski signs of meningeal irritation are often positive in children older than 12 months. In young infants, signs of meningeal inflammation may be minimal with only irritability, depressed mental status, and/or poor feeding present. Focal neurological signs, seizures, arthralgia, myalgia, petechial or purpuric lesions, sepsis, shock, and coma may occur. Symptoms of increased intracranial pressure include headache, diplopia, and vomiting; a bulging fontanelle may be present in infants. Papilledema is uncommon unless there is occlusion of the venous sinuses, subdural empyema, or brain abscess.

LABORATORY AND IMAGING STUDIES

If bacterial meningitis is suspected, a LP should be performed unless there is evidence of cardiovascular instability or of increased intracranial pressure (due to the risk of herniation). Routine CSF examination includes a white blood cell count with differential, protein and glucose levels, and Gram stain (Table 100.2). CSF should be cultured for bacteria and, when appropriate, fungi and mycobacteria. PCR is used to diagnose

TABLE 100.2 Cerebrospinal Fluid Findings in Various Central Nervous System Disorders

CONDITION	PRESSURE (cm H_2O)	LEUKOCYTES (cells/μL)	PROTEIN (mg/dL)	GLUCOSE (mg/dL)	COMMENTS
Normal	10-20	<5; 60-70% lymphocytes, 30-40% monocytes, 1-3% neutrophils	20-45	>50% of serum glucose	WBC up to 10-20 cells/μL can be normal in neonates
Acute bacterial meningitis	Usually elevated (>25)	>100; usually thousands; PMNs predominate	100-500	Usually <40 or <40% of serum glucose	Organisms may be seen on Gram stain and recovered by culture
Partially treated bacterial meningitis	Normal or elevated	1-10,000; PMNs usual but mononuclear cells may predominate if pretreated for extended period	>100	Depressed or normal	Organisms may be seen; pretreatment may render CSF sterile but bacteria may be detected by PCR
Tuberculous meningitis	Usually elevated; may be low because of CSF block in advanced stages	10-500; PMNs early but lymphocytes and monocytes predominate later	100-500; may be higher in presence of CSF block	Usually <50; decreases with time if treatment not provided	Acid-fast organisms may be seen on smear; organisms can be recovered in culture or by PCR. Adenine deaminase or gamma interferon levels can be used to aid in the diagnosis.
Fungal	Usually elevated	10-500; PMNs early; mononuclear cells predominate later	20-500	Usually <50; decreases with time if treatment not provided	Budding yeast may be seen; organisms may be recovered in culture; India ink preparation and antigen may be positive in cryptococcal disease
Viral meningitis or meningoencephalitis	Normal or slightly elevated	10-1,000; PMNs early; mononuclear cells predominate later	<50	Generally normal; may be depressed to 40 in some viral diseases (in 15-20% of mumps)	Viruses may be detected by PCR
Abscess (parameningeal infection)	Normal or elevated	0-100 PMNs unless rupture into CSF	20-200	Normal	Profile may be completely normal

CSF, Cerebrospinal fluid; *HSV,* herpes simplex virus; *PCR,* polymerase chain reaction; *PMNs,* polymorphonuclear leukocytes.

viral meningitis; it is more sensitive and rapid than viral culture. Peripheral leukocytosis is common, and blood cultures may be positive depending on the organism and whether there was antibiotic pretreatment. Ideally, CSF should be obtained prior to empiric therapy; however, antibiotics should not be delayed if there is an inability to perform an LP. If imaging is required prior to the LP, blood cultures should be sent and antibiotics started, prior to a computed tomography (CT) scan. Interpretation of CSF in children who received prior antibiotics is complicated. In meningococcal meningitis, CSF can rapidly become sterile, often within 1-2 hours, and most commonly with a single dose of therapy. Sterilization of the CSF in *S. pneumoniae* meningitis may also occur within a few hours.

DIFFERENTIAL DIAGNOSIS

Many disorders other than meningitis and encephalitis may show signs of meningeal irritation and increased intracranial pressure, including trauma, hemorrhage, rheumatic diseases, and malignancies. Seizures can be associated with central nervous system (CNS) infection or can be the sequelae of brain edema, cerebral infarction or hemorrhage, or vasculitis.

TREATMENT

Treatment of bacterial meningitis focuses on sterilization of the CSF by antibiotics (Table 100.3) and maintenance of adequate cerebral and systemic perfusion. Due to increasing *S. pneumoniae* resistance, an empiric third-generation cephalosporin *plus* vancomycin should be administered until culture results and antibiotic susceptibility testing are available. Cefotaxime or ceftriaxone are also adequate to treat *N. meningitidis, H. influenzae,* and some *E. coli.* For infants younger than 2 months of age, ampicillin is added to cover the possibility of *Listeria monocytogenes.* Duration of treatment is 5-7 days for *N. meningitidis,* 7-10 days for *H. influenzae,* and 10-14 days for *S. pneumoniae.* Meningitis caused by gram-negative bacilli should generally be treated a minimum of 21 days or 14 days beyond the first negative CSF culture, whichever is longer.

Dexamethasone as **adjunctive therapy** initiated just before or concurrently with the first dose of antibiotics, significantly diminishes the incidence of hearing loss resulting from *H. influenzae* meningitis. The role of adjuvant steroids for diminishing neurological sequelae and mortality for pneumococcal and meningococcal meningitis in children is less clear.

Supportive therapy involves treatment of dehydration, shock, disseminated intravascular coagulation, syndrome of inappropriate antidiuretic hormone (SIADH), seizures, increased intracranial pressure, apnea, arrhythmias, and coma. Adequate cerebral perfusion must be maintained in the presence of cerebral edema.

TABLE **100.3** Initial Antimicrobial Therapy by Age for Presumed Bacterial Meningitis

AGE	RECOMMENDED TREATMENT	ALTERNATIVE TREATMENTS
Newborns (0-28 days)	Cefotaxime plus ampicillin with or without gentamicin	Ampicillin plus gentamicin
Infants and toddlers (1 month to 4 years)	Ceftriaxone or cefotaxime plus vancomycin	
Children and adolescents (5-13 years) and adults	Ceftriaxone or cefotaxime plus vancomycin	Cefepime plus vancomycin

COMPLICATIONS AND PROGNOSIS

Decision-Making Algorithm
Available @ StudentConsult.com
Hearing Loss

SIADH may complicate meningitis and necessitates monitoring of urine output and fluid administration. Persistent fever is common during treatment but also may be related to ineffective treatment or immune complex-mediated pericardial or joint effusions, thrombophlebitis, drug fever, or nosocomial infection. A repeat LP after 48 hours of therapy should be considered for those whose condition has not improved or has worsened, gram-negative meningitis, and for those who received adjunct steroids, which can interfere with the ability to monitor clinical response. CNS imaging should be considered in children who demonstrate focal neurological signs or symptoms or persistently positive CSF cultures. CT with contrast, or magnetic resonance imaging, is used to detect subdural effusions with *S. pneumoniae* and *H. influenzae* meningitis or brain abscess associated with gram-negative organisms. *Citrobacter koseri* produces neonatal meningitis with a high incidence of brain abscess formation. Neurosurgery should be consulted to consider drainage if a brain abscess is present.

With current management, the mortality rate for bacterial meningitis in children remains significant, up to 15% depending on the organism and the study. Morbidity and mortality are highest with *S. pneumoniae.* Of survivors, up to 30% have sequelae, including deafness, seizures, blindness, paresis, ataxia, or hydrocephalus. All patients with meningitis should have a hearing evaluation before discharge and at follow-up. Learning disabilities and behavioral problems may be more subtle, long-term consequences of infection. Careful developmental follow-up is important. Poor prognosis is associated with young age, long duration of illness before effective antibiotic therapy, seizures, coma at presentation, shock, low or absent CSF white blood cell count in the presence of visible bacteria on CSF Gram stain, and immunocompromised status.

Rarely relapse may occur 3-14 days after treatment, possibly from parameningeal foci or resistant organisms. Recurrence may indicate an underlying immunological or anatomical defect that predisposes the patient to meningitis.

PREVENTION

Routine immunizations against *H. influenzae* and *S. pneumoniae* are recommended for children beginning at 2 months of age. Quadrivalent vaccines against *N. meningitidis* (serotypes A, C, Y, and W-135) are recommended at age 11 or 12 years with a booster dose at 16 years, and for children >2 months of age who are at high-risk of infection, including functional asplenia, complement deficiencies and travelers to or residents of hyperendemic areas. A newer vaccine against *N. meningitidis* serotype B is currently recommended for high-risk patients 10 years and older. **Chemoprophylaxis** with rifampin, ciprofloxacin, azithromycin, or ceftriaxone to eradicate the carrier state and decrease transmission is recommended both for index cases with *N. meningitidis* and for their close contacts. For invasive *H. influenzae* type B, prophylaxis consists of rifampin.

CHAPTER 101

Encephalitis

ETIOLOGY

Encephalitis is an inflammatory process of the brain parenchyma, which usually presents with fever, headache, and mental status changes. Encephalitis is a challenging diagnosis in many aspects, as determining its etiology is difficult and treatment options are quite limited. The term **meningoencephalitis** is used when meningeal inflammation is also present. Encephalitis is usually an acute infectious process, but also may be a postinfectious, autoimmune, part of a systemic disorder (lupus), or the result of an indolent viral infection. Encephalitis may be diffuse or localized. Organisms cause encephalitis by one of two mechanisms: (1) direct infection of the brain parenchyma via an extension of meningitis, secondary to viremia, or retrograde spread via peripheral nerves or (2) a postinfectious, immune-mediated response in the CNS that usually begins several days to weeks after clinical manifestations of the infection.

Viruses are the principal infectious causes of acute infectious encephalitis (Table 101.1). The most common viral causes of encephalitis in the United States are enteroviruses, arboviruses, and herpesviruses. Human immunodeficiency virus (HIV) is also an important cause of subacute encephalitis in children and adolescents and may present as an acute febrile illness but, more commonly, is insidious in onset (see Chapter 125). Other less common viral causes of encephalitis include measles, JC virus, lymphocytic choriomeningitis virus (LCMV), rabies, influenza, and Japanese encephalitis. Numerous other infectious etiologies for encephalitis are possible in the appropriate setting, including prion-diseases (e.g., Creutzfeldt-Jakob disease) and parasites such as amoeba, *Bartonella henselae, Mycobacterium tuberculosis, Plasmodium falciparum,* and *Mycoplasma pneumoniae.* Encephalitis also may result from metabolic, toxic, and neoplastic disorders. In many cases, the cause remains unknown.

Acute disseminated encephalomyelitis (ADEM) is the abrupt development of multiple neurological signs related to an inflammatory, demyelinating disorder of the brain and spinal cord. ADEM can follow childhood viral infections (such as measles and chickenpox) or vaccinations, and can clinically resemble multiple sclerosis.

Autoimmune encephalitis is a relatively common cause of encephalitis and is associated with specific autoantibodies directed to brain antigens, such as anti-N-methyl-D-aspartate receptor antibodies. The presentation is often subacute with psychological manifestations, cortical dysfunction, movement disorders, autonomic dysfunction, and seizures.

TABLE 101.1 Causes of Acute Encephalitis

VIRUSES	BACTERIA
Enteroviruses Parechoviruses	*Borrelia burgdorferi* (Lyme disease)
Herpes simplex viruses (types 1 and 2)	*Bartonella henselae* (cat-scratch disease)
EBV	*Mycoplasma pneumoniae*
Arboviruses (West Nile virus, St. Louis, Japanese, LaCrosse, Powassan and equine encephalitis viruses)	*Rickettsia rickettsii* (Rocky mountain spotted fever)
Cytomegalovirus	**PARASITES**
Human immunodeficiency virus	*Plasmodium falciparum*
Rabies virus	*Naegleria fowleri*
LCMV	*Acanthamoeba* spp
VZV	**FUNGI**
Influenza virus	*Cryptococcus neoformans*
Mumps virus	*Coccidioides* species
Measles virus	*Histoplasma capsulatum*

EBV, Epstein-Barr virus; *LCMV*, lymphocytic choriomeningitis virus; *VZV*, varicella-zoster virus.

EPIDEMIOLOGY

Arboviral and enteroviral encephalitides characteristically appear in clusters or epidemics that occur from midsummer to early fall, although sporadic cases of enteroviral encephalitis occur throughout the year. Herpesviruses and other infectious agents account for additional sporadic cases throughout the year.

Arboviruses tend to be limited to certain geographic areas, reflecting the reservoir and mosquito vector. In North America, West Nile virus and La Crosse encephalitis occur in the summer time, resulting in a range of manifestations from asymptomatic infection to severe neurological involvement. La Crosse virus is found in the Midwest and southeastern United States, whereas West Nile virus is more disseminated across the country. The principal vectors for West Nile virus are *Culex* mosquitoes, and a broad range of birds serves as its major reservoir.

Herpes simplex virus (HSV) encephalitis can occur in neonates with or without skin lesions via perinatal or postnatal transmission. Beyond the neonatal period, HSV encephalitis can result from primary or recurrent infection with HSV type 1. In the immunocompromised host, other herpes viruses, such as cytomegalovirus (CMV), Epstein-Barr virus (EBV), human herpesvirus-6 (HHV-6) and varicella-zoster virus (VZV), as well as *Toxoplasma gondii* and JC viruses can reactivate and cause encephalitis. Fungal infections of the CNS are rare but can also cause disease in this patient population.

CLINICAL MANIFESTATIONS

Decision-Making Algorithms
Available @ StudentConsult.com

Stiff or Painful Neck
Headaches
Ataxia
Altered Mental Status
Hearing Loss Query
Polyuria

Acute infectious encephalitis may be preceded by a prodrome of several days of nonspecific symptoms, such as sore throat, fever, headache, and abdominal complaints followed by the characteristic symptoms of progressive lethargy, behavioral changes, and neurological deficits. Seizures are common at presentation. Children with encephalitis also may have a maculopapular rash and severe complications, such as fulminant coma, transverse myelitis, anterior horn cell disease, or peripheral neuropathy.

Neonates with HSV encephalitis can present with fever, lethargy, and/or seizures. Vesicular skin lesions typical of cutaneous infection may or may not be present.

DIFFERENTIAL DIAGNOSIS

The diagnosis is established presumptively by the presence of characteristic neurological signs, typical epidemiological findings, and evidence of infection by cerebrospinal fluid (CSF) analysis, electroencephalogram (EEG), and brain imaging techniques. Encephalitis may result from infections with bacteria, *Mycoplasma, Rickettsia,* fungi, and parasites, and from many noninfectious diseases, including metabolic diseases (encephalopathy), such as Reye syndrome, hypoglycemia, collagen vascular disorders, drugs, hypertension, and malignancies.

Elucidating a careful history, including immunization record, travel, and geographic and social risk factors, may help to establish the etiology of encephalitis in a patient. If the patient is known to be or found to be immunocompromised, the differential diagnosis must be broadened accordingly.

LABORATORY AND IMAGING STUDIES

The diagnosis of viral encephalitis is supported by examination of the CSF, which typically shows a lymphocytic pleocytosis, a slight elevation in protein content, and a normal glucose level. The CSF occasionally may be normal. Extreme elevations of protein and reductions of glucose suggest tuberculosis, cryptococcal infection, or meningeal carcinomatosis. Blood can be sent for a complete blood count with differential and culture, as well as liver function tests and infectious serologies.

Neuroimaging studies are often required prior to a lumbar puncture (LP) in these children as they generally have altered mental status. Magnetic resonance imaging (MRI) is generally the study of choice in the diagnosis of encephalitis; however, computed tomography (CT) may be used to exclude contraindications to LP or if MRI is unavailable. Brain imaging may be normal or may show diffuse cerebral swelling of the parenchyma or focal abnormalities. EEG can show diffuse, slow wave activity, although focal changes may be present. A temporal lobe focus on EEG or brain imaging is a characteristic feature of HSV infection.

Serum and CSF testing may help determine an infectious etiology for encephalitis. Depending on the risk factors, serological studies should be obtained for arboviruses (including West Nile virus, if indicated by the patient risk factors), HIV, EBV, *M. pneumoniae, B. henselae,* and Lyme disease. Additional serological testing for less common pathogens should be performed as indicated by the travel, social, or medical history. In most cases of viral encephalitis, the virus is difficult to isolate from the CSF. Polymerase chain reaction (PCR) tests for HSV, enteroviruses, mycoplasma, West Nile virus, and other viruses are available and can be sent. Viral cultures of stool, throat, and a nasopharyngeal swab may also be obtained. CSF viral culture is not recommended. Even with extensive testing and the use of PCR assays, the cause of encephalitis remains undetermined in one third of cases. Both blood and CSF should be sent to detect brain-specific antibodies present in ~95% of patients with autoimmune encephalitis.

Brain biopsy is seldom performed and is generally recommended only if the etiology remains unknown and a patient continues to deteriorate. Rabies encephalitis and prion-related diseases (Creutzfeldt-Jakob disease and kuru) may be routinely diagnosed by culture or pathological examination of brain biopsy tissue. Brain tissue can be sent for pathology, culture, and PCR testing and may be helpful to identify arbovirus and enterovirus infections, tuberculosis, fungal infections, and noninfectious illnesses, particularly primary CNS vasculopathies and malignancies.

TREATMENT

With the exception of HSV, VZV, CMV, HHV-6, and HIV, there is no specific therapy for viral encephalitis. Management is supportive and frequently requires intensive care unit admission to facilitate aggressive therapy for seizures, timely detection of electrolyte abnormalities, and, when necessary, airway monitoring and protection or reduction of increased intracranial pressure and maintenance of adequate cerebral perfusion pressure.

Intravenous acyclovir is the treatment of choice for HSV and VZV infections. CMV disease is treated with ganciclovir. HHV-6 encephalitis in patients who are post–bone marrow transplant can also be treated with ganciclovir or foscarnet. HIV infections may be treated with a combination of antiretroviral agents. *M. pneumoniae* infections may be treated with doxycycline, fluoroquinolones, or macrolides, although the clinical value of treating encephalitis associated with *Mycoplasma* disease is uncertain.

ADEM has been treated with high-dose intravenous corticosteroids, but it is unclear whether the improved outcome with corticosteroids reflects milder cases recognized by MRI, fewer cases caused by measles (which can cause severe ADEM), or improved supportive care. Autoimmune encephalitis has been treated with steroids, intravenous immunoglobulin (IVIG), and rituximab.

COMPLICATIONS AND PROGNOSIS

Among survivors, symptoms usually resolve over several days to 2-3 weeks. Although most patients with epidemic forms of infectious encephalitis (St. Louis, California, West Nile, and enterovirus infections) in the United States recover without sequelae, severe cases leading to death or substantial neurological sequelae can occur with virtually any of these neurotropic viruses. Sequelae can include paresis or spasticity, cognitive impairment, weakness, ataxia, and recurrent seizures. Most patients gradually recover some or all of their function. The overall mortality for infectious encephalitis is low, depending on the etiology.

Disease caused by HSV, Eastern equine encephalitis, or *M. pneumoniae* is associated with a worse prognosis, especially in children younger than 1 year of age or with coma. Rabies, with very rare exceptions, is fatal.

Relapses of ADEM occur in 14%, usually within 1 year with the same or new clinical signs. Recurrences of ADEM may represent the onset of multiple sclerosis in childhood.

PREVENTION

The best prevention for arboviral encephalitis is to avoid mosquito-borne or tick-borne exposures and to remove ticks carefully (see Chapter 122). There are no vaccines in use in the United States for the prevention of arboviral infection or for enteroviruses except for poliomyelitis. There are no specific preventive measures for HSV encephalitis except for cesarean section for mothers with active genital lesions (see Chapter 65). Rabies can be prevented by preexposure or postexposure vaccination. Influenza encephalitis can be prevented by use of influenza vaccination. Reye syndrome can be prevented by avoiding use of aspirin or aspirin-containing compounds for children with fever as well as use of varicella and influenza vaccines.

CHAPTER 102

Upper Respiratory Tract Infection

ETIOLOGY

Upper respiratory tract infection (URI), also known as "the common cold," is a self-limited viral process with prominent symptoms of rhinorrhea and nasal congestion, absent or mild fever, and few systemic manifestations. URIs are the most common cause of human disease and are often a cause of missed work or school, as well as visits to primary care pediatricians. Young children are at highest risk for frequent URI due to their lack of immunity from previous infection and close contact with others who frequently shed virus.

The viruses most commonly associated with colds are rhinoviruses. Other viruses that cause URIs include respiratory syncytial virus (RSV), human metapneumovirus, coronaviruses, coxsackieviruses, influenza, parainfluenza, and adenoviruses. Viral infection of nasal epithelium causes an acute inflammatory response with mucosal infiltration by inflammatory cells and release of cytokines. The host inflammatory response is partly responsible for many of the symptoms.

EPIDEMIOLOGY

URIs occur throughout the year with peak incidence from fall through late spring, reflecting the seasonal prevalence of viral pathogens and confined habitation during colder months. Young children have an average of seven to eight viral infections each year. The number decreases with age, to two to three colds each year by adulthood. Children in out-of-home day care during the first year of life have 50% more URIs than children cared for at home only. With preschool attendance, it is not unusual for children to experience one infection/month of the respiratory virus season. This difference diminishes during subsequent years in day care.

CLINICAL MANIFESTATIONS

Decision-Making Algorithms
Available @ StudentConsult.com

Rhinorrhea
Sore Throat

URI symptoms typically develop 1-3 days after viral infection and include nasal congestion, rhinorrhea, sore or scratchy throat, and occasional nonproductive cough. Fever, although uncommon in adults, may occur in infants and young children. Symptoms usually persist for approximately 5-7 days, although it can be longer in preschool aged children. Constitutional symptoms such as fever, myalgia, and headaches generally are present only early in the illness. Respiratory symptoms tend to persist for the duration of the illness. There is often a change in the color or consistency of nasal secretions, which is not necessarily indicative of sinusitis or bacterial superinfection. Examination of the nasal mucosa may reveal swollen, erythematous nasal turbinates.

LABORATORY AND IMAGING STUDIES

Laboratory studies often are not helpful. A nasopharyngeal swab for respiratory virus polymerase chain reaction is sometimes obtained in the inpatient setting in immunocompromised patients or for infection prevention reasons. A **nasal smear** for eosinophils may be useful in the evaluation for allergic rhinitis (see Chapter 79).

DIFFERENTIAL DIAGNOSIS

The differential diagnosis of URI includes allergic rhinitis, foreign body (especially with unilateral nasal discharge), sinusitis, pertussis, and pharyngitis. Allergic rhinitis is characterized by absence of fever, eosinophils in the nasal discharge, and other manifestations, such as allergic shiners, nasal polyps, a transverse crease on the nasal bridge, and pale, edematous, nasal turbinate mucosa. Other, rare causes of chronic rhinorrhea are choanal atresia or stenosis, cerebrospinal fluid fistula, diphtheria, tumor, congenital syphilis (with *snuffles*), nasopharyngeal malignancy, and granulomatosis with polyangiitis.

TREATMENT

There is no specific therapy for URIs. Antibacterial therapy is not beneficial and instead may cause harm. Management consists of symptomatic therapies. Antihistamines and decongestants are not recommended for children younger than 6 years of age because of adverse effects and lack of benefits. Similarly, cough suppressants and expectorants have not been shown to be beneficial. Vitamin C and inhalation of warm, humidified air are no more effective than placebo. The benefit of zinc lozenges or sprays has been inconsistent.

COMPLICATIONS AND PROGNOSIS

Otitis media is the most common complication and occurs in about 5% of children with a URI (see Chapter 105). Other complications include bacterial sinusitis, which should be considered if rhinorrhea or daytime cough persists without improvement for at least 10-14 days or if severe signs of sinus involvement develop, such as high fever for more than 3 days, facial pain, or facial swelling (see Chapter 104). Viral infections may lead to exacerbation of asthma and may result in inappropriate antibiotic treatment.

PREVENTION

There are no proven methods for prevention of colds other than good handwashing and avoiding contact with infected persons. No significant effect of vitamin C or Echinacea for prevention of URIs has been confirmed.

CHAPTER 103

Pharyngitis

ETIOLOGY

Many infectious agents can cause pharyngitis (Table 103.1), viruses being the most common. **Group A streptococcus** ***(Streptococcus pyogenes)*** is the most common important bacterial cause of pharyngitis. Other bacterial organisms less often associated with pharyngitis include groups C and G streptococci (also β-hemolytic) and rarely *Arcanobacterium haemolyticum* (β-hemolytic, gram-positive rod) and *Francisella tularensis* (gram-negative coccobacillus and cause of tularemia). *Chlamydophila pneumonia* is associated with lower respiratory disease but can also cause sore throat. *Mycoplasma pneumoniae* is associated with atypical pneumonia and may cause mild pharyngitis without distinguishing clinical manifestations. *Neisseria gonorrhoeae* should be considered in a sexually active adolescent or adult with pharyngitis. Other bacteria, including *Staphylococcus aureus, Haemophilus influenzae,* and *S. pneumoniae,* are cultured frequently from the throats of children, but their role in causing pharyngitis is unclear.

Many viruses cause acute pharyngitis. Some viruses, such as adenoviruses, are more likely than others to cause pharyngitis as a prominent symptom, whereas other viruses, such as rhinoviruses, are more likely to cause pharyngitis as a minor part of an illness that primarily features other symptoms, such as rhinorrhea or cough. Epstein-Barr virus (EBV), enteroviruses (herpangina), herpes simplex virus (HSV), and primary human immunodeficiency virus (HIV) infection can also produce pharyngitis.

TABLE 103.1 Major Microbial Causes of Acute Pharyngitis

AGENT	SYNDROME OR DISEASE	ESTIMATED PROPORTION OF ALL PHARYNGITIS (%)
BACTERIAL		
Group A streptococcus (*Streptococcus pyogenes*)	Pharyngitis, tonsillitis, scarlet fever	15-30
Group C and G streptococcus	Pharyngitis, tonsillitis	1-5
Arcanobacterium haemolyticum	Pharyngitis (Scarlet fever-like syndrome)	0.5-3
Fusobacterium necrophorum	Lemierre syndrome	Unknown
Mycoplasma pneumoniae	Pharyngitis, pneumonia	Unknown
Other (e.g., *Neisseria gonorrhoeae, Corynebacterium diphtheriae, Francisella tularensis*)	Pharyngitis, laryngitis, tularemia	<5
VIRAL		
Rhinoviruses (>100 types)	URI	20
Coronaviruses (>4 types)	URI	>5
Adenoviruses (types 3, 4, 7, 14, 21)	Pharyngoconjunctival fever, acute respiratory disease	5
Herpes simplex viruses (types 1 and 2)	Gingivitis, stomatitis, pharyngitis	4
Parainfluenza viruses (types 1-4)	URI, croup	2
Influenza viruses (types A and B)	Influenza	2
Epstein-Barr virus	Mononucleosis	Unknown
Cytomegalovirus	Mononucleosis	Unknown
Coxsackie virus	Herpangina, hand, foot and mouth disease	Unknown
UNKNOWN		40

URI, Upper respiratory tract infection.
Modified from Hayden GF, Hendley JO, Gwaltney JM Jr. Management of the ambulatory patient with a sore throat. Curr Clin Top Infect Dis. *1988;9:62–75.*

EPIDEMIOLOGY

Sore throat is the primary symptom in approximately one third of upper respiratory tract illnesses. Streptococcal pharyngitis is relatively uncommon before 2-3 years of age, but the incidence increases in young school-age children and then declines in late adolescence and adulthood. Streptococcal pharyngitis occurs throughout the year in temperate climates. The illness often spreads to siblings and classmates. Viral infections generally spread via close contact with an infected person and peak during winter and spring. EBV or cytomegalovirus related **mononucleosis** (see Chapter 99) can feature pharyngitis as a prominent symptom and is most common in adolescents and young adults.

CLINICAL MANIFESTATIONS

Decision-Making Algorithms
Available @ StudentConsult.com

Sore Throat
Fever and Rash
Lymphadenopathy

Pharyngeal inflammation causes cough, sore throat, dysphagia, and fever. If involvement of the tonsils is prominent, the term **tonsillitis** or **tonsillopharyngitis** is often used.

The onset of streptococcal pharyngitis is often rapid and associated with prominent sore throat and moderate to high fever. Headache, nausea, vomiting, and abdominal pain are frequent. In a typical, florid case, the pharynx is distinctly red. The tonsils are enlarged and may be covered with a yellow, blood-tinged exudate. There may be petechiae on the soft palate and posterior pharynx and the uvula may be red, stippled, and swollen. Anterior cervical lymph nodes are enlarged and tender to touch. However, some children present with only mild pharyngeal erythema without tonsillar exudate or cervical lymphadenitis. Compared with classic streptococcal pharyngitis, the onset of viral pharyngitis is typically more gradual, and symptoms more often include rhinorrhea, cough, and diarrhea. Conjunctivitis, coryza, or oral ulcerations also suggest a viral etiology. The diagnosis of streptococcal pharyngitis cannot be made on clinical features alone.

In addition to sore throat and fever, some patients with streptococcal pharyngitis exhibit the stigmata of **scarlet fever:** circumoral pallor, strawberry tongue, and a fine diffuse erythematous macular-papular rash. The tongue initially has a white coating, but red and edematous lingual papillae later project through this coating, producing a **white strawberry tongue.** When the white coating peels off, the resulting **red strawberry tongue** is beefy red with prominent papillae. Patients infected with *A. haemolyticum* may present with similar findings.

Gingivostomatitis is characteristic of HSV type 1. **Herpangina** is an enteroviral infection with sudden onset of high fever, vomiting, headache, malaise, myalgia, poor intake, drooling, sore throat, and dysphagia. The oral lesions of herpangina may be nonspecific, but classically there are one or more small, tender, papular, or pinpoint vesicular lesions on an erythematous base scattered over the soft palate, uvula, and tongue. These vesicles enlarge from 1 to 4 mm over 3-4 days, rupture, and produce small, punched-out ulcers that persist for several days. Similar lesions may have been seen in hand, foot, and mouth disease caused by coxsackieviruses.

LABORATORY EVALUATION

The principal challenge is to distinguish pharyngitis caused by group A streptococcus from pharyngitis caused by viral organisms. A rapid streptococcal antigen test, a throat culture, or both should be performed to improve diagnostic precision and to identify children most likely to benefit from antibiotic therapy. Antigen-based rapid diagnostic tests for streptococcal pharyngitis have excellent specificity of 95-99%. However, the sensitivity of these rapid tests varies, and negative rapid tests should be confirmed by a throat culture. Throat culture or polymerase chain reaction (PCR) are the definitive diagnostic tests to establish the presence of streptococcal pharyngitis. However, as many as 20% of positive cultures in children during winter months represent chronic **streptococcal carriage** and not acute pharyngitis.

The predictive values of white blood cell count, erythrocyte sedimentation rate, and C-reactive protein are not sufficient to distinguish streptococcal from nonstreptococcal pharyngitis, and these tests are not routinely recommended. The white blood cell count in patients with infectious mononucleosis usually shows a predominance of atypical lymphocytes.

DIFFERENTIAL DIAGNOSIS

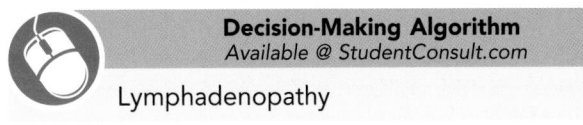

Decision-Making Algorithm
Available @ StudentConsult.com

Lymphadenopathy

The differential diagnosis of infectious pharyngitis includes other local infections of the oral cavity, retropharyngeal abscesses (*S. aureus*, streptococci, anaerobes), diphtheria (if unimmunized), peritonsillar abscesses (streptococci, anaerobes, or, rarely, *S. aureus*), and epiglottitis. In addition, neutropenic mucositis (leukemia, aplastic anemia), thrush (candidiasis secondary to T-cell immune deficiency), autoimmune ulceration (systemic lupus erythematosus, Behçet disease), and Kawasaki disease may cause pharyngitis. Pharyngitis can be a feature of the acute retrovirus syndrome associated with primary HIV infection (see Chapter 125).

Vincent angina or **trench mouth** refers to a virulent form of anaerobic gingivitis and pharyngitis; gray pseudomembranes are found on the tonsils. **Lemierre syndrome** is acute pharyngitis complicated by thrombosis of the internal jugular vein and septic pulmonary emboli. It primarily occurs in adolescents and is caused by *Fusobacterium necrophorum.* **Ludwig angina** is a mixed anaerobic bacterial cellulitis of the submandibular and sublingual regions. It is typically due to spreading from an abscess of the second or third mandibular molar. It also has been associated with tongue piercing. A propensity for rapid spread, glottic and lingual swelling, and consequent airway obstruction makes prompt intervention imperative.

A syndrome of **periodic fever, aphthous stomatitis, pharyngitis, and cervical adenitis (PFAPA)** is a rare cause of recurrent fever in children. The fevers begin at a young age (usually <5 years). Episodes last approximately 5 days, with a mean of 28 days between episodes. Episodes are shorter with oral prednisone and do not respond to nonsteroidal antiinflammatory drugs or antibiotics. Long-term sequelae do not develop.

TREATMENT

Even if untreated, most episodes of streptococcal pharyngitis resolve uneventfully over a few days. Early antimicrobial therapy accelerates clinical recovery by 24-48 hours. The major benefit of antimicrobial therapy is the prevention of acute rheumatic fever (see Chapter 146). Because the latent (incubation) period of **acute rheumatic fever** is relatively long (1-3 weeks), treatment instituted within 9 days of illness onset is virtually 100% successful in preventing rheumatic fever. Treatment begun after this period, although less than 100% successful, has some preventive value. Therefore antibiotic therapy should be started promptly in children with a positive rapid test or throat culture (or PCR) for group A streptococcus or a diagnosis of scarlet fever. In addition, a child who has symptomatic pharyngitis and a history of rheumatic fever, or a recent family history of rheumatic fever, or whose sibling has documented streptococcal infection should be treated.

A variety of antimicrobial agents can be used to treat streptococcal pharyngitis (Table 103.2). Penicillin or amoxicillin

TABLE 103.2 Antimicrobial Treatment of Group A Streptococcal Pharyngitis

Oral penicillin V (2-3 times daily for 10 days) 250-500 mg/dose
Intramuscular benzathine penicillin G (single dose)—For children ≤27 kg: 600,000 U; For larger children and adults: 1.2 million U
For persons allergic to penicillin
Cephalexin 25 mg/kg/dose BID, maximum dose 500 mg/dose × 10 days
Clindamycin 7 mg/kg/dose TID, maximum dose 300 mg/dose × 10 days
For persons allergic to β-lactams
Azithromycin, children: 12 mg/kg (maximum: 500 mg/dose) on day 1 followed by 6 mg/kg/dose (maximum: 250 mg/dose) OD on days 2 through 5

BID, Twice daily; *OD*, once daily; *TID*, three times daily.

remain first-line therapy. Ten days of treatment is recommended to prevent rheumatic fever. Intramuscular penicillin G can be used for children who cannot tolerate oral therapy. Cephalosporins have superior pharyngeal bacterial eradication rates compared to penicillin; however, they are only recommended as an alternative option. Five days of azithromycin is also an alternate treatment option for group A streptococcal pharyngitis, although rates of resistance to azithromycin are higher than those to penicillins. Test of cure for patients who respond clinically to treatment is not required. Children with recurrent episodes of group A streptococcal pharyngitis pose a particular problem. True treatment failure is rare. Recurrent infection may represent nonadherence, chronic streptococcal carriage in the setting of a viral pharyngitis, or reinfection. A second course of treatment can be administered. Amoxicillin-clavulanate or clindamycin can be effective for eliminating streptococcal carriage.

Specific antiviral therapy is unavailable for most cases of viral pharyngitis. Patients with primary herpetic gingivostomatitis benefit from early treatment with oral acyclovir.

COMPLICATIONS AND PROGNOSIS

Pharyngitis caused by streptococci or respiratory viruses usually resolves completely. The complications of group A streptococcal pharyngitis include local suppurative complications, such as parapharyngeal abscess and other infections of the deep fascial spaces of the neck, and nonsuppurative complications, such as acute rheumatic fever and acute postinfectious glomerulonephritis. Viral upper respiratory tract infections, including infections caused by influenza A, adenoviruses, parainfluenza type 3, and rhinoviruses, may predispose the patient to bacterial middle ear infections.

PREVENTION

Antimicrobial prophylaxis with daily oral penicillin V prevents recurrent streptococcal infections and is recommended to prevent recurrences of rheumatic fever in at-risk patients.

CHAPTER 104

Sinusitis

ETIOLOGY

Sinusitis is a suppurative infection of the paranasal sinuses and most commonly occurs as a complication of an upper respiratory tract infection (URI). Only the maxillary and ethmoid sinuses are present at birth, whereas the sphenoid sinuses are present by 5 years of age. Frontal sinuses begin to develop at 7 years of age and are not completely developed until adolescence. The ostia draining the sinuses are narrow (1-3 mm) and drain into the middle meatus in the **ostiomeatal complex.** The mucociliary system maintains the sinuses as normally sterile. Indwelling nasogastric and nasotracheal tubes predispose to nosocomial sinusitis.

Obstruction to mucociliary flow, such as mucosal edema resulting from a URI, impedes sinus drainage and predisposes to bacterial proliferation. The bacterial causes of most cases of acute sinusitis are *Streptococcus pneumoniae,* nontypable *Haemophilus influenzae,* and *Moraxella catarrhalis. Staphylococcus aureus* and anaerobes emerge as important pathogens in subacute and chronic sinusitis.

EPIDEMIOLOGY

The true incidence of sinusitis is unknown. In addition to predisposing URI, other risk factors include allergic rhinitis, cystic fibrosis, immunodeficiency, human immunodeficiency virus (HIV) infection, nasogastric or nasotracheal intubation, primary ciliary dyskinesia, nasal polyps, and nasal foreign body.

CLINICAL MANIFESTATIONS

Decision-Making Algorithms
Available @ StudentConsult.com

Rhinorrhea
Cough
Vomiting
Headaches

The most common presentation of acute bacterial sinusitis is persistent rhinorrhea, nasal congestion, and cough, especially at night. Symptoms should be persistent and not improving for >10 days to distinguish sinusitis from a URI. Less common symptoms include a nasal quality to the voice, halitosis, headache, and facial swelling and tenderness. Alternate presentations of acute bacterial sinusitis include high fever and purulent nasal discharge for at least 3 days or a biphasic illness where a patient has typical URI symptoms for up to a week but then worsens with increasing respiratory symptoms and new or recurrent fever.

Chronic sinusitis includes upper respiratory symptoms for >30 days, often accompanied by sore throat and/or headache. Fever is rare.

LABORATORY AND IMAGING STUDIES

Culture of the nasal mucosa is not useful. Sinus aspirate culture is the most accurate method of determining etiology but is not practical or necessary in immunocompetent patients.

Routine imaging is not recommended in uncomplicated infections. Plain x-ray, computed tomography (CT), and magnetic resonance imaging (MRI) may reveal sinus clouding, mucosal thickening, or air-fluid levels in the sinuses. However, abnormal radiographic findings do not differentiate infection from allergic disease and often show abnormalities in the sinuses of children with a simple viral URI. Conversely, normal imaging can have a high negative predictive value for bacterial sinusitis. Bony erosion may be seen on imaging studies in immunocompromised hosts.

TREATMENT

Amoxicillin for 10-14 days can be used as first-line therapy of uncomplicated sinusitis in children. Broadening therapy to amoxicillin-clavulanate is appropriate if there is no clinical response to amoxicillin within 2-3 days, if risk factors for resistant organisms are present (antibiotic treatment in the preceding 1-3 months, day care attendance, age <2 years), if there is chronic sinusitis, or if any amount of eye swelling is present.

COMPLICATIONS AND PROGNOSIS

Complications of bacterial sinusitis include orbital cellulitis, epidural or subdural empyema, brain abscess, dural sinus thrombosis, osteomyelitis of the frontal sinus **(Pott puffy tumor)**, and meningitis. These all should be managed with sinus drainage and broad-spectrum parenteral antibiotics. Sinusitis also may exacerbate bronchoconstriction in patients with asthma.

Orbital (postseptal) cellulitis is a serious complication of sinusitis that follows bacterial spread into the orbit through the wall of the infected sinus. It typically begins as ethmoid sinusitis and spreads through the **lamina papyracea**, a thin, bony plate that separates the medial orbit and the ethmoid sinus. Orbital involvement can lead to subperiosteal abscess, cavernous sinus thrombosis, and vision loss. Clinical manifestations of orbital cellulitis include a swollen edematous eye, eye pain, proptosis, chemosis, and limitations in extraocular muscle motion, diplopia, and reduced visual acuity. Infection of the orbit must be differentiated from that of the preseptal (anterior to the palpebral fascia) or periorbital space. **Preseptal (periorbital) cellulitis** is most common in young children; these patients do not have proptosis or ophthalmoplegia. Preseptal cellulitis may be associated with a skin lesion or trauma and usually is caused by *S. aureus* or group A streptococcus.

The diagnosis of orbital cellulitis is confirmed by a CT scan of the orbit, which helps determine the extent of orbital infection and the need for surgical drainage. Therapy for orbital cellulitis involves broad-spectrum parenteral antibiotics, such as vancomycin and ceftriaxone.

PREVENTION

The best means of prevention are good handwashing to minimize acquisition of URIs and management of allergic rhinitis.

CHAPTER 105

Otitis Media

ETIOLOGY

Otitis media (OM) is a suppurative infection of the middle ear cavity. Bacteria gain access to the middle ear when the normal patency of the eustachian tube is blocked by upper airway infection or hypertrophied adenoids. Air trapped in the middle ear is resorbed, creating negative pressure in this cavity and facilitating reflux of nasopharyngeal bacteria.

Bacteria are the most common pathogens in OM, most frequently as a co-infection with viruses. Viruses can be the sole pathogen in OM, but this is less common (<20%). The common bacterial pathogens are *Streptococcus pneumoniae*, nontypable *Haemophilus influenzae*, *Moraxella catarrhalis*, and, less frequently, group A streptococcus. *S. pneumoniae* that is **relatively resistant** to penicillin (minimal inhibitory concentration 2-8 μg/mL) or **highly resistant** to penicillin (minimal inhibitory concentration ≥8 μg/mL) is isolated with increasing frequency from young children, particularly those who attend day care or have recently received antibiotics.

EPIDEMIOLOGY

Diseases of the middle ear account for approximately one third of office visits to pediatricians. The peak incidence of acute otitis media (AOM) is between 6 and 15 months of life. By the second birthday, 90% of children will have experienced at least one episode of symptomatic or asymptomatic OM. OM is more common in younger children, children exposed to young children, and those with a positive family history. In most of the United States, OM is a seasonal disease with a distinct peak in late winter/early spring, which corresponds to the rhinovirus, respiratory syncytial virus, and influenza seasons.

Approximately 10% of children in the general population have **recurrent OM,** as defined by the presence of three or more AOM episodes in the preceding 6 months or four or more episodes in the preceding 12 months, with at least one episode in the past 6 months, and would be considered **otitis prone.** Craniofacial anomalies (cleft palate) and immunodeficiencies often are associated with recurrent OM, although most children with recurrent AOM are otherwise healthy.

CLINICAL MANIFESTATIONS

Decision-Making Algorithms
Available @ StudentConsult.com

Ear Pain
Strabismus
Abnormal Eye Movements
Diarrhea
Hearing Loss
Fever without a Source

In infants, the most frequent symptoms of AOM are nonspecific and include fever, irritability, and poor feeding. In older children and adolescents, AOM usually is associated with fever and

otalgia (acute ear pain). AOM also may present with **otorrhea** (ear drainage) after spontaneous rupture of the tympanic membrane. Signs of a common cold, which predisposes to AOM, are often present (see Chapter 102). A bulging tympanic membrane, air fluid level, or visualization of purulent material by otoscopy are reliable signs of infection (Table 105.1).

Examination of the ears is essential for diagnosis and should be part of the physical examination of any child with fever. The hallmark of OM is the presence of effusion in the middle ear cavity (see Table 105.1). The presence of an effusion does not confirm the presence of a bacterial OM, but it does define the need for appropriate diagnosis and therapy.

Pneumatic otoscopy, using an attachment to an otoscope, allows evaluation of ventilation of the middle ear and is a standard for clinical diagnosis. The tympanic membrane of the normal, air-filled middle ear has much greater compliance than if the middle ear is fluid-filled. With AOM, the tympanic membrane is often characterized by **hyperemia,** or red color rather than the normal pearly gray color, but may appear pink, white, or yellow depending on the degree of bulging (Fig. 105.1). The light reflex is lost, and the middle ear structures are obscured and difficult to distinguish. There should be poor or absent mobility to negative and positive pressure; this is a necessary finding for the diagnosis of OM. A hole in the tympanic membrane or purulent drainage confirms perforation. Occasionally bullae are present on the lateral aspect of the tympanic membrane, which characteristically are associated with severe ear pain.

TABLE 105.1 Definition of Acute Otitis Media

A diagnosis of acute otitis media (AOM) requires:
History of acute onset of signs and symptoms
Presence of middle ear effusion
Signs and symptoms of middle ear inflammation
The definition of AOM includes all of the following:
Recent, usually abrupt, onset of signs and symptoms of middle ear inflammation and middle ear effusion
The presence of middle ear effusion that is indicated by any of the following:
Bulging of the tympanic membrane
Limited or absent mobility of the tympanic membrane
Air-fluid level behind the tympanic membrane
Otorrhea
Signs or symptoms of middle ear inflammation as indicated by either:
Distinct erythema of the tympanic membrane
Distinct otalgia (discomfort clearly referable to the ear that results in interference with or precludes normal activity or sleep)

LABORATORY AND IMAGING STUDIES

Routine laboratory studies, including complete blood count and erythrocyte sedimentation rate, are not useful in the evaluation of OM. **Tympanometry** provides objective acoustic measurements of the tympanic membrane–middle ear system by reflection or absorption of sound energy from the external ear duct as pressure in the duct is varied. Measurements of the resulting **tympanogram** correlate well with the presence or absence of middle ear effusion.

Instruments using **acoustic reflectometry** are available for office use. Use of reflectometry as a screening test for AOM should be followed by examination with pneumatic otoscopy when abnormal reflectometry is identified.

Bacteria recovered from the nasopharynx do not correlate with bacteria isolated by tympanocentesis. Tympanocentesis and middle ear exudate culture are not always necessary, but they are required for accurate identification of bacterial pathogens and may be useful in neonates, immunocompromised patients, and patients not responding to therapy.

DIFFERENTIAL DIAGNOSIS

The major difficulty is differentiation of AOM from **OM with effusion (OME),** which also is referred to as **chronic OM.** AOM is accompanied by signs of acute illness, such as fever, pain, and upper respiratory tract inflammation. OME is the presence of effusion without any of the other signs and symptoms. OME may occur either as the sequel of AOM or eustachian tube dysfunction secondary to an upper respiratory tract infection. It may also predispose to the development of AOM. Because OME is not an acute infectious process, it is important to be able to differentiate between OME and AOM accurately to prevent overprescribing of antibiotics.

TREATMENT

Recommendations for treatment are based on age, certainty of diagnosis, and severity of illness (Table 105.2). The recommended first-line therapy for most children meeting criteria for antibiotic therapy is amoxicillin (80-90 mg/kg/day in two divided doses). Some children with mild illness or uncertain

TABLE 105.2 Recommendations for Initial Management of Confirmed Acute Otitis Media*

AGE	AOM WITH OTORRHEA	AOM WITH SEVERE SYMPTOMS†	BILATERAL AOM WITHOUT OTORRHEA	UNILATERAL AOM WITHOUT OTORRHEA
6 months to 2 years	Antibiotics	Antibiotics	Antibiotics	Antibiotics or additional observation‡
≥2 years	Antibiotics	Antibiotics	Antibiotics or additional observation	Antibiotics or additional observation

**Applies only to children with well-documented AOM with high certainty of diagnosis.*
†A toxic-appearing child, persistent otalgia for >48 hours, temperature ≥39°C (102.2°F) in the past 48 hours, or if there is uncertain follow-up.
‡Requires shared decision making with parents and close follow-up within 48-72 hours.
AOM, Acute otitis media.
Reproduced with permission from Lieberthal AS, Carroll AE, Chonmaitree T, et al. American academy of pediatrics clinical practice guideline: the diagnosis and management of acute otitis media. Pediatrics. 2013;131:e964–e999. Copyright 2013 by the AAP.

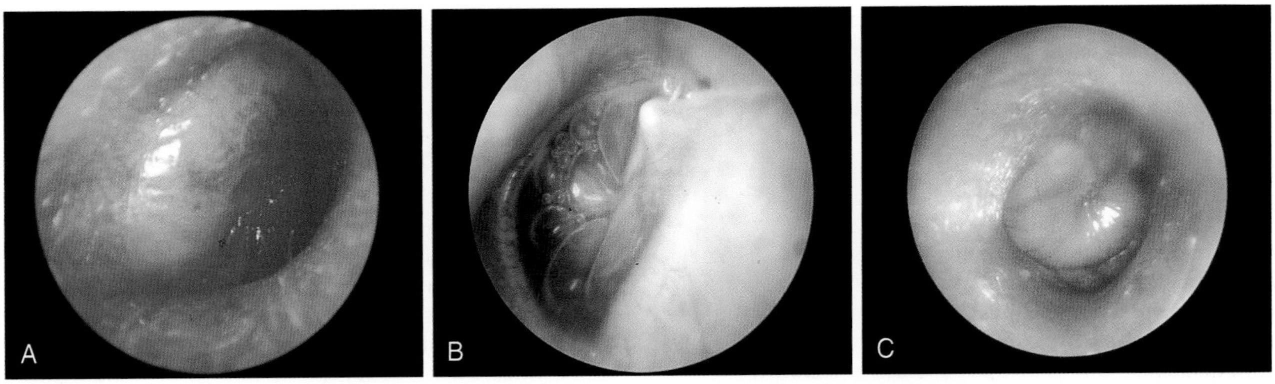

FIGURE 105.1 Appearance of tympanic membrane in acute otitis media. **(A)** Erythematous, opaque, bulging tympanic membrane. The light reflex is reduced, and the landmarks are partially obscured. Mobility markedly reduced. **(B)** Presence of air and fluid forming bubbles separated by grayish-yellow menisci. **(C)** Injection at the periphery. Yellow purulent effusion causing the inferior portion to bulge outward. Mobility markedly reduced. (From Yellon RF, Chi DH. Otolaryngology. In: Zitelli BJ, McIntire SC, Nowalk AJ, eds. *Atlas of Pediatric Physical Diagnosis.* 6th ed. Philadelphia: Saunders; 2012:923. Fig. 23–24.)

diagnosis may be observed if appropriate follow-up within 48-72 hours can be arranged with initiation of antibiotic therapy if symptoms do not self-resolve (Table 105.2). The failure of initial therapy with amoxicillin at 3 days suggests infection with β-lactamase-producing *H. influenza, M. catarrhalis,* or resistant *S. pneumoniae.* Recommended next-step treatments include high-dose amoxicillin-clavulanate (amoxicillin 80-90 mg/kg/day), cefdinir, or ceftriaxone (50 mg/kg intramuscularly in daily doses for 3 days). Intramuscular ceftriaxone is especially appropriate for children with vomiting that precludes oral treatment. Tympanocentesis may be required for patients who are difficult to treat or who do not respond to therapy. Acetaminophen and ibuprofen are recommended for fever. Decongestants or antihistamines are not effective.

COMPLICATIONS AND PROGNOSIS

Decision-Making Algorithms
Available @ StudentConsult.com

Ear Pain
Strabismus
Hearing Loss

The complications of OM are tympanic membrane perforation, chronic effusion, chronic otorrhea, hearing loss, cholesteatoma (mass-like keratinized epithelial growth), petrositis, intracranial extension (brain abscess, subdural empyema, or venous thrombosis), and mastoiditis. **Acute mastoiditis** is a suppurative complication of OM with inflammation and potential destruction of the mastoid air spaces. The disease progresses from a periostitis to an osteitis with mastoid abscess formation. Posterior auricular tenderness, swelling, and erythema, in addition to the signs of OM, are present. The pinna is displaced downward and outward. Computed tomography scan of the mastoid reveals clouding of the air cells, demineralization, or bone destruction. Treatment includes systemic antibiotics and drainage if the disease has progressed to abscess formation.

OME is the most frequent sequela of AOM and occurs most frequently in the first 2 years of life (up to 30-50% of children with AOM). **Persistent middle ear effusion** may last for many weeks or months in some children but usually resolves by 3 months following infection. Evaluating young children for this condition is an important part of all well-child examinations because, although not an infectious process, it is associated with hearing loss.

Conductive hearing loss should be assumed to be present with persistent middle ear effusion; the loss is mild to moderate and often is transient or fluctuating. In children at developmental risk or with frequent episodes of recurrent AOM, 3 months of persistent effusion with significant bilateral hearing loss is a reasonable indicator of need for intervention with insertion of pressure equalization tubes.

PREVENTION

Parents should be encouraged to continue exclusive breast feeding as long as possible and should be cautioned about the risks of *bottle-propping* and of children taking a bottle to bed. The home should be a smoke-free environment, and pacifier use should be limited.

The conjugate *S. pneumoniae* vaccine reduces pneumococcal OM caused by vaccine serotypes by 50%, all pneumococcal OM by 33%, and all OM by 6-10%. Annual immunization against influenza virus may be helpful in high-risk children.

CHAPTER 106

Otitis Externa

ETIOLOGY

Otitis externa, also known as **swimmer's ear,** is defined by inflammation and exudate in the external auditory canal in the absence of other disorders, such as otitis media or mastoiditis. The most common bacterial pathogens are *Pseudomonas aeruginosa*, especially in association with swimming in pools or lakes, and *Staphylococcus aureus.* Otitis externa develops in approximately 20% of children with **tympanostomy tubes,** associated with *S. aureus, Streptococcus pneumoniae, Moraxella catarrhalis, Proteus, Klebsiella,* and occasionally anaerobes.

Coagulase-negative staphylococci and *Corynebacterium* are isolated frequently from cultures of the external canal but represent normal flora. **Malignant otitis externa** is caused by *P. aeruginosa* in immunocompromised persons and adults with diabetes.

EPIDEMIOLOGY

Otitis externa cases peak in summer, in contrast to otitis media, which occurs primarily in colder seasons in association with viral upper respiratory tract infections. Cleaning of the auditory canal, swimming, and, in particular, diving disrupt the integrity of the cutaneous lining of the ear canal and local defenses, such as cerumen, predisposing to otitis externa.

CLINICAL MANIFESTATIONS

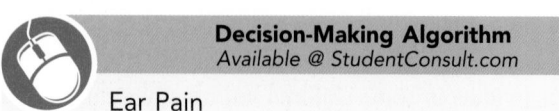

Decision-Making Algorithm
Available @ StudentConsult.com

Ear Pain

Pain, tenderness, and aural discharge are the characteristic clinical findings of otitis externa. Fever is notably absent, and hearing is unaffected. Tenderness with movement of the pinna, especially the tragus, and with chewing is particularly characteristic, which are symptoms notably absent in otitis media. Inspection usually reveals that the lining of the auditory canal is inflamed with mild to severe erythema and edema. Scant to copious discharge from the auditory canal may obscure the tympanic membrane. The most common symptoms of **malignant otitis externa** are similar, but facial nerve palsy occasionally occurs. The most common physical findings are swelling and granulation tissue in the canal, usually with a discharge from the external auditory canal.

LABORATORY AND IMAGING STUDIES

The diagnosis of uncomplicated otitis externa usually is established solely on the basis of the clinical symptoms and physical examination findings without the need for additional laboratory or microbiologic evaluation. Cultures are required to identify the etiological agent, which is usually *P. aeruginosa*, and the antimicrobial susceptibility.

DIFFERENTIAL DIAGNOSIS

Otitis media with tympanic perforation and discharge into the auditory canal may be confused with otitis externa. Pain on movement of the pinnae or tragus, typical of otitis externa, is absent. Local and systemic signs of mastoiditis indicate a process more extensive than otitis externa. **Malignancies** or cholesteatoma presenting in the auditory canal are rare in children but may present with discharge, unusual pain, or hearing loss.

TREATMENT

Topical antimicrobial/corticosteroid otic preparations (such as ofloxacin, ciprofloxacin with hydrocortisone or dexamethasone, and polymyxin B-neosporin-hydrocortisone) are sufficient in most cases of otitis externa. These preparations are equally effective and are active against *S. aureus* and most gram-negative bacteria, including *P. aeruginosa.* None of these antibiotics has any antifungal activity. Use of aminoglycosides such as neomycin should be avoided in cases of tympanic membrane rupture due to their ototoxicity. **Tympanostomy tube otorrhea** is best treated with quinolone otic drugs, which are considered less likely to be ototoxic.

Treatment with topical otic analgesics and ceruminolytics is usually unnecessary. It is important with any topical therapy to remove purulent discharge from the external auditory canal with a swab or with suction to permit instillation of the solution. Excess water should be removed after bathing and the ear canal dried using a hairdryer. The predisposing activity, such as swimming or diving, should be avoided until the inflammation has resolved.

Fungi such as *Aspergillus*, *Candida*, and dermatophytes are occasionally isolated from the external ear. It may be difficult to determine whether they represent normal flora or are the cause of inflammation. In most cases, local therapy and restoration of normal pH as recommended for bacterial otitis externa are sufficient.

Malignant otitis externa is treated by parenteral antimicrobials with activity against *P. aeruginosa*, such as an extended-spectrum penicillin (piperacillin-tazobactam), a cephalosporin with activity against *P. aeruginosa* (ceftazidime, cefepime), or a fluoroquinolone (ciprofloxacin).

COMPLICATIONS AND PROGNOSIS

Acute otitis externa usually resolves promptly without complications within 1-2 days of initiating treatment. Persistent pain, especially if severe or if accompanied by other symptoms (e.g., fever) should prompt re-evaluation for other conditions.

Complications of malignant otitis externa include invasion of the bones at the base of the skull, which may cause cranial nerve palsies. A mortality of 15-20% occurs in adults with malignant otitis media. Relapses within the first year after treatment are common.

PREVENTION

Overly vigorous cleaning of an asymptomatic auditory canal should be avoided. Drying the auditory canals with acetic acid (2%), Burow solution, or diluted isopropyl alcohol (rubbing alcohol) after swimming may be used prophylactically to help prevent the maceration that facilitates bacterial invasion. There is no role for prophylactic otic antibiotics.

CHAPTER 107

Croup (Laryngotracheobronchitis)

ETIOLOGY AND EPIDEMIOLOGY

Croup, or laryngotracheobronchitis, is the most common infection of the middle respiratory tract. The most common causes of croup are parainfluenza viruses (types 1, 2, 3, and 4) and respiratory syncytial virus (RSV). Laryngotracheal airway inflammation disproportionately affects children because a small decrease in diameter secondary to mucosal edema and inflammation exponentially increases airway resistance and the work of breathing. During inspiration, the walls of the subglottic space are drawn together, aggravating the obstruction and producing the **stridor** characteristic of croup. Croup is most common in children 6 months to 3 years of age, with a peak in fall and early winter. It typically follows a common cold. Symptomatic reinfection is common, yet reinfections are usually mild. In adolescents, it manifests as laryngitis.

CLINICAL MANIFESTATIONS

Decision-Making Algorithms
Available @ StudentConsult.com

Cough
Hoarseness
Stridor
Apnea

The manifestations of croup are a harsh cough described as **barking** or **brassy,** hoarseness, inspiratory stridor, low-grade fever, and respiratory distress that may develop slowly or quickly. **Stridor** is a harsh, high-pitched respiratory sound produced by turbulent airflow. It is usually inspiratory, but it may be biphasic and is a sign of upper airway obstruction. Signs of upper airway obstruction, such as labored breathing, cyanosis, and marked suprasternal, intercostal, and subcostal retractions, may be evident on examination (see Chapter 135). Wheezing may be present if there is associated lower airway involvement.

LABORATORY AND IMAGING STUDIES

Anteroposterior radiographs of the neck often show the diagnostic subglottic narrowing of croup known as the **steeple sign** (Fig. 107.1). Routine laboratory studies are not useful in establishing the diagnosis. Leukocytosis is uncommon and suggests epiglottitis or bacterial tracheitis. Many rapid tests (using polymerase chain reaction [PCR]) are available for parainfluenza viruses, RSV, and other less common viral causes of croup, such as influenza and adenoviruses.

DIFFERENTIAL DIAGNOSIS

The diagnosis of croup is usually established by clinical manifestations. The infectious differential diagnosis includes epiglottitis, bacterial tracheitis, and parapharyngeal abscess. Noninfectious causes of stridor include mechanical and anatomical causes (foreign body aspiration, laryngomalacia, subglottic stenosis, hemangioma, vascular ring, vocal cord paralysis). Stridor in infants younger than 4 months of age, positional stridor, or persistence of symptoms for longer than 1 week indicates an increased probability of another lesion and the need for imaging and direct laryngoscopy (see Chapter 135).

Epiglottitis is a medical emergency because of the risk of sudden airway obstruction. This illness is now rare and usually

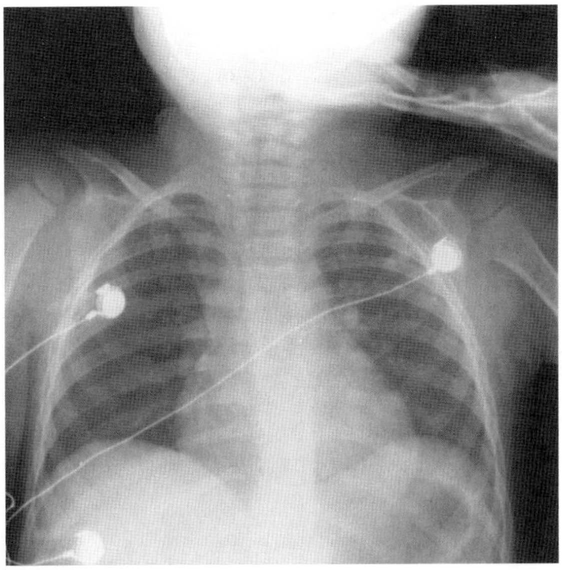

FIGURE 107.1 Croup (laryngotracheobronchitis). Radiograph of the airway and chest of a patient with croup, demonstrating the typical subglottic narrowing ("steeple sign"). (From Roosevelt GE. Acute inflammatory upper airway obstruction [croup, epiglottitis, laryngitis, and bacterial tracheitis]. In: Kliegman RM, Stanton BF, St. Geme III JW, Schor NF, eds. *Nelson Textbook of Pediatrics.* 20th ed. Philadelphia: Elsevier; 2016. Fig. 385-1.)

caused by group A streptococcus or *Staphylococcus aureus* or *Haemophilus influenzae* type b in unimmunized patients. Patients typically prefer sitting, often with the head held forward, the mouth open, and the jaw thrust forward **(sniffing position)**, and may appear distressed and toxic. Lateral radiograph reveals thickened and bulging epiglottis **(thumb sign)** and swelling of the aryepiglottic folds. The diagnosis is confirmed by direct observation of the inflamed and swollen supraglottic structures and swollen, cherry red epiglottitis. Direct observation of the larynx should only be performed in the operating room with an anesthesiologist and a competent surgeon prepared to place an endotracheal tube or perform a tracheostomy if needed. Epiglottitis requires antibiotic therapy and endotracheal intubation to maintain the airway. Both onset and clinical recovery are rapid, and most children can be extubated safely within 48-72 hours.

Bacterial tracheitis is a rare but serious superinfection of the trachea that may follow viral croup and is most commonly caused by *S. aureus.* Patients may be toxic appearing, and intubation may be required. **Spasmodic croup** describes sudden onset of croup symptoms, usually at night, but without a significant upper respiratory tract prodrome. These episodes may be recurrent and severe but usually are of short duration. Spasmodic croup has a milder course than viral croup and responds to relatively simple therapies, such as exposure to cool or humidified air. The etiology is not well understood and may be allergic.

TREATMENT

Oral or intramuscular dexamethasone for children with croup reduces symptoms and the need for hospitalization, and shortens hospital stays. Dexamethasone (0.6-1 mg/kg) may be given once intramuscularly or orally. Alternatively, prednisolone (2 mg/kg/day) may be given orally in two to three divided doses. For significant airway compromise, administration of aerosolized racemic (D- and L-)epinephrine reduces subglottic edema by adrenergic vasoconstriction, temporarily producing marked clinical improvement. The peak effect is within 10-30 minutes and fades within 60-90 minutes. A rebound effect may occur, with worsening of symptoms as the effect of the drug dissipates. Aerosol treatment may need to be repeated every 20 minutes (for no more than 1-2 hours) in severe cases.

Children should be kept as calm as possible to minimize forceful inspiration. One useful calming method is for a child with croup to sit on the parent's lap. Sedatives should be used cautiously and in the intensive care unit only. Cool mist administered by face mask may help prevent drying of the secretions around the larynx.

Hospitalization is often required for children with cyanosis, or stridor at rest. Children receiving aerosol treatment should be hospitalized or observed for at least 2-3 hours because of the risk of rebound airway obstruction. Decreased symptoms may indicate improvement or fatigue, and impending respiratory failure.

COMPLICATIONS AND PROGNOSIS

The most common complication of croup is viral pneumonia, which occurs in 1-2% of children. Parainfluenza virus pneumonia and secondary bacterial pneumonia are more common in immunocompromised patients. Bacterial tracheitis may also be a complication of croup.

The prognosis for croup is excellent. Illness usually lasts approximately 5 days. As children grow, they become less susceptible to the airway effects of viral infections of the middle respiratory tract.

PREVENTION

There are no licensed vaccines for parainfluenza or RSV.

CHAPTER 108

Pertussis

ETIOLOGY

Classic pertussis **(whooping cough)** is caused by *Bordetella pertussis*, a gram-negative pleomorphic bacillus with fastidious growth requirements. *B. pertussis* infects only humans and is transmitted person to person by coughing.

EPIDEMIOLOGY

The typical incubation period is 7-10 days but can range between 5 and 21 days. Patients are most contagious during the first 2 weeks of cough. The annual rate of pertussis was approximately 100-200 cases per 100,000 population in the prevaccination era; worldwide there continue to be an estimated 15 million cases of pertussis and 200,000 childhood deaths annually. In the United States the incidence of pertussis decreased after the introduction of vaccine, but it has increased steadily since the 1980s, with more than 18,000 cases reported in 2015. Pertussis incidence peaks among those less than 6 months of age—infants too young to be completely immunized and most likely to have severe complications—at approximately 150 cases per 100,000 population. Rates of infection in late childhood and adolescence have also been rising, likely due to a combination of waning immunity from previous vaccines, underimmunization, and improved diagnostics. Epidemics can occur in fully immunized patients because vaccine-induced immunity wanes.

CLINICAL MANIFESTATIONS

Decision-Making Algorithms
Available at StudentConsult.com

Cough
Cyanosis
Apnea

Classic pertussis is seen in children between 1 and 10 years old. The progression of the disease is divided into catarrhal, paroxysmal, and convalescent stages. The **catarrhal stage** is marked by nonspecific signs (increased nasal secretions and low-grade fever) lasting 1-2 weeks. The **paroxysmal stage** is the most distinctive stage of pertussis and lasts 2-4 weeks. Coughing occurs in **paroxysms** during expiration, causing young children to lose their breath. This pattern of coughing is needed to dislodge plugs of necrotic bronchial epithelial tissues and thick mucus. The forceful inhalation against a narrowed glottis that follows this paroxysm of cough produces the characteristic **whoop.** Posttussive emesis is common. The **convalescent stage** is marked by gradual resolution of symptoms over 1-2 weeks. Coughing becomes less severe, and the paroxysms and whoops slowly disappear. Although the disease typically lasts 6-8 weeks, residual cough may persist for months, especially with physical stress or respiratory irritants.

Infants may not display the classic findings, and the first sign in the neonate may be apnea. Young infants are unlikely to have the classic whoop, more likely to have central nervous system damage as a result of hypoxia, and more likely to have secondary bacterial pneumonia. Adolescents and adults with pertussis usually present with a prolonged bronchitic illness with persistent, nonproductive cough that often begins as a nonspecific upper respiratory tract infection. In general, adolescents and adults do not have a whoop with the cough, although they may have severe paroxysms.

LABORATORY AND IMAGING STUDIES

The diagnosis depends on isolation of *B. pertussis* or detection of its nucleic acids. Culture on specialized media is usually performed during the early phases of illness on specimens from nasopharyngeal swabs or aspirates, but this can be difficult to accomplish given the organism's fastidious nature. Polymerase chain reaction is available in many clinical laboratories. False-positive results can occur. Direct fluorescent antibody staining is not recommended. Serological tests are not useful for diagnosing acute infection but can be confirmatory in the convalescent phase of illness, though there are no commercial kits approved by the U.S. Food and Drug Administration.

Lymphocytosis is present in 75-85% of infants and young children but is not diagnostic. The white blood cell count may increase from 20,000/mm^3 to more than 50,000/mm^3, consisting primarily of mature lymphocytes. Physical examination and radiographic signs of segmental lung atelectasis may develop during pertussis, especially during the paroxysmal stage. Perihilar infiltrates are common and are similar to those seen in viral pneumonia.

DIFFERENTIAL DIAGNOSIS

For a young child with classic pertussis, the diagnosis based on the pattern of illness is quite accurate. The paroxysmal stage is the most distinctive part of the syndrome. Other causes of pertussis-like prolonged cough illnesses include *Bordetella parapertussis* and *Bordetella holmesii*—which cause a similar but milder illness and are not prevented by *B. pertussis* vaccination—*Mycoplasma pneumoniae, Chlamydophila pneumoniae*, adenoviruses, and respiratory syncytial virus.

TREATMENT

Macrolide antibiotics (azithromycin, clarithromycin, or erythromycin) are recommended for treatment. Azithromycin is preferred in neonates due to the association between erythromycin treatment and the development of pyloric stenosis. Treatment during the catarrhal phase eradicates nasopharyngeal carriage of organisms within 3-4 days and may lessen symptom severity. Treatment in the paroxysmal stage does not alter the course of illness but decreases the potential for spread to others. Trimethoprim-sulfamethoxazole is an alternative therapy among children older than 2 months, although studies of its use for this indication are limited.

COMPLICATIONS AND PROGNOSIS

Major complications are most common among infants and young children and include hypoxia, apnea, pneumonia, seizures, encephalopathy, malnutrition, and death. The most frequent complication is pneumonia caused by *B. pertussis* itself or resulting from secondary bacterial infection with *Streptococcus pneumoniae, Haemophilus influenzae*, and *Staphylococcus aureus.* Atelectasis may develop secondary to mucous plugs. The force of the paroxysm may produce pneumomediastinum, pneumothorax, or interstitial or subcutaneous emphysema; epistaxis; hernias; and retinal and subconjunctival hemorrhages. Otitis media and sinusitis may occur.

Most children recover normal pulmonary function with complete healing of the respiratory epithelium. Most permanent disability is a result of encephalopathy.

PREVENTION

Active immunity is induced with acellular pertussis components given as a vaccine in combination with the tetanus and diphtheria toxoids (DTaP). The acellular pertussis vaccines contain two to five antigens of *B. pertussis*, including pertussis toxin, pertactin, filamentous hemagglutinin, and fimbrial agglutinogens FIM-2 and FIM-3. DTaP vaccine is recommended at 2, 4, 6, and 15-18 months, with a booster at 4-6 years, and has an efficacy of 70-90%. A single booster dose of Tdap vaccine is recommended at 11-12 years or once for all adults. A booster dose of Tdap vaccine is recommended for pregnant women with each pregnancy, preferably in the third trimester, to provide higher levels of antibodies to the infant via transplacental transfer.

Macrolides are effective in preventing secondary cases in contacts exposed to pertussis. Underimmunized close contacts under 7 years of age should receive a booster dose of DTaP (unless a booster dose has been given within the preceding 3 years), whereas those 7-10 years of age should receive Tdap. All close contacts should receive prophylactic antibiotics for 5 days (azithromycin) or 7-14 days (clarithromycin or erythromycin, duration based on age).

CHAPTER 109

Bronchiolitis

ETIOLOGY

Bronchiolitis is a disease of small bronchioles with increased mucus production and occasional bronchospasm, sometimes leading to airway obstruction. It is most commonly caused by a viral lower respiratory tract infection. Bronchiolitis is most commonly seen in infants and young children, with most severe cases occurring among infants. Bronchiolitis is potentially life-threatening.

Respiratory syncytial virus (RSV) is a primary cause of bronchiolitis, followed in frequency by human metapneumovirus, parainfluenza viruses, influenza viruses, adenoviruses, rhinoviruses, coronaviruses, and, infrequently, *Mycoplasma pneumoniae.* Viral bronchiolitis is extremely contagious and is spread by contact with infected respiratory secretions. Although coughing produces aerosols, hand carriage of contaminated secretions is the most frequent mode of transmission.

EPIDEMIOLOGY

Bronchiolitis is a leading cause of hospitalization of infants. Bronchiolitis occurs almost exclusively during the first 2 years of life, with a peak age at 2-6 months. Many healthy children with bronchiolitis can be managed as outpatients; however, premature infants and children with chronic lung disease of prematurity, hemodynamically significant congenital heart disease, neuromuscular weakness, or immunodeficiency are at increased risk of severe, potentially fatal disease. Children acquire infection after exposure to infected family members, who typically have symptoms of an upper respiratory tract infection, or from infected children in day care. In the United States, annual peaks are usually in the late winter months from December through March.

CLINICAL MANIFESTATIONS

Decision-Making Algorithms
Available @ StudentConsult.com

Wheezing
Apnea

Bronchiolitis caused by RSV typically has an incubation period of 4-6 days. Bronchiolitis classically presents as a progressive respiratory illness similar to the common cold in its early phase, with cough and rhinorrhea. It progresses over 3-7 days to noisy, raspy breathing and audible wheezing. There is usually a low-grade fever accompanied by irritability, which may reflect the increased work of breathing. In contrast to the classic progression of disease, young infants infected with RSV may not have a prodrome and may have apnea as the first sign of infection.

Physical signs of bronchiolar obstruction include prolongation of the expiratory phase of breathing, nasal flaring, intercostal retractions, suprasternal retractions, and air trapping with hyperexpansion of the lungs. During the wheezing phase, percussion of the chest usually reveals only hyperresonance, but auscultation usually reveals diffuse wheezes and crackles throughout the breathing cycle. With more severe disease, grunting and cyanosis may be present.

LABORATORY AND IMAGING STUDIES

Routine laboratory tests are not required to confirm the diagnosis. It is important to assess oxygenation in severe cases of bronchiolitis. **Pulse oximetry** is adequate for monitoring oxygen saturation. Frequent, regular assessments and cardiorespiratory monitoring of infants are necessary because respiratory failure may develop precipitously in very tired infants even though blood gas values taken before rapid decompensation are reassuring.

Rapid viral diagnosis of nasopharyngeal secretions performed by polymerase chain reactions for RSV, parainfluenza viruses, influenza viruses, and adenoviruses are sensitive tests to confirm the infection. Identifying the viral agent is helpful for cohorting children with the same infection but is not necessary to make the diagnosis of bronchiolitis.

Chest radiographs are not always necessary but frequently show signs of lung hyperinflation, including increased lung lucency and flattened or depressed diaphragms. Areas of increased density may represent either viral pneumonia or localized atelectasis.

DIFFERENTIAL DIAGNOSIS

The major difficulty in the diagnosis of bronchiolitis is to differentiate other diseases associated with wheezing. It may be difficult to differentiate asthma from bronchiolitis by physical examination, but age of presentation, presence of fever, and absence of personal or family history of asthma are the major differential factors. Bronchiolitis occurs primarily in the first year of life and is accompanied by fever, whereas asthma usually presents in older children with previous wheezing episodes typically unaccompanied by fever unless a respiratory tract infection is the trigger for the asthma exacerbation.

Wheezing may also be due to an airway foreign body, congenital airway obstructive lesion, cystic fibrosis, exacerbation of chronic lung disease, viral or bacterial pneumonia, and other lower respiratory tract diseases (see Chapter 78). **Cardiogenic asthma**, which can be confused with bronchiolitis in infants, is wheezing associated with pulmonary congestion secondary to left-sided heart failure. Wheezing associated with gastroesophageal reflux is likely to be chronic or recurrent, and the patient may have a history of frequent emesis. Cystic fibrosis is associated with poor growth, chronic diarrhea, and a positive family history. A focal area on radiography that remains inflated despite changes in position suggests **foreign body aspiration.**

TREATMENT

Bronchiolitis treatment consists of supportive therapy, including respiratory monitoring, control of fever, hydration, upper airway suctioning, and, if needed, oxygen administration. Indications for hospitalization include moderate to marked respiratory distress, hypoxemia, apnea, inability to tolerate oral feeding, and lack of appropriate care available at home. Hospitalization of high-risk children with bronchiolitis should be considered. Among hospitalized infants, supplemental oxygen by nasal cannula is often necessary, but intubation and ventilatory assistance for respiratory failure or apnea are required in <10% of these infants. Bronchodilators, corticosteroids, chest physiotherapy, and hypertonic saline are seldom effective and are not generally recommended. Likewise, antibiotics should be avoided unless there is strong suspicion for concomitant bacterial infection.

COMPLICATIONS AND PROGNOSIS

Most hospitalized children show marked improvement in 2-5 days with supportive treatment alone. The course of the wheezing phase varies, however. Tachypnea and hypoxia may progress to respiratory failure requiring assisted ventilation. Apnea is a major concern for very young infants with bronchiolitis.

Most cases of bronchiolitis resolve completely, although minor abnormalities of pulmonary function and bronchial hyperreactivity may persist for several years. Recurrence is common but tends to be mild and should be assessed and treated similarly to the first episode. The incidence of asthma seems to be higher in children hospitalized for bronchiolitis as infants, but it is unclear whether this is causal or whether children prone to asthma are more likely to be hospitalized with bronchiolitis. There is a 1-2% mortality rate, highest among infants with preexisting cardiopulmonary or immunological impairment.

PREVENTION

Monthly injections of **palivizumab**, an RSV-specific monoclonal antibody, initiated just before the onset of the RSV season confers some protection from severe RSV disease. Palivizumab is indicated for some infants with prematurity (born before 29 weeks, 0 days' gestation), chronic lung disease of prematurity, and those with hemodynamically significant cyanotic and acyanotic congenital heart disease in the first year of life, and rarely in the second year of life. Immunization with influenza vaccine is recommended for all children older than 6 months and may prevent influenza-associated disease.

CHAPTER 110

Pneumonia

ETIOLOGY

Pneumonia is an infection of the lower respiratory tract that involves the airways and parenchyma, with consolidation of the alveolar spaces. The term **lower respiratory tract infection**

is often used to encompass bronchitis, bronchiolitis (see Chapter 109), pneumonia, or any combination of the three. **Pneumonitis** is a general term for lung inflammation that may or may not be associated with consolidation. **Lobar pneumonia** describes pneumonia localized to one or more lobes of the lung. **Atypical pneumonia** describes patterns typically more diffuse or interstitial than lobar pneumonia. **Bronchopneumonia** refers to inflammation of the lung that is centered in the bronchioles and leads to the production of a mucopurulent exudate that obstructs some of these small airways and causes patchy consolidation of the adjacent lobules. **Interstitial pneumonitis** refers to inflammation of the interstitium, which is composed of the walls of the alveoli, the alveolar sacs and ducts, and the bronchioles. Interstitial pneumonitis is characteristic of acute viral infections but may also be a chronic inflammatory or fibrosing process.

Defects in host defenses increase the risk of pneumonia. Lower airways and secretions are sterile as a result of a multifactorial system. Airway contaminants are caught in the mucus secreted by the goblet cells. Cilia on epithelial surfaces, composing the ciliary elevator system, beat synchronously to move particles upward toward central airways and into the throat, where they are swallowed or expectorated. Polymorphonuclear neutrophils from the blood and tissue macrophages ingest and kill microorganisms. IgA secreted into the upper airway fluid protects against invasive infections and facilitates viral neutralization.

Infectious agents that commonly cause community-acquired pneumonia vary by age (Table 110.1). *Streptococcus pneumoniae* is the most common bacterial cause of pneumonia (particularly **lobar** pneumonia) and occurs in children of any age outside the neonatal period. Other common causes include respiratory syncytial virus (RSV) in infants (see Chapter 109), other respiratory viruses (parainfluenza viruses, influenza viruses, human metapneumovirus, adenoviruses) in children younger than 5 years old, and *Mycoplasma pneumoniae* in children older than age 5 years. *M. pneumoniae* and *Chlamydophila pneumoniae* are principal causes of **atypical pneumonia**.

Chlamydia trachomatis and less commonly *Mycoplasma hominis, Ureaplasma urealyticum*, and cytomegalovirus (CMV) cause a similar respiratory syndrome in infants 2 weeks to 3 months of age, with subacute onset of an **afebrile pneumonia**; cough and hyperinflation are the predominant signs. These infections are difficult to diagnose and distinguish from each other. In adults these organisms are carried primarily as part of the genital mucosal flora. Women who harbor these agents may transmit them perinatally to newborns.

Additional agents occasionally cause pneumonia. **Severe acute respiratory syndrome (SARS)** is due to SARS-associated coronavirus (SARS-CoV). **Avian influenza (bird flu)** is a highly contagious viral disease of poultry and other birds caused by **influenza A (H5N1).** There were outbreaks among humans in Southeast Asia in 1997 and 2003-2004, with high mortality rates. A novel influenza A (H1N1) of swine origin began circulating in 2009. Other etiological agents to consider, based on specific exposure history, include *Staphylococcus aureus* and *Streptococcus pyogenes* (especially after influenza infection), *Mycobacterium tuberculosis, Francisella tularensis, Brucella* spp., *Coxiella burnetii, Chlamydophila psittaci, Legionella pneumophila,* hantavirus, *Histoplasma capsulatum, Coccidioides immitis, Blastomyces dermatitidis,* and oral flora or gram-negative bacilli (after aspiration).

Causes of pneumonia in immunocompromised persons include gram-negative enteric bacteria, mycobacteria (*M. avium* complex), fungi (aspergillosis), viruses (CMV), and *Pneumocystis jirovecii* (formerly *carinii*). Pneumonia in patients with cystic fibrosis is usually caused by *S. s aureus* in infancy and *Pseudomonas aeruginosa* or *Burkholderia cepacia* in older patients.

EPIDEMIOLOGY

Immunizations have markedly reduced the incidence of pneumonia caused by pertussis, diphtheria, measles, *Haemophilus influenzae* type b, and *S. pneumoniae.* Where used, bacille Calmette-Guérin (BCG) immunization for tuberculosis has also had some impact. Pneumonia is the single largest contributor of childhood mortality worldwide, killing an estimated 1 million children under 5 years of age annually. Risk factors for lower respiratory tract infections include gastroesophageal reflux, neurological impairment (aspiration), immunocompromised states, anatomical abnormalities of the respiratory tract, residence in residential care facilities, and hospitalization, especially in an intensive care unit.

CLINICAL MANIFESTATIONS

Decision-Making Algorithms
Available @ StudentConsult.com

Cough
Wheezing
Hemoptysis
Chest Pain
Abdominal Pain
Failure to Thrive
Acidemia

Age is a determinant in the clinical manifestations of pneumonia. Neonates may have fever or hypoxia only, with subtle or absent physical examination findings (see Chapter 65). With a young infant, apnea may be the first sign of pneumonia. Fever, chills, tachypnea, cough, malaise, pleuritic chest pain, retractions, and apprehension—because of difficulty breathing or shortness of breath—are common in older infants and children. Physical examination findings cannot reliably distinguish viral and bacterial pneumonias, but complete physical examination may help identify other foci of disease or associated findings to suggest an etiology.

Viral pneumonias are generally associated more often with cough, wheezing, or stridor; fever is less prominent than with bacterial pneumonia. Mucosal congestion and upper airway inflammation suggest a viral infection. Bacterial pneumonias are typically associated with higher fever, chills, cough, dyspnea, and auscultatory findings of lung consolidation. Atypical pneumonia in young infants is characterized by tachypnea, cough, and crackles on auscultation. Concomitant conjunctivitis may be present in infants with chlamydial pneumonia. Other signs of respiratory distress include nasal flaring, intercostal and subcostal retractions, and grunting.

Asymmetry or shallow breathing may be due to splinting from pain. Hyperexpansion, common in asthma but also frequently accompanying viral lower respiratory infections, may cause

TABLE 110.1 Etiological Agents and Empirical Antimicrobial Therapy for Pneumonia in Patients Without History of Recent Antibiotic Therapy

AGE GROUP	COMMON PATHOGENS* (IN APPROXIMATE ORDER OF FREQUENCY)*	LESS COMMON PATHOGENS	OUTPATIENTS (7-10 DAYS TOTAL DURATION OF TREATMENT)†	PATIENTS REQUIRING HOSPITALIZATION (10-14 DAYS TOTAL DURATION OF TREATMENT)‡	PATIENTS REQUIRING INTENSIVE CARE (10-14 DAYS TOTAL DURATION OF TREATMENT)*,‡
Neonates (up to 1 mo of age)	Group B streptococcus, *Escherichia coli*, other gram-negative bacilli, *Streptococcus pneumoniae*	Cytomegalovirus, Herpes simplex virus, *Listeria monocytogenes*, *Treponema pallidum*, *Haemophilus influenzae* (type b,§ nontypable)	Outpatient management not recommended	Ampicillin *plus* cefotaxime or an aminoglycoside *plus* an antistaphylococcal agent if *Staphylococcus aureus* is suspected	Ampicillin *plus* cefotaxime or an aminoglycoside *plus* an antistaphylococcal agent if *S. aureus* is suspected
1-3 mo					
Febrile pneumonia	Respiratory syncytial virus, other respiratory viruses (parainfluenza viruses, influenza viruses, adenoviruses), *S. pneumoniae*, *H. influenzae* (type b,§ nontypable)		Initial outpatient management not recommended	Amoxicillin or ampicillin if fully immunized for age for *S. pneumoniae* and *H. influenzae* type b. Alternatives: cefotaxime or ceftriaxone if not fully immunized or local *S. pneumoniae* penicillin resistance is significant, with clindamycin if MRSA suspected	Cefotaxime or ceftriaxone *plus* nafcillin, oxacillin, clindamycin, or vancomycin
Afebrile pneumonia	*Chlamydia trachomatis*, *Mycoplasma hominis*, *Ureaplasma urealyticum*, cytomegalovirus *Bordetella pertussis*		Erythromycin, azithromycin, or clarithromycin with close follow-up	Erythromycin, azithromycin, or clarithromycin	Erythromycin, azithromycin, or clarithromycin *plus* cefotaxime or ceftriaxone *plus* nafcillin, oxacillin, clindamycin, or vancomycin
3 mo to 5 yr	Respiratory syncytial virus, other respiratory viruses (parainfluenza viruses, influenza viruses, human metapneumovirus adenoviruses), *S. pneumoniae*, *H. influenzae* (type b,§ nontypable)	*C. trachomatis*, *Mycoplasma pneumoniae*, *Chlamydophila pneumoniae*, group A streptococcus, *S. aureus*, *Mycobacterium tuberculosis*	Amoxicillin *plus* erythromycin, azithromycin, or clarithromycin if atypical pneumonia suspected	Ampicillin Alternatives: cefotaxime or ceftriaxone if not fully immunized or local *S. pneumoniae* penicillin resistance is significant, with clindamycin if MRSA suspected; Add erythromycin, azithromycin, or clarithromycin if atypical pneumonia suspected	Cefuroxime or ceftriaxone *plus* azithromycin, erythromycin or clarithromycin *with or without* clindamycin or vancomycin
5-18 yr	*M. pneumoniae*, *S. pneumoniae*, *C. pneumoniae*	*H. influenzae* (type b,§ nontypable), influenza viruses, adenoviruses, other respiratory viruses	Amoxicillin *plus* erythromycin, azithromycin, or clarithromycin if atypical pneumonia suspected	Ampicillin *plus* erythromycin, azithromycin, or clarithromycin if atypical pneumonia suspected	Cefuroxime or ceftriaxone *plus* azithromycin, erythromycin or clarithromycin *with or without* clindamycin or vancomycin
≥18 yr§	*M. pneumoniae*, *S. pneumoniae*, *C. pneumoniae*, *H. influenzae* (type b,§ nontypable), influenza viruses, adenoviruses	*Legionella pneumophila*, *M. tuberculosis*	Amoxicillin, *or* erythromycin, azithromycin, clarithromycin, doxycycline, moxifloxacin, gatifloxacin, levofloxacin, or gemifloxacin‖ if atypical pneumonia suspected	Ampicillin *plus* erythromycin, azithromycin, or clarithromycin if atypical pneumonia suspected *or* moxifloxacin, gatifloxacin, levofloxacin, or gemifloxacin	Cefotaxime or ceftriaxone, *plus either* azithromycin or clarithromycin *with or without* clindamycin or vancomycin, *or* moxifloxacin, gatifloxacin, levofloxacin, or gemifloxacin *with or without* clindamycin or vancomycin

**Severe pneumonia, from* Streptococcus pneumoniae, Staphylococcus aureus, group A streptococcus, Haemophilus influenzae, *or* Mycoplasma pneumoniae *requiring admission to an intensive care unit. Antipseudomonal agents should be added if Pseudomonas is suspected.*

†*Oral administration.*

‡*Intravenous administration for inpatients except for the macrolides (erythromycin, azithromycin, and clarithromycin), which are given orally.*

§Haemophilus influenzae *type b infection is uncommon with universal* H. influenzae *type b immunization.*

‖*Fluoroquinolones are contraindicated for children younger than 18 years of age and pregnant or lactating women. Tetracyclines are not recommended for children younger than 9 years.*

MRSA, Methicillin-resistant *Staphylococcus aureus.*

a low diaphragm seen on a chest x-ray. Poor diaphragmatic excursion may indicate hyperexpanded lungs or an inability for expansion due to a large consolidation or effusion. Dullness to percussion may be due to lobar or segmental infiltrates or pleural fluid. Auscultation may be normal in early or very focal pneumonia, but the presence of localized crackles, rhonchi, and wheezes may help one detect and locate pneumonia. Distant breath sounds may indicate a large, poorly ventilated area of consolidation or pleural fluid.

LABORATORY AND IMAGING STUDIES

Bacterial flora of the upper respiratory tract do not accurately reflect flora present in lower respiratory tract infections, and high-quality sputum is rarely obtainable from children. In otherwise healthy children without life-threatening disease, invasive procedures to obtain lower respiratory tissue or secretions are seldom indicated. Serological tests are not useful for the most common causes of bacterial pneumonia.

The white blood cell (WBC) count with viral pneumonias is often normal or mildly elevated, with a predominance of lymphocytes, whereas with bacterial pneumonias the WBC count is elevated (>15-20,000/mm^3), with a predominance of neutrophils. Mild eosinophilia is characteristic of infant *C. trachomatis* pneumonia. Blood cultures should be performed on ill, hospitalized children to attempt to diagnose a bacterial cause of pneumonia. Blood cultures identify a bacterial respiratory pathogen in 5-10% of children hospitalized for pneumonia (and 10-20% of those with pneumonia with empyema or large effusion). Urinary antigen tests are especially useful for *L. pneumophila* (Legionnaires disease).

Viral respiratory pathogens can be diagnosed using polymerase chain reaction (PCR) or rapid viral antigen detection, but neither can rule out concomitant bacterial pneumonia. *M. pneumoniae* can be confirmed by *Mycoplasma* PCR. CMV pneumonitis can be diagnosed with PCR from bronchoalveolar lavage fluid. The diagnosis of *M. tuberculosis* is established by the tuberculin skin test, serum interferon-gamma release assay, or analysis of sputum or gastric aspirates by culture, antigen detection, or PCR.

The need to establish an etiological diagnosis of pneumonia is greater in immunocompromised patients, patients with recurrent pneumonia, or those with pneumonia unresponsive to empirical therapy. For these patients, bronchoscopy with bronchoalveolar lavage and brush mucosal biopsy, needle aspiration of the lung, and open lung biopsy are methods of obtaining material for microbiologic diagnosis.

When there is a pleural **effusion or empyema**, a thoracentesis to obtain pleural fluid can be diagnostic and therapeutic. Evaluation differentiates between empyema and a sterile parapneumonic effusion caused by irritation of the pleura contiguous with the pneumonia. Gram stain, bacterial culture, or broad-range bacterial PCR may lead to microbiologic diagnosis. The pleural fluid can also be cultured for mycobacteria and fungi. Removal of grossly purulent pleural fluid reduces the patient's toxicity and associated discomfort and may facilitate more rapid recovery. Drainage of large pleural accumulations also improves pulmonary mechanics and gas exchange by increasing the ability of the lung to expand.

Frontal and lateral radiographs are required to localize disease and adequately visualize retrocardiac infiltrates; they are recommended for diagnosis among hospitalized children but are not necessary to confirm the diagnosis in well-appearing outpatients. Although there are characteristic radiographic findings of pneumonia, radiography alone cannot provide a definitive microbiologic diagnosis. Bacterial pneumonia characteristically shows lobar consolidation or a round pneumonia, with pleural effusion in 10-30% of cases (Fig. 110.1). Viral pneumonia characteristically shows diffuse, streaky infiltrates of bronchopneumonia (Fig. 110.2) and hyperinflation. Atypical pneumonia, as with *M. pneumoniae* and *C. pneumoniae*, shows increased interstitial markings or bronchopneumonia. Chest radiographs may be normal in early pneumonia, with infiltrates appearing during treatment as hydration is restored. Hilar lymphadenopathy is uncommon with bacterial pneumonia but may be a sign of tuberculosis, endemic mycoses,

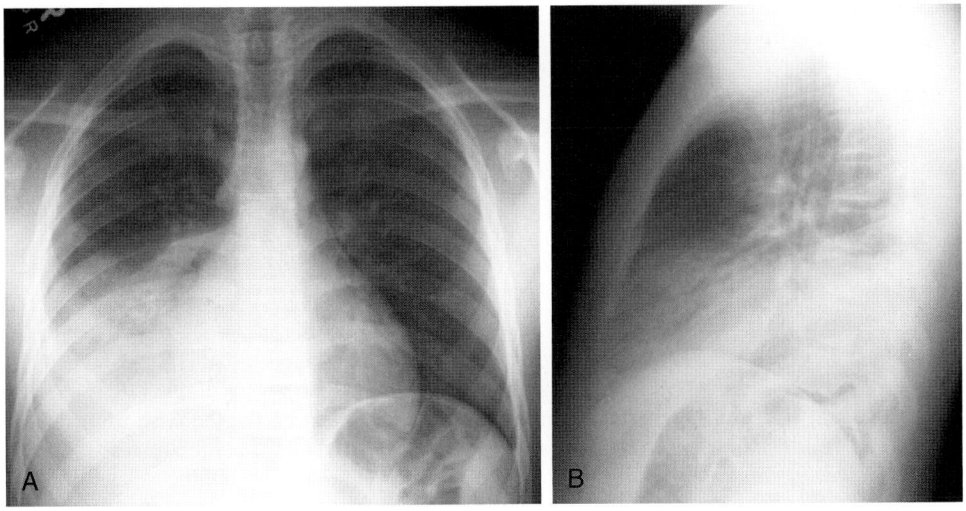

FIGURE 110.1 Acute lobar pneumonia of the right lower lobe in a 14-year-old boy with fever and cough. **(A)** Posteroanterior and **(B)** lateral chest radiographs demonstrate right-lower-lobe airspace consolidation, which obliterates the silhouette of the right heart border. (From Kelly MS, Sandora TJ. Community-acquired pneumonia. In: Kliegman RM, Stanton BF, St. Geme III JW, Schor NF, eds. *Nelson Textbook of Pediatrics*. 20th ed. Philadelphia: Elsevier; 2016. Fig. 400.3.)

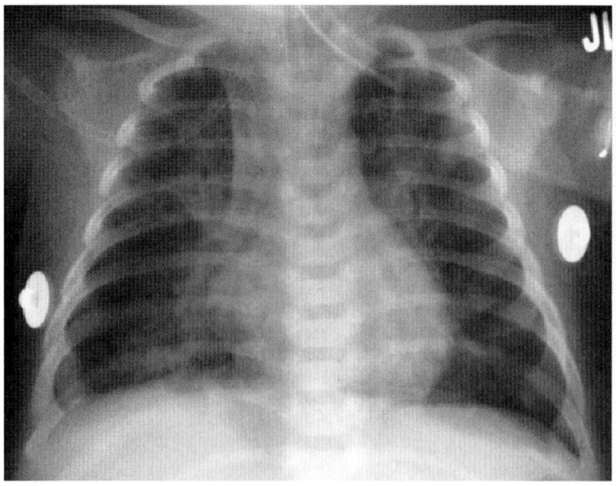

FIGURE 110.2 Diffuse respiratory syncytial virus pneumonia in a 6-month-old infant with tachypnea and fever. Anteroposterior chest radiograph shows bilateral, perihilar, peribronchial thickening and fine airspace disease with hyperinflation. (From Kelly MS, Sandora TJ. Community-acquired pneumonia. In: Kliegman RM, Stanton BF, St. Geme III JW, Schor NF, eds. *Nelson Textbook of Pediatrics*. 20th ed. Philadelphia: Elsevier; 2016. Fig. 400.2A.)

autoimmune conditions, or an underlying malignant neoplasm. Decubitus views or ultrasound should be used to assess the size of pleural effusions and whether they are freely mobile. Computed tomography (CT) is used to evaluate serious disease, lung abscesses, bronchiectasis, and effusion characteristics. Unusual etiologies or recurrent pneumonias require special considerations (Table 110.2). Lung abscesses, pneumatoceles, and empyema may require surgical management.

TABLE 110.2 Differential Diagnosis of Recurrent Pneumonia
HEREDITARY DISORDERS
Cystic fibrosis
Sickle cell disease
DISORDERS OF IMMUNITY
AIDS
Bruton agammaglobulinemia
Complement deficiency
Selective IgG subclass deficiencies
Common variable immunodeficiency syndrome
Severe combined immunodeficiency syndrome
DISORDERS OF LEUKOCYTES
Chronic granulomatous disease
Hyperimmunoglobulin E syndrome (Job syndrome)
Leukocyte adhesion defect
DISORDERS OF CILIA
Primary ciliary dyskinesia
Kartagener syndrome
ANATOMICAL DISORDERS
Sequestration
Lobar emphysema
Foreign body
Tracheoesophageal fistula (H type)
Congenital pulmonary airway malformation (cystic adenomatoid malformation)
Gastroesophageal reflux
Bronchiectasis
Aspiration (oropharyngeal incoordination)
NONINFECTIOUS MIMICS OF PNEUMONIA
Autoimmune diseases (e.g., granulomatosis with polyangiitis)
Hypersensitivity pneumonitis

DIFFERENTIAL DIAGNOSIS

Pneumonia must be differentiated from other acute pulmonary diseases, including allergic pneumonitis, asthma, and cystic fibrosis; cardiac diseases, such as pulmonary edema caused by heart failure; and autoimmune diseases, such as certain vasculitides and systemic lupus erythematosus. Radiographically pneumonia must be differentiated from lung trauma and contusion, hemorrhage, foreign body aspiration, and sympathetic effusion due to subdiaphragmatic inflammation.

TREATMENT

Decision-Making Algorithm
Available @ StudentConsult.com

Fever Without a Source

Therapy for pneumonia includes supportive and specific treatment and depends on the degree of illness, complications, and knowledge of the infectious agent likely causing the pneumonia. Most cases of pneumonia in healthy children can be managed on an outpatient basis. However, children with hypoxemia, inability to maintain adequate hydration, or moderate to severe respiratory distress should be hospitalized. Hospitalization should be considered in infants under 6 months with suspected bacterial pneumonia, those in whom there is a concern for a pathogen with increased virulence (e.g., methicillin-resistant *S. aureus*), or when concern exists about a family's ability to care for the child and to assess symptom progression.

Because viruses cause many community-acquired pneumonias in young children, not all children require empiric antibiotic treatment for pneumonia. Recommended therapies in those without recent antibiotic exposure are listed in Table 110.1. Exceptional situations include lack of response to empiric therapy, unusually severe presentations, nosocomial pneumonia, and immunocompromised children susceptible to infections with opportunistic pathogens (Table 110.3). Presumed pneumococcal pneumonia can be treated with high-dose ampicillin therapy even with high-level penicillin resistance. Ceftriaxone and/or vancomycin can be used if the isolate shows high-level resistance and the patient is severely ill. For infants 2-18 weeks old with afebrile pneumonia most likely caused by *C. trachomatis*, a macrolide is the recommended treatment. Oseltamivir or zanamivir should be used if influenza is identified or suspected, ideally within 48 hours of symptom onset.

TABLE 110.3 Antimicrobial Therapy for Pneumonia Caused by Specific Pathogens*

PATHOGEN	RECOMMENDED TREATMENT	ALTERNATIVE TREATMENT
Streptococcus pneumoniae with MIC for penicillin ≤2.0 μg/mL	Ampicillin or penicillin IV; amoxicillin PO	Ceftriaxone, cefotaxime, clindamycin, or vancomycin IV; Cefuroxime, cefpodoxime, levofloxacin,† or linezolid PO
S. pneumoniae with MIC for penicillin ≥4.0 μg/mL	Ceftriaxone IV; levofloxacin† or linezolid PO	Ampicillin, levofloxacin,† clindamycin, or vancomycin IV; clindamycin PO
Group A streptococcus	Penicillin or ampicillin IV; amoxicillin or penicillin PO	Ceftriaxone, cefotaxime, clindamycin, or vancomycin IV; clindamycin PO
Group B streptococcus	Penicillin or ampicillin IV; amoxicillin or penicillin PO	Ceftriaxone, cefotaxime, clindamycin, or vancomycin IV; clindamycin PO
Haemophilus influenzae	Ampicillin IV or amoxicillin PO if β-lactamase negative; ceftriaxone or cefotaxime IV or amoxicillin-clavulanate PO if β-lactamase positive	Ciprofloxacin† or levofloxacin† IV; cefdinir, cefixime, or cefpodoxime PO
Mycoplasma pneumoniae, Chlamydophila pneumoniae, or *Chlamydia trachomatis*	Azithromycin IV or PO	Erythromycin or levofloxacin IV; clarithromycin, erythromycin, doxycycline,† or a fluoroquinolone† PO
Staphylococcus aureus, methicillin susceptible (MSSA)	Cefazolin, oxacillin, or nafcillin IV; cephalexin PO	Clindamycin or vancomycin IV; clindamycin PO
S. aureus, methicillin resistant (MRSA)	Clindamycin or vancomycin IV; clindamycin PO	TMP-SMX or Linezolid IV or PO
Gram-negative aerobic bacilli (except *P. aeruginosa*)	Cefotaxime or ceftriaxone with or without an aminoglycoside IV; amoxicillin-clavulanate, cefdinir, or cefixime PO	Piperacillin-tazobactam plus an aminoglycoside‡; fluoroquinolone† PO
P. aeruginosa	Ceftazidime IV with or without an aminoglycoside‡; ciprofloxacin† if susceptible PO	Piperacillin-tazobactam IV with or without an aminoglycoside‡
Herpes simplex virus	Acyclovir IV	

*Oral outpatient therapy may be used for mild illness. Intravenous inpatient therapy should be used for moderate to severe illness.
†Appropriate respiratory fluoroquinolones include moxifloxacin, gatifloxacin, levofloxacin, and gemifloxacin. Fluoroquinolones are contraindicated for children younger than 18 years of age and pregnant or lactating women. Tetracyclines are not recommended for children younger than 9 years.
‡Aminoglycoside dosing should be guided by serum antibiotic concentrations after a steady state has been reached.
IV, Intravenous; *MIC*, minimum inhibitory concentration; *MRSA*, methicillin-resistant *Staphylococcus aureus*; *MSSA*, methicillin susceptible *Staphylococcus aureus*; *PO*, per os (orally); *TMP-SMX*, trimethoprim-sulfamethoxazole.

COMPLICATIONS AND PROGNOSIS

Bacterial pneumonias frequently cause inflammatory fluid to collect in the adjacent pleural space, causing a **parapneumonic effusion** or, if grossly purulent, an **empyema**. Small effusions may not require any special therapy. Large effusions may restrict breathing and require drainage. Air dissection within lung tissue results in a **pneumatocele**. Scarring of the airways and lung tissue may leave dilated bronchi, resulting in **bronchiectasis** and increased risk for recurrent infection.

Pneumonia that causes necrosis of lung tissue may evolve into a **lung abscess**. Lung abscess is an uncommon problem in children and is usually caused by aspiration, infection behind an obstructed bronchus, or certain virulent organisms. Anaerobic bacteria usually predominate, along with various streptococci, *Escherichia coli*, *Klebsiella pneumoniae*, *P. aeruginosa*, and *S. aureus*. Chest radiograph or CT scan reveals a cavitary lesion, often with an air-fluid level, surrounded by parenchymal inflammation. If the cavity communicates with the bronchi, organisms may be isolated from sputum. Diagnostic bronchoscopy may be indicated to exclude a foreign body and obtain microbiologic specimens. Lung abscesses usually respond to appropriate antimicrobial therapy with clindamycin, penicillin G, or ampicillin-sulbactam.

Most children recover from pneumonia rapidly and completely, although radiographic abnormalities may persist for 6-8 weeks. In a few children, symptoms may last longer than 1 month or may be recurrent. In such cases, the possibility of underlying disease must be investigated further, such as with the tuberculin skin test, sweat chloride determination for cystic fibrosis, serum immunoglobulin and IgG subclass determinations, bronchoscopy to identify anatomical abnormalities or foreign body, and barium swallow for gastroesophageal reflux.

Severe adenovirus pneumonia may result in **bronchiolitis obliterans**, a subacute inflammatory process in which the small airways are replaced by scar tissue, resulting in a reduction in lung volume and lung compliance. **Unilateral hyperlucent lung**, or **Swyer-James syndrome**, is a focal sequela of severe necrotizing pneumonia in which all or part of a lung has increased translucency radiographically; it has been linked to adenovirus type 21.

PREVENTION

Annual influenza vaccine is recommended for all children over 6 months of age (see Chapter 94). Trivalent or quadrivalent, inactivated influenza vaccines are licensed for use beginning at 6 months of age; live-attenuated vaccine can be used for persons 2-49 years of age. Universal childhood vaccination with conjugate vaccines for *H. influenzae* type b and *S. pneumoniae* has greatly diminished the incidence of these pneumonias. RSV infections can be prevented by use of palivizumab in some high-risk patients (see Chapter 109).

Reducing the duration of mechanical ventilation and administering antibiotics judiciously reduces the incidence of ventilator-associated pneumonias. The head of the bed should be raised to 30-45 degrees for intubated patients to minimize risk of aspiration, and all suctioning equipment and saline should be sterile. Handwashing before and after every patient contact and use of gloves for invasive procedures are important measures to prevent nosocomial transmission of infections. Hospital staff with respiratory illnesses or who are carriers of certain organisms, such as methicillin-resistant *S. aureus*, should comply with infection control policies to prevent transfer of organisms to patients. Treating sources of aerosols, such as air coolers, can prevent *L. pneumonia*.

CHAPTER 111
Infective Endocarditis

ETIOLOGY

Infective endocarditis (IE) is an infection on the endothelial surface of the heart, including the heart valves. The management of infections on the endothelial surfaces of blood vessels **(endovascular infections)** is very similar. Turbulent flow from congenital heart disease or an indwelling central venous catheter can result in endothelial damage. Fibrin and platelets gather at the site, forming a thrombus. In the setting of transient bacteremia, this lesion can become infected and can result in a **vegetation**, which usually occurs on a valve leaflet and is composed of microorganisms trapped in a fibrin mesh that extends into the bloodstream.

Many microorganisms have been reported to cause endocarditis, although there are only a few common causes in children (Table 111.1). *Streptococcus viridans* is the principal cause in children with congenital heart diseases without previous surgery. *Staphylococcus aureus* and coagulase-negative staphylococci (CONS) are important causes of endocarditis, especially following cardiac surgery and in the presence of prosthetic cardiac and endovascular materials. Gram-negative endocarditis is rare. *Candida* species can cause fungal endocarditis, especially in premature infants with central venous catheters and/or on parenteral nutrition.

TABLE 111.1 Pathogens Causing Infective Endocarditis in Children
BACTERIA
Viridans *Streptococcus* groups: *S. sanguis, S. mitis, S. mutan, S. anginosus, S. salivarius, S. bovis*
Staphylococcus aureus
Enterococcus
Coagulase-negative staphylococci
Streptococci: groups A, B (in neonates and elderly), *Streptococcus pneumoniae*
Gram-negative enteric bacilli
HACEK organisms (i.e., *Haemophilus aphrophilus, Aggregatibacter species, Cardiobacterium hominis, Eikenella corrodens,* and *Kingella kingae*)
Chlamydophila
Coxiella burnetii (Q fever)
FUNGI
Candida species
CULTURE NEGATIVE
Fastidious organisms (*Abiotrophia* or *Granulicatella* species)
Bartonella species
Tropheryma whipplei
Coxiella burnetii (Q fever)

EPIDEMIOLOGY

Rheumatic heart disease used to be a major risk factor for IE but has become much less common. Patients at highest risk for IE include those with prosthetic cardiac valves and children who have cyanotic congenital heart disease, either with or without repair. The risk in these patients is increased after dental and oral procedures, instrumentation, or surgical procedures of the respiratory, genitourinary, or gastrointestinal tracts. Use of central vascular catheters is a significant risk factor for native valve endocarditis. Approximately 8-10% of IE in children occurs without structural heart disease (normal native valve) or other obvious risk factors. *S. aureus* is the most likely infective organism in these cases.

CLINICAL MANIFESTATIONS

Decision-Making Algorithms
Available @ StudentConsult.com

Heart Murmurs
Fever and Rash

The most common early symptoms of IE are nonspecific and include fever, malaise, and weight loss. Tachycardia and a new or changed heart murmur are common findings. The subtle and nonspecific findings underscore the need to obtain blood cultures if endocarditis is suspected, especially for children with congenital heart disease and for unexplained illness after dental or surgical procedures. Endocarditis is often a subacute, slowly progressive process, but it can also present acutely with high fevers and a sepsis-like picture. Heart failure, splenomegaly, petechiae, glomerulonephritis, and embolic phenomena (Osler nodes, Roth spots, Janeway lesions, and splinter hemorrhages) may be present. In neonates, the signs and symptoms of IE may be especially subtle and variable, including feeding issues, respiratory distress, and hypotension, in addition to changes in the cardiac exam.

LABORATORY STUDIES AND IMAGING

The key to diagnosis is confirming continuous bacteremia or fungemia by culturing the blood. Multiple blood cultures should be obtained before initiating antibiotic therapy. For optimal sensitivity, adequate volumes of blood should be obtained, 1-3 mL for infants and young children and at least 5-7 mL for older children. If volumes are not adequate, emphasis should be placed on obtaining aerobic blood cultures, as anaerobic organisms rarely cause IE. If possible, in patients who are not critically ill, empiric antibiotic therapy should be held until at least three sets of blood cultures (from different venipuncture sites) are obtained. Patients who have recently been treated with antibiotics or who are currently receiving antibiotics should have additional serial cultures performed. Despite adequate blood culture techniques, the microbiologic diagnosis is not confirmed in 5-15% of cases, known as **culture-negative endocarditis.**

The agent in culture-negative endocarditis may be identified by antibody testing and examination of the valve tissue (following surgery) by polymerase chain reaction (PCR) for bacterial (16S) or fungal (18S) ribosomal RNA.

Erythrocyte sedimentation rate and C-reactive protein are often elevated. Leukocytosis, anemia, and hematuria are common laboratory findings.

Echocardiography should be performed in all cases where IE is suspected. It can be used to visualize vegetations and assess valvular regurgitation and conduit flow. Transesophageal echocardiography (TEE) is more sensitive than transthoracic echocardiography (TTE) for adolescents and adults and for patients with prosthetic valves, but it is often unnecessary in children.

DIFFERENTIAL DIAGNOSIS

IE must be differentiated from other causes of bacteremia and other cardiac conditions. The modified **Duke criteria** can be used to assist in the diagnosis of IE (Table 111.2). Noninfectious causes of endocardial vegetations must be excluded, such as sterile clots. Prolonged bacteremia can be caused by infectious endothelial foci outside of the heart, often associated with congenital vascular malformations, vascular trauma, an infected venous thrombosis, or previous vascular surgery.

TABLE 111.2 Modified Duke Clinical Criteria for Diagnosis of Infective Endocarditis

DEFINITE INFECTIVE ENDOCARDITIS
Histopathological Criteria
Microorganisms shown by culture or histopathological examination in a vegetation, emboli, intracardiac abscess. *or*
Active endocardial lesions on pathological examination
Clinical Criteria
Two major criteria *or* one major and three minor criteria *or* five minor criteria
Major Criteria
Positive blood cultures
Two or more separate cultures positive with typical organisms for infective endocarditis
Two or more positive cultures of blood drawn more than 12 hr apart or 4 positive blood cultures irrespective of timing of obtaining specimen
A positive blood culture for *Coxiella burnetii* or positive IgG titer >1:800
Evidence of endocardial involvement
Positive findings on echocardiogram (vegetation on valve or supporting structure, abscess, new valvular regurgitation)
Minor Criteria
Predisposition—predisposing heart condition or injection drug use
Fever—temperature >38°C (>100.4°F)
Vascular phenomena (major arterial emboli, septic pulmonary infarcts, mycotic aneurysm, intracranial hemorrhage, conjunctival hemorrhages, Janeway lesions)
Immunological phenomena (glomerulonephritis, Osler nodes, Roth spots, rheumatoid factor)
Microbiologic evidence (positive blood culture result, but not meeting major criteria, or serological evidence of active infection with organism consistent with infective endocarditis)
POSSIBLE INFECTIVE ENDOCARDITIS
Clinical Criteria
One major and one minor criteria or three minor criteria
REJECTED
Firm alternative diagnosis for manifestations of endocarditis *or*
Resolution of manifestations of endocarditis with antibiotic therapy for <4 days *or*
No pathological evidence of endocarditis at surgery or autopsy after antibiotic therapy of >4 days *or* does not meet criteria for possible endocarditis

Modified from Tissieres P, Gervaix A, Beghetti M, et al. Value and limitations of the van Reyn, Duke, and modified Duke criteria for the diagnosis of infective endocarditis in children. Pediatrics. *2003;112:e467–e471.*

TREATMENT

Severely ill patients must be stabilized with supportive therapies for cardiac failure, pulmonary edema, and low cardiac output (see Chapter 145). Empirical antibiotic therapy may be started for acutely ill patients after blood cultures are obtained. With subacute disease, awaiting results of blood cultures to confirm the diagnosis is recommended to direct therapy according to the susceptibility of the isolate. Because antibiotics must reach the organisms by passive diffusion through the fibrin mesh, high doses of bactericidal antibiotics are required for an extended period of treatment (4-8 weeks). Exact duration of therapy varies depending on the presence of prosthetic material and the causative organism. *Staphylococcus aureus* bacteremia can be persistent, and if associated with an indwelling catheter, requires line removal in most cases. Surgery is indicated if medical treatment is unsuccessful, if bacteremia is persistent, or if the pathogen is unusual or difficult to treat (e.g., fungal endocarditis). Surgical intervention may also be required with the presence of a valve annulus or myocardial abscess, rupture of a valve leaflet, valvular insufficiency with acute or refractory heart failure, recurrent serious embolic complications, or refractory prosthetic valve disease.

COMPLICATIONS AND PROGNOSIS

The major complications of IE are direct damage to cardiac tissue and function and distant complications secondary to **septic emboli** from vegetations. Damage to cardiac valves may cause regurgitation, defects in valve leaflets, abscess of the valve ring, or myocardial abscess. Cardiac function can decline, resulting in heart failure. These complications should be monitored by physical examination and echocardiography. Septic emboli can result in pneumonia, osteomyelitis, and abscesses in the brain, kidneys, and spleen.

The prognosis of IE varies depending on causative organism and underlying cardiac condition. Cardiovascular infections with gram-negative bacilli and fungi have the poorest prognosis.

PREVENTION

Good oral hygiene should be emphasized in all patients at risk for IE. In certain high-risk patients (unrepaired cyanotic heart disease, previous IE, repaired congenital heart disease with residual defects, cardiac transplantation), prophylactic antibiotics may be considered before certain dental and other invasive procedures of the respiratory tract and/or infected skin or muscle.

CHAPTER 112

Acute Gastroenteritis

ETIOLOGY AND EPIDEMIOLOGY

Acute gastroenteritis refers to a clinical syndrome of diarrhea (>3 stool episodes in 24 hours) with or without vomiting that generally lasts for several days. In general, diarrhea is caused by a variety of infectious or inflammatory processes in the intestine that directly affect enterocyte secretory and absorptive functions. Gastroenteritis or enteritis has many infectious causes, including viruses, bacteria, and parasites (Table 112.1). Based on pathogenesis, diarrhea can be classified as invasive or inflammatory, or it can be classified as secretory, producing either bloody stools with abdominal cramping and fever or large quantities of watery stool without other symptoms (Table 112.2).

Infectious diarrhea is a leading cause of morbidity and mortality in children around the world. Rates of disease and death vary with age and access to health care, clean water, and sanitation. Gastrointestinal infections are generally acquired via fecal-oral transmission or through ingestion of contaminated food or water. The patient's immune status and environmental exposures (i.e., food, water, travel, antibiotics, child care) help guide the differential diagnosis in the presence of acute gastrointestinal symptoms. Traveler's diarrhea occurs frequently, especially within the first 1-2 weeks of arrival. Epidemiology varies with destination, but in general children are at risk for the same illnesses that affect adult travelers.

Viral gastroenteritis is the most common cause of diarrhea in children globally. These illnesses may be associated with vomiting as well as diarrhea, have incubation periods of hours to days, and are usually self-limited illnesses lasting 3-7 days. **Rotavirus** is the most frequent cause of diarrhea in young children during the winter months. Primary infection with rotavirus may cause moderate to severe disease in infancy but is less severe later in life. The rotavirus vaccine has resulted in significant reductions in the incidence of acute gastroenteritis and hospitalizations due to rotavirus. **Norovirus** occurs in people of all ages, year round, and is the most common cause of outbreaks of acute gastroenteritis because it is highly contagious. Other viral causes of acute gastroenteritis include astroviruses, sapovirus, and enteric adenoviruses (serotypes 40 and 41).

Food-borne and water-borne diseases are important causes of acute gastroenteritis both for individual and public health

TABLE 112.1 Common Pathogenic Organisms Causing Diarrhea and Their Virulence Mechanisms

ORGANISMS	PATHOGENIC MECHANISM(S)
VIRUSES	
Rotaviruses	Damage to microvilli
Caliciviruses (noroviruses)	Mucosal lesion
Astroviruses	Mucosal lesion
Enteric adenoviruses (serotypes 40 and 41)	Mucosal lesion
BACTERIA	
Campylobacter jejuni	Invasion, enterotoxin
Clostridium difficile	Cytotoxin, enterotoxin
Escherichia coli	
Enteropathogenic (EPEC)	Adherence, effacement
Enterotoxigenic (ETEC) (traveler's diarrhea)	Enterotoxins (heat-stable or heat-labile)
Enteroinvasive (EIEC)	Invasion of mucosa
Enterohemorrhagic (EHEC) (includes O157: H7 causing HUS)	Adherence, effacement, cytotoxin
Enteroaggregative (EAEC)	Adherence, mucosal damage
Salmonella	Invasion, enterotoxin
Shigella	Invasion, enterotoxin, cytotoxin
Vibrio cholerae	Enterotoxin
Vibrio parahaemolyticus	Invasion, cytotoxin
Yersinia enterocolitica	Invasion, enterotoxin
PARASITES	
Entamoeba histolytica	Invasion, enzyme and cytotoxin production; cyst resistant to physical destruction
Giardia lamblia	Adheres to mucosa; cyst resistant to physical destruction
Spore-forming intestinal protozoa	Adherence, inflammation
Cryptosporidium parvum	
Isospora belli	
Cyclospora cayetanensis	
Microsporidia (*Enterocytozoon bieneusi, Encephalitozoon intestinalis*)	

HUS, Hemolytic uremic syndrome.

TABLE 112.2 Mechanisms of Infectious Diarrhea

PRIMARY MECHANISM	DEFECT	STOOL EXAMINATION	EXAMPLES	COMMENTS
Secretory	Decreased absorption, increased secretion: electrolyte transport	Watery, normal osmolality	Cholera, toxigenic *Escherichia coli* (EPEC, ETEC); carcinoid, *Clostridium difficile*, cryptosporidiosis (in AIDS)	Persists during fasting; bile salt malabsorption also may increase intestinal water secretion; no stool leukocytes
Mucosal invasion	Inflammation, decreased mucosal surface area and/or colonic reabsorption, increased motility	Blood and increased WBCs in stool	Celiac disease, *Salmonella* infection, shigellosis, amebiasis, yersiniosis, *Campylobacter* infection	Dysentery (blood, mucus, and WBCs)

WBCs, White blood cells; infection may also contribute to increased motility.
From Wyllie R. Major symptoms and signs of digestive tract disorders. In: Kliegman RM, Behrman RE, Jenson HB, eds. Nelson Textbook of Pediatrics. 18th ed. Philadelphia: Saunders; 2007:152. Table 303.7.

reasons. In the United States, the most common bacterial food-borne causes (in order of frequency) are nontyphoidal *Salmonella, Campylobacter, Shigella, Escherichia coli* O157:H7, *Yersinia, Listeria monocytogenes,* and *Vibrio cholerae.* Food-borne diarrhea can also result from ingestion of preformed enterotoxins produced by bacteria, such as *Staphylococcus aureus* and *Bacillus cereus,* which multiply in contaminated foods, and nonbacterial toxins such as from fish, shellfish, and mushrooms. After a short incubation period, vomiting and cramps are prominent symptoms, and diarrhea may or may not be present. Heavy metals that leach into canned food or drinks causing gastric irritation and emetic syndromes may mimic symptoms of acute infectious enteritis.

Nontyphoidal *Salmonella* produces diarrhea by invading the intestinal mucosa. The organisms are transmitted through contact with infected animals (chickens, iguanas, other reptiles, turtles) or from contaminated food products, such as dairy products, eggs, and poultry. A large inoculum of organisms is required for disease because *Salmonella* is killed by gastric acidity. The incubation period for gastroenteritis ranges from 6 to 72 hours but is usually less than 24 hours.

Shigella dysenteriae may cause disease by producing **Shiga toxin**. The incubation period is 1-7 days. Infected adults may shed organisms for 1 month. Infection is spread by person-to-person contact or by the ingestion of contaminated food with 10-100 organisms. The colon is selectively affected. High fever and febrile seizures may occur in addition to diarrhea.

Only certain strains of *E. coli* produce diarrhea. Strains associated with enteritis are classified by the mechanism of diarrhea: enterotoxigenic (ETEC), enterohemorrhagic (EHEC) or Shiga toxin–producing (STEC), enteroinvasive (EIEC), enteropathogenic (EPEC), or enteroaggregative (EAEC). ETEC strains produce **heat-labile (cholera-like) enterotoxin, heat-stable enterotoxin**, or both. ETEC is a frequent cause of **traveler's diarrhea**. ETEC adhere to the epithelial cells in the upper small intestine and produces disease by liberating toxins that induce intestinal secretion and limit absorption. EHEC or STEC, especially the *E. coli* O157:H7 strain, produces a **Shiga-like toxin** that is responsible for a hemorrhagic colitis and most cases of diarrhea associated with **hemolytic uremic syndrome (HUS),** which presents with microangiopathic hemolytic anemia, thrombocytopenia, and renal failure (see Chapter 164). STEC is associated with contaminated food, including unpasteurized fruit juices and especially undercooked beef, and can present with nonbloody diarrhea that then becomes bloody. EIEC invades the colonic mucosa, producing widespread mucosal damage with acute inflammation similar to *Shigella.* EIEC diarrhea is usually watery and is often associated with fever. EPEC causes mild watery diarrhea but can cause severe dehydration in young children in resource-poor countries in sporadic or epidemic patterns.

Campylobacter jejuni is spread by person-to-person contact and by contaminated water and food, especially poultry, raw milk, and cheese. The organism invades the mucosa of the jejunum, ileum, and colon. ***Yersinia enterocolitica*** is transmitted by pets and contaminated food, especially chitterlings. Infants and young children characteristically have a diarrheal disease, whereas older children usually have acute lesions of the terminal ileum or acute mesenteric lymphadenitis mimicking appendicitis or Crohn disease. Postinfectious arthritis, rash, and spondylopathy may develop.

Clostridium difficile causes diarrhea and/or colitis and is usually associated with prior antibiotic exposure. The organism produces spores that spread from person to person and also as fomites on surfaces. Infection is generally hospital-acquired, but community acquisition of infection is increasingly reported. Diagnosis is made by detection of toxin in the stool. Infants <12 months of age should not be tested for *C. difficile* as they are frequently asymptomatically colonized with the organism in their stool, possibly due to a lack of the receptor required for infection. Of note, patients on antibiotics often experience diarrhea related to alterations in their intestinal flora that are unrelated to *C. difficile* infection.

Important enteric parasites found in North America include *Entamoeba histolytica* (amebiasis), *Giardia lamblia,* and *Cryptosporidium parvum.* **Amebiasis** occurs in warmer climates, whereas giardiasis is endemic throughout the United States and is common among infants in daycare centers. *E. histolytica* infects the colon; amebae may pass through the bowel wall and invade the liver, lung, and brain. Diarrhea is of acute onset, is bloody, and contains leukocytes. ***G. lamblia*** is transmitted through ingestion of cysts, either from contact with an infected individual or from food or freshwater or well water contaminated with infected feces. The organism adheres to the microvilli of the duodenal and jejunal epithelium. Insidious onset of progressive anorexia, nausea, gaseousness, abdominal distention, watery diarrhea, secondary lactose intolerance, and weight loss is characteristic of giardiasis. ***Cryptosporidium*** causes mild, watery diarrhea in immunocompetent persons that resolves without treatment. It produces severe, prolonged diarrhea in persons with acquired immunodeficiency syndrome (AIDS; see Chapter 125).

CLINICAL MANIFESTATIONS

Decision-Making Algorithms
Available @ StudentConsult.com

Vomiting
Diarrhea
Edema
Eosinophilia

Gastroenteritis may be accompanied by systemic findings, such as fever, lethargy, myalgias, and abdominal pain. **Viral diarrhea** is characterized by watery stools with no blood or mucus. Vomiting may be present and dehydration may be prominent, especially in infants and younger children. Fever, when present, is low grade.

Dysentery is enteritis involving the colon and rectum, with blood and mucus, possibly foul-smelling stools, and fever. *Shigella* is the prototypical cause of dysentery, which must be differentiated from infection with EIEC, EHEC, *E. histolytica* **(amebic dysentery)**, *C. jejuni, Y. enterocolitica,* and nontyphoidal *Salmonella.* Gastrointestinal bleeding and blood loss may be significant.

A chief consideration in management of a child with diarrhea is assessing the degree of dehydration as evident from clinical signs and symptoms, ongoing losses, and daily requirements (see Chapter 33). The degree of dehydration dictates the urgency of the situation and the volume of fluid needed for rehydration. Mild to moderate dehydration can usually be treated with oral rehydration; severe dehydration usually requires intravenous rehydration and may even require admission to an intensive care unit.

LABORATORY AND IMAGING STUDIES

Initial laboratory evaluation of moderate to severe diarrhea includes electrolytes, blood urea nitrogen, creatinine, and urinalysis for specific gravity as an indicator of hydration. Stool specimens should be examined for mucus, blood, and leukocytes, which indicate colitis in response to bacteria that diffusely invade the colonic mucosa. Patients infected with Shiga toxin–producing *E. coli* and *E. histolytica* generally have minimal fecal leukocytes.

Viral polymerase chain reaction (PCR)—also called the nucleic and amplification test (NAAT)—assays may be used if the diagnosis will alter management. Bacterial stool cultures are recommended for patients with fever, profuse diarrhea, and dehydration or if HUS or pseudomembranous colitis is suspected. If the stool test result is negative for blood and leukocytes and there is no history to suggest contaminated food ingestion, a viral etiology is most likely. Stool evaluation for parasitic agents should be considered for acute dysenteric illness, especially in returning travelers, and in protracted cases of diarrhea in which no bacterial agent is identified. The diagnosis of *E. histolytica* is based on identification of the organism in the stool. Serological tests are useful for diagnosis of extraintestinal amebiasis, including amebic hepatic abscess. Giardiasis can be diagnosed by identifying trophozoites or cysts in stool, but this may require three specimens. More specific and sensitive fecal immunoassays and NAATs are the diagnostic tests of choice.

Positive blood cultures are uncommon with bacterial enteritis except for *Salmonella* and *E. coli* enteritis in very young infants. In typhoid fever, blood cultures are positive early in the disease, whereas stool cultures become positive only after the secondary bacteremia.

DIFFERENTIAL DIAGNOSIS

Decision-Making Algorithms
Available @ StudentConsult.com

Abdominal Pain
Vomiting
Diarrhea
Failure to Thrive

Diarrhea can be caused by infection, toxins, gastrointestinal allergy (including allergy to milk or soy proteins), malabsorption defects, inflammatory bowel disease, celiac disease, or any injury to enterocytes. Acute enteritis may mimic other acute diseases, such as intussusception and acute appendicitis, which are best identified by diagnostic imaging. Many noninfectious causes of diarrhea produce chronic diarrhea, with persistence for more than 14 days. Persistent or chronic symptoms may require tests for malabsorption or invasive studies, including endoscopy and small bowel biopsy.

TREATMENT

Most infectious causes of diarrhea in children are self-limited. Antibiotics are not generally useful and may be a risk factor in the development of HUS when *E. coli* O157:H7 is present. Management of viral and most bacterial causes of diarrhea is primarily supportive and consists of correcting dehydration and ongoing fluid and electrolyte deficits.

Hyponatremia is common; hypernatremia is less common. Metabolic acidosis results from losses of bicarbonate in stool, lactic acidosis results from shock, and phosphate retention results from transient prerenal-renal insufficiency. Traditionally therapy for 24 hours with oral rehydration solutions alone is effective for viral diarrhea. Therapy for severe fluid and electrolyte losses involves intravenous hydration. Less severe degrees of dehydration (<10%) in the absence of excessive vomiting or shock may be managed with oral rehydration solutions containing glucose and electrolytes. Ondansetron may be administered to reduce emesis when this is persistent.

Antibiotic therapy may be necessary for high-risk patients or those with severe disease or bacteremia. Antibiotic treatment of *Shigella* may reduce the duration of symptoms and decrease transmission of infection. Azithromycin is first-line oral therapy for children. Many *Shigella sonnei* isolates, the predominant strain affecting children, are resistant to amoxicillin and trimethoprim-sulfamethoxazole. Fluoroquinolone resistance in *Salmonella* and many other gram-negative organisms is increasing in many parts of the world. *Salmonella* is treated with antibiotics in children less than 3 months of age.

Treatment of traveler's diarrhea is generally supportive, although antibiotics can be indicated in instances of bloody diarrhea or a febrile illness, in which case azithromycin is a recommended choice for children. Due to lack of consistent access to health care in many areas, providing a prescription to a family in advance of travel to a high-risk area such as in Asia, Africa, or South America may be considered.

Treatment of *C. difficile* (pseudomembranous colitis) includes discontinuation of the inciting antibiotic and oral metronidazole or vancomycin. *E. histolytica* dysentery is treated with metronidazole followed by a luminal agent, such as iodoquinol. The treatment of *G. lamblia* is metronidazole, tinidazole, or nitazoxanide.

COMPLICATIONS AND PROGNOSIS

The major complication of gastroenteritis is dehydration and hypovolemic shock. Seizures may occur with high fever, especially with *Shigella*. Intestinal abscesses can form with *Shigella, Yersinia,* and *Salmonella* infections, leading to intestinal perforation, a life-threatening complication. Severe vomiting associated with gastroenteritis can cause esophageal tears or aspiration pneumonia.

Deaths resulting from diarrhea reflect the principal problem of disruption of fluid and electrolyte homeostasis, which can lead to dehydration, electrolyte imbalance, hemodynamic instability, and shock. Diarrheal diseases cause approximately 10% of childhood deaths worldwide.

PREVENTION

The most important means of preventing childhood diarrhea is the provision of clean, uncontaminated water and proper hygiene in growing, collecting, and preparing foods. Good hygienic measures, especially appropriate handwashing with soap and water, are the best means of controlling person-to-person spread of most organisms causing gastroenteritis. Poultry products should be considered potentially contaminated with *Salmonella* and should be handled and cooked appropriately. Families should also be aware of the risk of acquiring salmonellosis from household reptile pets. Transmission of *Salmonella* from reptiles can be prevented by thorough handwashing after handling the animals or their cages. Children under 5 years of age and immunocompromised persons should avoid contact with reptiles.

Immunization against rotavirus infection is recommended for all children beginning at 6 weeks of age, with the first dose by 14 weeks 6 days and the last dose by 8 months (see Chapter 94). Two typhoid vaccines are licensed in the United States: an oral live-attenuated vaccine (Ty21a) for children 6 years of age and older and a capsular polysaccharide vaccine (ViCPS) for intramuscular administration for children 2 years of age and older. These are recommended for travelers to endemic areas of developing countries or for household contacts of *S. typhi* chronic carriers.

The risk for traveler's diarrhea, caused primarily by ETEC, may be minimized by avoiding uncooked food and untreated drinking water. Symptomatic self-treatment for mild diarrhea with an **oral rehydration solution** is recommended for children at least 6 years of age and adults. Self-treatment of moderate diarrhea and fever with a fluoroquinolone is recommended in adults. Similarly, children can receive azithromycin. Prompt medical evaluation is indicated for disease persisting more than 3 days, bloody stools, fever above 102°F (38.9°C) or chills, persistent vomiting, or moderate to severe dehydration.

CHAPTER 113
Viral Hepatitis

ETIOLOGY

Acute hepatitis, or liver inflammation, can be the result of a number of infectious and noninfectious etiologies. Among infectious causes of hepatitis, viruses play an important role. The six primary hepatotropic viruses, hepatitis A to G, differ in their virological characteristics, transmission, severity, likelihood of persistence, and subsequent risk of causing hepatocellular carcinoma (Table 113.1). The cause of 10-15% of cases of acute hepatitis is unknown.

EPIDEMIOLOGY

Hepatitis A virus (HAV) is the most common cause of acute viral hepatitis and is spread by fecal-oral transmission. HAV is common in children globally, especially in areas of poor sanitation. Among U.S. children, infection due to HAV was often associated with childcare settings; however, rates have decreased since the introduction of routine vaccination. Hepatitis B virus (HBV), hepatitis C virus (HCV), and hepatitis D virus (HDV) infections can result in chronic hepatitis, or a chronic carrier state, which facilitates spread. HDV, also known as the **delta agent,** is a defective virus that requires HBV for spread and causes either coinfection with HBV or superinfection in chronic carriers of hepatitis B surface antigen (HBsAg). Routine vaccination has also been effective in reducing the rates of HBV infection, especially in children.

The major risk factors for HBV and HCV are injectable drug use, frequent exposure to blood products, and perinatal transmission from maternal infection. Hepatitis E virus (HEV) infection occurs following travel to endemic areas (South Asia) outside of the United States. Hepatitis G virus (HGV) is prevalent in HIV-infected persons. HBV and HCV cause chronic infection, which may lead to cirrhosis and hepatocellular carcinoma and represents a persistent risk of transmission.

CLINICAL MANIFESTATIONS

Decision-Making Algorithms
Available @ StudentConsult.com

Jaundice
Hepatomegaly
Fever Without a Source

Asymptomatic or mild, nonspecific illness without icterus is common with HAV, HBV, and HCV, especially in young children. When present, symptoms of acute infection are difficult to distinguish between these viruses. Younger children are often asymptomatic when infected with HAV, HBV, and HCV. Fulminant HAV infection is rare, and chronic infection does not

TABLE 113.1 Characteristics of Agents Causing Acute Viral Hepatitis

FEATURE	HAV	HBV	HCV	HDV	HEV	HGV
Viral structure	27-nm ssRNA virus	42-nm dsDNA virus	30- to 60-nm ssRNA virus	36-nm circular ssRNA hybrid particle with HBsAg coat	27- to34-nm ssRNA virus	50- to 100-nm ssRNA virus
Family	Picornavirus	Hepadnavirus	Flavivirus	Satellite	Flavivirus	Flavivirus
Transmission	Fecal-oral, rarely parenteral	Transfusion, sexual, inoculation, perinatal	Parenteral, transfusion, perinatal	Similar to HBV	Fecal-oral (endemic and epidemic)	Parenteral, transfusion
Incubation period	15-30 days	60-180 days	30-60 days	Coinfection with HBV	35-60 days	Unknown
Serum markers	Anti-HAV	HBsAg, HBcAg, HBeAg, anti-HBs, anti-HBc	Anti-HCV (IgG, IgM), RIBA, PCR assay for HCV RNA	Anti-HDV, RNA	Anti-HEV	RNA by RT-PCR assay
Fulminant liver failure	Rare	<1% unless coinfection with HDV	Uncommon	2-20%	20%	Probably no
Persistent infection	No	5-10% (90% with perinatal infection)	85%	2-70%	No	Persistent infection common; chronic disease rare
Increased risk of hepato-cellular carcinoma	No	Yes	Yes	No	No	Unknown
Prophylaxis	Vaccine: immune serum globulin	Vaccine: hepatitis B immunoglobulin (HBIG)				

dsDNA, Double-stranded DNA; *HAV*, hepatitis A virus; *HBV*, hepatitis B virus; *HCV*, hepatitis C virus; *HDV*, hepatitis D virus; *HEV*, hepatitis E virus; *HGV*, hepatitis G virus; *PCR*, polymerase chain reaction; *RIBA*, recombinant immunoblot assay; *RT-PCR*, reverse transcriptase–polymerase chain reaction; *ssDNA/ssRNA*, single-stranded DNA/RNA; *TTV*, transfusion-transmitted virus.

occur. In acute HBV infection the likelihood of symptoms increases with age, ranging from 1% of infants <12 months of age to 30-50% of people >5 years. In HBV infection, the **preicteric phase**, which lasts approximately 1 week, is characterized by headache, anorexia, malaise, abdominal discomfort, nausea, and vomiting; it usually precedes the onset of clinically detectable disease. Extrahepatic manifestations such as arthralgia, arthritis, rash, thrombocytopenia, glomerulonephritis, or papular acrodermatitis **(Gianotti-Crosti syndrome)** can occur early in the illness. Jaundice and tender hepatomegaly occur later and characterize the **icteric phase**. Prodromal symptoms, particularly in children, may abate during the icteric phase. Hepatic enzymes may increase 15- to 20-fold. Resolution of the hyperbilirubinemia and normalization of the transaminases may take 6-8 weeks.

LABORATORY AND IMAGING STUDIES

Alanine aminotransferase (ALT) and aspartate aminotransferase (AST) levels are elevated and generally reflect the degree of parenchymal inflammation. Alkaline phosphatase and total and direct (conjugated) bilirubin levels indicate the degree of cholestasis, which results from hepatocellular and bile duct damage. The prothrombin time is a good predictor of severe hepatocellular injury and progression to fulminant hepatic failure (see Chapter 130).

The diagnosis of viral hepatitis is confirmed by serological testing (see Table 113.1 and Fig. 113.1). The presence of IgM-specific antibody to HAV with low or absent IgG antibody is presumptive evidence of acute HAV infection.

The presence of HBsAg signifies acute or chronic infection with HBV. Antigenemia appears early in the illness and is usually transient but is characteristic of chronic infection. Maternal HBsAg status should always be determined when HBV infection is diagnosed in children younger than 1 year of age because of the likelihood of vertical transmission. Hepatitis B early antigen (HBeAg) appears in the serum with acute HBV. The continued presence of HBsAg and HBeAg in the absence of antibody to e antigen (anti-HBe) indicates high risk of transmissibility that is associated with ongoing viral replication. Clearance of HBsAg from the serum precedes a variable **window period**, followed by the emergence of the antibody to surface antigen (anti-HBs), which indicates development of lifelong immunity and is also a marker of immunization. Antibody to core antigen (anti-HBc) is a useful marker for recognizing HBV infection during the window phase (when HBsAg has disappeared but before the appearance of anti-HBs). Anti-HBe is useful in predicting a low degree of infectivity during the carrier state.

Seroconversion after HCV infection may occur 6 months after infection. A positive result of HCV enzyme-linked immunosorbent assay (ELISA) should be confirmed with the more specific recombinant immunoblot assay, which detects antibodies to multiple HCV antigens. Detection of HCV RNA by polymerase chain reaction (PCR) is a sensitive marker for active infection, and results may be positive just 3 days after inoculation.

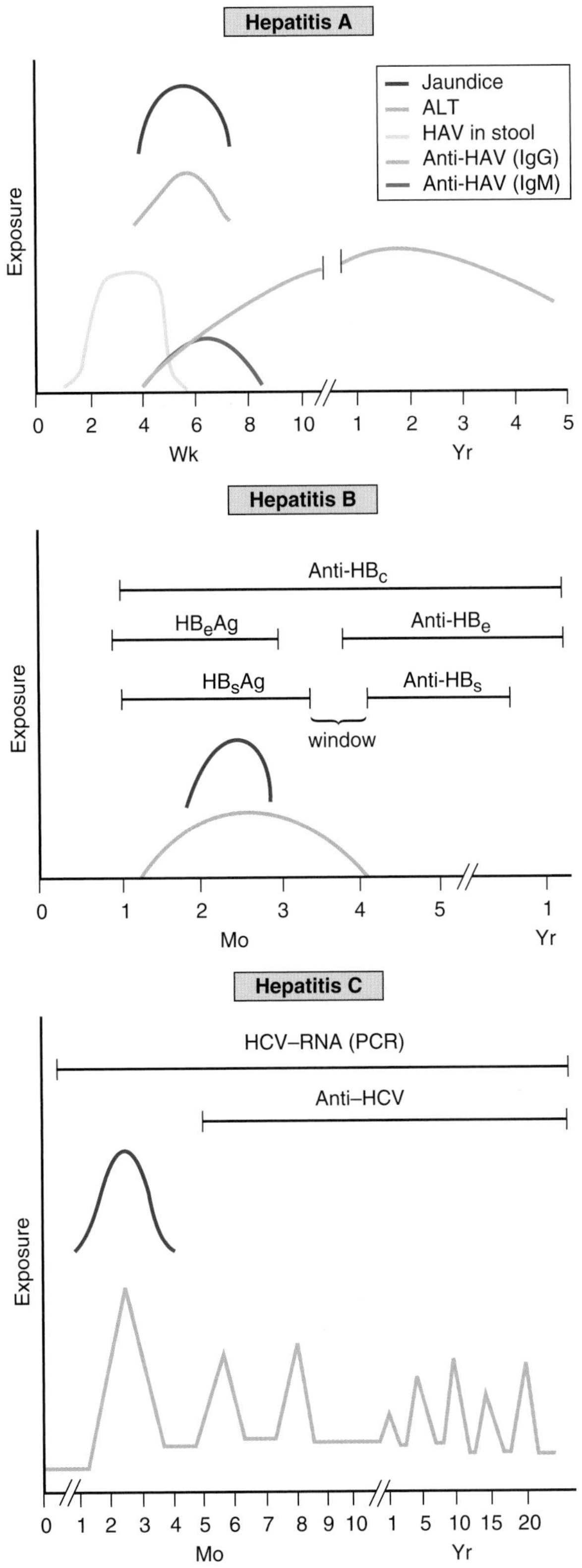

FIGURE 113.1 Clinical course and laboratory findings associated with hepatitis A, hepatitis B, and hepatitis C. *ALT*, Alanine aminotransferase; *HAV*, hepatitis A virus; *anti-HBc*, antibody to hepatitis B core antigen; *HBeAg*, hepatitis B early antigen; *anti-HBe*, antibody to hepatitis B early antigen; *HBsAg*, hepatitis B surface antigen; *anti-HBs*, antibody to hepatitis B surface antigen; *HCV*, hepatitis C virus; *PCR*, polymerase chain reaction.

DIFFERENTIAL DIAGNOSIS

Many other viruses may cause hepatitis as a component of systemic infection, including Epstein–Barr virus, cytomegalovirus, varicella-zoster virus, herpes simplex virus, and adenoviruses. Bacterial sepsis can also cause hepatic inflammation and dysfunction. Patients with cholecystitis, cholangitis, and choledocholithiasis may present with acute symptoms and jaundice. Other causes of acute liver disease in childhood include drugs (isoniazid, phenytoin, valproic acid, carbamazepine, oral contraceptives, acetaminophen), parenteral nutrition, toxins (ethanol, poisonous mushroom), Wilson disease, metabolic disease (galactosemia, tyrosinemia, mitochondrial disorders), α_1-antitrypsin deficiency, tumor, shock, anoxia, autoimmune hepatitis, hemophagocytic syndromes, and graft-versus-host disease (see Chapter 130).

TREATMENT

The treatment of acute hepatitis is largely supportive and involves rest, hydration, and adequate nutrition. Hospitalization is indicated for children with severe vomiting and dehydration, a prolonged prothrombin time, or signs of hepatic encephalopathy. When the diagnosis of viral hepatitis is established, attention should be directed toward preventing its spread to close contacts. For HAV, hygienic measures include handwashing and careful disposal of excreta, contaminated diapers or clothing, needles, and other blood-contaminated items.

The treatment of chronic HBV and HCV infections is evolving with the development of new antivirals. The decision to treat is based on the patient's age, viral genotype, and stage of viral infection.

COMPLICATIONS AND PROGNOSIS

Most cases of acute viral hepatitis resolve without specific therapy, with less than 0.1% of cases progressing to fulminant hepatic necrosis. HAV and HEV cause acute infection only. HBV, HCV, and HDV may persist as chronic infection, with chronic inflammation, fibrosis, and cirrhosis and the associated risk of hepatocellular carcinoma.

From 5 to 10% of adults with HBV develop persistent infection, defined by persistence of HBsAg in the blood for more than 6 months, compared with 90% of children who acquire HBV by perinatal transmission. Chronic HBsAg carriers are usually HBeAg-negative and have no clinical, biochemical, or serological evidence of active hepatitis unless there is superinfection with HDV. Approximately 10-15% of HBsAg carriers eventually clear HBsAg.

Approximately 85% of persons infected with HCV remain chronically infected, which is characterized by fluctuating transaminase levels (see Fig. 113.1). There is poor correlation of symptoms with ongoing liver damage. Approximately 20% of persons with chronic infection develop cirrhosis, and approximately 25% of those develop hepatocellular carcinoma. HIV infection and ethanol use increase the risk of HCV progression.

PREVENTION

Good hygienic practices significantly reduce the risk of fecal–oral transmission of HAV. HAV vaccine is recommended for routine immunization of all children beginning at 12 months.

Unvaccinated household and sexual contacts of persons with HAV should receive postexposure prophylaxis as soon as possible and within 2 weeks of the last exposure. A single dose of HAV vaccine at the age-appropriate dose is preferred for persons 12 months to 40 years of age. Immunoglobulin (0.02 mL/kg) given intramuscularly (IGIM) is preferred for children under 12 months of age, persons over 40 years of age, and immunocompromised persons. For preexposure prophylaxis, unvaccinated travelers to endemic regions who are 12 months of age or older should also receive a single dose of HAV vaccine administered at any time before departure. Infants <12 months of age, older adults, immunocompromised people, or those with chronic liver disease or other chronic medical conditions can receive IGIM along with the HAV vaccine dose to optimize protection. This regimen can also be considered for travel <2 weeks in the future.

HBV vaccine is recommended for routine immunization of all infants beginning at birth and for all children and adolescents through 18 years of age who have not been immunized previously (see Fig. 94.1). It is also recommended as a preexposure vaccination for older children and adults at increased risk of sexual, percutaneous, or mucosal exposure to HBV as well as those with chronic liver disease, human immunodeficiency virus (HIV), and travelers to areas of endemic HBV infection. Routine prenatal screening for HBsAg is recommended for all pregnant women in the United States. Infants born to HBsAg-positive mothers should receive HBV vaccine and hepatitis B immunoglobulin (HBIG; 0.5 mL) within 12 hours of birth, with subsequent vaccine doses at 1 and 6 months of age followed by testing for HBsAg and anti-HBs at 9-15 months of age. Infants born to mothers whose HBsAg status is unknown should receive vaccine within 12 hours of birth. If maternal testing is positive for HBsAg, the infant should receive HBIG as soon as possible (no later than 1 week of age). The combination of HBIG and vaccination is 99% effective in preventing vertical transmission of HBV. Vaccination alone without HBIG may prevent 75% of cases of perinatal HBV transmission and approximately 95% of cases of symptomatic childhood HBV infection.

Postexposure prophylaxis of unvaccinated persons using HBIG and vaccine is recommended following needle-stick injuries with blood from an HBsAg-positive patient and for sexual or needle-sharing contacts or victims of sexual abuse by an HBsAg-positive person. The screening of blood donors significantly reduces the risk of blood-borne transmission.

CHAPTER 114

Urinary Tract Infection

ETIOLOGY

Urinary tract infections (UTIs) include **cystitis** (infection localized to the bladder), **pyelonephritis** (infection of the renal parenchyma, calyces, and renal pelvis), and **renal abscess**, which may be intrarenal or perinephric. The urinary tract and urine are normally sterile. *Escherichia coli*, ascending from bowel (perineum) flora, accounts for 85% of first infections. Other bacteria commonly causing infection include *Klebsiella, Proteus, Enterococcus, Pseudomonas,* and *Enterobacter. Staphylococcus saprophyticus* is associated with UTI in some children and accounts for ≥15% of UTIs in adolescent girls. *Staphylococcus aureus* is an uncommon cause of UTI and usually represents bacteremic seeding of the urinary tract.

EPIDEMIOLOGY

Approximately 3% of girls and 1% of boys have a UTI during their prepubertal years with the highest incidence in the first year of life. It is only during the first year of life that the incidence of UTIs in males exceeds that in females; during this period uncircumcised boys are at 10-fold greater risk of developing a UTI compared to circumcised boys. After 12 months of age, UTI in healthy children usually is seen in girls.

A short urethra predisposes girls to UTIs. Obstruction to urine flow and urinary stasis is the major risk factor and may result from anatomical abnormalities, nephrolithiasis, renal tumor, indwelling urinary catheter, ureteropelvic junction obstruction, megaureter, extrinsic compression, and pregnancy. Severe vesicoureteral reflux, whether primary or secondary to urinary tract obstruction, predisposes to chronic infection and renal scarring. Scarring may also develop in the absence of reflux. Constipation or withholding urine also increases the risk of UTI.

CLINICAL MANIFESTATIONS

Decision-Making Algorithms
Available @ StudentConsult.com

Dysuria
Enuresis
Red Urine and Hematuria

The symptoms and signs of UTI vary markedly with age. Few have high positive predictive value in neonates, with failure to thrive, feeding problems, and fever as the most consistent symptoms. Infants 1 month to 2 years of age may present with feeding problems, failure to thrive, diarrhea, vomiting, or unexplained fever. The symptoms may masquerade as gastrointestinal illness, with colic, irritability, and crying periods. At 2 years of age, children begin to show the classic signs of UTI, such as urgency, dysuria, frequency, and abdominal or back pain. The presence of UTI should be suspected in all infants and young children with unexplained fever and in patients of all ages with fever and congenital anomalies of the urinary tract.

LABORATORY AND IMAGING STUDIES

The diagnosis of UTI in infants and young children requires the presence of both pyuria and at least 50,000 CFU/mL of a single pathogenic organism. For older children and adolescents, >100,000 CFU/mL indicates infection. It is appropriate to obtain urine cultures by midstream, clean-catch technique for older children and adolescents, whereas suprapubic bladder aspiration or transurethral catheterization is the appropriate method for younger children and infants. Perineal bags for urine collection are prone to contamination and are not recommended for urine collection for culture. If there is uncertainty about diagnosis of UTI in a younger child or infant, urine can be collected by the most convenient method for urinalysis, and if suggestive of infection, collect urine by catheterization prior to starting antibiotics.

Urinalysis showing **pyuria** (leukocyturia of >10 white blood cells [WBCs]/mm^3) suggests infection but is also consistent with urethritis, vaginitis, nephrolithiasis, glomerulonephritis, and interstitial nephritis. Other urinalysis findings suggestive of infection include any bacteria per high-powered field in the unstained uncentrifuged urinary sediment, positive urinary leukocyte esterase test, and positive urinary nitrite test. Combined testing for leukocyte esterase, nitrite, and microscopic bacteria has almost 100% sensitivity for detecting UTI by positivity of ≥1 of the three tests. The negative predictive value of a urinalysis is about 100% if all three tests are negative and may obviate the need for culture except in neonates, where urinalysis results are less reliable predictors of infection.

Ultrasonography of the bladder and kidneys is recommended for infants and non–toilet trained children with first-time febrile UTIs so as to exclude structural abnormalities or detect hydronephrosis. Voiding cystourethrogram (VCUG) is indicated if the ultrasound is abnormal (hydronephrosis, scarring, or other findings suggesting obstruction or congenital abnormality). Vesicoureteral reflux is the most common abnormality found and is ranked from grade I (ureter only) to grade V (complete gross dilation of the ureter and obliteration of caliceal and pelvic anatomy) (see Chapter 167). A technetium-99m dimercaptosuccinic acid (DMSA) scan can identify acute pyelonephritis and is most useful to define renal scarring as a late effect of UTI.

DIFFERENTIAL DIAGNOSIS

The diagnosis of a UTI is confirmed by a positive urine culture, but this does not distinguish between upper and lower tract infection. Localization of a UTI is important because upper Pyelonephritis is associated more frequently with bacteremia and anatomical abnormalities than is uncomplicated cystitis. The clinical manifestations of UTI do not reliably distinguish the site of infection in neonates, infants, and toddlers. Fever and abdominal pain may occur with either lower or upper UTI, although high fever, vomiting, costovertebral tenderness, leukocytosis on complete blood count (CBC), and bacteremia each suggest upper tract involvement.

The manifestations of UTI overlap with signs of sepsis seen in young children and with enteritis, appendicitis, mesenteric lymphadenitis, and pneumonia in older children. Dysuria may indicate pinworm infection, hypersensitivity to soaps or detergents, vaginitis, or sexual abuse and infection.

TREATMENT

Decision-Making Algorithm
Available @ StudentConsult.com
Fever Without a Source

Empirical therapy should be initiated for symptomatic children and for all children with a urine culture confirming UTI. For infants and children who do not appear ill but have a positive urine culture, oral antibiotic therapy should be initiated. For all young infants and any child with suspected UTI who appears toxic, appears dehydrated, or is unable to retain oral fluids, initial antibiotic therapy should be administered parenterally.

Neonates with UTI are treated for 7-14 days with parenteral antibiotics because UTIs in this age group are assumed to occur from hematogenous spread regardless of blood culture results. If a 7-day course of parental antibiotics is given, 7 additional days of enteral antibiotics are provided to complete a 14-day total course of therapy. Older children with UTI are treated for 7-14 days of enteral antibiotics or a combination of parenteral followed by enteral antibiotic therapy. Initial treatment with parenteral antibiotics in this age group is determined by clinical status. Parenteral antibiotics should be continued until there is clinical improvement (typically 24-48 hours), defined as resolution of fever and improved oral intake. Empiric antibiotic therapy should be guided by the local antimicrobial susceptibility patterns and the results of the patient's prior urine cultures because of increasing problems related to antimicrobial resistance. Definitive antibiotic therapy should be guided by the patient's urine culture results. Commonly used empiric parenteral antibiotics include cefazolin, ceftriaxone, or ampicillin plus gentamicin. Oral regimens include a cephalexin, amoxicillin plus clavulanic acid, or trimethoprim-sulfamethoxazole. Infants and children who do not show the expected clinical response within 2 days of starting antimicrobial therapy should be re-evaluated, have another urine specimen obtained for culture, and undergo imaging promptly to evaluate for renal abscess.

The degree of toxicity, dehydration, and ability to retain oral intake of fluids should be assessed carefully. Restoring or maintaining adequate hydration, including correction of electrolyte abnormalities that are often associated with vomiting or poor oral intake, is important.

COMPLICATIONS AND PROGNOSIS

Bacteremia occurs in approximately 5% of patients with pyelonephritis and is more likely in infants than in older children. Focal renal abscesses are an uncommon complication. Parents should be counseled to follow up for evaluation for subsequent fevers to determine the possibility of a recurrence of UTI. If a recurrent UTI is diagnosed, further imaging studies (VCUG) are indicated, if not already performed, to evaluate the possibility of vesicoureteral reflux (see Chapter 167).

PREVENTION

Primary prevention is achieved by promoting good perineal hygiene and managing underlying risk factors for UTI, such as chronic constipation, encopresis, and daytime and nighttime urinary incontinence. There is evidence that antibiotic prophylaxis may prevent more severe symptomatic recurrent infections, although the effect is small and is associated with the development of resistant organisms. The impact of secondary prophylaxis to prevent renal scarring is unknown. Acidification of the urine with cranberry juice is not recommended as the sole means of preventing UTI in children at high risk.

CHAPTER 115

Vulvovaginitis

ETIOLOGY

Vulvovaginitis, which is inflammation of the vulva or vagina or both, is the most common gynecological problem in prepubertal

TABLE 115.1 Characteristics of Vulvovaginitis

ETIOLOGY CONDITION/ DISORDER	PRESENTATION	DIAGNOSIS	TREATMENT
Physiological vaginal discharge (physiological leukorrhea)	Minimal, clear, thin discharge without pruritus or inflammation; occurs soon after birth and again at 6-12 mo before menarche	No pathogenic organisms on culture	Reassurance
Nonspecific vaginitis	Vaginal discharge, dysuria, pruritus; fecal soiling of underwear	Evidence of poor hygiene; no pathogenic organisms on culture	Improved hygiene, sitz baths 2-3 times/day
Bacterial vaginosis	Often asymptomatic; possible thin vaginal discharge with a "fishy" odor	≥3 of the following criteria: (1) thin, homogeneous vaginal discharge; (2) vaginal pH >4.5; (3) a fishy odor of volatile amines on the addition of a drop of 10% potassium hydroxide to a drop of vaginal discharge (the "whiff test"); and (4) the presence of clue cells on a saline wet mount of vaginal discharge	Metronidazole, clindamycin
Candidiasis	Pruritus, dysuria, white "cottage cheese" vaginal discharge that is usually not malodorous	*Candida* on KOH preparation of vaginal discharge	Topical antifungal (e.g., butoconazole, clotrimazole, miconazole, nystatin) Single oral dose fluconazole
Enterobiasis (pinworms)	Perineal pruritus (nocturnal); gastrointestinal symptoms; variable vulvovaginal contamination from feces; often recurrent symptoms	Adult worms in stool or eggs on perianal skin ("Scotch tape test")	Mebendazole or albendazole
Molluscum contagiosum	Vulvar lesions, nodules with central umbilication; white core of curd-like material	Clinical appearance; Isolation of poxvirus	Dermal curettage of umbilicated area
Phthirus pubis infection (pediculosis pubis)	Pruritus, excoriation, sky-blue macules; inner thigh or lower abdomen	Nits on hair shafts, lice on skin or clothing	1% permethrin
Sarcoptes scabiei infection (scabies)	Nocturnal pruritus, pruritic vesicles, pustules in runs	Mites; ova, black dots of feces (microscopic)	5% permethrin
Shigella infection	Bloody vaginal discharge; fever, malaise, fecal contamination, diarrhea; blood and mucus in stool, abdominal cramps	Stools: white blood cells and red blood cells, positive for *Shigella*	Oral third-generation cephalosporin
Staphylococcus, Streptococcus infection	Vaginal discharge, possibly bloody; hyperemic vulvar mucosa; spread from primary lesion	Isolation of causative organism on bacterial culture	First-generation cephalosporin or dicloxacillin; penicillin or amoxicillin for group A streptococcus infection
Foreign body	Foul-smelling vaginal discharge, sometimes bloody	Foreign body on physical examination	Removal of foreign body

KOH, Potassium hydroxide.

girls. Poor hygienic practices, close proximity of the vagina to the rectum, and low levels of estrogen predispose prepubertal girls to vulvovaginal irritation. Low levels of estrogen result in thin, atrophic vaginal epithelium that is susceptible to bacterial invasion. At puberty, estrogen increases, and the pH of the vagina becomes more acidic. Vulvovaginitis can be due to nonspecific and specific causes. **Nonspecific vaginitis** results from overgrowth of normal aerobic vaginal flora that is associated with poor hygiene. There are several specific causes of vulvovaginitis (Table 115.1), including sexually transmitted infections such as *Trichomonas vaginalis* and herpes simplex virus (see Chapter 116). **Bacterial vaginosis** is the most common cause of vaginitis in postpubertal women and represents disruption of the normal vaginal flora with reduction in *Lactobacillus* and overgrowth of organisms including *Gardnerella vaginalis*, *Bacteroides*, *Mobiluncus*, and *Peptostreptococcus*.

EPIDEMIOLOGY

Nonspecific vaginitis is the most common cause of vulvovaginitis in prepubertal girls. *G. vaginalis* is often present as part of the normal vaginal flora in prepubertal girls, and its role as a cause of vaginitis in this age group is uncommon. *Candida* is much less common in prepubertal girls than in women.

CLINICAL MANIFESTATIONS

Decision-Making Algorithms
Available @ StudentConsult.com

Abnormal Vaginal Bleeding
Vaginal Discharge

The primary symptoms of vulvovaginitis are vaginal discharge, erythema, foul smell, dysuria, and pruritus. Characteristics of specific etiologies are outlined in Table 115.1.

LABORATORY AND IMAGING STUDIES

Wet mount microscopic examination, prepared by mixing vaginal secretions with normal saline solution, and culture may be used to confirm a specific diagnosis (see Table 115.1). **Clue cells** are vaginal epithelial cells that are covered with *G. vaginalis* and have a granular appearance (Fig. 115.1). Vaginal cultures for *G. vaginalis* are not useful. *Candida* may be identified by KOH stain or by culture.

DIFFERENTIAL DIAGNOSIS

Noninfectious causes of vulvovaginitis include physical agents (foreign body, sand), chemical agents (bubble bath, soap, detergent), and vulvar skin disease (atopic dermatitis, seborrhea, psoriasis). Physiological vaginal discharge or **physiological leukorrhea** of desquamated vaginal cells and mucus occurs normally in females soon after birth, with discharge lasting for about 1 week, and appears again at 6-12 months before menarche. The discharge is minimal, clear, and thin without pruritus or inflammation. No treatment is necessary.

TREATMENT

The treatment of vulvovaginitis depends on the etiology (see Table 115.1). Treatment of nonspecific vaginitis focuses on improving perineal hygiene. Douching or vaginal irrigation is not beneficial and is not recommended.

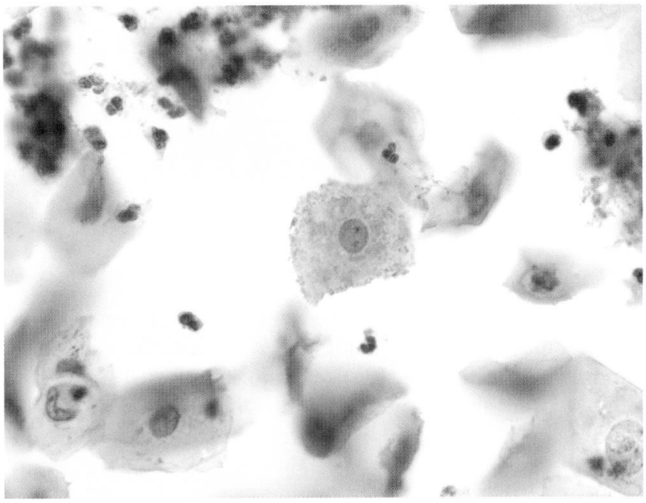

FIGURE 115.1 A film of coccobacilli covers squamous cells in a cervical cytology sample. This aspect is commonly referred to as "clue cells" and is associated with bacterial vaginosis (Papanicolaou stain, ×100). (*From Tambouret R. Gynecologic infections. In: Kradin RL, ed.* Diagnostic Pathology of Infectious Diseases. *Philadelphia: Elsevier; 2010.*)

COMPLICATIONS AND PROGNOSIS

Complications of nonspecific vulvovaginitis are rare, and prognosis is excellent. Bacterial vaginosis is associated with birth complications such as chorioamnionitis and preterm labor, but evidence regarding treatment of bacterial vaginosis to prevent these complications is conflicting.

PREVENTION

There are no recognized prophylactic measures for bacterial vaginosis or nonspecific vaginitis other than maintaining good perineal hygiene. Douching is not protective and reduces normal vaginal flora, which are protective against pathogenic organisms.

CHAPTER 116
Sexually Transmitted Infections

Decision-Making Algorithms
Available @ StudentConsult.com

Dysmenorrhea
Abnormal Vaginal Bleeding
Vaginal Discharge

Adolescents have the highest rates of sexually transmitted infections (STIs). Compared with adults, sexually active adolescents are more likely to believe they will not contract an STI, more likely to come into contact with an infected sexual partner, less likely to receive health care when an STI develops, and less likely to be compliant with treatment for an STI.

Although numerous organisms cause STIs, the diseases can be grouped by their characteristic clinical presentations. **Urethritis** and **endocervicitis** (Table 116.1) are characteristic of *Neisseria gonorrhoeae* and *Chlamydia trachomatis* and are the most common STIs. Note that 70% of new genital chlamydial infections occur in adolescents aged 15-24 years and most infections are asymptomatic. **Genital ulcers** (Table 116.2) are characteristic of syphilis *(Treponema pallidum)*, genital herpes simplex virus (HSV) infections, chancroid *(Haemophilus ducreyi)*, lymphogranuloma venereum (LGV; *C. trachomatis*), and granuloma inguinale, also known as *donovanosis (Klebsiella granulomatis)*. **Vaginal discharge** (Table 116.3) is a symptom of trichomoniasis *(Trichomonas vaginalis)* and is part of the spectrum of vulvovaginitis (see Chapter 115), which is not always associated with sexual activity. Human papillomavirus (HPV) causes **condylomata acuminata**, or **genital warts** (Table 116.4), and is the major risk factor for cervical, vulvar, and vaginal cancers.

STIs are associated with significant physiological and psychological morbidity. Early diagnosis and treatment are important for preventing medical complications and infertility. All STIs

TABLE 116.1 Features of Sexually Transmitted Infections Caused by *Chlamydia trachomatis* and *Neisseria gonorrhoeae**

FEATURE	*C. TRACHOMATIS*	*N. GONORRHOEAE*
Incubation period	7-21 days	2-7 days
Possible presentations	Conjunctivitis (including neonatal conjunctivitis), pneumonia, urethritis, cervicitis, proctitis, epididymitis, perihepatitis, lymphogranuloma venereum, reactive arthritis (arthritis, urethritis, and bilateral conjunctivitis)	Pharyngitis, conjunctivitis (including neonatal conjunctivitis), urethritis, cervicitis, proctitis, epididymitis, perihepatitis, disseminated disease (arthritis, dermatitis, endocarditis, meningitis)
SIGNS/SYMPTOMS OF COMMON SYNDROMES		
Urethritis	*Female* Dysuria, frequency >10 PMNs/hpf *Male* Penile discharge >10 PMNs/hpf	
Mucopurulent cervicitis	Cervical erythema, friability, with thick creamy discharge >10 PMNs/hpf Mild cervical tenderness Gram-negative intracellular diplococci	Cervical edema, erythema, or friability with purulent or mucopurulent discharge >10 PMNs/hpf Mild cervical tenderness Gram-negative diplococci
Pelvic inflammatory disease	Onset of symptoms within 7 days menstrual cycle Lower abdominal pain Adnexal tenderness, mass (5-50%) Pain on cervical motion (>95%) Fever (35%) Vaginal discharge (55%) Mucopurulent cervical discharge (80%) Menstrual irregularities (variable) Nausea, vomiting (variable) Weakness, syncope, dizziness (variable) Perihepatitis (5%)	
Diagnostic tests	NAAT, culture	NAAT, culture
Treatment	Ceftriaxone *plus* doxycycline *or* azithromycin If PID: cefotetan or cefoxitin *plus* doxycycline	

**Coinfection is common, and clinical presentations have significant overlap.*
hpf, High-power field; *NAAT*, nucleic acid amplification test; *PID*, pelvic inflammatory disease; *PMNs*, polymorphonuclear cells.

are preventable; primary prevention of STIs should be a goal of all health care providers for adolescents. Diagnosis of an STI necessitates evaluation or treatment for concomitant STIs and notification and treatment of sexual partners; some STIs are reportable to state health departments.

Many infections that are not traditionally considered STIs are sexually transmissible, including those caused by human immunodeficiency virus (HIV), human T-cell leukemia viruses types I and II, cytomegalovirus, Epstein-Barr virus, human herpes virus (HHV-6, HHV-7), hepatitis B virus, molluscum contagiosum virus, and *Sarcoptes scabiei.* The presence of any STI suggests behavior that increases risk for HIV (see Chapter 125), and HIV counseling and testing should be provided to all adolescents with STIs. Acquisition of gonorrhea, chlamydia, syphilis, genital HSV, and trichomoniasis in prepubertal children beyond the neonatal period indicates sexual contact and signifies the need to investigate for possible sexual abuse (see Chapter 22); diagnosis of STIs in infants can represent abuse or perinatal acquisition. The association of sexual abuse with vulvovaginitis and genital HPV infection, which may result from skin or genital HPV types, is less certain.

PELVIC INFLAMMATORY DISEASE

Direct extension of *N. gonorrhoeae* and/or *C. trachomatis* to the endometrium, fallopian tubes, and peritoneum causes **pelvic inflammatory disease (PID)**. Complications of PID include tubo-ovarian abscess, perihepatitis (**Fitz-Hugh-Curtis syndrome**, an inflammation of the liver capsule), and infertility. The differential diagnosis of PID includes ectopic pregnancy, septic abortion, ovarian cyst torsion or rupture, urinary tract infection, appendicitis, mesenteric lymphadenitis, and inflammatory bowel disease. Pelvic ultrasound may detect thickened adnexal structures and is the imaging study of choice to exclude other possible diagnoses. Minimum clinical criteria for diagnosis of PID are pelvic or lower abdominal tenderness with uterine,

TABLE 116.2 Features of Sexually Transmitted Infections Characterized by Genital Ulcers

	SYPHILIS	GENITAL HERPES	CHANCROID	GRANULOMA INGUINALE (DONOVANOSIS)
Agent	*Treponema pallidum*	HSV-1, HSV-2	*Haemophilus ducreyi*	*Klebsiella granulomatis*
Incubation	10-90 days	2-14 days	1-10 days	8-80 days
Systemic findings	Primary syphilis: Uncommon Secondary syphilis: Fever, rash, malaise, anorexia, arthralgia, lymphadenopathy	Headache, fever, malaise, myalgia (40-70%)	None	Local spread only
Inguinal lymphadenopathy	Late, bilateral, nontender, no suppuration	Early, bilateral, tender, no suppuration	Early, rapid, tender, and unilateral; suppuration likely (bubo)	Lymphatic obstruction
Primary lesion	Papule	Vesicle	Papule to pustule	Subcutaneous nodule
ULCER CHARACTERISTICS				
Number	>1	Multiple	<3	>1, may coalesce
Edges	Distinct	Reddened, ragged	Sharply demarcated, serpiginous borders	Rolled, distinct
Depth	Shallow	Shallow	Shallow	Raised
Base	Red, smooth	Red, smooth	Necrotic	Beefy red, clean
Secretion	Serous	Serous	Purulent	None
Induration	Firm	None	None	Firm
Pain	None	Usual	Often	None
Diagnosis				
Serology	MHA-TP or FTA-ABS; VDRL or RPR	Seroconversion (primary infection only)	None	None
Isolation	No in vitro test; rabbit testes inoculation	Culture	Swab of ulcer on selective medium, node aspirates usually sterile	None
Microscopic	Dark-field examination	PCR or fluorescent antibody staining	Gram-negative coccobacilli	Staining of ulcer biopsy material for donovan bodies
Treatment	*Early (primary, secondary and early latent)*: Benzathine penicillin G (2.4 million U IM) once *Late latent (>1 yr duration)*: Benzathine penicillin G (2.4 million U IM) weekly × 3 doses	Acyclovir *or* famciclovir *or* valacyclovir	Aspirate or excise fluctuant nodes Incision and drainage of buboes >5 cm Azithromycin *or* ceftriaxone *or* ciprofloxacin *or* erythromycin	Doxycycline *or* azithromycin

FTA-ABS, Fluorescent treponemal antibody–absorption; *HSV*, herpes simplex virus; *IM*, intramuscular; *MHA-TP*, microhemagglutination assay-*Treponema pallidum*; *PCR*, polymerase chain reaction; *RPR*, rapid plasma reagin; *VDRL*, Venereal Disease Research Laboratory.

adnexal, or cervical motion tenderness. Additional criteria that support the diagnosis are fever, mucopurulent cervical discharge or cervical friability, presence of abundant numbers of white blood cells (WBCs) on saline microscopy of vaginal fluid, elevated inflammatory markers, and documented infection with *N. gonorrhoeae* or *C. trachomatis*. Adolescents should be hospitalized for treatment if there is uncertainty about the diagnosis, pregnancy, no clinical response to oral therapy within 72 hours, inability to adhere to or tolerate oral therapy, a tubo-ovarian abscess, or severe illness with high fever, nausea, and vomiting. The recommended parenteral treatment for hospitalized patients is cefotetan or cefoxitin plus doxycycline orally. The recommended ambulatory treatment of PID is ceftriaxone (250 mg) in a single intramuscular (IM) dose, plus doxycycline (100 mg) orally twice a day for 14 days, with or without metronidazole (500 mg twice a day) orally for 14 days. Follow-up examination should be performed within 72 hours.

GONORRHEA *(NEISSERIA GONORRHOEAE)*

Neisseria gonorrhoeae, a gram-negative coccus, is often seen microscopically as diplococci. Gonorrhea is a common STI among adolescents. The highest incidence in the United States is in 15- to 24-year-olds, and incidence rates differ by race and gender, with more cases in men than in women. The organism causes infection at the site of acquisition, which

TABLE 116.3 Features of Sexually Transmitted Infections Characterized by Vaginal Discharge

FEATURE	PHYSIOLOGICAL LEUKORRHEA (NORMAL)	TRICHOMONIASIS	BACTERIAL VAGINOSIS
Agent	Normal flora	*Trichomonas vaginalis*	Reduction in *Lactobacillus* and overgrowth organisms including *Gardnerella vaginalis, Bacteroides, Mobiluncus,* and *Peptostreptococcus*
Incubation	—	5-28 days	Not necessarily sexually transmitted
Predominant Symptoms			
Pruritus	None	Mild to moderate	None to mild
Discharge	Minimal	Moderate to severe	Mild to moderate
Pain	None	Mild	Uncommon
Vulvar inflammation	None	Common	Uncommon
Characteristics of Discharge			
Amount	Small	Profuse	Moderate
Color	Clear, milky	Yellow-green or gray	Gray
Consistency	Flocculent	Frothy	Homogeneous
Viscosity	Thin	Thin	Thin
Foul odor	None	Possible	Yes
Odor with KOH	None	Possible	Characteristic fishy odor (amine)
pH	<4.5	>5.0	>4.5
Diagnosis			
Saline drop	Squamous and few WBCs	WBC; Motile flagellates, slightly larger than WBCs	Squamous cells studded with bacteria ("clue cells") and WBCs
Gram stain	Gram-positive and gram-negative rods and cocci	*Trichomonas*	Predominance of gram-negative rods and cocci with paucity of gram-positive rods
Culture	Mixed flora with *Lactobacillus* predominant	Culture generally not indicated; antibody and nucleic acid tests available	Culture not useful
Treatment	Reassurance	Metronidazole or tinidazole	Metronidazole or clindamycin

KOH, Potassium hydroxide; *WBCs*, white blood cells.

commonly results in mucopurulent cervicitis and urethritis (see Table 116.1), but infection of the rectum and pharynx can also occur. **Disseminated gonococcal infections** can occur with hematogenous spread and results in petechial or pustular acral skin lesions, asymmetric polyarthralgia, tenosynovitis or oligoarticular septic arthritis, and, occasionally, endocarditis or meningitis. Perinatal transmission of maternal infection can lead to neonatal sepsis, meningitis (see Chapter 65), and ophthalmia neonatorum (see Chapter 119).

Gonococcal infection is diagnosed by either culture of endocervical (women) or urethral (men) swab specimens or nucleic acid amplification tests (NAATs) of endocervical swabs, vaginal swabs, urethral swabs, throat specimens, and urine. Culture should be performed in cases of possible treatment failure to allow for antimicrobial susceptibility testing. In cases of suspected sexual abuse, culture is the preferred diagnostic method due to concerns regarding NAAT false-positive results from cross reaction with nongonococcal *Neisseria* species.

Treatment regimens should be effective against *N. gonorrhoeae* and *C. trachomatis* because of the high frequency of coinfection. Increasing rates of resistance to fluoroquinolones limit treatment options. A single IM dose of ceftriaxone (250 mg) in combination with a single oral dose of azithromycin (1 g) is recommended for uncomplicated gonococcal infections of the cervix, urethra, and rectum. The addition of azithromycin helps to prevent the emergence of resistance in *N. gonorrhoeae* and also serves as empirical *C. trachomatis* treatment. Hospitalization and treatment with ceftriaxone for 7-28 days, depending on the diagnosis, plus a single dose of azithromycin are recommended for disseminated gonococcal infections.

CHLAMYDIA *(CHLAMYDIA TRACHOMATIS)*

Decision-Making Algorithms
Available @ StudentConsult.com

Dysuria
Scrotal Pain
Abnormal Vaginal Bleeding
Vaginal Discharge

TABLE 116.4 Features of Sexually Transmitted Infections Characterized by Nonulcerative External Genital Symptoms

FEATURE	GENITAL WARTS	VULVOVAGINAL CANDIDIASIS	PEDICULOSIS PUBIS (CRABS)
Agent	Human papillomavirus	*Candida albicans*	*Phthirus pubis*
Incubation/transmission	Variable	Uncommon sexual transmission	5-10 days for eggs to hatch
Presenting complaints	Genital warts are seen or felt	Vulvar itching or discharge	Pubic itching; live organisms may be seen; sexual partner has "crabs"
Signs	Firm, gray-to-pink, single or multiple, fimbriated, painless excrescences on vulva, introitus, vagina, cervix, penis, perineum, anus	Inflammation of vulva, with thick, white, "cottage cheese" discharge, $pH < 4.5$; friable mucosa that easily bleeds	Eggs (nits) at base of pubic hairs, lice may be visible; excoriated, red skin secondary to infestation
Clinical associations	Cervical neoplasia, dysplasia	Oral contraceptives, diabetes, antibiotics	—
Diagnosis	Clinical appearance; most infections asymptomatic; acetowhite changes on colposcopy; enlarged cells with perinuclear halo and hyperchromatic nuclei	KOH (10%): pseudohyphae; Gram stain: gram-positive pseudohyphae; Nickerson or Sabouraud medium for culture	History and clinical appearance
Treatment	*Patient-applied therapies:* podofilox solution or gel *or* imiquimod cream	*Intravaginal agents:* butoconazole *or* clotrimazole *or* miconazole *or* nystatin *Oral agent:* fluconazole	Permethrin 1% cream *or* pyrethrin with piperonyl butoxide
	Provider-applied therapies: cryotherapy with liquid nitrogen or cryoprobe *or* topical podophyllin resin *or* trichloroacetic acid or bichloracetic acid *or* surgical removal		

KOH, Potassium hydroxide.

Chlamydiae are obligate intracellular bacteria with a biphasic life cycle, existing as relatively inert elementary bodies in their extracellular form and as reticulate bodies when phagocytosed and replicating within a phagosome. Reticulate bodies divide by binary fission and, after 48-72 hours, reorganize into elementary bodies that are released from the cell. Chlamydia infects nonciliated squamocolumnar cells and the transitional epithelial cells that line the mucosa of the urethra, cervix, rectum, and conjunctiva. The incidence of chlamydial infections is highest among persons <25 years of age, and annual screening is recommended for all sexually active women in this age group.

There are at least 18 *C. trachomatis* serovars. Serovars A through C cause trachoma, an ocular infection eventually leading to blindness from extensive local scarring; serovars B and D through K cause urethritis, cervicitis, PID, inclusion conjunctivitis in newborns, and infant pneumonia; serovars L13 cause LGV, an infrequent STI characterized by an ulcerative genital lesion followed by unilateral, painful inguinal lymphadenitis.

Chlamydia is the most frequently diagnosed bacterial STI in adolescents and accounts for most cases of **nongonococcal urethritis and cervicitis** (see Table 116.1). There is a 2.5:1 female-to-male ratio. Males often have dysuria and mucopurulent discharge, although asymptomatic infection also occurs. Women are more often asymptomatic or may have minimal symptoms, including dysuria, mild abdominal pain, or vaginal discharge. Prepubertal girls may have vaginitis. At least 30% of persons with gonococcal cervicitis, urethritis, proctitis, or epididymitis have *C. trachomatis* coinfection.

Chlamydia infection is usually diagnosed by NAAT detection of vaginal, cervical, urethral, and early-morning first-voided urine specimens. Amplification tests have supplanted less sensitive culture and enzyme-linked immunosorbent assay (ELISA) tests. NAAT can be used for vaginal and urine specimens from girls in the evaluation of sexual abuse. Culture is still preferred for detection of urogenital infection in boys and to evaluate for extragenital *C. trachomatis* in boys and girls.

Treatment regimens effective against *C. trachomatis* include a single oral dose of azithromycin (1 g) or doxycycline for 7 days. Individuals should be advised to avoid unprotected intercourse until all their sexual partners have been tested and treated. Tests of cure are not recommended unless therapeutic adherence is in question, symptoms persist, or reinfection is suspected.

SYPHILIS *(TREPONEMA PALLIDUM)*

Decision-Making Algorithms
Available @ StudentConsult.com

Vaginal Discharge
Fever and Rash
Lymphadenopathy
Petechiae/Purpura

Syphilis is caused by *T. pallidum,* a long, slender, coiled spirochete. It cannot be cultivated routinely in vitro but can be observed by dark-field microscopy. Untreated infection progresses through several clinical stages (see Table 116.2). **Primary syphilis** is manifested as a single, painless genital ulcer, or **chancre,** usually on the genitalia, that appears approximately 3 weeks after inoculation and spontaneously heals in a few weeks. **Secondary syphilis** follows 4-8 weeks later and is manifested as fever, generalized lymphadenopathy, and a disseminated maculopapular rash that is also present on the palms and soles. Plaque-like skin lesions, **condylomata lata**, and mucous membrane lesions occur, particularly in moist areas around the vulva and anus, and are infectious. Secondary syphilis resolves spontaneously within 3-12 weeks. **Tertiary syphilis** is a slowly progressive disease involving the cardiovascular, neurological, and musculoskeletal systems that manifests 15-30 years after initial infection. **Latent syphilis** is an asymptomatic infection detected by serological testing. Early latent syphilis indicates acquisition within the preceding year; all other cases of latent syphilis are designated as either late latent syphilis or latent syphilis of unknown duration. Infection can be passed from pregnant women to infect their infants, resulting in **congenital syphilis** (see Chapter 66).

The diagnosis of syphilis is based on serological testing. There are different types of serological tests for syphilis, and both are required to make a diagnosis: **nontreponemal antibody tests**: the **Venereal Disease Research Laboratory (VDRL)** test, the **rapid plasma reagin (RPR)** test; specific **treponemal antibody tests**: the **microhemagglutination assay–*T. pallidum*** (MHA-TP), the **fluorescent treponemal antibody-absorption** (FTA-ABS) test, various enzyme immunoassays (EIAs), and chemiluminescence immunoassays. The syphilis screening algorithm starts with a screening-specific treponemal EIA or chemiluminescence immunoassay. Screening with specific treponemal antibody tests will identify persons with active disease but will also be positive in persons who were previously adequately treated for syphilis, those with incompletely treated syphilis, and those with false-positive results. Positive treponemal screening antibody tests should be followed by a nontreponemal test with titer. The titer can help guide management, as it increases with increasing duration of infection and decreases in response to therapy. Negative nontreponemal tests should be confirmed with a different treponemal test to confirm the results of the initial treponemal test. A nonquantitative VDRL test can be performed on cerebrospinal fluid but is insensitive. Rheumatic disease and other infectious diseases may cause false-positive VDRL results. Dark-field examination of chancres, mucous membranes, or cutaneous lesions may reveal motile organisms.

The treatment of choice for all stages of syphilis is parenteral penicillin G. Primary syphilis, secondary syphilis, and early latent syphilis are treated with a single IM dose of benzathine penicillin G. Tertiary, late latent, and latent syphilis of unknown duration are treated with three doses at 1-week intervals. Neurosyphilis is treated with intravenous aqueous crystalline penicillin G for 10-14 days. A systemic, febrile **Jarisch-Herxheimer reaction** can occur within the first 24 hours of penicillin initiation in patients being treated for syphilis.

HERPES SIMPLEX VIRUS INFECTION

Decision-Making Algorithms
Available @ StudentConsult.com

Sore Throat
Dysuria
Vaginal Discharge
Vesicles and Bullae
Fever and Rash
Lymphadenopathy

HSV-1 and HSV-2 are large, double-stranded DNA viruses of the herpesvirus family with a linear genome contained within an icosahedral capsid. There is significant DNA homology between types 1 and 2. The virus initially infects mucosal surfaces and enters cutaneous neurons, where it migrates along the axons to sensory ganglia. As viral replication occurs in the ganglia, infectious virus moves along the axon to infect and destroy epithelial cells. Infection may disseminate to other organs in immunocompromised patients. Virus latency is maintained in the ganglia where it undergoes periodic reactivation and replication triggered by undefined events. Although either virus can be found in any site, HSV-1 more commonly occurs in the central nervous system, eyes, and mouth, whereas HSV-2 more commonly involves the genitalia. Reinfection can occur with exposure to the other type or even a second strain of the same type.

Primary genital herpes is characterized by multiple painful, grouped vesicles or ulcerative and crusted external genital lesions on an erythematous base (see Table 116.2). In females the cervix may also be involved. Symptoms may include fever, regional lymphadenopathy, discharge, and dysuria. Primary illness lasts 10-20 days. Asymptomatic primary infection may also occur. **Secondary, recurrent,** or **reactivation eruptions** are not as dramatic and are not associated with systemic symptoms. In primary infection, viral shedding lasts an average of 11 days, and the entire course from vesicle and ulcer onset resolves over 20 days. In recurrent disease, virus shedding lasts for an average of 4 days, and the course resolves over 9-10 days. Many persons experience 4-6 recurrences per year. Some primary and many recurrent episodes are asymptomatic.

Viral cultures and polymerase chain reaction (PCR) are the preferred methods of diagnosis; culture typically shows cytopathic effect in 1-3 days and seldom takes longer than 5 days. PCR assays have increased sensitivity over culture. Viral shedding is intermittent after primary infection, so both culture and PCR can fail to detect latent infection. Serological testing is useful for primary infection only (to show seroconversion between acute and convalescent sera), and positive serologies persist lifelong. Titers are not helpful in guiding management of recurrences.

Oral famciclovir and valacyclovir are effective treatments in reducing the severity and duration of symptoms in primary cases and may reduce recurrences. Once-daily suppressive therapy reduces the frequency of genital herpes recurrences by >75%, and lesions tend to be mild when they do occur. Local hygiene and sitz baths may relieve discomfort. The use of condoms provides some protection against sexual transmission of HSV.

TRICHOMONIASIS *(TRICHOMONAS VAGINALIS)*

Decision-Making Algorithms
Available @ StudentConsult.com

Abnormal Vaginal Bleeding
Vaginal Discharge

Trichomoniasis is caused by the protozoan *T. vaginalis* and often is associated with other STIs, such as gonorrhea and *Chlamydia*. Infection is asymptomatic in as many as 70-85% of infected persons. Symptomatic males can have urethritis.

Symptomatic females have vaginitis, with thin, malodorous, frothy yellow-green discharge, vulvar irritation, and cervical "strawberry hemorrhages" (see Table 116.3). Diagnosis is based on visualization of motile, flagellated protozoans in the urine or in a saline wet mount, which has a sensitivity of only 60-70% among symptomatic women. *T. vaginalis*–specific NAAT is available for testing vaginal, endocervical, and urine samples and is highly sensitive (95-100%) and specific (95-100%). Rapid point-of-care testing has become available in recent years, with a turnaround time of approximately 10 minutes. Treatment of sexual partners with oral metronidazole or tinidazole in a single dose is recommended.

GENITAL WARTS (HUMAN PAPILLOMAVIRUSES)

Decision-Making Algorithms
Available @ StudentConsult.com

Hoarseness
Vaginal Discharge

HPV, the cause of genital warts **(condylomata acuminata)**, is the most common STI in the United States, with the highest prevalence rates among 15- to 24-year-olds. Most HPV infections are asymptomatic or subclinical (90%) and self-resolve within 2 years. HPV types 6 and 11 cause 90% of genital warts and are nononcogenic. HPV types 16 and 18 are associated with 70% of cases of cervical cancer. HPV types 31, 33, 45, 52, and 58 are also oncogenic.

Genital warts can occur on the squamous epithelium or mucous membranes of the genital and perineal structures of females and males (see Table 116.4). Genital warts are usually multiple, firm, gray-to-pink excrescences. Untreated genital warts may remain unchanged, increase in size or number, or resolve spontaneously. Warts can become tender if macerated or secondarily infected. The diagnosis is usually established by appearance without biopsy. The differential diagnosis includes condylomata lata (secondary syphilis) and tumors.

The goal of treatment is removal of symptomatic warts to induce wart-free periods. Treatment modalities involve destruction of infected epithelium; patient-applied therapies include podofilox, sinecatechins, or imiquimod; and provider-applied therapies include cryotherapy with liquid nitrogen or cryoprobe and trichloroacetic acid or bichloroacetic acid. An alternative is surgical removal. Intralesional interferon and laser surgery have also been effective. Factors that may influence selection of treatment include wart number, size, anatomical sites, wart morphology, patient preference, treatment cost, convenience, adverse effects, and provider experience. Recurrences after treatment are common and are frequently asymptomatic.

PUBIC LICE *(PHTHIRUS PUBIS)*

Pubic lice, or pediculosis pubis, are caused by infestation with *Phthirus pubis,* the **pubic crab louse**. The louse is predominantly sexually transmitted and lives out its life cycle on pubic hair, where it causes characteristic, intense pruritus (see Table 116.4). Diagnosis can be made clinically; lice are visible to the naked eye. Erythematous papules and **egg cases (nits)** are not seen before puberty. Treatment consists of education regarding personal and environmental hygiene and the application of an appropriate pediculicide, such as permethrin 1% cream or pyrethrins with piperonyl butoxide. Bedding and clothing should be decontaminated (machine-washed and machine-dried using the heat cycle or dry cleaned) or removed from body contact for at least 72 hours. Fumigation of living areas is not necessary.

CHAPTER 117

Osteomyelitis

ETIOLOGY

Acute hematogenous osteomyelitis is the most common manifestation of osteomyelitis in children and evolves secondary to bacteremia. **Subacute osteomyelitis** may also follow local inoculation by penetrating trauma and is not associated with systemic symptoms; **chronic osteomyelitis** results from an untreated or inadequately treated (usually subacute) osteomyelitis.

In children beyond the newborn period and without hemoglobinopathies, bone infections occur almost exclusively in the metaphyses of long bones due to sluggish blood flow through tortuous vascular loops unique to this site. Preceding nonpenetrating trauma is often reported and may lead to local bone injury that predisposes to infection. Bone infections in children with sickle cell disease occur in the diaphyseal portion of the long bones, probably as a consequence of antecedent focal infarction. In children younger than 12-18 months of age, capillaries perforate the epiphyseal growth plate, permitting spread of infection across the epiphysis and leading to suppurative arthritis, whereas in older children, infection is contained in the metaphysis because these vessels no longer cross the epiphyseal plate (Fig. 117.1A and B).

Staphylococcus aureus is responsible for more than 80% of acute skeletal infections. Other common causes include group A streptococcus and *Streptococcus pneumoniae. Neisseria meningitidis, Mycobacterium tuberculosis, Bartonella henselae, Actinomyces* spp., and anaerobes are less common causes. Group B streptococcus and enteric gram-negatives are other major causes in neonates. Sickle cell disease and other hemoglobinopathies predispose to osteomyelitis caused by *Salmonella* and *S. aureus. Pasteurella multocida* osteomyelitis may follow cat or dog bites. The use of polymerase chain reaction (PCR) testing reveals that a significant proportion of **culture-negative osteomyelitis** is due to *Kingella kingae*, particularly in children under 5 years of age. Conjugate vaccine has greatly reduced the incidence of *Haemophilus influenzae* type b infections.

Subacute focal bone infections caused by *Pseudomonas aeruginosa* and *S. aureus* usually occur in ambulatory persons who sustain **puncture wounds** of the foot. *Pseudomonas* **chondritis** is strongly associated with puncture wounds through sneakers, which harbor *Pseudomonas* in the foam insole. *S. aureus* is the most common cause of chronic osteomyelitis. **Chronic recurrent multifocal osteomyelitis** is an autoinflammatory noninfectious syndrome characterized by recurrent episodes of fever, bone pain, and radiographic findings of osteomyelitis. Bones uncommonly involved in acute hematogenous osteomyelitis—such as

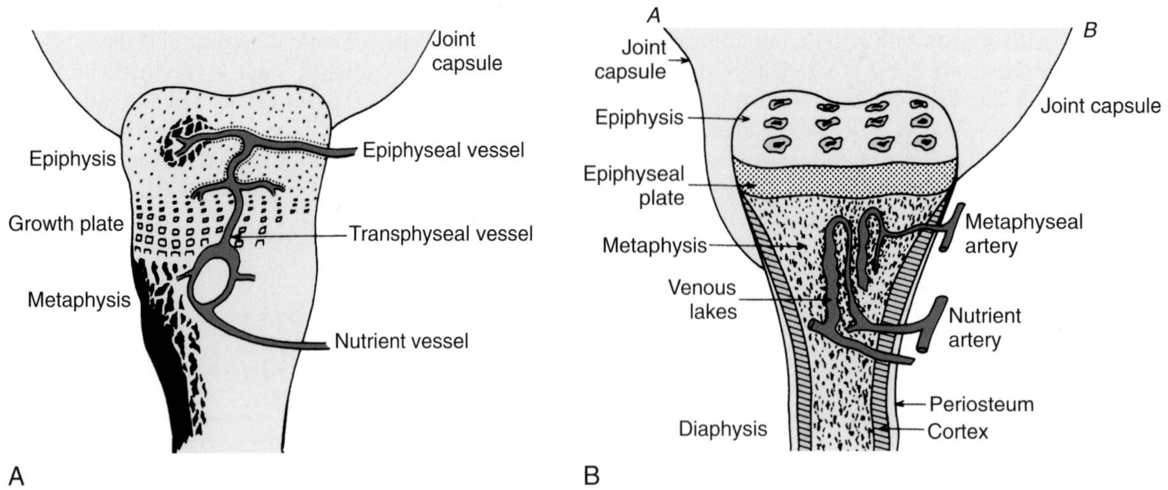

FIGURE 117.1 **(A)** Major structures of the bone of an infant before maturation of the epiphyseal growth plate. Note the transphyseal vessel, which connects the vascular supply of the epiphysis and metaphysis, facilitating spread of infection between these two areas. **(B)** Major structures of the bone of a child. Joint capsule *A* inserts below the epiphyseal growth plate, as in the hip, elbow, ankle, and shoulder. Rupture of a metaphyseal abscess in these bones is likely to produce pyarthrosis. Joint capsule *B* inserts at the epiphyseal growth plate, as in other tubular bones. Rupture of a metaphyseal abscess in these bones is likely to lead to a subperiosteal abscess but seldom to an associated pyarthrosis. (From Gutman LT. Acute, subacute, and chronic osteomyelitis and pyogenic arthritis in children. *Curr Probl Pediatr.* 1985;15:1–72.)

the clavicle, scapula, or small bones of the hands or feet—are often affected. Pathogens are not identified on culture and histopathology demonstrates plasmacytic infiltrates.

EPIDEMIOLOGY

Osteomyelitis may occur at any age but is most common in children 3-12 years of age; it affects boys twice as frequently as girls. Osteomyelitis from penetrating trauma or peripheral vascular disease is more common in adults.

CLINICAL MANIFESTATIONS

Decision-Making Algorithms
Available @ StudentConsult.com

Limp
Knee Pain
Extremity Pain
Stiff or Painful Neck
Fever Without a Source
Fever of Unknown Origin

The most common presenting complaints are focal pain, exquisite point tenderness over the bone, warmth, erythema, and swelling. Fever, anorexia, irritability, and lethargy may accompany the focal findings. Weight bearing and active and passive motion of the affected extremity are decreased, mimicking paralysis **(pseudoparalysis).** Muscle spasm may make the extremity difficult to examine. The adjacent joint space may be involved in young children, suggested by pain with minimal joint range of motion (see Chapter 118).

Usually only one bone is involved. The femur, tibia, or humerus is affected in approximately two thirds of patients. Approximately 15% of cases involve the bones of the hands or feet, and 10% involve the pelvis. Vertebral osteomyelitis is notable for an insidious onset, vague symptoms, backache, occasional spinal cord compression, and usually little associated fever or systemic toxicity. Patients with osteomyelitis of the pelvis may present with fever, limp, and vague abdominal, hip, groin, or thigh pain. **Pyomyositis** of pelvic muscles may mimic osteomyelitis.

LABORATORY AND IMAGING STUDIES

The presence of leukocytosis is inconsistent. Blood cultures are important but are negative in many cases. Elevated acute-phase reactants, erythrocyte sedimentation rate (ESR), and C-reactive protein (CRP) are sensitive but nonspecific findings. Serial determinations of ESR and CRP are helpful in monitoring the course of the illness and response to treatment. Direct subperiosteal or metaphyseal needle aspiration can definitively establish the diagnosis. Identification of bacteria in aspirated material by Gram stain can establish the diagnosis within hours of clinical presentation.

Plain radiographs can demonstrate soft tissue swelling such as the **loss of the periosteal fat line** within the first 3 days of symptoms, but bony lesions such as **periosteal elevation** and **bone destruction** are absent until after 10-14 days of symptoms. **Brodie abscess** is a subacute intraosseous abscess that does not drain into the subperiosteal space and is classically located in the distal tibia. **Sequestra,** portions of avascular bone that have separated from adjacent bone, frequently are covered with a thickened sheath, or **involucrum,** both of which are hallmarks of chronic osteomyelitis.

Radionuclide scanning for osteomyelitis has largely been supplanted by magnetic resonance imaging, which is sensitive to the inflammatory marrow changes even during the earliest

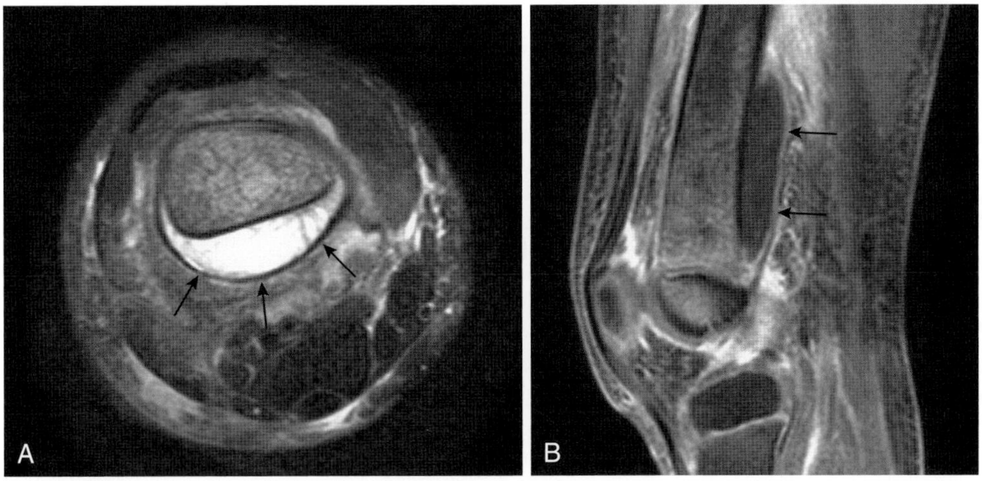

FIGURE 117.2 Acute osteomyelitis of the distal femur in a 5-year-old boy. **(A)** T2-weighted fat-saturated axial magnetic resonance imaging (MRI) shows a large subperiosteal abscess *(arrows)* at the posterior femur. Increased signal is seen within the bone, along with adjacent soft-tissue edema. **(B)** T1-weighted fat-saturated postgadolinium sagittal MRI demonstrates the longitudinal extent of the same subperiosteal abscess and its enhancing wall *(arrows)*. (From Kan JH, Azouz EM. Musculoskeletal infections. In: Coley BD, ed. *Caffey's Pediatric Diagnostic Imaging*. 12th ed. Philadelphia: Saunders; 2013. Fig. 138.13.)

stages of osteomyelitis (Fig. 117.2). Technetium-99m bone scans are useful for identifying multifocal disease.

DIFFERENTIAL DIAGNOSIS

Osteomyelitis must be differentiated from infectious arthritis (see Chapter 118), cellulitis, pyomyositis, fasciitis, diskitis, trauma, juvenile idiopathic arthritis, bone cysts, histiocytosis, and malignancy.

TREATMENT

Decision-Making Algorithm
Available @ StudentConsult.com

Fever Without a Source

Initial antibiotic therapy for osteomyelitis is based on the likely organism for the age of the child, Gram stain of bone aspirate, and associated diseases (Table 117.1). Initial therapy includes an antibiotic that targets *S. aureus* and *Kingella*, such as cefazolin or nafcillin. Clindamycin or vancomycin should be used if methicillin-resistant *S. aureus* is suspected based on patient factors or local *S. aureus* epidemiology. For patients with sickle cell disease, initial therapy should include an antibiotic with activity against *Salmonella* and *S. pneumoniae.*

Response to intravenous (IV) antibiotics usually occurs within 48 hours. Lack of improvement after 48 hours indicates that surgical drainage may be necessary or that an unusual pathogen may be present. Surgical drainage may be indicated for presence of extensive, severe, chronic, or atypical disease; presence of abscess; hip joint involvement; or **sequestrum** or spinal cord compression. Antibiotics are administered for a minimum of 4-6 weeks. After initial inpatient treatment and adequate clinical response, including decreases in CRP or ESR, transition to home therapy with oral or IV antibiotics may be considered if adherence is ensured. Home IV antibiotics are associated with increased adverse event rates and need for unscheduled medical visits.

TABLE 117.1 Recommended Antibiotic Therapy for Osteomyelitis in Children

COMMON PATHOGEN	RECOMMENDED TREATMENT*
ACUTE HEMATOGENOUS OSTEOMYELITIS	
Staphylococcus aureus	
Methicillin-sensitive	Nafcillin (or oxacillin) or cefazolin
Methicillin-resistant	Clindamycin or vancomycin or linezolid
Streptococcus pyogenes (group A streptococci)	Ampicillin/amoxicillin
Streptococcus pneumoniae	Ampicillin/amoxicillin or ceftriaxone/cefotaxime or vancomycin
SUBACUTE FOCAL OSTEOMYELITIS	
Pseudomonas aeruginosa	Ceftazidime or piperacillin-tazobactam or ciprofloxacin
Kingella kingae	Ampicillin/amoxicillin or cefotaxime

**Optimal specific therapy is based on susceptibilities of the organism that is isolated.*

COMPLICATIONS AND PROGNOSIS

Complications of acute osteomyelitis are uncommon and usually arise because of inadequate or delayed therapy or concomitant bacteremia. Vascular insufficiency, which affects delivery of antibiotics, and trauma are associated with higher rates of complications.

Hematogenous osteomyelitis has an excellent prognosis if treated promptly and if surgical drainage is performed when appropriate. The poorest outcomes are in neonates and in infants with involvement of the hip or shoulder joints (see Chapter 118). Approximately 2-4% of acute infections recur despite adequate therapy, and approximately 25% of these fail to respond to extensive surgical debridement and prolonged antimicrobial therapy, ultimately resulting in bone loss, sinus tract formation, or amputation (although rare). Sequelae related to skeletal growth disturbance are most common with neonatal osteomyelitis.

PREVENTION

There are no effective means of preventing hematogenous *S. aureus* osteomyelitis. Universal immunization of infants with conjugate *H. influenzae* type b vaccine has practically eliminated serious bacterial infections from this organism, including bone and joint infections.

Children with puncture wounds to the foot should receive prompt irrigation, cleansing, debridement, removal of any visible foreign body or debris, and tetanus prophylaxis. The value of oral prophylactic antibiotics for preventing osteomyelitis after penetrating injury is uncertain.

CHAPTER **118**

Infectious Arthritis

ETIOLOGY

Infectious arthritis **(suppurative** or **septic arthritis)** is a serious bacterial infection of the joint space resulting from hematogenous bacterial dissemination. Infectious arthritis less often results from contiguous spread of infection from surrounding soft tissues or direct inoculation into the joint (penetrating trauma). Spread of osteomyelitis into the joint space is more common in children under 18 months of age and occurs via organisms passing through transphyseal vessels to the epiphysis (see Fig. 117.1A). The bacteria causing infectious arthritis are similar to those causing osteomyelitis (Table 118.1). Lyme disease may also cause arthritis (see Chapter 122).

The arthritis of **disseminated gonococcal infections** includes both reactive and suppurative forms in early and late gonococcal disease, respectively. With untreated genital infection, gonococcemia may occur with fever and a polyarticular, symmetric arthritis and rash, known as the **arthritis-dermatitis syndrome**. Bacterial cultures of the synovium are sterile at this stage, despite a relatively high prevalence of bacteremia. Monarticular arthritis of large, weight-bearing joints develops days to weeks later. Cultures of affected synovial fluid at this stage often yield the pathogen.

Reactive arthritis is immune-mediated synovial inflammation that follows a bacterial or viral infection, especially with *Chlamydia trachomatis*, *Yersinia*, and other enteric infections. Reactive arthritis of the hip joints in children 3-6 years of age is known as **toxic** or **transient synovitis** (see Chapter 200).

EPIDEMIOLOGY

Infectious arthritis occurs most commonly in children younger than 5 years of age and adolescents.

TABLE 118.1 Pathogenic Organisms Causing Arthritis in Children

COMMON	UNCOMMON
YOUNG INFANT (<2 MO)	
Group B streptococci	*Neisseria gonorrhoeae*
Staphylococcus aureus	*Candida*
Escherichia coli	
Klebsiella pneumoniae	
OLDER INFANTS AND CHILDREN (2 MO TO MATURITY)	
S. aureus	Anaerobic bacteria
Streptococcus pneumoniae	*Pseudomonas aeruginosa*
Group A streptococci	*Enterobacteriaceae*
Kingella kingae	*Haemophilus influenzae type b**
N. gonorrhoeae	*Mycobacterium tuberculosis*
Borrelia burgdorferi (Lyme disease)	
REACTIVE ARTHRITIS	
Yersinia enterocolitica	
Campylobacter jejuni	
Shigella flexneri	
Chlamydia trachomatis	
Salmonella	
Group A streptococci	
Neisseria meningitidis	
Coccidioides immitis	
Rubella virus	

**The incidence of invasive infections caused by* Haemophilus influenzae type b *has diminished greatly with universal childhood Hib vaccination.*

CLINICAL MANIFESTATIONS

Decision-Making Algorithms
Available @ StudentConsult.com

Limp
Arthritis
Knee Pain
Extremity Pain

The typical features of suppurative arthritis include monarticular involvement with erythema, warmth, swelling, and tenderness over the affected joint with a palpable effusion and markedly decreased range of movement secondary to pain. The onset may be sudden or insidious with symptoms noted when the joint is moved only, such as during a diaper change, or if parents become aware of decreased voluntary movement of a joint or limb. Toddlers may exhibit a limp or refuse to walk. In septic arthritis of the hip, the lower limb may be preferentially held in external rotation and flexion to minimize pain from pressure on the joint capsule. Similarly, the knee and elbow joints are usually held in flexion. The joints of the lower extremity are most often involved: knees (40%), hips (20%), and ankles (14%).

Small joints, such as those of the hand, are usually involved after penetrating trauma or closed fist injuries.

Minor genital tract symptoms that have been ignored may precede development of the early arthritis–dermatitis syndrome associated with disseminated gonococcal infection. A history of febrile illness antedating the development of monarticular arthritis characterizes late gonococcal arthritis.

Reactive arthritis is typically symmetric and polyarticular, and it usually involves the large joints, especially the hips. Patients may have had a preceding episode of gastroenteritis or urethritis. Urethritis may appear with the arthritis.

LABORATORY AND IMAGING STUDIES

Leukocytosis and an elevated erythrocyte sedimentation rate (ESR) and C-reactive protein (CRP) are common. Arthrocentesis is important to distinguish among the causes of arthritis (Table 118.2). Adolescents with acute infectious arthritis should have urethral, cervical, rectal, and pharyngeal examinations and cultures or nucleic acid amplification tests performed for *Neisseria gonorrhoeae.*

Blood or joint cultures are positive in approximately 50% of cases. Joint fluid that exhibits the characteristics of pyogenic infection may not reveal bacterial pathogens, even in the absence of preceding antibiotic therapy, because of the bacteriostatic effects of synovial fluid. Gram stain should be performed and is often informative even if the cultures are negative. PCR testing for *Kingella* is essential in all culture-negative samples.

Ultrasound is especially useful for identifying joint effusions and is the initial diagnostic procedure of choice for evaluating suppurative infections of the hip. Plain radiographs typically add little information to the physical findings. Radiographs may show joint capsule swelling, a widened joint space, and displacement of adjacent normal fat lines. Radionuclide scans are of limited use, although magnetic resonance imaging may be helpful to exclude concurrent bone infection or deep abscesses.

DIFFERENTIAL DIAGNOSIS

The differential diagnosis of infectious arthritis in infants, children, and adolescents includes other infectious diseases, autoimmune disorders, rheumatic fever, malignancy, and trauma.

Suppurative arthritis must be distinguished from Lyme disease, osteomyelitis, suppurative bursitis, fasciitis, myositis, cellulitis, and soft tissue abscesses. Psoas muscle abscess often presents with fever and pain on hip flexion and rotation. Juvenile idiopathic arthritis, Kawasaki syndrome, Henoch–Schönlein purpura, other rheumatic disorders, and Crohn disease must be differentiated from infectious arthritis. In most of these diseases, the presence of symmetric or multiple joint involvement often excludes infectious arthritis. **Suppurative bursitis** with *Staphylococcus aureus* occurs most often in older boys and men and is usually a consequence of trauma or, less commonly, a complication of bacteremia.

TREATMENT

Initial antibiotic therapy for infectious arthritis is based on the likely organism for the age of the child and the Gram stain of joint fluid. Suppurative arthritis of the hip joint, especially, or shoulder joint necessitates prompt surgical drainage. With insertion of the joint capsule below the epiphysis in these

TABLE 118.2 Synovial Fluid Findings in Various Joint Diseases

CONDITION	APPEARANCE	WBC COUNT (mm^3/L)	PMNs (%)	MUCIN CLOT	SYNOVIAL FLUID–BLOOD GLUCOSE DIFFERENCE (mg/dL)	COMMENTS
Normal	Clear, yellow	0-200 (200)*	<10	Good	No difference	—
Trauma	Clear, turbid, or hemorrhagic	50-4,000 (600)	<30	Good	No difference	Common in hemophilia
Systemic lupus erythematosus	Clear or slightly turbid	0-9,000 (3,000)	<20	Good to fair	No difference	LE cell positive, complement decreased
Juvenile idiopathic arthritis, reactive arthritis, inflammatory bowel disease	Turbid	250-80,000 (19,000)	>70	Poor	30	Decreased complement
Infectious pyogenic infection	Turbid	10,000-250,000 (80,000)	>90	Poor	50-90	Positive culture result, positive Gram stain
Tuberculosis	Turbid	2,500-100,000 (20,000)	>60	Poor	40-70	Positive results on culture, PPD or interferon-gamma release assay testing, and acid-fast stain
Lyme arthritis	Turbid	500-100,000 (20,000)	>60	Poor	70	History of tick bite or erythema migrans and appropriate travel risk factors

*Average in parentheses.
LE, Lupus erythematosus; *PMN*, polymorphonuclear cell; *PPD*, purified protein derivative; *WBC*, white blood cell.

TABLE 118.3 Recommended Antibiotic Therapy for Infectious Arthritis in Children

AGE GROUP	COMMON PATHOGENS	RECOMMENDED TREATMENT*
Infants (younger than 2 mo of age)	Group B streptococci	Ampicillin *plus* aminoglycoside
	Escherichia coli	Cefotaxime *with or without* aminoglycoside
	Klebsiella pneumoniae	Cefotaxime *with or without* aminoglycoside
	Staphylococcus aureus	Nafcillin (*or* oxacillin *or* cefazolin), *or* clindamycin *or* vancomycin
Older infants and children	*S. aureus*	Nafcillin (*or* oxacillin *or* cefazolin), *or* clindamycin *or* vancomycin
	Streptococcus pneumoniae	Ampicillin *or* cefotaxime (*or* ceftriaxone) *or* vancomycin
	Group A streptococci	Penicillin G
	Kingella kingae	Amoxacillin, ampicillin, or cefotaxime
	Haemophilus influenzae type b[†]	Ampicillin *or* cefotaxime *or* ceftriaxone
	Neisseria gonorrhoeae: disseminated gonococcal infection	Ceftriaxone

**Use the narrowest-spectrum agent available based on organism's susceptibilities.*
[†]The incidence of invasive infections caused by Haemophilus influenzae *type b has diminished greatly with universal childhood* Haemophilus influenzae *type b vaccination.*

ball-and-socket joints, increased pressure in the joint space can adversely affect the vascular supply to the head of the femur or humerus, leading to avascular necrosis. Infections of the knee may be treated with repeated arthrocenteses in addition to appropriate parenteral antibiotics.

Several antimicrobial agents provide adequate antibiotic levels in joint spaces (Table 118.3). Initial therapy for neonates should include antibiotics such as nafcillin and cefotaxime with activity against *S. aureus*, group B streptococcus, and aerobic gram-negative rods. Initial therapy for children 3 months to 5 years old should include antibiotics with activity against *S. aureus.* Addition of appropriate antibiotics should be considered if the child is unimmunized against *Haemophilus influenzae* type b (Hib). Confirmed methicillin-susceptible *S. aureus* infections are best treated with nafcillin, oxacillin, or cefazolin initially; methicillin-resistant *S. aureus* infections are best treated with clindamycin if susceptible or vancomycin otherwise.

The duration of therapy depends on clinical resolution of fever and pain and decline of the ESR and CRP. Infection with virulent organisms, such as *S. aureus,* usually necessitates treatment for at least 21 days, although shorter courses of 10-14 days have been used in some circumstances. Treatment may be transitioned to oral antibiotics if adherence can be ensured. Oral agents with excellent activity against *S. aureus* that are often used to complete therapy include cephalexin, clindamycin, amoxicillin-clavulanate, dicloxacillin, and ciprofloxacin, though due to concerns about ciprofloxacin's side effects it should not be first-line.

COMPLICATIONS AND PROGNOSIS

The prognosis for the common forms of infectious arthritis encountered in infants and children is excellent. The major complications of neonatal, childhood, and gonococcal arthritis are loss of joint function resulting from damage to the articular surface. The highest incidence of these complications occurs with hip and shoulder infections, presumably resulting from avascular necrosis. The high incidence of concurrent suppurative arthritis with adjacent osteomyelitis in neonates places the epiphyseal growth plate at high risk for growth abnormalities. Neonates with osteomyelitis have an approximately 40-50% likelihood of growth disturbances with loss of longitudinal bone growth and ultimate limb shortening.

PREVENTION

There are no effective means of preventing hematogenous *S. aureus* arthritis. Universal immunization of infants with conjugate Hib vaccine has practically eliminated serious bacterial infections from this organism, including bone and joint infections.

CHAPTER 119

Ocular Infections

ETIOLOGY

Acute conjunctivitis is usually a viral or bacterial infection of the eye characterized by a rapid onset of symptoms that persist for a few days. Nontypable *Haemophilus influenzae, Streptococcus pneumoniae*, and *Moraxella catarrhalis* account for approximately two thirds of bacterial causes (Table 119.1). Other causes include *Neisseria gonorrhoeae* and *Pseudomonas aeruginosa*; the latter is associated with extended-wear soft contact lenses. *Bartonella henselae* can cause a granulomatous conjunctivitis associated with preauricular lymphadenopathy or **Parinaud oculoglandular syndrome**. Viral conjunctivitis most commonly is caused by adenoviruses, which cause **epidemic keratoconjunctivitis**, and less frequently by coxsackieviruses and other enteroviruses. **Keratitis**, or inflammation of the cornea, is not commonly associated with conjunctivitis but occurs with *N. gonorrhoeae,* herpes simplex virus (HSV), and adenovirus infections.

Neonatal conjunctivitis, or **ophthalmia neonatorum**, is purulent conjunctivitis during the first month of life, usually acquired during birth. The common causes of neonatal conjunctivitis, in order of decreasing prevalence, are chemical conjunctivitis secondary to silver nitrate gonococcal prophylaxis, *Chlamydia trachomatis*, common bacterial causes of conjunctivitis, *Escherichia coli*, other gram-negative enteric bacilli, HSV, and *N. gonorrhoeae*.

TABLE 119.1 Manifestations of Acute Conjunctivitis in Children

	CLINICAL CHARACTERISTICS	
FEATURE	**BACTERIAL**	**VIRAL**
Common pathogens	*Haemophilus influenzae* (usually nontypable)	Adenoviruses types 8, 19
	Streptococcus pneumoniae	Enteroviruses
	Moraxella catarrhalis	Herpes simplex virus
Incubation	24-72 hr	1-14 days
SYMPTOMS		
Photophobia	Mild	Moderate to severe
Blurred vision	Common with discharge	If keratitis is present
Foreign body sensation	Unusual	Yes
SIGNS		
Discharge	Purulent discharge	Mucoid/serous discharge
Palpebral reaction	Papillary response	Follicular response
Preauricular lymph node	Unusual for acute (<10%)	More common (20%)
Chemosis	Moderate	Mild
Hemorrhagic conjunctivae	Occasionally with pneumococcus or *Haemophilus* species	Frequent with enteroviruses
Treatment (topical)	Polymyxin B-trimethoprim *or* sulfacetamide 5% *or* erythromycin	Adenovirus: self-limited Herpes simplex virus: trifluridine 1% solution *or* ganciclovir 0.15% gel *or* acyclovir; ophthalmologic consultation
End of contagious period	24 hr after start of effective treatment	7 days after onset of symptoms

EPIDEMIOLOGY

Conjunctivitis is common in young children, especially if they come in contact with other children with conjunctivitis. Predisposing factors for bacterial infection include nasolacrimal duct obstruction, sinus disease, ear infection, and allergic disease when children rub their eyes frequently. Conjunctivitis occurs in 1-12% of neonates. Approximately 50% of infants born vaginally to infected mothers have neonatal acquisition of *C. trachomatis*, with which the risk of chlamydial conjunctivitis **(inclusion conjunctivitis)** is 25-50%.

CLINICAL MANIFESTATIONS

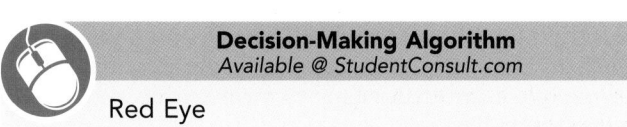

Decision-Making Algorithm
Available @ StudentConsult.com

Red Eye

Symptoms of ocular infection include redness, discharge, matted eyelids, and mild photophobia. Physical examination findings include chemosis, injection of the conjunctiva, and edema of the eyelids. Corneal involvement suggests gonococcal or herpetic infection. Herpetic corneal lesions appear as dendritic or ameboid ulcers or, more commonly, in recurrent infection, as a deep keratitis. Unilateral conjunctivitis with ipsilateral otitis media is often caused by nontypable *H. influenzae*.

The timing and manifestations of neonatal conjunctivitis are helpful in identifying the cause (Table 119.2). *N. gonorrhoeae* causes severe conjunctivitis with profuse purulent discharge. Chlamydial conjunctivitis usually occurs in the second week of life but may appear 3 days to 6 weeks after delivery. There is mild to moderate inflammation with purulent discharge issuing from one or both eyes.

LABORATORY AND IMAGING STUDIES

Cultures are not routinely obtained because bacterial conjunctivitis is usually self-limited or responds quickly to topical antibiotic treatment. If gonococcal conjunctivitis is suspected, especially in neonates, Gram stain and culture must be obtained. In these infants, blood and other sites of infection (such as cerebrospinal fluid) should also be cultured. Additional testing for *Chlamydia*, human immunodeficiency virus (HIV), and syphilis should be performed on the mother and infant as necessary.

DIFFERENTIAL DIAGNOSIS

Distinguishing bacterial from viral conjunctivitis by presentation and appearance is difficult (see Table 119.1). Vesicular lid lesions, if present, suggest HSV. **Hyperpurulent conjunctivitis** characterized by reaccumulation of purulent discharge within minutes is characteristic of *N. gonorrhoeae* infection. The differential diagnosis is delineated in Table 119.3.

Blepharitis is associated with staphylococcal infections, seborrhea, and meibomian gland dysfunction. The child complains of photophobia, burning, irritation, and a foreign body sensation that causes the child to rub the eyes. Eyelid hygiene with an **eyelid scrub** routine is the initial step in treatment.

Hordeola are acute suppurative nodular inflammatory lesions of the eyelids associated with pain and redness. **External hordeola** or **styes** occur on the anterior eyelid, in the Zeis glands, or in the lash follicles and usually are caused by staphylococci. **Internal hordeola** occur in the meibomian glands and may be infected with staphylococci or may be sterile. If the meibomian gland becomes obstructed, the gland secretions accumulate, and a **chalazion** develops. Hordeola usually respond spontaneously to local treatment measures, but may recur.

Dacryocystitis is an infection or inflammation of the lacrimal sac, which is usually obstructed, and is most commonly caused by *Staphylococcus aureus* or coagulase-negative staphylococci. A mucopurulent discharge can be expressed with gentle pressure on the nasolacrimal sac. Treatment usually requires probing of the nasolacrimal system to establish communication.

Endophthalmitis is an emergent, sight-threatening infection that usually follows trauma, surgery, or hematogenous spread from a distant focus. Causative organisms include coagulase-negative staphylococci, *S. aureus*, *S. pneumoniae*, *Bacillus cereus*, and *Candida albicans*. Examination is difficult because of severe

TABLE 119.2 Clinical Manifestations and Treatment of Neonatal Conjunctivitis

ETIOLOGICAL AGENT	CASES (%)	DISCHARGE AND EXTERNAL EXAMINATION	TYPICAL AGE AT ONSET	DIAGNOSIS	ASSOCIATED MANIFESTATIONS	TREATMENT
Chemical: silver nitrate	Variable (1%), depending on use of silver nitrate	Watery discharge	1-3 days	No organisms on smear or culture	None	None
Chlamydia trachomatis (inclusion conjunctivitis)	2-40	Scant discharge; mild swelling; hyperemia; follicular response; late corneal staining	4-19 days	Test of discharge with a DIF test or PCR assay	May presage *C. trachomatis* pneumonia (at 3 wk-3 mo of age)	Erythromycin (oral)
Bacterial: *Staphylococcus, Streptococcus, Pseudomonas, E. coli*	30-50	Purulent moderate discharge; mild lid and conjunctival swelling; corneal involvement with risk for perforation	2-7 days	Gram stain; culture on blood agar		Topical therapy
Neisseria gonorrhoeae	<1	Copious, purulent discharge; swelling of lids and conjunctivae; corneal involvement common; risk for perforation and corneal scar	1-7 days	Gram stain (gram-negative intracellular diplococci); culture on chocolate agar. Culture other sites including blood and CSF	May be associated with severe disseminated gonococcal infection	Ceftriaxone Hospitalize patient
HSV	<1	Clear or serosanguineous discharge; lid swelling; keratitis with cloudy cornea; dendrite formation	3 days-3 wk	Viral culture; DIF test, PCR assay	May be associated with disseminated perinatal HSV infection	Acyclovir (intravenous)

CSF, Cerebrospinal fluid; *DIF*, direct immunofluorescence; *HSV*, herpes simplex virus; *PCR*, polymerase chain reaction.

blepharospasm and extreme photophobia. A **hypopyon** and haze in the anterior chamber may be visible on examination.

TREATMENT

The lids should be treated as needed with warm compresses to remove accumulated discharge. Acute bacterial conjunctivitis is frequently self-limited, but topical antibiotics hasten resolution. Antibiotics are instilled between the eyelids four times a day until the discharge and chemosis subside. Recommended treatment includes topical trimethoprim-polymyxin B solution, sulfacetamide 5% solution, or erythromycin ointment. Ciprofloxacin solution should be restricted to corneal infections and resistant gram-negative infections in hospitalized patients. Gonococcal conjunctivitis in adults is treated with a single intramuscular (IM) dose of ceftriaxone (1 g) plus azithromycin (1 g in a single dose, to treat possible concomitant chlamydial infection and cover for the possibility of antimicrobial resistance to ceftriaxone).

The treatment of **ophthalmia neonatorum** depends on the cause (see Table 119.2). Gonococcal ophthalmia neonatorum is treated with a single dose of ceftriaxone (25-50 mg/kg intravenous [IV] or IM; maximum dose 125 mg). These infants should be hospitalized. Antibiotic treatment also is recommended for infants born to mothers with untreated gonorrhea. Chlamydial conjunctivitis is treated with oral erythromycin for 14 days, partly to reduce the risk of subsequent chlamydial pneumonia.

COMPLICATIONS AND PROGNOSIS

The prognosis for bacterial and viral conjunctivitis is excellent. The major complication is keratitis, which can lead to ulcerations and perforation, and is uncommon except with *N. gonorrhoeae* and HSV infections. Chlamydial conjunctivitis may progress in infants to chlamydial pneumonia, which typically develops from 2-18 weeks of age (see Chapter 110).

PREVENTION

Careful hand washing is important to prevent spread of conjunctivitis. Bacterial conjunctivitis is considered contagious for 24 hours after initiating effective treatment. Children may return to school, but treatment measures must be continued until there is complete clinical resolution.

All newborns, whether delivered vaginally or by cesarean section, should receive prophylaxis for gonococcal ophthalmia neonatorum as soon as possible after delivery. A single application of erythromycin 0.5% ointment is used most often. Alternative methods include tetracycline 1% ointment and silver nitrate 1% solution. These are equally effective in preventing gonococcal ophthalmia, but silver nitrate usually causes a chemical conjunctivitis. Neither silver nitrate solution nor tetracycline ophthalmic ointment is manufactured in the United States currently. Erythromycin ointment does not prevent chlamydial ophthalmia.

TABLE 119.3 Differential Diagnosis of Ocular Infections

CONDITION	ETIOLOGICAL AGENTS	SIGNS AND SYMPTOMS	TREATMENT
Bacterial conjunctivitis	*Haemophilus influenzae, Haemophilus aegyptius, Streptococcus pneumoniae, Neisseria gonorrhoeae*	Mucopurulent unilateral or bilateral discharge, normal vision, photophobia, conjunctival injection and edema (chemosis); gritty sensation	Topical antibiotics, parenteral ceftriaxone for gonococcus
Viral conjunctivitis	Adenovirus, echovirus, coxsackievirus	Same as for bacterial infection; may be hemorrhagic, unilateral	Self-limited
Neonatal conjunctivitis	*Chlamydia trachomatis,* gonococcus, chemical (silver nitrate), *Staphylococcus aureus*	Palpebral conjunctival follicle or papillae; same as for bacterial infection	Ceftriaxone for gonococcus and oral erythromycin for *C. trachomatis*
Allergic conjunctivitis	Seasonal pollens or allergen exposure	Itching, incidence of bilateral chemosis (edema) greater than that of erythema, tarsal papillae	Antihistamines, steroids, cromolyn
Keratitis	Herpes simplex, adenovirus, *S. pneumoniae, S. aureus, Pseudomonas, Acanthamoeba,* chemicals	Severe pain, corneal swelling, clouding, limbus erythema, hypopyon, cataracts; contact lens history with amebic infection	Specific antibiotics for bacterial/ fungal infections; keratoplasty, acyclovir for herpes
Endophthalmitis	*S. aureus, S. pneumoniae, Candida albicans,* associated surgery or trauma	Acute onset, pain, loss of vision, swelling, chemosis, redness; hypopyon and vitreous haze	Specific antibiotics for bacterial/ fungal infections
Anterior uveitis (iridocyclitis)	JIA, reactive arthritis, sarcoidosis, Behçet disease, inflammatory bowel disease	Unilateral/bilateral; erythema, ciliary flush, irregular pupil, iris adhesions; pain, photophobia, small pupil, poor vision	Topical steroids, plus therapy for primary disease
Posterior uveitis (choroiditis)	Toxoplasmosis, histoplasmosis, *Toxocara canis*	No signs of erythema, decreased vision	Specific therapy for pathogen
Episcleritis/scleritis	Idiopathic autoimmune disease (e.g., SLE, Henoch-Schönlein purpura)	Localized pain, intense erythema, unilateral; blood vessels bigger than in conjunctivitis; scleritis may cause globe perforation	Episcleritis is self-limiting; topical steroids for fast relief
Foreign body	Occupational or other exposure	Unilateral, red, gritty feeling; visible or microscopic size	Irrigation, removal; check for ulceration
Blepharitis	*S. aureus, Staphylococcus epidermidis,* seborrheic, blocked lacrimal duct; rarely molluscum contagiosum, *Phthirus pubis, Pediculus capitis*	Bilateral, irritation, itching, hyperemia, crusting, affecting lid margins	Topical antibiotics, warm compresses
Dacryocystitis	Obstructed lacrimal sac: *S. aureus, H. influenzae, S. pneumoniae*	Pain, tenderness, erythema and exudate in areas of lacrimal sac (inferomedial to inner canthus); tearing (epiphora); possible orbital cellulitis	Systemic, topical antibiotics; surgical drainage
Dacryoadenitis	*S. aureus, S. pneumoniae,* CMV, measles, EBV, enteroviruses; trauma, sarcoidosis, leukemia	Pain, tenderness, edema, erythema over gland area (upper temporal lid); fever, leukocytosis	Systemic antibiotics; drainage of orbital abscesses
Orbital cellulitis (postseptal cellulitis)	Paranasal sinusitis: *H. influenzae, S. aureus, S. pneumoniae,* other streptococci Trauma: *S. aureus* Fungi: *Aspergillus, Mucor* if immunodeficient	Rhinorrhea, chemosis, vision loss, painful extraocular motion, proptosis, ophthalmoplegia, fever, lid edema, leukocytosis	Systemic antibiotics; drainage of orbital abscesses
Periorbital cellulitis (preseptal cellulitis)	Trauma: *S. aureus,* other streptococci Bacteremia: pneumococcus, streptococci, *H. influenzae*	Cutaneous erythema, warmth, normal vision, minimal involvement of orbit; fever, leukocytosis, toxic appearance	Systemic antibiotics

CMV, Cytomegalovirus; *EBV,* Epstein-Barr virus; *JIA,* juvenile idiopathic arthritis; *SLE,* systemic lupus erythematosus.

CHAPTER 120

Infection in the Immunocompromised Person

ETIOLOGY

Many diseases or their treatments adversely affect the immune system, including primary immunodeficiencies, human immunodeficiency virus (HIV) infection and acquired immunodeficiency syndrome (AIDS), cancer, stem cell and organ transplantation, and immunosuppressive drugs used to treat cancer, autoimmune diseases, and transplant patients. These patients are at significant risk of life-threatening infections from invasive bacterial or fungal flora of the oropharynx, skin, and gastrointestinal tract; acquisition of exogenous infection from infected persons or the environment; and reactivation of latent infections until their immune function recovers (Table 120.1).

The infections seen in immunocompromised persons can often be predicted by which component of the immune system is abnormal. Episodes of fever and **neutropenia**, defined as an **absolute neutrophil count (ANC)** of less than 500/mm^3, are especially common in cancer and transplant patients and increase risk for bacterial and fungal infections. The use of **corticosteroids** and potent immunosuppressive drugs that

TABLE 120.1 Immunodeficiencies and Associated Prevalent Pathogens

DEFECT	PATHOGEN
Granulocytopenia	GRAM-POSITIVE COCCI
	Staphylococcus aureus
	Coagulase-negative staphylococci (*S. epidermidis, S. haemolyticus, S. hominis*)
	Viridans group streptococci (*S. mitis, S. oralis*)
	Granulicatella and *Abiotrophia* spp. (formerly nutritionally variant streptococci)
	Enterococci (*E. faecalis, E. faecium*)
	GRAM-NEGATIVE BACILLI
	Escherichia coli
	Pseudomonas aeruginosa
	Klebsiella pneumoniae
	Enterobacter and Citrobacter spp.
Damaged integument	
Skin and central venous catheter related	Coagulase-negative staphylococci (*S. epidermidis, S. haemolyticus, S. hominis*)
	Staphylococcus aureus
	Stenotrophomonas maltophilia
	Pseudomonas aeruginosa
	Acinetobacter spp.
	Corynebacteria
	Candida spp. (*C. albicans, C. parapsilosis*)
	Rhizopus spp.
Oral mucositis	Viridans group streptococci (*S. mitis, S. oralis*)
	Abiotrophia and *Granulicatella* species (nutritionally variant streptococci)
	Capnocytophaga spp.
	Fusobacterium spp.
	Rothia mucilaginosa
	Candida spp. (*C. albicans, C. tropicalis, C. glabrata*)
	Herpes simplex virus
Gut mucosal barrier injury	*Escherichia coli*
	Pseudomonas aeruginosa
	Coagulase-negative staphylococci
	Enterococci (*E. faecalis, E. faecium*)
	Candida spp.
Neutropenic enterocolitis	*Clostridium* spp. (*C. septicum, C. tertium*)
	Staphylococcus aureus
	Pseudomonas aeruginosa
Impaired cellular immunity	Herpesviruses
	Cytomegalovirus
	Respiratory viruses
	Listeria monocytogenes
	Nocardia spp.
	Mycobacterium tuberculosis
	Nontuberculous mycobacteria
	Pneumocystis jirovecii
	Aspergillus spp.
	Cryptococcus spp.
	Histoplasma capsulatum
	Coccidioides spp.
	Penicillium marneffei
	Toxoplasma gondii
Impaired humoral immunity	*Streptococcus pneumoniae*
	Haemophilus influenzae
COMPROMISED ORGAN FUNCTION	
Splenectomy	*Streptococcus pneumoniae*
	Haemophilus influenzae
	Neisseria meningitidis
Deferoxamine for iron overload	*Rhizopus* spp.
	Yersinia enterocolitica

From JP Donnelly. Infections in the immunocompromised host: general principles. In: Mandell GL, Bennett JE, Dolin R, eds. Mandell, Douglas, and Bennett's Principles and Practice of Infectious Diseases. *7th ed. Philadelphia: Elsevier; 2010:3782.*

impair the activation of T lymphocytes increases the risk for pathogens normally controlled by T cell–mediated responses, such as *Pneumocystis jiroveci* and *Toxoplasma gondii*, as well as intracellular pathogens, such as *Salmonella*, *Listeria*, and *Mycobacterium*. Lymphopenia also increases the risk of viral infections, either due to primary acquisition or reactivation of latent infection.

Immunocompromised patients also have increased risk for bacterial infection due to the presence of central indwelling catheters. Organisms most commonly isolated in this case include coagulase-negative staphylococci, *S. aureus*, gram-negative bacteria, *Enterococcus*, and *Candida* (see Chapter 121).

Fungal pathogens account for approximately 10% of all infections associated with childhood cancer. *Candida* species are the most common cause of all fungal infections, with *Aspergillus* being the second most common pathogen. Other risk factors for fungal infections include oropharyngeal and gastrointestinal mucositis facilitating systemic fungal invasion, presence of long-term indwelling intravascular catheters, parenteral nutrition, hyperglycemia, extreme prematurity, and broad-spectrum antibacterial therapy that promotes fungal colonization as a precursor to infection.

Infection with *T. gondii* represents reactivation of quiescent infection facilitated by cancer-associated or therapy-associated cellular immunodeficiency. *P. jirovecii* primarily causes pneumonitis in patients with leukemia, lymphoma, HIV, or those on long-term corticosteroids and can occasionally cause extrapulmonary disease (sinusitis, otitis media).

Viral opportunistic infections in patients with cancer usually represent symptomatic reactivation from latency facilitated by cancer or therapy-associated cellular immunodeficiency. Herpes simplex virus (HSV) can cause severe and prolonged mucocutaneous infection or disseminated disease. Cytomegalovirus (CMV) can also cause focal or systemic disease in immunocompromised persons, especially in transplant patients. Manifestations of CMV disease include retinitis, hepatitis, pneumonitis, esophagitis, encephalitis, and colitis. Reactivation of Epstein-Barr virus (EBV) is associated with **posttransplant lymphoproliferative disorder (PTLD)**. Varicella-zoster virus (VZV) can cause serious primary infection in susceptible persons, sometimes with accompanying encephalitis, hepatitis, or pneumonitis. VZV can also reactivate as shingles during chemotherapy and may cause disseminated infection.

EPIDEMIOLOGY

Chemotherapeutic agents target rapidly dividing cells, especially myeloproliferative cells, which causes myelosuppression. Children receiving allogeneic transplants are at greater risk for infection than children receiving autologous transplants. Prolonged time to hematological engraftment is a significant risk factor for infection in these patients (Fig. 120.1). Foreign bodies (shunts, central venous catheters) and mucositis interfere with cutaneous barriers against infection and, together with neutropenia and/or lymphopenia, increase the risk of bacterial or fungal infections. Multiple antimicrobial exposures put these patients at risk for resistant bacterial, fungal, and viral infections.

The relative rate of some infection in patients with cancer is 10-15%. The most frequently infected sites, in descending order, are the respiratory tract (lung, sinuses), the bloodstream, surgical wounds, and the urinary tract.

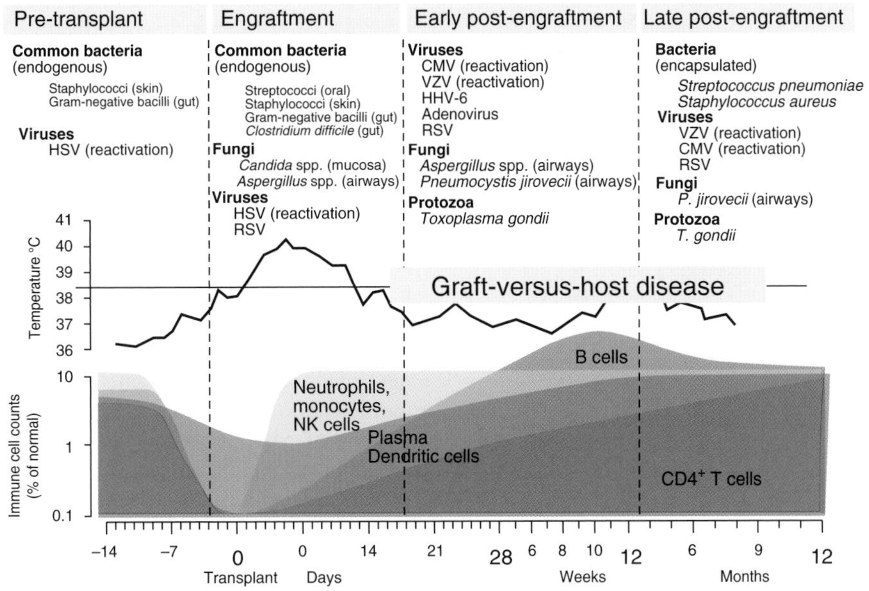

FIGURE 120.1 Infectious phases after transplant. The infectious complications that occur most commonly are set against the phases before and after an allogeneic hematopoietic stem cell transplant. Note the time scale progresses from days to weeks, then to months. The fluctuations in the different components of the immune system are represented at the bottom of the figure and show when severe deficiency coincides with the time of engraftment and begins to recover thereafter. The various classes of microorganism change during the different phases, but note that viruses and fungi can cause infections throughout the entire period. *CMV*, Cytomegalovirus; *HHV-6*, human herpesvirus 6; *HSV*, herpes simplex virus; *NK*, natural killer; *RSV*, respiratory syncytial virus; *VZV*, varicella-zoster virus. (From Donnelly JP, Blijlevens NMA, van der Velden WJFM. Infections in the immunocompromised host: general principles. In: Bennett JE, Dolin R, Blaser MJ, eds. *Mandell, Douglas, and Bennett's Principles and Practice of Infectious Diseases*. 8th ed. Philadelphia: Elsevier; 2015. Fig 309.6.)

CLINICAL MANIFESTATIONS

Decision-Making Algorithms
Available @ StudentConsult.com

Neutropenia
Pancytopenia
Fever Without a Source
Recurrent Infections

Fever is the most common, and sometimes the only, presenting symptom of serious infection in cancer and transplant patients. The presence of fever with neutropenia, even in the absence of other signs or symptoms, demands prompt evaluation and empiric antimicrobial therapy because of the potential for life-threatening infection. All symptoms and signs should be evaluated thoroughly. However, some symptoms may be absent based on the underlying immunodeficiency. In the absence of neutrophils to induce localized signs of inflammation, determination of the source of infection by physical examination is often difficult. For example, chest findings may be absent, despite pneumonia, and revealed only by chest radiograph at presentation or when the neutrophil count recovers.

LABORATORY TESTS AND IMAGING

Evaluation of fever and neutropenia in immunocompromised persons requires blood cultures for bacterial and fungal pathogens obtained by peripheral venipuncture and from all lumens of any indwelling vascular catheters (Table 120.2). A complete blood count with manual differential, C-reactive protein, complete chemistry panel, culture of urine, and Gram staining/culture of potential sites of specific infection found during history and physical should be performed. Chest radiographs are important to assess for the presence of pulmonary infiltrates. Specialized imaging studies, such as computed tomography (CT) or magnetic resonance imaging (MRI), can be useful in selected cases, such as with suspected sinusitis or intraabdominal infection, or to further delineate the location and extent of abnormalities seen on plain radiographs. Sinus infection with bacteria, *Aspergillus*, or Zygomycetes is common in neutropenic hosts and may be detected only on the CT scan. Viruses can be detected in blood, respiratory samples, cerebrospinal fluid, and skin lesions by polymerase chain reaction (PCR).

TABLE 120.2 Initial Diagnostic Evaluation of Children With Fever and Neutropenia

- Careful medical history
- Physical examination with attention to the skin, perirectal area, and other mucosal sites (which should be repeated at least daily in febrile neutropenic patients)
- Specimens for culture
    - Blood: peripheral venipuncture and specimens from every lumen or access port of intravascular catheters
    - Urine
    - Respiratory secretions: for bacteria and viruses if symptoms are present
    - Any site with clinical signs of infection, including Clostridium difficile toxin assay if diarrhea present and cerebral spinal fluid if headache, meningismus, or mental status change
- Chest radiograph
- Other imaging studies or diagnostic procedures as clinically indicated
    - Sinus radiograph or computed tomography
    - Abdominal ultrasonography or computed tomography
    - Head CT or MRI with contrast

Modified from Koh AY, Pizzo PA. Fever and Granulocytopenia. In: Long SS, ed. Principles and Practice of Pediatric Infectious Diseases. 4th ed. Philadelphia: Elsevier; 2012.

DIFFERENTIAL DIAGNOSIS

Initially the patient should have a complete physical examination, including careful scrutiny of the oropharynx, nares, external auditory canals, skin and axilla, groin, perineum, and rectal area. The exit site and subcutaneous tunnel of any indwelling vascular catheter should be examined closely for erythema and palpated for tenderness and expression of purulent material. Perirectal abscess is a potentially serious infection in neutropenic hosts, with tenderness being the only clue on examination. Any presumptive infection identified during the evaluation should direct appropriate cultures and tailor anti-infective therapy.

TREATMENT

Treatment should be provided as appropriate for focal infections identified by physical examination or diagnostic imaging. Select *low-risk* patients may be managed as outpatients. Empirical treatment of fever and neutropenia without an identified source should include an extended-spectrum penicillin or cephalosporin with activity against gram-negative bacilli, including *P. aeruginosa*. If the patient has an indwelling vascular catheter, vancomycin may be added because of the increasing prevalence of methicillin-resistant *S. aureus* (MRSA) but can be discontinued if *S. aureus* is not cultured after 48-72 hours. Specific antibiotic regimens should be guided by local antibiotic resistance patterns at each institution.

If no microbiologic cause is isolated, empirical broad-spectrum antibiotics are continued as long as the patient remains neutropenic, regardless of whether the fever resolves. Antibiotic therapy should be modified as indicated by new findings or if the patient's clinical status deteriorates. Further investigation for fungal infection and empirical treatment with antifungal agents is instituted in patients who have neutropenia and persistent fever without a focus, despite broad-spectrum antibacterial therapy for approximately 5 days.

PREVENTION

Current guidelines discourage the use of broad-spectrum prophylactic antibiotics to prevent fever and neutropenia because of lack of efficacy and concerns about development of antibiotic resistance. Administration of trimethoprim-sulfamethoxazole to prevent *P. jiroveci* infection is routine for patients undergoing intensive chemotherapy or immunosuppression for transplantation. Prophylaxis against *P. jiroveci* generally starts with initiation of chemotherapy and continued until 6 months after it has been completed. In select populations, such as patients undergoing hematopoietic stem cell transplantation, prophylactic antifungals such as fluconazole or voriconazole are beneficial. Patients at risk for viral reactivation with HSV, VZV, and/or CMV may be placed on antiviral prophylaxis with acyclovir or ganciclovir.

Immunocompromised susceptible persons exposed to chickenpox within 2 days before the onset of rash until 5 days after the onset of rash in the index case should receive varicella-zoster immune globulin (VZIG). Modified infection after VZIG may not result in protective immunity, and persons who receive VZIG prophylaxis should be considered still at risk with any subsequent exposures.

CHAPTER 121

Infections Associated With Medical Devices

Infections are a common and important complication of indwelling medical devices and are a major part of **health care–associated infections** (formerly known as **nosocomial infections**).

VASCULAR DEVICE INFECTIONS

Vascular catheters are inserted in most inpatients and used in many outpatients. The use of catheters for long-term access to the bloodstream has been an important advance for the care of persons who require parenteral nutrition, chemotherapy, or extended parenteral antibiotic therapy. The major complication of such catheters is infection. Short, peripheral intravenous (IV) catheters used for short-term access in stable patients are associated with a low rate of infection, especially in children. **Peripherally inserted central catheters (PICC)** are commonly used for medium-term venous access. **Central venous catheters** are commonly placed for extended vascular access, such as for chemotherapy, using tunneled silicone elastomer catheters (**Broviac** or **Hickman catheters**) that are surgically inserted into a central vein, passed through a subcutaneous tunnel before exiting the skin, and anchored by a subcutaneous cuff. Contamination of the catheter hub or any connection of the IV tubing is common and is a major predisposition to catheter-associated infection. Totally implanted venous access systems (Port-a-Cath, Infuse-a-Port) have a silicone elastomer catheter tunneled beneath the skin to a reservoir implanted in a subcutaneous pocket. Implanted catheters or ports decrease, but do not eliminate, the opportunity for microbial entry at the skin site.

Catheter-related thrombosis and catheter-related infection can develop separately or together. Ultrasound can identify thrombi, but infection can be identified by culture only. **Thrombophlebitis** is inflammation with thrombosis in a blood vessel. **Septic thrombophlebitis** is thrombosis with organisms embedded in the clot. **Central line associated bloodstream infection (CLABSI)** implies isolation of the same organism from a catheter and from peripheral blood of a patient with clinical symptoms of bacteremia and no other apparent source of infection. Confirmation requires quantitative colony counts of both samples, which is not routinely performed. Possible sources of the bacteremia include the infusate, contamination via tubing and catheter connections, or transient bacteremia seeding the catheter, which may or may not be clinically apparent. Infection may be associated with an **exit site infection** limited to the insertion site or may extend along the catheter tunnel of buried catheters to cause a **tunnel infection.** Given the proximity of central venous catheters to cardiac valves, persistent central infections can also be complicated by endocarditis. An echocardiogram should be considered in patients with persistent bacteremia related to a central line (see Chapter 111).

Many microorganisms cause catheter-related infections (Table 121.1). Gram-positive cocci, primarily staphylococci, cause more than 50% of CLABSIs and exit site infections. Other skin flora, such as coagulase-negative staphylococci, diphtheroids, and *Bacillus* are often involved. Gram-negative organisms also commonly cause infection. Polymicrobial infections of central venous catheters are common. Fungal catheter infections, usually *Candida* species, are most common among persons receiving broad-spectrum antibiotics or parenteral nutrition.

Risk factors for CLABSI include prematurity, burns and skin disorders that adversely affect the skin integrity, neutropenia, and other immunodeficiencies (see Chapter 120). Infection rates are lower for tunneled and implanted catheters. Catheters inserted in emergency settings are more likely to be infected than catheters placed electively.

Clinical signs of catheter-associated bacteremia or fungemia range from mild fever to overwhelming sepsis. Infection at the site of the central catheter entrance is manifested as a localized cellulitis with warmth, tenderness, swelling, erythema, and discharge. Tunnel infection is manifested by similar findings along the tunnel route. Thrombophlebitis is classically manifested as a warm, erythematous, tender palpable cord originating at the IV catheter site but may be subclinical or manifested only by persistent fever without signs of local inflammation.

Decision-Making Algorithm
Available @ StudentConsult.com
Fever and Rash

TABLE 121.1 Organisms Causing Catheter-Related Infections

CLASSIFICATION OF PATHOGEN	COMMON	UNCOMMON
Gram-positive organisms	Coagulase-negative staphylococci, *Staphylococcus aureus*, *Enterococcus*	Diphtheroids, *Bacillus*, Micrococcus
Gram-negative organisms	*Escherichia coli*, *Klebsiella*, *Pseudomonas aeruginosa*	*Acinetobacter*, *Enterobacter*, *Neisseria*
Fungi	*Candida* species	*Malassezia furfur*
Miscellaneous		Nontuberculous mycobacteria, *Lactobacillus*

The treatment of catheter-related infection depends on the site of the infection and the pathogen involved. CLABSI is optimally treated with catheter removal; however, in a stable patient or with certain organisms, antibiotic therapy alone may suffice. Infection with organisms of low virulence may be manifested by fever alone, and removal of the catheter frequently is followed by prompt defervescence and complete resolution of infection. Nonetheless many patients are dependent on the catheter and removal may be difficult. Empirical initial therapy for suspected infection should include antibiotics active against gram-negative organisms such as a broad-spectrum cephalosporin and against *S. aureus* and coagulase-negative staphylococci with vancomycin. Subsequently, antibiotic regimens should be tailored to the specific organism identified. If the patient is not critically ill and the pathogen is likely to be susceptible to antibiotic therapy, a trial of antibiotics is given through the infected catheter. The total duration of therapy depends on the pathogen and the duration of positive cultures and is usually 10-14 days after sterilization of the bloodstream. Catheter removal is indicated with sepsis, septic thrombophlebitis, clinical deterioration (despite appropriate therapy), persistently positive blood culture results after 48-72 hours of appropriate antimicrobial therapy, embolic lesions, or fungal infection because of poor response to antifungal therapy alone. Catheter removal is also recommended for infection with *Staphylococcus aureus* and *Pseudomonas aeruginosa*. Infection of the pocket around an implanted port is unlikely to respond to antibiotics alone, and removal of the foreign body is usually necessary.

Antibiotic-lock therapy is a method of sterilizing intravascular catheters by using high concentrations of antibiotics or ethanol infused into the portion of the catheter between the hub and the vessel entry. The solution is allowed to dwell within the catheter segment for several hours. It may be useful for treatment of catheter-associated infections in which line salvage is desired and/or for prevention of infection in patients at high risk.

Aseptic technique is essential during catheter insertion. Catheters that are placed during emergency situations should be replaced as soon as medically feasible. Care of indwelling catheters involves meticulous attention to sterile technique whenever the system is entered. Care of the catheter entry site commonly involves a topical antibiotic or disinfectant. Catheters that are no longer necessary should be removed.

VENTILATOR-ASSOCIATED PNEUMONIA

Intubation of the airway provides direct access to the lungs and bypasses normal host defenses. Organisms enter the lungs directly through the lumen of the tube or by descending around the tube, which may result in **ventilator-associated pneumonia**. Contaminated respiratory equipment, humidification systems, or condensate introduces bacteria directly into lower airways. The continuously open upper airway increases the risk of aspiration of oropharyngeal flora and reflux of gastric contents and interferes with clearance of the airway because an effective cough requires a closed glottis.

URINARY CATHETERS

The most important risk factors for urinary tract infections (UTIs) are the presence of catheters, instrumentation, and anatomical abnormalities (see Chapter 114). Organisms enter the bladder through the catheter by instillation of contaminated irrigation fluids, backflow of contaminated urine from the drainage bag, or ascent of bacteria around the meatus along the outside of the catheter. Indwelling catheters facilitate direct access to the bladder and should have a closed drainage system. After simple, straight catheterization, the incidence of UTI is 1-2%. Organisms that cause catheter-associated UTIs include fecal flora, such as gram-negative enteric bacilli, most commonly *Escherichia coli* and *Enterococcus*. With concomitant antibiotic treatment, resistant organisms predominate, and fungi may emerge as pathogens.

The most important aspect of prevention is to minimize the duration and use of catheterization. Intermittent catheterization is preferred over indwelling catheter drainage whenever feasible. Insertion of catheters must be performed with aseptic technique, and the drainage system must remain closed at all times, with sterile technique used whenever the system is entered. Drainage bags always should be dependent to avoid backflow of urine into the bladder.

PERITONEAL DIALYSIS–ASSOCIATED INFECTIONS

Indwelling catheters used for peritoneal dialysis may develop exit site infections, tunnel infections, or lead to peritonitis. The usual route of infection is from the skin surface along the tunnel and into the peritoneum. The most common pathogens are skin flora, including *Staphylococcus* species; organisms that contaminate water, such as *Pseudomonas* and *Acinetobacter*; enteric flora, such as *E. coli* and *Klebsiella*; and fungi, such as *C. albicans*. Peritonitis may present with fever, vague abdominal pain, and cloudy dialysate. The diagnosis is established on clinical manifestations and confirmed by culture of the dialysate. Prevention of infection requires careful planning of the location of the exit site to minimize contamination, aseptic insertion of the catheter, meticulous care of the catheter site, securing of the catheter to avoid tension and motion, and aseptic technique during dialysis.

CENTRAL NERVOUS SYSTEM SHUNTS

Important risk factors of health care–associated central nervous system (CNS) infections are surgery, presence of a ventriculoperitoneal shunt (VPS), and cerebrospinal fluid (CSF) leaks. Infection of a VPS results from contamination of the system at the time of placement, breakdown of overlying skin, or from hematogenous seeding. Externalized ventricular drains and subdural bolts allow direct access of skin flora to the CSF. For these devices, the rates of infection increase with the duration of catheterization, especially beyond 5 days. Device-related CNS infections can be diagnosed in the same way as other types of meningitis or ventriculitis with assessment of the CSF for pleocytosis, protein, glucose, and gram stain and culture.

The most common pathogens causing shunt infections are coagulase-negative staphylococci and *S. aureus*. After skull fracture or cranial surgery, a CSF leak may facilitate ascending infection from the nasopharynx, especially with *Streptococcus pneumoniae*, which frequently colonizes the nasopharynx. Patients with shunt infections may present with only fever and headache or may present with typical signs and symptoms of meningitis (see Chapter 100). Infections caused by coagulase-negative staphylococci or *Propionibacterium acnes* typically present with insidious onset of fever, malaise, headache, and vomiting. Empirical therapy is with vancomycin, with additional antibiotics if gram-negative bacteria are suspected.

Antibiotics frequently are used perioperatively during placement of shunts and other neurosurgical procedures. It is not clear that antibiotics decrease infection rates in these clean procedures, especially beyond one dose. External ventricular drains should be maintained as closed systems with aseptic technique and removed as soon as possible. Drainage bags always should be dependent to avoid backflow.

CHAPTER 122

Zoonoses and Vector Borne Infections

Zoonoses are classically defined as infections that are transmitted in nature between vertebrate animals and humans. Many zoonotic pathogens are maintained in nature by means of an **enzootic cycle**, in which mammalian hosts and arthropod vectors reinfect each other. Humans frequently are only incidentally infected. Of the more than 150 different human zoonotic diseases that have been described (Table 122.1), Lyme disease *(Borrelia burgdorferi)* is the most common tick-borne infection in the United States. Other common pathogens include *Rickettsia rickettsii* (Rocky Mountain spotted fever [RMSF]), ehrlichiosis *(Ehrlichia chaffeensis)*, West Nile virus, and anaplasmosis *(Anaplasma phagocytophilum)*. The epidemiology of zoonoses is related to the geographic distribution of the hosts and, if vector-borne, the distribution and seasonal life cycle of the vector.

Many zoonoses are spread by ticks, including Lyme disease, RMSF, ehrlichiosis, tularemia, tick typhus, and babesiosis. Preventive measures to avoid tick-borne diseases include using insect repellents that contain **DEET** (*N,N*-diethyl-*m*-toluamide) on skin and insect repellents that contain **permethrin** on clothing; avoiding tick-infested habitats (thick scrub oak, briar, poison ivy sites); avoiding excretory products of wild animals; wearing appropriate protective clothing (closed-toe shoes, long pants); and promptly removing ticks.

Ticks are best removed using blunt forceps or tweezers to grasp the tick as close to the skin as possible to pull the tick steadily outward. Squeezing, twisting, or crushing the tick should be avoided because the tick's bloated abdomen can act like a syringe if squeezed. Transmission of infection seems to be most efficient after 24-48 hours of nymphal tick attachment for human granulocytic ehrlichiosis, after 36 hours for *B. burgdorferi*, and after 36-48 hours for *Babesia*. Prophylactic antimicrobial therapy after a tick bite or exposure is not recommended.

TABLE 122.1 Major Zoonotic Infections*

DISEASE	CAUSATIVE AGENT	COMMON ANIMAL RESERVOIRS	VECTORS/MODES OF TRANSMISSION	GEOGRAPHIC DISTRIBUTION	COMMON CLINICAL PRESENTATIONS†
BACTERIAL DISEASES					
Anthrax	*Bacillus anthracis*	Cattle, goats, sheep	Aerosol inhalation of spores in hides and other animal by-products, direct contact with infected animals or their carcasses	Worldwide; rare in United States	**Cutaneous**: ulcerative lesion with central eschar **Inhalation**: multiorgan failure, widened mediastinum **Gastrointestinal**: intestinal or oropharyngeal involvement
Brucellosis	*Brucella*	Cattle, sheep, goats, swine, elk, bison, deer, dogs	Aerosol inhalation, direct contact, ingestion of contaminated goat cheese and milk	Worldwide	Nonspecific symptoms, prolonged fever, hepatosplenomegaly, osteomyelitis
Campylobacteriosis	*Campylobacter jejuni*	Poultry, dogs (puppies), kittens, hamsters	Direct contact, ingestion of contaminated food or water	Worldwide	Diarrhea
Capnocytophaga canimorsus		Dogs, cats (rare)	Bites, scratches	Worldwide	Wound infection
Cat-scratch disease	*Bartonella henselae*	Cats, dogs (rare)	Bites and scratches	Worldwide	Regional lymphadenopathy/ lymphadenitis, follicular conjunctivitis with ipsilateral preauricular lymphadenopathy (Parinaud oculoglandular syndrome), sepsis, prolonged fever, hepatosplenomegaly

Continued

TABLE 122.1 Major Zoonotic Infections*—cont'd

DISEASE	CAUSATIVE AGENT	COMMON ANIMAL RESERVOIRS	VECTORS/MODES OF TRANSMISSION	GEOGRAPHIC DISTRIBUTION	COMMON CLINICAL PRESENTATIONS†
Erysipeloid	*Erysipelothrix rhusiopathiae*	Sheep, swine, cattle, horses, birds, fish	Direct contact	Worldwide	Mild localized cutaneous eruption, generalized cutaneous disease or septicemia ± endocarditis
Listeriosis	*Listeria monocytogenes*	Cattle, fowl, goats, sheep	Ingestion of contaminated food, unpasteurized cheese and dairy products	Worldwide	Gastroenteritis, neonatal sepsis/meningitis, spontaneous abortion
Pasteurella multocida		Cats, dogs	Bites, scratches, licks	Worldwide	Wound infection
Plague	*Yersinia pestis*	Wild and domestic rodents, cats, prairie dogs	Direct contact, flea bite	New Mexico, Arizona, Utah, Colorado, California	Buboes, sepsis, pneumonia
Psittacosis	*Chlamydophila psittaci*	Pet birds, poultry	Aerosol inhalation		Pneumonia
Rat-bite fever (streptobacillary or Haverhill fever)	*Streptobacillus moniliformis*	Rodents (especially rats), cats, gerbils	Bites, ingestion of contaminated food or water	Japan, Asia; rare in United States	Relapsing fever, rash, migratory polyarthritis
Salmonellosis	Nontyphoidal *Salmonella*	Poultry, dogs, cats, reptiles, amphibians	Direct contact, ingestion of contaminated food or water	Worldwide	Gastroenteritis, bacteremia
Tularemia	*Francisella tularensis*	Rabbits, sheep, cattle, cats	Aerosol inhalation, direct contact, ingestion of contaminated meat, tick bite, deerfly bite	California, Utah, Arkansas, Oklahoma	Ulcerative lymphadenopathy
Yersiniosis	*Yersinia enterocolitica, Yersinia pseudotuberculosis*	Rodents, cattle, goats, sheep, swine, birds, horses	Direct contact, ingestion of contaminated food or water	Worldwide	Gastroenteritis, pseudoappendicitis syndrome (RLQ pain)
MYCOBACTERIAL DISEASES					
Mycobacteriosis	*Mycobacterium marinum, Mycobacterium fortuitum, Mycobacterium kansasii*	Fish, aquarium	Direct contact, scratches	Worldwide	Wound infection
SPIROCHETAL DISEASES					
Leptospirosis	*Leptospira* species	Dogs, rodents, livestock	Direct contact, contact with water or soil contaminated by urine of infected animals	Worldwide	Sepsis, liver and/or renal failure
Lyme disease	*Borrelia burgdorferi*	Rodents	Tick bite *(Ixodes scapularis, Ixodes pacificus)*	Northeast and Midwest United States, California	Erythema migrans, arthritis, carditis, neurological symptoms
Rat-bite fever	*Spirillum minus* (Asia); *Streptobacillus moniliformis* (U.S.)	Mice, rats, hamsters	Bites, ingestion of contaminated food or water	Japan, Asia; United States	Rash, ulcer at bite site
Relapsing fever	*Borrelia* (e.g., *Borrelia hermsii*)	Rodents	Soft tick bite	Western and southern United States	Relapsing fever, rash
Southern tick-associated rash illness	*Unknown*	Deer, rodents	Tick bite	Southeastern and south-central U.S.	Erythema migrans-like rash

TABLE 122.1 Major Zoonotic Infections*—cont'd

DISEASE	CAUSATIVE AGENT	COMMON ANIMAL RESERVOIRS	VECTORS/MODES OF TRANSMISSION	GEOGRAPHIC DISTRIBUTION	COMMON CLINICAL PRESENTATIONS†
RICKETTSIAL DISEASES					
Spotted Fever Group					
Rocky Mountain spotted fever	*Rickettsia rickettsii*	Dogs, rodents	Tick bite	Western hemisphere	Nonspecific febrile illness, rash, shock, multiorgan failure
Mediterranean spotted fever (Boutonneuse fever)	*Rickettsia conorii*	Dogs, rodents	Tick bite	Africa, Mediterranean region, India, Middle East	Eschar (usually single), regional adenopathy, rash on extremities
African tick-bite fever	*Rickettsia africae*	Cattle, possibly goats	Tick bite	Sub-Saharan Africa, Caribbean	Eschar, rash
Rickettsialpox	*Rickettsia akari*	Mice	Mite bite	North America, Russia, Ukraine, Adriatic region, Korea, South Africa	Eschar, rash
Murine typhus–like illness	*Rickettsia felis*	Opossums, cats	Flea bite	Western hemisphere, Europe	Rash
Typhus Group					
Typhus, flea-borne endemic	*Rickettsia typhi*	Rats, cats	Rat flea or cat flea feces	Worldwide	Rash
Typhus, louse-borne endemic	*Rickettsia prowazekii*	Flying squirrels	Lice or fleas of flying squirrel, person-to-person via body louse	United States	Headache, myalgias, rash, altered mental status
Scrub Typhus					
Scrub typhus	*Orientia tsutsugamushi*	Rodents	Chigger bite	Southern Asia, Japan, Indonesia, Australia, Korea, Asiatic Russia, India, China	Headaches, myalgias, eschar, rash
Ehrlichiosis and Anaplasmosis					
Human monocytic ehrlichiosis	*Ehrlichia chaffeensis*	Deer, dogs	Tick bite	United States, Europe, Africa	Acute febrile illness, rash, respiratory distress syndrome, meningitis
Anaplasmosis (human granulocytic ehrlichiosis)	*Anaplasma phagocytophilum*	Rodents, deer, ruminants	Tick bite	United States, Europe	Acute febrile illness, respiratory distress syndrome, meningitis
Ehrlichiosis ewingii	*Ehrlichia ewingii*	Dogs	Tick bite	United States	Same as *E. chaffeensis*
Sennetsu ehrlichiosis	*Neorickettsia sennetsu*	Unknown	Unknown; possibly ingestion of raw fish	Japan, Malaysia	Same as *E. chaffeensis*
Q Fever					
Q fever	*Coxiella burnetii*	Cattle, sheep, goats, cats, wild rodents	Inhalation of infected aerosols, ingestion of contaminated dairy products, direct contact with excreta	Worldwide	**Acute:** nonspecific febrile illness **Chronic:** osteomyelitis, endocarditis
VIRAL DISEASES					
Colorado tick fever	Colorado tick fever virus	Rodents	Tick bite	Rocky Mountains, Pacific northwest, western Canada	Nonspecific febrile illness, rash
Hantavirus cardiopulmonary syndrome	Hantavirus	Rodents, mice	Aerosol inhalation of infected excreta	Southwestern United States	Noncardiogenic pulmonary edema
Herpesvirus B infection	Herpesvirus B	Macaque monkeys	Animal bite	Africa, Asia (and primate centers worldwide)	Encephalitis and death

Continued

TABLE 122.1 Major Zoonotic Infections*—cont'd

DISEASE	CAUSATIVE AGENT	COMMON ANIMAL RESERVOIRS	VECTORS/MODES OF TRANSMISSION	GEOGRAPHIC DISTRIBUTION	COMMON CLINICAL PRESENTATIONS†
Lymphocytic choriomeningitis	Lymphocytic choriomeningitis virus	Rodents, hamsters, mice	Aerosol inhalation, direct contact, bite	Worldwide	Meningitis
Monkeypox	Monkeypox virus	Prairie dogs, African rodents	Direct contact, bite, scratch	Central and west Africa	Lymphadenopathy, rash
Orf	Orf virus	Sheep, goats	Direct contact with infected saliva	Worldwide	Nodular or ulcerative skin lesions
Rabies	Rabies virus	Skunks, bats, raccoons, foxes, cats, dogs	Bites and scratches	Worldwide	Encephalitis and death
Vesicular stomatitis	Vesicular stomatitis virus	Horses, cattle, swine	Direct contact	Americas	Flu-like illness
PROTOZOAN DISEASES					
African Trypanosomiasis					
East African sleeping sickness	*Trypanosoma brucei rhodesiense*	Wild animals (antelope, bush buck, and hartebeest), rarely cattle	Insect bite (tsetse fly)	East Africa	Acute febrile illness with multiorgan failure and meningoencephalitis
West African sleeping sickness	*Trypanosoma brucei gambiense*	Humans are main reservoir, wild and domestic animals	Insect bite (tsetse fly)	West Africa	Nonspecific febrile illness, posterior cervical lymphadenopathy (Winterbottom sign), neurological compromise 1-2 yr later
American trypanosomiasis (Chagas disease)	*Trypanosoma cruzi*	Raccoons, opossums, rodents, dogs	Insect bite (reduviid bug); contact with fecal material of reduviid bug	South America, Central America, south Texas	**Acute:** mild nonspecific symptoms, red indurated nodule (chagoma), periorbital edema (Romaña sign) **Chronic:** asymptomatic, cardiomyopathy, achalasia
Babesiosis	*Babesia*	White-footed mouse	Tick bite, blood transfusion	Worldwide	Often asymptomatic or mild disease but can cause life-threatening hemolytic anemia in asplenic, elderly or immunocompromised persons
Leishmaniasis, mucocutaneous and cutaneous	*Leishmania*	Rodents, dogs	Sandfly bite	Tropics	Nodular or ulcerative lesion (cutaneous), destruction of naso-oropharyngeal mucosa (mucocutaneous)
Leishmaniasis, visceral	*Leishmania donovani* complex	Rodents, dogs	Sandfly bite	Tropics	Multiorgan involvement (spleen, liver, bone marrow), grayish skin discoloration (kala-azar)
Toxoplasmosis	*Toxoplasma gondii*	Cats, livestock	Ingestion of oocysts in fecally contaminated material or ingestion of tissue cysts in undercooked meat	Worldwide	Congenital infection, mononucleosis-like illness, reactivation in the central nervous system in immunocompromised hosts

Many helminths are also zoonotic (see Tables 123.4 and 123.5).
†*In addition to fever.*
RLQ, Right lower quadrant.
From Kimberlin DW, Brady MT, Jackson MA, et al. Red Book: 2015 Report of the Committee on Infectious Diseases. *30th ed. Elk Grove Village, IL: American Academy of Pediatrics; 2015:1015–1022. Copyright 2015 American Academy of Pediatrics. Reproduced with permission.*

LYME DISEASE (*BORRELIA BURGDORFERI*)

Etiology

Lyme disease is a tick-borne infection caused by the spirochete, *B. burgdorferi*. The vector in the eastern and midwestern United States is *Ixodes scapularis*, the **black-legged tick** that is commonly known as the **deer tick**. The vector on the Pacific coast is *Ixodes pacificus*, the **western black-legged tick**. Ticks usually become infected by feeding on the white-footed mouse (*Peromyscus leucopus*), which is a natural reservoir for *B. burgdorferi*. The larvae are dormant over winter and emerge the following spring in the nymphal stage, the stage of the tick that is most likely to transmit the infection to humans.

Epidemiology

Over 20,000 cases are reported annually in the United States, with >90% of cases reported from New England and the eastern parts of the middle Atlantic states (Fig. 122.1). In Europe most cases occur in Scandinavian countries and central Europe. Because exposure to ticks is more common in warm months, Lyme disease is noted predominantly in spring and summer. The incidence is highest among children 5-9 years old, at almost twice the incidence among adolescents and adults.

Clinical Manifestations

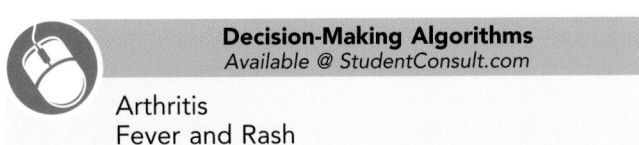

Decision-Making Algorithms
Available @ StudentConsult.com

Arthritis
Fever and Rash

Reported Cases of Lyme Disease in the United States, 2014.

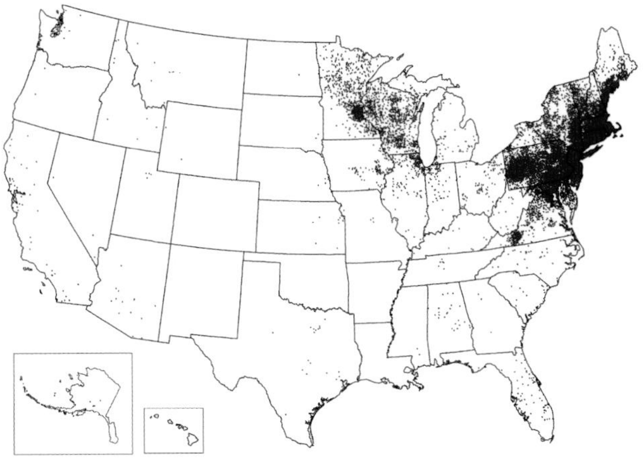

1 dot placed randomly within county
of residence for each confirmed case

FIGURE 122.1 The geographic distribution of 25,359 confirmed cases of Lyme disease in the United States in 2014. The risk for acquiring Lyme disease varies by the distribution of *Ixodes scapularis* and *Ixodes pacificus*, the proportion of infected ticks for each species at each stage of the tick's life cycle, and the presence of grassy or wooded locations favored by white-tailed deer. (From Centers for Disease Control and Prevention: Lyme Disease—United States, 2014. Available from the CDC website: http://www.cdc.gov/lyme/resources/reportedcasesoflymedisease_2014.pdf.)

The clinical manifestations are divided into early and late stages. Early infection may be localized or disseminated. **Early localized disease** develops 7-14 days after a tick bite as the site forms an erythematous papule that expands to form a red, raised border, often with central clearing (Fig. 122.2). The lesion, **erythema migrans**, is pruritic or painful, harbors *B. burgdorferi*, and, without treatment, may expand to as much as 15 cm in diameter. Systemic manifestations may include malaise, lethargy, fever, headache, arthralgias, stiff neck, myalgias, and lymphadenopathy. The skin lesions and early manifestations resolve without treatment over 2-4 weeks. Not all patients with Lyme disease recall a tick bite or develop erythema migrans.

Approximately 25% of children with Lyme disease are initially diagnosed with **early disseminated disease**, which is a consequence of bacteremic dissemination of *B. burgdorferi* to multiple sites. Early disseminated disease is characterized by multiple secondary skin lesions, aseptic meningitis, pseudotumor, papilledema, neuropathies including Bell palsy, polyradiculitis, peripheral neuropathy, mononeuritis multiplex, or transverse myelitis. Carditis with various degrees of heart block rarely may develop during this stage. Neurological manifestations usually resolve by 3 months but may recur or become chronic.

Late disease begins weeks to months after infection and is diagnosed in approximately 7% of children at initial presentation. Arthritis is the usual manifestation and may develop in 50-60% of untreated patients. The knee is involved in greater than 90% of cases, but any joint may be affected. Symptoms may resolve over 1-2 weeks but often recur in other joints. **Neuroborreliosis**, the late manifestations of Lyme disease involving the central nervous system (CNS), is rarely reported in children.

Laboratory and Imaging Studies

Antibody tests during early, localized Lyme disease may be negative and are not useful. Additionally, patients appropriately treated for their early, localized Lyme disease may not develop a positive antibody test. The diagnosis of late disease is confirmed

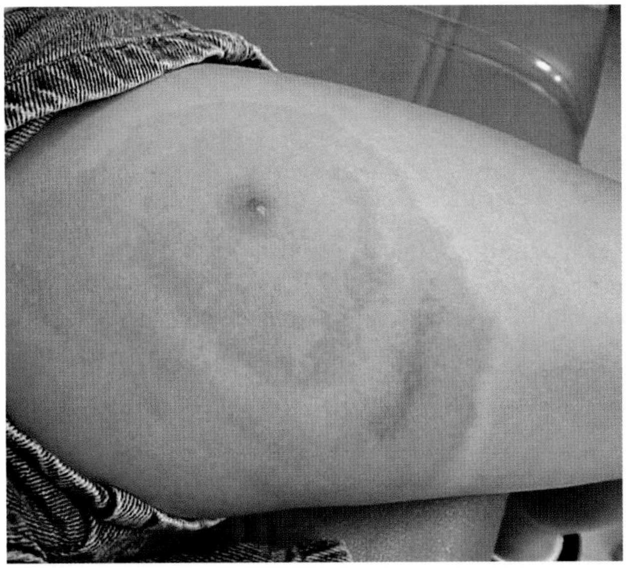

FIGURE 122.2 Expanding annular lesion of erythema migrans at the site of a tick bite. (Courtesy Dr. Jay Capra, Abilene, Texas.)

by serological tests specific for *B. burgdorferi*. The sensitivity and specificity of serological tests for Lyme disease vary substantially. A positive enzyme-linked immunosorbent assay or immunofluorescence assay result must be confirmed by immunoblot showing antibodies against at least either two to three (for IgM) or five (for IgG) proteins of *B. burgdorferi* (at least one of which is one of the more specific, low molecular weight, outer-surface proteins).

In late disease, the erythrocyte sedimentation rate is elevated and complement may be reduced. The joint fluid shows an inflammatory response with total white blood cell count of 25,000-125,000 cells/mm^3, often with a polymorphonuclear predominance (see Table 118.2). The rheumatoid factor and antinuclear antibody are negative, but the Venereal Disease Research Laboratory test may be falsely positive. With CNS involvement, the cerebrospinal fluid shows a lymphocytic pleocytosis with normal glucose and slightly elevated protein.

Differential Diagnosis

A history of a tick bite and the classic rash is helpful but is not always present. Erythema migrans of early, localized disease may be confused with nummular eczema, tinea corporis, granuloma annulare, an insect bite, or cellulitis. **Southern tick-associated rash illness (STARI)**, which is similar to erythema migrans but not associated with any of the disseminated complications of Lyme disease, occurs in southeastern and south-central states and is associated with the bite of *Amblyomma americanum*, the lone star tick, which is abundant in the southern states and incapable of transmitting *B. burgdorferi*.

During early, disseminated Lyme disease, multiple lesions may appear as erythema multiforme or urticaria. The aseptic meningitis is similar to viral meningitis, and the seventh nerve palsy is indistinguishable from herpetic or idiopathic Bell palsy. Lyme carditis is similar to viral myocarditis. Monarticular or pauciarticular arthritis of late Lyme disease may mimic suppurative arthritis, juvenile idiopathic arthritis, or rheumatic fever (see Chapter 89). The differential diagnosis of neuroborreliosis includes degenerative neurological illness, encephalitis, and depression.

Treatment

Early localized disease and early disseminated disease, including facial nerve palsy (or other cranial nerve palsy) and carditis with first-degree or second-degree heart block, is treated with doxycycline or amoxicillin for 14-21 days. Early disseminated disease with carditis with third-degree heart block or meningitis and late neurological disease are treated with intravenous or intramuscular ceftriaxone or intravenous penicillin G for 14-28 days. Arthritis is treated with doxycycline (for children ≥8 years of age) or amoxicillin for 28 days. If there is recurrence, treatment should be with a repeated oral regimen or with the regimen for late neurological disease.

Complications and Prognosis

Carditis, especially conduction disturbances, and arthritis are the major complications of Lyme disease. Even untreated, most cases eventually resolve without sequelae. Lyme disease is readily treatable and curable. The long-term prognosis is excellent for treated early and late disease. Early treatment of erythema migrans almost always prevents progression to later stages. Recurrences of arthritis after treatment occur in 5-10% of patients. The most common reason patients "recur" or do not respond to treatment is that the initial diagnosis was incorrect.

Prevention

Measures to minimize exposure to tick-borne diseases are the most reasonable means of preventing Lyme disease. Postexposure prophylaxis is not routinely recommended because the overall risk of acquiring Lyme disease after a tick bite is only 1-3% even in endemic areas, and treatment of the infection, if it develops, is highly effective. Nymphal stage ticks must feed for >36 hours before the risk of transmission of *B. burgdorferi* from infected ticks becomes substantial. In hyperendemic regions, prophylaxis of adults with doxycycline, 200 mg as a single dose, within 72 hours of a nymphal tick bite is effective in preventing Lyme disease.

ROCKY MOUNTAIN SPOTTED FEVER (*RICKETTSIA RICKETTSII*)

Etiology

The cause of RMSF is *R. rickettsii*, gram-negative coccobacillary organisms that resemble bacteria but have incomplete cell walls and require an intracellular site for replication. The organism invades and proliferates within the endothelial cells of blood vessels of all major organs and tissues, causing vasculitis and resulting in increased vascular permeability, edema, and, eventually, decreased vascular volume, altered tissue perfusion, and widespread organ failure. Many tick species are capable of transmitting *R. rickettsii*. The principal ticks are the **American dog tick** *(Dermacentor variabilis)* in the eastern United States and Canada, the **wood tick** *(Dermacentor andersoni)* in the western United States and Canada, the **brown dog tick** *(Rhipicephalus sanguineus)* in Mexico and southwestern United States, and *Amblyomma cajennense* in Central and South America.

Epidemiology

RMSF is the most common rickettsial illness in the United States, occurring primarily in the eastern coastal, southeastern, and south-central states. Most cases occur from April to September after outdoor activity in wooded areas. RMSF occurs more commonly in adults, but the case fatality rate is highest in children 5-9 years of age. In approximately 50% of pediatric cases of RMSF there is no recall of a tick bite.

Clinical Manifestations

Decision-Making Algorithms
Available @ StudentConsult.com

Hepatomegaly
Fever and Rash
Petechiae/Purpura
Fever Without a Source

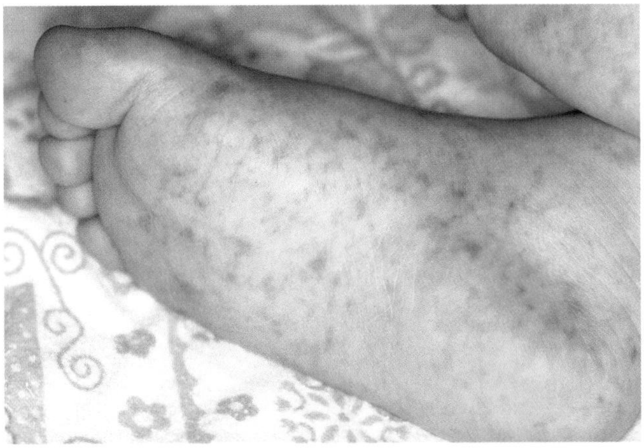

FIGURE 122.3 Petechial and purpuric rash of Rocky Mountain Spotted Fever. (From McQuiston JH, Regan JJ, Paddock CD. Rickettsia rickettsii [Rocky Mountain Spotted Fever]. In: Long SS, Pickering LK, Prober CG, eds. *Principles and Practice of Pediatric Infectious Diseases*. 4th ed. Philadelphia: Churchill Livingstone; 2012. Fig. 178.4B.)

The incubation period of RMSF is 2-14 days, with an average of 7 days. The onset is nonspecific with headache, malaise, and fever. A pale, rose-red macular or maculopapular rash appears in 90% of cases usually 2-5 days after fever onset. The early rash blanches on pressure and is accentuated by warmth. It progresses over hours or days to a petechial and purpuric eruption that appears first on the feet and ankles, then the wrists and hands, and progresses centripetally to the trunk and head. A hallmark feature is the involvement of the palms and soles (Fig. 122.3). Myalgias, especially of the lower extremities, and intractable headaches are common. Severe cases progress with splenomegaly, myocarditis, renal impairment, pneumonitis, and shock.

Laboratory and Imaging Studies

Thrombocytopenia, anemia, hyponatremia, hypoalbuminemia, and elevated hepatic transaminase levels are common laboratory findings. Organisms can be detected in skin biopsy specimens by fluorescent antibodies or polymerase chain reaction, although this test is not widely available. Serological testing is used to confirm the diagnosis. Approximately 50% of patients will not have detectable antibody until the second week of illness, and treatment should not be withheld pending confirmation.

Differential Diagnosis

The differential diagnosis includes meningococcemia, bacterial sepsis, toxic shock syndrome, leptospirosis, ehrlichiosis, measles, enteroviruses, infectious mononucleosis, collagen vascular diseases, Henoch-Schönlein purpura, and idiopathic thrombocytopenic purpura. The diagnosis of RMSF should be suspected with fever and petechial rash, especially with a history of a tick bite or outdoor activities during spring and summer in endemic regions. Delayed diagnosis and late treatment usually result from atypical initial symptoms and late appearance of the rash.

Treatment

Therapy for suspected RMSF should not be postponed pending results of diagnostic tests. Doxycycline is the drug of choice, even for young children, despite the theoretical risk of dental staining in children younger than 8 years of age.

Complications and Prognosis

In severe infections, capillary leakage results in noncardiogenic pulmonary edema (acute respiratory distress syndrome), hypotension, disseminated intravascular coagulation, circulatory collapse, and multiple organ failure, including encephalitis, myocarditis, hepatitis, and renal failure.

Untreated illness may persist for 3 weeks and progress to multisystem involvement. The mortality rate is 20-80% without treatment, which is reduced to 1-3% with treatment. Permanent sequelae are common after severe disease.

Prevention

Preventive measures to avoid tick-borne infections and careful removal of ticks are recommended.

EHRLICHIOSIS *(EHRLICHIA CHAFFEENSIS)* AND ANAPLASMOSIS *(ANAPLASMA PHAGOCYTOPHILUM)*

Etiology

The term **ehrlichiosis** often is used to refer to all forms of infection with *Ehrlichia*. **Human monocytic ehrlichiosis** is caused by *E. chaffeensis*, which infects predominantly monocytic cells and is transmitted by the tick *A. americanum* (lone star tick). Disease may also be caused by *Ehrlichia ewingii* (granulocytes) and *Ehrlichia muris*–like agent (unknown, suspected monocytes). **Human anaplasmosis** is caused by *A. phagocytophilum* and is transmitted by the tick *I. scapularis* (black-legged tick) or *I. pacificus* (western black-legged tick).

Epidemiology

Human monocytic ehrlichiosis occurs in broad areas across the southeastern, south-central, and mid-Atlantic United States in a distribution that parallels that of RMSF. Anaplasmosis is found mostly in the northeastern and upper midwestern United States, but infections have been identified in northern California, the mid-Atlantic states, and broadly across Europe. Ehrlichiosis due to *E. muris*–like agents have been reported only from Wisconsin and Minnesota.

Clinical Manifestations

Human monocytic ehrlichiosis, anaplasmosis, and *Ehrlichiosis ewingii* cause similar acute febrile illnesses characterized by fever, malaise, headache, myalgias, anorexia, and nausea. Rash occurs more commonly in ehrlichiosis than anaplasmosis but even so is uncommon in adults. In contrast to adult patients, nearly two thirds of children with human monocytic ehrlichiosis present with a macular or maculopapular rash, although petechial lesions may occur. Symptoms usually last for 1-2 weeks.

Laboratory and Imaging Studies

Characteristic laboratory findings include leukopenia, lymphocytopenia, thrombocytopenia, anemia, and elevated hepatic transaminases. Morulae are found infrequently in circulating monocytes of persons with human monocytic ehrlichiosis, but are found in 20-60% of persons with anaplasmosis (Fig. 122.4). Seroconversion or fourfold rise in antibody titer confirms the diagnosis; this requires acute and convalescent samples and is not helpful during the acute illness. Polymerase chain reaction (PCR) tests for both ehrlichiosis and anaplasmosis are available and can confirm diagnosis during the acute illness.

Differential Diagnosis

Ehrlichiosis is clinically similar to other arthropod-borne infections, including RMSF, tularemia, babesiosis, early Lyme disease, murine typhus, relapsing fever, and Colorado tick fever. The differential diagnosis also includes infectious mononucleosis, Kawasaki disease, endocarditis, viral infections, hepatitis, leptospirosis, Q fever, collagen vascular diseases, and leukemia.

Treatment

As with RMSF, therapy for suspected ehrlichiosis should not be postponed pending results of diagnostic tests. Ehrlichiosis and anaplasmosis are treated with doxycycline.

Complications and Prognosis

Severe pulmonary involvement with acute respiratory distress syndrome has been reported in several cases. Other reported severe complications include meningoencephalitis and myocarditis. Most patients improve within 48 hours. Failure to respond to doxycycline within 3 days suggests either misdiagnosis or co-infection with another organism.

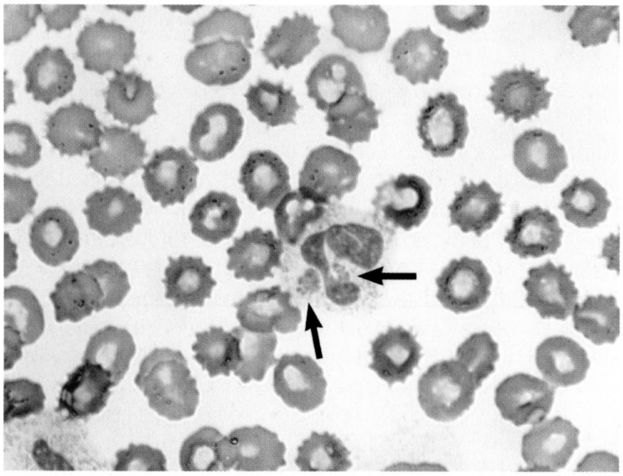

FIGURE 122.4 Intracellular inclusion within a neutrophil of a patient with human granulocytic anaplasmosis *(arrows)*. *Ehrlichia chaffeensis* and *Anaplasma phagocytophilum* have similar morphologies but are serologically and genetically distinct. (Wright stain, original magnification ×1,000.) (From Dumler JS, Walker DH. *Ehrlichia chaffeensis* [human monocytotropic ehrlichiosis], *Anaplasma phagocytophilum* [human granulocytotropic anaplasmosis], and other Anaplasmataceae. In: Bennett JE, Dolin R, Blaser MJ, eds. *Mandell, Douglas, and Bennett's Principles and Practice of Infectious Diseases*. 8th ed. Philadelphia: Elsevier; 2015. Fig. 194.2.)

Prevention

Preventive measures to avoid tick-borne infections and careful removal of ticks are recommended.

WEST NILE VIRUS (see Chapter 101)

Dengue Fever

There are four dengue fever virus types (flaviviruses) transmitted to humans predominantly by the *A. aegypti* mosquito vector. Enzootic transmission via monkeys may occur, but person (viremic) to mosquito to person is the most frequent mechanism of viral infection. Dengue virus is most prevalent in the tropics, and endogenous infections have been reported in Florida and Texas.

Infected patients may have subclinical disease or a self-limited febrile illness. Dengue hemorrhagic fever, the most severe manifestation of the illness, occurs in patients who have had a previous Dengue virus infection (different serotype) and who manifest an exaggerated immunological response to the new Dengue virus serotype.

Dengue viremia usually precedes the influenza-like illness characterized by fever, myalgias, musculoskeletal pain **(break bone fever)**, headaches, macular rash, elevated liver enzymes, acute respiratory distress syndrome, and peripheral cytopenias. Shock may occur with third space fluid losses, which may be associated with an increasing hematocrit. Epistaxis, hemoptysis, gastrointestinal, and uterine bleeding may occur.

Diagnosis is based on the geographic epidemiology, clinical presentation, and detection of dengue virus by PCR. Therapy requires good supportive care with fluid and blood replacement as needed.

Ebola Virus

Ebola virus is a filovirus producing a severe and often lethal hemorrhagic fever syndrome. It is transmitted by direct person-to-person contact, particularly body fluids; the fruit bat may be the animal reservoir for ebola and the related marburg virus. Ebola is most often seen in central Africa, although imported cases have been reported in persons traveling from endemic or epidemic regions.

Clinical manifestations may begin with a sudden onset of fever, myalgias, diarrhea, and malaise, but are then followed by significant hemorrhagic manifestations. Leukopenia, lymphopenia, thrombocytopenia, elevated liver enzymes, and prolonged clotting times are common. The diagnosis is confirmed by the presence of IgM and IgG antibodies to the virus. Treatment is supportive, including replacement of blood and fluid losses.

Chikungunya Virus

Chikungunya virus (CHIK) is an alphavirus in the togavirus family and is transmitted by most *Aedes* species of mosquitos in Africa and Latin America. Nonhuman primates may be the animal reservoir.

CHIK fever is characterized by a sudden illness with high fever, rash, and severe arthralgias. Fever may abate but return in the "saddleback" pattern. Polyarthralgias involve the small joints, which are exquisitely tender, and may persist for several weeks. The rash appears as facial flushing but evolves to a maculopapular occasionally pruritic eruption on the trunk, extremities, soles, and palms. Children may have CNS symptoms (irritability, seizures). Leukopenia, lymphocytosis, and an elevated erythrocyte sedimentation rate (ESR) or C-reactive protein (CRP) are common.

The diagnosis is confirmed by PCR or antibody responses. Treatment is supportive, particularly for the incapacitating joint manifestations. Tumor necrosis factor (TNF)-blocking agents may be beneficial for severe and persistent arthritis.

Zika Virus

Zika virus, a member of the flavivirus group, is transmitted by many *Aedes* mosquito species and is prevalent in equatorial regions of South America and Asia. Monkeys may be the animal reservoir. Zika virus infection is manifest with fever, rash, arthralgia, nonpurulent conjunctivitis, and headache. Infection in children and adults is usually self-limited; the greatest concern is infection during pregnancy resulting in transplacental transmission to the fetus with subsequent severe microcephaly and other congenital malformation.

Diagnosis is confirmed by Zika virus antibody titers or PCR.

CHAPTER 123

Parasitic Diseases

PROTOZOAL DISEASES

Protozoa are the simplest organisms of the animal kingdom. They are unicellular. Most are free-living, but some have a commensal or parasitic existence. Protozoal diseases include malaria, toxoplasmosis, babesiosis, and the intestinal protozoal diseases, amebiasis, cryptosporidiosis, and giardiasis.

Malaria

Etiology

Malaria is caused by obligate intracellular protozoa of the genus *Plasmodium*, including *P. falciparum*, *P. malariae*, *P. ovale*, *P. vivax*, and *P. knowlesi*. *Plasmodium* has a complex life cycle that enables survival in different cellular environments in the human host and in the mosquito vector. There are two major phases in the life cycle, an **asexual phase (schizogony)** in humans and a **sexual phase (sporogony)** in mosquitoes. The **erythrocytic phase** of *Plasmodium* asexual development begins when the merozoites released from exoerythrocytic schizonts in the liver penetrate erythrocytes. When inside the erythrocyte, the parasite transforms into the **ring form**, which enlarges to become a **trophozoite**. These latter two forms can be identified with Giemsa stain on blood smear, which is the primary means of confirming the diagnosis of malaria.

The parasites usually are transmitted to humans by female *Anopheles* mosquitoes. Malaria also can be transmitted through blood transfusion, via contaminated needles, and transplacentally to a fetus.

Epidemiology

Malaria is a worldwide problem with transmission in more than 100 countries with a combined population of more than 3.2 billion people. Malaria is an important cause of fever and morbidity in the tropical world. The principal areas of transmission are sub-Saharan Africa, southern Asia, Southeast Asia, and Central and South America. Approximately 1,500-2,000 imported cases are recognized annually in the United States, with most cases occurring among infected foreign civilians from endemic areas who travel to the United States and among U.S. citizens who travel to endemic areas without appropriate chemoprophylaxis.

Clinical Manifestations

Decision-Making Algorithm
Available @ StudentConsult.com
Fever of Unknown Origin

The clinical manifestations of malaria range from asymptomatic infection to fulminant illness and death, depending on the virulence of the infecting malaria species and the host immune response. The incubation period ranges from 7-30 days, depending on the *Plasmodium* species (Table 123.1). The most characteristic clinical feature of malaria, which is seldom noted with other infectious diseases, is **febrile paroxysms** alternating with periods of fatigue but otherwise relative wellness. The classic symptoms of the febrile paroxysms of malaria include high fever, rigors, sweats, and headache. Paroxysms coincide with the ruptures of schizonts that occur every 48 hours with *P. vivax* and *P. ovale* (**tertian periodicity**), every 72 hours with *P. malariae* (**quartan periodicity**), and every 24 hours with *P. knowlesi*. Periodicity can be tertian with *P. falciparum* infections but is often irregular.

Short-term relapse describes the recurrence of symptoms after a primary attack that is due to the survival of erythrocyte forms in the bloodstream. **Long-term relapse** describes the renewal of symptoms long after the primary attack, usually due to the release of merozoites from an exoerythrocytic source in the liver. Long-term relapse occurs with *P. vivax* and *P. ovale* because of persistence in the liver (Fig. 123.1).

Laboratory and Imaging Studies

The diagnosis of malaria is established by the identification of organisms on stained smears of peripheral blood. In nonimmune persons, symptoms typically occur 1-2 days before parasites are detectable on blood smear. Although *P. falciparum* is most likely to be identified from blood during a febrile paroxysm, the timing of the smears is less important than obtaining smears several times each day over 3 successive days. Both thick and thin blood smears should be examined. The concentration of erythrocytes on a **thick smear** is approximately 20-40 times greater than that on a **thin smear**. Thick smears are used to scan large numbers of erythrocytes quickly. Thin smears allow for positive identification of the malaria species and determination of the percentage of infected erythrocytes, called parasitemia, which also is useful in following the response to therapy. **Rapid diagnostic tests** are available as point-of-care tests. Such tests provide results in 15-20 minutes and are particularly useful in areas where reliable microscopic diagnosis is not available. The rapid tests are able to detect *P. falciparum* but are unable to

TABLE 123.1 Characteristics of *Plasmodium* Species Causing Malaria

CHARACTERISTIC	*P. FALCIPARUM*	*P. VIVAX*	*P. OVALE*	*P. MALARIAE*	*P. KNOWLESI*
Exoerythrocytic cycle	5.5-7 days	6-8 days	12 days	9 days	16 days
Erythrocytic cycle	43-52 hr	48 hr	48 hr	72 hr	24 hr
Usual incubation period (range)	13-14 days	13-14 days	13-14 days	35 days	Unknown
Erythrocyte preference	Can infect all	Reticulocytes	Older erythrocytes	Reticulocytes	Can infect all
Usual parasite load (% erythrocytes infected)	High	Low	Low	Low	May be high
Secondary exoerythrocytic cycle (hypnozoites) and relapses	Absent	Present	Present	Absent	Absent
Severity of primary attack	Can be severe	Mild to severe	Mild	Mild—severe disease in a patient suspected of having *P. malariae* should raise the suspicion of *P. knowlesi*	Mild to severe
Usual periodicity of febrile attacks	None	48 hr	48 hr	72 hr	24 hr

Modified from Taylor T, Agbenyega T. Malaria. In: Magill AJ, Edward R, Tom S, David H, eds. Hunter's Tropical Medicine and Emerging Infectious Disease. *9th ed. Philadelphia: Saunders; 2013:700.*

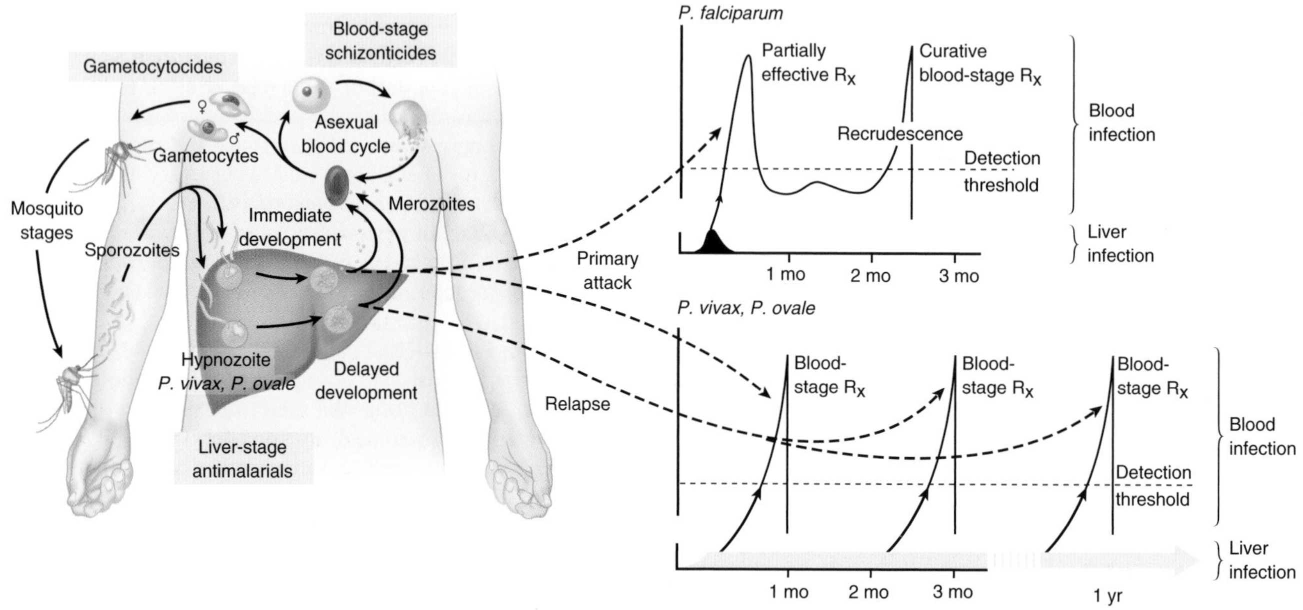

FIGURE 123.1 The *Plasmodium* life cycle and disease patterns of recrudescence and relapse. Anopheline mosquitoes transmit malaria by injecting sporozoites into the human host. The sporozoites then invade hepatocytes, in which they develop into schizonts. Each infected hepatocyte ruptures to liberate 10,000-30,000 merozoites that invade circulating erythrocytes. Growth and development of the parasites in red cells result in subsequent waves of merozoite invasion. This asexual blood cycle repeats every 24 *(Plasmodium knowlesi)*, 48 *(Plasmodium falciparum, Plasmodium vivax, Plasmodium ovale)*, or 72 *(Plasmodium malariae)* hours, leading to amplification of parasite density; paroxysms of chills, fevers, and sweats; and other manifestations of disease. Malaria symptoms are typically experienced 2-4 weeks after the mosquito bite. If the parasites are not cleared (e.g., patient receives partially effective therapy), recrudescence of parasitemia and malaria symptoms can occur. Eradicating parasites with an effective drug regimen cures malaria. Some *P. vivax* and *P. ovale* parasites can postpone their development in the liver, persisting as latent forms called hypnozoites. Hypnozoites are not eradicated by standard therapy (e.g., chloroquine) directed against blood stages. Resumption of hypnozoite development months to years after initial infection can lead to malaria relapse that requires an additional round of drug therapy to treat recurrent symptoms and eradicate blood-stage parasites. A course of primaquine can prevent relapses of malaria, but this treatment may not always be successful because of inadequate patient compliance, interindividual variations of drug metabolism, or variable parasite responses to low or high drug doses. (From Fairhurst RM, Wellems TE. Malaria [*Plasmodium* species]. In: Bennett JE, Dolin R, Blaser MJ, eds. *Mandell, Douglas, and Bennett's Principles and Practice of Infectious Diseases.* 8th ed. Philadelphia: Elsevier; 2015. Fig. 276.2.)

differentiate between *P. vivax*, *P. ovale*, and *P. malariae*. Sensitivity is low for non-*falciparum* species and in patients with low-level parasitemia. For these reasons as well as to guide management decisions, all rapid tests should be followed by microscopic examination regardless of the results.

Differential Diagnosis

The most important aspect of diagnosing malaria in children is to consider the possibility of malaria in any child who has fever, chills, splenomegaly, anemia, or decreased level of consciousness with a history of recent travel or residence in an endemic area, regardless of the use of chemoprophylaxis. The differential diagnosis is broad and includes many infectious diseases, such as typhoid fever, tuberculosis, brucellosis, relapsing fever, infective endocarditis, influenza, poliomyelitis, yellow fever, trypanosomiasis, kala-azar, and amebic liver abscess.

Treatment

Oral chloroquine is the recommended treatment except for chloroquine-resistant *P. falciparum*. Either atovaquone-proguanil, mefloquine, or artemether-lumefantrine is an appropriate first-line therapy for malaria acquired in areas of chloroquine resistance. Specific treatment should be guided by where the patient acquired the infection and the local resistance patterns. Patients with malaria usually require hospitalization and may require intensive care unit admission. Quinidine gluconate is the only drug available in the United States that is used for parenteral treatment. Artesunate is available from the Centers for Disease Control and Prevention as an investigational new drug.

Complications and Prognosis

Cerebral malaria is a complication of *P. falciparum* infection and a frequent cause of death (10-40% of cases), especially among children and nonimmune adults. Similar to other complications, cerebral malaria is more likely to occur among patients with intense parasitemia (>5% of erythrocytes on a blood smear). Other complications include splenic rupture, renal failure, severe hemolysis **(blackwater fever)**, pulmonary edema, hypoglycemia, thrombocytopenia, and **algid malaria** (sepsis syndrome with vascular collapse).

Death may occur with any of the malarial species but is most frequent with complicated *P. falciparum* malaria. The likelihood of death is increased in children with pre-existing health problems, such as measles, intestinal parasites, schistosomiasis, anemia, and malnutrition. Death is much more common in developing countries.

Prevention

There are two components of malaria prevention: reduction of exposure to infected mosquitoes and chemoprophylaxis. Mosquito protection is necessary because no prophylactic regimen can guarantee protection in every instance due to the widespread development of resistant organisms.

Chemoprophylaxis is necessary for all visitors to, and residents of, the tropics who have not lived there since infancy. Children of nonimmune women should have chemoprophylaxis from birth. Children of women from endemic areas have passive immunity until 3-6 months of age, after which they are increasingly likely to acquire malaria. Specific chemoprophylaxis should be guided by the distribution of resistance pattern and determined before making specific recommendations (http://www.cdc.gov/malaria/travelers/country_table/a.html). Mefloquine, doxycycline, chloroquine, and atovaquone-proguanil are commonly prescribed medications.

Toxoplasmosis

Decision-Making Algorithms
Available @ StudentConsult.com

Splenomegaly
Lymphadenopathy
Petechiae/Purpura
Fever of Unknown Origin

Toxoplasmosis is a zoonosis caused by *Toxoplasma gondii*, an intracellular protozoan parasite. Infection is acquired by infectious oocysts, such as those excreted by newly infected cats, which play an important role in amplifying the organism in nature, or from ingesting cysts in contaminated, undercooked meat. Less commonly, transmission occurs transplacentally during acute infection of pregnant women. In the United States, the incidence of congenital infection is 1-10 per 10,000 live births.

Acquired toxoplasmosis is usually asymptomatic. Symptomatic infection is typically a heterophile-negative mononucleosis syndrome that includes lymphadenopathy, fever, and hepatosplenomegaly. Disseminated infection, including myocarditis, pneumonia, and central nervous system (CNS) toxoplasmosis, is more common among immunocompromised persons, especially persons with acquired immunodeficiency syndrome (AIDS). Among women infected during pregnancy, 50-60% give birth to an infected infant. The later in pregnancy that infection occurs, the more likely it is that the fetus will be infected, but the less severe the illness (see Chapter 66). Serological diagnosis can be established by a fourfold increase in antibody titer or seroconversion, a positive IgM antibody titer, or positive polymerase chain reaction for *T. gondii* in peripheral white blood cells, cerebrospinal fluid (CSF), serum, or amniotic fluid.

Treatment includes pyrimethamine and sulfadiazine, which act synergistically against *Toxoplasma*. Because these compounds are folic acid inhibitors, they are used in conjunction with folinic acid. Spiramycin, which is not licensed in the United States but can be obtained from the manufacturer at no cost as an investigational new drug, is also used in therapy of pregnant women with toxoplasmosis. Corticosteroids are reserved for patients with acute CNS or ocular infection.

Ingesting only well-cooked meat and avoiding cats or soil in areas where cats defecate are prudent measures for pregnant or immunocompromised persons. Administration of spiramycin to infected pregnant women has been associated with lower risks of congenital infection in their offspring.

HELMINTHIASES

Helminths are divided into three groups: roundworms, or nematodes, and two groups of flatworms, the trematodes (flukes) and the cestodes (tapeworms).

Hookworm Infections

Hookworm infection is caused by several species of hookworms, with *Ancylostoma duodenale* and *Necator americanus* being the most important (Table 123.2). There are more than 600 million humans worldwide infected with hookworms. *Ancylostoma duodenale* is the predominant species in the Mediterranean region, northern Asia, and certain areas of South America. *N. americanus* predominates in the Western hemisphere, sub-Saharan Africa, and Southeast Asia. Optimal soil conditions and fecal contamination are found in many agrarian tropical countries and in the southeastern United States. Infection typically occurs in young children, especially during the first decade of life. The larvae are found in warm, damp soil and infect humans by penetrating the skin. They migrate to the lungs, ascend the trachea, are swallowed, and reside in the intestine. The worms mature and attach to the intestinal wall, where they suck blood and shed eggs.

Infections are usually asymptomatic. Intense pruritus *(ground itch)* occurs at the site of larval penetration, usually the soles of the feet or between the toes, and may include papules and vesicles. Migration of larvae through the lungs usually is asymptomatic. Symptoms of abdominal pain, anorexia, indigestion, fullness, and diarrhea occur with hookworm infestation. The major manifestation of infection is anemia. Examination of fresh stool for hookworm eggs is diagnostic. Therapy includes anthelmintic treatment with albendazole, mebendazole, or pyrantel pamoate and treatment for anemia. Eradication depends on sanitation of the patient's environment and treatment with antiparasitics.

Ascariasis

Ascariasis is caused by *Ascaris lumbricoides*, a large nematode. It is the most prevalent helminthiasis, affecting more than 800 million people (see Table 123.2). After humans ingest the eggs, larvae are released and penetrate the intestine, migrate to the lungs, ascend the trachea, and are swallowed. On entering the intestines again, they mature and produce eggs that are excreted in the stool and are deposited in the soil, where they survive for prolonged periods.

Manifestations may be the result of migration of the larvae to other sites of the body or the presence of adult worms in the intestine. **Pulmonary ascariasis** occurs as the larvae migrate through the lung, producing cough, blood-stained sputum, eosinophilia, and transient infiltrates on chest x-ray films. Adult larvae in the small intestine may cause abdominal pain and distention. Intestinal obstruction from adult worms can occur, particularly in children due to the small diameter of their intestinal lumens and their propensity to acquire large worm burdens. Migration of worms into the bile duct may rarely cause acute biliary obstruction. Examination of fresh stool for characteristic eggs is diagnostic. Effective control depends on adequate sanitary treatment and disposal of infected human feces.

Visceral Larva Migrans

Visceral larva migrans is a systemic nematodiasis caused by ingestion of the eggs of the dog tapeworm, *Toxocara canis*, or, less commonly, the cat tapeworm, *Toxocara cati*, or the raccoon

TABLE 123.2 Major Pediatric Syndromes Caused by Parasitic Nematodes

SYNDROME	ETIOLOGICAL AGENT	TRANSMISSION	TREATMENT
Hookworm iron deficiency	*Ancylostoma duodenale*	Larval ingestion and penetration	Albendazole *or* mebendazole *or* pyrantel pamoate
	Necator americanus	Larval penetration	
Cutaneous larva migrans	*Ancylostoma braziliense* (a zoonotic hookworm)	Larval penetration (and failure to migrate)	Generally self-limited; albendazole *or* ivermectin
Trichuris dysentery or colitis	*Trichuris trichiura*	Egg ingestion	Mebendazole *or* albendazole *or* ivermectin
Intestinal ascariasis	*Ascaris lumbricoides*	Ingestion of *Ascaris* eggs	Albendazole *or* mebendazole *or* ivermectin
Visceral larva migrans	*Toxocara canis* *Toxocara cati* *Baylisascaris procyonis*	Egg ingestion	Albendazole *or* mebendazole *or* ivermectin
Ocular larva migrans	*Toxocara canis* *Toxocara cati* *Baylisascaris procyonis*	Egg ingestion	Albendazole *or* mebendazole *or* ivermectin
Diarrhea, malabsorption (celiac-like)	*Strongyloides stercoralis*	Larval penetration	Ivermectin
Pinworm	*Enterobius vermicularis*	Egg ingestion	Albendazole *or* mebendazole *or* pyrantel pamoate
Trichinellosis	*Trichinella spiralis*	Ingestion of infected undercooked meat	Albendazole *or* mebendazole *plus* corticosteroids for severe symptoms
Abdominal angiostrongyliasis	*Angiostrongylus costaricensis*	Ingestion of contaminated food	Albendazole *or* mebendazole
Eosinophilic meningitis	*Angiostrongylus cantonensis* (rat lungworm)	Ingestion of undercooked contaminated seafood	Albendazole

tapeworm, *Baylisascaris procyonis* (see Table 123.2). These organisms also cause **ocular larva migrans.**

Visceral larva migrans is most common in young children with pica who have dogs or cats as pets. Ocular toxocariasis occurs in older children. The eggs of these roundworms are produced by adult worms residing in the dog and cat intestine. Ingested eggs hatch into larvae that penetrate the gastrointestinal tract and migrate to the liver, lung, eye, CNS, and heart, where they die and calcify.

Symptoms of visceral larva migrans are the result of the number of migrating larvae and the associated immune response. Light infections are often asymptomatic. Symptoms include fever, cough, wheezing, and seizures. Physical findings may include hepatomegaly, crackles, rash, and lymphadenopathy. Visual symptoms may include decreased acuity, strabismus, periorbital edema, or blindness. Eye examination may reveal granulomatous lesions near the macula or disc. Ocular larva migrans is generally characterized by isolated, unilateral ocular disease and no systemic findings.

Eosinophilia and hypergammaglobulinemia associated with elevated isohemagglutinin levels suggest the diagnosis, which is confirmed by serology (enzyme-linked immunosorbent assay) or, less commonly, by biopsy. This is usually a self-limited illness. In severe disease, albendazole or mebendazole is used. Deworming puppies and kittens, major excreters of eggs, decreases the risk of infection.

Enterobiasis (Pinworm)

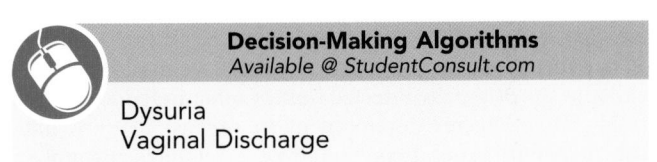

Decision-Making Algorithms
Available @ StudentConsult.com

Dysuria
Vaginal Discharge

Pinworm is caused by *Enterobius vermicularis*, a nematode that is distributed worldwide. Enterobiasis affects individuals at all socioeconomic levels, especially children. Crowded living conditions predispose to infection. Humans ingest the eggs carried on hands, present in house dust or on bedclothes. The eggs hatch in the stomach, and the larvae migrate to the cecum and mature. At night the females migrate to the perianal area to lay their eggs (up to 10,000 eggs), which remain infective in the indoor environment for 2-3 weeks.

The most common symptoms are nocturnal anal pruritus **(pruritus ani)** and sleeplessness, presumably resulting from the migratory female worms. Vaginitis and salpingitis may develop secondary to aberrant worm migration. The eggs are detected by microscopically examining adhesive cellophane tape pressed against the anus in the morning to collect eggs. Less commonly, a worm may be seen in the perianal region. Treatment is with albendazole or pyrantel pamoate each given as a single oral dose and repeated in 2 weeks.

Schistosomiasis

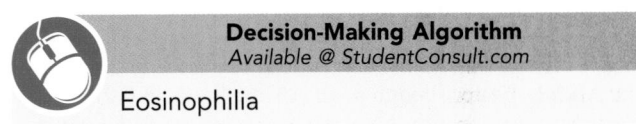

Decision-Making Algorithm
Available @ StudentConsult.com

Eosinophilia

Schistosomiasis (bilharziasis) is caused by flukes that parasitize the bloodstream, including *Schistosoma haematobium*, *S. mansoni*, *S. japonicum*, and, rarely, *S. intercalatum* and *S. mekongi* (Table 123.3). Schistosomiasis affects more than 190 million people. Humans are infected by cercariae in contaminated water that emerge in an infectious form from snails and penetrate intact skin. Each adult worm migrates to specific sites: *S.*

TABLE 123.3 Major Pediatric Syndromes Caused by Parasitic Trematodes

SYNDROME	ETIOLOGICAL AGENT	TRANSMISSION	TREATMENT
Schistosomiases		Freshwater contact with penetration through the skin	
Intestinal or hepatic schistosomiasis	*Schistosoma mansoni* *Schistosoma japonicum* *Schistosoma mekongi*		Praziquantel *or* oxamniquine
Urinary schistosomiasis	*Schistosoma haematobium*		
Parasitoses due to other trematodes		Ingestion of raw or inadequately cooked foods	
Clonorchiasis	*Clonorchis sinensis* (Chinese liver fluke)		Praziquantel *or* albendazole
Fascioliasis	*Fasciola hepatica* (sheep liver fluke)		Triclabendazole
Fasciolopsiasis	*Fasciolopsis buski*		Praziquantel
Heterophyiasis	*Heterophyes heterophyes*		Praziquantel
Metagonimiasis	*Metagonimus yokogawai*		Praziquantel
Metorchiasis	*Metorchis conjunctus* (North American liver fluke)		Praziquantel
Nanophyetiasis	*Nanophyetus salmincola* (salmon fluke)		Praziquantel
Opisthorchiasis	*Opisthorchis viverrini* (Southeast Asian liver fluke)		Praziquantel *or* albendazole
Paragonimiasis	*Paragonimus westermani, P. kellicotti, P. uterobilateralis, P. skjabini, P. heterotremus, P. africanus* (lung flukes)		Praziquantel *or* triclabendazole

TABLE 123.4 Major Pediatric Syndromes Caused by Parasitic Cestodes

SYNDROME	ETIOLOGICAL AGENT	TRANSMISSION	TREATMENT
Echinococcosis		Ingestion of *Echinococcus* eggs	
Unilocular	*E. granulosus*		Surgical resection *plus* albendazole
Alveolar echinococcosis	*E. multilocularis*		Surgical resection is only reliable means of treatment; some reports suggest adjunct use of albendazole or mebendazole
Neurocysticercosis	Larval stage of *Taenia solium* (cysticerci)	Ingestion of eggs through direct fecal-oral contact or ingestion of fecally contaminated foods	Albendazole *or* praziquantel
Adult tapeworm infections	*T. solium* (pork tapeworm)	Ingestion of contaminated raw/ undercooked pork	Praziquantel
	Hymenolepis diminuta	Ingestion of infected insect	Praziquantel
	Hymenolepis nana	Fecal-oral	Praziquantel

haematobium to the **bladder plexus** and *S. mansoni* and *S. japonicum* to the **mesenteric vessels**. The eggs are deposited by the adult flukes in urine *(S. haematobium)* or stool (*S. mansoni* and *S. japonicum*). *S. haematobium* is prevalent in Africa and the Middle East; *S. mansoni* in Africa, the Middle East, the Caribbean, and South America; *S. japonicum* in China, the Philippines, and Indonesia; *S. mekongi* in Cambodia and Laos; and *S. intercalatum* in West and Central Africa.

The manifestations of schistosomiasis result from eggs that are trapped at the site of deposition or at metastatic locations. Within 4-8 weeks of infection, while the worms are maturing, a syndrome of fever, malaise, cough, abdominal pain, hepatosplenomegaly, eosinophilia, and rash can occur **(Katayama fever)**. This syndrome is followed by a resultant inflammatory response that leads to further symptoms. Eggs may be found in the urine *(S. haematobium)* or stool (*S. mansoni* and *S. japonicum*) of infected individuals. Sanitary measures, molluscacides, and therapy for infected individuals may help control the illness.

Echinococcosis

Echinococcosis includes **hydatid or unilocular cyst disease**, caused by *Echinococcus granulosus* (the **minute dog tapeworm**), polycystic disease, caused by *Echinococcus vogeli*, and **alveolar cyst disease**, caused by *Echinococcus multilocularis* (Table 123.4). Dogs become infected with tapeworms by eating infected sheep or cattle viscera and excrete eggs in their stools. Humans acquire echinococcosis by ingesting eggs and become an intermediate host. The eggs hatch in the intestinal tract, and the larva **(oncospheres)** penetrate the mucosa and enter the circulation to pass to the liver and other visceral organs, forming cysts.

E. granulosus has a worldwide distribution and is endemic in sheep-raising and cattle-raising areas of Australia, South America, South Africa, the former Soviet Union, and the Mediterranean region. The prevalence is highest in children. Symptoms caused by *E. granulosus* result from space-occupying cysts. Pulmonary cysts may cause hemoptysis, cough, dyspnea, and respiratory distress. Brain cysts appear as tumors; liver cysts cause problems as they compress and obstruct blood flow. Ultrasonography identifies cystic lesions, and the diagnosis is confirmed by serological testing. Large or asymptomatic granulosa cysts are removed surgically. Treatment with albendazole has shown some benefit.

Neurocysticercosis

Neurocysticercosis is caused by infection with the embryonated eggs of the **pork tapeworm**, *Taenia solium*, and is the most frequent helminthic infection of the CNS (see Table 123.4). Humans are infected after consuming cysticerci in raw or undercooked larva-containing pork. Infected humans then pass *T. solium* eggs in their feces. Fecal-oral transmission of eggs, either to the originally infected host or other individuals, then results in cysticerci development in organs; in particular, subcutaneous tissues, brain, and eyes. *T. solium* is endemic in Asia, Africa, and Central and South America.

Cysts typically enlarge slowly, causing no or minimal symptoms for years or decades until the organism begins to die. The cyst then begins to swell, and leakage of antigen incites an inflammatory response, resulting in the presenting signs of focal or generalized seizures and calcified cerebral cysts identified by computed tomography or magnetic resonance imaging. The CSF shows lymphocytic or eosinophilic pleocytosis. The diagnosis is confirmed by serological testing. Neurocysticercosis is treated with albendazole or praziquantel, corticosteroids for concomitant cerebral inflammation from cyst death, and anticonvulsant drugs.

CHAPTER 124

Tuberculosis

ETIOLOGY

Mycobacterium tuberculosis bacilli are pleomorphic, weakly gram-positive curved rods that are **acid fast**, which is the capacity to form stable mycolate complexes with arylmethane dyes. *M tuberculosis* grows slowly; culture from clinical specimens on solid synthetic media usually takes 3-6 weeks. Drug-susceptibility testing requires an additional 4 weeks. Growth can be detected in 1-3 weeks in selective liquid media using radiolabeled nutrients. Polymerase chain reaction (PCR) of clinical specimens allows rapid diagnosis in many laboratories.

EPIDEMIOLOGY

It is estimated that one third of the world's population is infected with tuberculosis (TB). Most of these are latent infections. Without treatment, tuberculosis *disease* develops in 5-10% of immunologically normal adults with tuberculosis *infection* at some time during their lives; the risk is higher in infants, those who are immunocompromised, and especially HIV-positive individuals. An estimated 9 million new cases of tuberculosis occur each year worldwide, including 1 million children. One to 2 million deaths are attributed to the disease annually. Almost 10,000 TB cases were reported in the United States in 2014.

Transmission of *M. tuberculosis* is from person to person, usually by respiratory droplets that become airborne when a symptomatic individual coughs, sneezes, laughs, or even breathes. Infected droplets dry and become droplet nuclei, which may remain suspended in the air for hours, long after the infectious person has left the environment.

Several patient-related factors are associated with an increased chance of transmission. Of these, a positive acid-fast smear of the sputum most closely correlates with infectivity. Children with primary pulmonary tuberculosis disease rarely, if ever, infect others because tubercle bacilli are relatively sparse in the endobronchial secretions of children with pulmonary tuberculosis. In addition, when young children cough, they rarely produce sputum, lacking the tussive force necessary to project and suspend infectious particles of the requisite size. Hospitalized patients with suspected pulmonary tuberculosis should be placed initially in airborne isolation. Most infectious patients become noninfectious within 2 weeks of starting effective treatment. Cavitary disease, nonadherence to treatment, and resistant infection increase the risk of transmission.

In North America, tuberculosis rates are highest in foreign-born persons from high-prevalence countries, residents of prisons, residents of nursing homes, homeless persons, users of illegal drugs, persons who are poor and without health care, health care workers, and children exposed to adults in high-risk groups. Most children are infected with *M. tuberculosis* from household contacts, but outbreaks of childhood tuberculosis centered in schools, daycares, churches, school buses, and stores still occur. A high-risk adult working in the area has been the source of the outbreak in most cases. Immunodeficiency, especially from HIV infection or from immunosuppressive drugs, is an important risk factor. Certain biological response modifiers (anti-tumor necrosis factor [TNF] antibodies), often used for inflammatory conditions, can increase risk of development of tuberculosis disease.

CLINICAL MANIFESTATIONS

Decision-Making Algorithms
Available @ StudentConsult.com

Cough
Hemoptysis
Back Pain
Fever and Rash
Lymphadenopathy
Fever of Unknown Origin

Latent tuberculosis describes the asymptomatic stage of infection with *M. tuberculosis.* The tuberculin skin test (TST) or interferon-gamma release assay (IGRA) is positive, but the chest radiograph is normal or shows healed infection (calcification). **Tuberculosis disease** occurs when there are clinical signs and symptoms and/or an abnormal chest radiograph or other extrapulmonary manifestation. The interval between latent tuberculosis and the onset of disease may be several weeks in children or many decades in adults. In young children, tuberculosis usually develops as an immediate complication of the primary infection, and the distinction between infection and disease may be less obvious.

Primary tuberculosis in children is often an asymptomatic infection. Often the disease is manifested by a positive TST or IGRA with mild abnormalities on the chest radiograph, such as atelectasis or an infiltrate accompanied by hilar or other adenopathy **(Ghon complex)**. Malaise, low-grade fever, erythema nodosum, or symptoms resulting from lymph node enlargement may occur after the development of delayed hypersensitivity. **Progressive primary disease** is characterized by a primary pneumonia that develops shortly after initial infection. Progression to disseminated miliary disease or central nervous system (CNS) infection occurs most commonly in the first year of life. Cavitation is rare in children but more typical with reactivation pulmonary TB in adolescents and adults.

Tuberculous pleural effusion, which may accompany primary infection, generally represents the immune response to the organisms and most commonly occurs in older children or adolescents. Pleurocentesis reveals lymphocytes and an increased protein level, but the pleural fluid usually does not contain bacilli.

Reactivation pulmonary tuberculosis, common in adolescents and typical in adults, usually is confined to apical segments of upper lobes or superior segments of lower lobes. There is usually little lymphadenopathy and no extrathoracic infection. This is a manifestation of a secondary expansion of infection at a site seeded years previously during primary infection. Advanced disease is associated with cavitation and endobronchial spread of bacilli. Symptoms include fever, night sweats, malaise, and weight loss. A productive cough and hemoptysis often herald cavitation and bronchial erosion.

Miliary tuberculosis refers to widespread hematogenous dissemination to multiple organs. The lesions are of roughly the same size as a millet seed, from which the name *miliary* is derived. Miliary tuberculosis is characterized by fever, general malaise, weight loss, lymphadenopathy, night sweats, and hepatosplenomegaly. Diffuse bilateral pneumonitis is common, and meningitis may be present. The chest radiograph reveals bilateral miliary infiltrates, showing overwhelming infection. The TST may be nonreactive as a result of **anergy**. Liver or bone marrow biopsy may be useful for diagnosis.

Tuberculous meningitis most commonly occurs in children <5 years of age or immunocompromised patients and often within 6 months of primary infection. Tubercle bacilli that seed the meninges during the primary infection replicate, triggering an inflammatory response. This condition may have an insidious onset, initially characterized by low-grade fever, headache, and subtle personality change. Progression of the infection results in basilar meningitis with impingement of the cranial nerves and is manifested by meningeal irritation and, eventually, increased intracranial pressure, deterioration of mental status, and coma. Computed tomography (CT) scans show hydrocephalus, edema, periventricular lucencies, and infarctions. Cerebrospinal fluid (CSF) analysis reveals pleocytosis (50-500 leukocytes/mm^3), which early in the course of disease may be either lymphocytes or polymorphonuclear leukocytes. Glucose is low, and protein is significantly elevated. Acid-fast bacilli are not detected frequently in the CSF by either routine or fluorescent staining procedures. Although culture is the standard for diagnosis, PCR for *M. tuberculosis* may be useful to confirm meningitis, but lacks sensitivity.

Skeletal tuberculosis results from either hematogenous seeding or direct extension from a caseous lymph node. This is usually a chronic disease with an insidious onset that may be mistaken for chronic osteomyelitis. Radiographs reveal cortical destruction. Biopsy and culture are essential for proper diagnosis. Tuberculosis of the spine, **Pott disease**, is the most common skeletal site.

Other forms of tuberculosis include **abdominal tuberculosis** that occurs from swallowing infected material. This is a relatively uncommon complication in developed nations where dairy herds are inspected for bovine tuberculosis. Gastrointestinal TB can present with signs and symptoms similar to inflammatory bowel disease. **Tuberculous peritonitis** is associated with abdominal tuberculosis and presents as fever, anorexia, ascites, and abdominal pain. **Urogenital tuberculosis** is a late reactivation complication and is rare in children. Symptomatic illness presents as dysuria, frequency, urgency, hematuria, and *sterile* pyuria. Tuberculosis may also result in extrathoracic lymphadenitis in the cervical, supraclavicular, and submandibular areas **(scrofula)**.

Congenital tuberculosis can mimic neonatal sepsis or present at days to weeks of age with hepatosplenomegaly and respiratory disease.

LABORATORY AND IMAGING STUDIES

Two types of tests are used to detect the immune response to *M. tuberculosis* and are used to screen patients for latent tuberculosis and investigation of active tuberculosis. The TST response to tuberculin antigen is a manifestation of a T cell–mediated delayed hypersensitivity. The **Mantoux test**, an intradermal injection of 5 TU (tuberculin units) of **purified protein derivative standard (PPD-S)**, usually on the volar surface of the forearm, is the standard TST. It is usually positive 2-6 weeks after onset of infection (up to 3 months) and at the time of symptomatic illness. This test is preferred in children less than 5 years of age (Table 124.1). False-negative responses may occur early in the illness, with overwhelming TB infection, with concomitant viral infection, or as a result of immunosuppression (secondary to underlying illness, HIV, or malnutrition). Tests with questionable results should be repeated after several weeks. All internationally adopted children with an initially negative TST should have a repeat TST after 3 months in the United States. The TST is interpreted based on the host status and size of induration (Table 124.2). In general, interpretation of TST in people who have had previous **bacille Calmette-Guérin** (BCG) vaccine can be difficult, given the cross reaction of TST with antigens present in the vaccine. However, in situations when a tuberculosis exposure has occurred, the TST should be read and interpreted as if no vaccine had been given.

An **IGRA** is a whole blood test that measures interferon-gamma production by T lymphocytes in response to antigens from the *M. tuberculosis* complex, which includes *M. bovis* but not antigens found in the BCG vaccine. An IGRA is the recommended diagnostic test for persons older than 5 years of age in the United States. It has similar sensitivity to the TST but improved specificity because it is unaffected by prior BCG vaccination. It is also practically easier to obtain, as it requires only one visit to complete. As with the TST, in immunocompromised persons and in active tuberculosis, IGRA findings may be indeterminate.

The ultimate diagnostic confirmation relies on culture of the organism. Sputum is an excellent source for diagnosis in pulmonary disease in adults but is difficult to obtain in young children. Induced sputum or gastric fluid obtained via an indwelling nasogastric tube with samples taken before or immediately on waking contains swallowed sputum and provides alternate samples in young children. Large volumes of fluid (CSF, pericardial fluid) yield a higher rate of recovery of organisms, but slow growth of the mycobacteria makes culture less helpful in acute illness. Even with optimal collection, cultures are positive

TABLE 124.1 Tuberculin Skin Test Recommendations for Infants, Children, and Adolescents*

CHILDREN FOR WHOM IMMEDIATE TST OR IGRA IS INDICATED†:
• Contacts of people with confirmed or suspected contagious tuberculosis (contact investigation) • Children with radiographic or clinical findings suggesting tuberculosis disease • Children immigrating from countries with endemic infection (e.g., Asia, Middle East, Africa, Latin America, countries of the former Soviet Union), including international adoptees • Children with travel histories to countries with endemic infection and substantial contact with indigenous people from such countries
CHILDREN WHO SHOULD HAVE ANNUAL TST OR IGRA‡:
• Children infected with HIV infection (TST only)
CHILDREN AT INCREASED RISK OF PROGRESSION OF LTBI TO TUBERCULOSIS DISEASE:
• Children with other medical conditions, including diabetes mellitus, chronic renal failure, malnutrition, and congenital or acquired immunodeficiencies, deserve special consideration. Without recent exposure, these people are not at increased risk of acquiring tuberculosis infection. Underlying immune deficiencies associated with these conditions theoretically would enhance the possibility for progression to severe disease. Initial histories of potential exposure to tuberculosis should be included for all of these patients. If these histories or local epidemiological factors suggest a possibility of exposure, immediate and periodic TST or IGRA should be considered. **A TST or IGRA should be performed before initiation of immunosuppressive therapy, including prolonged steroid administration, organ transplantation, use of tumor necrosis factor-alpha antagonists or blockers, or other immunosuppressive therapy in any child requiring these treatments.**

**Bacille Calmette-Guérin immunization is not a contraindication to a TST.*
†Beginning as early as 3 months of age.
‡If the child is well, the TST or IGRA should be delayed for up to 10 weeks after return.
HIV, Human immunodeficiency virus; *IGRA*, interferon-gamma release assay; *LTBI*, latent tuberculosis infection; *TST*, tuberculin skin test.
From Recommendations from American Academy of Pediatrics. Tuberculosis. In: Kimberlin DW, Brady MT, Jackson MA, Long SS, eds. Red Book: 2015 Report of the Committee on Infectious Diseases. *30th ed. Elk Grove Village, IL: American Academy of Pediatrics; 2015. Copyright 2015 American Academy of Pediatrics. Reproduced with permission.*

TABLE 124.2 Criteria for Positive Tuberculin Skin Test Results in Clinically Defined Pediatric Populations*

POSITIVE RESULT	POPULATION(S)
Induration ≥5 mm	Children in close contact with persons with known or suspected contagious tuberculosis disease
	Children suspected to have tuberculosis disease
	Findings on chest radiograph consistent with active or previously active tuberculosis
	Clinical evidence of tuberculosis disease†
	Children receiving immunosuppressive therapy‡ or with immunosuppressive conditions, including HIV infection
Induration ≥10 mm	Children at increased risk for disseminated disease
	Children <4 yr of age
	Children with other medical conditions, including Hodgkin disease, lymphoma, diabetes mellitus, chronic renal failure, and malnutrition
	Children with increased exposure to tuberculosis disease
	Children born, or whose parents were born, in high-prevalence regions of the world
	Children frequently exposed to adults who are HIV-infected, homeless, users of illicit drugs, residents of nursing homes, incarcerated or institutionalized, or migrant farm workers
	Children who travel to high-prevalence regions of the world
Induration ≥15 mm	Children ≥4 yr of age without any risk factors

*These criteria apply regardless of previous BCG immunization. Erythema at tuberculin skin test site does not indicate a positive test result. Tuberculin reactions should be read at 48-72 hours after placement.
†Evidence by physical examination or laboratory assessment that would include tuberculosis in the working differential diagnosis (e.g., meningitis).
‡Including immunosuppressive doses of corticosteroids.
BCG, Bacille Calmette-Guérin; *HIV*, human immunodeficiency virus.

in less than half of children with tuberculosis. When the organism is grown, drug susceptibilities should be determined because of the increasing incidence of resistant organisms. Utilization of culture and susceptibility results from the source case is often necessary given the difficulty of obtaining timely results.

PCR testing for mycobacteria has expedited diagnosis, especially with CNS disease. However, these assays have limited sensitivity and provide no susceptibility data. Most experts would recommend that young infants <12 months of age with suspected tuberculosis undergo lumbar puncture for evaluation of CNS involvement.

Diagnostic Imaging

Because many cases of pulmonary tuberculosis in children are clinically relatively silent, radiography is a cornerstone for the diagnosis of disease (Figs. 124.1 and 124.2). All lobar segments of the lung are at equal risk of being the focus of the initial infection. In 25% of cases, two or more lobes of the lungs are involved, although disease usually occurs at one site only. Spread of infection to regional lymph nodes occurs early. Hilar lymphadenopathy is inevitably present with childhood tuberculosis. Partial bronchial obstruction caused by external compression from the enlarging nodes can cause air trapping, hyperinflation, and lobar emphysema. Occasionally children have a picture of lobar pneumonia without impressive hilar lymphadenopathy. If the infection is progressively destructive, liquefaction of the lung parenchyma leads to formation of a thin-walled primary tuberculous cavity. Adolescents with pulmonary tuberculosis may develop segmental lesions with hilar lymphadenopathy or the apical infiltrates, with or without cavitation, that are typical of adult reactivation tuberculosis.

Radiographic studies aid greatly in the diagnosis of **extrapulmonary tuberculosis** in children. Plain radiographs, CT, and magnetic resonance imaging (MRI) of the tuberculous spine usually show collapse and destruction of the vertebral body with narrowing of the involved disk spaces. Radiographic findings in bone and joint tuberculosis range from mild joint effusions and small lytic lesions to massive destruction of the bone. CT or MRI of the brains of patients with CNS involvement may be normal during early stages of the infection. As disease progresses, basilar enhancement and communicating hydrocephalus with signs of cerebral edema or early focal ischemia are the most common findings.

Granulomas on pathology of tissue can also help to establish the diagnosis of tuberculosis on samples from lymph nodes and other biopsies.

DIFFERENTIAL DIAGNOSIS

The differential diagnosis of tuberculosis includes a multitude of diagnoses because tuberculosis may affect any organ, and in early disease the symptoms and signs may be nonspecific. In pulmonary disease, tuberculosis may appear similar to bacterial or fungal pneumonia, malignancy, and any systemic disease in which generalized lymphadenopathy occurs. The diagnosis of tuberculosis should be suspected if the TST or IGRA is positive or if there is history of tuberculosis exposure.

The differential diagnosis of tuberculous lymphadenopathy includes infections caused by atypical mycobacteria, *Bartonella*, fungi, viruses, and bacteria, as well as toxoplasmosis, sarcoidosis, drug reactions, and malignancy.

TREATMENT

Combination therapy is the backbone of therapy for tuberculosis disease to prevent the emergence of resistance. The treatment of tuberculosis is affected by the presence of naturally occurring drug-resistant organisms in large bacterial populations, even before therapy is initiated, and the fact that mycobacteria replicate slowly and can remain dormant in the body for prolonged periods. Patients with latent tuberculosis infection have small bacterial populations, and a single drug, such as **isoniazid (INH)**, can be given for 9 months. Therapy for latent infection is aimed at eradicating organisms sequestered within macrophages and suppressed by normal T-cell activity. Children with primary pulmonary tuberculosis and patients with extrapulmonary tuberculosis have medium-sized populations in which significant numbers of drug-resistant organisms may or may not be present. In general these patients are treated

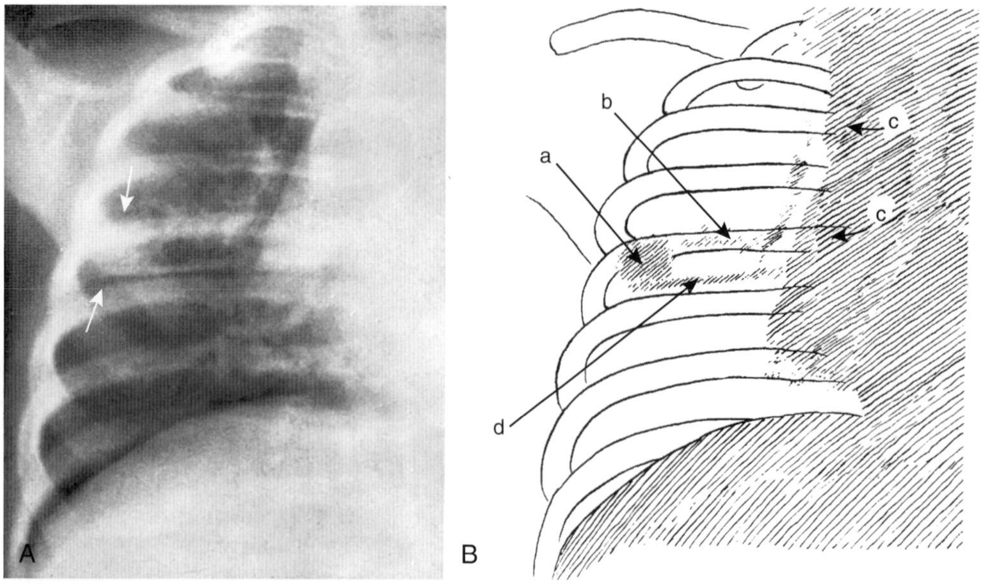

FIGURE 124.1 Fresh primary tuberculous complex in an infant 4 months of age. The pulmonary focus is the small shadow of increased density *(arrows)* in the inferolateral segment of the right upper lobe. **(A)** Roentgenogram. **(B)** Schematic drawing: *a*, primary focus; *b*, lymphangitis; *c*, enlarged hilar and mediastinal nodes; *d*, loculated pleural exudate. (From Silverman FN, Kuhn JP, et al. *Essentials of Caffey's Pediatric X-Ray Diagnosis*. Philadelphia: Saunders; 1990:292. Fig. 11.23.)

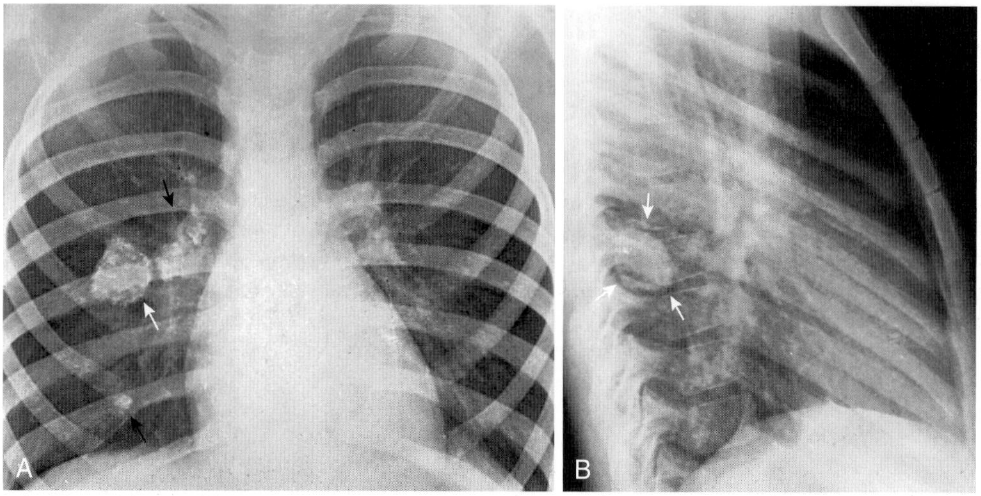

FIGURE 124.2 Huge calcifying primary tuberculous focus in the right lower lobe that dwarfs the rest of the complex in an asymptomatic girl 6 years of age. The healing and calcification of this huge necrotic focus without manifest clinical disease at any time demonstrates the often benign clinical aspects of severe structural tuberculous disease. In **(A)**, a frontal projection, the large calcifying focus appears to be perihilar, but in **(B)**, a lateral projection, this focus lies far behind the lung root in a dorsal sub-segment of the right lower lobe near the dorsal pleura. (From Silverman FN, Kuhn JP, et al. *Essentials of Caffey's Pediatric X-Ray Diagnosis*. Philadelphia: Saunders; 1990:293. Fig. 11.26.)

with at least two drugs (Table 124.3) for a prolonged course, typically 6-9 months, depending on the type of disease. Isoniazid and **rifampin (RIF)** are bactericidal for *M. tuberculosis*. Along with pyrazinamide ± ethambutol, they form the backbone of the antimicrobial treatment of tuberculosis. Other drugs and prolonged regimens are used in special circumstances, such as CNS infection and multidrug-resistant **(MDR)** or extensively drug-resistant (**XDR**) tuberculosis, which are unfortunately increasing in prevalence in some parts of the world, and are associated with increased treatment failure and mortality.

In the United States, drug-susceptible pulmonary tuberculosis is treated with 2 months of four drugs and then completed with INH and RIF for an additional 4 months. Noncompliance, or nonadherence, is a major problem in tuberculosis control because of the long-term nature of treatment and the sometimes difficult social circumstances of the patients. As treatment regimens become shorter, adherence assumes an even greater importance. Improvement in compliance occurs with **directly observed therapy (DOT)**, which requires a health care worker to witness the administration of medications and is the standard of care in most settings.

TABLE 124.3 Recommended Treatment Regimens for Drug-Susceptible Tuberculosis in Infants, Children, and Adolescents

INFECTION OR DISEASE CATEGORY	REGIMEN	COMMENTS
LATENT TUBERCULOSIS INFECTION (POSITIVE TEST RESULT, NO DISEASE)		
Isoniazid-susceptible	9 mo of isoniazid, once a day	If daily therapy is not possible, DOT twice a week can be used for 9 mo.
Isoniazid-resistant	6 mo of rifampin, once a day	
Isoniazid-rifampin–resistant	Consult a tuberculosis specialist	
Pulmonary and extrapulmonary (except meningitis)	2 mo of isoniazid, rifampin, and pyrazinamide daily, followed by 4 mo of isoniazid and rifampin twice weekly under DOT	If possible drug resistance is a concern, another drug (ethambutol or an aminoglycoside) is added to the initial three-drug therapy until drug susceptibilities are determined. DOT is highly desirable.
		If hilar lymphadenopathy only, a 6-mo course of isoniazid and rifampin is sufficient.
		Drugs can be given 2 or 3 times per week under DOT in the initial phase if nonadherence is likely.
Meningitis	2 mo of isoniazid, rifampin, pyrazinamide, and an aminoglycoside or ethionamide, once a day, followed by 7-10 mo of isoniazid and rifampin, once a day or twice a week (9-12 mo total)	A fourth drug, usually an aminoglycoside, is given with initial therapy until drug susceptibility is known.
		For patients who may have acquired tuberculosis in geographic areas where resistance to streptomycin is common, capreomycin, kanamycin, or amikacin may be used instead of streptomycin.

DOT, Directly observed therapy; *TST*, tuberculin skin test.
From Recommendations from Kimberlin DW, Brady MT, Jackson MA, Long SS, et al. Red Book: 2015 Report of the Committee on Infectious Diseases. *30th ed. Elk Grove Village, IL: American Academy of Pediatrics; 2015. Copyright 2015 American Academy of Pediatrics. Reproduced with permission.*

COMPLICATIONS AND PROGNOSIS

The prognosis of tuberculosis in infants, children, and adolescents is excellent with early recognition and effective chemotherapy. In most children with pulmonary tuberculosis, the disease completely resolves, and ultimately radiographic findings are normal. The prognosis for children with bone and joint tuberculosis and tuberculous meningitis depends directly on the stage of disease at the time antituberculosis medications are started. Tuberculosis of the spine may result in angulation or **gibbus** formation that requires surgical correction after the infection is cured. Most childhood tuberculous meningitis occurs in developing countries, where the prognosis is poor. Resistant organisms are more difficult to treat and worsen prognosis.

PREVENTION

Tuberculosis control programs work on case finding and treatment, which interrupts secondary transmission of infection from close contacts. Infected close contacts are identified by positive TST or IGRA testing and can be started on appropriate treatment to prevent transmission.

Prevention of transmission in health care settings involves appropriate physical ventilation of the air around the source case. Offices, clinics, and hospital rooms used by adults with possible tuberculosis should have adequate ventilation, with air exhausted to the outside (**negative-pressure ventilation**). Health care providers should have annual screening with a TST or IGRA.

The only available vaccine against tuberculosis is the BCG vaccine. The original vaccine organism was a strain of attenuated *Mycobacterium bovis*. The preferred route of administration is intradermal injection with a syringe and needle because this is the only method that permits accurate measurement of an individual dose. The official recommendation of the World Health Organization is a single dose administered during infancy. This vaccine is not routinely used in the United States. Some studies show BCG provides 80-90% protection from tuberculosis, and other studies show no protective efficacy at all. In general it is thought that vaccination reduces the incidence of miliary disease and TB meningitis in infants. Many who receive BCG vaccine never have a positive TST reaction. When a reaction does occur, the induration size is usually less than 10 mm, and variably wanes after several years. BCG vaccination does not affect results of an IGRA.

CHAPTER 125

Human Immunodeficiency Virus and Acquired Immunodeficiency Syndrome

ETIOLOGY

The cause of acquired immunodeficiency syndrome (AIDS) is the human immunodeficiency virus (HIV), a single-stranded

RNA virus of the retrovirus family that produces a reverse transcriptase enabling the viral RNA to act as a template for DNA transcription and integration into the host genome. HIV-1 causes 99% of all human cases. HIV-2, which is less virulent, causes 1-9% of cases in parts of Africa and is very rare in the United States.

HIV infects **helper T cells (CD4 cells)** and cells of monocyte-macrophage lineage via interaction of viral protein gp120 with the CD4 molecule and chemokines (CXCR4 and CCR5) that serve as coreceptors. Interaction with these molecules facilitates membrane fusion and cell entry by the virus. HIV infection directly and indirectly depletes CD4 T cells. Because helper T cells are important for delayed hypersensitivity, T cell–dependent B-cell antibody production, and T cell–mediated lymphokine activation of macrophages, their destruction produces a profound combined (B and T cell) immunodeficiency. A lack of T-cell regulation and unrestrained antigenic stimulation result in polyclonal hypergammaglobulinemia with nonspecific and ineffective globulins. Other cells bearing CD4, such as microglia, astrocytes, oligodendroglia, and placental tissues, also may be infected with HIV.

HIV infection is a continuously progressive process with a variable period of clinical latency before development of AIDS-defining conditions. All untreated patients have evidence of ongoing viral replication and progressive CD4 lymphocyte depletion. There are no overt manifestations of immunodeficiency until CD4 cell numbers decline to critical threshold levels. Quantitation of the viral load (HIV-1 RNA level) has become an important parameter in management.

Horizontal transmission of HIV is by sexual contact (vaginal, anal, or orogenital), percutaneous contact (from contaminated needles or other sharp objects), or mucous membrane exposure to contaminated blood or body fluid. Transmission by contaminated blood and blood products has been eliminated in developed countries by screening donated blood products, but still occurs in developing countries. **Vertical transmission** of HIV from mother to infant may occur transplacentally in utero, during birth, or via breast feeding. Risk factors for perinatal transmission include prematurity, prolonged rupture of membranes, and high maternal HIV viral load at delivery. In non–breast feeding infants, perinatal transmission can be decreased from approximately 25% to less than 8% with administration of intravenous (IV) zidovudine during labor and postnatal treatment of the infant with oral zidovudine. Maternal treatment during pregnancy with combination antiretroviral therapy (cART) can reduce the risk of transmission to <1%. Breast feeding by HIV-infected mothers increases the risk of vertical transmission. In developing countries where breast feeding is associated with increased survival and decreased morbidity from malnutrition, diarrheal diseases, and other infections, continued administration of either cART for the mother or postnatal prophylactic ART for the infant can reduce transmission risk from breast feeding. In untreated infants, the mean incubation interval for development of an AIDS-defining condition after vertical transmission is 5 months (range, 1-24 months) compared with a longer incubation period after horizontal transmission of 7-10 years.

EPIDEMIOLOGY

Worldwide, as of 2015, approximately 36.7 million persons are living with HIV, and 3.4 million of them are children. There were 2.1 million new infections in 2015 with approximately 150,000 new infections in children. Approximately 70% of all people living with HIV reside in sub-Saharan Africa. Worldwide, 1.1 million people died from HIV-related illnesses in 2015. In 2012 the estimated number of people over the age of 13 years and living with HIV in the United States was 1.2 million, and approximately 2,000 children have perinatally-acquired infection. Vertical transmission is much less common than previously, and approximately 100 infants each year in the United States acquire HIV perinatally. Most pediatric cases in the United States occur in adolescents who engage in unprotected sexual activities. Worldwide the number of deaths related to HIV and the numbers of children infected with HIV have steadily decreased in large part due to treatment with antiretroviral therapy.

CLINICAL MANIFESTATIONS

Decision-Making Algorithms
Available @ StudentConsult.com

Neck Masses
Hoarseness
Diarrhea
Arthritis
Fever and Rash
Lymphadenopathy
Anemia
Petechiae/Purpura
Failure to Thrive

In adolescents and adults, primary infection results in the **acute retroviral syndrome** (resembling mononucleosis) that develops after an incubation period of 2-6 weeks and consists of fever, malaise, weight loss, pharyngitis, lymphadenopathy, and often a maculopapular rash. The risk of opportunistic infections and other AIDS-defining conditions is related to the depletion of CD4 T cells. A combination of CD4 cell count and percentage and clinical manifestations is used to classify HIV infection in children (Tables 125.1 and 125.2).

Initial symptoms with vertical transmission vary and may include failure to thrive, neurodevelopmental delay, lymphadenopathy, hepatosplenomegaly, chronic or recurrent diarrhea, interstitial pneumonitis, or oral thrush. These findings may be subtle and remarkable only by their persistence. Manifestations that are more common in children than adults with HIV infection include recurrent bacterial infections, lymphoid hyperplasia, chronic parotid swelling, lymphocytic interstitial pneumonitis, and earlier onset of progressive neurological deterioration. Pulmonary manifestations of HIV infection are common and include *Pneumocystis jiroveci* pneumonia, which can present early in infancy as a primary pneumonia characterized by hypoxia, tachypnea, retractions, elevated serum lactate dehydrogenase, and fever.

In the United States, most pregnant women are screened and, if indicated, treated for HIV infection. Women with high HIV viral loads at delivery will be offered a cesarean section. All infants born to HIV-infected mothers are bathed prior to receiving their newborn hepatitis B vaccine and vitamin K injection, receive antiretroviral prophylaxis, are exclusively formula

TABLE 125.1 2014 Human Immunodeficiency Virus Pediatric Classification System: Immune Categories

	LABORATORY CRITERIA					
	<12 MO		1 TO <6 YR		≥6 YR	
IMMUNE CATEGORY	CD4+ CELLS/MM³	% TOTAL LYMPHOCYTES	CD4+ CELLS/MM³	% TOTAL LYMPHOCYTES	CD4+ CELLS/MM³	% TOTAL LYMPHOCYTES
Category 1 (no suppression)	≥1,500	≥34	≥1,000	≥30	≥500	≥26
Category 2 (moderate suppression)	750-1,499	26-33	500-999	22-29	200-499	14-25
Category 3 (severe suppression)	<750	<26	<500	<22	<200	<14

From Centers for Disease Control and Prevention. Revised Surveillance Case Definition for HIV Infection—United States, 2014. MMWR. 2014;63(No. RR-3):1–10.

TABLE 125.2 Human Immunodeficiency Virus–Related Symptoms

MILD HIV-RELATED SYMPTOMS

Children with two or more of the conditions listed but none of the conditions listed in Moderate Symptoms category:

- Lymphadenopathy (≥0.5 cm at more than 2 sites; bilateral at 1 site)
- Hepatomegaly
- Splenomegaly
- Dermatitis
- Parotitis
- Recurrent or persistent upper respiratory tract infection, sinusitis, or otitis media

MODERATE HIV-RELATED SYMPTOMS

- Anemia (hemoglobin <8 g/dL), neutropenia (white blood cell count <1,000/µL), and/or thrombocytopenia (platelet count <100 × 10³/µL) persisting for ≥30 mo
- Bacterial meningitis, pneumonia, or sepsis (single episode)
- Candidiasis, oropharyngeal (thrush), persisting (>2 mo) in children older than age 6 mo
- Cardiomyopathy
- Cytomegalovirus infection, with onset before 1 mo
- Diarrhea, recurrent or chronic
- Hepatitis
- Herpes simplex virus (HSV) stomatitis, recurrent (>2 episodes within 1 yr)
- HSV bronchitis, pneumonitis, or esophagitis with onset before 1 mo
- Herpes zoster (shingles) involving at least 2 distinct episodes or more than 1 dermatome
- Leiomyosarcoma
- Lymphoid interstitial pneumonia or pulmonary lymphoid hyperplasia complex
- Nephropathy
- Nocardiosis
- Persistent fever (lasting >1 mo)
- Toxoplasmosis, onset before 1 mo
- Varicella, disseminated (complicated chickenpox)

STAGE-3-DEFINING OPPORTUNISTIC ILLNESSES IN HIV INFECTION

- Bacterial infections, multiple or recurrent*
- Candidiasis of bronchi, trachea, or lungs
- Candidiasis of esophagus
- Cervical cancer, invasive†
- Coccidioidomycosis, disseminated or extrapulmonary
- Cryptococcosis, extrapulmonary
- Cryptosporidiosis, chronic intestinal (>1 mo duration)
- Cytomegalovirus disease (other than liver, spleen, or nodes), onset at age >1 mo
- Cytomegalovirus retinitis (with loss of vision)
- Encephalopathy attributed to HIV
- HSV: chronic ulcers (>1 mo duration) or bronchitis, pneumonitis, or esophagitis (onset at age >1 mo)
- Histoplasmosis, disseminated or extrapulmonary
- Isosporiasis, chronic intestinal (>1 mo duration)
- Kaposi sarcoma
- Lymphoma, Burkitt (or equivalent term)
- Lymphoma, immunoblastic (or equivalent term)
- Lymphoma, primary, of brain
- *Mycobacterium avium* complex or *Mycobacterium kansasii*, disseminated or extrapulmonary
- *Mycobacterium tuberculosis* of any site, pulmonary, disseminated, or extrapulmonary
- *Mycobacterium*, other species or unidentified species, disseminated or extrapulmonary
- *Pneumocystis jirovecii* (previously known as *Pneumocystis carinii*) pneumonia
- Pneumonia, recurrent†
- Progressive multifocal leukoencephalopathy
- *Salmonella* septicemia, recurrent
- Toxoplasmosis of brain, onset at age >1 mo
- Wasting syndrome attributed to HIV

Only among children aged <6 years.
†*Only among adults, adolescents, and children aged ≥6 years.*
HIV, Human immunodeficiency virus; *HSV*, herpes simplex virus.
From the Panel on Antiretroviral Therapy and Medical Management of HIV-Infected Children. Guidelines for the Use of Antiretroviral Agents in Pediatric HIV Infection. Available at http://aidsinfo.nih.gov/contentfiles/lvguidelines/pediatricguidelines.pdf. *[Table 6].*

fed, and are prospectively tested for infection. The diagnosis of HIV infection in most infants born in the United States is confirmed before development of clinical signs of infection.

LABORATORY AND IMAGING STUDIES

HIV infection can be diagnosed definitively in non–breast fed infants by 1 month of age and in virtually all infected infants by 6 months of age using viral diagnostic assays (RNA polymerase chain reaction [PCR] or DNA PCR). Maternal antibodies may be detectable until 12-15 months of age, and a positive serological test in the infant is not considered diagnostic until 18 months of age. HIV PCR (RNA or DNA) is the preferred method for diagnosing HIV infection during infancy and identifies ~50% of infected newborns at 48 hours and ~90% at 28 days. Timing of diagnostic viral testing varies depending on specific risk factors but typically involves testing at 1-2 weeks of age, at 1-2 months of age, and at 4-6 months of age. Testing at birth should be considered for infants at high risk for in utero infection (high maternal HIV viral load at delivery). HIV RNA PCR has 25-60% sensitivity during the first weeks of life, increasing to 90-100% by 2-3 months of age.

HIV infection of an exposed infant is confirmed if virological tests are positive on two separate occasions. HIV infection can be reasonably excluded in non–breast fed infants with at least two virological tests performed at older than 1 month of age, with one test being performed after 4 months of age. Loss of HIV antibody combined with negative HIV DNA PCR confirms absence of HIV infection. Persistence of a positive HIV antibody test after 18 months of age indicates HIV infection.

DIFFERENTIAL DIAGNOSIS

The differential diagnosis of AIDS in infants includes primary immunodeficiency syndromes and intrauterine infections such as cytomegalovirus (CMV) and syphilis. Prominence of individual symptoms, such as diarrhea, may suggest other etiologies.

TABLE 125.3 Indications for Initiation of Therapy in Antiretroviral Naive Children Infected With Human Immunodeficiency Virus

AGE	CRITERIA	RECOMMENDATION
<12 mo	Regardless of clinical symptoms, immune status, or viral load	Urgent treatment
1 to <6 yr	CDC Stage 3-defining opportunistic illnesses CDC Stage 3 immunodeficiency. CD4 <500 cells/mm^3	Urgent treatment
	Moderate HIV-related symptoms CD4 cell count 500-999 cells/mm^3	Treat within 1-2 wk, including an expedited discussion on adherence
	Asymptomatic or mild symptoms **and** CD4 cell count ≥1,000 cells/mm^3	Treat*
≥6 yr	CDC Stage 3-defining opportunistic illnesses CDC Stage 3 immunodeficiency. CD4 <200 cells/mm^3	Urgent treatment
	Moderate HIV-related symptoms CD4 cell count 200-499 cells/mm^3	Treat within 1-2 wk, including an expedited discussion on adherence
	Asymptomatic or mild symptoms **and** CD4 cell count ≥500 cells/mm^3	Treat*

**More time can be taken to fully assess and address issues associated with adherence with the caregivers and the child prior to initiating therapy. Patients/caregivers may choose to postpone therapy, and on a case-by-case basis, providers may elect to defer therapy based on clinical and/or psychosocial factors.*

From the Panel on Antiretroviral Therapy and Medical Management of HIV-Infected Children. Guidelines for the Use of Antiretroviral Agents in Pediatric HIV Infection. Available at http://aidsinfo.nih.gov/contentfiles/lvguidelines/pediatricguidelines.pdf. *[page F-2].*

TREATMENT

Management of HIV infection in children and adolescents is evolving and complex. It should be directed by a specialist in the treatment of HIV infection. cART is recommended for all HIV-infected children; however, urgency of cART initiation is based on age, the severity of HIV disease as indicated by AIDS-defining conditions, and the risk of disease progression as indicated by CD4 cell count (Table 125.3). Initiation of antiretroviral therapy while the patient is still asymptomatic may preserve immune function and prevent clinical progression but incurs the adverse effects of therapy and may facilitate emergence of drug-resistant virus if medication adherence is poor.

Urgent initiation of therapy (see Table 125.3) is recommended for infants less than 12 months of age regardless of symptoms of HIV disease or HIV RNA level. Urgent initiation of therapy is recommended for all children >1 year of age with AIDS or significant HIV-related symptoms or severe immunosuppression (CD4 below 500 cells/mm^3 for children ages 1 to ≤6 years and below 200 cells/mm^3 for children >6 years of age), regardless of symptoms or HIV RNA level. For all other children not meeting criteria for urgent cART initiation, more time can be taken to fully assess and address issues associated with adherence prior to initiating therapy.

Effective cART significantly reduces viral loads and leads to the amelioration of clinical symptoms and opportunistic infections. Combination therapy that includes either a non-nucleoside reverse transcriptase inhibitor (NNRTI), a protease inhibitor (PI), or an integrase inhibitor depending on the child's age plus a dual–nucleoside/nucleotide reverse transcriptase inhibitor (NRTI) backbone is recommended for initial treatment of all HIV infected children. The goal of therapy is to reduce the HIV viral load to below the level of detection and normalize or preserve the patient's immune status. The most recent specific recommendations for treatment regimens (http://aidsinfo.nih.gov/guidelines/) should be consulted before initiating therapy for any patient.

The ability of HIV to develop resistance to antiretroviral agents rapidly and the development of cross-resistance to several classes of agents simultaneously are major problems. Determination of HIV viral load, CD4 cell count, and HIV resistance genotype is essential for monitoring and modifying antiretroviral treatment.

Routine immunizations are recommended but may result in suboptimal immune responses. In addition to 13-valent pneumococcal conjugate vaccine, 23-valent pneumococcal polysaccharide vaccine is recommended for HIV-infected children at 2 years of age and adolescents and adults with CD4 counts at or above 200/mm^3. Because of the risk of fatal measles in children with AIDS, children without severe immunosuppression should receive their first dose of MMR at 12 months of age and the second dose at 4-6 years of age. Varicella-zoster virus (VZV) vaccine should be given only to asymptomatic, nonimmunosuppressed children beginning at 12 months of age as two doses of vaccine at least 3 months apart. Inactivated split influenza virus vaccine should be administered annually to all HIV-infected children at or after 6 months of age.

COMPLICATIONS

The approach to the numerous opportunistic infections in HIV-infected patients involves treatment and prophylaxis for infections likely to occur as CD4 cells are depleted. With potent antiretroviral therapy and immune reconstitution, routine prophylaxis for common opportunistic infections depends on the child's age and CD4 count. Infants born to HIV-infected mothers receive prophylaxis for *P. jiroveci* pneumonia with trimethoprim-sulfamethoxazole (TMP-SMX) beginning at 4-6 weeks of age and continued for the first year of life or until HIV infection has been excluded. TMP-SMX prophylaxis for *P. jiroveci* pneumonia for older children and adolescents is provided if CD4 cell counts are less than 500 cells/mm^3 or CD4 percentage <15% for children 1 to <6 years of age, or less than 200 cells/mm^3 or CD4 percentage <15% for children <6 years of age. Clarithromycin prophylaxis for *Mycobacterium avium* complex infection is provided if CD4 cell counts are below 750 cells/mm^3 for children <1 year of age, below 500 cells/mm^3 for children 1 to <2 years of age, below 75 cells/mm^3 for children 2 to <6 years of age, and below 50 cells/mm^3 for children ≥6 years of age.

P. jiroveci pneumonia is treated with high-dose TMP-SMX and corticosteroids. Oral and gastrointestinal candidiasis is common in children and usually responds to fluconazole therapy. VZV infection may be severe and should be treated with acyclovir or other antivirals. Recurrent herpes simplex virus (HSV) infections also may require long-term antiviral prophylaxis. Other common infections in HIV-infected patients include toxoplasmosis, CMV, Epstein-Barr virus infection, salmonellosis, and tuberculosis.

PROGNOSIS

The availability of cART has improved the prognosis for HIV and AIDS dramatically. Risk of death is directly related to the degree of immunosuppression, viral load, and young age. Children less than 1 year of age with very low CD4 percentiles and high viral loads have the poorest prognosis.

PREVENTION

Identification of HIV-infected women before or during pregnancy is crucial to providing optimal therapy for infected women and their infants and to preventing perinatal transmission. Prenatal HIV counseling and testing with consent should be provided for all pregnant women in the United States.

The rate of vertical transmission is reduced to less than 8% by chemoprophylaxis with a regimen of oral zidovudine to the mother started during pregnancy, continued during delivery with IV zidovudine, and then administered orally to the newborn for the first 6 weeks of life. Administration of maternal cART throughout pregnancy to achieve viral suppression (viral load <1,000 copies/mL) with postnatal antiretroviral prophylaxis to the infant reduces the risk of transmission even further to <1% in non–breast feeding infants. The current recommendations for the United States include a 4- to -6-week prophylactic regimen with zidovudine for the infant in combination with maternal intrapartum therapy. The maternal regimen includes continuation or initiation of antiretroviral therapy. In high-risk situations (e.g., mother's viral load is >1,000 copies/mL or is unknown, mother did not receive cART during pregnancy), intravenous zidovudine during delivery is administered and additional antiretrovirals may be given to the infant postnatally (http://aidsinfo.nih.gov/contentfiles/lvguidelines/peri_recommendations.pdf). Scheduled cesarean section at 38 weeks to prevent vertical transmission is recommended for women with HIV RNA levels greater than 1,000 copies/mL, but it is unclear whether cesarean section is beneficial when viral load is less than 1,000 copies/mL or when membranes have already ruptured.

Preventing HIV infection in adults decreases the incidence of infection in children. Adult prevention results from behavior changes such as safe-sex practices, decrease in intravenous drug use, and needle exchange programs. Screening of blood donors has almost eliminated the risk of HIV transmission from blood products. HIV infection almost never is transmitted in a casual or nonsexual household setting.

Suggested Readings

Bennett JE, Dolin R, Blaser MJ. *Mandell, Douglas, and Bennett's Principles and Practice of Infectious Diseases.* 8th ed. Philadelphia: Elsevier; 2015.

Cherry JD, Harrison GJ, Kaplan SL, et al. *Textbook of Pediatric Infectious Diseases.* 7th ed. Philadelphia: Saunders; 2014.

Isaacs D. *Evidence-Based Pediatric Infectious Disease.* Malden, MA: Blackwell Publishing; 2007.

Kimberlin DW, Brady MT, Jackson MA, et al. *Red Book: 2015 Report of the Committee on Infectious Diseases.* 30th ed. Elk Grove Village, IL: American Academy of Pediatrics; 2015.

Kliegman RM, Stanton B, St Geme JW, et al. *Nelson Textbook of Pediatrics.* 20th ed. Philadelphia: Elsevier; 2016.

Long SS, Pickering LK, Prober CG. *Principles and Practice of Pediatric Infectious Diseases.* 4th ed. Philadelphia: Churchill Livingstone; 2012.

Plotkin SA, Orenstein WA, Offit PA. *Vaccines.* 6th ed. Philadelphia: Saunders; 2013.

PEARLS FOR PRACTITIONERS

CHAPTER 93

Infectious Disease Assessment

- A complete infectious diseases history should include environmental exposures, sick contacts, travel, immune status, and immunization history.
- Routine screening tests may include complete blood count with differential, inflammatory markers, transaminases, urinalysis and culture, lumbar puncture, or blood culture.
- A microbiologic diagnosis of infection may be confirmed or suggested by rapid antigen tests, cultures, serological tests, or molecular tests (e.g., polymerase chain reaction).

CHAPTER 94

Immunization and Prophylaxis

- Purified polysaccharide vaccines are poor immunogens for children <2 years of age. Conjugation of a polysaccharide to a protein carrier creates immunogenic vaccines for *Haemophilus influenzae* type b, *Streptococcus pneumoniae*, and *Neisseria meningitidis* for this age group.
- Contraindications to vaccination include anaphylaxis to prior immunization and immunocompromised patients (live-virus vaccines).
- Administration of blood products and immunoglobulin can diminish response to live-virus vaccines if administered before the recommended interval.

CHAPTER 95

Antiinfective Therapy

- Obtain relevant cultures prior to initiating empiric antibiotics.
- Use of broad-spectrum empiric therapy is recommended for critically ill or immunocompromised patients.
- Sites with poor antimicrobial drug penetration may need drainage (abscess, osteomyelitis).
- Use targeted antimicrobial therapy to employ the least toxic, most narrow-spectrum agent effective against the causative pathogen.

CHAPTER 96

Fever Without a Focus

- Children <1 month of age with fever should have a complete evaluation of blood, urine, and cerebrospinal fluid (CSF) and should receive empiric antibiotics.
- Urinary tract infection is the most common serious bacterial infection in children <6 months of age.
- Children 3-36 months with fever should have a careful history and physical exam. Those without localizing signs or symptoms may need urine and blood cultures.
- Children with sickle cell anemia are at increased risk of bacteremia with encapsulated organisms.
- Children with unexplained fevers >14 days have fever of unknown origin. Among these episodes of fever of unknown origin, infections cause ~40-50%, inflammatory diseases ~20%, and malignancy ~10%.

CHAPTER 97

Infections Characterized by Fever and Rash

- Common childhood causes of febrile illnesses with rash include measles, rubella, human herpesvirus type 6 (HHV-6), parvovirus B19, and varicella.
- Chickenpox is characterized by fever and a pruritic vesicular rash that comes in crops; secondary staphylococcal on streptococcal skin infection is a common complication.
- Measles is characterized by cough, coryza, conjunctivitis, fever, rash, and Koplik spots on the buccal mucosa.
- Congenital rubella syndrome is characterized by intrauterine growth restriction, retinitis, blueberry muffin rash, and patent ductus arteriosus.
- Roseola (due to human herpes viruses 6 and 7) is characterized by an abrupt onset of a rash that appears after defervescence.
- Erythema infectiosum (due to parvovirus B19) is characterized by fever, malaise, a slapped cheek rash, and transient aplastic crisis in children with sickle cell anemia.

CHAPTER 98

Cutaneous Infections

- Many childhood cutaneous infections are caused by *Staphylococcus aureus* or group A streptococci.
- Crusted impetigo is often caused by *S. aureus*.
- Necrotizing fasciitis is a surgical emergency and is suggested by rapid extension of lesions, pain out of proportion to lesions, toxic appearance, or crepitus.
- Common viral causes of superficial skin infections include herpes simplex virus (HSV), human papillomavirus (HPV), and molluscum contagiosum virus.

CHAPTER 99

Lymphadenopathy

- Cervical lymphadenitis is the most common childhood regional lymphadenitis; common causes include streptococcal pharyngitis, respiratory viruses, Epstein-Barr virus (EBV), and cytomegalovirus (CMV).
- The differential diagnosis of cervical adenitis should include Kawasaki disease, cat-scratch disease, atypical tuberculosis, mononucleosis, human immunodeficiency virus (HIV), and lymphoma.

CHAPTER 100

Meningitis

- The organisms that most commonly cause neonatal meningitis are group B streptococcus, *Escherichia coli*, and Listeria monocytogenes. Older children are more likely to have *Streptococcus pneumoniae* and *Neisseria meningitidis* as a cause of meningitis.
- Partially treated bacterial meningitis may decrease the ability to grow the organism; polymerase chain reaction (PCR) is useful to detect the pathogen but does not provide antimicrobial pathogen sensitivities.
- Enteroviruses and parechovirus are common causes of viral meningitis.
- Herpes simplex may produce meningoencephalitis and requires treatment with intravenous acyclovir.
- Presumptive therapy for neonatal meningitis includes ampicillin and cefotaxime and for older children should be ceftriaxone and vancomycin.

CHAPTER 101

Encephalitis

- Viruses are the most common infectious cause of aseptic meningitis and encephalitis. Intravenous (IV) acyclovir should be used empirically if HSV or varicella-zoster virus (VZV) are suspected.
- Autoimmune encephalitis should be considered in all patients with encephalitis; diagnosis is by detecting brain-specific autoantibodies in blood and CSF.

CHAPTER 102

Upper Respiratory Tract Infection

- Young children typically have multiple upper respiratory tract infections (URIs) each year, up to 8-12. Antibiotics are not beneficial in treating these episodes and may instead cause harm.
- Complications of a URI include otitis media, sinusitis, and exacerbation of asthma.

CHAPTER 103

Pharyngitis

- Viruses are the most common cause of pharyngitis. However, if group A streptococcus is isolated by rapid antigen test or culture, it should be treated in order to prevent acute rheumatic fever. Penicillin or amoxicillin are first-line therapies.
- A major reason to treat streptococcal pharyngitis is to prevent rheumatic fever. Streptococcal pharyngitis is relatively uncommon in young children <3 years of age.

CHAPTER 104

Sinusitis

- The bacterial causes of acute sinusitis mirror those of otitis media and are *Streptococcus pneumoniae*, nontypable *Haemophilus influenzae*, and *Moraxella catarrhalis*.
- Complications of sinusitis include orbital cellulitis, Potts puffy tumor, and brain abscess.

CHAPTER 105

Otitis Media

- Poor or absent tympanic membrane mobility to negative and positive pressure using pneumatic otoscopy is a necessary finding for the diagnosis of acute otitis media (AOM).
- Complications of AOM include persistent middle ear effusion, hearing loss, mastoiditis, brain abscess, perforated tympanic membrane, and cholesteatoma.
- Otitis media (OM) with effusion is the most frequent sequela of AOM and may result in persistent middle ear effusion, which may be associated with hearing loss.
- Not all episodes of AOM require antibiotic treatment.

CHAPTER 106

Otitis Externa

- Otitis externa is most frequently caused by *Pseudomonas aeruginosa*.

CHAPTER 107

Croup (Laryngotracheobronchitis)

- Croup (laryngotracheobronchitis) is the most common infection of the middle respiratory tract; it is typically caused by parainfluenza virus and presents with stridor.
- The differential diagnosis of croup includes a foreign body, tracheitis, epiglottitis, tracheomalacia, and a vascular ring.

CHAPTER 108

Pertussis

- Pertussis typically lasts 6-8 weeks; it is marked by catarrhal, paroxysmal, and convalescent stages and can lead to apnea and severe respiratory distress in infants.
- Pertussis is associated with lymphocytosis and post-tussive emesis.

CHAPTER 109

Bronchiolitis

- Bronchiolitis is a common lower respiratory infection in children <2 years of age, is typically caused by respiratory syncytial virus (RSV), and requires only supportive treatment.
- The differential diagnosis of bronchiolitis includes asthma, heart failure, pneumonia, foreign body, and congenital airway or lung anomalies.

CHAPTER 110

Pneumonia

- *Streptococcus pneumoniae* is the most common bacterial cause of pneumonia outside the neonatal period and is the target of antibiotic selection for community-acquired pneumonia.
- Diagnostic evaluation for children hospitalized for pneumonia often includes complete blood count (CBC), blood culture, chest radiography, and occasionally rapid viral diagnostic testing.
- Amoxicillin or ampicillin are first-line antibiotics selections for community-acquired pneumonia in children.

CHAPTER 111

Infective Endocarditis

- Streptococci are the most common cause of native valve endocarditis in children, whereas staphylococci are more common in those with prosthetic material.
- If infectious endocarditis is suspected, multiple optimal-volume blood cultures should be obtained prior to starting antimicrobial therapy.

CHAPTER 112

Acute Gastroenteritis

- Management of acute gastroenteritis should include supportive care (correcting dehydration and electrolyte abnormalities) and not antibiotics in most circumstances.
- Enterohemorrhagic *Escherichia. coli* producing Shiga-toxin causes hemolytic uremic syndrome characterized by microangiopathic hemolytic anemia, thrombocytopenia, and acute kidney injury.
- Nucleic and amplification tests (NAAT) are the tests of choice for the most common causes of viral and bacterial gastroenteritis.
- When indicated, first-line therapy for traveler's diarrhea in children is azithromycin.

CHAPTER 113

Viral Hepatitis

- Various types of viral hepatitis are difficult to distinguish during acute infection; most have a nonspecific prodromal phase followed by an icteric phase. Often acute illness with hepatitis A virus (HAV), HBV, and HCV is mild or even asymptomatic in children.
- Vaccines are available to prevent HAV and HBV infection.
- HBV and HCV infection may become chronic with a risk for cirrhosis or hepatic cancer.

CHAPTER 114

Urinary Tract Infection

- *Escherichia coli* accounts for the vast majority of pediatric urinary tract infections.
- A renal ultrasound should be performed in young children to detect scaring, reflux, and congenital renal anomalies.
- Urinary tract infection (UTI) diagnosis requires a positive urine culture.
- Urine leukocyte esterase and nitrite testing aids in the diagnosis of a UTI.
- Nonspecific vaginitis is the most common cause of vulvovaginitis in prepubertal girls.

CHAPTER 115

Vulvovaginitis

- **Bacterial vaginosis** represents disruption of the normal vaginal flora with reduction in lactobacillus and overgrowth of other organisms.
- Nonspecific vaginitis is the most common cause of vulvovaginitis in prepubertal girls.

CHAPTER 116

Sexually Transmitted Infections

- There is increasing antibiotic resistance in *Neisseria gonorrhoeae.* Outpatient treatment of gonococcal urethritis or endocervicitis should include a single intramuscular (IM) dose of ceftriaxone in combination with a single oral dose of azithromycin 1 g to treat potential co-infection with *Chlamydia trachomatis* and prevent the emergence of resistance in *N. gonorrhoeae.*
- Chlamydia is the most frequently diagnosed bacterial sexually transmitted infection (STI) in adolescents and accounts for most cases of nongonococcal urethritis and cervicitis.
- Chlamydial cervicitis is often asymptomatic.

CHAPTER 117

Osteomyelitis

- *Staphylococcus aureus* is the most common bacterial cause of osteomyelitis and is the target of antibiotic selection for this condition.
- Magnetic resonance imaging is the most sensitive diagnostic imaging test for osteomyelitis and will identify lesions early in the course of disease.
- An antistaphylococcal agent (nafcillin, oxacillin, or cefazolin) is the preferred empiric therapy for osteomyelitis in areas where methicillin-resistant *S. aureus* rates are low.

CHAPTER 118

Infectious Arthritis

- *Staphylococcus aureus* is the most common bacterial cause of septic arthritis and is the target of antibiotic selection for this condition.
- Diagnostic evaluation for septic arthritis should include joint aspirate for cell count, Gram stain, and culture.
- An antistaphylococcal agent (nafcillin, oxacillin, or cefazolin) is the preferred empiric therapy for septic arthritis in areas where methicillin-resistant *S. aureus* rates are low.

CHAPTER 119

Ocular Infections

- All newborns should receive prophylaxis for ophthalmia neonatorum, typically with erythromycin 0.5% ointment, which will prevent gonococcal but not chlamydial ophthalmia.
- Chlamydia conjunctivitis in the newborn is treated with oral antibiotics to prevent chlamydial pneumonia.
- Neonatal conjunctivitis due to gonococcus is treated with IM or IV ceftriaxone.
- Conjunctivitis and or keratitis in patients who use contact lenses may be due to pseudomonas.

CHAPTER 120

Infection in the Immunocompromised Person

- The presence of fever with neutropenia, even in the absence of other symptoms, demands prompt and thorough evaluation and empiric antimicrobial therapy.
- Fever is often the only sign of serious infection in immunocompromised patients.
- Rectal tenderness or pain on defecation may suggest a perianal abscess.
- The central line exit site and subcutaneous track should be inspected and blood drawn for culture from each lumen to detect line infections.
- Pneumonia, sinusitis, and bacteremia are the most common sites of infection in patients with fever and neutropenia.

CHAPTER 121

Infections Associated With Medical Devices

- The major complication of indwelling medical devices such as central lines, ventriculo-peritoneal shunts, and urinary catheters is infection (health care–associated infections).
- Antibiotic-lock therapy may be used to aid in treatment or prevention of catheter line infections.

CHAPTER 122

Zoonoses and Vector Borne Infections

- Lyme disease *(Borrelia burgdorferi)* is the most common tick-borne infection in the United States.
- Early treatment of erythema migrans almost always prevents progression to later stages of Lyme disease. The most common reason patients "recur" or do not respond to treatment is that the initial diagnosis was incorrect.
- Ehrlichiosis and anaplasmosis presents like Rocky Mountain Spotted fever.
- Rocky Mountain Spotted Fever is a severe life-threatening illness that has a 20-80% case fatality rate if untreated.
- Dengue hemorrhagic fever is seen in patients with a previous infection with Dengue virus.

CHAPTER 123

Parasitic Diseases

- Chemoprophylaxis for malaria is necessary for all visitors to and residents of the tropics who have not lived there since infancy.
- Malaria is characterized by febrile paroxysms.
- Long-term relapse with malaria occurs because of persistent hepatic infection with either *Plasmodium vivax* or *P. ovale.*

CHAPTER 124

Tuberculosis

- The diagnosis of Mycobacterium tuberculosis infection can be difficult. Young children under 5 should have a purified protein derivative (PPD) test, whereas older children can have a PPD or interferon-gamma release assay (IGRA). Both may not be positive during active infection.
- Pulmonary tuberculosis initially presents as a pulmonary infiltrate with hilar adenopathy.
- Bone or brain involvement with tuberculosis (TB) occurs due to hematogenous spread following primary pulmonary TB.
- Reactivation of TB occurs most often in adolescents and patients exposed to corticosteroids or anti-TNF antibodies.

CHAPTER 125

Human Immunodeficiency Virus and Acquired Immunodeficiency Syndrome

- Vertical transmission of HIV, from mother to child, is now an uncommon occurrence in the United States due to the effectiveness of preventative measures including early maternal diagnosis, maternal treatment during pregnancy and delivery, postnatal prophylactic treatment of the infant, and avoidance of breast feeding.
- Perinatal acquired HIV presents with failure to thrive, lymphadenopathy, hepatosplenomegaly, parotitis, diarrhea, and opportunistic infections.
- Sexually active adolescents are the highest risk group of becoming HIV positive.

DIGESTIVE SYSTEM

Warren P. Bishop | Dawn R. Ebach

CHAPTER 126

Digestive System Assessment

HISTORY

After identifying the major gastrointestinal (GI) symptom, the onset and progression should be determined (improved, unchanged, worsening). Characterization of signs and symptoms should identify factors that trigger or alleviate the symptom; the timing, frequency, and duration of symptoms; relationship to meals and defecation; and associated symptoms (e.g., fever or weight loss). Other key history includes exposures to others (family, school contacts, pets), travel, environmental exposure, and impact of illness on the child (school absences, weight loss).

PHYSICAL EXAMINATION

The history may suggest a diagnosis and direct the evaluation, which should include a full examination as well as a thorough abdominal examination. Extraintestinal disorders may produce GI manifestations (e.g., emesis with group A streptococcal pharyngitis, abdominal pain with lower lobe pneumonia). The examination should begin with a careful external inspection for abdominal distention, bruising or discoloration, abnormal abdominal veins, jaundice, surgical scars, and ostomies. Abnormalities of intensity and pitch of bowel sounds can occur with bowel obstruction. When palpating for tenderness, the examiner should note location, facial expression, guarding, and rebound tenderness. Palpation can also detect enlargement of the liver or spleen as well as feces and masses. If detected, organomegaly should be measured (with a tape measure), noting abnormal firmness or contour. A rectal examination, including inspection for fissures, skin tags, abscesses, and fistulous openings, should be performed for children with history suggesting constipation, GI bleeding, abdominal pain, chronic diarrhea, and suspicion of inflammatory bowel disease (IBD). Digital rectal examination should include assessment of anal sphincter tone, anal canal size and elasticity, tenderness, extrinsic masses, presence of fecal impaction, and caliber of the rectum. Stool should be tested for occult blood.

SCREENING TESTS

A **complete blood count** may provide evidence for inflammation (white blood cell [WBC] and platelet count), poor nutrition or bleeding (hemoglobin, red blood cell volume, reticulocyte count), and infection (WBC number and differential, presence of toxic granulation). Serum electrolytes, blood urea nitrogen (BUN), and creatinine help define hydration status. Tests of liver dysfunction include total and direct bilirubin, alanine aminotransferase, aspartate aminotransferase for evidence of hepatocellular injury, and γ-glutamyltransferase or alkaline phosphatase for evidence of bile duct injury. **Hepatic synthetic function** can be assessed by coagulation factor levels, prothrombin time, and albumin level. Pancreatic enzyme tests (amylase, lipase) provide evidence of pancreatic injury or inflammation. Urinalysis can gauge dehydration and identify a possible source of protein loss.

DIAGNOSTIC IMAGING

Radiology

A plain abdominal x-ray to document excessive retained stool when history is consistent with constipation and encopresis is not necessary, as physical examination alone can confirm the diagnosis.

Endoscopy

Endoscopy permits the direct visualization of the interior of the gut. **Video endoscopes** may be used even in very small infants by pediatric gastroenterologists. **Wireless capsule endoscopy** (Fig. 126.1) enables visualization of lesions beyond the reach of conventional endoscopes.

Consultation with a pediatric gastroenterologist for endoscopy is recommended for further evaluation of suspected esophageal or gastric inflammation unresponsive to medications, to confirm the diagnosis of eosinophilic esophagitis or celiac disease, to evaluate GI bleeding, to investigate suspected IBD, or to screen for polyp disorders. In addition, a trained endoscopist can remove esophageal and gastric foreign bodies and place feeding tubes.

COMMON MANIFESTATIONS OF GASTROINTESTINAL DISORDERS

Abdominal Pain

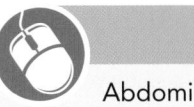

Decision-Making Algorithm
Available @ StudentConsult.com

Abdominal Pain

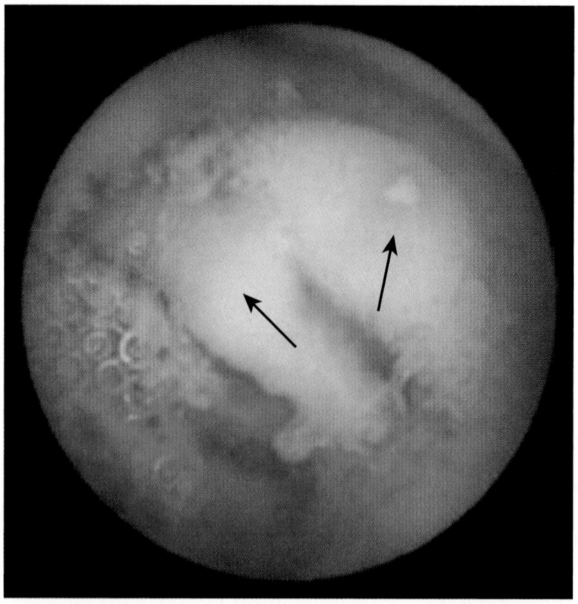

FIGURE 126.1 Wireless capsule endoscopy: Aphthous ulcers *(arrows)* in jejunum diagnostic of Crohn disease in patient with negative findings on upper endoscopy and colonoscopy.

General Considerations

Abdominal pain can result from injury to the intraabdominal organs or overlying somatic structures in the abdominal wall, or from extraabdominal diseases. **Visceral pain** results when autonomic nerves within the gut detect injury, transmitting sensation by nonmyelinated fibers. The pain is vague, dull, slow in onset, and poorly localized. A variety of stimuli, including normal peristalsis and various intraluminal chemical and osmotic states, activate these fibers to some degree. Regardless of the stimulus, visceral pain is perceived when a threshold of intensity or duration is crossed. Lower degrees of activation may result in perception of nonpainful or perhaps vaguely uncomfortable sensations, whereas more intensive stimulation of these fibers results in pain. Overactive sensation may be the basis of some kinds of abdominal pain, such as **functional abdominal pain** and **irritable bowel syndrome (IBS)**.

In contrast to visceral pain, **somatic pain** results when overlying body structures are injured. Somatic structures include the parietal peritoneum, fascia, muscles, and skin of the abdominal wall. In contrast to pain emanating from visceral injury, somatic nociceptive fibers are myelinated and are capable of rapid transmission of well-localized painful stimuli. When intraabdominal processes cause inflammation or injury to the parietal peritoneum or abdominal wall structures, poorly localized visceral pain becomes well-localized somatic pain. For example, in acute appendicitis, the initial activation of visceral nociceptive fibers yields poorly localized discomfort in the midabdomen. When the inflammatory process extends to the overlying parietal peritoneum, the pain becomes severe and localizes to the right lower quadrant. This is called **somatoparietal pain.**

Referred pain is a painful sensation in a body region distant from the true source of pain. The location of referred pain is predictable based on the locus of visceral injury. Stomach pain is referred to the epigastric and retrosternal regions, and liver and pancreas pain is referred to the epigastric region. Gallbladder pain often is referred to the region below the right scapula. Somatic pathways stimulated by small bowel visceral afferents affect the periumbilical area, and colonic injury results in infraumbilical referred pain.

Acute Abdominal Pain

Distinguishing Features

Acute abdominal pain can signal the presence of a dangerous intraabdominal process (e.g., appendicitis or bowel obstruction) or may originate from extraintestinal sources (e.g., lower lobe pneumonia or urinary tract stone). Not all episodes of acute abdominal pain require emergency intervention. Appendicitis and volvulus, for example, must be ruled out as quickly as possible. Few patients presenting with acute abdominal pain actually have a surgical emergency, but they must be separated from cases that can be managed conservatively.

Initial Diagnostic Evaluation

Table 126.1 lists a diagnostic approach to acute abdominal pain in children. Events that occur with a discrete, abrupt onset, such as passage of a stone, perforation of a viscus, or infarction, result in a sudden **onset of pain**. Gradual onset of pain is common with infectious or inflammatory causes, such as appendicitis and IBD.

A standard group of laboratory tests usually is performed for acute abdominal pain (see Table 126.1). An abdominal x-ray series evaluates for bowel obstruction, fecalith, or nephrolithiasis. Ultrasound or computed tomography (CT) can visualize the appendix if appendicitis is suspected but the diagnosis remains in doubt. If the initial evaluation suggests intussusception, a barium or pneumatic (air) enema may be used to diagnose and treat this condition (see Chapter 129).

Differential Diagnosis

Table 126.2 lists the differential diagnosis of acute abdominal pain in children. The urgent task of the clinician is to rule out surgical emergencies. In young children, malrotation with volvulus, incarcerated hernia, congenital anomalies, and intussusception are common concerns. In older children and teenagers, appendicitis is more common. An acute surgical abdomen is characterized by signs of peritonitis, including tenderness, abdominal wall rigidity, guarding, and absent or diminished bowel sounds. Helpful characteristics of onset, location, referral, and quality of pain are noted in Table 126.3.

Functional Abdominal Pain and Irritable Bowel Syndrome

Decision-Making Algorithms
Available @ StudentConsult.com

Abdominal Pain
Vomiting

Recurrent abdominal pain is a common problem, affecting more than 10% of all children. The peak incidence occurs between ages 7 and 12 years. Although the differential diagnosis of recurrent abdominal pain is fairly extensive (Table 126.4), most children do not have a serious (or even identifiable) underlying illness causing the pain.

TABLE 126.1 Diagnostic Approach to Acute Abdominal Pain

HISTORY	
Onset	Sudden or gradual, prior episodes, association with meals, history of injury
Nature	Sharp versus dull, colicky or constant, burning
Location	Epigastric, periumbilical, generalized, right or left lower quadrant, change in location over time
Associated symptoms	Fever, vomiting (bilious?), diarrhea (bloody?), abdominal distention
Extraintestinal symptoms	Cough, dyspnea, dysuria, urinary frequency, flank pain
Course of symptoms	Worsening or improving, change in nature or location of pain, aggravating and alleviating factors, last menstrual period
PHYSICAL EXAMINATION	
General position	Growth and nutrition, general appearance, hydration, degree of discomfort, body position
Abdominal	Tenderness, distention, bowel sounds, rigidity, guarding, mass
Genitalia	Testicular torsion, hernia, pelvic inflammatory disease, ectopic pregnancy
Surrounding structures	Breath sounds, rales, rhonchi, wheezing, flank tenderness, tenderness of abdominal wall structures, ribs, costochondral joints
Rectal examination	Perianal lesions, stricture, tenderness, fecal impaction, blood
LABORATORY	
CBC, C-reactive protein, ESR	Evidence of infection or inflammation
AST, ALT, GGT, bilirubin	Biliary or liver disease
Amylase, lipase	Pancreatitis
Urinalysis	Urinary tract infection; bleeding due to stone, trauma, or obstruction
Pregnancy test (older females)	Ectopic pregnancy
RADIOLOGY	
Plain flat and upright abdominal films	Bowel obstruction, appendiceal fecalith, free intraperitoneal air, kidney stones, constipation, mass
CT scan	Intraabdominal or pelvic abscess, appendicitis, Crohn disease, pancreatitis, gallstones, kidney stones
Barium enema	Intussusception, malrotation
Ultrasound	Gallstones, appendicitis, intussusception, pancreatitis, kidney stones
Endoscopy	Colitis
Upper endoscopy	Suspected peptic ulcer or esophagitis

ALT, Alanine aminotransferase; *AST*, aspartate aminotransferase; *CBC*, complete blood count; *CT*, computed tomography; *ESR*, erythrocyte sedimentation rate; *GGT*, γ-glutamyltransferase.

TABLE 126.2 Differential Diagnosis of Acute Abdominal Pain

TRAUMATIC
Duodenal hematoma
Ruptured spleen
Perforated viscus
Traumatic pancreatitis
FUNCTIONAL
Constipation*
Irritable bowel syndrome*
Dysmenorrhea*
Mittelschmerz (ovulation)*
Infantile colic*
Abdominal migraine
INFECTIOUS
Appendicitis*
Viral or bacterial gastroenteritis/adenitis*
Abscess
Spontaneous bacterial peritonitis
Pelvic inflammatory disease
Cholecystitis
Urinary tract infection*
Pneumonia
Bacterial typhlitis
Hepatitis
GENITAL
Testicular torsion
Ovarian torsion
Ruptured ovarian cyst
Ectopic pregnancy
GENETIC
Sickle cell crisis*
Familial Mediterranean fever
Porphyria
Hereditary angioedema
METABOLIC
Diabetic ketoacidosis
Fabry disease
INFLAMMATORY
Inflammatory bowel disease
Vasculitis
Henoch-Schönlein purpura*
Pancreatitis
OBSTRUCTIVE
Intussusception*
Malrotation with volvulus
Ileus*
Incarcerated hernia

Continued

TABLE 126.2	Differential Diagnosis of Acute Abdominal Pain—cont'd
Postoperative adhesion	
Meconium ileus equivalent (cystic fibrosis)	
Duplication cyst	
Congenital stricture	
BILIARY	
Gallstone	
Gallbladder hydrops	
Biliary dyskinesia	
PEPTIC	
Gastric or duodenal ulcer	
Gastritis*	
Esophagitis	
RENAL	
Kidney stone	
Hydronephrosis/ureteropelvic junction obstruction	

*Common.

Differential Diagnosis

Children with **functional abdominal pain** characteristically have pain almost daily. The pain is not associated with meals or relieved by defecation and is often associated with a tendency toward anxiety and perfectionism. Symptoms often result from stress at school or in novel social situations. The pain often is worst in the morning and often prevents or delays children from attending school. **IBS** is a subset of functional abdominal pain, characterized by onset of pain at the time of a change in stool frequency or consistency, a stool pattern fluctuating between diarrhea and constipation, and relief of pain with defecation. Symptoms in IBS are linked to gut motility. Pain is commonly accompanied in both groups of children by school avoidance, secondary gains, anxiety about imagined causes, lack of coping skills, and disordered peer relationships (Table 126.5).

Distinguishing Features

One needs to distinguish between functional pain/IBS and more serious underlying disorders. **Warning signs** for underlying illness are listed in Table 126.6. If present, further investigation is necessary. Some laboratory evaluation is warranted even in

TABLE 126.3 Distinguishing Features of Abdominal Pain in Children

DISEASE	ONSET	LOCATION	REFERRAL	QUALITY	COMMENTS
Functional: irritable bowel syndrome	Recurrent	Periumbilical, splenic and hepatic flexures	None	Dull, crampy, intermittent; duration 2 hr	Family stress, school phobia, diarrhea and constipation; hypersensitive to pain from distention
Esophageal reflux	Recurrent, after meals, at bedtime	Substernal	Chest	Burning	Sour taste in mouth; Sandifer syndrome
Duodenal ulcer	Recurrent, before meals, at night	Epigastric	Back	Severe burning, gnawing	Relieved by food, milk, antacids; family history important; gastrointestinal bleeding
Pancreatitis	Acute	Epigastric-hypogastric	Back	Constant, sharp, boring	Nausea, emesis, marked tenderness
Intestinal obstruction	Acute or gradual	Periumbilical–lower abdomen	Back	Alternating cramping (colic) and painless periods	Distention, obstipation, bilious emesis, increased bowel sounds
Appendicitis	Acute	Periumbilical or epigastric; localizes to right lower quadrant	Back or pelvis if retrocecal	Sharp, steady	Nausea, emesis, local tenderness, ± fever, avoids motion
Meckel diverticulum	Recurrent	Periumbilical–lower abdomen	None	Sharp	Hematochezia; painless unless intussusception, diverticulitis, or perforation
Inflammatory bowel disease	Recurrent	Depends on site of involvement		Dull cramping, tenesmus	Fever, weight loss, ±hematochezia
Intussusception	Acute	Periumbilical–lower abdomen	None	Cramping, with painless periods	Guarded position with knees pulled up, currant jelly stools, lethargy
Lactose intolerance	Recurrent with milk products	Lower abdomen	None	Cramping	Distention, gaseousness, diarrhea
Urolithiasis	Acute, sudden	Back	Groin	Severe, colicky pain	Hematuria
Pyelonephritis	Acute, sudden	Back	None	Dull to sharp	Fever, costochondral tenderness, dysuria, urinary frequency, emesis
Cholecystitis and cholelithiasis	Acute	Right upper quadrant	Right shoulder	Severe, colicky pain	Hemolysis ± jaundice, nausea, emesis

Modified from Andreoli TE, Carpenter CJ, Plum F, et al: Cecil Essentials of Medicine. *Philadelphia: WB Saunders; 1986.*

TABLE 126.4 Differential Diagnosis of Recurrent Abdominal Pain

Functional abdominal pain*
Irritable bowel syndrome*
Chronic pancreatitis
Gallstones
Peptic disease
Duodenal ulcer
Gastric ulcer
Esophagitis
Lactose intolerance*
Fructose malabsorption
Inflammatory bowel disease*
Crohn disease
Ulcerative colitis
Constipation*
Obstructive uropathy
Congenital intestinal malformation
Malrotation
Duplication cyst
Stricture or web
Celiac disease*
Abdominal migraine
Eosinophilic esophagitis*

*Common.

the absence of warning signs. The initial evaluation recommended in Table 126.7 is a sensible approach, avoiding unnecessary testing and providing ample sensitivity for most serious underlying disorders. While waiting for laboratory and ultrasound results, a 3-day trial of a lactose-free diet can evaluate for lactose intolerance. If tests are normal and no warning signs are present, testing should be stopped. If there are warning signs, progression of symptoms, or laboratory abnormalities that suggest a specific diagnosis, additional investigation may be warranted.

Treatment of Recurrent Abdominal Pain

A child who is repeatedly kept home from school because of pain receives reinforcement in the form of being excused from responsibilities and withdraws from full social functioning. This tends to both increase anxiety and prolong the course. To break the cycle of pain and disability, the child with functional pain must be assisted in **returning to normal activities** immediately. Instead of being sent home from school with stomachaches, a child may be allowed to take a short break from class until symptoms abate. The child and parents should be informed that pain is likely to be worse on the day the child returns to school as anxiety worsens dysmotility and enhances pain perception. Medications may be helpful. **Fiber supplements** may help to manage symptoms of IBS. Probiotics and peppermint oil can be beneficial in treating IBS. In difficult and persistent cases, cognitive behavioral therapy, amitriptyline, or a selective serotonin reuptake inhibitor may be helpful. When

TABLE 126.5 Rome III Criteria for Pediatric Functional Gastrointestinal Syndromes

A. DIAGNOSTIC CRITERIA FOR CHILDHOOD FUNCTIONAL ABDOMINAL PAIN

Must include all of the following:*
1. Episodic or continuous abdominal pain
2. Insufficient criteria for other functional gastrointestinal diseases
3. No evidence of an inflammatory, anatomical, metabolic, or neoplastic process that explains the subject's symptoms

*Criteria fulfilled at least once per week for at least 2 mo before diagnosis

B. DIAGNOSTIC CRITERIA FOR CHILDHOOD FUNCTIONAL ABDOMINAL PAIN SYNDROME

Must include functional abdominal pain at least 25% of the time and 1 or more of the following:*
1. Some loss of daily functioning
2. Additional somatic symptoms such as headache, limb pain, or difficulty sleeping

*Criteria fulfilled at least once per week for at least 2 mo before diagnosis

C. DIAGNOSTIC CRITERIA FOR IRRITABLE BOWEL SYNDROME

Must include all of the following:*
1. Abdominal discomfort (an uncomfortable sensation not described as pain) or pain associated with 2 or more of the following at least 25% of the time:
   a. improved with defecation
   b. onset associated with change in frequency of stool
   c. onset associated with a change in form (appearance) of stool
2. No evidence of an inflammatory, anatomical, metabolic, or neoplastic process that explains the subject's symptoms

*Criteria fulfilled at least once per week for at least 2 mo before diagnosis

D. DIAGNOSTIC CRITERIA FOR ABDOMINAL MIGRAINE

Must include all of the following:*
1. Paroxysmal episodes of intense, acute periumbilical pain that lasts for 1 hr or more
2. Intervening periods of usual health lasting weeks to months.
3. The pain interferes with normal activities
4. The pain is associated with 2 or more of the following:
   a. anorexia
   b. nausea
   c. vomiting
   d. headache
   e. photophobia
   f. pallor
5. No evidence of an inflammatory, anatomical, metabolic, or neoplastic process considered that explains the subject's symptoms

*Criteria fulfilled 2 or more times in the preceding 12 mo

E. DIAGNOSTIC CRITERIA FOR CYCLIC VOMITING SYNDROME

Must include all of the following:
1. Two or more periods of intense nausea and unremitting vomiting or retching lasting hours to days
2. Return to usual state of health lasting weeks to months

F. FUNCTIONAL DIARRHEA

Must include all of the following
1. Daily painless, recurrent passage of three or more large, unformed stools
2. Symptoms lasting more than 4 wk
3. Onset of symptoms that begins between 6 and 36 mo of age
4. Passage of stools that occur during waking hours
5. There is no failure to thrive if caloric intake is adequate

Courtesy of the Rome Foundation.

TABLE 126.6	Warning Signs of Underlying Illness in Recurrent Abdominal Pain

Vomiting
Abnormal screening laboratory study (anemia, hypoalbuminemia, inflammatory markers)
Fever
Bilious emesis
Growth failure
Pain awakening child from sleep
Weight loss
Location away from periumbilical region
Blood in stools or emesis
Delayed puberty
Nocturnal diarrhea
Dysphagia
Arthritis
Perianal disease
Family history of inflammatory bowel disease, celiac disease, or peptic ulcer disease

TABLE 126.7	Suggested Evaluation of Recurrent Abdominal Pain

INITIAL EVALUATION	FOLLOW-UP EVALUATION*
Complete history and physical examination	CT scan of the abdomen and pelvis with oral, rectal, and intravenous contrast
Ask about "warning signs" (see Table 126.6)	Celiac disease serology—endomysial antibody or tissue transglutaminase antibody
Determine degree of functional impairment (e.g., missing school)	Barium upper GI series with small bowel follow-through
CBC	Endoscopy of the esophagus, stomach, and duodenum
ESR	Colonoscopy
Amylase, lipase	
Urinalysis	
Abdominal ultrasound—examine liver, bile ducts, gallbladder, pancreas, kidneys, ureters	
Trial of 3-day lactose-free diet	

*Consider *using one or more of these to investigate warning signs, abnormal laboratory tests, or specific or persistent symptoms.*
CBC, Complete blood count; *CT*, computed tomography; *ESR*, erythrocyte sedimentation rate; *GI*, gastrointestinal.

significant anxiety or social dysfunction persists, a mental health professional should be consulted.

Vomiting

Decision-Making Algorithm
Available @ StudentConsult.com
Vomiting

Vomiting is a coordinated, sequential series of events that leads to forceful oral emptying of gastric contents. It is a common problem in children and has many causes. Vomiting should be distinguished from **regurgitation** of stomach contents, also known as gastroesophageal reflux (GER), chalasia, or "spitting up." Although the end result of vomiting and regurgitation is similar, they have completely different characteristics. Vomiting is usually preceded by nausea and is accompanied by forceful gagging and retching. Regurgitation, on the other hand, is effortless and not preceded by nausea.

Differential Diagnosis

In neonates with true vomiting, congenital obstructive lesions should be considered. Allergic reactions to formula in the first 2 months of life may present with vomiting. **Infantile GER** ("spitting up") occurs in most infants and can be large in volume, but is effortless, and these infants do not appear ill. **Pyloric stenosis** occurs in the first months of life and is characterized by steadily worsening, forceful vomiting that occurs immediately after feedings. A visibly distended stomach, often with visible peristaltic waves, is often seen before vomiting. Pyloric stenosis is more common in male infants; the family history may be positive. Other obstructive lesions, such as intestinal duplication cysts, atresias, webs, and midgut malrotation, should be considered. Metabolic disorders (e.g., organic acidemias, galactosemia, urea cycle defects, adrenogenital syndromes) may present with vomiting in infants. In older children with acute vomiting, viruses and food poisoning are common. Other infections, especially streptococcal pharyngitis, urinary tract infections, and otitis media, commonly result in vomiting. When vomiting is chronic, central nervous system (CNS) causes (increased intracranial pressure, migraine) must be considered. **Cyclic vomiting syndrome** or migraine may be the etiology of recurrent vomiting. When abdominal pain or bilious emesis accompanies vomiting, evaluation for bowel obstruction, peptic disorders, and appendicitis must be immediately initiated.

Distinguishing Features

Table 126.8 lists common diagnoses that must be considered and their important historical features. Given the frequency of viral gastroenteritis as the etiology, it is important to be alert for unusual features that suggest another diagnosis. Viral gastroenteritis usually is not associated with severe abdominal pain or headache and does not recur at frequent intervals.

Physical examination should include assessment of the child's hydration status, including examination of capillary refill, moistness of mucous membranes, and skin turgor (see Chapter 38). The chest should be auscultated for evidence of rales or other signs of pulmonary involvement. The abdomen must be examined carefully for distention, organomegaly, bowel sounds, tenderness, and guarding. A rectal examination and testing stool for occult blood should be considered.

Laboratory evaluation of vomiting should include serum electrolytes, tests of renal function, complete blood count, amylase, lipase, and liver function tests. Additional testing may be required immediately when history and examination suggest a specific etiology. Ultrasound is useful to look for pyloric stenosis, gallstones, renal stones, hydronephrosis, biliary obstruction, pancreatitis, malrotation, intussusception, and other anatomical abnormalities. CT may be indicated to rule out appendicitis or to observe structures that cannot be visualized well by ultrasound. Barium studies can show obstructive or inflammatory lesions of the gut and can be therapeutic, as in the use of contrast enemas for intussusception (see Chapter 129).

TABLE 126.8 Differential Diagnosis and Historical Features of Vomiting

DIFFERENTIAL DIAGNOSIS	HISTORICAL CLUES
Viral gastroenteritis	Fever, diarrhea, sudden onset, absence of pain
Gastroesophageal reflux	Effortless, not preceded by nausea, chronic
Hepatitis	Jaundice, history of exposure
Extragastrointestinal infections	
Otitis media	Fever, ear pain
Urinary tract infection	Dysuria, unusual urine odor, frequency, incontinence
Pneumonia	Cough, fever, chest discomfort
Allergic	
Milk or soy protein intolerance (infants)	Associated with particular formula or food, blood in stools
Other food allergy (older children)	
Peptic ulcer or gastritis	Epigastric pain, blood or coffee-ground material in emesis, pain relieved by acid blockade
Appendicitis	Fever, abdominal pain migrating to the right lower quadrant, tenderness
Pancreatitis	Severe epigastric abdominal pain
Anatomical obstruction	
Intestinal atresia	Neonate, usually bilious, polyhydramnios
Midgut malrotation	Pain, bilious vomiting, GI bleeding, shock
Intussusception	Colicky pain, lethargy, vomiting, currant jelly stools, mass occasionally
Duplication cysts	Colic, mass
Pyloric stenosis	Nonbilious vomiting, postprandial, <4 mo old, hunger, progressive weight loss
Bacterial gastroenteritis	Fever, often with bloody diarrhea
CNS	
Hydrocephalus	Large head, altered mental status, bulging fontanelles
Meningitis	Fever, stiff neck
Migraine syndrome	Attacks scattered in time, relieved by sleep; headache
Cyclic vomiting syndrome	Similar to migraine, usually no headache
Brain tumor	Morning vomiting, accelerating over time, headache, diplopia
Motion sickness	Associated with travel in vehicle
Labyrinthitis	Vertigo
Metabolic disease	Presentation early in life, worsens when catabolic or exposure to substrate
Pregnancy	Morning, sexually active, cessation of menses
Drug reaction or side effect	Associated with increased dose or new medication
Cancer chemotherapy	Temporarily related to administration of chemotherapeutic drugs
Eosinophilic esophagitis	May have dysphagia or abdominal pain

CNS, Central nervous system; *GI*, gastrointestinal.

Treatment needs to address the consequences and the causes of the vomiting. Dehydration must be treated with fluid resuscitation. This can be accomplished in most cases with oral fluid-electrolyte solutions, but intravenous (IV) fluids may be required. Electrolyte imbalances should be corrected by appropriate choice of fluids. Underlying causes should be treated when possible.

The use of **antiemetic medications** is controversial. These drugs should not be prescribed until the etiology of the vomiting is known, and then only for severe symptoms. Anticholinergics (e.g., scopolamine) and antihistamines (e.g., dimenhydrinate) are useful for the prophylaxis and treatment of motion sickness. Drugs that block serotonin 5-HT_3 receptors, such as ondansetron and granisetron, are frequently used for viral gastroenteritis and can improve tolerance of oral rehydration therapy. They are helpful for chemotherapy-induced vomiting, often combined with dexamethasone. No antiemetic should be used in patients with surgical emergencies or when a specific treatment of the underlying condition is possible. Correction of dehydration, ketosis, and acidosis is helpful to reduce vomiting in most patients with viral gastroenteritis.

Acute and Chronic Diarrhea

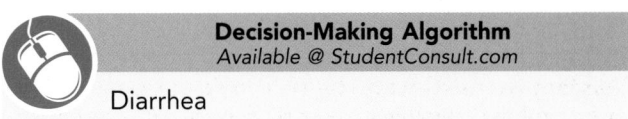

Decision-Making Algorithm
Available @ StudentConsult.com

Diarrhea

Diarrhea is a major cause of childhood morbidity and mortality worldwide. Deaths from diarrhea are rare in industrialized countries but are common elsewhere. **Acute diarrhea** is a major problem when it occurs with malnutrition or in the absence of basic medical care (see Chapter 30). In North America, most acute diarrhea is viral and is self-limited, requiring no diagnostic testing or specific intervention. Bacterial agents tend to cause much more severe illness and typically are seen in food-associated outbreaks or in regions with poor public sanitation. Bacterial enteritis should be suspected when there is **dysentery** (bloody diarrhea with fever) and whenever severe symptoms are present. These infections can be diagnosed by stool culture or other assays for specific pathogens. **Chronic diarrhea** lasts more than 2 weeks and has a wide range of possible causes, including serious and benign conditions that are more difficult to diagnose.

Parents use the word *diarrhea* to describe loose or watery stools, excessively frequent stools, or stools that are large in volume. Constipation with overflow incontinence can be mislabeled as diarrhea. A more exact definition of diarrhea is excessive daily stool liquid volume (>10 mL stool/kg body weight/day). Stool texture, volume, and frequency help to characterize the episode of diarrhea.

Differential Diagnosis

Diarrhea may be classified by etiology or by physiological mechanisms (secretory or osmotic). Etiological agents include viruses, bacteria or their toxins, chemicals, parasites, malabsorbed substances, and inflammation. Table 126.9 lists common causes of diarrhea in childhood. **Secretory diarrhea** occurs when the intestinal mucosa directly secretes fluid and electrolytes into the stool and is the result of inflammation (e.g., IBD, chemical stimulus). Secretion also is stimulated by mediators of inflammation and by various hormones, such as vasoactive intestinal peptide secreted by a neuroendocrine tumor. Cholera is a secretory diarrhea stimulated by the enterotoxin of *Vibrio cholerae*, which causes increased levels of cyclic adenosine monophosphate (cAMP) within enterocytes and leads to secretion into the small-bowel lumen.

Osmotic diarrhea occurs after malabsorption of an ingested substance, which "pulls" water into the bowel lumen. A classic example is the diarrhea of lactose intolerance. Osmotic diarrhea also can result from generalized maldigestion, such as that seen with pancreatic insufficiency or with intestinal injury. Certain nonabsorbable laxatives, such as polyethylene glycol and milk of magnesia, also cause osmotic diarrhea. Fermentation of malabsorbed substances (e.g., lactose) often occurs, resulting

TABLE 126.9 Differential Diagnosis of Diarrhea

	INFANT	CHILD	ADOLESCENT
ACUTE			
Common	Gastroenteritis* Systemic infection Antibiotic associated (?)	Gastroenteritis* Food poisoning Systemic infection Antibiotic associated	Gastroenteritis* Food poisoning Antibiotic associated
Rare	Primary disaccharidase deficiency Hirschsprung toxic colitis Adrenogenital syndrome		Hyperthyroidism
CHRONIC			
Common	Postinfectious secondary lactase deficiency Cow's milk/soy protein intolerance Chronic nonspecific diarrhea of infancy (toddler's diarrhea) Celiac disease Cystic fibrosis AIDS enteropathy	Postinfectious secondary lactase deficiency Irritable bowel syndrome Celiac disease Lactose intolerance Giardiasis Inflammatory bowel disease	Irritable bowel syndrome Inflammatory bowel disease Lactose intolerance Giardiasis Laxative abuse (anorexia nervosa) Celiac disease
Rare	Primary immune defects Familial villous atrophy (?) Secretory tumors Congenital chloridorrhea Acrodermatitis enteropathica Lymphangiectasia Abetalipoproteinemia Eosinophilic gastroenteritis Short-bowel syndrome Autoimmune enteropathy/IPEX-like disorders Factitious	Acquired immune defects Secretory tumor Pseudo-obstruction Factitious AIDS enteropathy	Secretory tumors Primary bowel tumor AIDS enteropathy

*Gastroenteritis includes viral (rotavirus, norovirus, astrovirus) and bacterial (*Salmonella, Shigella, Escherichia coli, Clostridium difficile, Yersinia, Campylobacter*, other) agents.*

AIDS, Acquired immunodeficiency syndrome; *IPEX*, immune dysregulation, polyendocrinopathy, enteropathy, X-linked.

in gas, cramps, and acidic stools. A common cause of chronic loose stools in early childhood is **functional diarrhea**, commonly known as **toddler's diarrhea**. This condition is defined by frequent watery stools in the setting of normal growth and weight gain and is caused by excessive intake of sweetened liquids overwhelming the disaccharide absorptive capacity of the intestine. Diarrhea typically improves tremendously when the child's beverage intake is reduced or changed.

Distinguishing Features

Decision-Making Algorithm
Available @ StudentConsult.com
Diarrhea

Stools are isosmotic, even in osmotic diarrhea, because of the relatively free exchange of water across the intestinal mucosa. Osmoles present in the stool are a mixture of electrolytes and other osmotically active solutes. To determine whether the diarrhea is osmotic or secretory, the **osmotic gap** is calculated:

$$\text{Osmotic gap} = 290 - 2([\text{Na}^+] + [\text{K}^+])$$

Assuming the stool is isosmotic (an osmolarity of 290 mOsm/L), the measured stool sodium and potassium (and their associated anions, accounting for an equal amount) accounts for much of the osmolality. Secretory diarrhea is characterized by an osmotic gap of less than 50. A number significantly higher than 50 defines osmotic diarrhea and indicates that malabsorbed substances other than electrolytes account for fecal osmolarity.

Another way to differentiate between osmotic and secretory diarrhea is to stop all feedings (in hospitalized patients receiving IV fluids). If the diarrhea stops completely while the child is NPO (nothing by mouth), the patient has osmotic diarrhea. A child with a pure secretory diarrhea would continue to have massive stool output. Neither method for classifying diarrhea works perfectly, because most diarrheal illnesses are a mixture of secretory and osmotic components. Viral enteritis damages the intestinal lining, causing malabsorption and osmotic diarrhea. The associated inflammation results in release of mediators that cause excessive secretion. A child with viral enteritis may have decreased stool volume while NPO, but the secretory component of the diarrhea persists until the inflammation resolves.

The **history** should include the onset of diarrhea, number and character of stools, estimates of stool volume, and presence of other symptoms, such as blood in the stool, fever, and weight loss. Recent travel and exposures should be documented, dietary factors should be investigated, and a list of medications recently used should be obtained. Factors that seem to worsen or improve the diarrhea should be determined. **Physical examination** should be thorough, evaluating for abdominal distention, tenderness, quality of bowel sounds, presence of blood in the stool or a large fecal mass on rectal examination, and anal sphincter tone.

Laboratory testing should include stool culture and complete blood count if bacterial enteritis is suspected. If diarrhea occurs after a course of antibiotics, a *Clostridium difficile* toxin assay should be ordered; if stools are reported to be oily or fatty, fecal fat content or fecal elastase to test for pancreatic insufficiency should be measured. Tests for specific diagnoses should be sent when appropriate (e.g., serum antibody tests for celiac disease; colonoscopy for suspected ulcerative colitis). A trial of lactose restriction for several days or lactose breath hydrogen testing is helpful in the evaluation of lactose intolerance.

Constipation and Encopresis

Decision-Making Algorithm
Available @ StudentConsult.com
Constipation

Constipation is a common problem in childhood. When a child is thought to be constipated, his parents may be concerned about straining with defecation, hard stool consistency, large stool size, decreased stool frequency, fear of passing stools, or any combination of these. Physicians define **constipation** as *two or fewer stools per week or passage of hard, pellet-like stools for at least 2 weeks.* A common pattern of constipation is **functional constipation**, which is characterized by two or fewer stools per week, voluntary withholding of stool, and infrequent passage of large-diameter, often painful stools. Children with functional fecal retention often exhibit "retentive posturing" (standing or sitting with legs extended and stiff or crossed legs) and have associated fecal incontinence caused by leakage of retained stool (**encopresis**).

Differential Diagnosis

The differential diagnosis is listed in Table 126.10. **Functional constipation** commonly occurs during toilet training, when the child is unwilling to defecate on the toilet. Retained stool becomes harder and larger over time, leading to painful defecation. This aggravates voluntary withholding of stool, with perpetuation of the constipation.

Hirschsprung disease is characterized by delayed meconium passage in newborns, abdominal distention, vomiting, occasional fever, and foul-smelling stools. This condition is caused by failure of ganglion cells to migrate into the distal bowel, resulting in spasm and functional obstruction of the aganglionic segment. Only about 6% of infants with Hirschsprung disease pass meconium in the first 24 hours of life, compared with 95% of normal infants. Most affected babies rapidly become ill with symptoms of enterocolitis or obstruction. Affected older children do not pass large-caliber stools because of rectal spasm, and they do not have encopresis. Other causes of constipation include spinal cord abnormalities, hypothyroidism, drugs, cystic fibrosis, and anorectal malformations (see Table 126.10). A variety of systemic disorders affecting metabolism or muscle function can result in constipation. Children with **developmental disabilities** have a great propensity for constipation because of diminished capacity to cooperate with toileting, reduced effort or control of pelvic floor muscles during defecation, and diminished perception of the need to pass stool.

Distinguishing Features

Table 126.10 includes typical characteristics of the common causes of constipation. Congenital malformations usually cause symptoms from birth. Functional constipation is overwhelmingly the most common diagnosis in older patients. Constipation in older children often begins after starting school, when free and private access to toilets may be restricted. Use of some drugs,

TABLE 126.10 Common Causes of Constipation and Characteristic Features

CAUSES OF CONSTIPATION	CLINICAL FEATURES
Hirschsprung disease	*History:* Failure to pass stool in first 24 hr, abdominal distention, vomiting, symptoms of enterocolitis (fever, foul-smelling diarrhea, megacolon). Not associated with large-caliber stools or encopresis *Examination:* Snug anal sphincter, empty, contracted rectum. May have explosive release of stool as examiner's finger is withdrawn *Laboratory:* Absence of ganglion cells on rectal suction biopsy specimen, absent relaxation of the internal sphincter, "transition zone" from narrow distal bowel to dilated proximal bowel on barium enema
Functional constipation	*History:* No history of significant neonatal constipation, onset at potty training, large-caliber stools, retentive posturing, may have encopresis *Examination:* Normal or reduced sphincter tone, dilated rectal vault, fecal impaction, soiled underwear, palpable fecal mass in left lower quadrant *Laboratory:* No abnormalities, barium enema would show dilated distal bowel
Anorectal and colonic malformations Anal stenosis Anteriorly displaced anus Imperforate anus Colonic stricture	*History:* Constipation from birth due to abnormal anatomy *Examination:* Anorectal abnormalities are shown easily on physical examination Anteriorly displaced anus is found chiefly in females, with a normal-appearing anus located close to the posterior fourchette of the vagina *Laboratory:* Barium enema shows the anomaly
Multisystem disease Muscular dystrophy Cystic fibrosis Diabetes mellitus Developmental delay Celiac disease	*History:* Presence of other symptoms or prior diagnosis *Examination:* Specific abnormalities may be present that directly relate to the underlying diagnosis *Laboratory:* Tests directed at suspected disorder confirm the diagnosis
Spinal cord abnormalities Meningomyelocele Tethered cord Sacral teratoma or lipoma	*History:* History of swelling or exposed neural tissue in the lower back, history of urinary incontinence *Examination:* Lax sphincter tone due to impaired innervation, visible or palpable abnormality of lower back usually (but not always) present *Laboratory:* Bony abnormalities often present on plain x-ray. Magnetic resonance imaging (MRI) of spinal cord reveals characteristic abnormalities
Drugs Narcotics Psychotropics	*History:* Recent use of drugs known to cause constipation (lead poisoning, opiates) *Examination:* Features suggest functional constipation *Laboratory:* No specific tests available

especially opiates and some psychotropic medications, also is associated with constipation.

For a few specific causes of constipation, directed diagnostic testing can make the diagnosis. A narrowed, aganglionic distal bowel and dilated proximal bowel on barium enema suggests Hirschsprung disease. Rectal suction biopsy confirms the absence of ganglion cells in the rectal submucosal plexus, with hypertrophy of nerve fibers. Lack of internal anal sphincter relaxation can be shown by anorectal manometry in Hirschsprung disease. Hypothyroidism is diagnosed by examination and by thyroid function testing. Anorectal malformations are easily detected by rectal examination. Cystic fibrosis (meconium ileus) is diagnosed by sweat chloride determination or *CFTR* gene mutation analysis (see Chapter 137). Most children with constipation have functional constipation and do not have any laboratory abnormality. Examination reveals normal or reduced anal sphincter tone (owing to stretching by passage of large stools). Fecal impaction is usually present, but a large-caliber, empty rectum may be found if a stool has just been passed.

Evaluation and Treatment of Functional Constipation

In most cases of constipation, the history is consistent with functional constipation—absence of neonatal constipation, active fecal retention, and infrequent, large stools with soiling. In these patients, no testing other than a good physical examination is necessary. Young children with painful defecation must have a prolonged course of stool softener therapy to alleviate fear of defecation. The child should be asked to sit on the toilet for a few minutes on awakening in the morning and immediately after meals, when the colon is most active and it is easiest to pass a stool. Use of a positive reinforcement system for taking medication and sitting on the toilet is helpful for younger children. The stool softener chosen should be non–habit forming, safe, and palatable. Polyethylene glycol and milk of magnesia are the most commonly used agents.

Gastrointestinal Bleeding

Decision-Making Algorithm
Available @ StudentConsult.com

Gastrointestinal Bleeding

GI tract bleeding can be an emergency when large-volume bleeding is present, but even the presence of small amounts of blood in stool or emesis is sufficient to cause concern. Evaluation of bleeding should include confirmation that blood truly is present, estimation of the amount of bleeding, stabilization of the patient's intravascular blood volume, localization of the source of bleeding, and appropriate treatment of the underlying cause. When bleeding is massive, it is crucial that the patient receive adequate resuscitation with fluid and blood products before moving ahead with diagnostic testing.

Differential Diagnosis

GI bleeding has different causes at different ages (Table 126.11).

Distinguishing Features

Red substances in foods, beverages, or medications (such as cefdinir) occasionally can be mistaken for blood. A test for occult blood is worth performing whenever the diagnosis is in doubt.

The GI tract may not be the source of the observed fecal blood. A history of cough and examination of the mouth, nostrils, and lungs is needed to exclude these as a source of hematemesis. Blood in the toilet or diaper may be coming from the urinary tract, vagina, or even a severe diaper rash. If the bleeding is GI, it is important to determine the source as high in the GI tract or distal to the ligament of Treitz. Vomited blood is always proximal. Rectal bleeding may be coming from anywhere in the gut. When dark clots or melena are seen mixed with stool, a higher location is suspected, whereas bright red blood on the surface of stool probably is coming from lower in the colon. When upper GI tract bleeding is suspected, a nasogastric tube may be placed and gastric contents aspirated for evidence of recent bleeding.

The location and hemodynamic significance of the bleeding can also be assessed by history and examination. The parents should be asked to quantify the bleeding. Details of associated symptoms should be sought. Assessment of the vital signs including orthostatic changes when bleeding volume is large, pulses, capillary refill, and assessment of pallor of the mucous membranes provides valuable information. Laboratory assessment and imaging studies should be ordered as indicated (Table 126.12).

Treatment

Treatment of GI bleeding should begin with an initial assessment, rapid stabilization, and a logical sequence of diagnostic tests. When a treatable cause is identified, specific therapy should

TABLE 126.11 Causes and Distinguishing Characteristics of Gastrointestinal Bleeding

AGE	TYPE OF BLEEDING	CHARACTERISTICS
NEWBORN		
Ingested maternal blood*	Hematemesis or rectal, large	Apt test indicates adult hemoglobin is present, cracked maternal nipples
Peptic disease	Hematemesis, amount varies	Blood found in stomach on lavage
Coagulopathy	Hematemesis or rectal, bruising, other sites	History of home birth (no vitamin K)
Allergic colitis*	Streaks of bloody mucus in stool	Eosinophils in feces and in rectal mucosa
Necrotizing enterocolitis	Rectal	Sick infant with tender and distended abdomen
Duplication cyst	Hematemesis	Cystic mass in abdomen on imaging study
Volvulus	Hematemesis, hematochezia	Acute tender, distended abdomen
INFANCY TO 2 YEARS OLD		
Peptic disease	Usually hematemesis, rectal possible	Epigastric pain, coffee-ground emesis
Esophageal varices	Hematemesis	History or evidence of liver disease
Intussusception*	Rectal bleeding	Crampy pain, distention, mass
Meckel diverticulum*	Rectal	Massive, bright red bleeding; no pain
Bacterial enteritis*	Rectal	Bloody diarrhea, fever
NSAID injury	Usually hematemesis, rectal possible	Epigastric pain, coffee-ground emesis
>2 YEARS OLD		
Peptic disease	See above	See above
Esophageal varices	See above	See above
NSAID injury*	See above	See above
Inflammatory bowel disease	Usually rectal	Crampy pain, poor weight gain, diarrhea
Bacterial enteritis*	See above	See above
Pseudomembranous colitis	Rectal	History of antibiotic use, bloody diarrhea
Juvenile polyp	Rectal	Painless, bright red blood in stool; not massive
Meckel diverticulum*	See above	See above
Nodular lymphoid hyperplasia	Rectal	Streaks of blood in stool, no other symptoms
Mallory-Weiss syndrome*	Hematemesis	Bright red or coffee-ground, follows retching
Hemolytic uremic syndrome	Rectal	Thrombocytopenia, anemia, uremia
Hemorrhoids	Rectal	Dilated external veins, blood with wiping

*Common.
NSAID, Nonsteroidal antiinflammatory drug.

TABLE 126.12 Evaluation of Gastrointestinal Bleeding

LABORATORY INVESTIGATION	Meckel scan
All Patients	Mesenteric arteriogram
CBC and platelet count	Video capsule endoscopy
Coagulation tests: prothrombin time, partial thromboplastin time	**INITIAL RADIOLOGIC EVALUATION**
Tests of liver dysfunction: AST, ALT, GGT, bilirubin	**All Patients**
Occult blood test of stool or vomitus	Abdominal x-ray series
Blood type and crossmatch	**Evaluation of Hematemesis**
Evaluation of Bloody Diarrhea	Barium upper GI series if endoscopy not available
Stool culture, *Clostridium difficile* toxin	**Evaluation of Bleeding With Pain and Vomiting (Bowel Obstruction)**
Sigmoidoscopy or colonoscopy	Abdominal x-ray series
CT with contrast	Pneumatic or contrast enema
Evaluation of Rectal Bleeding With Formed Stools	Upper GI series
External and digital rectal examination	
Sigmoidoscopy or colonoscopy	

ALT, Alanine aminotransferase; *AST*, aspartate aminotransferase; *CBC*, complete blood count; *CT*, computed tomography; *GGT*, γ-glutamyltransferase; *GI*, gastrointestinal.

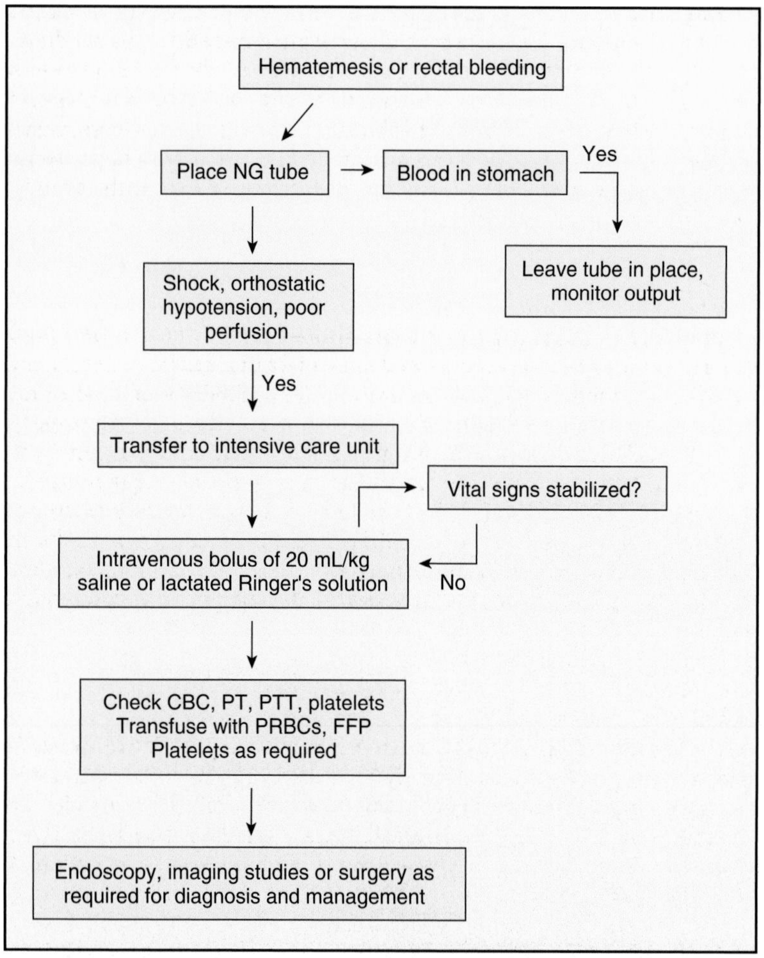

FIGURE 126.2 Initial management of gastrointestinal bleeding. *CBC*, Complete blood count; *FFP*, fresh frozen plasma; *NG*, nasogastric; *PRBCs*, packed red blood cells; *PT*, prothrombin time; *PTT*, partial thromboplastin time.

be started. In many cases, the amount of blood is small, and no resuscitation is required. For children with large-volume bleeds, the **ABCs** of resuscitation (airway, breathing, circulation) should be addressed first (see Chapters 38 and 40). Oxygen should be administered and the airway protected with an endotracheal tube if massive hematemesis is present. Fluid boluses and transfusion with packed red blood cells as required should be administered through two large-bore IVs. Frequent reassessment should continue to ensure maintenance of physiological stability (Fig. 126.2).

CHAPTER 127

Oral Cavity

EFFECTS OF SYSTEMIC DISEASE ON THE ORAL CAVITY

Medications taken for a variety of conditions may cause oral abnormalities. Drugs with anticholinergic properties diminish saliva production and increase the risk of dental caries and parotitis. Tetracyclines taken before the eruption of the permanent teeth stain the enamel. Excessive fluoride in vitamin preparations or in drinking water can result in mottled teeth. Gingival hypertrophy may be caused by cyclosporine, phenytoin, and calcium channel blockers.

Gastroesophageal reflux disease (GERD) can lead to substantial enamel erosion and caries. Neonatal hyperbilirubinemia can result in discoloration of the deciduous teeth. Renal failure is associated with mottled enamel of the permanent teeth. Congenital syphilis causes marked abnormalities in the shape of teeth, especially incisors and molars. Celiac disease can result in enamel defects. Crohn disease is associated with oral aphthous ulcers. Abnormal pigmentation of the lips and buccal mucosa is seen with Peutz-Jeghers syndrome and Addison disease. Candidiasis is seen commonly with immunodeficiency disorders and diabetes. Leukemic infiltrates result in gum hyperplasia and bleeding; treatment of neoplastic conditions can cause severe mucositis. Some tumors, including lymphoma, may present as mass lesions of the buccal cavity.

Osteogenesis imperfecta is associated with abnormal dentin and risk of caries. Children with *ectodermal dysplasias* commonly have malformed or missing teeth. Pierre Robin and Stickler syndromes are associated with micrognathia and cleft palate. Disorders resulting in facial dysmorphism can have a profound effect on dental occlusion and mandibular function. Examples include mandibulofacial dysostosis, Crouzon syndrome, conditions associated with dwarfism, and others.

DECIDUOUS AND PRIMARY TEETH

Most infants are born without teeth. *Natal teeth* are present at birth, are usually supernumerary, and may be poorly attached. Usually, no treatment is necessary, but removal by a dentist may be needed if they are causing difficulties with feeding or injuries to the tongue. Table 127.1 presents the ages when normal **deciduous teeth** are acquired. The lower central incisors are typically the first to erupt, followed by the upper central incisors, lateral incisors, first molars, and bicuspids. **Delayed eruption** may occur in association with hypopituitarism, hypothyroidism, osteopetrosis, Gaucher disease, Down syndrome, cleidocranial dysplasia, and rickets. Deciduous teeth begin to be replaced by the permanent teeth at around age 6 years. The sequence of replacement is similar to that of the appearance of deciduous teeth.

DENTAL CARIES

Etiology

Dental caries, commonly referred to as "cavities," occurs as a result of interactions between the tooth enamel, dietary carbohydrates, and oral flora. There is increased susceptibility if the enamel is abnormal or hypoplastic. Bacteria (*Streptococcus mutans*) that can adhere to and colonize the teeth, survive at low pH, and produce acids during fermentation of carbohydrates cause dental caries. The diet has a significant role. A classic example is "bottle mouth," or **baby bottle caries.** This condition results when infants are allowed to have a bottle in the mouth for prolonged periods, especially during sleep, and with sweet beverages or milk in the bottle. Bacteria then have continuous substrate for acid production and can destroy multiple teeth, especially the upper incisors. Sticky sweet foods, such as candy, have the same effect.

TABLE 127.1 Time of Eruption of the Primary and Permanent Teeth

	PRIMARY, AGE (mo)		PERMANENT, AGE (yr)	
TOOTH TYPE	UPPER	LOWER	UPPER	LOWER
Central incisor	6 ± 2	7 ± 2	7-8	6-7
Lateral incisor	9 ± 2	7 ± 2	8-9	7-8
Cuspids	18 ± 2	16 ± 2	11-12	9-10
First bicuspids	—	—	10-11	10-12
Second bicuspids	—	—	10-12	11-12
First molars	14 ± 2	12 ± 2	6-7	6-7
Second molars	24 ± 2	20 ± 2	12-13	11-13
Third molars	—	—	17-21	17-21

Epidemiology and Treatment

Risk of caries is associated with lack of dental care and poor socioeconomic status and, predictably, is greatest in developing countries. Baby bottle caries are seen in 50-70% of low-income infants. Treatment of caries is with dental restorative surgery. The carious portion is removed and filled with silver amalgam or plastic. If the damage is severe, a protective crown may be required; extraction of the tooth may be necessary when not salvageable. If not properly treated, dental decay results in inflammation and infection of the dental pulp and surrounding alveolar bone, which can lead to abscess and facial space infections.

Prevention

Avoiding inappropriate use of bottles and excessive sweets is a commonsense remedy for baby bottle caries. Oral hygiene offers some protection, but young children (<8 years old) do not have the ability to brush their own teeth adequately; brushing should be done by the parents. Fluoride supplementation of community water supplies to a concentration of 1 ppm is highly effective in reducing dental caries. Home water supplies, such as from a well, should have the fluoride content tested before supplements are prescribed. If the child spends part of the day at another location, the total fluoride concentration from all sources must be considered before prescribing any oral supplements. Excessive fluoride supplementation causes fluorosis, a largely cosmetic defect of chalky white marks and brown staining of the teeth.

The American Academy of Pediatrics recommends that primary care physicians apply fluoride varnish to the teeth of all children every 3-6 months, starting at the emergence of the first tooth. Fluoride varnish is a concentrated fluoride preparation that adheres to the teeth on contact with saliva. It is painted onto the teeth with a small brush, after first drying the tooth with a gauze pad, and has a prolonged cavity-prevention effect.

CLEFT LIP AND PALATE

Epidemiology

Cleft lip and palate occur separately or together and affect approximately 1 in 700 infants. It is more common in Asians (1:500) and least common in Africans (1:2,500). Clefting occurs with two possible patterns: isolated soft tissue cleft palate or cleft lip with or without associated clefts of the hard palate. Isolated cleft palate is associated with a higher risk of other congenital malformations. The combined cleft lip/palate type has a male predominance.

Etiology

Cleft lip is due to hypoplasia of the mesenchymal tissues with subsequent failure of fusion. There is a strong genetic component; the risk is highest in children with affected first-degree relatives. Monozygotic twins are affected with only 60% concordance, suggesting other nongenomic factors. Environmental factors during gestation also increase risk, including drugs (phenytoin, valproic acid, thalidomide), maternal alcohol and tobacco use, dioxins and other herbicides, and possibly high altitude. Chromosomal and nonchromosomal syndromes are associated with clefting, as are specific genes in some families.

Clinical Manifestations and Treatment

Cleft lip can be unilateral or bilateral and associated with cleft palate and defects of the alveolar ridge and dentition. When present, palatal defects allow direct communication between the nasal and oral cavities, creating problems with speech and feeding. Management includes squeeze-bottle feedings, special nipples, nipples with attached shields to seal the palate, and gastrostomy in severe cases. Surgical closure of the cleft lip is usually done by 3 months of age. Closure of the palate follows, usually before 1 year of age. Missing teeth are replaced by prostheses. Cosmetic results are often good, but depend on the severity of the defect.

Complications

Speech is nasal as a result of the cleft palate. Surgical treatment is effective, but sometimes does not restore palatal function completely. Speech therapy or, occasionally, the use of a speech-assisting appliance may help. Frequent episodes of otitis media are common, as are defects of teeth and the alveolar ridge.

THRUSH

Epidemiology

Oropharyngeal *Candida albicans* infection, or thrush, is common in healthy neonates. The organism may be acquired in the birth canal or from the environment. Persistent infection is common in breast fed infants as a result of colonization or infection of the mother's nipples. Thrush in healthy older patients can occur but should suggest the possibility of an immunodeficiency, broad-spectrum antibiotic or inhaled steroid use, or diabetes.

Clinical Manifestations

Thrush is easily visible as white plaques, often with a "fuzzy" appearance, on oral mucous membranes. When scraped with a tongue depressor, the plaques are difficult to remove and the underlying mucosa is inflamed and friable. Clinical diagnosis is usually adequate but may be confirmed by fungal culture or potassium hydroxide smear. Oropharyngeal candidiasis is sometimes painful (especially if associated with esophagitis) and can interfere with feeding.

Treatment

Thrush is treated with topical nystatin or an azole antifungal agent such as fluconazole. When the mother's breasts are infected and painful, consideration should be given to treating her at the same time. Because thrush is commonly self-limited in newborns, withholding therapy in asymptomatic infants and treating only persistent or severe cases is a reasonable approach.

CHAPTER 128

Esophagus and Stomach

GASTROESOPHAGEAL REFLUX

Etiology and Epidemiology

Decision-Making Algorithms
Available @ StudentConsult.com

Cough
Wheezing
Abdominal Pain
Vomiting
Gastrointestinal Bleeding

Gastroesophageal reflux (GER) is defined as the effortless retrograde movement of gastric contents upward into the esophagus or oropharynx. In infancy, GER is not always an abnormality. **Physiological GER** ("spitting up") is normal in infants younger than 8-12 months old. Nearly half of all infants are reported to spit up between 2 and 4 months of age. Infants who regurgitate meet the criteria for physiological GER so long as they maintain adequate nutrition and have no signs of respiratory complications or esophagitis. Contributing factors of infantile GER include liquid diet; horizontal body position; short, narrow esophagus; small, noncompliant stomach; frequent, relatively large-volume feedings; and an immature lower esophageal sphincter (LES). As infants grow, they spend more time upright, eat more solid foods, develop a longer and larger diameter esophagus, have a larger and more compliant stomach, and experience lower caloric needs per unit of body weight. As a result, most infants stop spitting up by 9-12 months of age.

Gastroesophageal reflux *disease* (GERD) occurs when GER leads to troublesome symptoms or complications such as poor growth, pain, or breathing difficulties. GERD occurs in a minority of infants but is often implicated as the cause of fussiness. GERD is seen in fewer than 5% of older children. In older children, normal protective mechanisms against GER include antegrade esophageal motility, tonic contraction of the LES, and the geometry of the gastroesophageal junction. Abnormalities that cause GER in older children and adults include reduced tone of the LES, transient relaxations of the LES, esophagitis (which impairs esophageal motility), increased intraabdominal pressure, cough, respiratory difficulty (asthma or cystic fibrosis), and hiatal hernia.

Clinical Manifestations

Decision-Making Algorithms
Available @ StudentConsult.com

Cough
Hoarseness
Wheezing
Abdominal Pain
Failure to Thrive

The presence of GER is easy to observe in an infant who spits up. In older children, the refluxate is usually kept down by reswallowing, but GER may be suspected by associated symptoms, such as heartburn, cough, epigastric abdominal pain, dysphagia, wheezing, aspiration pneumonia, hoarse voice, failure to thrive, and recurrent hiccoughs or belching. In severe cases of esophagitis, there may be laboratory evidence of anemia and hypoalbuminemia secondary to esophageal bleeding and inflammation.

When esophagitis develops as a result of acid reflux, esophageal motility and LES function are impaired further, creating a cycle of reflux and esophageal injury.

Laboratory and Imaging Studies

A clinical diagnosis is often sufficient in children with classic effortless regurgitation and no complications. Diagnostic studies are indicated if there are persistent symptoms or complications or if other symptoms suggest the possibility of GER in the absence of regurgitation. A child with recurrent pneumonia, chronic cough, or apneic spells without overt emesis may have occult GER. A **barium upper gastrointestinal (GI) series** helps to rule out gastric outlet obstruction, malrotation, or other anatomical contributors to GER. Because of the brief nature of the examination, a negative barium study does *not* rule out GER, nor does it rule it in as it is normal to have some reflux into the esophagus many times per day. A **24-hour esophageal pH probe monitoring** uses a pH electrode placed transnasally into the distal esophagus, with continuous recording of esophageal pH. Data typically are gathered for 24 hours and analyzed for the number and temporal pattern of acid reflux events. **Esophageal impedance monitoring** records the migration of electrolyte-rich gastric fluid in the esophagus. **Endoscopy** is useful to evaluate for esophagitis, esophageal stricture, and anatomical abnormalities.

Treatment

In otherwise healthy young infants, no treatment is necessary. For infants with complications of GER, an H_2 blocker or proton-pump inhibitor may be offered (Table 128.1), but these have

TABLE 128.1 Treatment of Gastroesophageal Reflux

THERAPIES	COMMENTS
CONSERVATIVE THERAPIES	
Towel on caregiver's shoulder	Cheap, effective; useful only for physiological reflux
Thickened feedings	Reduces number of episodes, enhances nutrition
Smaller, more frequent feedings	Can help some; be careful not to *underfeed* child
Avoidance of tobacco smoke and alcohol	Always a good idea; may help reflux symptoms
Abstaining from caffeine	Inexpensive, offers some benefit
Positional therapy—upright in seat, elevate	Prone positioning with head of crib or bed up is helpful, but *not* for young infants because of risk of SIDS
Weight loss when indicated	Increased weight (especially abdominal) increases intraabdominal pressure, leading to reflux
MEDICAL THERAPY	
Proton pump inhibitor	Effective medical therapy for heartburn and esophagitis
H_2-receptor antagonist	Reduces heartburn, less effective for healing esophagitis
Metoclopramide	Enhances stomach emptying and LES tone; real benefit is often minimal
SURGICAL THERAPY	
Nissen or other fundoplication procedure	For life-threatening or medically unresponsive cases
Feeding jejunostomy	Useful in child requiring tube feeds; delivering feeds downstream eliminates GERD

GERD, Gastroesophageal reflux disease; *LES*, lower esophageal sphincter; *SIDS*, sudden infant death syndrome.

shown little benefit in infants with uncomplicated GER and/or fussiness. Prokinetic drugs, such as metoclopramide, occasionally are helpful by enhancing gastric emptying and increasing LES tone, but they are seldom effective and may lead to complications. When severe symptoms persist despite medication, or if life-threatening aspiration is present, surgical intervention may be required. Fundoplication procedures, such as the Nissen operation, are designed to enhance the antireflux anatomy of the LES. In children with a severe neurological defect who cannot tolerate oral or gastric tube feedings, placement of a feeding jejunostomy may be considered as an alternative to fundoplication. In older children, lifestyle changes should be discussed, including cessation of smoking, weight loss, not eating before bed or exercise, and limiting intake of caffeine, carbonation, and high-fat foods. However, proton pump inhibitor therapy is more effective in reducing symptoms and supports healing.

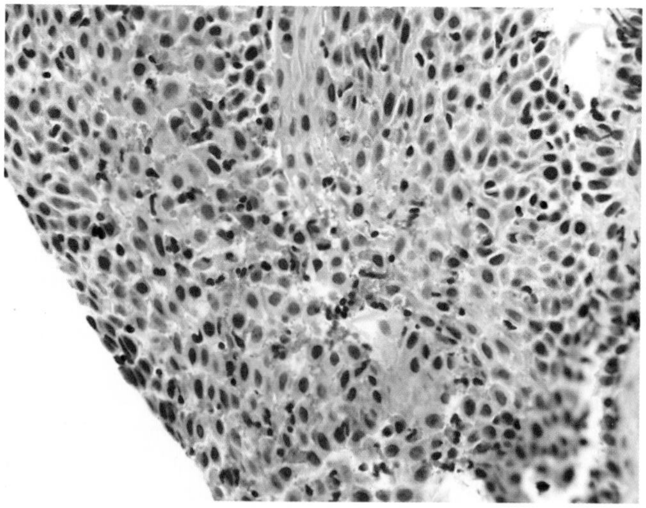

FIGURE 128.1 Histological image of eosinophilic esophagitis. Note the large number of eosinophils within the lamina propria.

EOSINOPHILIC ESOPHAGITIS

Etiology and Epidemiology

This chronic immune-mediated disorder is characterized by infiltration of eosinophils into the mucosa of the esophagus. It is thought to be triggered by non–immunoglobulin (Ig) E-mediated allergic reactions to ingested foods or aeroallergens. Eosinophilic esophagitis (EoE) may have a familial component; no specific gene has yet been identified. Incidence appears to be increasing with estimated prevalence of more than 4 per 10,000 children. It may be more common in males than females and in patients with history of atopy.

Clinical Manifestations

The presentation of EoE often varies with age. In young children, it may present with oral aversion, vomiting, and failure to thrive. In school-age children, it may present with vague abdominal pain or vomiting. In adolescents and adults, it presents with dysphagia and food impactions. These symptoms are attributed to the inflammatory response in the esophagus leading to edema and poor esophageal motility.

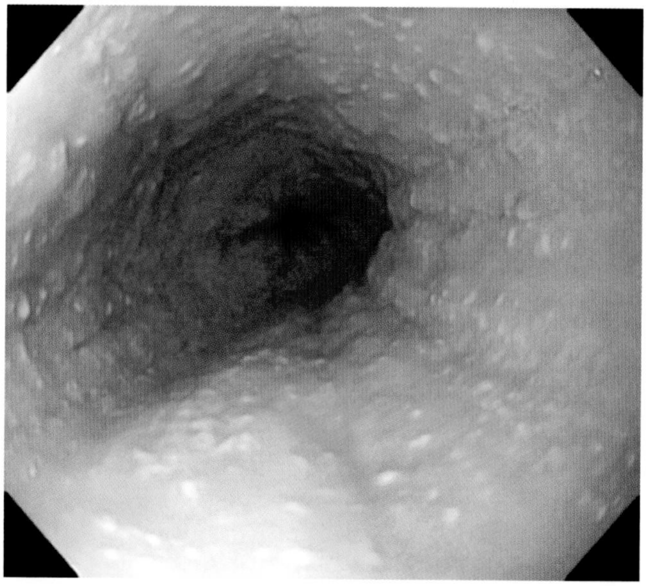

FIGURE 128.2 Endoscopic picture of eosinophilic esophagitis. White plaques on the surface are collections of eosinophils (eosinophilic abscesses). Linear furrowing is also seen.

Laboratory and Imaging Studies

Diagnosis requires multilevel esophageal biopsies via flexible endoscopy with the finding of more than 15 eosinophils per high-power field (Fig. 128.1). Treatment with high-dose proton pump inhibitor therapy is recommended to exclude the possibility that findings are secondary to severe acidic esophageal injury or by evaluating for acid reflux by pH probe testing. Gross findings at endoscopy may include normal appearance, or esophageal furrowing, trachealization, and eosinophilic abscesses (Fig. 128.2). A barium study may reveal a food impaction in an acutely symptomatic patient or esophageal stricture in someone with chronic disease.

Treatment and Prognosis

Exposure to identified causative antigens needs to be eliminated. Identification can be difficult, as typical allergy testing (skin prick, RAST, and immunocap assays) only identifies IgE-mediated antigens. Atopic patch testing may be more reliable but is not standardized and can be difficult to perform. One approach is to eliminate cow's milk, soy, wheat, eggs, peanuts, and fish/shellfish from the diet ("Six food elimination diet"), as these are the most common causative dietary antigens. Repeat endoscopies are often necessary to document efficacy of these eliminations. An elemental diet can also be used and is very effective, but often requires either nasogastric or gastrotomy administration because of its poor palatability.

Systemic glucocorticoids can decrease symptoms, but long-term use is discouraged due to concerns for potential complications. Swallowed "topical" glucocorticoids administered via a metered-dose inhaler (fluticasone) or mixed as a slurry (budesonide) have shown benefit. *Candida* esophagitis or oral thrush are the most common side effects.

Endoscopy can be used to relieve food impactions and to dilate esophageal strictures secondary to EoE. The prognosis for EoE is largely unknown. Symptoms tend to wax and wane over time.

Complications

Failure to thrive or weight loss may be seen due to difficulty in eating. Food impactions are a common complication in the older child and may require endoscopic removal. Chronic inflammation of the esophagus can predispose to esophageal strictures and possibly dysplasia.

ESOPHAGEAL ATRESIA AND TRACHEOESOPHAGEAL FISTULA

Etiology and Epidemiology

The esophagus and trachea develop in close proximity to each other during weeks 4-6 of fetal life. Defects in the mesenchyme separating these two structures result in a tracheoesophageal fistula (TEF), often in association with other anomalies (renal, heart, spine, limbs). This defect occurs in about 1 in 3,000 live births. TEF is not thought to be a genetic defect.

Clinical Manifestations

The most common forms of TEF occur with esophageal atresia; the "H-type" TEF without atresia is uncommon, as is esophageal atresia without TEF (Fig. 128.3). Associated defects include the **VACTERL** association—vertebral anomalies (70%), **a**nal atresia (imperforate anus) (50%), **c**ardiac anomalies (30%), **TE**F (70%), **r**enal anomalies (50%), and **l**imb anomalies (polydactyly, forearm defects, absent thumbs, syndactyly) (70%). A single-artery umbilical cord is often present. Infants with esophageal atresia have a history of polyhydramnios, exhibit drooling, and have mucus and saliva bubbling from the nose and mouth. Patients with a TEF are vulnerable to aspiration pneumonia. When TEF is suspected, the first feeding should be delayed until a diagnostic study is performed.

Laboratory and Imaging Studies

The simplest test for TEF is to gently attempt to place a 10F or larger tube via the mouth into the stomach. The passage of the tube is blocked at the level of the atresia. A chest x-ray reveals the tube coiled in the esophageal pouch. Air can be injected through the tube to outline the atretic pouch. Barium should not be used because of extreme risk of aspiration, but a tiny amount of dilute water-soluble contrast agent can be given carefully, then suctioned when the defect is clearly shown.

Treatment and Prognosis

The treatment of TEF is surgical. The fistula is divided and ligated. The esophageal ends are approximated and anastomosed. In some cases, primary anastomosis cannot be performed because of a long gap between the proximal and distal esophagus. Various techniques have been described to treat this problem, including pulling up the stomach, elongating the esophagus by myotomy, and simply delaying esophageal anastomosis and providing continuous suction to the upper pouch while allowing for growth.

Complications

The surgically reconstructed esophagus is not normal and is prone to poor motility, GER, anastomotic stricture, recurrent fistula, and leakage. The trachea also is malformed; tracheomalacia and wheezing are common.

ESOPHAGEAL FOREIGN BODIES

Etiology and Epidemiology

Young children often place nonfood items in their mouths. When these items are swallowed, they may become lodged

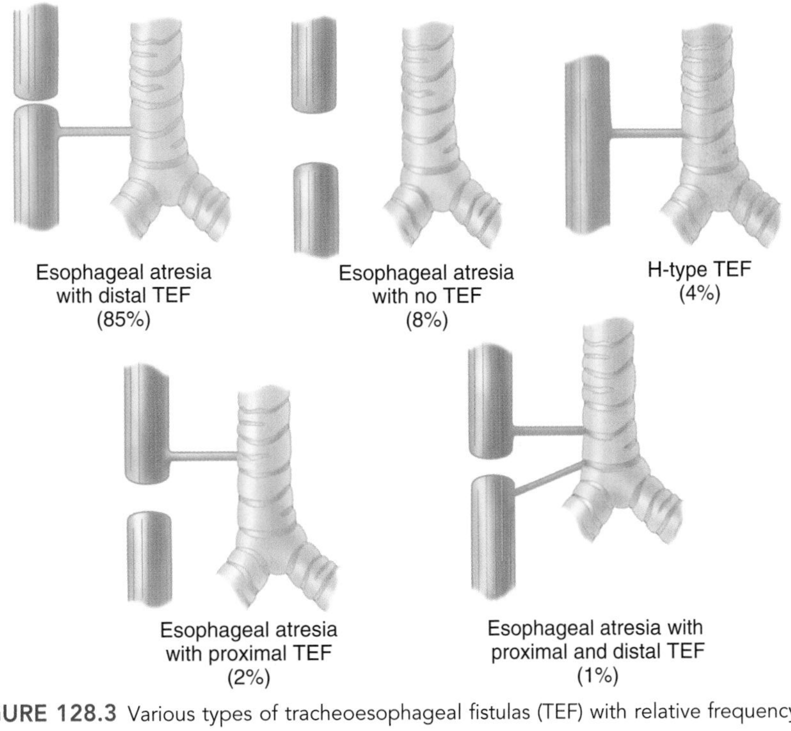

FIGURE 128.3 Various types of tracheoesophageal fistulas (TEF) with relative frequency (%).

in the esophagus at the thoracic inlet or at the LES. The most common objects are coins. Smaller coins may pass harmlessly into the stomach, where they rarely cause symptoms. Other common esophageal foreign bodies include food items, small toys or toy parts, disk batteries, and other small household items. Children with a prior history of esophageal atresia or with poor motility secondary to GER or EoE are more prone to food impactions, which seldom occur in the normal esophagus.

Clinical Manifestations

Some children are asymptomatic, but most exhibit some degree of drooling, food refusal, or chest discomfort. Older children usually can point to the region of the chest where they feel the object to be lodged. Respiratory symptoms tend to be minimal, but cough or wheezing may be present, especially when the esophagus is completely blocked by a large object, such as a piece of meat, which presses on the trachea.

Diagnosis

Plain chest and abdominal radiographs should be taken when foreign body ingestion is suspected. Metallic objects are easily visualized. A plastic object often can be seen if the child is given a small amount of dilute x-ray contrast material to drink, although endoscopy is probably safer and more definitive.

Treatment

Endoscopy is ultimately necessary in most cases to remove a retained esophageal foreign body. Various devices can be used to remove the object, depending on its size, shape, and location. Coins usually are grasped with special-purpose forceps and removed. Nets, baskets, and snares also are available. Whenever objects that may threaten the airway are being recovered, endoscopy should be performed with endotracheal intubation and under general anesthesia. Removal is usually not necessary if the object is small and in the stomach as it will most likely pass without complication. Endoscopy is emergent for removal of any esophageal foreign body if symptomatic or if the ingested foreign body is a suspected disc battery in the esophagus or multiple magnets located in the upper intestinal tract.

Complications

Sharp objects may lacerate or perforate the esophagus; smooth objects present for a long time also may result in perforation due to ulceration. Corrosive objects, such as zinc-containing pennies and disc batteries, can cause considerable local tissue injury and esophageal perforation. Magnets can lead to perforation and fistula formation when they connect between adjacent loops of bowel.

CAUSTIC INJURIES AND PILL ULCERS

Etiology and Epidemiology

In adolescents, caustic ingestion injuries are usually the result of suicide attempts. In toddlers, ingestion of household cleaning products typically is accidental. Injurious agents include drain cleaners, toilet bowl cleaners, dishwasher and laundry detergents, and powerful bleaching agents. Childproof lids for commercial products offer some protection, but have not eliminated the problem. Lye-based drain cleaners, especially liquid products, cause the worst injuries because they are swallowed easily and liquefy tissue rapidly. Full-thickness burns can occur in seconds. Granular products are less likely to cause esophageal injury during accidental exposures because they burn the tongue and lips and often are expelled before swallowing. Less caustic agents, such as bleach and detergents, cause less serious injury. **Pill ulcers** occur when certain medications (tetracyclines and nonsteroidal antiinflammatory drugs [NSAIDs]) are swallowed without sufficient liquids, allowing prolonged direct contact of the pill with the esophageal mucosa.

Clinical Manifestations

Caustic burns cause immediate and severe mouth pain. The child cries out, drools, spits, and usually drops the container immediately. Burns of the lips and tongue are visible almost immediately. These burns clearly indicate the possibility of esophageal involvement, although esophageal injury can occur in the absence of oral burns. Symptoms may not be present; further evaluation by endoscopy usually is indicated with any significant history of caustic ingestion. Pill injury causes severe chest pain and often prominent odynophagia (painful swallowing) and dysphagia.

Laboratory and Imaging Studies

A chest x-ray should be obtained to rule out aspiration and to inspect for mediastinal air. The child should be admitted to the hospital and given intravenous (IV) fluids until endoscopy. The true extent of burns may not be endoscopically apparent immediately, but delayed endoscopy can increase the risk of perforation. Most endoscopists perform the initial endoscopy soon after injury, when the patient has been stabilized. The extent of injury and severity of the burn should be carefully determined. Risk of subsequent esophageal strictures is related to the degree of burn and whether the injury is circumferential.

Treatment

A nasogastric tube can be placed over a guide wire at the time of the initial endoscopy to provide a route for feeding and to stent the esophagus. Systemic steroid use has not been found to be beneficial in reducing stricture formation. Broad-spectrum antibiotics should be prescribed if infection is suspected.

Complications

Esophageal strictures, if they occur, usually develop within 1-2 months and can be treated with endoscopic dilation. There is a risk of perforation during dilation. When esophageal destruction is severe, surgical reconstruction of the esophagus using stomach or intestine may be necessary.

PYLORIC STENOSIS

Etiology and Epidemiology

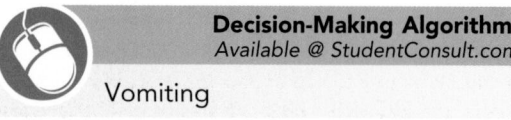

Decision-Making Algorithm
Available @ StudentConsult.com

Vomiting

Pyloric stenosis is an acquired condition caused by hypertrophy and spasm of the pyloric muscle, resulting in gastric outlet obstruction. It occurs in 6-8 per 1,000 live births, has a 5-to-1 male predominance, and is more common in first-born children. Its cause is unknown.

Clinical Manifestations

Infants with pyloric stenosis typically begin vomiting during the first weeks of life, but onset may be delayed. The emesis becomes increasingly frequent and forceful as time passes. Vomiting differs from spitting up because of its extremely forceful and often projectile nature. The vomited material never contains bile, because the gastric outlet obstruction is proximal to the duodenum. This feature differentiates pyloric stenosis from most other obstructive lesions of early childhood. Affected infants are ravenously hungry early in the course of the illness but become more lethargic with increasing malnutrition and dehydration. The stomach becomes massively enlarged with retained food and secretions, and gastric **peristaltic waves** are often visible in the left upper quadrant. A hypertrophied pylorus (the "olive") may be palpated. As the illness progresses, very little of each feeding is able to pass through the pylorus, and the child becomes progressively thinner and more dehydrated.

Laboratory and Imaging Studies

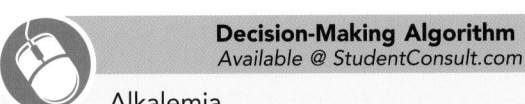

Decision-Making Algorithm
Available @ StudentConsult.com
Alkalemia

Repetitive vomiting of purely gastric contents results in loss of hydrochloric acid; the classic laboratory finding is a **hypochloremic, hypokalemic metabolic alkalosis** with elevated blood urea nitrogen (BUN) secondary to dehydration. Jaundice with unconjugated hyperbilirubinemia may also occur. Plain abdominal x-rays typically show a huge stomach and diminished or absent gas in the intestine (Fig. 128.4). Ultrasound examination shows marked elongation and thickening of the pylorus (Fig. 128.5). A barium upper GI series also may be obtained whenever doubt about the diagnosis exists; this shows a "string sign" caused by barium moving through an elongated, constricted pyloric channel.

Treatment

Treatment of pyloric stenosis includes IV fluid and electrolyte resuscitation followed by surgical pyloromyotomy. Before surgery, dehydration and hypochloremic alkalosis must be corrected, generally with an initial normal saline fluid bolus followed by infusions of half-normal saline containing 5% dextrose and potassium chloride when urine output is observed. In pyloromyotomy (often by laparoscope), the pyloric muscle is incised longitudinally to release the constriction.

PEPTIC DISEASE

Etiology and Epidemiology

Acid-related injury can occur in the esophagus, stomach, or duodenum. Table 128.2 lists risk factors for **peptic ulcer disease**

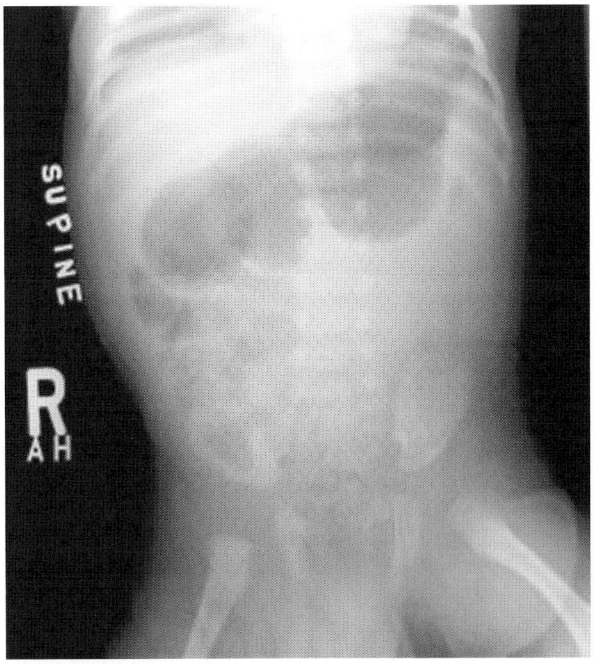

FIGURE 128.4 Pyloric Stenosis. Note the huge, gas-filled stomach extending across the midline, with minimal air in the intestine downstream. (Courtesy Warren Bishop, MD.)

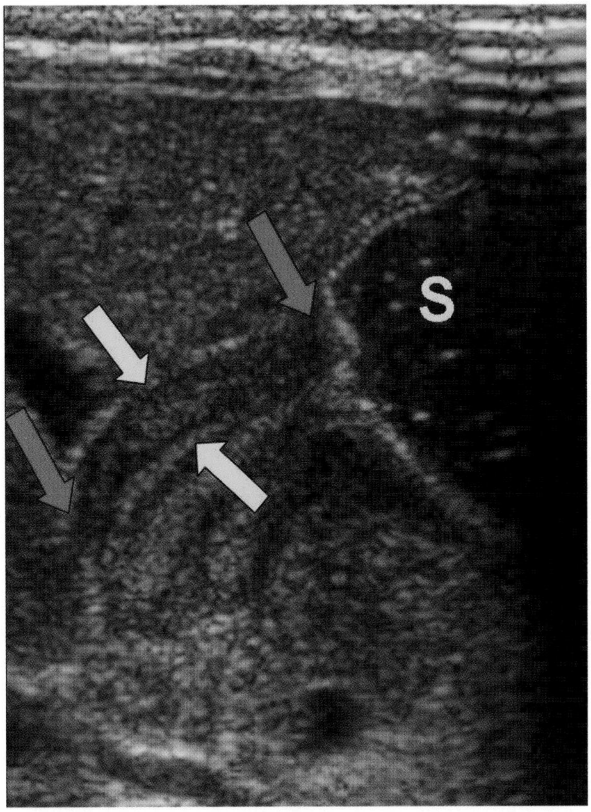

FIGURE 128.5 Ultrasound image of infant with pyloric stenosis. Large, fluid-filled stomach *(S)* is seen at right, with an elongated, thickened pylorus. The length of the pylorus is marked by the *red arrows*; the wall thickness is marked by the *yellow arrows*.

TABLE 128.2 Risk Factors for Peptic Ulcer Disease

Helicobacter pylori infection
Drugs
NSAIDs, including aspirin
Tobacco use
Bisphosphonates
Potassium supplements
Family history
Sepsis
Head trauma
Burn injury
Hypotension

NSAIDs, Nonsteroidal antiinflammatory drugs.

in children. ***Helicobacter pylori*** is responsible for more than half of ulcers in the stomach and duodenum in adults. *H. pylori* plays a significant but lesser role in childhood ulcer disease. Risk factors for acquisition of *H. pylori* are low socioeconomic status and poor sanitation, with the highest incidence in developing countries. **Nonulcer dyspepsia** includes upper abdominal symptoms (pain, bloating, nausea, early satiety) in the absence of gastric or duodenal ulceration. Nonulcer dyspepsia is *not* associated with *H. pylori* infection. GER (see Chapter 128) allows acidic gastric contents to injure the esophagus, resulting in **esophagitis.** Esophagitis is characterized by retrosternal and epigastric burning pain and is best diagnosed by endoscopy. It can range from minimal, with only erythema and microscopic inflammation on biopsy, to superficial erosions and finally, to frank ulceration.

Clinical Manifestations

Typical symptoms are listed in Table 128.3. The presence of recurrent burning epigastric and retrosternal pain is a risk factor for esophagitis. With duodenal ulcers, pain typically occurs several hours after meals and often awakens patients at night. Eating tends to relieve the pain. Gastric ulcers differ in that pain is commonly aggravated by eating, resulting in weight loss. GI bleeding from either can occur. Many patients report symptom relief with antacids or acid blockers.

Laboratory and Imaging Studies

Endoscopy can be used to diagnose the underlying condition. Empiric therapy with H_2 blockers or proton pump inhibitors can be used but may delay diagnosis of conditions such as *H. pylori.* For patients with chronic epigastric pain, the possibilities of inflammatory bowel disease, anatomical abnormality such as malrotation, pancreatitis, and biliary disease should be ruled out by appropriate testing when suspected (see Chapter 126 and Table 128.3 for recommended studies). Testing for *H. pylori* can be performed by biopsy during endoscopy with use of a urease test or presence histologically on tissue. If endoscopy is not done, noninvasive tests for infection can be done with reasonable accuracy with *H. pylori* fecal antigen and ^{13}C urea breath tests.

TABLE 128.3 Peptic Disorders, Symptoms, and Clinical Investigation

SYNDROME AND ASSOCIATED SYMPTOMS	CLINICAL INVESTIGATION
ESOPHAGITIS	
Retrosternal and epigastric location Burning pain Sensation of regurgitation Dysphagia, odynophagia	Endoscopy Therapeutic trial of acid-blocker therapy pH probe study
NONULCER DYSPEPSIA	
Upper abdominal location Fullness Bloating Nausea	Endoscopy Therapeutic trial of acid-blocker therapy Upper GI series to ligament of Treitz—rule out malrotation CBC, ESR, amylase, lipase, abdominal ultrasound
PEPTIC ULCER DISEASE	
"Alarm" symptoms Weight loss Hematemesis Melena, heme-positive stools Chronic vomiting Microcytic anemia Nocturnal pain Other symptoms—same as for esophagitis and nonulcer dyspepsia	Endoscopy—mandatory with alarm symptoms Test for *Helicobacter pylori* CBC, ESR, amylase, lipase, abdominal ultrasound

CBC, Complete blood count; *ESR,* erythrocyte sedimentation rate; *GI,* gastrointestinal.

Treatment

If *H. pylori* is present in association with ulcers, it should be treated with a multidrug regimen, such as omeprazole-clarithromycin-metronidazole, omeprazole-amoxicillin-clarithromycin, or omeprazole-amoxicillin-metronidazole, given twice daily for 1-2 weeks. Other proton pump inhibitors may be substituted when necessary. Bismuth compounds are effective against *H. pylori* and can be considered. In North America, only the subsalicylate salt is available, the use of which raises some concerns about Reye syndrome and potential salicylate toxicity. Tetracycline is useful in adults but should be avoided in children less than 8 years of age. In the absence of *H. pylori,* esophagitis and peptic ulcer disease are treated with a proton-pump inhibitor, which yields higher rates of healing than H_2 receptor antagonists. Gastric and duodenal ulcers heal in 4-8 weeks in at least 80% of patients. Esophagitis requires 4-5 months of proton pump inhibitor treatment for optimal healing.

CYCLIC VOMITING SYNDROME

Etiology and Epidemiology

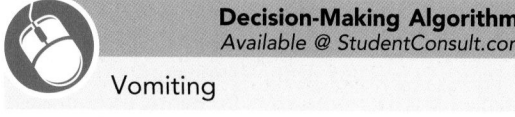

Decision-Making Algorithm
Available @ StudentConsult.com

Vomiting

Cyclic vomiting syndrome (CVS) presents with intermittent episodes of prolonged nausea and vomiting with periods of health in between. It can occur at any age but is diagnosed most frequently in preschool to school-age children. It is thought to be a migraine variant; many patients have a positive family history of migraines, and some with CVS will eventually develop migraine headaches. Triggers to an episode often include viral illnesses, lack of sleep, stressful or exciting events (holidays, birthdays, vacations), physical exhaustion, and menses.

Clinical Manifestations

Episodes can start at any time but will often start in the early morning hours. Episodes are similar to each other in timing and duration. Repetitive vomiting can last hours to days. Patients can also have abdominal pain, diarrhea, and headaches. Those affected are typically pale, listless, and prefer to be left alone. They may have photo- or phonophobia.

Laboratory and Imaging Studies

There are no specific tests for CVS, which is diagnosed based on the history and the exclusion of other disorders. Diagnoses that should be considered include malrotation with intermittent volvulus, uteropelvic junction (UPJ) obstruction, EoE, intracranial mass lesions, and metabolic disorders. Rome III criteria for diagnosis are outlined in Table 126.5.

Treatment

For the acute episode, supportive treatment includes hydration; dark, quiet environment; and antiemetics such as ondansetron. In addition, abortive therapy using antimigraine medications such as NSAIDs and triptans can be used. For those with frequent or prolonged episodes, prophylactic therapy can be used, such as cyproheptadine, tricyclic antidepressants, beta blockers, or topiramate.

CHAPTER 129

Intestinal Tract

MALROTATION

Etiology and Epidemiology

During early fetal life, the midgut is attached to the yolk sac and loops outward into the umbilical cord. Beginning at around 10 weeks' gestation, the bowel re-enters the abdomen and rotates counterclockwise around the superior mesenteric artery until the cecum arrives in the right lower quadrant. The duodenum rotates behind the artery and terminates at the **ligament of Treitz** in the left upper quadrant. The base of the mesentery becomes fixed along a broad attachment posteriorly, running from the cecum to the ligament of Treitz (Fig. 129.1A). When

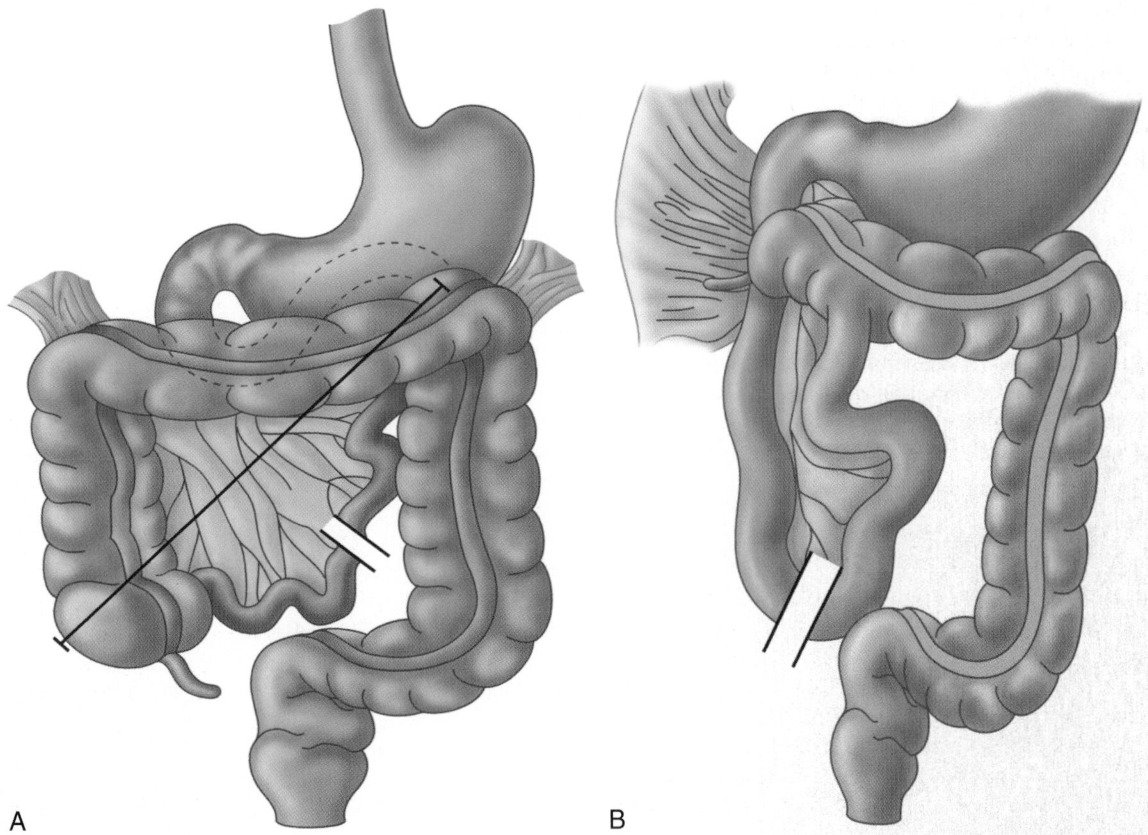

FIGURE 129.1 **(A)** Normal rotation of the midgut. Note the long axis of mesenteric attachment *(line)*. **(B)** Midgut malrotation. Note the narrow mesentery, which predisposes to volvulus, and the presence of Ladd bands extending across the duodenum from the abnormally elevated cecum. (From Donellan WJ, ed. *Abdominal Surgery of Infancy and Childhood*. Luxembourg: Harwood Academic; 1996:43/6, 43/8.)

rotation is incomplete or otherwise abnormal, "malrotation" is present. Incomplete rotation occurs when the cecum stops near the right upper quadrant and the duodenum fails to move behind the mesenteric artery; this results in an extremely narrow mesenteric root (see Fig. 129.1B) that makes the child susceptible to midgut **volvulus**, causing intestinal obstruction or mesenteric artery occlusion and intestinal infarction (Fig. 129.2). It is also common for abnormal mesenteric attachments (Ladd bands) to extend from the cecum across the duodenum, causing partial obstruction.

Clinical Manifestations

Decision-Making Algorithms
Available @ StudentConsult.com

Abdominal Pain
Vomiting
Gastrointestinal Bleeding

About 60% of children with malrotation present with symptoms of bilious vomiting during the first month of life. The remaining 40% presents later in infancy or childhood. The emesis initially may be due to obstruction by Ladd bands without volvulus. When midgut volvulus occurs, the venous drainage of the gut is impaired; congestion results in ischemia, pain, tenderness, and often bloody emesis and stools. The bowel undergoes ischemic necrosis, and the child may appear septic. Physicians must be alert to the possibility of volvulus in patients with vomiting and fussiness or abdominal pain.

Laboratory and Imaging Studies

Plain abdominal x-rays generally show evidence of obstruction. Abdominal ultrasound may show evidence of malrotation. An upper gastrointestinal (GI) series shows the absence of a typical duodenal "C-loop," with the duodenum instead remaining on the right side of the abdomen. Abnormal placement of the cecum on follow-through (or by contrast enema) confirms the diagnosis. Laboratory studies are nonspecific, showing evidence of dehydration, electrolyte loss, or evidence of sepsis. A decreasing platelet count is a common indicator of bowel ischemia.

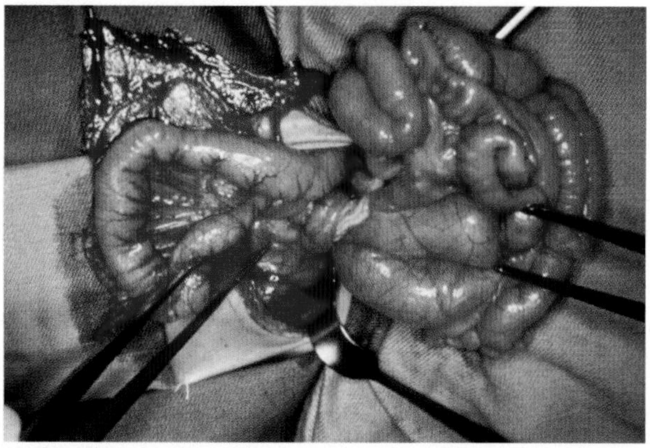

FIGURE 129.2 Malrotation with volvulus. Midgut is twisted around the mesentery, with an area of darker, ischemic intestine visible. (Courtesy Robert Soper, MD.)

Treatment

Treatment is surgical. The bowel is untwisted, and Ladd bands and other abnormal membranous attachments are divided. The mesentery is spread out and flattened against the posterior wall of the abdomen by moving the cecum to the left side of the abdomen. Sutures may be used to hold the bowel in position, but postoperative adhesions tend to hold the mesentery in place, resulting in a broad attachment and eliminating the risk of recurrent volvulus. Necrotic bowel is resected and, at times, results in short gut syndrome.

INTESTINAL ATRESIA

Etiology and Epidemiology

Decision-Making Algorithms
Available @ StudentConsult.com

Abdominal Pain
Vomiting

Congenital partial or complete blockage of the intestine is a developmental defect that occurs in about 1 in 1,500 live births. Atresia occurs in several forms (Fig. 129.3). One or more segments of bowel may be missing completely, there may be varying degrees of obstruction caused by webs or stenosis, or there may be obliteration of the lumen in cordlike bowel remnants. The end result is obstruction with upstream dilation of the bowel and small, disused intestine distally. When obstruction is complete or high grade, bilious vomiting and abdominal distention are present in the newborn period. In lesser cases, as in "windsock" types of intestinal webs, the obstruction is partial, and symptoms are more subtle. Duodenal atresia is associated with other anomalies in more than half of infants. Down syndrome is the most common associated disorder but can also be associated with biliary, cardiac, renal, or vertebral anomalies. Jejunal and ileal atresia can be seen in meconium ileus secondary to cystic fibrosis.

Clinical Manifestations

Intestinal atresia presents with a history of polyhydramnios, abdominal distention, and bilious vomiting in the neonatal period. If intestinal perforation is present, peritonitis and sepsis may develop.

Laboratory and Imaging Studies

Plain abdominal x-rays may localize the area of atresia and identify evidence of perforation, such as free air or calcifications typical of meconium peritonitis. Duodenal atresia appears as a double-bubble sign (gas in the stomach and enlarged proximal duodenum), with no gas distally. Atresias of the distal intestine are characterized by longer segments of dilated, air-filled bowel. Contrast studies are helpful if plain films are not sufficient. Atresia may be a complication of **meconium ileus** associated with cystic fibrosis. Laboratory evaluation for **cystic fibrosis** (see Chapter 137) is indicated in cases of small bowel atresia. A complete blood count, serum electrolytes, liver functions, and amylase should be measured to identify dehydration, pancreatitis, and other complications.

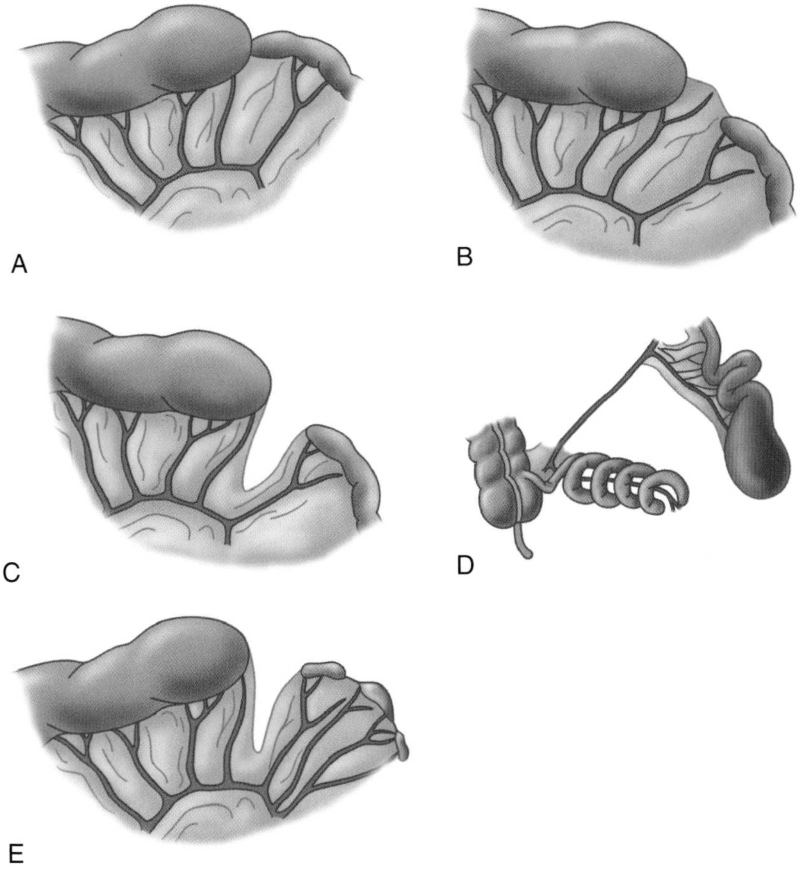

FIGURE 129.3 Types of intestinal atresia. **(A)** Internal web; **(B)** cordlike remnant connecting proximal and distal bowel; **(C)** interrupted bowel with V-shaped mesenteric defect; **(D)** "apple peel" atresia with surviving bowel spiraling around a marginal artery; **(E)** multiple atresias. (From Grosfeld JL, Ballantine TVN, Shoemaker R. Operative management of intestinal atresia based on pathologic findings. *J Pediatr Surg*. 1979;14:368–375.)

Treatment

The treatment of intestinal atresia is surgical, but surgery must be preceded by adequate hemodynamic stabilization of the patient. Intravenous (IV) fluids, nasogastric suction, and broad-spectrum antibiotics should be given.

OTHER CONGENITAL DISORDERS

Gastroschisis is an abdominal wall defect, not involving the umbilicus, through which intestinal contents have herniated. In contrast to omphalocele, the bowel is not covered by peritoneum or amniotic membrane. As a result, prolonged contact with the amniotic fluid typically causes a thick, exudative covering (a "peel") on the exposed bowel. Gastroschisis is not associated with extraintestinal anomalies, but segments of intestinal atresia are common. After surgical reduction of the defect, return of normal bowel function may be slow and requires prolonged parenteral nutrition for infants with long atretic segments (short-bowel syndrome) and infants with a thick peel.

Omphalocele is an abdominal wall defect through the umbilicus caused by failure of the intestine to return to the abdomen during fetal life. The bowel remains within the umbilical cord and is covered by peritoneum and amniotic membranes. This defect is associated with other congenital anomalies, especially cardiac defects, **Beckwith-Wiedemann syndrome**, and intestinal complications. Treatment is surgical closure, which sometimes must be performed in stages to fit the bowel into a congenitally small abdominal cavity.

Anorectal malformations, including imperforate anus and its variants, are embryological defects recognized at birth by the absence of a normal anal opening. Evaluation of these infants should include observation for emergence of meconium from the urethra or fistulas on the perineum. A urinary catheter should be placed if urinary distention is present. In low lesions, a fistulous opening that drains meconium is present on the perineum. Low lesions commonly are associated with fistulization between the bowel and bladder, vagina, or urethra. Lateral plain x-rays show the level of the defect and show gas in the bladder caused by a fistula. Initial treatment is a colostomy to divert the fecal flow, with subsequent reconstruction. The internal sphincter muscle is functionally absent in high lesions, and continence after repair is difficult to achieve. All children with imperforate anus require magnetic resonance imaging (MRI) of the lumbosacral spinal cord because of high incidence of tethered spinal cord. Urological dysfunction is common and should be evaluated.

Hirschsprung disease is a motility defect caused by failure of ganglion cell precursors to migrate into the distal bowel during fetal life. The aganglionic distal segment does not exhibit normal motility and is functionally obstructed secondary to spasm. In 75% of cases, the involved segment is limited to the rectosigmoid; total colonic involvement is seen in 8%. Rarely, long segments of small bowel also are aganglionic. "Ultrashort" segment involves only a few centimeters of distal rectum. About 95% of normal infants pass stool spontaneously by 24 hours of age; 95% of infants with Hirschsprung disease do not. Symptoms of distal bowel obstruction occur with distention and bilious vomiting. If the diagnosis is not made quickly, **enterocolitis** can result, associated with a high rate of mortality. Diagnosis is based on examination and one or more diagnostic studies. Abdominal distention is present in most cases. Digital rectal examination reveals an empty rectum that clenches around the examiner's finger, giving the impression of an elongated sphincter. When the finger is withdrawn, a powerful gush of retained stool is often expelled. A deep **rectal biopsy** specimen obtained surgically or by using a suction biopsy instrument is required for diagnosis. When no ganglion cells are shown in the submucosal plexus, accompanied by nerve trunk hyperplasia, the diagnosis is certain. **Barium enema** and **anorectal manometry** may be used before biopsy, but false-negative and false-positive results can occur. Therapy is surgical. When the bowel is markedly distended or inflamed, an initial colostomy usually is performed above the aganglionic segment, followed weeks later by one of several definitive repair procedures. The transanal pull-through excises the aganglionic bowel and creates a primary colorectal anastomosis without laparotomy. This procedure can be considered in patients with uncomplicated involvement limited to the rectosigmoid region.

Meckel diverticulum is a remnant of the fetal omphalomesenteric duct and is an outpouching of the distal ileum present in 1-2% of the population. Although most diverticula are asymptomatic throughout life, some cause massive, painless GI bleeding. Ectopic gastric tissue within the diverticulum causes ulceration of mucosa in the adjacent ileum. Meckel diverticulum may be a lead point for intussusception or may enable twisting (volvulus) of neighboring bowel around its vascular supply. Diverticulitis mimics appendicitis. Diagnosis may be made in most cases by technetium scan (Meckel scan), which labels the acid-producing mucosa. Because not all diverticula are seen, ultrasound, barium enteroclysis, or video capsule endoscopy may be useful. When the level of suspicion is high, surgical or laparoscopic investigation is warranted. The treatment is surgical excision.

INFLAMMATORY BOWEL DISEASE

Epidemiology and Etiology

Decision-Making Algorithms
Available @ StudentConsult.com

Abdominal Pain
Diarrhea
Fever and Rash
Pubertal Delay

The peak incidence of inflammatory bowel disease (IBD) in children is in the second decade of life. IBD includes Crohn disease (CD), which can involve any part of the gut, and ulcerative colitis (UC), which affects only the colon. The incidence of IBD is increasing, especially in industrialized countries, for reasons that are unclear. It is more common in northern latitudes. IBD is uncommon in tropical and Third World countries. It is more common in Jewish than in other ethnic populations. Genetic factors play a role in susceptibility, with significantly higher risk if there is a family history of IBD. Having a first-degree relative with IBD increases the risk about 30-fold. Susceptibility has been linked to some human leukocyte antigen (HLA) subtypes, and linkage analysis has identified multiple other susceptibility loci on several chromosomes. Environmental factors (not yet identified) also seem to play a role because there is often nonconcordance among monozygotic twins. Dietary and infectious triggers have been proposed but not yet proven. Smoking increases the risk as well as the severity of CD and decreases the risk for UC.

Clinical manifestations depend on the region of involvement. UC involves only the colon, whereas CD can include the entire gut from mouth to anus. **Colitis** from either condition results in diarrhea; blood and mucus in the stool; urgency; and *tenesmus*, a sensation of incomplete emptying after defecation. When colitis is severe, the child often awakens from sleep to pass stool. **Toxic megacolon** is a life-threatening complication characterized by fever, abdominal distention and pain, massively dilated colon, anemia, and low serum albumin owing to fecal protein losses. Symptoms of colitis always are present in UC and usually suggest the diagnosis early in its course. Extraintestinal manifestations of UC occur in a few patients and may include primary sclerosing cholangitis, arthritis, uveitis, and pyoderma gangrenosum (Table 129.1).

Symptoms can be subtle in CD. **Small bowel involvement** in CD is associated with loss of appetite, crampy postprandial pain, poor growth, delayed puberty, fever, anemia, and lethargy. Symptoms may be present for some time before the diagnosis is made. Severe CD with fibrosis may cause partial or complete

TABLE 129.1 Comparison of Crohn Disease and Ulcerative Colitis

FEATURE	CROHN DISEASE	ULCERATIVE COLITIS
Malaise, fever, weight loss	Common	Sometimes
Rectal bleeding	Sometimes	Usual
Abdominal mass	Common	Rare
Abdominal pain	Common	Common
Perianal disease	Common	Rare
Ileal involvement	Common	None (backwash ileitis)
Strictures	Common	Unusual
Fistula	Common	Very rare
Skip lesions	Common	Not present
Transmural involvement	Usual	Not present
Crypt abscesses	Variable	Usual
Intestinal granulomas	Common	Rarely present
Risk of cancer*	Increased	Greatly increased
Erythema nodosum	Common	Less common
Mouth ulceration	Common	Rare
Osteopenia at onset	Yes	No
Autoimmune hepatitis	Rare	Yes
Sclerosing cholangitis	Rare	Yes

Colonic cancer, cholangiocarcinoma, lymphoma in Crohn disease.

small bowel obstruction. Perineal abnormalities, including skin tags and fistulas, are another feature distinguishing CD from UC. Other extraintestinal manifestations of CD include arthritis, erythema nodosum, and uveitis or iritis.

Laboratory and Imaging Studies

Blood tests should include complete blood count, albumin, erythrocyte sedimentation rate, and C-reactive protein (Table 129.2). Anemia and elevated platelet counts are typical. Testing for abnormal serum antibodies can be helpful in diagnosing IBD and in discriminating between the colitis of CD and UC. Serological testing for IBD may be considered but is not recommended for screening due to poor sensitivity. Elevated fecal calprotectin or positive lactoferrin testing indicates intestinal inflammation. These tests have a high negative predictive value but are not specific to IBD.

In patients with suspected IBD, upper endoscopy and colonoscopy are recommended. Colonoscopic findings in UC include diffuse carpeting of the distal or entire colon with tiny ulcers and loss of haustral folds. Within the involved segment, no skip areas are present. In CD, ulcerations tend to be much larger and deeper with a linear, branching, or aphthous appearance; skip areas are usually present. **Upper endoscopy** cannot evaluate the jejunum and ileum, but is more sensitive than contrast studies in identifying proximal CD involvement. Other methods to detect small bowel involvement include **video capsule endoscopy**; upper GI series with small bowel follow through; computed tomography (CT) scanning, which can detect small bowel disease as well as abscesses; and **MR enterography**, which has the advantage of no radiation and good sensitivity for finding active bowel disease.

TABLE 129.2 Diagnostic Studies for Inflammatory Bowel Disease

STUDIES	INTERPRETATION
BLOOD TESTS	
CBC with WBC differential	Anemia, elevated platelets suggest IBD
ESR	Elevated in many, but not all, IBD patients
C-reactive protein	Elevated in many, but not all, IBD patients
Albumin	May be low in IBD due to fecal loss
ASCA	Found in about 50% of CD patients and few UC patients
Atypical p-ANCA	Found in most UC patients and few CD patients
Anti-OmpC	Found in some UC and CD patients, rare in non-IBD
Anti-C Bir1	Found in about 50% of CD patients
STOOL STUDIES	
Fecal calprotectin and lactoferrin	Elevated in IBD and can differentiate from functional disorders
IMAGING STUDIES	
Upper GI series with SBFT	Evaluate for ileal and jejunal CD
CT scan	Used to detect abscess, small bowel involvement
Magnetic resonance enterography	Used to detect bowel thickening, inflammation, and strictures as well as abscesses and fistulas
ENDOSCOPY	
Upper endoscopy	Evaluate for CD of esophagus, stomach, and duodenum; obtain tissue for histological diagnosis
Colonoscopy	Show presence or absence of colitis and terminal ileal CD; obtain tissue for histology
Video capsule endoscopy	Emerging role in diagnosis of small bowel CD, more sensitive than upper GI series with SBFT

Anti-OmpC, Antibody to outer membrane protein C; *ASCA,* anti–*Saccharomyces cerevisiae* antibody; atypical p-ANCA, atypical perinuclear staining by antineutrophil cytoplasmic antibody; *CBC,* complete blood count; *CD,* Crohn disease; *CT,* computed tomography; *ESR,* erythrocyte sedimentation rate; *GI,* gastrointestinal; *IBD,* inflammatory bowel disease; *SBFT,* small bowel follow-through; *UC,* ulcerative colitis; *WBC,* white blood cell.

Treatment

Ulcerative Colitis

UC is treated with the aminosalicylate drugs, which deliver **5-aminosalicylic acid** (5-ASA) to the distal gut. Because it is rapidly absorbed, pure 5-ASA (mesalamine) must be specially packaged in coated capsules or pills or taken as a suppository to be effective in the colon. Other aminosalicylates (sulfasalazine, olsalazine, and balsalazide) use 5-ASA covalently linked to a carrier molecule. Sulfasalazine is the least expensive, but side effects resulting from its sulfapyridine component are common. When aminosalicylates alone cannot control the disease, steroid therapy may be required to induce remission. Whenever possible, steroids should not be used for long-term therapy. An immunosuppressive drug, such as **6-mercaptopurine** or **azathioprine,** is useful to spare excessive steroid use in difficult cases. More potent immunosuppressives, such as cyclosporine or anti–tumor necrosis factor (TNF) agents such as infliximab, may be used as rescue therapy when other treatments fail. Surgical colectomy with ileoanal anastomosis is an option for unresponsive severe disease or electively to end chronic symptoms and to reduce the risk of colon cancer, which is increased in patients with UC.

Crohn Disease

Inflammation in CD typically responds less well to aminosalicylates; oral or IV steroids are more important in inducing remission. To avoid the need for repetitive steroid therapy, immunosuppressive drugs, usually either azathioprine, 6-mercaptopurine, or methotrexate, are often started soon after diagnosis. CD that is difficult to control may be treated with agents that block the action of TNFα such as infliximab or adalimumab. Other antibodies that inhibit white blood cell (WBC) migration or action, such as vedolizumab, also show promise. Exclusive enteral nutrition can be an effective therapy for CD. Patients take formula as their sole source of nutrition for months as a steroid-sparing therapy. Other diets such as the specific carbohydrate diet continue to be studied as a possible therapy. As with UC, surgery is sometimes necessary, usually because of obstructive symptoms, abscess, or severe, unremitting symptoms. Because surgery is not curative in CD, its use must be limited, and the length of bowel resection must be minimized.

CELIAC DISEASE

Etiology and Epidemiology

Celiac disease is an injury to the mucosa of the small intestine caused by the ingestion of **gluten** (a protein component) from wheat, rye, barley, and related grains. In its severe form, celiac disease causes malabsorption and malnutrition. The availability of more sensitive and specific serological testing has revealed many patients with few or no GI symptoms who have early, attenuated, or latent disease. Incidence of celiac disease is estimated at 1%, but only a small proportion has been diagnosed. The disease is seen in association with type 1 diabetes, thyroiditis, Turner syndrome, and trisomy 21.

Clinical Manifestations

Decision-Making Algorithms
Available @ StudentConsult.com

Diarrhea
Pubertal Delay
Failure to Thrive

Symptoms can begin at any age when gluten-containing foods are given. Diarrhea, abdominal bloating, failure to thrive, irritability, decreased appetite, and ascites caused by hypoproteinemia are classic. Children may be minimally symptomatic or may be severely malnourished. Constipation is found in a few patients, probably because of reduced intake. A careful inspection of the child's growth curve and evaluation for reduced subcutaneous fat and abdominal distention are crucial. Celiac disease should be considered in any child with chronic abdominal complaints, short stature, poor weight gain, or delayed puberty. Extraintestinal manifestations include osteopenia, arthritis or arthralgias, ataxia, dental enamel defects, elevated liver enzymes, dermatitis herpetiformis, and erythema nodosum.

Laboratory and Imaging Studies

Serological markers include IgA antiendomysial antibody and IgA tissue transglutaminase antibody. Because IgA deficiency is common in celiac disease, total serum IgA also must be measured to document the accuracy of these tests. In the absence of IgA deficiency, either test yields a sensitivity and specificity of 95%. An endoscopic **small bowel biopsy** is essential to confirm the diagnosis and should be performed while the patient is still ingesting gluten. The biopsy specimen shows various degrees of villous atrophy (short or absent villi), mucosal inflammation, crypt hyperplasia, and increased numbers of intraepithelial lymphocytes. When there is any question about response to treatment, a repeat biopsy specimen may be obtained several months later. Other laboratory studies should be performed to rule out complications, including complete blood count, calcium, phosphate, vitamin D, iron, total protein and albumin, and liver function tests. Mild elevations of the transaminases are common and should normalize with dietary therapy.

Treatment

Treatment consists of complete elimination of gluten from the diet. Consultation with a dietitian experienced in celiac disease is helpful, as is membership in a celiac disease support group. Lists of prepared foods that contain hidden gluten are particularly important for patients to use. Starchy foods that are safe include rice, soy, tapioca, buckwheat, potatoes, and (pure) oats. Many resources also are available via the Internet to help families cope with the large changes in diet that are required. Most patients respond clinically within a few weeks with weight gain, improved appetite, and improved sense of well-being. Histological improvement lags behind clinical response, requiring several months to normalize.

MILK AND SOY PROTEIN INTOLERANCE (ALLERGIC COLITIS)

See Chapter 34.

INTUSSUSCEPTION

Etiology and Epidemiology

Intussusception is the "telescoping" of a segment of proximal bowel (the intussusceptum) into downstream bowel (the intussuscipiens). Most cases occur in infants 1-2 years old; in this age group, nearly all cases are idiopathic. Viral-induced lymphoid hyperplasia may produce a lead point in these children. In older children, the proportion of cases caused by a pathological lead point increases. In young children, **ileocolonic** intussusception is common; the ileum invaginates into the colon, beginning at or near the ileocecal valve. When pathological lead points are present, the intussusception may be ileoileal, jejunoileal, or jejunojejunal.

Clinical Manifestations

Decision-Making Algorithms
Available @ StudentConsult.com

Abdominal Pain
Gastrointestinal Bleeding
Irritable Infant

An infant with intussusception has sudden onset of crampy abdominal pain; the infant's knees draw up, and the infant cries out and exhibits pallor with a colicky pattern occurring every 15-20 minutes. Feedings are refused. As the intussusception progresses and obstruction becomes prolonged, bilious vomiting becomes prominent and the dilated, fatigued intestine generates less pressure and less pain. As the intussuscepted bowel is pulled further and further into the downstream intestine by motility, the mesentery is pulled with it and becomes stretched and compressed. The venous outflow from the intussusceptum is obstructed, leading to edema, weeping of fluid, and congestion with bleeding. Third space fluid losses and "currant jelly" stools result. Another unexpected feature of intussusception is **lethargy**. Between episodes of pain, the infant is glassy-eyed and groggy and appears to have been sedated. A sausage-shaped mass caused by the swollen, intussuscepted bowel may be palpable in the right upper quadrant or epigastrium.

Laboratory and Imaging Studies

The diagnosis depends on the direct demonstration of bowel-within-bowel. A simple way of showing this is by abdominal ultrasound. If the ultrasound is positive, or if good visualization has not been achieved, a pneumatic or contrast enema under fluoroscopy is indicated. This is a potentially useful way to both identify and **treat** intussusception. Air and barium can show the intussusception quickly and, when administered with controlled pressure, usually can reduce it completely. The success rate for pneumatic reduction is higher than for hydrostatic reduction with barium and approaches 90%, if done when symptoms have been present for less than 24 hours. The pneumatic enema has the additional advantages over barium of not preventing subsequent radiologic studies and having no risk of causing barium peritonitis if perforation occurs. Nonoperative reduction should not be attempted if the patient is unstable or has evidence of pre-existing perforation or peritonitis.

Treatment

Therapy must begin with placement of an IV catheter and a nasogastric tube. Before radiologic intervention is attempted, the child must have adequate **fluid resuscitation** to correct the often severe dehydration caused by vomiting and third space losses. Ultrasound may be performed before the fluid resuscitation is complete. Surgical consultation should be obtained early as the surgeon may prefer to be present during nonoperative reduction. If pneumatic or hydrostatic reduction is successful, the child should be admitted to the hospital for overnight observation of possible recurrence (risk is 5-10%). If reduction is not complete, emergency surgery is required. The surgeon attempts gentle manual reduction but may need to resect the involved bowel after failed radiologic reduction because of severe edema, perforation, a pathological lead point (polyp, Meckel diverticulum), or necrosis.

APPENDICITIS

Etiology and Epidemiology

Appendicitis is the most common surgical emergency in childhood. The prevalence of appendicitis varies by age with the peak in the second decade. Appendicitis begins with obstruction of the lumen, most commonly by fecal matter (fecalith), but appendiceal obstruction also can occur secondary to hyperplasia of lymphoid tissue associated with viral infections or, rarely, the presence of neoplastic tissue, such as an appendiceal carcinoid tumor. Trapped bacteria proliferate and begin to invade the appendiceal wall, inducing inflammation and secretion. The obstructed appendix becomes engorged, its blood supply is compromised, and it finally ruptures. The entire process is rapid, with appendiceal rupture usually occurring within 48 hours of the onset of symptoms.

Clinical Manifestations

Decision-Making Algorithms
Available @ StudentConsult.com

Abdominal Pain
Vomiting

Classic appendicitis begins with **visceral pain**, localized to the periumbilical region. Nausea and vomiting occur soon after, triggered by the appendiceal distention. As the inflammation begins to irritate the parietal peritoneum adjacent to the appendix, **somatic pain** fibers are activated, and the pain localizes to the right lower quadrant. Examination of the patient reveals a tender right lower quadrant. Voluntary guarding is present initially, progressing to rigidity, then to rebound tenderness with rupture and peritonitis. These classic findings may not be present, especially in young children or if the appendix is retrocecal, covered by omentum, or in another unusual location. Clinical prediction rules have been developed for the diagnosis of appendicitis. The Alvarado/MANTRELS rule is scored by 1 point for each of the following: migration of pain to the right lower quadrant, anorexia, nausea/vomiting, rebound pain, temperature of at least 37.3°C, and WBC shift to greater than 75% neutrophils; 2 points are given for each of tenderness in the right lower quadrant and leukocytosis greater than 10,000/μL. Children with a score of 4 or less are unlikely to have appendicitis; a score of 7 or greater increases the likelihood that the patient has appendicitis. When classic history and physical examination findings are present, the patient is taken to the operating room. When doubt exists, imaging is helpful to rule out complications (right lower quadrant abscess, liver disease) and other disorders, such as mesenteric adenitis and ovarian or fallopian tube disorders. If the evaluation is negative and some doubt remains, the child should be admitted to the hospital for close observation and serial examinations.

Laboratory and Imaging Studies

The history and examination are often enough to make the diagnosis, but laboratory and imaging studies are helpful when the diagnosis is uncertain (Table 129.3). A WBC count greater than 10,000/mm^3 is found in 89% of patients with appendicitis and 93% with perforated appendicitis. This criterion is met by 62% of abdominal pain patients without appendicitis. Urinalysis is done to rule out urinary tract infection, and x-rays of the chest or the kidney-ureter-bladder (KUB) rule out lower lobe pneumonia masquerading as abdominal pain. Amylase, lipase, and liver enzymes are done to look for pancreatic or liver and gallbladder disease. The plain abdominal x-ray may reveal a calcified fecalith, which strongly suggests the diagnosis. When these studies are inconclusive, imaging is indicated with an abdominal ultrasound or CT scan, which may reveal the presence of an enlarged, thick-walled appendix with surrounding fluid. A diameter of more than 6 mm is considered diagnostic.

TABLE 129.3 Diagnostic Studies in Suspected Appendicitis

INITIAL LABORATORY TESTING
CBC with differential
Urinalysis
Amylase and lipase
ALT, AST, GGT
Flat and upright abdominal radiographs (KUB)
FOLLOW-UP STUDIES*
Abdominal ultrasound
CT scan of abdomen

*Perform when diagnosis remains in doubt.
ALT, Alanine aminotransferase; *AST*, aspartate aminotransferase; *CBC*, complete blood count; *CT*, computed tomography; *GGT*, γ-glutamyltransferase; *KUB*, kidney-ureter-bladder.

Treatment

Treatment of appendicitis is usually surgical. Laparoscopic appendectomy is curative if performed before perforation. With perforation, a course of postoperative IV antibiotics is required. Broad-spectrum coverage is necessary to cover the mixed bowel flora. In low-risk patients with nonperforated appendicitis, some centers have a nonsurgical approach and use high dose broad-spectrum intravenous antibiotics in a hospital setting.

CHAPTER 130

Liver Disease

CHOLESTASIS

Etiology and Epidemiology

Cholestasis is defined as reduced bile flow and is characterized by elevation of the conjugated, or direct, bilirubin fraction. This condition must be distinguished from physiological neonatal jaundice, in which the direct bilirubin is never elevated (see Chapter 62). Neonatal jaundice that is secondary to unconjugated hyperbilirubinemia is the result of immature hepatocellular excretory function or hemolysis, which increases the production of bilirubin. When direct bilirubin is elevated, many potentially serious disorders must be considered (Fig. 130.1, Table 130.1). Emphasis must be placed on the rapid diagnosis of treatable and potentially imminently lethal disorders, especially biliary atresia and metabolic disorders, such as galactosemia or tyrosinemia.

Clinical Manifestations

Decision-Making Algorithm
Available @ StudentConsult.com

Jaundice

The jaundice of **extrahepatic biliary atresia** (biliary atresia) usually is not evident immediately at birth, but develops in the first week or two of life. The reason is that extrahepatic bile ducts are usually present at birth but are then destroyed by an idiopathic inflammatory process. Aside from jaundice, these infants do not initially appear ill. The liver injury progresses rapidly to cirrhosis; symptoms of portal hypertension with splenomegaly, ascites, muscle wasting, and poor weight gain are evident by a few months of age. If surgical drainage is not performed successfully early in the course (ideally by 2 months), progression to liver failure is inevitable.

Neonatal hepatitis is characterized by an ill-appearing infant with an enlarged liver and jaundice. There is no specific diagnostic test. If liver biopsy is performed, the presence of hepatocyte giant cells is characteristic. Cytomegalovirus, herpes simplex virus, and syphilis must be ruled out. Hepatobiliary scintigraphy typically shows slow hepatic uptake with eventual excretion of isotope into the intestine. These infants have a good prognosis overall, with spontaneous resolution occurring in most.

α_1-Antitrypsin deficiency presents with clinical findings indistinguishable from neonatal hepatitis. Only about 10-20% of all infants with the genetic defect exhibit neonatal cholestasis. Of these affected infants, about 20-30% develop chronic liver disease, which may result in cirrhosis and liver failure. Life-threatening α_1-antitrypsin deficiency occurs in only 3-5% of affected pediatric patients. α_1-Antitrypsin deficiency is the leading metabolic disorder requiring liver transplantation.

Alagille syndrome is characterized by chronic cholestasis with the unique liver biopsy finding of *paucity of bile ducts* in the portal triads. Associated abnormalities in some (syndromic) types include peripheral pulmonic stenosis or other cardiac anomalies; hypertelorism; unusual facies with deep-set eyes, prominent forehead, and a pointed chin; butterfly vertebrae; and a defect of the ocular limbus *(posterior embryotoxon)*. Cholestasis is variable but is usually lifelong and associated with hypercholesterolemia and severe pruritus. Progression to end-stage liver disease is uncommon. Liver transplantation sometimes is performed electively to relieve severe and uncontrollable pruritus.

Laboratory and Imaging Studies

The laboratory approach to diagnosis of a neonate with cholestatic jaundice is presented in Table 130.2. Noninvasive studies may aid a rapid diagnosis. Early imaging studies are performed to evaluate for biliary obstruction and other anatomical lesions that may be surgically treatable. When necessary to rule out biliary atresia or to obtain prognostic information, liver biopsy is a final option (Fig. 130.2).

Treatment

Treatment of extrahepatic biliary atresia is the surgical **Kasai procedure,** in which the fibrotic extrahepatic bile duct remnant is removed and replaced with a roux-en-Y loop of jejunum. This operation must be performed before 3 months of age to have the best chance of success. Even so, the success rate is low; many children require liver transplantation. Some metabolic causes of neonatal cholestasis are treatable by dietary manipulation (galactosemia) or medication (tyrosinemia); all affected patients require supportive care. This includes fat-soluble vitamin supplements (vitamins A, D, E, and K) and formula containing medium-chain triglycerides, which can be absorbed without bile salt–induced micelles. Choleretic agents, such as ursodeoxycholic acid, may improve bile flow in some conditions.

VIRAL HEPATITIS

See Chapter 113.

FULMINANT LIVER FAILURE

Etiology and Epidemiology

Fulminant liver failure is defined as severe liver disease with onset of hepatic encephalopathy within 8 weeks after initial symptoms, in the absence of chronic liver disease. Etiology includes viral hepatitis, metabolic disorders, autoimmune hepatitis, ischemia, neoplastic disease, and toxins (Table 130.3).

JAUNDICE

- **Unconjugated Hyperbilirubinemia**
  - **Hemolysis and Reticulocytosis**
    - *Positive Coombs test*
      - ABO and Rh incompatibility
      - Autoimmune, systemic lupus erythematosus
      - Drug-induced and idiopathic acquired hemolytic anemia
    - *Negative Coombs test*
      - RBC enzyme defect (G6PD deficiency)
      - Hemoglobinopathy (sickle cell anemia)
      - RBC membrane defect (hereditary spherocytosis)
      - Hemolytic-uremic syndrome
      - Wilson disease
  - **No Hemolysis**
    - Gilbert syndrome
    - Physiological jaundice of the newborn
    - Breast milk jaundice
    - Crigler-Najjar syndrome
    - Hypothyroidism
    - Pyloric stenosis
    - Internal hemorrhage
- **Conjugated Hyperbilirubinemia**
  - **Obstructive**
    - Alagille syndrome
    - Nonsyndromic paucity of intrahepatic bile ducts
    - Biliary atresia
    - Choledochal cyst
    - Cholelithiasis
    - Tumor/neoplasia
    - Bile duct stenosis
    - Spontaneous bile duct perforation
    - Bile-mucus plug
    - Congenital hepatic fibrosis
  - **Infectious**
    - Hepatitis A, B, C, D, E, G
    - Cytomegalovirus
    - Herpes simplex 1, 2, 6
    - Epstein-Barr virus
    - Coxsackievirus
    - ECHO virus
    - Measles
    - Varicella
    - Syncytial giant cell (paramyxovirus)
    - Human parvovirus B19
    - Toxoplasmosis
    - Syphilis
    - Leptospirosis
    - Bacterial sepsis/urinary tract infection (especially gram-negative)
    - Cholecystitis
    - Curtis–Fitz-Hugh syndrome
  - **Metabolic**
    - Progressive familial intrahepatic cholestasis
    - Wilson disease
    - α_1-Antitrypsin deficiency
    - Galactosemia
    - Tyrosinemia
    - Fructosemia
    - Niemann-Pick disease
    - Gaucher disease
    - Zellweger syndrome
    - Wolman disease
    - Cystic fibrosis
    - Neonatal iron storage disease
    - Indian childhood cirrhosis
    - Defects in bile acid synthesis
  - **Toxic**
    - Total parenteral nutrition
    - Acetaminophen
    - Ethanol
    - Salicylates
    - Iron
    - Halothane
    - Isoniazid
    - Valproic acid
    - Venoocclusive disease (cyclophosphamide)
    - Herbal teas
    - Volatile hydrocarbons
    - *Bacillus cereus* toxin
    - Phenytoin
    - Estradiol
    - Methyldopa
  - **Idiopathic**
    - Idiopathic neonatal hepatitis
    - Familial benign recurrent cholestasis
    - Cholestasis with lymphedema (Aagenaes syndrome)
    - Cholestasis with hypopituitarism
    - Familial erythrophagocytic lymphohistiocytosis
    - Shock
  - **Autoimmune**
    - Autoimmune chronic hepatitis
    - Sclerosing cholangitis
    - Graft-versus-host disease

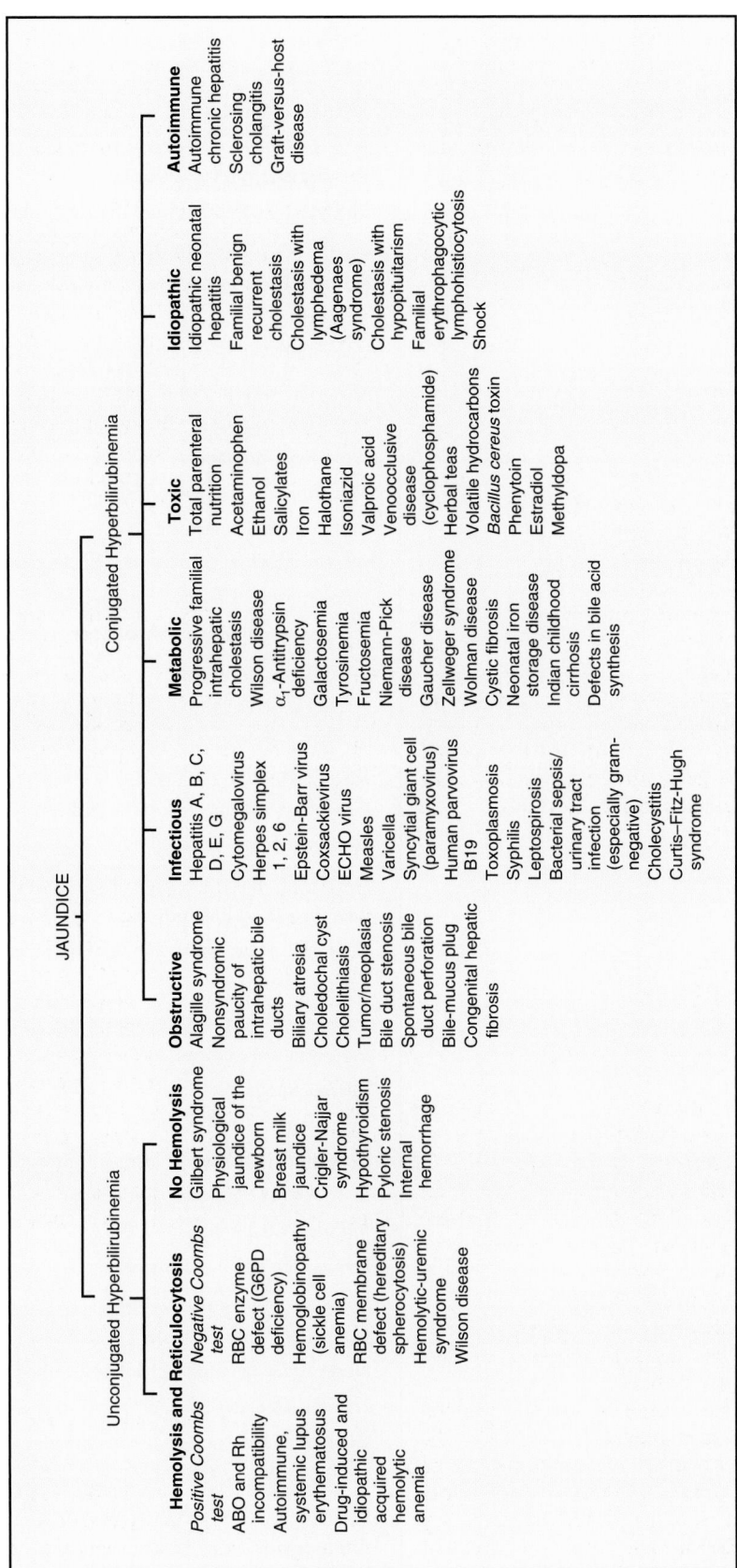

FIGURE 130.1 Differential diagnosis of jaundice in childhood. *G6PD*, Glucose-6-phosphate dehydrogenase; *RBC*, red blood cell.

TABLE 130.1 Differential Diagnosis of Conjugated Hyperbilirubinemia in Infants

OBSTRUCTIVE/ANATOMICAL DISORDERS
Biliary atresia
Choledochal cyst
Caroli disease (cystic dilatation of intrahepatic ducts)
Congenital hepatic fibrosis
Neonatal sclerosing cholangitis
Bile duct stenosis
Spontaneous bile duct perforation
Anomalous choledocho-pancreatico-ductal junction
Cholelithiasis
Inspissated bile or mucous
Mass or neoplasia
INFECTIONS
Bacterial (gram negative) sepsis
Urinary tract infection
Listeriosis
Syphilis
Toxoplasmosis
Tuberculosis
Cytomegalovirus
Herpesvirus (herpes simplex, herpes zoster, human herpesvirus 6)
Rubella virus
Hepatitis B virus
Human immunodeficiency virus (HIV)
Coxsackievirus
Echovirus
Parvovirus B19
Adenovirus
Measles
METABOLIC DISORDERS
α_1-Antitrypsin deficiency
Cystic fibrosis
Citrin deficiency
Neonatal hemochromatosis (neonatal iron storage disease)
ENDOCRINE DISORDERS
Panhypopituitarism
Hypothyroidism
DISORDERS OF CARBOHYDRATE METABOLISM
Galactosemia
Hereditary fructose intolerance (fructosemia)
Glycogen storage disease type IV
DISORDERS OF AMINO ACID METABOLISM
Tyrosinemia
Hypermethioninemia
DISORDERS OF LIPID METABOLISM
Wolman disease
Cholesterol ester storage disease
Farber disease
Niemann-Pick disease
Beta-oxidation defects
Gaucher disease
DISORDERS OF BILE ACID SYNTHESIS AND METABOLISM
Primary Enzyme Deficiencies
3β-Hydroxy-$\Delta 5$-C27-steroid dehydrogenase/isomerase
$\Delta 4$-3-Oxosteroid 5β-reductase
Oxysterol 7α-hydroxylase
Secondary
Zellweger syndrome (cerebrohepatorenal syndrome)
Infantile Refsum disease
Smith-Lemli-Opitz syndrome
Other enzymopathies
Mitochondrial disorders (respiratory chain)
Intrahepatic Cholestasis
Alagille syndrome (arteriohepatic dysplasia)
Nonsyndromic paucity of intrahepatic bile ducts
Progressive familial intrahepatic cholestasis (PFIC)
Type 1: Byler disease
Type 2: Defect in the bile salt export pump
Type 3: Defect in canalicular phospholipid transporter
Benign recurrent intrahepatic cholestasis
Greenland familial cholestasis (Nielsen syndrome)
North American Indian cirrhosis
Hereditary cholestasis with lymphedema (Aagenaes syndrome)
Toxin- or Drug-Related
Cholestasis associated with total parenteral nutrition
Chloral hydrate
Home remedies/herbal medicines
Venoocclusive disease
Miscellaneous
Idiopathic neonatal hepatitis
Autoimmune hemolytic anemia with giant cell hepatitis
Shock or hypoperfusion (including cardiac disease)
Intestinal obstruction
Langerhans cell histiocytosis
Neonatal lupus erythematosus
Dubin-Johnson syndrome
North American Indian childhood cirrhosis
Trisomies (18, 21)
Congenital disorders of glycosylation
Kabuki syndrome
Donahue syndrome (leprechaunism)
Arthrogryposis, cholestatic pigmentary disease, renal dysfunction syndrome
Familial hemophagocytic lymphohistiocytosis

Modified from Balistreri WF. Liver disease in infancy and childhood. In: Schiff ER, Sorrell MF, Maddrey WC, eds. Schiff's Diseases of the Liver. *8th ed. Philadelphia: Lippincott-Raven; 1999:1370; Suchy FJ. Approach to the infant with cholestasis. In: Suchy FJ, Sokol RJ, Balistreri WF, eds.* Liver Disease in Children. *2nd ed. Philadelphia: Lippincott Williams & Wilkins; 2001:188.*

TABLE 130.2 Laboratory and Imaging Evaluation of Neonatal Cholestasis

EVALUATION	RATIONALE
INITIAL TESTS	
Total and direct bilirubin	Elevated direct fraction confirms cholestasis
AST, ALT	Hepatocellular injury
GGT	Biliary obstruction/injury
RBC galactose-1-phosphate uridyltransferase	Galactosemia
α_1-Antitrypsin level	α_1-Antitrypsin deficiency
Urinalysis and urine culture	Urinary tract infection can cause cholestasis in neonates
Blood culture	Sepsis can cause cholestasis
Serum amino acids	Aminoacidopathies
Urine organic acids	Organic acidurias
Very-long-chain fatty acids	Zellweger syndrome, peroxisomal disorders
Carnitine profile	Mitochondrial and fatty acid oxidation disorders
Sweat chloride or CF mutation analysis	Cystic fibrosis
Urine culture for cytomegalovirus	Congenital cytomegalovirus infection
INITIAL IMAGING STUDY	
Abdominal ultrasound	Choledochal cyst, gallstones, mass lesion, Caroli disease
SECONDARY IMAGING STUDY	
Hepatobiliary scintigraphy	Evaluate for biliary atresia
Pathology	
Percutaneous liver biopsy	Biliary atresia, idiopathic giant cell hepatitis, α_1-antitrypsin deficiency

ALT, Alanine aminotransferase; *AST*, aspartate aminotransferase; *CF*, cystic fibrosis; *GGT*, γ-glutamyltransferase; *RBC*, red blood cell.

Clinical Manifestations

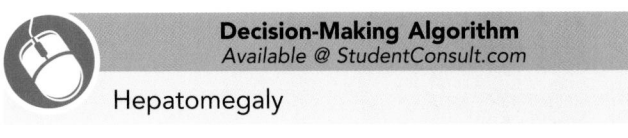

Decision-Making Algorithm
Available @ StudentConsult.com

Hepatomegaly

Liver failure is a multisystem disorder with complex interactions among the liver, kidneys, vascular structures, gut, central nervous system (CNS), and immune function. Hepatic encephalopathy is characterized by varying degrees of impairment (Table 130.4). Respiratory compromise occurs as severity of the failure increases and requires early institution of ventilatory support. Hypoglycemia resulting from impaired glycogenolysis and gluconeogenesis must be prevented. Renal function is impaired, and frank renal failure, or **hepatorenal syndrome**, may occur. This syndrome is characterized by low urine output, azotemia, and low urine sodium content. Ascites develops secondary to hypoalbuminemia and disordered regulation of fluid and electrolyte homeostasis. Increased risk of infection occurs and may cause death. Esophageal varices may cause significant hemorrhage, whereas hypersplenism from portal hypertension may produce thrombocytopenia.

Laboratory and Imaging Studies

Coagulation tests and serum albumin are used to follow hepatic synthetic function. These tests are confounded by administration of blood products and clotting factors. Vitamin K should be administered to maximize the liver's ability to synthesize factors II, VII, IX, and X. In addition to monitoring prothrombin time and partial thromboplastin time, many centers measure factor V serially as a sensitive index of synthetic function. Renal function tests, electrolytes, serum ammonia, blood counts, and urinalysis also should be followed. In the setting of acute liver failure, liver biopsy may be indicated to ascertain the nature and degree of injury and estimate the likelihood of recovery. In the presence of coagulopathy, biopsy must be done using a transjugular or surgical approach.

Treatment

Because of the life-threatening and complex nature of this condition, management must be carried out in an intensive care unit at a liver transplant center. Treatment of acute liver failure is supportive; the definitive lifesaving therapy is liver transplantation. Supportive measures are listed in Table 130.5. Efforts are made to treat metabolic derangements, avoid hypoglycemia, support respiration, minimize hepatic encephalopathy, and support renal function.

CHRONIC LIVER DISEASE

Etiology and Epidemiology

Chronic liver disease in childhood is characterized by the development of cirrhosis and its complications, and by progressive hepatic failure. Causative conditions may be congenital or acquired. Major congenital disorders leading to chronic disease include biliary atresia, tyrosinemia, untreated galactosemia, and α_1-antitrypsin deficiency. In older children, hepatitis B or C virus, autoimmune hepatitis, Wilson disease, primary sclerosing cholangitis, cystic fibrosis, and biliary obstruction secondary to choledochal cyst are leading causes.

Clinical Manifestations

Decision-Making Algorithms
Available @ StudentConsult.com

Gastrointestinal Bleeding
Jaundice
Abdominal Masses
Bleeding

Chronic liver disease is characterized by the consequences of portal hypertension, impaired hepatocellular function, and cholestasis. **Portal hypertension** caused by cirrhosis results in risk of gastrointestinal bleeding, ascites, and reduced hepatic

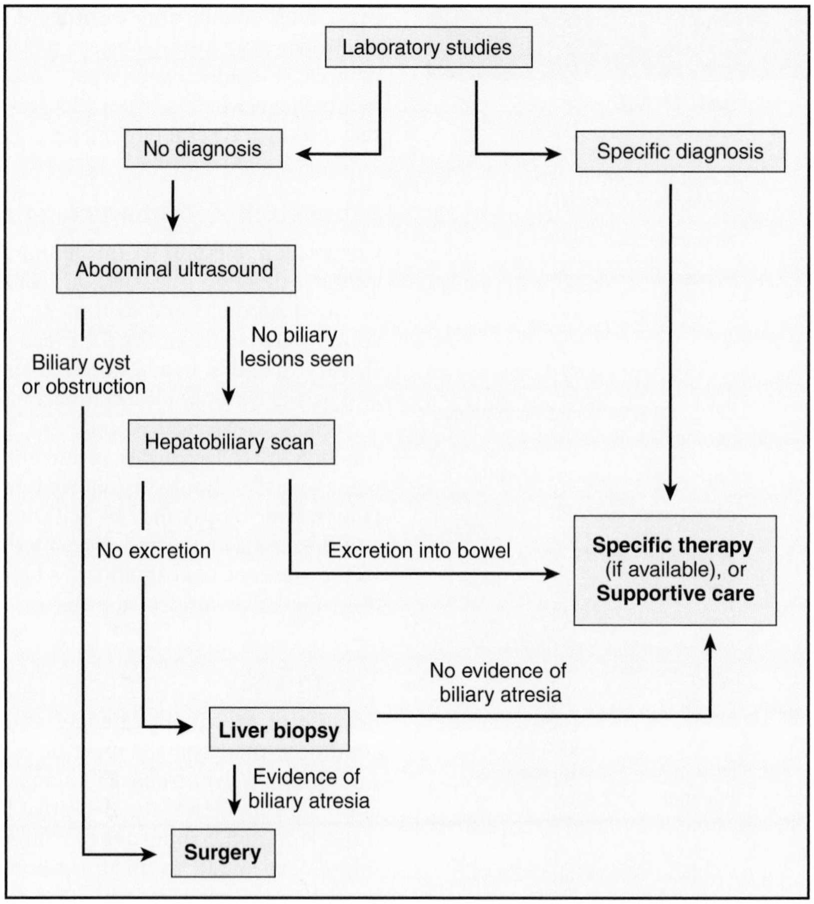

FIGURE 130.2 Flow chart for evaluation of neonatal cholestasis.

blood flow. Blood entering the portal vein from the splenic and mesenteric veins is diverted to collateral circulation that bypasses the liver, enlarging these previously tiny vessels in the esophagus, stomach, and abdomen. **Esophageal varices** are particularly prone to bleed, but bleeding also can occur from hemorrhoidal veins, engorged gastric mucosa, and gastric varices. **Ascites** develops as a result of weeping of a high-pressure ultrafiltrate from the surfaces of the viscera and is at risk of becoming infected (spontaneous bacterial peritonitis); ascites can often be massive and interfere with patient comfort and respiration. The spleen enlarges secondary to impaired splenic vein outflow, causing excessive scavenging of platelets and white blood cells; this increases the patient's susceptibility to bleeding and infection.

Impaired hepatocellular function is associated with coagulopathy unresponsive to vitamin K, low serum albumin, elevated ammonia, and **hepatic encephalopathy**. The diversion of portal blood away from the liver via collateral circulation worsens this process. Malaise develops and contributes to poor nutrition, leading to muscle wasting and other consequences.

Chronic cholestasis causes debilitating pruritus and deepening jaundice. The reduced excretion of bile acids impairs absorption of fat calories and fat-soluble vitamins, which contributes to the poor nutritional state. Deficiency of vitamin K impairs production of clotting factors II, VII, IX, and X and increases the risk of bleeding. Vitamin E deficiency leads to hematological and neurological consequences unless corrected.

Laboratory and Imaging Studies

Laboratory studies include specific tests for diagnosis of the underlying illness and testing to monitor the status of the patient. Children presenting for the first time with evidence of chronic liver disease should have a standard investigation (Table 130.6). Monitoring should include coagulation tests, electrolytes and renal function testing, complete blood count with platelet count, transaminases, alkaline phosphatase, and γ-glutamyltransferase at appropriate intervals. Frequency of testing should be tailored to the pace of the patient's illness. Ascites fluid can be tested for infection by culture and cell count and generally is found to have an albumin concentration lower than that of serum.

Treatment

Treatment of chronic liver disease is complex. Supportive care for each of the many problems encountered in these patients is outlined in Table 130.7. Ultimately, survival depends on the availability of a donor liver and the patient's candidacy for transplantation. When transplantation is not possible or is delayed, palliative procedures, such as portosystemic shunts, can be considered. The transjugular intrahepatic portosystemic shunt is an expandable stent placed between the hepatic vein and a branch of the portal vein within the hepatic parenchyma. This procedure is performed using catheters inserted via the jugular vein and is entirely nonsurgical. All portosystemic shunts carry increased risk of hepatic encephalopathy.

TABLE 130.3 Causes of Fulminant Liver Failure in Childhood
METABOLIC
Neonatal hemochromatosis
Electron chain transport and other mitochondrial defects
Disorders of fatty acid oxidation
Galactosemia
Tyrosinemia
Hereditary fructose intolerance
Bile acid synthesis disorders
Wilson disease
CARDIOVASCULAR
Shock, hypotension
Congestive heart failure
Budd-Chiari syndrome
INFECTIOUS
Hepatitis virus A, B
Echovirus
Coxsackievirus
Adenovirus
Parvovirus
Cytomegalovirus
Sepsis
Herpes simplex
NEOPLASTIC
Acute leukemia
Lymphoproliferative disease
TOXIC
Acetaminophen
Valproic acid
Phenytoin
Isoniazid
Halothane
Amanita mushrooms
IMMUNOLOGICAL
Autoimmune hepatitis
Familial hemophagocytic lymphohistiocytosis

TABLE 130.4 Stages of Hepatic Encephalopathy
STAGE I
Alert and awake
Agitated and distractible
Infants and young children—irritable and fussy
Normal reflexes
Tremor, poor handwriting
Obeys age-appropriate commands
STAGE II
Confused and lethargic
Combative or inappropriate euphoria
Hyperactive reflexes
Asterixis present
Purposeful movements, but may not obey commands
STAGE III
Stuporous but arousable
Sleepy
Incoherent speech
Motor response to pain
Hyperreflexic
Hyperventilation
Asterixis present
STAGE IV
Unconscious, not arousable
Unresponsive or responds nonpurposefully to pain
Reflexes hyperactive
Irregular respirations
Pupil response sluggish
STAGE V
Unconscious
Hypoactive reflexes
Flaccid muscle tone
Apneic
Pupils fixed

SELECTED CHRONIC HEPATIC DISORDERS

Wilson Disease

Decision-Making Algorithms
Available @ StudentConsult.com

Jaundice
Hepatomegaly
Involuntary Movements
Hypocalcemia

Wilson disease is characterized by abnormal storage of copper in the liver, leading to hepatocellular injury, CNS dysfunction, and hemolytic anemia. It is an autosomal recessive trait caused by mutations in the *ATP7B* gene. The encoded protein of this gene functions as an ATP-driven copper pump. The **diagnosis** is made by identifying depressed serum levels of ceruloplasmin, elevated 24-hour urine copper excretion, the presence of Kayser-Fleischer rings in the iris, evidence of hemolysis, and elevated hepatic copper content. In any single patient, one or more of these measures may be normal. **Clinical presentation** also varies, but seldom occurs before age 3 years. Neurological abnormalities may predominate, including tremor, decline in school performance, worsening handwriting, and psychiatric disturbances. Anemia may be the first noted symptom. Hepatic presentations include appearance of jaundice, spider hemangiomas, portal

TABLE 130.5 Treatment of Fulminant Liver Failure

Hepatic encephalopathy	Avoid sedatives
	Lactulose via nasogastric tube—start with 1-2 mL/kg/day, adjust dose to yield several loose stools per day
	Rifaximin or neomycin
	Enemas if constipated
	Mechanical ventilation if stage III or IV
Coagulopathy	Fresh frozen plasma only if active bleeding, monitor coagulation studies frequently
	Platelet transfusions as required
Hypoglycemia	Intravenous glucose supplied with ≥10% dextrose solution, electrolytes as appropriate
Ascites	Restrict fluid intake to 50-60% maintenance
	Restrict sodium intake to 0.5-1 mEq/kg/day
	Monitor central venous pressure to maintain adequate intravascular volume (avoid renal failure)
Renal failure	Maintain adequate intravascular volume, give albumin if low
	Diuretics
	Vasoconstrictors
	Dialysis or hemofiltration
	Exchange transfusion
	Liver transplantation

hypertension and its consequences, and fulminant hepatic failure. **Treatment** consists of administration of copper-chelating drugs (penicillamine or trientine), with monitoring of urine copper excretion at intervals. Zinc salts often replace chelating agents after chelation therapy has successfully reduced excessive body copper stores. Adequate therapy must be continued for life to prevent liver and CNS deterioration.

Autoimmune Hepatitis

Immune-mediated liver injury may be primary or occur in association with other autoimmune disorders, such as inflammatory bowel disease or systemic lupus erythematosus. **Diagnosis** is made on the basis of elevated serum total IgG and the presence of an autoantibody, most commonly anti-nuclear, anti–smooth muscle, or anti–liver-kidney microsomal antibody. Liver biopsy specimen shows the presence of a plasma cell–rich portal infiltrate with piecemeal necrosis. **Treatment** consists of corticosteroids initially, usually with the addition of an immunosuppressive drug after remission is achieved. Steroids are tapered gradually as tolerated to minimize glucocorticoid side effects. Many patients require lifelong immunosuppressive therapy, but some may be able to stop medications after several years under careful monitoring for recurrence.

TABLE 130.6 Laboratory and Imaging Investigation of Chronic Liver Disease

METABOLIC TESTING	AST, ALT, GGT, alkaline phosphatase
Serum α_1-antitrypsin level	Total and direct bilirubin
α_1-Antitrypsin phenotype if low serum level	Serum cholylglycine or bile acids
Serum ceruloplasmin	Serum cholesterol
Sweat chloride, CF gene tests if CF suspected	Ultrasound examination of liver and bile ducts
Testing for other specific conditions as indicated by clinical/laboratory findings	Doppler ultrasound of hepatic vessels*
VIRAL HEPATITIS	Magnetic resonance cholangiography*
HBsAg	Magnetic resonance angiography of hepatic vessels*
Hepatitis B viral DNA, HBeAg if HBsAg positive	Percutaneous or endoscopic cholangiography*
Hepatitis C antibody	Liver biopsy*
Hepatitis C antibody confirmatory test if positive	**ANATOMICAL EVALUATION**
Hepatitis C viral RNA, genotype if antibody confirmed	Ultrasound of liver, pancreas, and biliary tree
AUTOIMMUNE HEPATITIS	Consider magnetic resonance cholangiography or ERCP if evidence of biliary process
Antinuclear antibody	Liver biopsy—as required for diagnosis or prognosis
Liver-kidney microsomal antibody	**TESTS TO EVALUATE NUTRITIONAL STATUS**
Anti–smooth muscle antibody	Height, weight, skinfold thickness
Antineutrophil cytoplasmic antibody	25-Hydroxyvitamin D level
Total serum IgG (usually elevated)	Vitamin A level
TESTS TO EVALUATE LIVER FUNCTION AND INJURY	Vitamin E level
Prothrombin time and partial thromboplastin time	Prothrombin time and partial thromboplastin time before and after vitamin K administration
Serum ammonia	Serum albumin and prealbumin
CBC with platelet count	
Serum albumin	

**Perform when indicated to obtain specific anatomical information.*

ALT, Alanine aminotransferase; *AST,* aspartate aminotransferase; *CBC,* complete blood count; *CF,* cystic fibrosis; *ERCP,* endoscopic retrograde cholangiopancreatography; *GGT,* γ-glutamyltransferase; *HBeAg,* hepatitis B early antigen; *HBsAg,* hepatitis B surface antigen; *Ig,* immunoglobulin.

TABLE 130.7 Management of Chronic Liver Disease

PROBLEM	CLINICAL MANIFESTATIONS	DIAGNOSTIC TESTING	TREATMENT
Gastrointestinal variceal bleeding*	Hematemesis, rectal bleeding, melena, anemia	CBC, coagulation tests, Doppler ultrasound, magnetic resonance angiography, endoscopy	Somatostatin (octreotide) infusion, variceal band ligation or sclerotherapy, propranolol to reduce portal pressure, acid-blocker therapy, TIPSS or surgical portosystemic shunt if transplant not possible
Ascites	Abdominal distention, shifting dullness and fluid wave, respiratory compromise, spontaneous bacterial peritonitis	Abdominal ultrasound, diagnostic paracentesis; measure ascites fluid albumin (and serum albumin), cell count, WBC differential, culture fluid in blood culture bottles	Restrict sodium intake to 0.5-1 mEq/kg/day, restrict fluids, monitor renal function, treat peritonitis and portal hypertension Central portosystemic shunt may be required
Nutritional compromise	Muscle wasting, fat-soluble vitamin deficiencies, poor or absent weight gain, fatigue	Coagulation studies, serum albumin, 25-hydroxyvitamin D level, vitamin E level, vitamin A level	Fat-soluble vitamin supplements: vitamins A, D, E, and K; use water-soluble form of vitamins. Supplemental feedings—nasogastric or parenteral if necessary
Hepatic encephalopathy	Irritability, confusion, lethargy, somnolence, coma	Serum ammonia	Lactulose orally or via nasogastric tube, avoid narcotics and sedatives, liver transplantation

**May also have peptic ulcerations.*
CBC, Complete blood count; *TIPSS*, transjugular intrahepatic portosystemic shunt; *WBC*, white blood cell.

Nonalcoholic Fatty Liver Disease

Nonalcoholic fatty liver disease is characterized by the presence of macrovesicular fatty change in hepatocytes on biopsy. Varying degrees of inflammation and portal fibrosis may be present. This disorder occurs in obese children, sometimes in association with insulin-resistant (type 2) diabetes and hyperlipidemia. Children with marked obesity, with or without type 2 diabetes, who have elevated liver enzymes and no other identifiable liver disease are likely to have this condition. Nonalcoholic fatty liver disease can progress to significant fibrosis. Treatment is with weight loss and exercise. Vitamin E may have some benefit. Efforts should be made to control blood glucose and hyperlipidemia and promote weight loss. In general, the rate of progression to end-stage liver disease is slow.

CHAPTER 131

Pancreatic Disease

PANCREATIC INSUFFICIENCY

Etiology and Epidemiology

The cause of inadequate pancreatic digestive function in 95% of cases is **cystic fibrosis** (see Chapter 137). The defect in *CFTR* chloride channel function results in thick secretions in the lungs, intestines, pancreas, and bile ducts. In the pancreas, there is destruction of pancreatic function, often before birth. Some mutations result in less severe defects in *CFTR* function and later onset of lung disease and pancreatic insufficiency. Less common causes of pancreatic insufficiency are *Shwachman-Diamond* syndrome and *Pearson* syndrome in developed countries and severe malnutrition in developing countries.

Clinical Manifestations

Decision-Making Algorithm
Available @ StudentConsult.com
Failure to Thrive

Children with pancreatic exocrine insufficiency have many bulky, foul-smelling stools each day, usually with visible oil or fat. They typically have voracious appetites because of massive malabsorption of calories from fat, complex carbohydrates, and proteins. Failure to thrive is uniformly present if diagnosis and treatment are not accomplished rapidly. It is important to distinguish children with malabsorption due to pancreatic disease from children with intestinal disorders that interfere with digestion or absorption. Appropriate testing should be performed to rule out conditions such as celiac disease and inflammatory bowel disease if any doubt about the state of pancreatic sufficiency exists.

Laboratory and Imaging Studies

Testing of pancreatic function is difficult. Direct measurement of enzyme concentrations in aspirated pancreatic juice is not routine and is technically difficult. Stools can be tested for the presence of maldigested fat, which usually indicates poor fat digestion. Measuring fecal fat can give either a qualitative assessment of fat absorption (fecal Sudan stain) or a semiquantitative measurement (72-hour fecal fat determination) of fat maldigestion. Another way to assess pancreatic function is to test for the presence of pancreatic enzymes in the stool. Of these, measuring **fecal elastase-1** by immunoassay seems to be the most accurate method of assessment. Depressed fecal elastase-1 concentration correlates well with the presence of pancreatic insufficiency.

Treatment

Replacement of missing pancreatic enzymes is the best available therapy. Pancreatic enzymes are available as capsules containing enteric-coated microspheres. The coating on these spheres is designed to protect the enzymes from gastric acid degradation. For children unable to swallow capsules, the contents may be sprinkled on a spoonful of soft food, such as applesauce. Excessive use of enzymes must be avoided because high doses (usually >6,000 U/kg/meal) can cause colonic fibrosis. In infants, typical dosing is 2,000-4,000 U of lipase/120 mL of formula. In children younger than 4 years old, 1,000 U/kg/meal is given. For older children, 500 U/kg/meal is usual. This dose may be adjusted upward as required to control steatorrhea, but a dose of 2,500 U/kg/meal should not be exceeded. Use of H_2-receptor antagonists or proton pump inhibitors can increase the efficacy of pancreatic enzymes by enhancing their release from the microspheres and reducing inactivation by acid.

ACUTE PANCREATITIS

Etiology and Epidemiology

The exocrine pancreas produces numerous proteolytic enzymes, including trypsin, chymotrypsin, and carboxypeptidase. These are produced as inactive proenzymes to protect the pancreas from autodigestion. Trypsin is activated after leaving the pancreas by enterokinase, an intestinal brush border enzyme. After activation, trypsin cleaves other proteolytic proenzymes into their active states. Protease inhibitors found in pancreatic juice inhibit early activation of trypsin; the presence of self-digestion sites on the trypsin molecule allows for feedback inactivation. Pancreatitis occurs when digestive enzymes are activated inside the pancreas, causing injury. Triggers for acute pancreatitis differ between adults and children. In the adult patient, most episodes are related to alcohol abuse or gallstones. In children, most cases are idiopathic or due to medications. Some cases are caused by pancreatic sufficient cystic fibrosis, hypertriglyceridemia, biliary microlithiasis, trauma, or viral infection. Collagen vascular disorders and parasite infestations are responsible for the remainder (Table 131.1).

TABLE 131.1 Causes of Acute Pancreatitis in Children
OBSTRUCTIVE
Cholelithiasis and biliary sludge
Choledochal cyst
Pancreas divisum
Anomalous junction of biliary and pancreatic ducts
Annular pancreas
Ampullary obstruction (mass, inflammation from Crohn disease)
Ascaris infection
MEDICATIONS AND TOXINS
L-Asparaginase
Valproic acid
Azathioprine and 6-mercaptopurine
Didanosine
Pentamidine
Tetracycline
Opiates
Mesalamine
Sulfasalazine
Alcohol
Cannabis
SYSTEMIC DISEASES
Inflammatory bowel disease
Hemolytic uremic syndrome
Diabetic ketoacidosis
Collagen vascular disease
Kawasaki disease
Shock
Sickle cell disease
INFECTIOUS
Sepsis
Mumps
Coxsackievirus
Cytomegalovirus
Varicella-zoster
Herpes simplex
Mycoplasma
Ascaris
GENETIC
Cystic fibrosis—*CFTR* mutations
Hereditary pancreatitis—*SPINK*, *PRSS1*, and *CTRC* mutations
OTHER
Trauma
Hyperlipidemia
Hypercalcemia
Autoimmune

Clinical Manifestations

Decision-Making Algorithms
Available @ StudentConsult.com

Abdominal Pain
Vomiting
Hyponatremia
Hypocalcemia

Acute pancreatitis presents with relatively rapid onset of pain, usually in the epigastric region. The pain may radiate to the back and is nearly always aggravated by eating. The patient moves frequently to find a position of comfort. Nausea and vomiting occur in most cases. Pain is typically continuous and quite severe, usually requiring narcotics. Severe pancreatitis can lead to hemorrhage, visible as ecchymoses in the flanks (Grey Turner sign) or periumbilical region (Cullen sign). Rupture of a minor pancreatic duct can lead to development of a pancreatic pseudocyst, characterized by persistent severe pain and tenderness and a palpable mass. With necrosis and fluid collections, patients experiencing severe pancreatitis are prone to infectious complications, and the clinician must be alert for fever and signs of sepsis.

Laboratory and Imaging Studies

The diagnosis of acute pancreatitis is based on 2 of the following 3 criteria: abdominal pain consistent with the disease (severe epigastric pain typically), serum amylase and/or lipase greater than 3 time the upper limit of normal, and/or characteristic findings on imaging. Acute pancreatitis can be difficult to diagnose. Pancreatic enzymes are released into the blood during pancreatic injury. Nonspecific elevations of the enzymes are common. As acute pancreatitis progresses, the amylase level tends to decline faster than lipase, making the latter a good choice for diagnostic testing late in the course of the disease.

Because enzyme levels are not 100% sensitive or specific, imaging studies are important for the diagnosis of pancreatitis. In acute pancreatitis, edema is present in all but the mildest cases. Ultrasound is capable of detecting this edema and should be performed as part of the overall diagnostic approach. If overlying bowel gas obscures the pancreas, a computed tomography (CT) scan allows complete visualization of the gland. CT scans should be done with oral and intravenous (IV) contrast agents to facilitate interpretation. Ultrasound and CT also can be used to monitor for the development of **pseudocysts** and for evidence of ductal dilation secondary to obstruction. The other important reason to perform imaging studies early in the course of pancreatitis is to rule out gallstones; the liver, gallbladder, and common bile duct all should be visualized. Magnetic resonance cholangiopancreatography may be used to detect anatomical variants causing pancreatitis.

Treatment

There are no proven specific therapies for acute pancreatitis. If a predisposing etiology is found, such as a drug reaction or a gallstone obstructing the sphincter of Oddi, this should be specifically treated. Fluid resuscitation is necessary because of vomiting and third space losses. Pain relief should be provided. Oral, nasogastric, or nasojejunal feedings can begin early if tolerated and may improve outcome. If this is not possible, parenteral nutrition is an option. Fewer complications and more rapid recovery occur with enteral feedings compared with parenteral nutrition. Antibiotics should be considered if the patient is febrile, has extensive pancreatic necrosis, or has laboratory evidence of infection. A broad-spectrum antibiotic, such as imipenem, is considered the best choice.

CHRONIC PANCREATITIS

Etiology and Epidemiology

Chronic pancreatitis is defined as recurrent or persistent attacks of pancreatitis, which have resulted in irreversible morphological changes in pancreatic structure. These include scarring of the ducts with irregular areas of narrowing and dilation (beading), fibrosis of parenchyma, and loss of acinar and islet tissue. Pancreatic exocrine insufficiency and diabetes mellitus may result from unremitting chronic pancreatitis. Most patients have discrete attacks of acute symptoms occurring repeatedly, but chronic pain may be present. The causes of chronic pancreatitis include hereditary pancreatitis and milder phenotypes of cystic fibrosis associated with pancreatic sufficiency. Familial disease is caused by one of several known mutations in the trypsinogen gene. These mutations obliterate autodigestion sites on the trypsin molecule, inhibiting feedback inhibition of trypsin digestion. Genetic testing is readily available for these mutations. Genetic testing for cystic fibrosis can be performed, but must include screening for the less common mutations associated with pancreatic sufficiency. Sweat chloride testing is less expensive and is abnormal in most. Less commonly, mutations in the *SPINK1* gene, which codes for pancreatic trypsin inhibitor, and *PRSS1*, a mutation of cationic trypsinogen, or *CTRC*, a mutation in chymotrypsin C are found.

Clinical Manifestations

Children with chronic pancreatitis initially present with recurring attacks of acute pancreatitis. Injury to the pancreatic ducts predisposes these children to continued attacks owing to scarring of small and large pancreatic ducts, stasis of pancreatic secretions, stone formation, and inflammation. Loss of pancreatic exocrine and endocrine tissue over time can lead to exocrine and endocrine deficiency. More than 90% of the pancreatic mass must be destroyed before exocrine deficiency becomes clinically apparent; this is a late complication that does not occur in all cases. Chronic pain is a serious problem in most affected individuals. These patients have many episodes; many do not require hospitalization.

Laboratory and Imaging Studies

Laboratory diagnosis of chronic pancreatitis is similar to acute pancreatitis, but with more severe loss of pancreatic tissue, it becomes less likely that the patient presents with elevation of amylase or lipase. Monitoring also should include looking for consequences of chronic injury, including diabetes mellitus and compromise of the pancreatic and biliary ducts. Pancreatic and biliary imaging has been accomplished by endoscopic retrograde cholangiopancreatography (ERCP). ERCP offers the possibility of therapeutic intervention to remove gallstones, dilate strictures, and place stents to enhance flow of pancreatic juice. Magnetic resonance cholangiopancreatography is an alternative to ERCP. Plain abdominal x-rays may show pancreatic calcifications. Diagnostic testing for the etiology of chronic pancreatitis should include genetic testing for hereditary pancreatitis and cystic fibrosis and sweat chloride determination.

Treatment

Treatment is largely supportive. Potential but unproven therapies include the use of daily pancreatic enzyme supplements, octreotide (somatostatin) to abort early attacks, low-fat diets, and daily antioxidant therapy. Care must be taken that extreme diets do not result in nutritional deprivation. Interventional ERCP to dilate large strictures and remove stones and surgical pancreatic drainage procedures to decompress dilated pancreatic ducts by creating a side-to-side pancreaticojejunostomy may have some value.

CHAPTER 132

Peritonitis

ETIOLOGY AND EPIDEMIOLOGY

The peritoneum consists of a single layer of mesothelial cells that covers all intraabdominal organs. The portion that covers the abdominal wall is derived from the underlying somatic structures and is innervated by somatic nerves. The portion covering the viscera is derived from visceral mesoderm and is innervated by nonmyelinated visceral afferents. Inflammation of the peritoneum, or peritonitis, usually is caused by infection but may result from exogenous irritants introduced by penetrating injuries or surgical procedures, radiation, and endogenous irritants such as meconium. Infectious peritonitis can be an acute complication of intestinal inflammation and perforation, as in appendicitis, or it can occur secondary to contamination of pre-existing ascites associated with renal, cardiac, or hepatic disease. In this setting, when there is no other intraabdominal source, it is referred to as **spontaneous bacterial peritonitis**. Spontaneous bacterial peritonitis is usually due to pneumococcus and less often to *Escherichia coli.*

CLINICAL MANIFESTATIONS

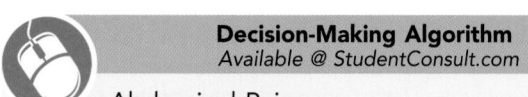

Decision-Making Algorithm
Available @ StudentConsult.com

Abdominal Pain

Peritonitis is characterized on examination by marked abdominal tenderness. Rebound tenderness also generally is quite pronounced. The patient tends to move very little owing to intense peritoneal irritation and pain. Fever is not always present, and absence of fever should not be regarded as contradictory to the diagnosis. Patients who are taking corticosteroids for an underlying condition, such as nephrotic syndrome, are likely to have little fever and reduced tenderness.

LABORATORY AND IMAGING STUDIES

Blood tests should focus on identifying the nature of the inflammation and its underlying cause. An elevated white blood cell count, erythrocyte sedimentation rate, and C-reactive protein suggest infection. In children older than 5 years, appendicitis is the leading cause. Total serum protein, albumin, and urinalysis should be ordered to rule out nephrotic syndrome. Liver function tests should be performed to rule out chronic liver disease causing ascites. The best way to diagnose suspected peritonitis is to sample the peritoneal fluid with a needle or catheter (paracentesis). Peritoneal fluid in spontaneous bacterial peritonitis has a high neutrophil count of greater than 250 cells/mm^3. Other tests that should be run on the peritoneal fluid include amylase (to rule out pancreatic ascites), culture, albumin, and lactate dehydrogenase concentration. For culture, a large sample of fluid should be placed into aerobic and anaerobic blood culture bottles immediately on obtaining the sample.

Appendicitis may be identified by ultrasound or computed tomography (CT) scan. When other intraabdominal emergencies are suspected, such as midgut volvulus, meconium ileus, peptic disease, or any other condition predisposing to intestinal perforation, specific testing should be performed.

TREATMENT

Peritonitis caused by an intraabdominal surgical process, such as appendicitis or a penetrating wound, must be managed surgically. Spontaneous bacterial peritonitis should be treated with a broad-spectrum antibiotic with good coverage of resistant pneumococcus and enteric bacteria. Cefotaxime is generally effective as initial therapy while awaiting culture and sensitivity results. Anaerobic coverage with metronidazole should be added whenever a perforated viscus is suspected.

Suggested Readings

Belsha D, Bremner R, Thomson M. Indications for gastrointestinal endoscopy in childhood. *Arch Dis Child.* 2016;101(12):1153–1160.

Brown LK, Beattie RM, Tighe MP. Practical management of functional abdominal pain in children. *Arch Dis Child.* 2015;101(7):677–683.

Clark MB, Slayton RL, Segura A, et al. Fluoride use in caries prevention in the primary care setting. *Pediatrics.* 2014;134(3):626–633.

Davies I, Burman-Roy S, Murphy MS, et al. Gastro-oesophageal reflux disease in children. *BMJ.* 2015;350:g7703.

Ediger TR, Hill ID. Celiac disease. *Pediatr Rev.* 2014;35(10):409–415. PMID:25274968.

Fell JM, Muhammed R, Spray C, et al. Management of ulcerative colitis. *Arch Dis Child.* 2016;101(5):469–474. PMID:26553909.

Gailey DG. Feeding infants with cleft and the postoperative cleft management. *Oral Maxillofac Surg Clin North Am.* 2016;28(2):153–159.

Gottesman LE, Del Vecchio MT, Aronoff SC. Etiologies of conjugated hyperbilirubinemia in infancy: a systematic review of 1692 subjects. *BMC Pediatr.* 2015;15:192.

Horslen S. Acute liver failure and transplantation in children. *S Afr Med J.* 2014;104(11 Pt 2):808–812.

Kammermeier J, Morris MA, Garrick V, et al. Management of Crohn's disease. *Arch Dis Child.* 2016;101(5):475–480. PMID:26553907.

Khalaf R, Phen C, Karjoo S, et al. Cholestasis beyond the neonatal and infancy periods. *Pediatr Gastroenterol Hepatol Nutr.* 2016;19(1):1–11.

Kim JS. Acute abdominal pain in children. *Pediatr Gastroenterol Hepatol Nutr.* 2013;16(4):219–224.

Koletzko S, Jones NL, Goodman KJ, et al. Evidence-based guidelines from ESPGHAN and NASPGHAN for Helicobacter pylori infection in children. *J Pediatr Gastroenterol Nutr.* 2011;53(2):230–243.

Kulik DM, Uleryk EM, Maguire JL. Does this child have appendicitis? A systematic review of clinical prediction rules for children with acute abdominal pain. *J Emerg Med.* 2013;66(1):95–104.

Li BU, Lefevre F, Chelimsky GG, et al. North American Society for Pediatric Gastroenterology, Hepatology, and Nutrition consensus statement on the diagnosis and management of cyclic vomiting syndrome. *J Pediatr Gastroenterol Nutr.* 2008;47(3):379–393.

Moyer VA. Prevention of dental caries in children from birth through age 5 years: U.S. Preventive Services Task Force recommendation statement. *Pediatrics.* 2014;133(6):1102–1111.

Neidich GA, Cole SR. Gastrointestinal bleeding. *Pediatr Rev.* 2014;35(6):243–253, quiz 254.

Papadopolou A, Koletzo S, Heuschkel R, et al. Management guidelines of eosinophilic esophagitis in childhood. *J Pediatr Gastroenterol Nutr.* 2014;58:107–118.

Pinto RB, Schneider AC, da Silveira TR. Cirrhosis in children and adolescents: an overview. *World J Hepatol.* 2015;7(3):392–405.

Pohl JF, Uc A. Paediatric Pancreatitis. *Curr Opin Gastroenterol.* 2015;31(5):380–386. PMID:26181572.

Preece ER, Athan E, Watters DA, et al. Spontaneous bacterial peritonitis: a rare mimic of acute appendicitis. *ANZ J Surg.* 2012;82(4):283–284.

Reilly S, Reid J, Skeat J, et al. ABM clinical protocol #18: guidelines for breastfeeding infants with cleft lip, cleft palate, or cleft lip and palate, revised 2013. *Breastfeed Med.* 2013;8(4):349–353.

Sahn B, Bitton S. Lower gastrointestinal bleeding in children. *Gastrointest Endosc Clin N Am.* 2016;26(1):75–98.

Saito JM. Beyond appendicitis: evaluation and surgical treatment of pediatric acute abdominal pain. *Curr Opin Pediatr.* 2012;24(3):357–364.

Schwimmer JB. Clinical advances in pediatric nonalcoholic fatty liver disease. *Hepatology*. 2016;63(5):1718–1725.
Somaraju UR, Solis-Moya A. Pancreatic enzyme replacement for people with cystic fibrosis. *Cochrane Database Syst Rev*. 2014;(10):CD008227, PMID:25310479.
Srinath AI, Lowe ME. Pediatric pancreatitis. *Pediatr Rev*. 2013;34(2):79–90. PMID: 23378615.
Tabbers MM, DiLorenzo C, Berger MY, et al. Evaluation and treatment of functional constipation in infants and children: evidence-based recommendations from ESPGHAN and NASPGHAN. *J Pediatr Gastroenterol Nutr*. 2014;58(2):258–274.
Teo S, Walker A, Steer A. Spontaneous bacterial peritonitis as a presenting feature of nephrotic syndrome. *J Paediatr Child Health*. 2013;49(12):1069–1071.
van Heurn LW, Pakarinen MP, Wester T. Contemporary management of abdominal surgical emergencies in infants and children. *Br J Surg*. 2014;101(1):e24–e33.
Verkade HJ, Bezerra JA, Davenport M, et al. Biliary atresia and other cholestatic childhood diseases: advances and future challenges. *J Hepatol*. 2016;65(3):631–642.

PEARLS FOR PRACTITIONERS

CHAPTER 126

Digestive System Assessment

- Take a careful history and perform a thorough but focused physical examination, using your findings to form a diagnostic hypothesis and plan.
- Surgical emergencies, such as bowel obstruction or appendicitis, must be identified rapidly in children with acute abdominal pain. Common distinguishing characteristics include pain that is accompanied by vomiting, tenderness, abdominal wall rigidity, or guarding.
- Extraintestinal disorders (lower lobe pneumonia, pyelonephritis) may produce abdominal pain.
- When evaluating recurrent abdominal pain, a complete work-up must include not only a medical evaluation, but also assessment of functional impairment, such as missing school, and consideration of psychosocial factors influencing the pain.
- Recurrent abdominal pain is seen in 10% of school age children and is often functional.
- For patients with emesis, remember to distinguish between true vomiting (forceful retching, preceded usually by nausea) from regurgitation (effortless, usually no nausea) when considering the differential diagnosis.
- Emesis in a neonate suggests a gastrointestinal (GI) obstruction such as pyloric stenosis or volvulus; an inborn error of metabolism should be considered in the presence of acidosis, hypoglycemia, or hyperammonemia.
- When treating a patient with significant gastrointestinal bleeding, focus on fluid resuscitation and tissue oxygenation/perfusion as your first priority.
- Acute diarrhea is often due to viral gastroenteritis (rotavirus, norovirus). Dysentery often presents with fever, pain, and diarrhea with blood and mucus.
- Painless rectal bleeding in a 2-year-old would suggest a Meckel diverticulum; older patients may also have a polyp.

CHAPTER 127

Oral Cavity

- Many systemic disorders affect the oral cavity, which careful examination can demonstrate. Examples include Peutz-Jeghers syndrome, Crohn disease, gastroesophageal reflux disease (GERD), Addison disease, and leukemia.
- Deciduous teeth erupt in a predictable sequence and age. Significant delayed eruption may be associated with hypothyroidism, Down syndrome, and other disorders.
- Cleft lip and palate are common birth defects; combined cleft lip and palate is more common in males and isolated cleft palate is more likely to be associated with other congenital malformations.

CHAPTER 128

Esophagus and Stomach

- As many as half of infants will have physiological reflux. The majority of infants do not benefit from acid reduction therapy.
- Gastroesophageal reflux *disease* occurs when there are complications of reflux such as poor growth, esophagitis, abdominal or chest pain, or respiratory problems.
- Reflux cannot be diagnosed based on imaging as this is only a snapshot in time. Upper gastrointestinal series evaluates for anatomical abnormalities.
- In an older child who has not improved with lifestyle changes, a trial with a proton pump inhibitor is recommended.
- Eosinophilic esophagitis should be considered in children with poor feeding or growth, chronic abdominal pain or vomiting, and in children with dysphagia or recurrent food impactions.
- Diagnosis of eosinophilic esophagitis requires endoscopy and biopsy. Overlap of findings is seen with gastroesophageal reflux disease.
- Treatment of eosinophilic esophagitis includes dietary changes or topical glucocorticoid therapy.
- The six food elimination diet (cow milk, soy, wheat, egg, peanuts, fish/shellfish) has been recommended as an approach to eosinophilic esophagitis (EoE).
- A neonate with poor feeding and drooling with a nasogastric tube on x-ray coiled in the neck most likely has a tracheoesophageal fistula.
- Button batteries in the esophagus must be removed immediately. Two or more ingested magnets should be removed as soon as possible due to risk of perforation.

- Infants with pyloric stenosis develop hypochloremic, hypokalemic metabolic alkalosis.
- The diagnosis of pyloric stenosis may be made with abdominal ultrasonography.
- *Helicobacter pylori* cannot be reliably tested by blood tests. Urea breath hydrogen testing, endoscopy with biopsies, and fecal antigen testing can be considered.
- Cyclic vomiting syndrome is a migraine variant that leads to repeated bouts of repetitive vomiting over hours to days.

CHAPTER 129

Intestinal Tract

- Bile-stained emesis in an infant may suggest a volvulus.
- Intestinal malrotation may lead to a volvulus with subsequent intestinal infarction.
- Passage of first meconium after 24 hours of life should raise suspicion for Hirschsprung disease.
- Hirschsprung disease is diagnosed by suction rectal biopsy.
- Duodenal atresia is associated with trisomy 21 and prematurity. There may also be polyhydramnios.
- Suspect Crohn disease in a child with poor growth, delayed puberty, fatigue, and abdominal pain. Initial testing may show anemia, thrombocytosis, elevated sedimentation rate and C-reactive protein, and hypoalbuminemia, but can be normal.
- Fecal calprotectin is an inflammatory marker of intestinal inflammation. Normal fecal calprotectin makes inflammatory bowel disease diagnosis unlikely.
- Recommended serological testing for celiac disease is the tissue transglutaminase antibody immunoglobulin A (IgA). Confirmation of the diagnosis by duodenal biopsy is recommended prior to initiating a gluten-free diet.
- Celiac disease is associated with type 1 diabetes, thyroiditis, Turner syndrome, and trisomy 21.
- Intussusception is a common cause of acute colicky abdominal pain in toddlers; there may also be rectal bleeding and intestinal obstruction.
- The diagnosis of intussusception is suggested by abdominal ultrasonography but confirmed and treated by barium or air enema.
- Appendicitis can occur at any age but is most common in adolescents and young adults.
- Periumbilical pain followed by nausea followed by right lower quadrant pain is suggestive of appendicitis.

CHAPTER 130

Liver Disease

- Infants with jaundice that persists beyond a few weeks of life should have both total and direct (conjugated) bilirubin measured to assure that cholestasis is not missed.
- Neonatal giant cell hepatitis may be due to cytomegalovirus (CMV), herpes simplex, or syphilis.
- Alpha 1 antitrypsin deficiency may present like neonatal hepatitis.
- Alagille syndrome presents with chronic cholestasis due to paucity of bile ducts and is associated with itch, butterfly vertebra, and ocular posterior embryotoxon.
- Cholestasis in infants requires prompt investigation to identify treatable causes such as biliary atresia, choledochal cyst, and certain disorders of metabolism.
- Work-up of hepatitis in children requires consideration of more than just the classic hepatitis viruses and should include evaluation for autoimmune hepatitis, Wilson disease, and biliary obstruction, as well as measures of liver function.
- Wilson disease is associated with low serum ceruloplasmin and elevated urine copper.
- Consultation with a major referral center should be sought for any child with acute severe hepatitis or chronic hepatitis.

CHAPTER 131

Pancreatic Disease

- Fecal elastase is the preferred test for pancreatic insufficiency.
- Cystic fibrosis is the most common cause of pancreatic insufficiency in the United States.
- The diagnosis of acute pancreatitis is based on symptoms of severe epigastric abdominal pain and tenderness, increase of amylase and/or lipase more than three times the upper limit of normal, and/or imaging findings of pancreatic inflammation.
- Complications of pancreatitis include shock, pancreatic pseudocyst formation, and pancreatic abscess.
- Patients with pancreatitis may feed enterally if tolerated.
- In patients with recurrent pancreatitis, consider hereditary disorders such as cystic fibrosis or familial pancreatitis involving mutations in *CFTR*, *PRSS1*, *SPINK1* or *CTRC*.

CHAPTER 132

Peritonitis

- Acute abdominal pain must be investigated rapidly with a comprehensive history and physical examination.
- When peritonitis is suspected, appropriate laboratory and imaging studies should be ordered to reveal underlying conditions, such as appendicitis.
- Nephrotic syndrome, heart failure, and chronic liver disease are associated with an increased risk of spontaneous bacterial peritonitis due to chronic presence of ascites.
- Spontaneous bacterial peritonitis is most commonly caused by *Streptococcus pneumoniae* or by *Escherichia coli*.
- Paracentesis is required to accurately diagnose pancreatitis.
- Analysis of ascites fluid obtained with a needle should include culture, cell count with differential, amylase, albumin, and lactate dehydrogenase.

RESPIRATORY SYSTEM

Amanda Striegl | Thida Ong | Susan G. Marshall

Acute and chronic respiratory diseases are common in pediatrics. Children with respiratory problems typically present with symptoms, although abnormal imaging may at times precede physical findings. The underlying etiology of childhood respiratory diseases includes the following: genetic abnormalities (e.g., cystic fibrosis); anatomical differences (e.g., laryngomalacia); incomplete maturation (e.g., bronchopulmonary dysplasia); iatrogenic effects (e.g., ventilator-associated injury); immunological disorders (e.g., severe combined immunodeficiency); infectious diseases (e.g., croup or pneumonia); environmental exposures (e.g., pollutants); and extrapulmonary consequences (e.g., congenital heart disease). The optimal functioning of the entire respiratory system allows children not only to survive but to thrive.

CHAPTER 133

Respiratory System Assessment

ANATOMY OF THE RESPIRATORY SYSTEM

Air enters the **nose** and passes over the large surface area of the **nasal turbinates**, which warm, humidify, and filter the inspired air. Secretions draining from the paranasal sinuses are carried to the **pharynx** by the mucociliary action of the ciliated respiratory epithelium. Enlarged lymphoid tissue can obstruct airflow through the nasopharynx (adenoids) or the posterior pharynx (tonsils).

The **epiglottis** protects the larynx during swallowing by deflecting material toward the esophagus. The **arytenoid cartilages**, which assist in opening and closing the vocal folds, are less prominent in children than in adults. The opening formed by the vocal folds (the **glottis**) is V-shaped, with the apex of the V being anterior. Below the vocal folds, the walls of the **subglottic space** converge toward the cricoid portion of the trachea. In children under 3 years of age, the cricoid ring is the narrowest portion of the airway. In older children and adults it is the glottis. C-shaped cartilage, extending approximately 320 degrees around the airway circumference, supports the **trachea** and **mainstem bronchi**. The posterior wall of the trachea is membranous, allowing airway caliber to change during inspiration and expiration. Beyond the lobar bronchi, cartilaginous support of the airways becomes discontinuous but persists until the terminal **bronchioles**. Airway formation and branching is complete at birth, although length and caliber continue to increase until final adult height is achieved.

The right lung has three lobes (upper, middle, lower) and comprises approximately 55% of the total lung volume. The left lung has two lobes (upper, lower); the inferior division of the left upper lobe, the lingula, is analogous to the right middle lobe. The **lung parenchyma**, where gas exchange occurs, is comprised of the respiratory bronchioles, alveolar ducts, and alveoli. **Oxygen** (O_2) and **carbon dioxide** (CO_2) must traverse alveolar and capillary membranes and the **interstitium** to maintain adequate oxygenation and ventilation to meet the metabolic demands of the body.

The pediatric lung has tremendous capacity for growth. A full-term infant has approximately 25 million alveoli; an adult nearly 300 million alveoli. The growth of new alveoli occurs during the first 2 years of life and is complete by 8 years of age. After this time, lung volume increases primarily by increase in alveolar dimensions, with new alveoli rarely formed.

PULMONARY PHYSIOLOGY

Pulmonary Mechanics

The major function of the lungs is to exchange O_2 and CO_2 between the atmosphere and the blood. The anatomy of the airways, mechanics of the respiratory muscles and rib cage, nature of the alveolar-capillary interface, pulmonary circulation, tissue metabolism, and neuromuscular control of ventilation all influence gas exchange.

Air enters the lungs when intrathoracic pressure is less than atmospheric pressure. Negative intrathoracic pressure is generated by contraction and lowering of the **diaphragm** during normal inspiration. The accessory muscles of inspiration (**external intercostal**, **scalene**, and **sternocleidomastoid muscles**) are not used during quiet breathing but are recruited during exercise or in disease states to raise and enlarge the rib cage. Exhalation is normally passive, but with active exhalation the **abdominal** and **internal intercostal muscles** are recruited.

During normal breathing at rest, lung volumes are usually in the midrange of inflation (Fig. 133.1). **Tidal volume (TV)** is the amount of air inspired with each *relaxed* breath. The volume of gas retained in the lung at the end of a *relaxed* exhalation is the **functional residual capacity (FRC)**. This gas volume maintains exchange of O_2 between breaths. **Total lung capacity (TLC)** is the volume of gas in the lungs at the end of *maximal* inhalation and **residual volume (RV)** is the volume of gas left in the lungs at the end of a *maximal* exhalation. **Vital capacity (VC)** is the maximal amount of air that can be forcibly expelled from the lungs and is the difference between TLC and RV.

Airway resistance is influenced by the diameter and length of the conducting airways, the viscosity of gas, and the nature of the airflow. During quiet breathing, airflow in the smaller airways is laminar (streamlined). At higher flow rates, turbulent flow increases resistance. Resistance is inversely proportional to the fourth power of the radius of the airway, so relatively small changes in airway diameter can result in large changes in airway resistance. Excessive airway secretions, bronchospasm, mucosal edema, stenosis, foreign bodies, loss of airway wall integrity (bronchiectasis), and airway compression may all produce symptomatic increases in airway resistance. Diseases that impact airway resistance, particularly lower airway resistance, fall into the category of **obstructive airways disease**.

Lung compliance (change in volume for a given change in pressure) is a measure of the ease with which the lung can be inflated. Processes that decrease lung compliance (surfactant deficiency, pulmonary fibrosis, pulmonary edema) may lead to **restrictive lung disease**. Restrictive lung disease can also result from respiratory muscle weakness, pleural disease (effusion, inflammation, or mass), thoracic stiffness (scoliosis), and abdominal distention.

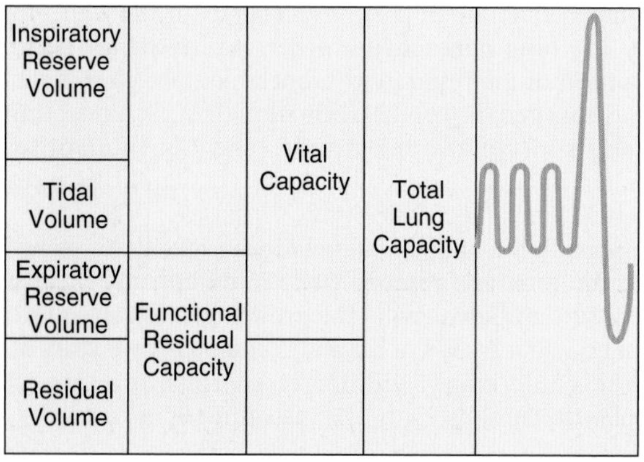

FIGURE 133.1 Lung volumes and capacities. Vital capacity and its subdivisions can be measured by spirometry, but calculation of residual volume requires measurement of functional residual capacity by body plethysmography, helium dilution, or nitrogen washout. (From Andreoli TE, Bennett JC, Carpenter CJ, et al., eds. *Cecil Essentials of Medicine*. 4th ed. Philadelphia: WB Saunders; 1997:127.)

Respiratory Gas Exchange

Alveolar ventilation is defined as the exchange of CO_2 between the alveoli and ambient air. Normally, about 30% of each tidal breath fills the conducting airways **(anatomical dead space)**. Because the anatomical dead space is relatively constant, increasing the TV generally increases the efficacy of ventilation. Conversely, if TV decreases, then the dead space/TV ratio increases and alveolar ventilation decreases.

Gas exchange depends on alveolar ventilation, **pulmonary capillary blood flow**, and the **diffusion** of gases across the alveolar-capillary membrane. Exchange of CO_2 is determined by alveolar ventilation, whereas the exchange of O_2 is influenced primarily by the regional matching of ventilation (V) with pulmonary blood flow (Q) (V/Q matching). V/Q matching is maintained, in part, by **hypoxic pulmonary vasoconstriction** (local constriction of the pulmonary vessels in areas that are underventilated). There are five causes of **hypoxemia** (Table 133.1). Disorders resulting in **V/Q mismatching** (such as pneumonia and atelectasis) are the most common causes of hypoxemia in children.

Lung Defense Mechanisms

The lungs are constantly exposed to particles and infectious agents. The **nose** is the primary filter for large particles. Particles less than 10 μm in diameter may reach the trachea and bronchi and deposit on the mucosa. Particles less than 1 μm may reach the alveoli. **Ciliated epithelium** lining the airways from the larynx to the bronchioles continuously propels a thin layer of mucus toward the mouth. **Alveolar macrophages** and **polymorphonuclear cells** engulf particles and pathogens that have been opsonized by locally secreted immunoglobulin (Ig)A antibodies or transudated serum antibodies.

TABLE 133.1 Causes of Hypoxemia

CAUSE	EXAMPLE(S)	PaO_2	$PaCO_2$	PaO_2 IMPROVES WITH SUPPLEMENTAL OXYGEN
Ventilation-perfusion mismatch	Asthma Bronchopulmonary dysplasia Pneumonia Atelectasis	↓	Normal, ↓, or ↑	Yes
Hypoventilation	Apnea Narcotic overdose Neuromuscular disease	↓	↑	Yes
Extrapulmonary shunt	Cyanotic heart disease	↓	Normal or ↑	No
Intrapulmonary shunt	Pulmonary arteriovenous malformation Atelectasis	↓	Normal or ↑	No
Low FiO_2	High altitude	↓	↓	Yes
Diffusion defect	Scleroderma Hepatopulmonary syndrome Pulmonary fibrosis	↓	Normal	Yes

FiO_2, Fraction of inspired oxygen; *$Paco_2$*, arterial partial pressure of carbon dioxide; *Pao_2*, arterial partial pressure of oxygen.

Cough is a critically important mechanism for protecting the lungs from infection. It may be voluntary or generated by reflex irritation of the nose, sinuses, pharynx, larynx, trachea, bronchi, or bronchioles. Cough is a rapid, forceful expiration intended to clear the airways of debris and secretions. Effective cough requires the ability to (1) inhale to near TLC, (2) close and open the glottis, and (3) contract abdominal muscles to forcibly exhale. Loss of the ability to cough, as with neuromuscular weakness, results in poor secretion clearance and predisposes to atelectasis and pneumonia. Persistent cough suggests chronic irritation at any of these sites due to infectious (e.g., chronic bronchitis), allergic (e.g., postnasal drip, asthma), or chemical (e.g., inhalation or aspiration) triggers.

HISTORY

Common respiratory complaints in children include cough, labored or noisy breathing, chest pain, and exercise intolerance. The complete respiratory history includes **onset**, **duration**, and **frequency** of symptoms. It is important to obtain information concerning severity (hospitalizations, missed school days) and pattern (acute, chronic, or intermittent), including factors leading to worsening or improvement. Exposure to others with respiratory illness and **environmental factors** (such as pet dander, tobacco smoke, or chemical fumes) should be reviewed. For infants, a **feeding history** should be obtained, including questions of coughing or choking with eating or drinking. Family history should include questions about asthma and atopy, immune deficiencies, and cystic fibrosis.

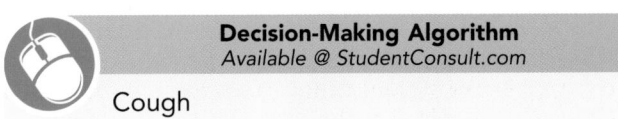

Decision-Making Algorithm
Available @ StudentConsult.com

Cough

Cough

A thorough history focused on the factors above is perhaps the most useful tool in determining the underlying etiology of cough. Morning cough may be due to the accumulation of excessive secretions during the night from sinusitis, allergic rhinitis, or bronchial infection. Nighttime cough is a hallmark of asthma and can also be caused by gastroesophageal reflux disease or postnasal drip. Cough with exercise is highly suggestive of exercise-induced asthma/bronchospasm. Habit cough can masquerade as organic disease but should disappear when children are distracted or during sleep. Paroxysmal cough (especially associated with cyanosis) suggests pertussis, whereas a repetitive, staccato cough occurs in chlamydial infections in infants. A harsh, brassy, seal-like cough suggests croup, tracheomalacia, or psychogenic (habit) cough. Sudden onset of cough after a choking episode suggests foreign body aspiration.

PHYSICAL EXAMINATION

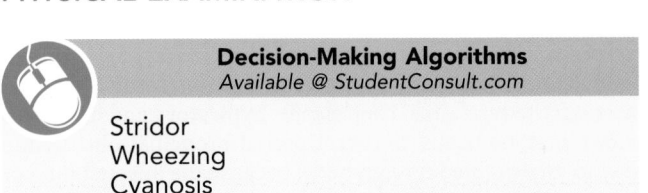

Decision-Making Algorithms
Available @ StudentConsult.com

Stridor
Wheezing
Cyanosis

Clothing should be removed from the upper half of the child's body so that the thorax may be inspected while maintaining modesty for adolescents. It is optimal to observe the respiratory pattern, rate, and work of breathing while the child is quiet, noting the shape and symmetry of the chest wall and the anteroposterior (AP) diameter.

Any factor that impairs respiratory mechanics is likely to increase the **respiratory rate**. However, nonrespiratory causes of tachypnea include fever, pain, and anxiety. Respiratory rates vary with age (Table 133.2).

It is important to observe the respiratory **pattern** and **degree of effort** (work of breathing). Abnormal respiratory patterns are detailed in Table 133.3. Increased work of breathing can be described as inspiratory (**intercostal, supraclavicular,** or **substernal retractions, nasal flaring**) or expiratory (use of abdominal muscles to actively exhale). Causes of increased work

TABLE 133.2 Normal Respiratory Rates by Age

AGE	RESPIRATORY RATE (BREATHS PER MINUTE)
Birth-9 months	30-60
9 months-2 years	24-40
2-5 years	20-36
5-12 years	14-26
12 years-adult	12-20

TABLE 133.3 Abnormal Breathing Patterns

PATTERN	FEATURES	CAUSES
Tachypnea	Respiratory rate > normal for age	Restrictive physiology, fever, increased metabolic demands, stress
Bradypnea	Respiratory rate < normal for age	Sleep, sedating medications, CNS injury, metabolic alkalosis
Hyperpnea	Increased depth of breathing, normal rate	Stress, exercise, metabolic acidosis
Periodic breathing	Brief pauses (<10 sec) followed by rapid, shallow breaths	Normal variant for preterm and term infants, prominent in sleep
Kussmaul respiration	Increased rate, increased tidal volume, regular deep respiration	Metabolic acidosis, especially diabetic ketoacidosis, uremia
Cheyne-Stokes respiration	Cyclic pattern of waxing and waning of depth of breathing interposed with apnea	CNS injury (brainstem), elevated intracranial pressure, heart failure, uremia
Biot respiration	Rapid, deep respiration followed by apnea	CNS injury or infection
Apneustic respiration	Long inspiration with short or staccato expiration	Brainstem lesion
Agonal respiration	Slow rate, variable tidal volume	Shock, sepsis, or asphyxia

CNS, Central nervous system.

TABLE 133.4 Physical Signs of Pulmonary Disease

DISEASE PROCESS	MEDIASTINAL DEVIATION	CHEST MOTION	VOCAL FREMITUS	PERCUSSION	BREATH SOUNDS	ADVENTITIOUS SOUNDS	VOICE SIGNS
Consolidation	No	Reduced over area	Increased	Dull	Bronchial or reduced	None or crackles	Egophony* Pectoriloquy†
Bronchospasm	No	Hyperexpansion with limited motion	Normal or decreased	Hyperresonant	Normal to decreased	Wheezes, crackles	Normal to decreased
Atelectasis	Shift toward affected side	Reduced over area	Decreased	Dull	Reduced	None or crackles	None
Pneumothorax	With tension: shift to the opposite side	Reduced over PMI	None	Resonant	None	None	None
Pleural effusion	If large: shift to opposite side	Reduced over area	None or reduced	Dull	None	Egophony Friction rub	Muffled
Interstitial process	No	Reduced	Normal to increased	Normal	Normal	Inspiratory crackles	None

*In egophony, e sounds like a (may be a sign of consolidation but also is associated with moderate-sized pleural effusions).
†In pectoriloquy, words/voice sounds clearer over the affected site (associated with consolidation and cavitary lesions).
PMI, Point of maximum impulse.
Modified from Andreoli TE, Bennett JC, Carpenter CJ, et al., eds. Cecil Essentials of Medicine. *4th ed. Philadelphia: WB Saunders; 1997:115.*

of breathing during inspiration include extrathoracic airway obstruction (laryngomalacia, croup, subglottic stenosis) and/or decreased pulmonary compliance (e.g., pneumonia, pulmonary edema). Increased expiratory work of breathing usually indicates intrathoracic airway narrowing (e.g., asthma, tracheomalacia). **Grunting** (forced expiration against a partially closed glottis) is often seen in small children with respiratory distress but may also be a manifestation of pain.

When attempting to determine the cause of a respiratory complaint, it is useful to auscultate over all potential sites of pathology, including the nose and mouth, neck, large airways (central chest and back), and all lobes of both lungs (anterior and posterior, upper and lower, as well as lateral chest wall).

Stridor is a harsh, monophonic sound caused by a partially obstructed large airway, more commonly heard on inspiration and localized to the neck. **Wheezing** is produced by partial obstruction of the smaller lower airways, more commonly heard during exhalation and localized to the chest. Wheezes can be monophonic and low-pitched (usually from large, central airways) or high-pitched and musical (from small peripheral airways). Secretions in the intrathoracic airways may produce wheezing but more commonly result in irregular sounds called **rhonchi**. Fluid or secretions in small airways may produce sounds characteristic of crumpling cellophane (**crackles** or **rales**). Having the child take a deep breath and exhale forcefully will accentuate many abnormal lung sounds. **Decreased, absent, or asymmetric breath sounds** may be due to atelectasis, lobar consolidation (pneumonia), thoracic mass, or a pleural effusion. Observation of respiratory rate, work of breathing, tracheal and cardiac deviation, and chest wall motion, combined with percussion and auscultation, help to identify intrathoracic disease (Table 133.4).

Digital clubbing (Fig. 133.2) is seen in cystic fibrosis and in other, less common chronic pulmonary diseases (such as interstitial lung disease). It is not associated with asthma, so its presence should heighten concern for other diagnoses. Clubbing may also be present in nonpulmonary chronic diseases (cardiac, gastrointestinal, or hematological) or, rarely, as a familial trait.

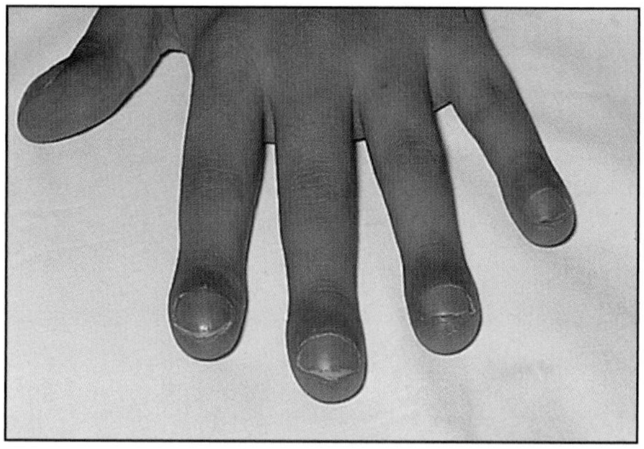

FIGURE 133.2 Clubbing of the fingers. There is increased curvature and loss of nail angle. This child has cystic fibrosis. (From Lissauer T, Clayden G, eds. *Illustrated Textbook of Pediatrics.* 4th ed. London: Mosby; 2012. Fig 2.6a.)

DIAGNOSTIC MEASURES

Imaging Techniques

Chest radiographs are useful in assessing respiratory disease in children. In addition to determining lung abnormalities, they provide information about the bony thorax (rib or vertebral abnormalities), the heart (cardiomegaly, pericardial effusion), and the great vessels (right aortic arch/vascular rings, rib notching). Chest radiographs should be obtained in both the posteroanterior (PA) and lateral projections and, if possible, following a full inspiration. Estimation of lung hyperinflation based on a single PA view is unreliable; flattened diaphragms and an increased AP diameter on lateral projection are a better indicator of hyperinflation. Increased density on chest radiograph can usually be classified as *blood, water, pus,* or *tissue,* with clinical features (e.g., fever or known cardiac disease) necessary to reach final conclusions. **Expiratory** and **decubitus views** may be useful to detect partial bronchial obstruction due to an aspirated foreign body, because the affected lung or lobe does not deflate on exhalation. Decubitus films can also help to differentiate pleural effusion from alveolar infiltrate.

A **barium esophagram** may be valuable in diagnosing disorders of swallowing (dysphagia) and esophageal motility, vascular rings (esophageal compression), tracheoesophageal fistulas, and, to a lesser extent, gastroesophageal reflux. When evaluating for a tracheoesophageal fistula, contrast material must be instilled under pressure via a catheter with the distal tip situated in the esophagus (see Chapter 128).

Computed tomography (CT) of the chest is the imaging tool of choice for evaluating masses, interstitial lung disease, and bronchiectasis, as well as delineating pleural from parenchymal lesions. CT scans with intravenous contrast provide excellent information about the pulmonary vasculature and great vessels, are useful for characterizing congenital pulmonary malformations, and can detect pulmonary embolism. The speed of current CT scanners makes it possible to scan most children without sedating them; however, sedation may be required in infants and toddlers to decrease motion artifact. **Magnetic resonance imaging (MRI)**, useful in visualizing cardiac and great vessel anatomy and mediastinal lesions, is less useful for evaluation of pulmonary parenchymal lesions. **Ultrasonography** can be used to delineate some intrathoracic masses and is the imaging procedure of choice for assessing size and character of parapneumonic effusion/empyema. It is also useful for assessing diaphragmatic motion in small children.

Measures of Respiratory Gas Exchange

A properly performed **arterial blood gas** analysis provides information about the effectiveness of both oxygenation and ventilation. As arterial samples are difficult to obtain, capillary and venous blood samples are more commonly used. Capillary or venous samples should not be used to assess oxygenation. The partial pressure of carbon dioxide (Pco_2) from a capillary sample is similar to that from arterial blood. The Pco_2 in venous samples is approximately 6 mm Hg higher than arterial Pco_2.

There are both respiratory and metabolic causes of acidosis (see Chapter 37). In the presence of an alkalosis or acidosis, respiratory compensation (altering Pco_2 to maintain a normal pH) can occur within minutes, but renal compensation (altering the serum bicarbonate level) may not be complete for several days. Since both the respiratory and metabolic compensation are incomplete, pH will remain on the side of the primary insult (whether acidosis or alkalosis).

Pulse oximetry measures the O_2 saturation of hemoglobin by measuring the blood absorption of two or more wavelengths of light. It is noninvasive, easy to use, and reliable. Because of the shape of the oxyhemoglobin dissociation curve, O_2 saturation does not decrease much until the partial pressure of oxygen (Po_2) reaches approximately 60 mm Hg. Pulse oximetry may not accurately reflect true O_2 saturation when abnormal hemoglobin is present (carboxyhemoglobin, methemoglobin), when perfusion is poor, or if no light passes through to the photodetector (nail polish).

The measurement of Pco_2 is accomplished most reliably by blood gas analysis. However, there are noninvasive monitors that record exhaled Pco_2 (**end-tidal CO_2**), which is representative of alveolar Pco_2. End-tidal Pco_2 measurements are most commonly used in intubated and mechanically ventilated patients, but some devices can measure Pco_2 at the nares. **Transcutaneous electrodes** can be used to monitor Pco_2 at the skin surface, but are less accurate. Noninvasive techniques of CO_2 measurement are best suited for detecting trends rather than for providing absolute values.

Pulmonary Function Testing

Measurement of lung volumes and airflow rates using **spirometry** are important in assessing pulmonary disease. Most children above 6 years of age can perform spirometry. The patient inhales to TLC and then forcibly exhales until no more air can be expelled. During the forced expiratory maneuver, **forced vital capacity (FVC)**, **forced expired volume in the first second (FEV_1)**, and **forced expiratory flow (FEF)** rates are measured. These are compared to predicted values based on patient age, gender, and race, but rely mostly on height. Severity of disease is quantified by calculated percentage of predicted values. The **peak expiratory flow rate (PEFR)** can be obtained with a simple hand-held device and may be useful for home monitoring of older children with asthma; however, it is *highly dependent on patient effort*, and values must be interpreted with caution. Measurement of **TLC, FRC**, and **RV** require **body plethysmography**. Helium dilution can also measure TLC and RV by determining the magnitude of dilution of inhaled helium in the air within the lung, but may underestimate air trapping.

Abnormal results on pulmonary function testing can be used to categorize **obstructive** (low flow rates and/or increased RV) or a **restrictive lung disease** (low FVC and TLC, with relative preservation of flow rates). When the FEV_1 is decreased to a greater extent than the FVC (**FEV_1/FVC ratio** <80%), obstructive lung disease is diagnosed. The mean midexpiratory flow rate (**$FEF_{25-75\%}$**) is a more sensitive measure of small airways disease than the FEV_1, but is also more variable. Spirometry can detect reversible airway obstruction characteristics of asthma when a significant improvement in FEV_1 (>12%) or in $FEF_{25-75\%}$ (>25%) following inhalation of a bronchodilator is measured. **Inhalation challenge tests** using methacholine, histamine, or cold, dry air are used to assess airway hyperreactivity but require sophisticated equipment and special expertise and should only be performed in a pulmonary function laboratory with experienced technicians.

Endoscopic Evaluation of the Airways

Endoscopic evaluation of the upper airways (**nasopharyngoscopy**) is performed with a flexible fiberoptic nasopharyngoscope to assess adenoid size, patency of the nasal passages, and abnormalities of the glottis. It is especially useful in evaluating stridor and assessing vocal cord motion/function and does not require sedation. Endoscopic evaluation of the subglottic space and intrathoracic airways can be done with either a flexible or rigid bronchoscope under anesthesia. **Flexible bronchoscopy** is useful in identifying dynamic or static airway abnormalities (stenosis, malacia, endobronchial lesions, excessive secretions) and to obtain airway samples for culture (**bronchoalveolar lavage**). **Rigid bronchoscopy** is the method of choice for removing foreign bodies from the airways and performing other interventions, such as airway dilation. Transbronchial biopsies are rarely performed in children.

Examination of Sputum

Sputum specimens may be useful in evaluating lower respiratory tract infections but are difficult to obtain in children. Specimens containing large numbers of squamous epithelial cells or heavily contaminated with upper airway secretions may yield misleading results. Sputum in patients with lower respiratory tract bacterial infections often contains polymorphonuclear leukocytes and one predominant organism on culture. If sputum cannot be obtained, then bronchoalveolar lavage may be necessary for microbiologic diagnosis in selected situations. In patients with CF who are unable to expectorate sputum, specially processed throat cultures are used as surrogates for lower airway cultures.

Lung Biopsy

When less invasive methods fail to provide diagnoses in patients with pulmonary disease, a lung biopsy may be required. Concern for childhood interstitial lung disease, atypical infection (especially in an immunocompromised host), and evaluation of a mass/malformation are the most common indications for biopsy. CT-guided **needle biopsy** performed by an interventional radiologist is an option if limited histology is needed and the lesion is amenable to percutaneous approach (e.g., fungal nodules). Either a **thoracoscopic procedure** or a **thoracotomy** is preferred if thorough histological evaluation is desired.

THERAPEUTIC MEASURES

Oxygen Administration

Any child in respiratory distress should be treated with **supplemental oxygen** at concentration sufficient to maintain *acceptable* O_2 saturation levels. Normal O_2 saturation is greater than 95%; however, lower saturations may be appropriate in certain clinical scenarios, such as preterm birth or congenital heart disease. It is not necessary to achieve 100% saturation. Patients requiring supplemental O_2 should be monitored with pulse oximetry, intermittently or continuously, or with arterial blood gas measurements of Po_2 to allow titration to the lowest required O_2 concentration. The actual fraction of inspired oxygen **(FiO_2)** delivered to the patient can be quite variable and is affected by the delivery device used, device position, the child's size, and respiratory pattern.

For long-term administration of O_2, a **nasal cannula** is the most widely used device, as it enables patients to eat and speak unhindered by the O_2 delivery system. **Humidified high flow nasal cannula** (HFNC) allows the provider to deliver greater flow rates of blended gas at a specific FiO_2. Though its use began in neonates as an alternative to continuous positive airway pressure (CPAP), it is now commonly used across the pediatric age spectrum. Depending on the size of the patient, the type of cannulae and device used, HFNC can deliver modest positive pressure, relieve dyspnea, and purge CO_2 from anatomical dead space to improve alveolar ventilation in addition to providing oxygenation. There are very limited options for provision of HFNC outside the hospital at this time. Supplemental O_2 may also be delivered by a variety of mask systems including a **simple mask** (delivers O_2 in L/min), a **Venturi mask** (blends to a specific FiO_2), and a **non-rebreather mask** with reservoir that can provide nearly 100% O_2.

Aerosol Therapy

Therapeutic agents such as bronchodilators, corticosteroids, and antibiotics can be delivered to the lower respiratory tract by **dry powder inhaler** (DPI), **metered-dose inhaler** (MDI), or **nebulizer**. All of these devices are designed to generate small particles that can bypass the filtering action of the upper airway and deposit in the lower airways. Many factors influence drug deposition including patient technique, device used, age of the child, and breathing pattern. Nebulizers should be used with a face mask (infants) or mouthpiece (children and teens) to minimize loss of drug to ambient air. Plastic holding chambers **(spacers)** are available for all ages and should always be used with MDIs. DPIs require a single rapid, deep inhalation for optimal drug delivery, which is difficult for children under 6 years of age. MDIs and nebulizers are equally effective in delivering medications only if the technique is correct, so it is important to review this frequently and carefully with families (Fig 133.3).

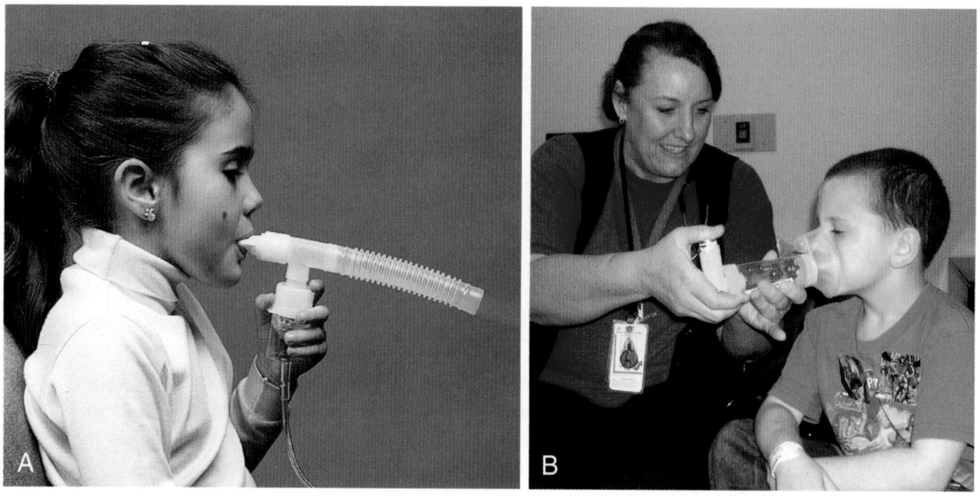

FIGURE 133.3 Inhaled drug delivery in children. *A*, Proper use of a nebulizer with mouthpiece and *B*, Metered-dose inhaler with space and face mask. (*A*, From Hopper T. *Mosby's Pharmacy* Technician. 2nd ed. St Louis: Mosby; 2007. Fig 25.7; *B*, From Hockenberry MJ, Wilson D, eds. *Wong's Essentials of Pediatric* Nursing. 8th ed. St Louis: Mosby; 2009. Fig 23.5.)

Chest Physiotherapy and Clearance Techniques

When disease processes impair normal ciliary and cough function, **airway clearance therapy** may help maintain airway patency and secretion mobilization. Most methods work by moving secretions toward the central airways, from which they can be expectorated. **Chest percussion** or **pneumatic vests** are often used in young or neurologically impaired children; whereas older children can operate hand-held devices that generate expiratory back-pressure and vibration (*TheraPEP, Flutter, Acapella*, and *Aerobika*). Pneumatic (therapy) vests may also be used in older children and adolescents, especially those with cystic fibrosis. Children who are too weak to generate an effective cough benefit from the use of a mechanical insufflation-exsufflation device (CoughAssist), used in conjunction with chest physiotherapy. Chest physiotherapy is generally not beneficial for patients with asthma or pneumonia, and its effectiveness in patients with atelectasis has not been clearly established.

Intubation

If the upper airway is obstructed or mechanical ventilation is needed, it may be necessary to provide the patient with an **artificial airway**. This is best done by placing an endotracheal tube via the mouth or nose into the trachea **(intubation)**. **Endotracheal tubes** can damage the larynx and the airways if the tubes are of improper size and are not carefully maintained. The cricoid ring is the narrowest segment of a child's airway and is completely surrounded by cartilage, which makes it vulnerable to damage and subglottic stenosis. If the pressure created by the tube against the airway mucosa exceeds capillary filling pressure (roughly 35 cm H_2O), mucosal ischemia develops, leading to necrosis. Therefore a small air leak should always be maintained around the endotracheal tube to minimize the risk of mucosal damage. No clear guidelines are available regarding how long pediatric patients can be intubated without sustaining airway damage or when conversion to tracheostomy is indicated.

Intubation alters the physiology of the respiratory tract in many ways, not all of which are beneficial. It interferes with the humidification, warming, and filtration of inspired air and stimulates secretion production. Providing adequate humidification of inspired air and appropriate suctioning of the tube reduce the probability of occlusion by secretions. In addition to endotracheal tubes, the **laryngeal mask airway (LMA)** can be used to provide mechanical ventilation. This device consists of a tube with a soft mask at the distal end that is placed over the larynx, creating a seal without the trachea being instrumented. Although less invasive, the LMA is less secure, so it is generally limited to procedural anesthesia.

Tracheostomy

Tracheostomy is the surgical placement of an artificial airway into the trachea below the larynx. Congenital or acquired upper airway obstruction (see Chapter 135) is the most common indication for tracheostomy in children. In addition, if prolonged mechanical ventilation is required, elective tracheostomy can be performed to increase patient comfort and facilitate nursing care. Many children with tracheostomy tubes can be cared for at home, provided the caregivers are well trained and adequately equipped. Because the tracheostomy tube hampers the ability to phonate and may become occluded with secretions, leading to life-threatening airway obstruction, the child must be monitored carefully at all times.

Mechanical Ventilation

Patients who are unable to maintain adequate gas exchange may require **mechanical ventilation**. Most modes of mechanical ventilation involve inflation of the lungs with gas using positive pressure. The inspiratory phase is active (air is pushed in), and exhalation is passive.

Mechanical ventilation often requires an artificial airway, although it can be provided *noninvasively* via tight-fitting nasal or full face masks. **Noninvasive ventilation** is particularly useful in patients with obstructive sleep apnea and neuromuscular disease who require support only part of the day or night, but it can also be used to assist ventilation continuously for patients in acute respiratory failure from a variety of causes.

No method of mechanical ventilation truly simulates natural breathing. All methods have their drawbacks and complications. Positive pressure is transmitted to the entire thorax and may impede venous return to the heart. The airways and lung parenchyma may be damaged by inflation pressures and high concentrations of inspired O_2. In general, inflation pressures should be limited to those necessary to provide sufficient lung expansion for adequate ventilation and the prevention of atelectasis. Pressure-cycled and volume-cycled ventilators (conventional ventilation) are the most widely used modalities in pediatrics. High-frequency jet ventilation and high-frequency oscillatory ventilation are used often in neonatology and may be used in patients with severe lung disease who are failing conventional mechanical ventilation.

CHAPTER 134

Control of Breathing

Ventilation is controlled primarily by **central chemoreceptors** located in the medulla that respond to intracellular pH and P_{CO_2} levels (Fig. 134.1). To a lesser extent, ventilation is modulated by **peripheral receptors** located in the carotid and aortic bodies which respond predominantly to P_{O_2}. The central receptors are quite sensitive. Small acute changes in Pa_{CO_2} normally result in significant changes in **minute ventilation**. The ventilatory drive is not increased when the P_{CO_2} is chronically elevated, as the intracellular pH returns to normal levels following compensatory increases in the bicarbonate level. The peripheral receptors do not stimulate ventilation until the Pa_{O_2} decreases to approximately 60 mm Hg. These receptors become important in patients with chronic Pa_{CO_2} elevation who may have a blunted ventilatory response to CO_2.

The output of the central respiratory center also is modulated by reflex mechanisms. Full lung inflation temporarily inhibits inspiratory effort in infants (**Hering-Breuer reflex**) through vagal afferent fibers. Other reflexes from the airways and intercostal muscles may influence the depth and frequency of respiratory efforts (see Fig. 134.1).

APNEA

Decision-Making Algorithm
Available @ StudentConsult.com

Apnea

Etiology

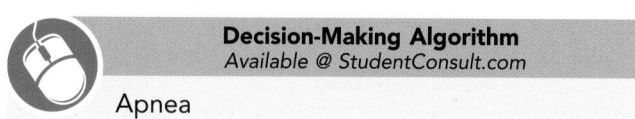

Apnea is defined as the cessation of airflow due to either: lack of respiratory effort (**central apnea**) or upper airway obstruction (**obstructive apnea**; Table 134.1). Central apnea is more common in infants, and obstructive apnea, especially during sleep, is more common in older children.

Central apnea lasting less than 10 seconds is common in healthy infants and can be present in normal children during sleep, especially after a sigh breath. Central pauses lasting longer than 15-20 seconds are considered abnormal. Premature infants can have **apnea of prematurity**, which consists of recurrent apneic episodes that are often of central origin, although they can be mixed central/obstructive. Apnea of prematurity should resolve by 44 weeks postconceptional age. Central apnea outside of infancy is a rare occurrence and warrants evaluation.

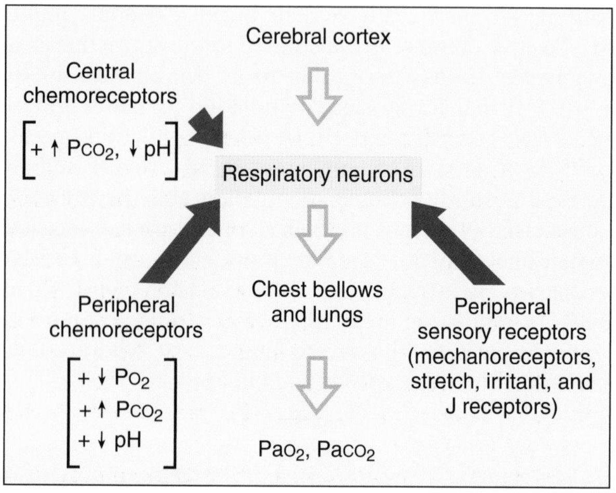

FIGURE 134.1 Schematic representation of the respiratory control system. The respiratory neurons in the brainstem receive information from the chemoreceptors, peripheral sensory receptors, and cerebral cortex. This information is integrated, and the resulting neural output is transmitted to the diaphragms and lungs. The sign denotes stimulation of the receptor. (From Andreoli TE, Bennett JC, Carpenter CJ, et al, eds. *Cecil Essentials of Medicine*. 4th ed. Philadelphia: WB Saunders; 1997:171.)

Congenital central hypoventilation syndrome **(CCHS)** is a rare genetic disorder in which there is profound loss of respiratory control during sleep leading to primary central apnea, hypercarbia, and hypoxemia. Most patients with CCHS have a defect in the ***PHOX2B*** gene, which is necessary for autonomic nervous system development. Infants with CCHS typically have respiratory difficulties within the first several weeks of life although it can also present later in childhood. CCHS is associated with an increased risk of Hirschsprung disease and neural crest tumors (neuroblastoma). Other genetic syndromes associated with abnormal central respiratory control include Rett, Joubert, and Prader-Willi syndromes and tuberous sclerosis. Secondary causes of central apnea and hypoventilation are more common and include medications impairing central respiratory drive (narcotics), increased intracranial pressure, central nervous system (CNS) tumors, myelomeningocele and/or Arnold-Chiari malformation, and mitochondrial/metabolic disorders.

Breath holding spells are a form of apnea occurring when a young child is awake, usually triggered by emotional stress. They often follow a sustained exhalation, so can be associated with cyanosis and loss of consciousness that is quite alarming. The return of spontaneous breathing usually occurs quickly. Most breath holding spells are benign and lessen over time, but seizures and disorders of central respiratory control should be considered.

Obstructive sleep apnea syndrome (OSA) affects 2-3% of young children with peak prevalence at 2-8 years of age. It is caused by complete or partial upper airway obstruction during sleep. Control of breathing is usually preserved, although infants and others with immature respiratory control may have obstructive and central apnea together. Restless sleep, behavioral problems, and inattention/hyperactivity are more common in young children than the classic adult findings of daytime hypersomnolence and loud snoring. Some children experience poor somatic growth due to interruption of normal growth hormone production during deep sleep. A small subset can have significant hypoxemia and hypercarbia leading to morning headaches, and if untreated, pulmonary hypertension and cor pulmonale. Not all children who snore have OSA, and not all

TABLE 134.1 Categories of Apnea

DISEASE	EXAMPLE(S)	MECHANISM	SIGNS	TREATMENT
Apnea of prematurity	Premature (<36 wk)	Central control, upper airway obstruction	Apnea, bradycardia	Caffeine, HFNC, CPAP, intubation
Central apnea/ hypoventilation	CCHS, Arnold-Chiari malformation	Abnormal central control	Apnea	Mechanical ventilation or BiPAP
Obstructive sleep apnea	Obesity, adenotonsillar hypertrophy, Pierre Robin sequence, Down syndrome, cerebral palsy	Upper airway obstruction due to excess tissue, loss of pharyngeal tone, or crowded anatomy	Snoring, restless sleep, poor school performance, behavior problems, mouth breathing	Adenotonsillectomy, CPAP or BiPAP, uvulopalatoplasty, tracheostomy
Breath holding spells	<3 yr old who turns blue after crying, may have syncope	Prolonged expiratory apnea; reflex anoxic seizures	Cyanosis, syncope, brief tonic-clonic movements after cyanosis	Reassurance; condition is self-limiting. Must exclude seizure disorder

BiPAP, Bi-level positive airway pressure; *CCHS*, congenital central hypoventilation syndrome; *CPAP*, continuous positive airway pressure; *HFNC*, high flow nasal cannula.

children who have OSA snore. Thus when the diagnosis is in question, it should be confirmed with a polysomnogram (PSG).

PSG is the only definitive test for evaluation of obstructive and central sleep apnea. It involves continuous recording of electroencephalogram (EEG) and electrooculogram for sleep staging, oronasal airflow and pressure, audible snore, chest and abdominal wall excursion, leg and chin electromyogram, electrocardiogram, pulse oximetry, and capnography. The measured score from a PSG is the **apnea-hypopnea index** (AHI) or number of times in an hour of sleep that the child has cessation or reduction of airflow of a significant magnitude to negatively affect oxygenation or sleep stage. An AHI less than 1 is the generally accepted norm for pediatric patients although the decision to treat often hinges on the severity of daytime impairment. Measured AHI is typically worse in rapid eye movement (REM) sleep and when the child is supine, so an ideal study captures all sleep stages and positions.

Adenotonsillar hypertrophy is the most common cause of OSA in young children, with peak age 2-5 years. Other risk factors for OSA include obesity, premature birth, craniofacial malformations, trisomy 21, and neuromuscular diseases. Treatment of OSA starts with determining whether the child will benefit from adenoidectomy, with or without tonsillectomy. If surgical intervention is not indicated or fails to alleviate the problem, then the use of continuous positive airway pressure **(CPAP)** or bi-level positive airway pressure **(BiPAP)** via nasal interfaces can be used to distend the upper airway during sleep. This requires a tight-fitting nasal mask, which may not be well tolerated in young children. Supplemental oxygen can blunt hypoxemia in milder cases of OSA but does not alter obstruction and sleep fragmentation. In extreme cases, especially those associated with craniofacial abnormalities or hypotonia, tracheostomy may be indicated.

BRIEF RESOLVED UNEXPLAINED EVENTS

A **brief resolved unexplained event (BRUE)** is defined as a <1 minute, self-limited episode with one or more of the following features: (1) cyanosis or pallor, (2) absent or irregular breathing, (3) change in tone, or (4) altered level of responsiveness in an infant <1 year of age. Importantly, BRUE differs from the previously used diagnostic term *apparent life-threatening event (ALTE)* in that it includes only episodes with cyanosis (not rubor) and/or altered responsiveness and does not include caregiver perception of the event as "life-threatening." The label BRUE should be used only when no other explanation for the event is identified on detailed history and physical examination. Historical data suggests that a cause could be identified in >50% of ALTE events, thus the new category of BRUE is quite small. History and exam should focus on the most common identifiable causes of abnormal breathing episodes in infancy including gastroesophageal reflux, CNS pathology (seizures, intracranial bleeding from accidental or nonaccidental trauma), and infection (respiratory syncytial virus [RSV], pertussis, and serious bacterial infections). Cardiovascular events (arrhythmia) and metabolic derangements are among diagnoses that may not be recognized on initial history and examination; however, these are quite uncommon.

Infants >2 months of age and born at >32 weeks gestation who experience a single, <1 minute, self-limited (no cardiopulmonary resuscitation [CPR] required) BRUE are considered at *low risk* for undiagnosed serious condition or repeat event. An electrocardiogram and pertussis screening may be considered in this low-risk group. Additional diagnostic tests (e.g., metabolic panel, complete blood count, imaging, polysomnography [PSG], and EEG) and hospital admission for cardiorespiratory monitoring are not recommended. Offering parents infant CPR instruction and attempting to alleviate anxiety surrounding the event are recommended. There is no consensus on evaluation and management of the high-risk infant with BRUE at this time. Careful history and physical examination should be used to guide differential diagnosis and assessment. Cardiorespiratory monitoring for 12-24 hours in the hospital can provide more detailed information on respiratory and cardiac patterns while allowing time to gather additional history and perform repeat examinations.

Of note, PSG in infants previously categorized as ALTE generally show nonspecific differences compared to control groups; thus it is not considered a useful tool for diagnosis unless clinical suspicion of OSA is high. PSG, home oximetry, and home cardiorespiratory monitoring are not helpful in predicting risk or preventing sudden infant death syndrome (SIDS) so should not be recommended for this purpose.

SUDDEN INFANT DEATH SYNDROME

Etiology and Epidemiology

SIDS is defined as the *unexpected* death of an infant younger than 1 year of age in which the cause remains *unexplained* after autopsy, death scene investigation, and review of clinical history. The risk of SIDS is higher in male, premature, and low birth weight infants; infants born to impoverished mothers; and mothers who smoke cigarettes or have abused drugs. The risk of SIDS is increased threefold to fivefold in siblings of infants who have died of SIDS and is highest during the winter. SIDS is rare before 4 weeks or after 6 months of age and is most common between 2 and 4 months. The incidence of SIDS has decreased dramatically since the 1980s.

A variety of unproven mechanisms have been proposed to explain SIDS. Current theories for a predisposition to SIDS include cellular brainstem abnormalities and maturational delay related to neural or cardiorespiratory control. Prone (chest down) position during sleep and exposure to maternal smoking both alter heart rate variability and arousal response, which may contribute to the risk of SIDS. A portion of SIDS deaths may be due to prolongation of the Q-T interval, abnormal CNS control of respiration, and CO_2 rebreathing from sleeping face down (especially in soft bedding). Importantly, there is no association between BRUE/ALTE and SIDS.

Differential Diagnosis

See Table 134.2 for the differential diagnosis of SIDS.

Prevention

SIDS is associated with prone position during sleep, especially on soft bedding, excess insulation, and bed sharing. There has been a significant decline in SIDS with the **back-to-sleep program** and avoiding soft bedding. Thus all parents should be instructed to place their infants in the supine position (on their backs/chest up) unless there are medical contraindications. All loose, soft bedding should be excluded from sleep space, and parents who share beds with their infants should be

TABLE 134.2 Differential Diagnosis of Sudden Infant Death Syndrome
INFECTIOUS DISEASE
Fulminant infection[*,†]
Infant botulism[*]
NEUROLOGICAL
Seizure disorder[†]
Brain tumor[*]
Intracranial hemorrhage due to accidental or nonaccidental trauma[*,‡]
Drug intoxication[‡]
METABOLIC
Hypoglycemia[†]
Medium-chain acyl-coenzyme A dehydrogenase deficiency[†]
Carnitine deficiency[*,‡]
Urea cycle defect[‡]
RESPIRATORY
Laryngospasm
Accidental suffocation[†]
Hemosiderosis/pulmonary hemorrhage syndrome
CARDIOVASCULAR
Cardiac arrhythmia
GASTROINTESTINAL
Gastroesophageal reflux[*,‡]
Midgut volvulus/shock[*]

**Obvious or suspected at autopsy.*
†Relatively common.
‡Diagnostic test required.

counseled on the risks, especially if consuming alcohol. Counseling for cessation of maternal cigarette smoking, both during and after pregnancy, is recommended. Breast feeding, pacifier use, and sharing a room (in separate beds) have been identified as protective. Though there are many commercial devices marketed for prevention, such as sleep positioners and home oximeters, none have been proven to reduce SIDS risk.

CHAPTER 135

Upper Airway Obstruction

ETIOLOGY

Upper airway obstruction (UAO), which is defined as blockage of any part of the airway located above the thoracic inlet, ranges from nasal obstruction due to the common cold to life-threatening obstruction of the larynx or upper trachea. In children, nasal obstruction is usually more of a nuisance than a danger because the mouth can serve as an airway, but it may be a serious problem for neonates, who breathe predominantly through their noses. The differential diagnosis of airway obstruction varies with patient age and can also be subdivided into **supraglottic**, **glottic**, and **subglottic** causes (Tables 135.1 to 135.3).

TABLE 135.1 Age-Related Differential Diagnosis of Sub-Acute Upper Airway Obstruction
NEWBORN
Choanal atresia
Rhinitis neonatorum
Micrognathia (Pierre Robin syndrome, Treacher Collins syndrome, DiGeorge syndrome)
Macroglossia (Beckwith-Wiedemann syndrome, hypothyroidism, Pompe disease, trisomy 21)
Pharyngeal collapse
Laryngeal web
Vocal cord paralysis/paresis (idiopathic, birth trauma or central nervous system pathology)
Congenital subglottic stenosis
Nasal encephalocele
INFANCY
Chronic or recurrent rhinitis (infection, acid reflux, irritant)
Laryngomalacia (most common)
Subglottic stenosis (congenital or acquired, e.g., after intubation)
Laryngeal web or cyst
Laryngeal papillomatosis
Airway hemangioma
Vascular rings/slings
TODDLERS
Chronic or recurrent rhinitis (infection, allergy, irritant)
Hypertrophied tonsils and adenoids (most common)
Spasmodic croup
Laryngeal papillomatosis
Vascular rings/slings
OLDER CHILDREN
Chronic or recurrent rhinitis (infection, allergic, irritants)
Hypertrophied tonsils and adenoids (most common)
Paradoxical vocal fold movement
Infectious mononucleosis

CLINICAL MANIFESTATIONS

Decision-Making Algorithms
Available @ StudentConsult.com

Hoarseness
Stridor

UAO is more pronounced during inspiration because the negative pressure generated collapses the upper airway, increasing resistance and turbulent airflow that creates an inspiratory noise. Children with UAO may have increased inspiratory work of breathing manifested by **suprasternal retractions**. The respiratory noise most commonly associated with UAO is **stridor**, a harsh sound caused by the vibration of the airway structures. Stridor often decreases during sleep because of lower inspiratory flow rates, and increases during feeding, excitement, and agitation because of higher flow rates. Occasionally stridor may also be present on exhalation. Hoarseness or aphonia with stridor suggests **vocal cord** involvement. **Stertor** is a low-pitched sound like a snore and suggests implosion of pharyngeal soft tissue structures.

TABLE 135.2 Common Causes of Acute Upper Airway Obstruction

DIAGNOSIS	AGE	HISTORY	EXAM	IMAGING AND LABS	TREATMENT
INFECTIOUS					
Croup (*parainfluenza* and other viruses)	6 mo-3 yr	Fever, URI	Nontoxic, stridor, barky cough, hoarse	Steeple sign	Aerosolized epinephrine, systemic steroids, cool mist
Epiglottitis (*Streptococcus pneumoniae, Haemophilus influenza*; respiratory viruses)	2-6 yr	High fever, rapid onset, no cough, unable to swallow	Toxic, agitated, tripod sitting, drooling, stridor	Thumb sign Leukocytosis	Intubation, antibiotics
Bacterial tracheitis (*Staphylococcus aureus, Moraxella catarrhalis*)	Any age	High fever, rapid onset, no URI symptoms	Toxic, anxious, ± stridor, ± cough	Ragged tracheal border Leukocytosis	Intubation, antibiotics
Retropharyngeal abscess (*S. aureus, Group A strep., oral anaerobes*)	<6 yr	Fever, insidious onset, sore throat, no URI/cough	Moderately toxic, drooling, arched neck, inflamed pharynx	Thickened retropharyngeal space Leukocytosis	Antibiotics, surgical drainage
Peritonsillar abscess (*Group A strep., oral anaerobes*)	>8 yr	Fever, sudden worsening, sore throat, trismus	Moderately toxic, "hot potato" voice, drooling, asymmetric tonsil swelling	Imaging not needed Leukocytosis	Antibiotics, surgical drainage
NONINFECTIOUS					
Angioedema	Any age	No fever, sudden onset, urticarial, facial swelling, ± allergen exposure	Nontoxic (unless anaphylaxis), ± stridor, hoarse, facial edema	Steeple sign	Aerosolized or intradermal epinephrine, systemic steroids, antihistamines
Spasmodic croup	6 mo-6 yr	Sudden onset, no fever/URI, recurrent, often nocturnal	Nontoxic, ± stridor, hoarse, barky cough	Often normal	Aerosolized epinephrine, antihistamines, antacids, systemic steroids
Foreign body	6 mo-5 yr	Sudden onset, cough and choke	Nontoxic, anxious, stridor, aphonic, brassy cough	Radiopaque object may be seen	Rigid bronchoscopy

URI, Upper respiratory tract infection (with coryza, sneezing).

TABLE 135.3 Differentiating Supraglottic From Subglottic Causes of Acute Airway Obstruction

FEATURE	SUPRAGLOTTIC OBSTRUCTION	SUBGLOTTIC OBSTRUCTION
Common clinical syndromes	Epiglottitis, peritonsillar and retropharyngeal abscess	Croup, angioedema, foreign body, bacterial tracheitis
Stridor	Quiet	Loud
Voice	Muffled	Hoarse
Dysphagia	Yes	No
Tripod or arching posture	Yes	No
Barking cough	No	Yes
Toxic	Yes	No, unless tracheitis
Trismus	Some	No
Drooling	Yes	No

Modified from Davis H, Gartner JC, Galvis AG, et al. Acute upper airway obstruction: croup and epiglottitis. Pediatr Clin North Am. *1981;28:859–880.*

DIAGNOSTIC STUDIES

Radiographic evaluation of a child with stridor is rarely helpful. On anteroposterior (AP) views of the neck taken with the head in extension, the subglottic space should be symmetrical and the lateral walls of the airway should fall away steeply. Asymmetry suggests subglottic stenosis or a mass lesion, whereas tapering suggests subglottic edema. However, these findings may be subtle. In the child with stertor or snoring, lateral views of the neck and nasopharynx may provide information about tonsil or adenoid hypertrophy. Computed tomography (CT) scans of the upper airway can help delineate the site of the obstruction when soft tissue mass (e.g., tonsillar abscess) is suspected, but may require sedation in younger children. Flexible nasopharyngoscopy/laryngoscopy, which can be done without sedation, is extremely useful in assessing airway patency, the presence of adenoid tissue or vocal cord and other airway lesions, and laryngomalacia.

DIFFERENTIAL DIAGNOSIS

Choanal Stenosis (Atresia)

Choanal stenosis/atresia is a congenital problem presenting in the neonatal period. It may be bilateral or unilateral and is relatively rare. Neonates are generally obligate nose breathers, so obstruction of nasal passages can cause significant respiratory distress, especially when feeding. Crying bypasses the obstruction because crying infants breathe through their mouths. Inability to easily pass a small catheter through the nostrils should raise the suspicion of choanal atresia. The diagnosis is confirmed by CT scan and by inspecting the area directly with a flexible nasopharyngoscope. An oral airway may be useful in the short term, but the definitive treatment is surgery.

Croup (Laryngotracheobronchitis)

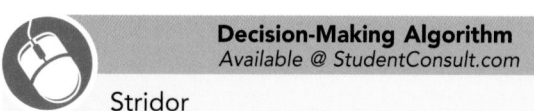

Decision-Making Algorithm
Available @ StudentConsult.com
Stridor

See Chapter 107.

Epiglottitis

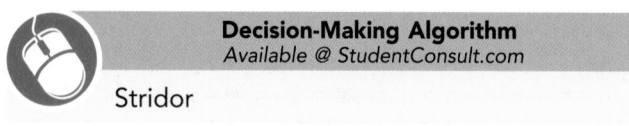

Decision-Making Algorithm
Available @ StudentConsult.com
Stridor

See Chapter 107.

Bacterial Tracheitis

See Chapter 107.

Laryngomalacia

Decision-Making Algorithm
Available @ StudentConsult.com
Stridor

Etiology

Laryngomalacia is due to exaggerated collapse of the glottic structures, especially the epiglottis and arytenoid cartilages, during inspiration. It is the most common cause of stridor in infants. It may be due to decreased muscular tone of the larynx and surrounding structures or to immature cartilaginous structures. It usually does not result in significant respiratory distress, but occasionally it is severe enough to cause apnea, hypoventilation, hypoxemia, and difficulty feeding.

Clinical Manifestations

The primary sign of laryngomalacia is **inspiratory stridor** with little or no expiratory component. The stridor is typically loudest when the infant is feeding or active and decreases when the infant is relaxed or placed prone, or when the neck is flexed. Any condition that increases upper airway inflammation will exacerbate laryngomalacia, including viral respiratory infections, dysphagia (swallowing dysfunction), and gastroesophageal reflux. Laryngomalacia normally peaks by 3-5 months of age and resolves between 6 and 12 months of age. However, occasionally it can persist in otherwise normal children up until 24 months of age, and even longer in children with underlying conditions, especially those with neurological diseases affecting control of upper airway muscles (such as cerebral palsy).

Diagnostic Studies

In many infants with presumed laryngomalacia, the diagnosis can be tentatively established by history and physical examination. If the patient follows the typical course for laryngomalacia, then no further work-up is necessary. However, to firmly establish the diagnosis, which is important in more severe or atypical cases, the patient should undergo flexible nasopharyngoscopy to assess the patency and dynamic movement (collapse) of the larynx and surrounding structures. This procedure can also identify vocal cord abnormalities and airway lesions above the vocal cords.

Treatment

In most cases, no therapy is required for laryngomalacia. The infant should be observed closely during times of respiratory infection for evidence of respiratory compromise. Infants with severe laryngomalacia resulting in hypoventilation, hypoxia, or growth failure may benefit from a surgical procedure (aryepiglottoplasty) or, in extreme cases, a tracheostomy to bypass the upper airway.

Subglottic Stenosis

Decision-Making Algorithm
Available @ StudentConsult.com
Stridor

Etiology

Subglottic stenosis is the narrowing of the portion of the trachea immediately below the vocal cords. It may be congenital but more often is acquired. Endotracheal intubation, especially prolonged or repeated intubation required in some premature infants, can lead to inflammation and scarring of the subglottic space.

Clinical Manifestations

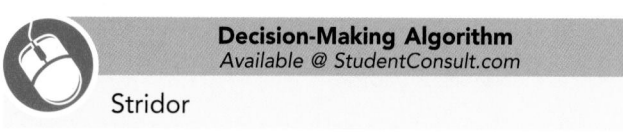

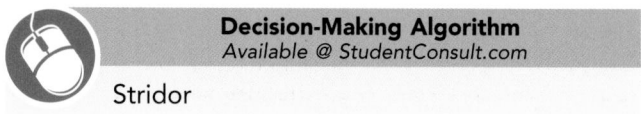

Subglottic stenosis can present as stridor that is **biphasic** (on both inspiration and expiration) but usually more prominent on inspiration. With increasing respiratory effort, the stridor becomes louder. Very small infants may not be able to breathe with enough force to generate a sound. Subglottic stenosis may also be associated with a barky cough similar to that noted with croup. Respiratory infections can cause subglottic edema, exacerbating the clinical manifestations of subglottic stenosis.

Diagnostic Studies

Definitive diagnosis requires endoscopic evaluation, either by flexible or rigid bronchoscopy.

Treatment

Mild subglottic stenosis can be managed conservatively and may improve sufficiently with airway growth alone. More severe cases require surgical intervention. Depending on the nature of the lesion, endoscopic laser treatment may be effective. Other surgical options include tracheoplasty and cricoid split procedures. A tracheostomy tube may be required to bypass the subglottic space until the airway is patent enough to allow adequate airflow.

Mass Lesions

Upper airway mass lesions are relatively uncommon. The most common laryngeal tumor in childhood is the **hemangioma**, which usually presents before 6 months of age and is often able to be treated medically (see Chapter 194). Definitive diagnosis requires endoscopy. If the obstruction is severe, a tracheostomy tube may be needed until the lesion spontaneously involutes or improves with therapy.

Laryngeal webs are the result of failed recanalization of the glottic airway in utero, whereas **laryngeal cysts** typically occur as a consequence of airway trauma (intubation). Both can produce biphasic stridor and are best identified by bronchoscopy. **Foreign body** should be considered in any infant or child capable of ingesting small objects who develops acute onset of stridor.

Juvenile laryngeal papillomatosis is a rare condition of benign tumors caused by human papillomavirus (HPV)-6 and HPV-11 acquired at birth from maternal genital warts. Clinical manifestations usually start in infancy and include biphasic stridor and hoarse voice/cry. The lesions are most commonly located in the larynx, but they can spread distally into the trachea, large bronchi, and even to the lung parenchyma. Treatment options, which are limited and rarely curative, include laser therapy and interferon. Tracheostomy may be required to ensure an adequate airway but should be avoided if possible as there is risk of seeding of the distal airways with tumor.

Vocal Cord Paralysis

Decision-Making Algorithm
Available @ StudentConsult.com

Stridor

Etiology

Vocal cord paralysis is an important cause of laryngeal dysfunction. Paralysis may be unilateral or bilateral and is more often caused by damage to the recurrent laryngeal nerve than by a central lesion. The left recurrent laryngeal nerve passes around the aortic arch and is more susceptible to damage than the right laryngeal nerve. Peripheral nerve injury may be caused by trauma (neck traction during delivery of infants or thoracic surgical procedures) and mediastinal lesions. Central causes include Arnold-Chiari malformation (meningomyelocele), hydrocephalus, and intracranial hemorrhage.

Clinical Manifestations

Vocal cord paralysis presents as biphasic stridor and alterations in voice and cry, including a weak cry (in infants), hoarseness, and aphonia. Children with vocal cord paralysis are at risk for aspiration, often manifested as coughing/choking with drinking and coarse airway sounds audibly and by auscultation.

Treatment and Prognosis

Patients with traumatic injury to the recurrent laryngeal nerve often have spontaneous improvement over time, usually within 3-6 months. If the paralyzed vocal cord has not recovered within 1 year of the injury, then it is likely to be permanently damaged. In some cases, Gelfoam injection of a paralyzed vocal cord can reposition the cord to improve phonation and airway protection. Patients with vocal cord paralysis resulting in severe airway obstruction and aspiration may require tracheostomy tube placement.

Adenoidal and Tonsillar Hypertrophy

Etiology

The most common cause of chronic UAO in children is hypertrophy of the adenoids and tonsils. Adenoidal and tonsillar hyperplasia may be aggravated by recurrent infection, allergy, and inhaled irritants.

Clinical Manifestations

The signs of adenoidal and tonsillar hypertrophy are mouth breathing, snoring, and, in some patients, obstructive sleep apnea (see Chapter 134). The eustachian tubes enter the nasopharynx at the choanae and can be obstructed by enlarged adenoids, predisposing to recurrent or persistent otitis media.

Diagnostic Studies

Adenoidal hypertrophy is assessed by a lateral radiograph of the nasopharynx or by flexible nasopharyngoscopy.

Treatment

If the adenoids or tonsils are large and thought to be significantly contributing to UAO, then the most effective treatment is removal. Because the adenoids are not a discrete organ but rather consist of lymphoid tissue, regrowth is possible, especially in preschool children. If the tonsils are large and the obstruction is severe, then removing the tonsils in addition to the adenoids may be necessary.

CHAPTER 136

Lower Airway, Parenchymal, and Pulmonary Vascular Diseases

ETIOLOGY

There are many causes of lower airway diseases (Table 136.1). Lower airway diseases often result in airway obstruction. The

TABLE 136.1 Causes of Wheezing in Childhood
ACUTE
Asthma
Exercise-induced asthma
Hypersensitivity reactions
Infection (e.g., bronchiolitis)
Inhalation of irritant gases or particulates
Descending aspiration
Foreign body (airway or esophageal)
Aspiration of gastric contents (ascending aspiration)
CHRONIC OR RECURRENT
Asthma (see under acute)
Hypersensitivity reactions, allergic bronchopulmonary aspergillosis (seen only in children with either asthma or cystic fibrosis)
Vocal cord dysfunction
Recurrent aspiration/swallowing dysfunction (dysphagia)
Retained foreign body
Gastroesophageal reflux
Bronchopulmonary dysplasia
Bronchitis, bronchiectasis
Cystic fibrosis
Primary ciliary dyskinesia
Bronchiolitis obliterans
Pulmonary edema (congestive heart failure)
Bronchomalacia/tracheomalacia
Vascular ring
Pulmonary artery dilatation (absent pulmonary valve)
Bronchial or pulmonary cysts/masses
Lymph nodes (tuberculosis, lymphoma)
Endobronchial masses/tumors (carcinoid)
Bronchial or tracheal stenosis
Cardiomegaly

most common lower airway disease in children is **asthma**, which results in variable and recurring symptoms, diffuse bronchial obstruction from airway inflammation, and hyperresponsiveness of bronchial smooth muscle leading to airway constriction. Virus-induced wheezing episodes are common, especially in children under 3 years of age. Wheezing that is localized to one area of the chest suggests focal airway obstruction (foreign body aspiration or extrinsic compression).

CLINICAL MANIFESTATIONS

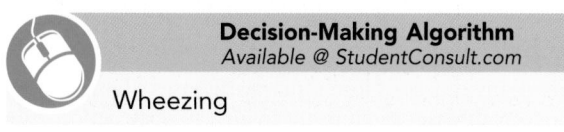

Decision-Making Algorithm
Available @ StudentConsult.com
Wheezing

A wheeze is a continuous sound that is produced by vibration of airway walls and generally has a more musical quality than does stridor. In contrast to upper airway obstruction, obstruction below the thoracic inlet causes more wheezing on expiration than on inspiration. Intrathoracic pressure is increased relative to atmospheric pressure during exhalation, which collapses the intrathoracic airways and accentuates airway narrowing on expiration. Expiratory airflow through obstructed intrathoracic airways leads to wheeze, prolonged expiratory phase, and increased abdominal work of breathing. In patients with chronic airway infection (e.g., cystic fibrosis), the bronchi become permanently damaged and dilated (bronchiectasis). Patients with bronchiectasis have episodes of cough, often productive of purulent sputum, and may have inspiratory crackles.

DIAGNOSTIC STUDIES

When asthma is suspected, empiric trials of therapy (bronchodilators, short courses of oral corticosteroids, long-term use of inhaled corticosteroids) are useful in arriving at a diagnosis. In children older than 6 years, pulmonary function tests (spirometry) can assess airflow obstruction and response to bronchodilators. **Radiographic evaluation** is not needed with each episode of wheezing, but those with significant respiratory distress, fever, history consistent with foreign body aspiration, or focal auscultatory findings should have posteroanterior (PA) and lateral chest radiographs obtained. Generalized **hyperinflation**, indicated by flattening of the diaphragms and an increased anteroposterior (AP) chest diameter, suggests diffuse obstruction of the small airways. Localized hyperinflation, especially on expiratory views, suggests localized bronchial obstruction (foreign body or an anatomical anomaly). Dysphagia leading to aspiration and airway inflammation can present with persistent wheezing. This is best assessed with a **videofluoroscopic swallowing study**. Gastroesophageal reflux may aggravate asthma and may lead to wheezing in very young children, especially if it is associated with aspiration. Infants with persistent wheezing despite empiric treatment with asthma therapy may benefit from an airway evaluation with **flexible bronchoscopy**.

DIFFERENTIAL DIAGNOSIS

Asthma

Decision-Making Algorithm
Available @ StudentConsult.com
Wheezing

See Chapter 78.

Tracheomalacia

Etiology

Tracheomalacia is a floppy trachea due to lack of structural integrity of the tracheal wall. The tracheal cartilaginous rings normally extend through an arc of approximately 320 degrees, maintaining rigidity of the trachea during changes in intrathoracic pressure. With tracheomalacia, the cartilaginous rings may not extend as far around the circumference (leaving the membranous posterior trachea wider than usual), may be completely absent, or may be present but damaged. These abnormalities can result in excessive collapse of the trachea, most pronounced during expiration. Tracheomalacia is the most common congenital tracheal abnormality and may be congenital (tracheoesophageal fistula or bony dysplasia syndromes) or acquired (long-term mechanical ventilation). Tracheomalacia must be differentiated from extrinsic tracheal compression by masses or vascular structures. Localized tracheomalacia may persist after the trachea has been relieved of extrinsic compression.

Clinical Manifestations

With tracheomalacia, the tracheal collapse may only be apparent during forced exhalation or with cough. It is commonly aggravated by respiratory infections. The airway collapse causes a harsh, monophonic wheeze compared to the polyphonic wheeze more often seen in asthma. Secretions may be retained behind the segment of malacia, predisposing to infection. Infants with severe tracheomalacia may completely collapse their tracheas during agitation, resulting in cyanotic episodes that resemble breath holding spells. The voice is normal, as is inspiratory effort. In older children, the hallmark sign is a brassy, barky cough due to the vibration of the tracheal walls. The expiratory noises of tracheomalacia are often mistakenly ascribed to asthma or bronchiolitis, and the barky cough is often misdiagnosed as croup.

Treatment

Infants with mild to moderate tracheomalacia usually require no intervention. Tracheomalacia improves with airway growth as the lumen increases in diameter and the tracheal wall becomes more firm. The treatment of older symptomatic children is geared toward treating the precipitating cause for cough and providing supportive care. Antibiotics may be necessary to treat concurrent infection. Children, especially infants, with severe tracheomalacia may require tracheostomy tubes to administer continuous positive airway pressure (CPAP), which serves to stent open the airway. Custom-length tracheostomy tubes are used to bypass the site of collapse. Surgical techniques such as slide tracheoplasty may benefit short segments of severe malacia. Aortopexy has been used to limit anterior collapse but does not treat posterior tracheal membrane collapse. Historically, surgically placed airway stents have been problematic in children because airway stents may erode and migrate, do not grow with children, and serve as a source of fixed stenosis and obstruction. Newer absorbable airway external splints and internal stents with 3D-printing technology are under active investigation for treatment of severe pediatric tracheomalacia.

Tracheoesophageal Fistula

See Chapter 128.

Extrinsic Tracheal Compression

Compression of the trachea by vascular structures or masses can cause significant respiratory compromise. Tracheal compression by aberrant great vessels (aorta, innominate artery) may cause wheezing, stridor, cough, and dyspnea. Incomplete vascular rings are often asymptomatic and incidentally found, but anterior tracheal compression can occur from an **anomalous innominate artery** that arises more distally than normal from the aortic arch. This usually results in mild respiratory symptoms. Surgical correction is rarely necessary. Complete vascular rings, which compress the esophagus posteriorly and the trachea anteriorly, include the double aortic arch and a right aortic arch with a persistent ligamentum arteriosum (most common). Both lesions have right-sided aortic arches, which may be visible on chest radiograph. In addition to respiratory symptoms, complete vascular rings may cause dysphagia as a result of esophageal compression. The diagnosis of vascular anomalies can often be made by a barium swallow, which identifies the esophageal compression (Fig 136.1). Bronchoscopy will identify a pulsatile compression of the airway, but the diagnostic procedures of choice are a computed tomography (CT) angiogram of the chest and great vessels or magnetic resonance angiogram (MRA). Definitive treatment of vascular rings requires surgical repair. Other causes of extrinsic tracheal compression include enlarged mediastinal lymph nodes (tuberculosis), mediastinal masses (teratoma, lymphoma, thymoma, germ cell tumors), and, rarely, cystic hygromas.

Foreign Body Aspiration

Epidemiology

Aspiration of foreign bodies into the trachea and bronchi is relatively common. The majority of children who aspirate foreign bodies are under 3 years of age. Patients with developmental delay or with older siblings are at increased risk. Because the right mainstem bronchus takes off at a less acute angle than the left mainstem bronchus, foreign bodies tend to lodge in right-sided airways. Some foreign bodies, especially nuts, can also lodge more proximally in the larynx or subglottic space,

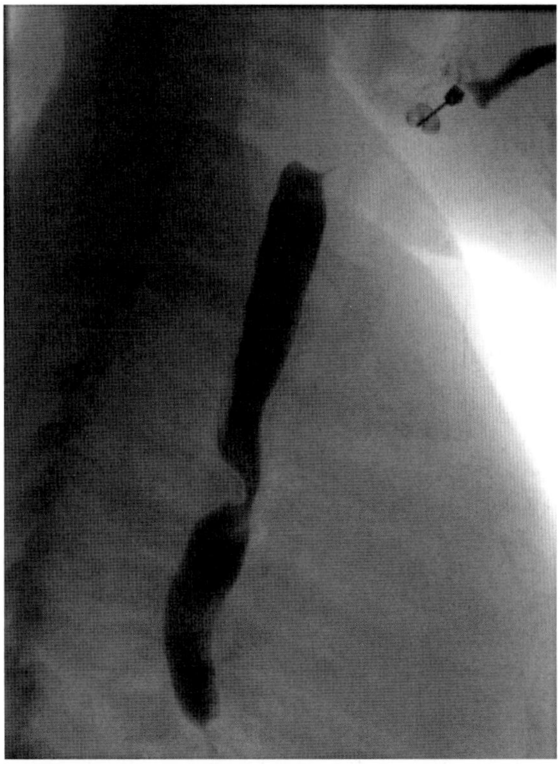

FIGURE 136.1 Vascular ring. Indentation of the posterior esophagus seen on barium swallow, lateral view. This child had a double aortic arch.

totally occluding the airway. Many foreign bodies are not radiopaque, which makes them difficult to detect radiographically. The most common foreign bodies aspirated by young children are food (especially nuts) and small toys. Coins more often lodge in the esophagus than in the airways. Older children have been known to aspirate rubber balloons, which can be life threatening.

Clinical Manifestations

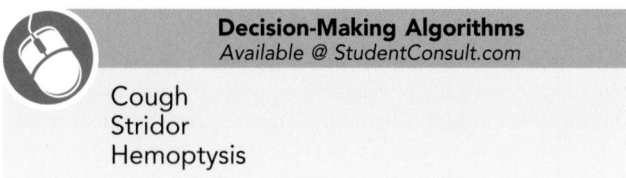

Decision-Making Algorithms
Available @ StudentConsult.com

Cough
Stridor
Hemoptysis

Many children who aspirate foreign bodies have clear histories of choking, witnessed aspiration, or physical or radiographic evidence of foreign body aspiration. However, a proportion of patients have a negative history because the aspiration went unrecognized. Physical findings observed with acute foreign body aspiration may include cough, localized wheezing, unilateral absence of breath sounds, stridor, and, rarely, bloody sputum.

Most foreign bodies are small and quickly expelled, but some may remain in the lung for long periods of time and may come to medical attention because of persistent cough, sputum production, or recurrent unilateral pneumonia. Foreign body aspiration should be in the differential diagnosis of patients with persistent wheezing unresponsive to bronchodilator therapy, persistent atelectasis, recurrent or persistent pneumonia, or chronic cough without another explanation. Foreign bodies may also lodge in the esophagus and compress the trachea, thus producing respiratory symptoms. Therefore esophageal foreign bodies should be included in the differential diagnosis of infants or young children with persistent cough, stridor, or wheezing, particularly if dysphagia is present.

Diagnostic Studies

Radiographic studies will reveal the presence of radiopaque objects and can also identify focal air trapping, especially on expiratory views or decubitus films. Many foreign bodies are not radiopaque. Thus when foreign body aspiration is suspected, expiratory or lateral decubitus chest radiographs may identify air trapping on the affected, dependent side. If history or exam is suggestive of foreign body aspiration, the patient should undergo rigid bronchoscopy, typically performed by an otolaryngologist. Flexible bronchoscopy can be used to locate an aspirated foreign body and may be useful when the presentation is not straightforward, but foreign body removal is best performed via rigid bronchoscopy.

Prevention

Common foods, including peanuts or other nuts, popcorn, uncooked carrots, or any foods difficult to break into small pieces, are at risk to be aspirated by infants and children, particularly before molar teeth have erupted. Older siblings should be counseled to keep small toys separate and not present younger children with small parts.

Bronchiolitis

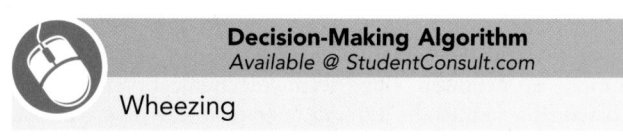

Decision-Making Algorithm
Available @ StudentConsult.com

Wheezing

See Chapter 109.

Bronchopulmonary Dysplasia

See Chapter 61.

Congenital Lung Anomalies

Congenital lobar emphysema (congenital lobar overinflation) consists of hyperinflation of one or more lobes of the lung. This overdistention may cause severe respiratory distress in the neonatal period due to compression of surrounding normal lung tissue, but it can also be asymptomatic and remain undiagnosed for years. Radiographically, it may be mistaken for a pneumothorax. Lobectomy may be required if respiratory distress is severe or progressive, but if the patient is asymptomatic, then surgical resection may not be indicated.

Congenital pulmonary airway malformations (CPAMs) are a spectrum of lesions arising during early lung development with histological appearance ranging from simplified bronchial to complex cystic alveolar tissue, connected to the tracheobronchial tree. They are often first identified on antenatal ultrasound, and after birth can be inconspicuous on chest radiograph. CPAMs are nonfunctioning lung tissue and can have hybrid features of **pulmonary sequestration** (presence of systemic circulation connections). Although CPAM lesions can be stand-alone lesions, a substantial proportion of pulmonary sequestrations are hybrid CPAM lesions. Sequestrations without hybrid features are separate from the tracheobronchial tree and are classified as intrapulmonary (located in a normal lobe without its own pleura) and extrapulmonary (outside normal lung). CPAMs and sequestrations can coexist with other chest lesions including **congenital diaphragmatic hernia**. Sequestration is also associated with **Scimitar syndrome** (partial anomalous pulmonary venous return). Symptomatic neonates with respiratory distress, large lesions, or family history of features concerning for malignancy require further imaging. Though large malformations can cause neonatal respiratory distress, many are asymptomatic. Chest CT with contrast is the diagnostic test of choice (Fig 136.2) but may be delayed if the child is asymptomatic with close clinical follow-up for symptom development. Surgical resection is curative, but risk of infection or malignancy is not completely understood in these children. Conservative management with observation is a reasonable option for families with low risk.

Pulmonary hypoplasia, or a relative decrease in amount of alveoli, may be the result of a number of congenital insults, such as **congenital diaphragmatic hernia** (see Chapter 61) or unilateral congenital absence of a pulmonary artery. Alveolar growth occurs after birth, predominantly up to 3 years, but has been documented beyond 8 years of age.

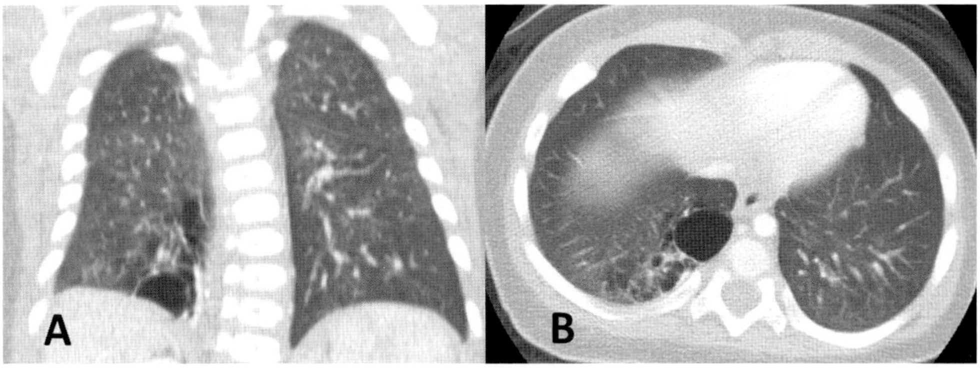

FIGURE 136.2 Congenital pulmonary airway malformation. Coronal *(A)* and axial *(B)* computed tomography images of a right lower lobe congenital pulmonary airway malformation in a child who presented with recurrent pneumonias. The entire left lung and upper and middle lobes of the right lung are normal.

Primary Ciliary Dyskinesia

Etiology

Primary ciliary dyskinesia (PCD, immotile cilia syndrome) is an inherited disorder in which there is absent or disordered movement of the cilia leading to a spectrum of clinical manifestations. This disorder affects approximately 1 in 15,000-20,000 live births, although the actual incidence may be higher because of a limited ability to definitively diagnose affected patients.

Clinical Manifestations

Clinical manifestations include neonatal respiratory distress, chronic cough, chronic nasal congestion, middle ear effusions, chronic pansinusitis, laterality defects (e.g., situs inversus), infertility, and bronchiectasis. Kartagener syndrome, the triad of **situs inversus**, **pansinusitis**, and **bronchiectasis**, accounts for approximately 50% of cases. Males are infertile as a result of immotile sperm. Because the cilia fail to beat normally, secretions accumulate in the airways, and endobronchial infection results. Chronic infection, if untreated, leads to bronchiectasis by early adulthood.

Diagnostic Studies

PCD diagnosis has historically relied on a combination of clinical features and ultrastructural analysis of respiratory cilia by electron microscopy, obtained from scrapings/biopsy of nasal or airway epithelium. Results may be difficult to interpret as chronic infection and inflammation may also lead to ultrastructural abnormalities in nasal cilia. The most common ultrastructural defect is the absence of dynein arms. A third of affected individuals have normal ciliary ultrastructure. The measurement of nasal nitric oxide has been used as a screening tool for PCD. Low nasal nitric oxide values (<77 nL/min) are consistent with PCD. High-speed video microscopy assesses ciliary beat frequency and pattern but requires specialized equipment and, currently, there is an absence of standardized reporting methods. PCD is generally autosomal recessive. Currently 31 genes have been identified to explain approximately 60% of cases. The association of genetic defects and clinical phenotype is unknown.

Treatment

Treatment is geared toward treating infections and improving clearance of respiratory secretions. High-resolution chest CT scans are useful to confirm and monitor bronchiectasis. Surveillance cultures help identify organisms involved and guide antibiotic therapy. Sinus surgical procedures are often done to manage chronic sinusitis, but their benefit is questionable. Most children require placement of pressure equalization (PE) tubes for management of recurrent otitis media. Chest physiotherapy and prompt treatment of bacterial infections are helpful, but the course of the disease tends to be slowly progressive. Inhaled hypertonic saline may improve cough clearance and has been shown in the short term to improve lung function. Antiinflammatory antibiotics, such as low-dose macrolides, may reduce the number of exacerbations per year.

Pneumonia

Decision-Making Algorithms
Available @ StudentConsult.com

Cough
Wheezing
Hemoptysis
Abdominal Pain
Acidemia

See Chapter 110.

Pulmonary Edema

Etiology

Pulmonary edema is the seepage of fluid into the alveolar and interstitial spaces. Capillary hydrostatic forces and interstitial osmotic pressures tend to push fluid into the air spaces, whereas plasma osmotic pressures and tissue mechanical forces tend to move fluid away from the air spaces. Under normal circumstances, the sum of these forces favors absorption, so the alveolar and interstitial spaces remain dry. Fluid entering the alveoli is normally removed by pulmonary lymphatics. Pulmonary edema forms when transcapillary fluid flux exceeds lymphatic drainage. Reduced left ventricular function leads to pulmonary venous hypertension and increased capillary hydrostatic pressure, and fluid moves into the interstitial space and alveoli. Fluid initially enters the interstitial space around the terminal bronchioles, alveoli, and arterioles **(interstitial edema)**, causing increased lung stiffness and premature closure of bronchioles on expiration. If the process continues, fluid then enters the alveoli, further reducing compliance and resulting in **intrapulmonary shunting** (alveolar units that are perfused but not ventilated). Decreased ventilation (hypercarbia) is a late finding.

Pulmonary edema is most commonly due to heart failure from left ventricular or biventricular dysfunction. Pulmonary hypertension (PH) and associated cor pulmonale (right ventricular dysfunction) do not usually cause pulmonary edema as the increased vascular resistance is proximal to the capillary bed. Increased capillary permeability, seen in disease states such as sepsis and acute respiratory distress syndrome, can lead to pulmonary edema. Pulmonary edema may also occur with excessive swings in intrathoracic pressure, as seen after tracheal foreign body aspiration or severe obstruction from hypertrophied tonsils and adenoids **(postobstructive pulmonary edema)**. Pulmonary edema may also be present in conditions with decreased serum oncotic pressure (hypoalbuminemia); after administration of large volumes of intravenous (IV) fluids, especially if there is capillary injury; with ascent to high altitude **(high-altitude pulmonary edema)**; and after central nervous system injury **(neurogenic pulmonary edema)**.

Clinical Manifestations

Decision-Making Algorithm
Available @ StudentConsult.com

Cough

The clinical manifestations of pulmonary edema are **dyspnea**, tachypnea, and cough (can occur with frothy, pink-tinged sputum). As the edema worsens, there is increased work of breathing and hypoxemia; diffuse inspiratory crackles can be heard on auscultation.

Diagnostic Studies

Chest radiographs may reveal diffuse hazy infiltrates, classically in a perihilar pattern, but these findings may be obscured by underlying lung disease. Interstitial edema **(Kerley B lines)** may be seen, especially at the lung bases.

Treatment and Prognosis

Treatment and prognosis depend on the cause of the pulmonary edema and response to therapy. Patients should be positioned in an upright posture and given supplemental O_2. Diuretic therapy and rapidly acting IV inotropic agents may be helpful in cardiogenic pulmonary edema. CPAP or intubation with positive pressure ventilation using high positive end-expiratory pressures (PEEP) may be required.

Acute Respiratory Distress Syndrome

See Chapter 39.

Pulmonary Arterial Hypertension and Cor Pulmonale

Etiology

PH is defined as a mean pulmonary artery pressure ≥25 mm Hg in children >3 months of age at sea level. Pediatric PH is categorized into five groups based on the World Health Organization classification, similar to adult PH. Group 1 is pulmonary arterial hypertension (PAH) due to diseases within veins and small pulmonary muscular arteries such as persistent PH of the newborn, congenital heart disease (including those with excessive pulmonary blood flow due to left-to-right cardiac shunting), exposure to various drugs (e.g., cocaine, amphetamines), and **idiopathic pulmonary arterial hypertension** (IPAH, previously called primary PH). Hereditary IPAH is also in this group and has been linked with the bone morphogenetic receptor-2 *(BMPR2)* gene. Group 2 is caused by dysfunction of the left heart such as valvular disease. Group 3 is secondary to lung disease or chronic hypoxia, including upper airway obstruction resulting in obstructive sleep apnea and hypoxemia. In Group 4, PH is secondary to chronic pulmonary thromboembolism. Group 5 includes PH of unclear but multifactorial diseases, including some autoimmune diseases and metabolic diseases. The Panama Classification is a new pediatric-specific system that includes ten categories to capture the heterogeneity of pulmonary hypertensive vascular disease from the fetus to adolescent (e.g., perinatal pulmonary vascular maladaptation, multifactorial pulmonary hypertensive vascular disease in congenital malformation syndromes, diffuse pediatric lung disease). This classification system is promising, but has yet to be tested and validated for utility and accuracy.

Prolonged PH may lead to irreversible changes in the intima and media of the pulmonary arterioles. PH strains the right side of the heart, which leads to hypertrophy and dilation of the right ventricle. Altered structure and/or function of the right heart from PH is known as **cor pulmonale**. The most common causes of cor pulmonale in children are chronic lung diseases, especially severe bronchopulmonary dysplasia and severe, untreated obstructive sleep apnea (with chronic hypoxia).

Clinical Manifestations and Diagnostic Studies

PAH should be suspected with developmental anatomical abnormalities or historical exposures (e.g., congenital diaphragmatic hernia, prolonged hypoxemia). Exertional dyspnea and unexplained syncope are presenting symptoms. In addition to the other physical findings associated with pulmonary and cardiac diseases, an accentuated pulmonary component of the second heart sound may be heard. Definitive diagnosis is made by cardiac catheterization, but echocardiography may confirm the presence of right ventricular hypertrophy, ventricular dysfunction, interventricular septal flattening, and tricuspid insufficiency, which can be used to estimate the pulmonary artery pressures. Cardiac magnetic resonance imaging can be useful in diagnosis and to assess changes in ventricular function and size. Lung biopsy may be considered for children with PAH suspected of diffuse lung disease, pulmonary venoocclusive disease, or vasculitis.

Treatment and Prognosis

Treatment should focus on the underlying condition of known causes of PH, such as lung volume optimization in persistent PH of the newborn, or therapy with diuretics and salt/fluid restriction in heart failure. In all conditions of PH and PAH, the relief of hypoxemia with supplemental O_2 therapy can be therapeutic as a pulmonary vasodilator. Medications for pulmonary vasodilation such as short-term inhaled nitric oxide may be helpful in some patients. Continuous infusions of prostacyclin may be helpful, both acutely and chronically, and is available in inhaled, subcutaneous, and IV forms. Endothelium antagonists may be beneficial. Unfortunately, many patients with the idiopathic form of PAH have progressive courses, and lung or heart-lung transplantation may be the only treatment option.

Pulmonary Hemorrhage

Etiology

Pulmonary hemorrhage is a rare but potentially life-threatening condition in children. It can be due to bleeding from the airways (hemangiomas, bronchial vessel bleeds) or from diffuse capillary bleeding (alveolar hemorrhage). Alveolar hemorrhage is usually due to diffuse capillary disruption/inflammation caused by autoimmune disorders but can occur in isolation without systemic manifestations **(pulmonary capillaritis)**. Airway bleeding can be due to airway hemangiomas, pulmonary arteriovenous malformations (e.g., hereditary hemorrhagic telangiectasia), and bronchial artery collaterals, which develop in some patients with chronic lung infections (e.g., cystic fibrosis). **Idiopathic pulmonary hemosiderosis** is a rare disorder characterized by recurrent alveolar bleeding, iron deficiency anemia, and hemosiderin-laden macrophages in the lung, which can be identified microscopically with the use of special iron-staining techniques in bronchoalveolar lavage or lung biopsy specimens. Although the term *hemosiderosis* is sometimes used interchangeably with pulmonary hemorrhage, it is a pathological finding that results from bleeding anywhere in the lung, airway, pharynx, nasopharynx, or mouth leading to hemosiderin accumulation in the lung. **Pulmonary hemorrhage** is a preferable term for bleeding from an intrathoracic source.

Clinical Manifestations

Decision-Making Algorithm
Available @ StudentConsult.com
Hemoptysis

The presentation of pulmonary hemorrhage is variable with a spectrum of asymptomatic radiographic abnormalities to life-threatening respiratory failure. **Hemoptysis,** although experienced by most children with pulmonary hemorrhage, can be absent in a third of individuals. It is important to rule out extrapulmonary sources of bleeding, including hematemesis and bleeding from the nasopharynx or mouth, as these are more common than true pulmonary hemorrhage. In addition to hemoptysis, the presenting signs and symptoms of pulmonary hemorrhage include cough, wheeze, shortness of breath, pallor, fatigue, cyanosis, and fever. Episodic pulmonary hemorrhage frequently manifests as recurrent respiratory symptoms associated with pulmonary infiltrates on chest radiographs. Symptomatic **airway hemorrhage** may result in significant hemoptysis with few radiographic changes, whereas **alveolar bleeding** often causes profound respiratory symptoms, hypoxemia, diffuse infiltrates on radiographs, and minimal hemoptysis. Some patients experience a localized bubbling sensation in the chest, which may be helpful in differentiating local from diffuse sources of pulmonary bleeding. Physical examination findings may include locally or diffusely decreased breath sounds, cyanosis, and crackles on auscultation.

The **differential diagnosis** of pulmonary hemorrhage includes alveolar and airway bleeding. The causes of alveolar (capillary) bleeding can be divided into immune-mediated and non–immune-mediated categories. Immune-mediated causes include antineutrophil cytoplasmic autoantibodies (ANCA)-associated vasculitides, isolated pulmonary capillaritis, antiglomerular basement membrane disease, drug-induced vasculitis, and other connective tissue diseases. Nonimmune mediated causes include idiopathic pulmonary hemosiderosis, clotting disorders, infection, inhalation injury, and cardiac conditions associated with elevated pulmonary venous and capillary pressures (Table 136.2). Alveolar hemorrhage following bone

TABLE 136.2 Differential Diagnosis of Hemoptysis-Pulmonary Hemorrhage

CARDIOVASCULAR DISORDERS
Heart failure with pulmonary edema
Pulmonary hypertension with Eisenmenger syndrome
Mitral stenosis
Venoocclusive disease
Arteriovenous malformation (Osler-Weber-Rendu syndrome)
Pulmonary embolism
Portal vein obstruction
PULMONARY DISORDERS
Bronchogenic cyst
Bronchopulmonary sequestration
Pneumonia (bacterial, mycobacterial, fungal, parasitic, or viral)
Bronchiectasis (cystic fibrosis, primary ciliary dyskinesia, immunodeficiency, retained foreign body)
Tracheobronchitis
Lung abscess
Tumor (adenoma, carcinoid, hemangioma, metastasis)
Trauma (contusion, laceration)
IMMUNE DISORDERS
Henoch-Schönlein purpura
Pulmonary capillaritis
Idiopathic pulmonary hemosiderosis
Antiglomerular basement membrane disease (Goodpasture)
Granulomatosis with polyangiitis (formerly known as Wegener granulomatosis)
Systemic lupus erythematosus
Polyarteritis nodosa
OTHER CONDITIONS/FACTORS
Coagulopathy (Von Willebrand)
Toxic inhalation (nitrogen dioxide, pesticides, crack cocaine)
Post–bone marrow transplantation
Catamenial hemoptysis (females)

marrow transplant can occur from immune-mediated causes and from complications of diffuse alveolar damage. Rarely, a previously well infant will present with life-threatening acute alveolar hemorrhage. Often no cause is found, and, once the acute episode resolves, the infant returns to normal. Most of these infants never have a second bleeding episode. Hemoptysis can have cardiovascular, pulmonary, or immunological causes (see Table 136.2).

Diagnostic Studies

It is important to perform a thorough upper airway examination to rule out epistaxis. Sometimes this requires nasopharyngoscopy. If extrapulmonary sources of bleeding have been excluded, then a chest radiograph, CT angiogram of the chest, bronchoscopy, echocardiogram, and evaluation for rheumatologic/autoimmune diseases follow, especially to consider antiglomerular basement membrane disease, granulomatosis with polyangiitis, Henoch-Schönlein purpura, and systemic lupus erythematosus.

Treatment

The management of acute episodes of pulmonary bleeding includes the administration of supplemental O_2, blood transfusions, and, often with acute alveolar hemorrhages, mechanical ventilation with PEEP to tamponade the bleeding. Treatment is directed toward the underlying disorders and providing supportive care. In bronchial arterial bleeding, arteriography with vessel embolization has been shown to be successful.

Pulmonary Embolism

Etiology

Pulmonary embolism is rare in children. When it occurs, it is often associated with indwelling central venous catheters, oral contraceptives, or hypercoagulable states. Other risk factors, such as trauma, surgery, immobilization, systemic lupus erythematosus, and cancer, may lead to deep vein thromboses (DVTs) and pulmonary embolism.

Clinical Manifestations

Because the pulmonary vascular bed is distensible, small emboli, even if multiple, may be asymptomatic unless they are infected (septic emboli) and cause pulmonary infection. Large emboli may cause acute dyspnea, pleuritic chest pain, cough, and hemoptysis. Tachypnea, tachycardia, and unilateral calf swelling may be present. **Hypoxia** is common, as are nonspecific ST-segment and T-wave changes on the electrocardiogram (ECG). The P_2 heart sound may be increased.

Diagnostic Studies

Although the chest x-ray is usually normal, atelectasis or cardiomegaly may be seen. The measurement of D dimers can be used as a screening test, but it must be interpreted in light of the probability of a pulmonary embolism. If the D dimer is normal and the probability for embolism is low, then no further work-up may be necessary. However, if the D dimer is elevated, or if it is normal but the probability of embolism is moderate or high, then the diagnostic test of choice is a **CT angiogram of the chest**. Ventilation-perfusion scans may reveal defects in perfusion without matching ventilation defects, but they are difficult to perform in young children. Doppler or compression ultrasonography can be useful in assessing patients for lower extremity DVTs. For definitive diagnosis of pulmonary embolism, the gold standard is still **pulmonary angiography**, although with the improvement in CT angiography, angiograms are now rarely necessary. Children with pulmonary embolism without an obvious cause should be evaluated for hypercoagulable states, the most common of which is factor V Leiden.

Treatment

To treat pulmonary embolism, the patient should be anticoagulated, usually with low-molecular-weight heparin or unfractionated heparin. Although rare, if pulmonary embolism is extensive and hemodynamically compromising, thrombolytic agents such as tissue plasminogen activator should be considered. All patients should receive supplemental O_2, and it is important to treat the predisposing factors.

CHAPTER 137

Cystic Fibrosis

ETIOLOGY AND EPIDEMIOLOGY

Cystic fibrosis (CF) is a life-shortening autosomal recessive disorder that affects over 70,000 individuals worldwide. Although found predominantly in people of European descent, CF is reported among all races and ethnicities. The gene for CF, located on the long arm of chromosome 7, encodes for the **cystic fibrosis transmembrane conductance regulator (CFTR)**, a chloride channel located on the apical surface of epithelial cells. CFTR is important for the proper movement of salt and water across cell membranes and maintaining the appropriate composition of various secretions, especially in the airways, liver, and pancreas. The most common mutation is a deletion of three base pairs resulting in the absence of phenylalanine at the 508 position (Phe508del, F508del). Nearly 2,000 mutations of the *CFTR* gene have been identified to date.

The secretory and absorptive characteristics of epithelial cells are affected by abnormal CFTR, resulting in the clinical manifestations of CF. The altered chloride ion conductance in the sweat gland results in excessively high sweat sodium and chloride levels. This is the basis for the sweat chloride test, which is still the standard diagnostic test for this disorder. It is positive (elevated sweat chloride ≥60 mEq/L) in 99% of patients with CF. Abnormal airway secretions make the airway more prone to colonization with bacteria. Defects in CFTR may also reduce the function of airway defenses and promote bacterial adhesion to the airway epithelium. This ultimately leads to chronic airway infections and eventually to bronchial damage (bronchiectasis).

CLINICAL MANIFESTATIONS

Decision-Making Algorithms
Available @ StudentConsult.com

Hemoptysis
Constipation
Hepatomegaly
Failure to Thrive
Hyponatremia

CF is a chronic progressive disease that can present with protein and fat malabsorption (failure to thrive, hypoalbuminemia, steatorrhea), liver disease (cholestatic jaundice), or chronic respiratory infection (Table 137.1). Many infants in the United States are currently diagnosed by newborn screening (available in all 50 states and the District of Columbia since 2010). Older children have traditionally presented with pulmonary manifestations such as chronic cough, poorly controlled asthma, and chronic respiratory infections, but recurrent pancreatitis, nasal polyps, and chronic sinusitis can also be presenting manifestations. The respiratory epithelium of patients with CF exhibits marked impermeability to chloride and an excessive reabsorption of sodium. This leads to thicker airway secretions, resulting in airway obstruction and impaired mucociliary transport. This, in turn, leads to endobronchial colonization with bacteria, especially *Staphylococcus aureus* and *Pseudomonas aeruginosa.* Chronic bronchial infection results in persistent or recurrent cough that is often productive of sputum, especially in older children. Chronic airway infection leads to airway obstruction and bronchiectasis and, eventually, to pulmonary insufficiency and premature death. The median age of survival is currently >40 years. **Digital clubbing** is common in patients with CF, even in those without significant lung disease. Chronic sinusitis and **nasal polyposis** are common.

Pulmonary infections with *P. aeruginosa* and some strains of *Burkholderia cepacia* are difficult to treat and may be associated with accelerated clinical deterioration. **Allergic bronchopulmonary aspergillosis (ABPA)** is a hypersensitivity reaction to *Aspergillus* in the CF airways. It causes airway inflammation/obstruction and aggravates CF lung disease. The treatment for ABPA is systemic corticosteroids (prednisone) and antifungal agents (itraconazole). Minor hemoptysis is usually due to airway infection, but major hemoptysis is often caused by bleeding from bronchial artery collateral vessels in damaged/chronically infected portions of the lung. Pneumothoraces can occur in patients with advanced lung disease.

Ninety percent of patients with CF are born with **exocrine pancreatic insufficiency**. The inspissation of mucus and subsequent destruction of the pancreatic ducts result in the inability to excrete pancreatic enzymes into the intestine. This leads to malabsorption of proteins, sugars (to a lesser extent), and especially fat. Fat malabsorption manifests clinically as **steatorrhea** (large, foul-smelling stools), deficiencies of fat-soluble vitamins (A, D, E, and K), and failure to thrive. Protein malabsorption can present early in infancy as hypoproteinemia and peripheral edema. Approximately 10% of patients with CF are born with intestinal obstruction caused by inspissated meconium **(meconium ileus)**. In older patients, intestinal obstruction may result from thick inspissated mucus in the intestinal lumen **(distal intestinal obstruction syndrome [DIOS])**. In adolescent or adult patients, progressive pancreatic damage can lead to enough islet cell destruction to cause **insulin deficiency**. This initially presents as glucose intolerance, but true diabetes that requires insulin therapy **(CF-related diabetes)** may develop. The failure of the sweat ducts to conserve sodium and chloride may lead to hyponatremia and hypochloremic metabolic alkalosis, especially in infants. Inspissation of mucus in the reproductive tract leads to reproductive dysfunction in both males and females. In males, congenital absence of the vas deferens and azoospermia are nearly universal. In females, secondary amenorrhea is often present as a result of chronic illness and reduced body weight. Fertility can be diminished by malnutrition and abnormal cervical mucus, but women with CF can conceive.

All infants with a positive newborn screen and/or with meconium ileus should be evaluated for CF. The diagnosis of CF should be seriously considered in any infant presenting with failure to thrive, cholestatic jaundice, chronic respiratory symptoms, or electrolyte abnormalities (hyponatremia, hypochloremia, metabolic alkalosis). CF should be in the differential diagnosis of children with chronic respiratory or gastrointestinal symptoms, especially if there is digital clubbing. Any child with nasal polyps, especially those younger than 12

TABLE 137.1 Complications of Cystic Fibrosis

RESPIRATORY COMPLICATIONS
Bronchiectasis, bronchitis, bronchiolitis, pneumonia
Hemoptysis
Pneumothorax
Nasal polyps
Sinusitis
Cor pulmonale (associated with chronic hypoxemia)
Respiratory failure
Atypical mycobacterial infection
Allergic bronchopulmonary aspergillosis
GASTROINTESTINAL COMPLICATIONS
Pancreatic insufficiency
Meconium ileus/peritonitis (infants)
Intestinal atresia (infants)
Distal intestinal obstruction syndrome (non-neonatal obstruction)
Rectal prolapse
Fibrosing colonopathy (strictures)
Recurrent pancreatitis
Hepatic cirrhosis (portal hypertension, esophageal varices, hypersplenism)
Neonatal obstructive jaundice
Hepatic steatosis
Gastroesophageal reflux
Cholelithiasis
Growth failure (malabsorption)
Fat-soluble vitamin deficiency states (vitamins A, K, E, D)
Cystic fibrosis–related diabetes
Malignancy (rare)
OTHER COMPLICATIONS
Infertility
Delayed puberty
Dehydration–heat exhaustion
Electrolyte disturbances (hyponatremic hypochloremic metabolic alkalosis)
Hypertrophic osteoarthropathy–arthritis
Pseudotumor cerebri
Digital clubbing

years, should be evaluated for CF. All siblings of patients with CF should also be evaluated.

DIAGNOSTIC STUDIES

Readily available commercial DNA tests detect many CF mutations, but because there are nearly 2,000 identified mutations (and some of unknown clinical significance), DNA analysis will not detect all cases of CF. All U.S. states have newborn screening for CF, based either on elevated immunoreactive trypsinogen (IRT) levels or DNA tests, identifying the majority of infants with CF, but there are both false-positive and false-negative results. Therefore the diagnostic test of choice is still the sweat test. Indications for performing a **sweat test** are listed in Table 137.2. The following criteria should be met to establish the diagnosis of CF:

TABLE 137.2 Indications for Sweat Testing
RESPIRATORY
Chronic or recurrent cough
Chronic or recurrent pneumonia
Recurrent bronchiolitis
Recurrent wheezing/difficult to control asthma
Recurrent or persistent atelectasis
Hemoptysis
Pseudomonas aeruginosa in the respiratory tract (if not explained by other factors, e.g., tracheostomy or prolonged intubation)
GASTROINTESTINAL
Meconium ileus
Neonatal intestinal obstruction (meconium plug, atresia)
Steatorrhea, malabsorption
Hepatic cirrhosis in childhood (including any manifestations such as esophageal varices or portal hypertension)
Cholestatic jaundice in infancy
Pancreatitis
Rectal prolapse
Fat-soluble vitamin deficiency states (A, D, E, K)
Hypoproteinemia, hypoalbuminemia, peripheral edema unexplained by other causes
Prolonged, direct-reacting neonatal jaundice
MISCELLANEOUS
Positive newborn screen (sweat testing performed after 2 wk of age and >2 kg if asymptomatic)
Digital clubbing
Failure to thrive
Family history of cystic fibrosis (e.g., in sibling or cousin)
Salty taste of skin (typically noted by parent on kissing affected child—from salt crystals formed after evaporation of sweat)
Hyponatremic hypochloremic alkalosis in infants
Nasal polyps
Recurrent sinusitis
Aspermia
Absent vas deferens

- The presence of one or more typical clinical features of CF (chronic pulmonary disease, characteristic gastrointestinal and nutritional abnormalities, salt loss syndromes, or obstructive azoospermia) AND
- Two elevated sweat chloride tests performed at an accredited CF Foundation certified laboratory (positive if the value is ≥60 mEq/L, borderline if 30-59 mEq/L, and negative if <30 mEq/L, with adequate sweat collection) OR
- Two mutations known to cause CF identified by DNA analysis OR
- A characteristic abnormality in ion transport across nasal epithelium demonstrated in vivo (nasal potential difference testing)

For those identified by positive newborn screening or because a sibling has CF, positive sweat chloride testing or the presence of known disease-causing DNA mutations are the only criteria required for diagnosis, as clinical symptoms may not be manifested early in life.

Although the sweat test is both specific and sensitive for CF, it is subject to technical problems with both false-positive and false-negative results (Table 137.3). Cutoff diagnostic measurements evolve as more disease-causing DNA mutations are identified. Other supportive tests include the measurement of bioelectrical potential differences across nasal epithelium (not widely available) and measurement of fecal elastase levels. Low fecal elastase levels indicate exocrine pancreatic insufficiency. CF genotyping done by commercial laboratories identifies approximately 95% of patients with CF, but there are mutations that are not identified by standard testing. Not all mutations in CFTR are considered disease-causing, and some have uncertain prognostic consequences. Some infants identified by newborn screening with borderline sweat tests and mutations of uncertain

TABLE 137.3 Causes of False-Positive and False-Negative Results on Sweat Testing
FALSE-POSITIVE
Adrenal insufficiency
Eczema
Ectodermal dysplasia
Nephrogenic diabetes insipidus
Hypothyroidism
Fucosidosis
Mucopolysaccharidosis
Dehydration
Malnutrition
Poor technique/inadequate sweat collection
Type I glycogen storage disease
Panhypopituitarism
Pseudohypoaldosteronism
Hypoparathyroidism
Prostaglandin E_1 administration
FALSE-NEGATIVE
Edema
Poor technique/inadequate sweat collection

consequence are considered to have CFTR-related metabolic syndrome (CRMS). Older children that present with atypical clinical features and borderline sweat tests may be considered nonclassic CF or mild variant CF.

Identification of carriers (heterozygotes) and prenatal diagnosis of children with the ΔF508 and other common mutations is offered at most medical centers. Prenatal testing techniques can identify more than 90% of carriers. Prenatal detection of a known CF genotype may be accomplished by amniocentesis or chorionic villus sampling.

TREATMENT

The treatment of CF is multifactorial. Most maintenance therapies are directed toward the gastrointestinal and pulmonary complications. Presently, there is no effective single cure for CF. Precision therapies, known as CFTR modulators, target genotype-specific functional defects of the CFTR protein. Ivacaftor, the first CFTR modulator approved by the U.S. Food and Drug Administration (FDA), is a small molecule potentiator that improves CFTR function in a small group of CF individuals who have an abnormal gating mechanism of their CFTR protein, contributing to sustained health improvements including lung function. The second FDA-approved medication is a combination of ivacaftor and lumacaftor, approved for individuals with two copies of the most common CFTR mutation, F508del. It has been associated with a modest but significant improvement in lung function, improved body mass index, and a decrease in hospitalizations for pulmonary exacerbations. Clinical trials are actively underway for the next generation of CFTR modulators.

Treatment with CFTR modulator therapy does not preclude management of pulmonary complications. Management of pulmonary exacerbations is directed toward facilitating clearance of secretions from the airways and minimizing the effects of chronic bronchial infection. Airway secretion clearance techniques **(chest physiotherapy)** help remove mucus from the airways, and aerosolized DNAse and 7% hypertonic saline, both delivered by nebulizer, decrease the viscosity of mucus. **Antibiotic therapy** is important in controlling chronic infection. Monitoring pulmonary bacterial flora via airway cultures and providing aggressive therapy with appropriate antibiotics (oral, aerosolized, and intravenous [IV]) help to slow the progression of lung disease. Patients often require 2-3–week courses of high-dose IV antibiotics and aggressive chest physiotherapy to treat pulmonary exacerbations. Antibiotics are selected based on organisms identified by sputum culture. If patients are unable to provide sputum, then a throat culture for CF pathogens can be used to direct therapy. Common infecting organisms include *P. aeruginosa* and *S. aureus.*

Exocrine pancreatic insufficiency is treated with enteric-coated pancreatic enzyme capsules, which contain lipase and proteases. Patients with CF are encouraged to follow high-calorie diets, often with the addition of nutritional supplements. Even with optimal pancreatic enzyme replacement, stool losses of fat and protein may be high. Fat should not be withheld from the diet, even when significant steatorrhea exists. Rather, pancreatic enzyme doses should be titrated to optimize fat absorption, although there is a limit to the doses that should be used. Lipase dosages exceeding 2,500 U/kg per meal are concerning because they have been associated with **fibrosing colonopathy.** Fat-soluble vitamins (A, D, E, and K) are recommended, preferably in a water-miscible form.

Newborns with **meconium ileus** may require surgical intervention, but some can be managed with contrast (Gastrografin) enemas. Intestinal obstruction in CF patients beyond the neonatal period is often due to DIOS, which may need to be treated with courses of oral laxatives (polyethylene glycol) or, in more refractory cases, with Gastrografin enemas. Pancreatic enzyme dosage adjustment, adequate hydration, and dietary fiber may help prevent recurrent episodes. Patients with CF-related diabetes are treated with insulin, primarily to improve nutrition and prevent dehydration, as ketoacidosis is rare. Although transaminase elevation is common in patients with CF, only 1-3% of patients have progressive cirrhosis resulting in portal hypertension. Cholestasis may be treated with the bile salt ursodeoxycholic acid. Portal hypertension and esophageal varices due to cirrhosis of the liver are managed, when necessary, with portal vein shunting procedures or liver transplantation. Patients with symptomatic sinus disease and nasal polyps not responding to medical management may require surgical intervention.

The management of CF is complex and is best coordinated by medical teams at accredited CF centers. More than 50% of the CF population are now adults, highlighting the importance of a successful transition of pediatric patients to adult centers. As with other severe chronic diseases, management of CF patients requires a multidisciplinary team working with patients and their families to maintain an optimistic, comprehensive, and aggressive approach to treatment.

CHAPTER 138
Chest Wall and Pleura

Thoracic scoliosis, when it is severe (curve >60 degrees), can be associated with chest wall deformity and limitation of chest wall movement (see Chapter 202). This, in turn, can lead to decreased lung volumes (restrictive lung disease), ventilation-perfusion mismatching, hypoventilation, and even respiratory failure (see Chapter 39). Surgical correction of scoliosis may prevent further loss of lung function, but it rarely improves pulmonary function beyond presurgical levels.

PECTUS EXCAVATUM AND CARINATUM

Pectus Excavatum

Sternal concavity **(pectus excavatum)**, a common chest wall deformity in children, is usually not associated with significant pulmonary compromise. Patients with pectus excavatum generally come to medical attention because of concerns over the appearance of the chest. However, occasionally, if severe, it may result in restrictive lung disease, obstructive defects, and/or decreased cardiac function. Adolescents with pectus excavatum may complain of exercise intolerance. Routine spirometry is often normal but may show decreased vital capacity consistent with restrictive lung disease. The main reason for surgical correction is generally to improve appearance (cosmetic reasons), although in some cases surgical repair is justified to improve cardiac function and exercise tolerance.

Pectus Carinatum

Pectus carinatum is an abnormality of chest wall shape in which the sternum bows out. It is not associated with abnormal pulmonary function. Underlying pulmonary disease may contribute to the deformity. It can be observed after cardiac surgery performed via midsternal approach. Surgical correction of this condition is rarely indicated, but occasionally is done for cosmetic purposes.

PNEUMOTHORAX

Etiology

Pneumothorax, which is the accumulation of air in the pleural space, may result from external trauma or from leakage of air from the lungs or airways. **Spontaneous primary pneumothorax** (no underlying cause) occurs in teenagers and young adults, more commonly in tall, thin males and smokers. Factors predisposing to **secondary pneumothorax** (underlying cause identified) include barotrauma from mechanical ventilation, asthma, cystic fibrosis, trauma to the chest, and severe necrotizing pneumonia.

Clinical Manifestations

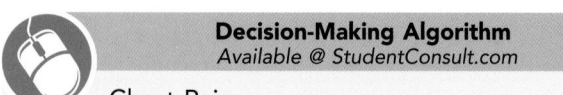

Decision-Making Algorithm
Available @ StudentConsult.com
Chest Pain

The most common signs and symptoms of pneumothorax are chest and shoulder pain and dyspnea. If the pneumothorax is caused by air that enters the pleural space during inspiration and cannot escape, mediastinal shift and functional lung compression may occur, resulting in **tension pneumothorax** with severe respiratory distress and hemodynamic changes (reduced venous return to the heart). Subcutaneous emphysema may result when the air leak communicates with the mediastinum. Physical findings associated with pneumothorax include decreased breath sounds on the affected side, a tympanitic percussion note, and evidence of mediastinal shift (deviation of the point of maximal impact [PMI] and trachea away from the side of the pneumothorax). If the pneumothorax is small, there may be few or no clinical findings. However, the patient's clinical condition can deteriorate rapidly if the pneumothorax expands, especially if the air in the pleural space is under pressure **(tension pneumothorax)**. This is a life-threatening condition that can result in death if the pleural space is not decompressed by evacuation of the pleural air.

Diagnostic Studies

The presence of a pneumothorax can usually be confirmed by upright chest radiographs. Computed tomography (CT) scans of the chest are useful in quantifying the size of pneumothoraces and differentiating air within the lung parenchyma (cystic lung disease) from air in the pleural space and for identifying subpleural blebs that may be present in spontaneous recurrent pneumothoraces. However, CT scans are generally not necessary unless chest x-rays suggest the need for further evaluation. In infants, transillumination of the chest wall may be of some use in making a rapid diagnosis of pneumothorax.

Treatment

The type of intervention depends on the size of the pneumothorax and the nature of the underlying disease. Small pneumothoraces (<20% of thorax occupied with pleural air) may not require intervention as they often resolve spontaneously. Inhaling high concentrations of supplemental O_2 may enhance reabsorption of pleural air by washing out nitrogen from the blood. Larger pneumothoraces and any tension pneumothorax require immediate drainage of the air, preferably via chest tube. In an emergency situation, a simple needle aspiration may suffice, although placement of a chest tube is often required for resolution. In patients with recurrent or persistent pneumothoraces, sclerosing the pleural surfaces to obliterate the pleural space (pleurodesis) may be necessary. This can be done either chemically, by instilling talc or sclerosis agents (doxycycline) through the chest tube, or mechanically, by surgical abradement. Surgical approaches, such as open thoracotomy and video-assisted thoracoscopic surgery (VATS), enable visualization of the pleural space and resection of pleural blebs, when indicated. Airline travel and spirometry may be restricted for a period of time (2 weeks or longer) following radiographic resolution of the pneumothorax to minimize risk of recurrence.

PNEUMOMEDIASTINUM

Pneumomediastinum results from the dissection of air from the pulmonary parenchyma into the mediastinum. It is usually a mild, self-limited process that does not require aggressive intervention. The most common causes in children are severe forceful coughing and acute asthma exacerbations. Common symptoms are chest pain and dyspnea. There are often no physical findings, although a crunching noise over the sternum can sometimes be appreciated on auscultation and subcutaneous emphysema may be detected about the neck. The diagnosis is confirmed by chest radiograph, and treatment is directed toward the underlying lung disease.

PLEURAL EFFUSION

Etiology

Fluid accumulates in the pleural space when the local hydrostatic forces that are pushing fluid out of the vascular space exceed the oncotic forces that are drawing fluid back into the vascular space. Pleural effusions can be transudates (intact membrane but abnormal hydrostatic or oncotic forces) or exudates (decreased integrity of the membrane due to inflammatory processes or impaired lymphatic drainage). There are relatively few causes of transudates, the primary ones being congestive heart failure and hypoproteinemia states, whereas the causes of exudates are numerous. Almost any pulmonary inflammatory process can result in pleural fluid accumulation. Among the most common causes of exudates are infection (e.g., tuberculosis, bacterial pneumonia), collagen vascular diseases (e.g., systemic lupus erythematosus), and malignancy. Chylous pleural effusions (elevated triglyceride levels) are seen with thoracic duct injury and abnormalities of lymphatic drainage (lymphangiomyomatosis, lymphangiectasia). Bacterial pneumonia can lead to an accumulation of pleural fluid **(parapneumonic effusion)**. When this fluid is purulent or infected, then it is called an **empyema**, although often the terms parapneumonic effusion and empyema are used interchangeably. Parapneumonic effusion/empyema is the most common reason for effusion in children. Upright and decubitus chest radiograph (Fig. 138.1) can be useful for identifying parapneumonic effusion; however, chest ultrasound or CT is necessary for accurate estimates of fluid volume and organization (loculation) if surgical drainage is being considered. Most parapneumonic effusions are due to pneumonia caused by *Streptococcus pneumoniae*, group A streptococci, or *Staphylococcus aureus*.

Clinical Manifestations

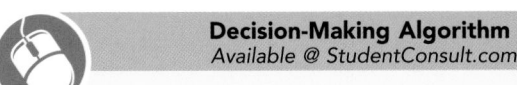

Decision-Making Algorithm
Available @ StudentConsult.com
Chest Pain

Small pleural effusions may be asymptomatic, but if they are large enough to compress lung tissue, then they can cause dyspnea, tachypnea, and occasionally chest pain. Effusions due to infection are usually associated with fever, malaise, poor appetite, pleuritic chest pain, and splinting. Physical findings include tachypnea, decreased breath sounds, dullness to percussion, and decreased tactile fremitus. Large effusions may occupy more than half the hemithorax and cause a mediastinal shift away from the affected side, compromising respiratory status, particularly in young children.

Diagnostic Studies

The presence of pleural fluid can often be confirmed by chest radiograph. In addition to anteroposterior and lateral projections, a decubitus view should be done to assess for layering of fluid. Chest ultrasonography is useful for confirming the presence of the effusion and quantifying its size. CT scans of the chest can help differentiate pleural fluid from parenchymal lesions and pleural masses. Both ultrasonography and CT scans can determine whether parapneumonic effusions contain loculations (fibrous strands that compartmentalize the effusion).

The analysis of pleural fluid is useful in differentiating a transudate from an exudate. Routine tests on pleural fluid such as cell count, pH, protein, lactose dehydrogenase, and glucose characterize the effusions. Triglyceride levels, cytology, hematocrit, gram and acid-fast bacilli stain, culture, and adenosine deaminase levels can be useful in diagnosing chylous, malignant, and tuberculous effusions (Table 138.1). However, the yield of pleural fluid cultures is low. Transudative pleural effusions have a low specific gravity (<1.015) and protein content (<2.5 g/dL), low lactate dehydrogenase activity (<200 IU/L), and a low white blood cell (WBC) count with few polymorphonuclear cells. In contrast, exudates are characterized by high specific gravity and high protein (>3 g/dL) and lactate dehydrogenase

TABLE 138.1 Pleural Fluid Analysis

EXUDATIVE EFFUSION BY LIGHT'S TRADITIONAL CRITERIA
Pleural fluid protein/serum protein ratio >0.5 **OR**
Pleural fluid LDH/serum LDH ratio >0.6 **OR**
Pleural fluid LDH >two thirds the upper limits of laboratory's normal serum LDH
CHYLOTHORAX
Triglycerides >110 mg/dL
TUBERCULOUS
Positive acid-fast bacilli stain, culture
Pleural fluid protein >4 g/dL
Pleural fluid adenosine deaminase level >35-50 U/L
Pleural fluid glucose 30-50 mg/dL
HEMOTHORAX
Pleural fluid hematocrit/serum hematocrit >0.5

LDH, Lactate dehydrogenase.

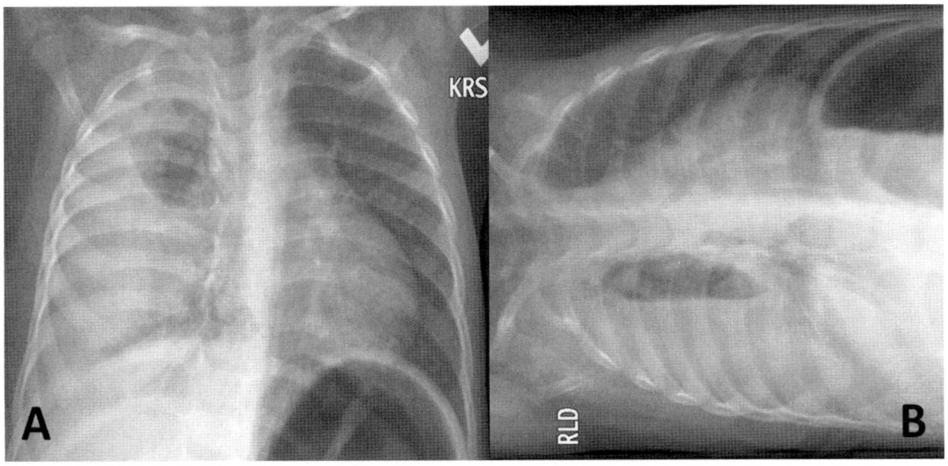

FIGURE 138.1 Parapneumonic effusion. *A*, Posterior-anterior chest radiograph showing dense opacification of the right hemithorax. *B*, On decubitus view, some of the density forms a horizontal layer indicating that there is pleural fluid in addition to pneumonia.

(>250 IU/L) levels. They may also have a low pH (<7.2), low glucose level (<40 mg/dL), and a high WBC count with many lymphocytes or polymorphonuclear leukocytes.

Treatment

Therapy is directed at the underlying condition causing the effusion and at relief of the mechanical consequences of the fluid collection. For small effusions, especially if they are transudates, no pleural drainage is required. Large effusions that are causing respiratory compromise should be drained. Transudates and most exudates, other than parapneumonic effusions, can be drained with a **chest tube**. With parapneumonic effusions/empyema, a chest tube alone is often not sufficient because the fluid may be thick and loculated. In such cases, pleural drainage is best achieved with either the administration of fibrinolytic agents via chest tubes or **VATS**. Approaches to parapneumonic effusions vary widely. Small effusions can be managed conservatively with intravenous antibiotics alone. Both fibrinolytic therapy via chest tubes and VATS can reduce morbidity and length of hospital stay, and many patients with moderate-sized parapneumonic effusions can be treated with chest tube drainage and intravenous antibiotics.

Suggested Readings

Levitzky MG. *Pulmonary Physiology*. 8th ed. McGraw-Hill: New York; 2013.

Respiratory system. In: Kliegman RM, Stanton BF, St. Geme JW, et al, eds. *Nelson Textbook of Pediatrics*. 20th ed. Philadelphia: Saunders; 2016.

Taussig LN, Landau LI. *Pediatric Respiratory Medicine*. 2nd ed. Philadelphia: Mosby; 2008.

Wilmott RW, Boat TF, Bush A, et al, eds. *Kendig and Chernick's Disorders of the Respiratory Tract in Children*. 8th ed. Philadelphia: Saunders; 2012.

PEARLS FOR PRACTITIONERS

CHAPTER 133

Respiratory System Assessment

- Airway branching is complete at birth; alveolar number increases through childhood.
- Resistance increases with reduction of airway diameter, leading to obstructive lung disease.
- Pulmonary compliance is reduced when lungs, pleura, or chest wall become stiff, leading to restrictive lung disease.
- Ventilation-perfusion (V/Q) mismatch is the most common cause of hypoxemia in children.
- A chest radiograph can provide valuable information about parenchymal, pleural, and airway disease and is recommended as first-line imaging for most patients with respiratory complaints.
- Spirometry is the pulmonary function test of choice for diagnosing asthma and other obstructive lung diseases; body plethysmography is needed to confirm restrictive lung disease.
- Flexible bronchoscopy is useful for evaluation of airway anatomy and obtaining lower respiratory samples; rigid bronchoscopy is required for foreign body removal.

CHAPTER 134

Control of Breathing

- Ventilation and oxygenation are regulated by central and peripheral chemoreceptors, with signal origin in the deep brainstem.
- Central apnea is more likely secondary (drugs, central nervous system tumor, or trauma) than primary (genetic syndrome).
- Apnea of prematurity should resolve by 44 weeks postmenstrual age.
- A brief resolved unexplained event (BRUE) is defined as a <1 minute, self-limited episode with cyanosis or pallor, irregular breathing, change in tone, or altered level of responsiveness occurring in an infant <1 year of age.
- The risk of sudden infant death syndrome (SIDS) is associated with preterm birth, maternal smoking, prone sleep position, and overinsulation.
- Obstructive sleep apnea is most commonly caused by adenotonsillar hypertrophy in children.
- Polysomnogram is the diagnostic test of choice for obstructive and central apnea.

CHAPTER 135

Upper Airway Obstruction

- Upper airway obstruction at the level of the glottis or subglottis produces stridor, typically worse when the child is awake and active.
- The most common cause of *noninfectious* stridor in infants is laryngomalacia.
- The most common cause of *infectious* stridor in infants and young children is croup (laryngotracheobronchitis).
- Upper airway obstruction at the level of the pharynx is usually due to soft tissue collapse or enlargement, leading to mouth breathing and snoring that is typically worse during sleep.
- The most common cause of *noninfectious* soft tissue upper airway obstruction in young children is adenotonsillar hypertrophy.
- Common infectious causes of soft tissue upper airway obstruction include retropharyngeal abscess and peritonsillar abscess.

CHAPTER 136

Lower Airway, Parenchymal, and Pulmonary Vascular Diseases

- The most common cause of lower airway disease in children is asthma.
- Asthma is a clinical disease of variable and recurring symptoms with airway inflammation and bronchial hyperresponsiveness.
- A wheeze is a continuous sound produced by small airway narrowing and is most pronounced on exhalation.
- Tracheomalacia is the most common tracheal abnormality, can be congenital or acquired, and often improves with growth.
- Vascular rings can be complete or incomplete, causing extrinsic tracheal compression, leading to wheezing, stridor, cough, or dyspnea.
- Foreign body aspiration typically occurs in children 1-4 years of age, often with nonradiopaque material such as food (e.g., nuts).
- Primary ciliary dyskinesia (PCD) is associated with chronic sinusitis, chronic otitis media, and recurrent pulmonary infections. Kartagener syndrome (situs inversus, pansinusitis, bronchiectasis) is seen in approximately 50% of cases of PCD.
- Pulmonary hypertension may lead to irreversible pulmonary vascular changes that strain the right heart and lead to cor pulmonale.
- Cor pulmonale is commonly caused by chronic lung disease, particularly severe bronchopulmonary dysplasia and untreated severe obstructive sleep apnea.
- Hemoptysis from pulmonary sources can occur from airway hemorrhage or alveolar bleeding.

CHAPTER 137

Cystic Fibrosis

- Cystic fibrosis (CF) is an autosomal recessive genetic disorder.
- The gene for CF encodes for a polypeptide, the cystic fibrosis transmembrane conductance regulator (CFTR), a chloride channel located on the apical surface of epithelial cells.
- Defects in the CFTR gene result in abnormal movement of salt and water across cell membranes leading to thick secretions impacting multiple organ systems.
- Clinical manifestations of CF include chronic cough, recurrent pulmonary infections, failure to thrive, poor growth and weight gain, recurrent sinusitis, nasal polyposis, steatorrhea, recurrent pancreatitis, and rectal prolapse.
- Common pathogens in CF sputum are *Staphylococcus aureus* and *Pseudomonas aeruginosa.*
- Sweat chloride testing is the diagnostic test of choice and confirms diagnosis with newborn screening, genetic testing, and clinical symptoms.
- Management of CF includes enhancing airway clearance, medications to decrease mucus viscosity, treating airway infections, and improving nutritional status with pancreatic enzyme replacement therapy and nutritional supplements.
- Newer therapies are genotype-specific and improve the function of CFTR protein for some individuals with CF.

CHAPTER 138

Chest Wall and Pleura

- Severe thoracic scoliosis can lead to chest wall deformity that limits lung volumes and causes restrictive lung disease.
- Pectus excavatum (sternal concavity) and pectus carinatum (sternal extrusion) are common chest wall deformities that are typically not associated with significant pulmonary compromise.
- Pneumothorax is an accumulation of air in the pleural space that can occur spontaneously from leakage of air from the lung or airways.
- Pleural effusions can be transudative (e.g., heart failure) or exudative (e.g., infection/empyema).
- Parapneumonic effusion in children is commonly associated with infection from *Streptococcus pneumoniae*, group A streptococci, or *Staphylococcus aureus*.

CARDIOVASCULAR SYSTEM

Daniel S. Schneider

CHAPTER 139

Cardiovascular System Assessment

HISTORY

A **maternal history** of medication, drug, or alcohol use or excessive smoking may contribute to cardiac and other systemic findings. The **prenatal history** may reveal a maternal infection early in pregnancy (possibly teratogenic) or later in pregnancy (causing myocarditis or myocardial dysfunction in infants). Infants with heart failure exhibit poor **growth**, with weight being more significantly affected than height and head circumference.

Heart failure may present with **fatigue** or **diaphoresis** with feeds or fussiness. **Tachypnea** without significant dyspnea may be present. Older children with heart failure may have easy fatigability, **shortness of breath** on exertion, and, sometimes, orthopnea. Not keeping up with other children during play or exercise is a sign of **exercise intolerance**. Heart failure may be misdiagnosed as recurrent pneumonia, bronchitis, wheezing, or asthma.

A history of a **heart murmur** is important, but many well children have an innocent murmur at some time in their lives. Other cardiac symptoms include cyanosis, palpitations, chest pain, syncope, and near-syncope. A review of systems assesses for possible systemic diseases or congenital malformation syndromes that may cause cardiac abnormalities (Tables 139.1 and 139.2). Current and past medication use as well as history of drug use is important. **Family history** should be reviewed for hereditary diseases, early atherosclerotic heart disease, congenital heart disease, sudden unexplained deaths, thrombophilia, rheumatic fever, hypertension, and hypercholesterolemia.

PHYSICAL EXAMINATION

A complete cardiovascular examination starts in the supine position and includes evaluation in sitting and standing positions, when possible. **Inspection** is supplemented by **palpation** and **auscultation** to provide a complete examination.

The examination starts with vital signs. The normal **heart rate** varies with age and activity. Newborn resting heart rates are approximately 120 beats per minute, slightly higher in infants 3-6 months of age, and then gradually declining through adolescence to near 80 beats per minute. The range of normal for any given age is approximately 30 beats per minute above or below the average. Tachycardia may be a manifestation of anemia, dehydration, shock, heart failure, or dysrhythmia. Bradycardia can be a normal finding in patients with high vagal tone (athletes) but may be a manifestation of atrioventricular block. The **respiratory rate** of infants is best assessed while the infant is quiet. Respiratory rate may be increased when there is a left-to-right shunt or pulmonary venous congestion.

Normal **blood pressure** also varies with age. A properly sized cuff should have a bladder width that is at least 90% and a length that is 80-100% of the arm circumference. Initially, blood pressure in the right arm is measured. If elevated, measurements in the left arm and legs are indicated to evaluate for possible coarctation of the aorta. The **pulse pressure** is determined by subtracting the diastolic pressure from the systolic pressure. It is normally below 50 mm Hg or half the systolic pressure, whichever is less. A wide pulse pressure may be seen with aortopulmonary connections (patent ductus arteriosus [PDA], truncus arteriosus, arteriovenous malformations), aortic insufficiency, or relative intravascular volume depletion (anemia, vasodilation with fever or sepsis). A narrow pulse pressure is seen with pericardial tamponade, aortic stenosis, and heart failure.

Inspection includes general appearance, nutritional status, circulation, and respiratory effort. Many chromosomal abnormalities and syndromes associated with cardiac defects have dysmorphic features or failure to thrive (see Table 139.2). Skin color must be assessed for **cyanosis** and pallor. Central cyanosis (tongue, lips) is associated with arterial desaturation; isolated peripheral cyanosis (hands, feet) is associated with normal arterial saturation and increased peripheral extraction of oxygen. Perioral cyanosis is a common finding, especially in pale infants or when infants and toddlers become cold. Chronic arterial desaturation results in **clubbing** of the fingernails and toenails. Inspection of the chest may reveal asymmetry or a prominent left precordium, suggesting chronic cardiac enlargement.

After inspection, **palpation** of pulses in all four extremities, the precordial activity, and the abdomen is performed. Pulses are assessed for rate, regularity, intensity, symmetry, and timing between upper and lower extremities. A good pedal pulse with normal right arm blood pressure effectively rules out coarctation of the aorta. The precordium should be assessed for apical impulse, **point of maximum impulse**, hyperactivity, and presence of a **thrill**. Abdominal palpation assesses liver and spleen size. The liver size provides an assessment of intravascular volume and is enlarged with systemic venous congestion. The spleen may be enlarged with infective endocarditis.

TABLE **139.1** Cardiac Manifestations of Systemic Diseases

SYSTEMIC DISEASE	CARDIAC COMPLICATIONS
Hunter-Hurler syndrome	Valvular insufficiency, heart failure, hypertension
Duchenne dystrophy	Cardiomyopathy, heart failure
Pompe disease	Short PR interval, cardiomegaly, heart failure, arrhythmias
Kawasaki disease	Coronary artery aneurysm, thrombosis, myocardial infarction, myocarditis
Marfan syndrome	Aortic and mitral insufficiency, dissecting aortic aneurysm
Juvenile rheumatoid arthritis	Pericarditis
Systemic lupus erythematosus	Pericarditis, Libman-Sacks endocarditis, congenital AV block
Lyme disease	Arrhythmias, myocarditis, heart failure
Graves disease (hyperthyroidism)	Tachycardia, arrhythmias, heart failure
Tuberous sclerosis	Cardiac rhabdomyoma
Neurofibromatosis	Pulmonic stenosis, coarctation of aorta

AV, Atrioventricular.

TABLE **139.2** Congenital Malformation Syndromes Associated With Congenital Heart Disease

SYNDROME	CARDIAC FEATURES
Trisomy 21 (Down syndrome)	Endocardial cushion defect, VSD, ASD, PDA
Trisomy 18	VSD, ASD, PDA, PS
Trisomy 13	VSD, ASD, PDA, dextrocardia
XO (Turner syndrome)	Coarctation of aorta, aortic stenosis
CHARGE association (coloboma, heart, atresia choanae, retardation, genital and ear anomalies)	TOF, aortic arch and conotruncal anomalies*
22q11 (DiGeorge) syndrome	Aortic arch anomalies, conotruncal anomalies*
VACTERL association† (vertebral, anal, cardiac, tracheoesophageal, radial, renal, limb anomalies)	VSD
Marfan syndrome	Dilated and dissecting aorta, aortic valve regurgitation, mitral valve prolapse
William syndrome	Supravalvular aortic stenosis, peripheral pulmonary stenosis
Infant of diabetic mother	Hypertrophic cardiomyopathy, VSD, conotruncal anomalies
Asplenia syndrome	Complex cyanotic heart lesions, anomalous pulmonary venous return, dextrocardia, single ventricle, single AV valve
Polysplenia syndrome	Azygos continuation of inferior vena cava, pulmonary atresia, dextrocardia, single ventricle
Fetal alcohol syndrome	VSD, ASD
Fetal hydantoin syndrome	TGA, VSD, TOF

**Conotruncal—tetralogy of Fallot, pulmonary atresia, truncus arteriosus, transposition of great arteries.*

†VACTERL association is also known as VATER association, in which the limb anomalies are not included.

ASD, Atrial septal defect; *AV*, atrioventricular; *PDA*, patent ductus arteriosus; *PS*, pulmonic stenosis; *TGA*, transposition of great arteries; *TOF*, tetralogy of Fallot; *VSD*, ventricular septal defect.

Auscultation is the most important part of the cardiovascular examination, but should supplement what already has been found by inspection and palpation. Systematic listening in a quiet room allows assessment of each portion of the cardiac cycle. In addition to heart rate and regularity, the heart sounds, clicks, and murmurs need to be timed and characterized.

Heart Sounds

$\mathbf{S_1}$ is associated with closure of the mitral and tricuspid valves, is usually single, and is best heard at the lower left sternal border (LLSB) or apex (Fig. 139.1). Although it can normally be split, if a split $\mathbf{S_1}$ is heard, the possibility of an ejection click or, much less commonly, an $\mathbf{S_4}$ should be considered. $\mathbf{S_2}$ is associated with closure of the aortic and pulmonary valves. It should normally split with inspiration and be single with exhalation. Abnormalities of splitting and intensity of the pulmonary component are associated with significant anatomical and physiological abnormalities (Table 139.3). $\mathbf{S_3}$ is heard in early diastole and is related to rapid ventricular filling. It is best heard at the LLSB or apex and may be a normal sound, but a loud $\mathbf{S_3}$ is abnormal and heard in conditions with dilated ventricles. $\mathbf{S_4}$ occurs late in diastole just before $\mathbf{S_1}$; it is best heard at the LLSB/apex and is associated with decreased ventricular compliance. It is rare and is always abnormal.

Clicks

A click implies a valvular abnormality or dilated great artery. It may be ejection or midsystolic in timing and may or may not be associated with a murmur. A midsystolic click is associated with mitral valve prolapse. **Ejection clicks** occur early in systole. Pulmonary ejection clicks are best heard at the left upper sternal border and vary in intensity with respiration. Aortic clicks are often louder at the apex, left midsternal border, or right upper sternal border and do not vary with respiration.

Murmurs

Decision-Making Algorithm
Available @ StudentConsult.com
Heart Murmurs

Murmur evaluation should determine timing, duration, location, intensity, radiation, and frequency or pitch of the murmur. The timing determines a murmur's significance and can be used to develop a differential diagnosis (see Fig. 139.1). Murmurs should be classified as **systolic, diastolic**, or **continuous.** Most murmurs are systolic and can be divided further into systolic ejection murmurs or holosystolic (also called pansystolic or

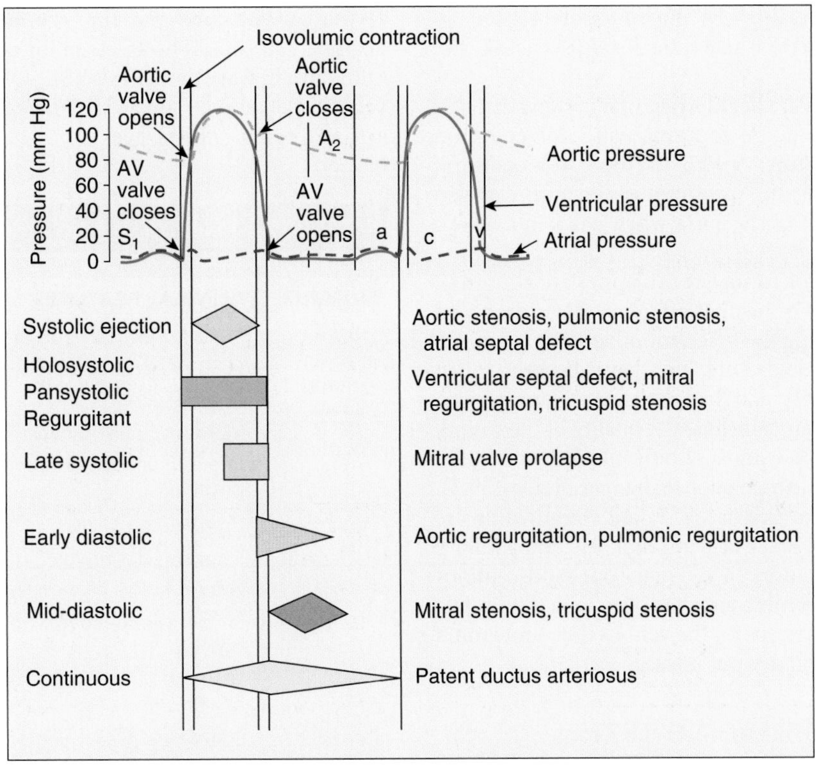

FIGURE 139.1 Timing of heart murmurs. *AV*, Atrioventricular.

TABLE 139.3 Abnormal Second Heart Sound

SINGLE S_2
Pulmonary hypertension (severe)
One semilunar valve (aortic atresia, pulmonary atresia, truncus arteriosus)
Malposed great arteries (d-TGA, l-TGA)
Severe aortic stenosis
WIDELY SPLIT S_2
Increased flow across valve (ASD, PAPVR)
Prolonged flow across valve (pulmonary stenosis)
Electrical delay (right bundle branch block)
Early aortic closure (severe mitral regurgitation)
PARADOXICALLY SPLIT S_2
Severe aortic stenosis
ABNORMAL INTENSITY OF P2
Increased in pulmonary hypertension
Decreased in severe pulmonary stenosis, tetralogy of Fallot

ASD, Atrial septal defect; *d-TGA*, dextro-transposition of the great arteries; *l-TGA*, levo-transposition of the great arteries; *PAPVR*, partial anomalous pulmonary venous return.

TABLE 139.4 Heart Murmur Intensity

GRADE	DESCRIPTION
Grade I	Very soft, heard in quiet room with cooperative patient
Grade II	Easily heard but not loud
Grade III	Loud but no thrill
Grade IV	Loud with palpable thrill
Grade V	Loud with thrill, audible with stethoscope at 45-degree angle
Grade VI	Loud with thrill, audible with stethoscope off chest 1 cm

regurgitant) murmurs. **Ejection murmurs** are crescendo-decrescendo with a short time between S_1 and the onset of the murmur (isovolumic contraction). Systolic ejection murmurs require the ejection of blood from the ventricle and may occur with aortic stenosis, pulmonary stenosis, atrial septal defects (ASDs), and coarctation of the aorta. **Holosystolic murmurs** have their onset with S_1. The murmur has a plateau quality and may be heard with ventricular septal defects (VSDs) and mitral or tricuspid regurgitation. A *late regurgitant* murmur may be heard after a midsystolic click in mitral valve prolapse.

Murmurs are often heard along the path of blood flow. Ejection murmurs usually are best heard at the base of the heart, whereas holosystolic murmurs are louder at the LLSB and apex. Pulmonary ejection murmurs radiate to the back and axilla. Aortic ejection murmurs radiate to the neck. The **intensity** or loudness of a heart murmur is assessed as grade I through VI (Table 139.4). The **frequency** or pitch of a murmur provides information regarding the pressure gradient. The higher the pressure gradient across a narrowed area (valve, vessel, or defect), the faster the flow and higher the frequency of the murmur. Low-frequency murmurs imply low-pressure gradients and mild obstruction or less restriction to flow.

Diastolic murmurs are much less common than systolic murmurs and should be considered abnormal. Early diastolic murmurs occur when there is regurgitation through the aortic or pulmonary valve. Mid-diastolic murmurs are caused by increased flow (ASD, VSD) or anatomical stenosis across the mitral or tricuspid valves.

Continuous murmurs are heard when there is flow through the entire cardiac cycle and are abnormal with one common exception, the **venous hum.** A PDA is the most common abnormal continuous murmur. Continuous murmurs can also be heard with coarctation of the aorta when collateral vessels are present.

Normal physiological or **innocent murmurs** are common, occurring in at least 80% of normal infants and children and are heard most often during the first 6 months of life, from 3-6 years of age, and in early adolescence. They have also been called benign, functional, vibratory, and flow murmurs. Characteristic findings of innocent murmurs include the quality of the sound, a lack of significant radiation, and a significant alteration in the intensity of the murmur with positional changes (Table 139.5). Most important, the cardiovascular history and examination are otherwise normal. The presence of symptoms, including failure to thrive or dysmorphic features, should make one more cautious about diagnosing a *normal* murmur. Diastolic, holosystolic, late systolic, and continuous (except for the venous hum) murmurs and the presence of a thrill are not normal.

LABORATORY AND IMAGING TESTS

Pulse Oximetry

Mild desaturation that is not clinically apparent may be the only early finding in complex congenital heart defects. Comparing pulse oximetry between the right arm and a lower extremity may allow diagnosis of a ductal-dependent lesion in which desaturated blood flows right to left across a PDA to perfuse the lower body. This is now becoming a routine screening test in newborn infants to rule out congenital heart disease.

Electrocardiography

The 12-lead electrocardiogram (ECG) provides information about the **rate**, **rhythm**, **depolarization**, and **repolarization** of the cardiac cells and the size and wall thickness of the chambers. It should be assessed for rate, rhythm, axis (P wave, QRS, and T wave), intervals (PR, QRS, QTc; Fig. 139.2), and voltages (left atrial, right atrial, left ventricular, right ventricular) adjusted for the child's age.

TABLE 139.5 Normal or Innocent Heart Murmurs

MURMUR	CLINICAL FEATURES	USUAL AGE WHEN HEARD
Still's murmur/ vibratory murmur	Systolic ejection murmur LLSB or between LLSB and apex Grades I-III/VI Vibratory, musical quality Intensity decreases in upright position	3-6 yr
Venous hum	Continuous murmur Infraclavicular region (right > left) Grades I-III/VI Louder with patient in upright position Changes with compression of jugular vein or turning head	3-6 yr
Carotid bruit	Systolic ejection murmur Neck, over carotid artery Grade I-III/VI	Any age
Adolescent ejection murmur	Systolic ejection murmur LUSB Grade I-III/VI Usually softer in upright position Does not radiate to back	8-14 yr
Normal peripheral pulmonary stenosis murmur	Systolic ejection murmur Axilla and back, LUSB/RUSB Grade I-III/VI Harsh, short, high-frequency	Newborn-6 mo

LLSB, Left lower scapular border; *LUSB*, left upper scapular border; *RUSB*, right upper scapular border.

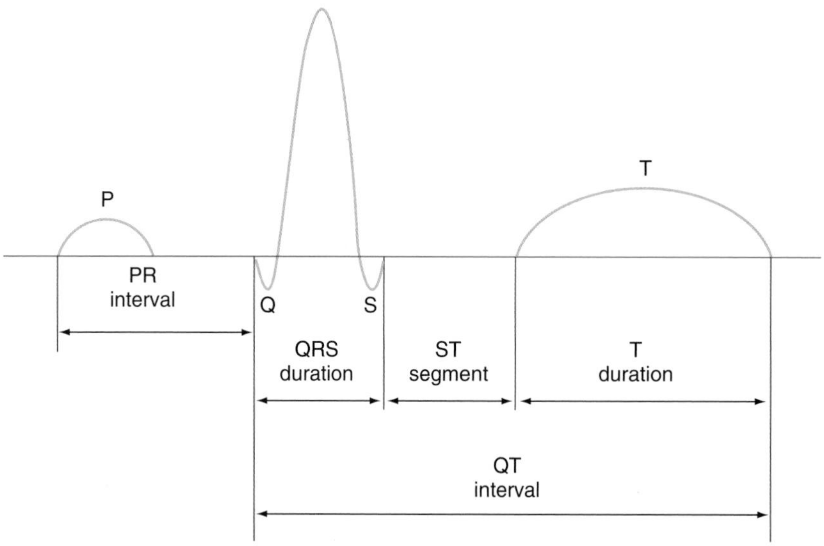

FIGURE 139.2 Nomenclature of electrocardiogram waves and intervals.

The **P wave** represents atrial depolarization. A criterion for right atrial enlargement is an increase of the amplitude of the P wave, reflected best in lead II. The diagnosis of left atrial enlargement is made by prolongation of the second portion of the P wave, exhibited best in the chest leads.

The **PR interval**, measured from the beginning of the P wave to the beginning of the QRS complex, increases with age. Conduction time is shortened when the conduction velocity is increased (glycogen storage disease) or when the atrioventricular node is bypassed (Wolff-Parkinson-White syndrome). A prolonged PR interval usually indicates slow conduction through the atrioventricular node. Diseases in the atrial myocardium, the bundle of His, or the Purkinje system may also contribute to prolonged PR intervals.

The **QRS complex** represents ventricular depolarization. A greater ventricular volume or mass causes a greater magnitude of the complex. The proximity of the right ventricle to the chest surface accentuates that ventricle's contribution to the complex. Changes in the normal ECG occur with age. Normative data for each age group must be known to make a diagnosis from the ECG.

The **QT interval** is measured from the beginning of the QRS complex to the end of the T wave. The corrected QT interval (corrected for rate) should be less than 0.45 second ($QTc = QT/\sqrt{\text{preceding R to R interval}}$). The interval may be prolonged in children with hypocalcemia or severe hypokalemia. It is also prolonged in a group of children at risk for severe ventricular arrhythmias and sudden death **(prolonged QT syndrome)**. Drugs such as quinidine and erythromycin may prolong the QT interval.

Chest Radiography

A systematic approach to reading a chest radiograph includes assessment of extracardiac structures, the shape and size of the heart, and the size and position of the pulmonary artery and aorta (Fig. 139.3). Assessment of the location and size of the heart and **cardiac silhouette** may suggest a cardiac defect. On a good inspiratory film, the cardiothoracic ratio should be less than 55% in infants under 1 year of age and less than 50% in older children and adolescents. An enlarged heart may be due to an increased volume load (left-right shunt) or due to myocardial dysfunction (dilated cardiomyopathy). The shape of the heart may suggest specific congenital heart defects. The most common examples are the *boot-shaped* heart seen with tetralogy of Fallot, the *egg-on-a-string* seen with dextroposed transposition of the great arteries, and the "snowman" seen with supracardiac total anomalous pulmonary venous return. The chest x-ray can aid in the assessment of **pulmonary blood flow**. Defects associated with left-to-right shunting have increased pulmonary blood flow *(shunt vascularity)* on x-ray. Right-to-left shunts have decreased pulmonary blood flow.

Echocardiography

Echocardiography has become the most important noninvasive tool in the diagnosis and management of cardiac disease, providing a full anatomical evaluation in most congenital heart defects (Fig. 139.4). Physiological data on the direction of blood flow can be obtained with the use of pulsed, continuous wave, and color flow Doppler. Imaging from multiple views provides

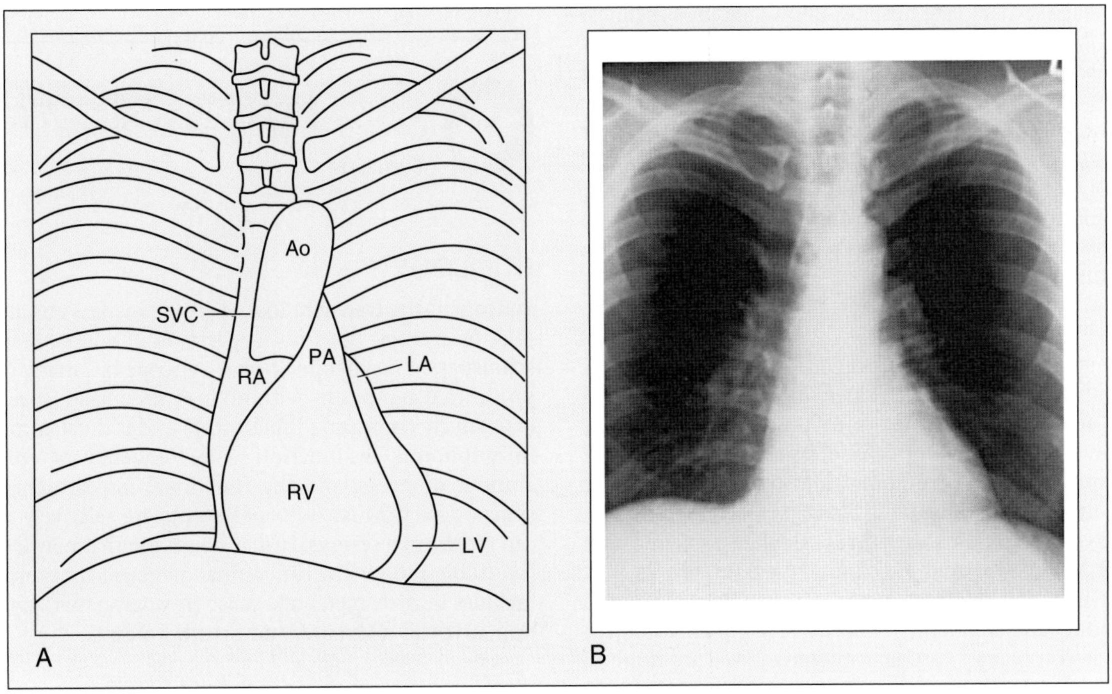

FIGURE 139.3 **A,** Parts of the heart whose outlines can be identified on a routine chest x-ray. **B,** Routine posteroanterior x-ray of the normal cardiac silhouette. *Ao,* Aorta; *LA,* left atrium; *LV,* left ventricle; *PA,* pulmonary artery; *RA,* right atrium; *RV,* right ventricle; *SVC,* superior vena cava. (From Andreoli TE, Carpenter CCJ, Plum F, et al, eds. *Cecil Essentials of Medicine*. 2nd ed. Philadelphia: WB Saunders; 1990.)

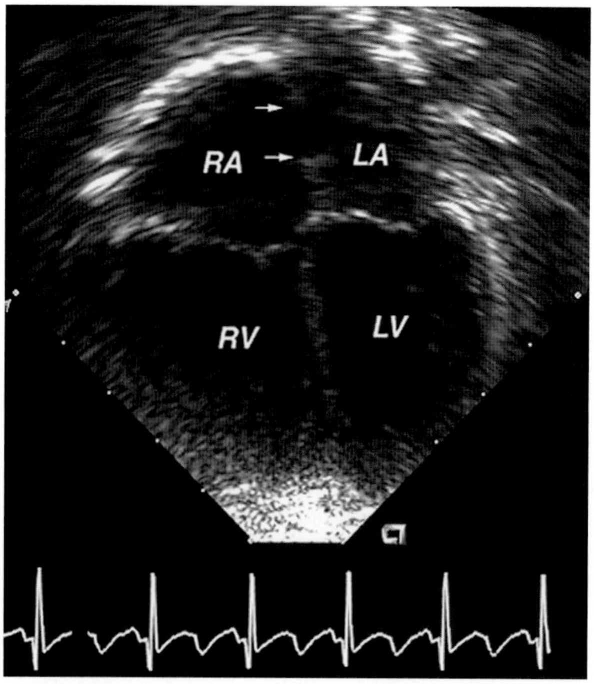

FIGURE 139.4 Four-chamber echocardiogram of an atrial septal defect. The defect margins are identified by the two *arrows*. *LA*, Left atrium; *LV*, left ventricle; *RA*, right atrium; *RV*, right ventricle.

an assessment of spatial relationships. Three-dimensional (3D) and four-dimensional (4D) imaging now allows reconstruction of the heart and manipulation of the images to provide more detail, especially with regard to valve structure and function. Prenatal or fetal echocardiography can diagnose congenital heart disease by 18 weeks of gestation and allows for delivery of the infant at a tertiary care hospital, improving the timeliness of therapy. Many congenital heart defects now are surgically repaired based on the echocardiogram without need for cardiac catheterization.

Transesophageal echocardiography (TEE) provides better imaging when transthoracic imaging is inadequate. It is used intraoperatively to assess results and cardiac function after surgery. TEE and intracardiac echocardiography are used to guide interventional catheterization and radiofrequency ablation of dysrhythmias.

Cardiac Catheterization

Cardiac catheterization is performed in patients who need additional anatomical information or precise hemodynamic information before operating or establishing a management plan. Pressures, oxygen saturations, and oxygen content are measured in each chamber and blood vessel entered (Fig. 139.5). This information is used to calculate systemic and pulmonary blood flow and resistance. Angiography is performed by injecting contrast material into selected sites to define anatomy and supplement noninvasive information. An increasing percentage of cardiac catheterizations are done to perform an intervention, including balloon dilation of stenotic valves and vessels, ballooning and stenting of stenotic lesions, closure of collateral vessels by coil embolization, and device closure of PDAs, secundum ASDs, patent foramen ovales, and muscular VSDs. Catheterization with electrophysiological studies allows for precise mapping of the electrical activity, can assess the risk of abnormal heart rhythms, and, often, is done in anticipation of radiofrequency ablation of the site of a dysrhythmia.

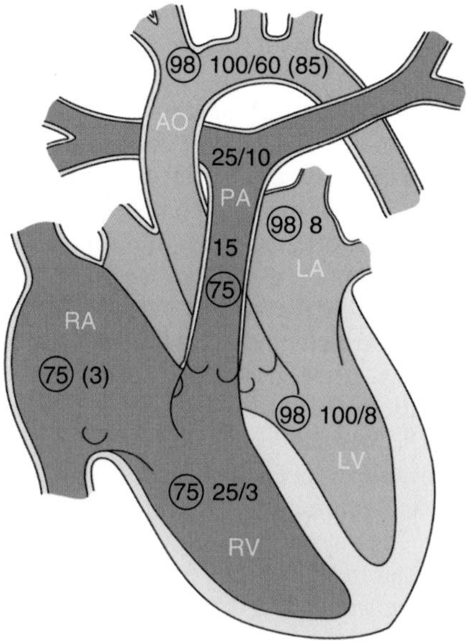

FIGURE 139.5 The normal heart. *Circled* values are oxygen saturations. *Ao*, Aorta; *LA*, left atrium; *LV*, left ventricle; *PA*, pulmonary artery; *RA*, right atrium; *RV*, right ventricle.

CHAPTER 140

Syncope

Decision-Making Algorithm
Available @ StudentConsult.com

Syncope

ETIOLOGY

Syncope is the transient loss of consciousness and muscle tone that, by history, does not suggest other altered states of consciousness. Presyncope or near-syncope has many or all of the prodromal symptoms without loss of consciousness. Syncope is relatively common (Table 140.1) and is most commonly due to autonomic dysfunction. The frequency of episodes, the amount of stress, and the functional impairment caused by syncope vary. Most syncopal events are relatively benign but can represent a serious cardiac condition that may lead to death (see Table 140.1). The differential diagnosis for typical syncope includes seizure, metabolic cause (hypoglycemia), hyperventilation, atypical migraine, and breath holding.

CLINICAL MANIFESTATIONS

Typical syncopal events usually occur in the upright position or are related to changing position. Syncope may be associated

TABLE 140.1 Syncope and Dizziness: Etiology

DIAGNOSIS	HISTORY	SIGNS/ SYMPTOMS	DESCRIPTION	HEART RATE/ BLOOD PRESSURE	DURATION	POSTSYNCOPE	RECURRENCE
Neurocardiogenic (vasodepressor)	At rest	Pallor, nausea, visual changes	Brief ± convulsion	↓/↓	<1 min	Residual pallor, sweaty, hot; recurs if child stands	Common
OTHER VAGAL							
Micturition	Postvoiding	Pallor, nausea	Brief; convulsions rare	↓/↓	<1 min		(+)
Hair grooming	Standing getting hair done or ears touched	Pallor, nausea, visual changes, lightheaded	Brief		<1 min	Residual pallor, sweaty, hot, can recur if stands too soon	(+)
Cough (deglutition)	Paroxysmal cough	Cough	Abrupt onset	May not change	<5 min	Fatigue or baseline	(+)
Carotid sinus	Tight collar, turned head	Vague, visual changes	Sudden onset, pallor	Usually ↓/↓	<5 min	Fatigue or baseline	(+)
CARDIAC SYNCOPE							
LVOT obstruction	Exercise	± Chest pain, SOB	Abrupt during or after exertion, pallor	↑/↓	Any duration	Fatigue, residual pallor, and sweating	(+)
Pulmonary hypertension	Any time, especially exercise	SOB	Cyanosis and pallor	↑/↓	Any duration	Fatigue, residual cyanosis	(+)
Myocarditis	Post–viral infection exercise	SOB, chest pain, palpitations	Pallor	↑/↓	Any duration	Fatigue	(+)
Tumor or mass	Recumbent, paroxysmal	SOB ± chest pain	Pallor	↑/↓	Any duration	Baseline	(+)
Coronary artery disease	Exercise	SOB ± chest pain	Pallor	↑/↓	Any duration	Fatigue, chest pain	(+)
Dysrhythmia	Any time	Palpitations ± chest pain	Pallor	↑ or ↑/↓	Usually <10 min	Fatigue or baseline	(+)

LVOT, Left ventricular outflow tract; *SOB*, shortness of breath; *±*, with or without; *(+)*, yes but not consistent or predictable.
From Lewis DA. Syncope and dizziness. In: Kliegman RM, ed. Practical Strategies in Pediatric Diagnosis and Therapy. *Philadelphia: WB Saunders; 1996.*

with anxiety, pain, blood drawing or the sight of blood, fasting, a hot environment, or crowded places. The patient often appears pale. A prodrome, consisting of dizziness, lightheadedness, nausea, diaphoresis, visual changes (blacking out), or possibly palpitations, warns the patient and often prevents injury. Unconsciousness lasts for less than 1 minute. A return to normal consciousness occurs relatively quickly. Most of these syncopal episodes are vasovagal or neurocardiogenic in origin. The physical examination is normal.

DIAGNOSTIC STUDIES

Syncopal episodes may require no more than reassurance to the patient and family. If the episodes have a significant impact on daily activities, further evaluation may be indicated. An electrocardiogram (ECG) should be obtained with attention to the QTc and PR intervals (see Chapter 139). Although reassurance and increasing fluid and salt intake may be adequate to treat most cases of syncope, medical management is sometimes indicated.

CHAPTER 141 Chest Pain

Decision-Making Algorithm
Available @ StudentConsult.com

Chest Pain

ETIOLOGY

Chest pain in the pediatric patient often generates a significant amount of patient and parental concern. Although chest pain is rarely cardiac in origin in children, common knowledge about atherosclerotic heart disease raises concerns about a child experiencing chest pain. Most diagnosable chest pain in childhood is musculoskeletal in origin. However, a significant amount remains idiopathic. Knowledge of the complete differential diagnosis is necessary to make an accurate assessment (Table 141.1).

TABLE 141.1 Differential Diagnosis of Pediatric Chest Pain

COMMON
Musculoskeletal
Costochondritis
Trauma or muscle overuse/strain
Pulmonary
Asthma (often exercise induced)
Severe cough
Pneumonia
Gastrointestinal
Reflux esophagitis
Psychogenic
Anxiety, hyperventilation
Miscellaneous
Precordial catch syndrome (Texidor twinge)
Sickle cell vasoocclusive crisis
Idiopathic
UNCOMMON/RARE
Cardiac
Ischemia (coronary artery abnormalities, severe AS or PS, HOCM, cocaine)
Infection/inflammation (myocarditis, pericarditis, Kawasaki disease)
Dysrhythmia
Musculoskeletal
Abnormalities of rib cage/thoracic spine
Tietze syndrome
Slipping rib
Tumor
Pulmonary
Pleurisy
Pneumothorax, pneumomediastinum
Pleural effusion
Pulmonary embolism
Gastrointestinal
Esophageal foreign body
Esophageal spasm
Psychogenic
Conversion symptoms
Somatization disorders
Depression

AS, Aortic stenosis; *HOCM*, hypertrophic obstructive cardiomyopathy; *PS*, pulmonary stenosis.

CLINICAL MANIFESTATIONS

Assessment of a patient with chest pain includes a thorough history to determine activity at the onset; the location, radiation, quality, and duration of the pain; what makes the pain better and worse during the time that it is present; and any associated symptoms. A family history and assessment of how much anxiety the symptom is causing are important and often revealing. A careful general physical examination should focus on the chest wall, heart, lungs, and abdomen. A history of chest pain associated with exertion, syncope, or palpitations or acute onset associated with fever suggests a cardiac etiology. Cardiac causes of chest pain are generally ischemic, inflammatory, or arrhythmic in origin.

DIAGNOSTIC STUDIES

Tests rarely are indicated based on the history. A chest x-ray, electrocardiogram (ECG), 24-hour Holter monitoring, echocardiogram, and exercise stress testing may be obtained based on history and examination. Referral to a pediatric cardiologist is based on the history, physical examination findings, family history, and, frequently, the level of anxiety in the patient or family members regarding the pain.

CHAPTER 142
Dysrhythmias

Decision-Making Algorithm
Available @ StudentConsult.com

Palpitations

ETIOLOGY AND DIFFERENTIAL DIAGNOSIS

Cardiac dysrhythmias or abnormal heart rhythms are uncommon in pediatrics but may be caused by infection and inflammation, structural lesions, metabolic abnormalities, and intrinsic conduction abnormalities (Table 142.1). Many pediatric dysrhythmias are normal variants that do not require treatment or even further evaluation.

Sinus rhythm originates in the sinus node and has a normal axis P wave (upright in leads I and aVF) preceding each QRS complex. Because normal rates vary with age, sinus bradycardia and sinus tachycardia are defined based on age. **Sinus arrhythmia** is a common finding in children and represents a normal variation in the heart rate associated with breathing. The heart rate increases with inspiration and decreases with expiration, producing a recurring pattern on the electrocardiogram (ECG) tracing. Sinus arrhythmia is normal and does not require further evaluation or treatment.

Atrial Dysrhythmias

A **wandering atrial pacemaker** is a change in the morphology of the P waves with variable PR interval and normal QRS complex. This is a benign finding, requiring no further evaluation or treatment.

TABLE 142.1 Etiology of Dysrhythmias
DRUGS
Intoxication (cocaine, tricyclic antidepressants, and others)
Antiarrhythmic agents (proarrhythmic agents [quinidine])
Sympathomimetic agents (caffeine, theophylline, ephedrine, and others)
Digoxin
INFECTION AND POSTINFECTION
Myocarditis
Lyme disease
Endocarditis
Diphtheria
Guillain-Barré syndrome
Rheumatic fever
METABOLIC-ENDOCRINE
Electrolyte disturbances (↓↑K^+, ↓↑Ca^{2+}, ↓Mg^{2+})
Cardiomyopathy
Thyrotoxicosis
Uremia
Pheochromocytoma
Porphyria
Mitochondrial myopathies
STRUCTURAL LESIONS
Congenital heart defects
Ventricular tumor
Ventriculotomy
Arrhythmogenic right ventricle (dysplasia)
OTHER CAUSES
Adrenergic-induced
Prolonged QT interval
Maternal systemic lupus erythematosus
Idiopathic
Central venous catheter

Premature atrial contractions are relatively common prenatally and in infants. A premature P wave, usually with an abnormal axis consistent with its ectopic origin, is present. The premature atrial activity may be blocked (no QRS following it), conducted normally (normal QRS present), or conducted aberrantly (a widened, altered QRS complex). Premature atrial contractions are usually benign and, if present around the time of delivery, usually disappear during the first few weeks of life.

Atrial flutter and **atrial fibrillation** are uncommon dysrhythmias in pediatrics and usually present after surgical repair of complex congenital heart disease. They may also be seen in patients with myocarditis or in association with drug toxicity.

Supraventricular tachycardia (SVT) is the most common symptomatic dysrhythmia in pediatric patients. The rhythm has a rapid, regular rate with a narrow QRS complex. SVT in infants is often 280-300 beats per minute with slower rates for older children and adolescents. The tachycardia has an abrupt onset and termination. In a child with a structurally normal heart, most episodes are relatively asymptomatic other than a pounding heartbeat. If there is structural heart disease or the episode is prolonged (>12 hours), there may be an alteration in the cardiac output and development of symptoms of heart failure. Although most patients with SVT have structurally normal hearts and normal baseline ECGs, some children have Wolff-Parkinson-White syndrome or preexcitation as the cause of the dysrhythmia.

Ventricular Dysrhythmias

Premature ventricular contractions (PVCs) are less common than premature atrial contractions in infancy but more common in older children and adolescents (Table 142.2). The premature beat is not preceded by a P wave, and the QRS complex is wide and bizarre. If the heart is structurally normal, and the PVCs are singleton, uniform in focus, and disappear with increased heart rate, they are usually benign and require no treatment. Any deviation from the presentation (history of syncope or a family history of sudden death) requires further investigation and possibly treatment with antiarrhythmic medications.

Ventricular tachycardia, defined as three or more consecutive PVCs, is also relatively rare in pediatric patients. Although there are multiple causes of ventricular tachycardia, it usually is a sign of serious cardiac dysfunction or disease. Rapid-rate ventricular tachycardia results in decreased cardiac output and cardiovascular instability. Treatment in symptomatic patients is synchronized cardioversion. Medical management with lidocaine or amiodarone may be appropriate in a conscious asymptomatic patient. Complete evaluation of the etiological picture is necessary, including electrophysiological study.

Heart Block

First-degree heart block is the presence of a prolonged PR interval. It is asymptomatic and, when present in otherwise normal children, requires no evaluation or treatment. **Second-degree heart block** is when some, but not all, of the P waves are followed by a QRS complex. Mobitz type I (also known as Wenckebach) is characterized by a progressive prolongation of the PR interval until a QRS complex is dropped. It is often seen during sleep, usually does not progress to other forms of heart block, and does not require further evaluation or treatment in otherwise normal children. Mobitz type II is present when the PR interval does not change, but a QRS is intermittently dropped. This form may progress to complete heart block and may require pacemaker placement. **Third-degree heart block**, whether congenital or acquired, is present when there is no relationship between atrial and ventricular activity. The ventricular rate is much slower than the atrial rate. **Congenital complete heart block** is associated with maternal collagen vascular disease (such as systemic lupus erythematosus or Sjögren syndrome) or congenital heart disease. The acquired form most often occurs after cardiac surgery but may be secondary to infection, inflammation, or drugs.

TREATMENT

Most atrial dysrhythmias require no intervention. Treatment of SVT depends on presentation and symptoms. Acute treatment of SVT in infants usually consists of **vagal maneuvers,** such

TABLE 142.2 Dysrhythmias in Children

TYPE	ELECTROCARDIOGRAM CHARACTERISTICS	TREATMENT
Supraventricular tachycardia	Rate usually >220 beats/min (range, 180-320 beats/min); abnormal atrial rate for age; P waves may be present and are related to QRS complex; normal, narrow QRS complexes unless aberrant conduction is present	Increase vagal tone (bag of ice water to face, Valsalva maneuver); adenosine; digoxin; sotalol; electrical cardioversion if acutely ill; catheter ablation
Atrial flutter	Atrial rate usually 300 beats/min, with varying degrees of block; sawtooth flutter waves	Digoxin, sotalol, cardioversion
Premature ventricular contraction	Premature, wide, unusually shaped QRS complex, with large inverted T wave	None if normal heart and if premature ventricular contractions disappear on exercise; lidocaine, procainamide
Ventricular tachycardia	>3 Premature ventricular beats; AV dissociation; fusion beats, blocked retrograde AV conduction; sustained if >30 sec; rate 120-240 beats/min	Lidocaine, amiodarone, procainamide, propranolol, cardioversion
Ventricular fibrillation	No distinct QRS complex or T waves; irregular undulations with varied amplitude and contour, no conducted pulse	Nonsynchronized cardioversion
Complete heart block	Atria and ventricles have independent pacemakers; AV dissociation; escape-pacemaker is at atrioventricular junction if congenital	Awake rate <55 beats/min in neonate or <40 beats/min in adolescent, or hemodynamic instability requires permanent pacemaker
First-degree heart block	Prolonged PR interval for age	Observe, obtain digoxin level if on therapy
Mobitz type I (Wenckebach) second-degree heart block	Progressive lengthening of PR interval until P wave is not followed by conducted QRS complex	Observe, correct underlying electrolyte or other abnormalities
Mobitz type II second-degree heart block	Sudden nonconduction of P wave with loss of QRS complex without progressive PR interval lengthening	Consider pacemaker
Sinus tachycardia	Rate <240 beats/min	Treat cause (fever), remove sympathomimetic drugs

AV, Atrioventricular.

TABLE 142.3 Classification of Drugs for Antiarrhythmia

CLASS	ACTION	EXAMPLE(S)
I	Depression of phase of depolarization (velocity of upstroke of action potential); sodium channel blockade	
Ia	Prolongation of QRS complex and QT interval	Quinidine, procainamide, disopyramide
Ib	Significant effect on abnormal conduction	Lidocaine, mexiletine, phenytoin, tocainide
Ic	Prolongation of QRS complex and PR interval	Flecainide, propafenone, moricizine?
II	β blockade; slowing of sinus rate; prolongation of PR interval	Propranolol, atenolol, acebutolol
III	Prolongation of action potential; prolongation of PR, QT intervals, QRS complex; sodium and calcium channel blockade	Bretylium, amiodarone, sotalol
IV	Calcium channel blockade; reduction in sinus and AV node pacemaker activity and conduction; prolongation of PR interval	Verapamil and other calcium channel blocking agents

AV, Atrioventricular.

as the application of cold (ice bag) to the face. Intravenous (IV) **adenosine** usually converts the dysrhythmia because the atrioventricular node forms a part of the re-entry circuit in most patients with SVT. In patients with cardiovascular compromise at the time of presentation, **synchronized cardioversion** is indicated using 1-2 J/kg. In patients with palpitations, it is important to document heart rate and rhythm during their symptoms before considering therapeutic options. The frequency, length, and associated symptoms during the episodes, as well as what is required to convert the rhythm, determine the need for ongoing treatment. Some patients require only education regarding the dysrhythmia and follow-up. Ongoing pharmacological management with either digoxin or a β-blocker is usually the first choice when treatment is needed. However, digoxin is contraindicated in patients with Wolff-Parkinson-White syndrome. Additional antiarrhythmic medications are rarely needed. In patients who are symptomatic or for those not wanting to take daily medications, **radiofrequency ablation** may be performed.

A variety of antiarrhythmic agents are used to treat ventricular dysrhythmias that require intervention (Table 142.3). Management of third-degree heart block depends on the ventricular rate and presence of symptoms. Treatment, if needed, often requires placement of a pacemaker.

CHAPTER 143
Acyanotic Congenital Heart Disease

Decision-Making Algorithm
Available @ StudentConsult.com
Heart Murmurs

ETIOLOGY AND EPIDEMIOLOGY

Congenital heart disease occurs in 8 per 1,000 births. The spectrum of lesions ranges from asymptomatic to fatal. Although most cases of congenital heart disease are multifactorial, some lesions are associated with chromosomal disorders, single gene defects, teratogens, or maternal metabolic disease (see Table 139-2).

Congenital heart defects can be divided into three pathophysiological groups (Table 143.1).

1. Left-to-right shunts
2. Right-to-left shunts
3. Obstructive, stenotic lesions

Acyanotic congenital heart disease includes left-to-right shunts resulting in an increase in pulmonary blood flow (patent ductus arteriosus [PDA], ventricular septal defect [VSD], atrial septal defect [ASD]) and obstructive lesions (aortic stenosis, pulmonary stenosis, coarctation of the aorta), which usually have normal pulmonary blood flow.

VENTRICULAR SEPTAL DEFECT

Etiology and Epidemiology

The ventricular septum is a complex structure that can be divided into four components. The largest component is the **muscular septum**. The inlet or posterior septum comprises **endocardial cushion tissue**. The subarterial or **supracristal septum** comprises conotruncal tissue. The **membranous septum** is below the aortic valve and is relatively small. VSDs occur when any of these components fail to develop normally (Fig. 143.1). VSD, the most common congenital heart defect, accounts for 25% of all congenital heart disease. **Perimembranous VSDs** are the most common of all VSDs (67%).

TABLE 143.1 Classification of Congenital Cardiac Defects

	SHUNTING		
STENOTIC	**RIGHT → LEFT**	**LEFT → RIGHT**	**MIXING**
Aortic stenosis	Tetralogy	Patent ductus arteriosus	Truncus
Pulmonary stenosis	Transposition	Ventricular septal defect	TAPVR
Coarctation of the aorta	Tricuspid atresia	Atrial septal defect	HLH

HLH, Hypoplastic left heart syndrome; *TAPVR*, total anomalous pulmonary venous return.

Although the location of the VSD is important prognostically and in approach to repair, the amount of flow crossing a VSD depends on the size of the defect and the pulmonary vascular resistance. Large VSDs are not symptomatic at birth because the pulmonary vascular resistance is normally elevated at this time. As the pulmonary vascular resistance decreases over the first 6-8 weeks of life, the amount of shunt increases, and symptoms may develop.

Clinical Manifestations

Small VSDs with little shunt are often asymptomatic but have a loud murmur. Moderate to large VSDs result in pulmonary overcirculation and heart failure. The typical physical finding with a VSD is a **pansystolic murmur**, usually heard best at the lower left sternal border. There may be a thrill. Large shunts increase flow across the mitral valve causing a **mid-diastolic murmur** at the apex. The splitting of S_2 and intensity of P_2 depend on the pulmonary artery pressure.

Imaging Studies

Electrocardiogram (ECG) and chest x-ray findings depend on the size of the VSD. Small VSDs usually have normal studies. Larger VSDs cause volume overload to the left side of the heart, resulting in ECG findings of left atrial and ventricular enlargement and hypertrophy. A chest x-ray may reveal cardiomegaly, enlargement of the left ventricle, an increase in the pulmonary artery silhouette, and increased pulmonary blood flow. Pulmonary hypertension due to either increased flow or increased pulmonary vascular resistance may lead to right ventricular enlargement and hypertrophy.

Treatment

Approximately one third of all VSDs close spontaneously. Small VSDs usually close spontaneously and, if they do not close, surgical closure may not be required. Initial treatment for moderate to large VSDs includes **diuretics** with some practitioners using **digoxin** and/or **afterload reduction**. Continued

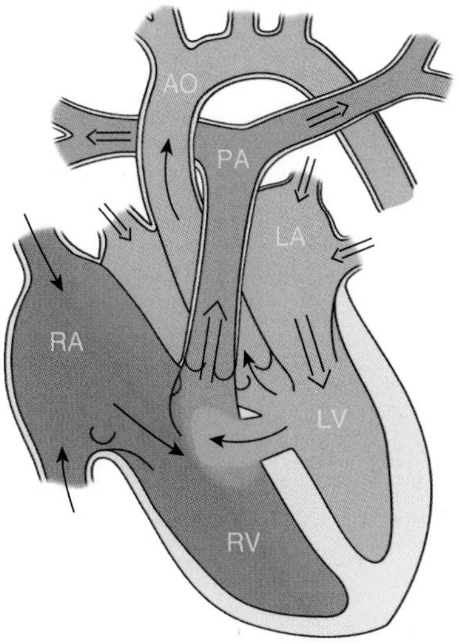

FIGURE 143.1 Ventricular septal defect. *AO*, Aorta; *LA*, left atrium; *LV*, left ventricle; *PA*, pulmonary artery; *RA*, right atrium; *RV*, right ventricle.

poor growth or pulmonary hypertension despite therapy requires closure of the defect. Most VSDs are closed surgically, but some VSDs, especially muscular defects, can be closed with **devices** placed at cardiac catheterization.

ATRIAL SEPTAL DEFECT

Etiology and Epidemiology

During the embryological development of the heart, a septum grows toward the endocardial cushions to divide the atria. Failure of septal growth or excessive reabsorption of tissue leads to ASDs (Fig. 143.2). ASDs represent approximately 10% of all congenital heart defects. A secundum defect, with the hole in the region of the foramen ovale, is the most common ASD. A **primum ASD**, located near the endocardial cushions, may be part of a complete atrioventricular canal defect or may be present with an intact ventricular septum. The least common ASD is the **sinus venosus defect**, which may be associated with anomalous pulmonary venous return.

Clinical Manifestations

The pathophysiology and amount of shunting depend on the size of the defect and the relative compliance of the both ventricles. Even with large ASDs and significant shunts, infants and children are rarely symptomatic. A prominent **right ventricular impulse** at the left lower sternal border (LLSB) often can be palpated. A soft (grade I or II) **systolic ejection murmur** in the region of the right ventricular outflow tract and a **fixed split S_2** (due to overload of the right ventricle with prolonged ejection into the pulmonary circuit) are often audible. A larger shunt may result in a mid-diastolic murmur at the LLSB as a result of the increased volume passing across the tricuspid valve.

Imaging Studies

ECG and chest x-ray findings reflect the **increased blood flow** through the right atrium, right ventricle, pulmonary arteries, and lungs. The ECG may show **right axis deviation** and **right ventricular enlargement**. A chest radiograph may show cardiomegaly, right atrial enlargement, and a prominent pulmonary artery.

Treatment

Medical management is rarely indicated. If a significant shunt is still present at around 3 years of age, closure is usually recommended. Many secundum ASDs can be closed with an ASD **closure device** in the catheterization laboratory. Primum and sinus venosus defects require **surgical closure**.

PATENT DUCTUS ARTERIOSUS

Etiology and Epidemiology

The ductus arteriosus allows blood to flow from the pulmonary artery to the aorta during fetal life. Failure of the normal closure of this vessel results in a PDA (Fig. 143.3). With falling pulmonary vascular resistance after birth, left-to-right shunting of blood and increased pulmonary blood flow occur. Excluding premature infants, PDAs represent approximately 5-10% of congenital heart disease.

Clinical Manifestations

Symptoms depend on the amount of pulmonary blood flow. The magnitude of the shunt depends on the size of the PDA (diameter, length, and tortuosity) and the pulmonary vascular resistance. Small PDAs are asymptomatic; moderate to large shunts can produce the symptoms of heart failure as the pulmonary vascular resistance decreases.

The physical examination findings depend on the size of the shunt. A **widened pulse pressure** is often present as a result of the runoff of blood into the pulmonary circulation during diastole. A **continuous, machine-like murmur** can be heard at the left infraclavicular area, radiating along the pulmonary arteries and often well heard over the left side of the back. Larger shunts with increased flow across the mitral valve may result

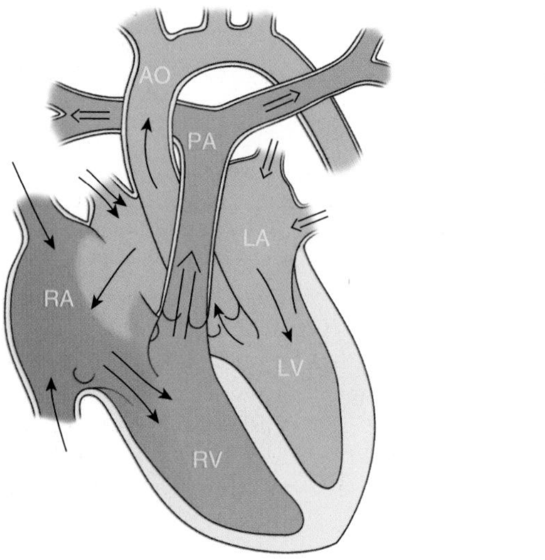

FIGURE 143.2 Atrial septal defect. *AO*, Aorta; *LA*, left atrium; *LV*, left ventricle; *PA*, pulmonary artery; *RA*, right atrium; *RV*, right ventricle.

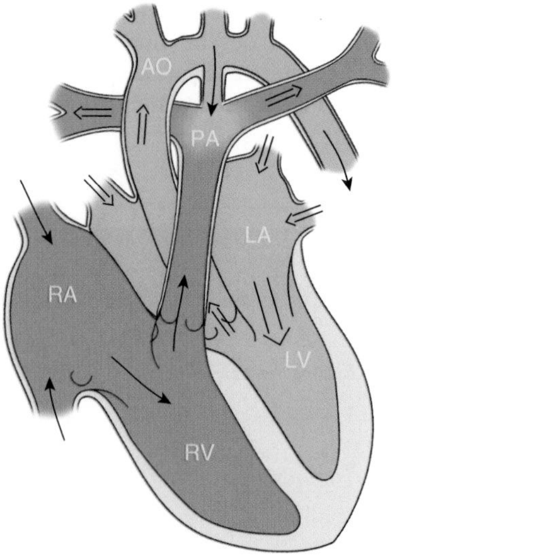

FIGURE 143.3 Patent ductus arteriosus. *AO*, Aorta; *LA*, left atrium; *LV*, left ventricle; *PA*, pulmonary artery; *RA*, right atrium; *RV*, right ventricle.

in a mid-diastolic murmur at the apex and a **hyperdynamic precordium**. Splitting of S_2 and intensity of P_2 depend on the pulmonary artery pressure. A thrill may be palpable.

Imaging Studies

ECG and chest x-ray findings are normal with small PDAs. Moderate to large shunts may result in a **full pulmonary artery silhouette** and **increased pulmonary vascularity**. ECG findings vary from normal to evidence of left ventricular hypertrophy. If pulmonary hypertension is present, there is also right ventricular hypertrophy.

Treatment

Spontaneous closure of a PDA after a few weeks of age is uncommon in full-term infants. Moderate and large PDAs may be managed initially with **diuretics**, but they eventually require closure. Elective closure of small, hemodynamically insignificant PDAs is controversial. Most PDAs can be closed in the catheterization laboratory by either **coil embolization** or a PDA **closure device**.

ENDOCARDIAL CUSHION DEFECT

Etiology and Epidemiology

Endocardial cushion defects, also referred to as **atrioventricular canal defects** or atrioventricular septal defects, may be complete (Fig. 143.4), partial, or transitional. Abnormal development of the endocardial cushion tissue results in failure of the septum to fuse with the endocardial cushion; this results in **abnormal atrioventricular valves** as well. The complete defect results in a primum ASD, a posterior or inlet VSD, and a common atrioventricular valve with anterior and posterior bridging leaflets. Partial and transitional defects have two separate atrioventricular valves, usually with a "cleft" in the anterior leaflet of the left-sided valve. In addition to left-to-right shunting at both levels, there may be **atrioventricular valve insufficiency**.

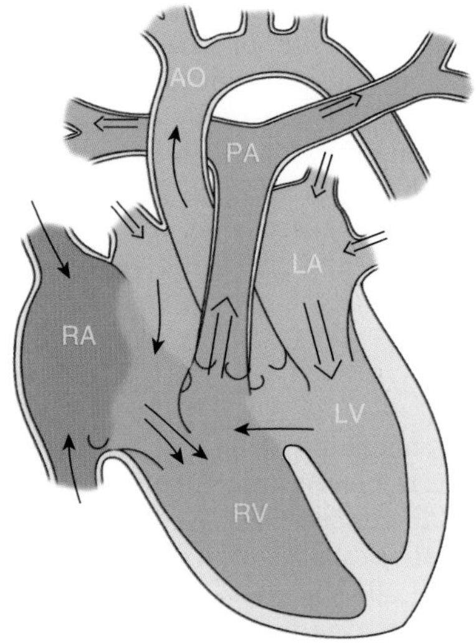

FIGURE 143.4 Atrioventricular canal defects. *AO*, Aorta; *LA*, left atrium; *LV*, left ventricle; *PA*, pulmonary artery; *RA*, right atrium; *RV*, right ventricle.

Clinical Manifestations

The symptoms of heart failure usually develop as the pulmonary vascular resistance decreases over the first 6-8 weeks of life. Symptoms may be earlier and more severe with significant atrioventricular valve insufficiency. Pulmonary hypertension is present due to the increased pulmonary blood flow and pulmonary vascular obstructive disease may develop early, especially in patients with Trisomy 21. The presence of murmurs varies depending on the amount of shunting at both atrial and ventricular levels. If there is a large VSD component, S_2 will be single. Growth is usually poor. This is the most common congenital heart defect in children with Trisomy 21.

Imaging Tests

The diagnosis usually is made with echocardiography. A chest radiograph reveals cardiomegaly with enlargement of all chambers and the presence of **increased vascularity**. An ECG reveals **left axis deviation** and **combined ventricular hypertrophy** and may show combined atrial enlargement.

Treatment

Initial management includes diuretics. Some practitioners use afterload reduction for treatment of heart failure but, ultimately, surgical repair of the defect is required.

PULMONARY STENOSIS

Etiology

Pulmonary stenosis accounts for approximately 10% of all congenital heart disease and can be **valvular**, **subvalvular**, or **supravalvular** in nature. Pulmonary stenosis results from the failure of the development, in early gestation, of the three leaflets of the valve, insufficient resorption of infundibular tissue, or insufficient canalization of the peripheral pulmonary arteries.

Clinical Manifestations

Symptoms depend on the degree of obstruction present. Mild pulmonary stenosis is asymptomatic. Moderate to severe stenosis results in **exertional dyspnea** and easy **fatigability**. Newborns with severe stenosis may be more symptomatic and even cyanotic because of right-to-left shunting at the atrial level.

Pulmonary stenosis causes a systolic ejection murmur at the second left intercostal space, which radiates to the back. A thrill may be present. S_2 may be widely split with a quiet pulmonary component. With more severe pulmonary stenosis, an impulse at the lower left sternal border results from **right ventricular hypertrophy**. Valvular stenosis may result in a **click** that varies with respiration. Worsening stenosis causes an increase in the duration of the murmur and a higher frequency of the sound. The systolic ejection murmurs of **peripheral pulmonary stenosis** are heard distal to the site of obstruction in the pulmonary circulation, including radiation to the axillae and back.

Imaging Tests

ECG and chest x-ray findings are normal in mild stenosis. Moderate to severe stenosis results in **right axis deviation** and **right ventricular hypertrophy**. The heart size is usually normal on chest x-ray, although **dilation of the main pulmonary artery** may be seen. Echocardiography provides assessment of the site of stenosis, degree of hypertrophy, valve morphology, as well as an estimate of the pressure gradient.

Treatment

Valvular pulmonary stenosis usually does not progress, especially if it is mild. **Balloon valvuloplasty** is usually successful in reducing the gradient to acceptable levels for more significant or symptomatic stenosis. **Surgical repair** is required if balloon valvuloplasty is unsuccessful or when subvalvular (muscular) stenosis is present.

AORTIC STENOSIS

Etiology and Epidemiology

Valvular, **subvalvular**, or **supravalvular** aortic stenosis represents approximately 5% of all congenital heart disease. Lesions result from failure of development of the three leaflets or failure of resorption of tissue around the valve.

Clinical Manifestations

Mild to moderate obstructions cause no symptoms. More severe stenosis results in easy fatigability, exertional chest pain, and syncope. Infants with critical aortic stenosis may present with symptoms of heart failure.

A **systolic ejection murmur** is heard at the right second intercostal space along the sternum and radiating into the neck. The murmur increases in length and becomes higher in frequency as the degree of stenosis increases. With valvular stenosis, a **systolic ejection click** often is heard, and a thrill may be present at the right upper sternal border or in the suprasternal notch. The aortic component of S_2 may be decreased in intensity.

Imaging Studies

ECG and chest x-ray findings are normal with mild degrees of stenosis. **Left ventricular hypertrophy** develops with moderate to severe stenosis and is detected on the ECG and chest x-ray. **Dilation** of the ascending aorta or aortic knob due to an intrinsic aortopathy may be seen on chest radiographs. Echocardiography shows the site of stenosis, valve morphology, and the presence of left ventricular hypertrophy, and it allows an estimate of the pressure gradient.

Treatment

The degree of aortic stenosis frequently progresses with growth and age. Aortic insufficiency often develops or progresses. Serial follow-up with echocardiography is indicated. **Balloon valvuloplasty** is usually the first interventional procedure for significant stenosis. It is not as successful as pulmonary balloon valvuloplasty and has a higher risk of significant valvular insufficiency. **Surgical management** is necessary when balloon valvuloplasty is unsuccessful or significant valve insufficiency develops.

COARCTATION OF THE AORTA

Etiology and Epidemiology

Coarctation of the aorta occurs in approximately 10% of all congenital heart defects. It is almost always **juxtaductal** in position. During development of the aortic arch, the area near the insertion of the ductus arteriosus fails to develop correctly, resulting in a narrowing of the aortic lumen.

Clinical Manifestations

Timing of presentation depends on the severity of obstruction and associated cardiac defects. Infants presenting with coarctation of the aorta frequently have hypoplastic aortic arches, abnormal aortic valves, and VSDs. They may be dependent on a PDA to provide descending aortic flow. Symptoms develop when the aortic ampulla of the ductus closes. Less severe obstruction causes no symptoms.

Symptoms, including poor feeding, respiratory distress, and shock, may develop before 2 weeks of age. Classically, the **femoral pulses** are weaker and delayed compared with the right radial pulse. The blood pressure in the lower extremities is lower than that in the upper extremities. However, if cardiac function is poor, these differences may not be as apparent until appropriate resuscitation is accomplished. In this situation, there may be no murmur, but an $\mathbf{S_3}$ is often present.

Older children presenting with coarctation of the aorta are usually asymptomatic. There may be a history of **leg discomfort** with exercise, headache, or epistaxis. Decreased or absent lower extremity pulses, **hypertension** (upper extremity), or a murmur may be present. The murmur is typically best heard in the left interscapular area of the back. If significant collaterals have developed, continuous murmurs may be heard throughout the chest. An abnormal aortic valve is present approximately 50% of the time, causing a systolic ejection click and systolic ejection murmur of aortic stenosis.

Imaging Studies

The ECG and chest x-ray show evidence of right ventricular enlargement and hypertrophy in infantile coarctation with marked **cardiomegaly** and **pulmonary edema**. Echocardiography shows the site of coarctation and associated lesions. In older children, the ECG and chest x-ray usually show left ventricular hypertrophy and a mildly enlarged heart. **Rib notching** may also be seen in older children (>8 years of age) with large collaterals. Echocardiography shows the site and degree of coarctation, the presence of left ventricular hypertrophy, and the aortic valve morphology and function.

Treatment

Management of an infant presenting with cardiac decompensation includes intravenous infusion of **prostaglandin** $\mathbf{E_1}$ (chemically opens the ductus arteriosus), inotropic agents, diuretics, and other supportive care. **Balloon angioplasty** has been done, especially in critically ill infants, but **surgical repair** of the coarctation is most commonly performed. Ballooning and stenting of older patients with coarctation has become more accepted as primary therapy, but surgical repair remains a common form of management.

CHAPTER 144
Cyanotic Congenital Heart Disease

Decision-Making Algorithms
Available @ StudentConsult.com

Cyanosis
Heart Murmurs

Cyanotic congenital heart disease occurs when some of the systemic venous return crosses from the right side of the heart to the left and returns to the body without going through the lungs **(right-to-left shunt)**. **Cyanosis**, the visible sign of this shunt, occurs when approximately 5 g/100 mL of reduced hemoglobin is present in systemic blood. Thus a polycythemic patient appears cyanotic with a higher oxygen saturation than a normocythemic patient. A patient with anemia requires a higher percentage of reduced hemoglobin (lower saturation) for the recognition of cyanosis.

The most common cyanotic congenital heart defects are the five *Ts*:
1. Tetralogy of Fallot
2. Transposition of the great arteries
3. Tricuspid atresia
4. Truncus arteriosus
5. Total anomalous pulmonary venous return

Other congenital heart defects that allow complete mixing of systemic and pulmonary venous return can present with cyanosis depending on the amount of pulmonary blood flow that is present. Many cyanotic heart lesions present in the neonatal period (Table 144.1).

TETRALOGY OF FALLOT

Etiology and Epidemiology

Tetralogy of Fallot is the most common cyanotic congenital heart defect, representing about 10% of all congenital heart defects (Fig. 144.1). There are four structural defects: **ventricular septal defect (VSD), pulmonary stenosis, overriding aorta,** and **right ventricular hypertrophy**. Tetralogy of Fallot is due to abnormal septation of the truncus arteriosus into the aorta and pulmonary artery that occurs early in gestation (3-4 weeks). The VSD is large, and the pulmonary stenosis is most commonly subvalvular or infundibular. It may also be valvular, supravalvular, or, frequently, a combination of levels of obstruction.

Clinical Manifestations

Infants initially may be acyanotic. A **pulmonary stenosis murmur** is the usual initial abnormal finding. The amount of right-to-left shunting at the VSD (and the degree of cyanosis) increases as the degree of pulmonary stenosis increases. With increasing severity of pulmonary stenosis, the murmur becomes shorter and softer. In addition to varying degrees of cyanosis and a murmur, a **single S_2** and **right ventricular impulse** at the left sternal border are typical findings.

TABLE 144.1 Categories of Presenting Symptoms and Signs in the Neonate

SYMPTOM/SIGN	PHYSIOLOGICAL CATEGORY	ANATOMICAL CAUSE	LESION
Cyanosis with respiratory distress	Increased pulmonary blood flow	Transposition	d-Transposition with or without associated lesions
Cyanosis without respiratory distress	Decreased pulmonary blood flow	Right heart obstruction	Tricuspid atresia
			Ebstein anomaly
			Pulmonary atresia
			Pulmonary stenosis
			Tetralogy of Fallot
Hypoperfusion	Poor cardiac output	Left heart obstruction	Total anomalous pulmonary venous return with obstruction
			Aortic stenosis
			Hypoplastic left heart syndrome
	Poor cardiac function	Normal anatomy	Cardiomyopathy
			Myocarditis
Respiratory distress with desaturation (not visible cyanosis)	Bidirectional shunting	Complete mixing	Truncus arteriosus
			AV canal
			Complex single ventricle (including heterotaxias) without pulmonary stenosis
Respiratory distress with normal saturation	Left-to-right shunting	Simple intracardiac shunt	ASD
			VSD
			PDA
			Aortopulmonary window
			AVM

ASD, Atrial septal defect; *AV*, atrioventricular; *AVM*, arteriovenous malformation; *PDA*, patent ductus arteriosus; *VSD*, ventricular septal defect.

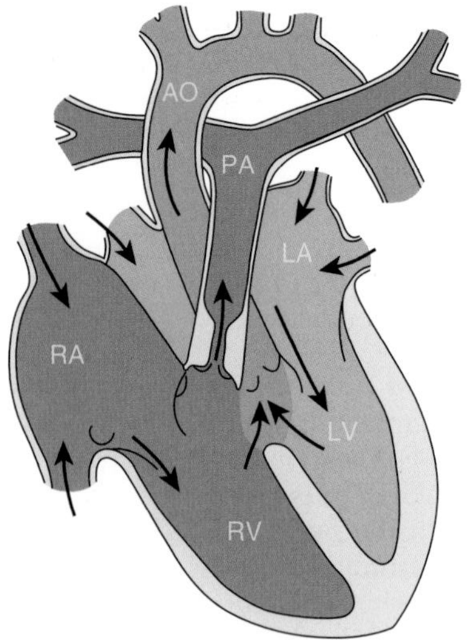

FIGURE 144.1 Tetralogy of Fallot. *AO*, Aorta; *LA*, left atrium; *LV*, left ventricle; *PA*, pulmonary artery; *RA*, right atrium; *RV*, right ventricle.

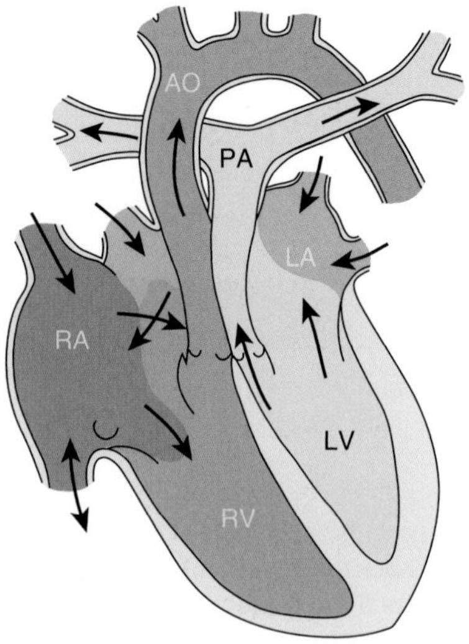

FIGURE 144.2 Transposition of the great vessels. *AO*, Aorta; *LA*, left atrium; *LV*, left ventricle; *PA*, pulmonary artery; *RA*, right atrium; *RV*, right ventricle.

When **hypoxic (Tet) spells** occur, they are usually progressive. During a spell, the child typically becomes restless and agitated and may cry inconsolably. An ambulatory toddler may squat. Hyperpnea occurs with gradually increasing cyanosis and loss of the murmur. In severe spells, prolonged unconsciousness and convulsions, hemiparesis, or death may occur. Independent of hypoxic spells, patients with unrepaired tetralogy of Fallot are at increased risk for cerebral thromboembolism and cerebral abscesses resulting, in part, from their right-to-left intracardiac shunt.

Imaging Studies

The electrocardiogram (ECG) usually has **right axis deviation** and **right ventricular hypertrophy**. The classic chest x-ray finding is a **boot-shaped heart** created by the small main pulmonary artery and upturned apex secondary to right ventricular hypertrophy. Echocardiography shows the anatomical features, including the anatomical level and quantification of pulmonary stenosis. Coronary anomalies, most commonly a left anterior descending coronary artery arising from the right coronary artery and crossing the anterior surface of the right ventricular outflow tract, are present in 5% of patients with tetralogy of Fallot.

Treatment

The natural history of tetralogy of Fallot is progression of pulmonary stenosis and cyanosis. Treatment of hypoxic spells consists of oxygen administration and placing the child in the knee-chest position (to increase venous return). Traditionally, morphine sulfate is given (to relax the pulmonary infundibulum and for sedation). If necessary, the systemic vascular resistance can be increased acutely through the administration of an α-adrenergic agonist (phenylephrine). The occurrence of a cyanotic spell is an indication to proceed with surgical repair.

Complete surgical repair with VSD closure and removal or patching of the pulmonary stenosis can be performed in infancy. Occasionally, **palliative shunt surgery** between the subclavian artery and pulmonary artery is performed for complex forms of tetralogy of Fallot and more complete repair is done at a later time. **Subacute bacterial endocarditis prophylaxis** is indicated until 6 months after complete repair unless there is a residual VSD. Prophylaxis is then continued as long as there is a residual VSD.

TRANSPOSITION OF THE GREAT ARTERIES

Etiology and Epidemiology

Although dextroposed transposition of the great arteries represents only about 5% of congenital heart defects, it is the most common cyanotic lesion to present in the newborn period (Fig. 144.2). Transposition of the great arteries is ventriculoarterial discordance secondary to abnormalities of septation of the truncus arteriosus. In dextroposed transposition, the aorta arises from the right ventricle, anterior and to the right of the pulmonary artery, which arises from the left ventricle. This results in desaturated blood returning to the right side of the heart and being pumped back out to the body, while well-oxygenated blood returning from the lungs enters the left side of the heart and is pumped back to the lungs. Without mixing of the two circulations, death occurs quickly. Mixing can occur at the atrial (patent foramen ovale/atrial septal defect [ASD]), VSD, or great vessel (patent ductus arteriosus [PDA]) level.

Clinical Manifestations

A history of **cyanosis** is always present, although it depends on the amount of mixing. **Quiet tachypnea** and a **single S_2** are typically present. If the ventricular septum is intact, there may be no murmur.

Children with transposition and a large VSD have improved intracardiac mixing and less cyanosis. They may present with signs of heart failure. The heart is hyperdynamic, with palpable left and right ventricular impulses. A loud VSD murmur is heard. S_2 is single.

Imaging Studies

ECG findings typically include **right axis deviation** and **right ventricular hypertrophy**. The chest x-ray reveals **increased pulmonary vascularity**, and the cardiac shadow is classically an **egg on a string** created by the narrow superior mediastinum. Echocardiography shows the transposition of the great arteries, the sites and amount of mixing, and any associated lesions.

Treatment

Initial medical management includes **prostaglandin E_1** to maintain ductal patency. If significant hypoxia persists on prostaglandin therapy, a **balloon atrial septostomy** improves mixing between the two circulations. Complete surgical repair is most often an **arterial switch**. The arterial switch usually is performed within the first 2 weeks of life, when the left ventricle can still maintain systemic pressure.

TRICUSPID ATRESIA

Etiology and Epidemiology

Tricuspid atresia accounts for approximately 2% of all congenital heart defects (Fig. 144.3). The absence of the tricuspid valve results in a **hypoplastic right ventricle**. All systemic venous return must cross the atrial septum into the left atrium. A PDA or VSD is necessary for pulmonary blood flow and survival.

Clinical Manifestations

Infants with tricuspid atresia are usually **severely cyanotic** and have a **single S_2**. If a VSD is present, there may be a murmur. A diastolic murmur across the mitral valve may be audible. Frequently there is no significant murmur.

Imaging Studies

The ECG shows **left ventricular hypertrophy** and a **superior QRS axis** (between 0 and −90 degrees). The chest x-ray reveals a normal or mildly enlarged cardiac silhouette with **decreased pulmonary blood flow**. Echocardiography shows the anatomy, associated lesions, and source of pulmonary blood flow.

Treatment

Management initially depends on the presence of a VSD and the amount of antegrade blood flow to the lungs. If there is no VSD, or it is small, prostaglandin E_1 maintains pulmonary blood flow until surgery. Surgery is staged with an initial subclavian artery-to-pulmonary shunt **(Blalock-Taussig procedure)** typically followed by a two-stage procedure: **bidirectional cavopulmonary shunt (bidirectional Glenn)** and **Fontan procedure**. These surgeries direct systemic venous return directly to the pulmonary arteries.

TRUNCUS ARTERIOSUS

Etiology and Epidemiology

Truncus arteriosus occurs in less than 1% of all cases of congenital heart disease (Fig. 144.4). It results from the failure of septation of the truncus during the first 3-4 weeks of gestation. A single arterial trunk arises from the heart with a large VSD immediately below the truncal valve. The pulmonary arteries arise from the single arterial trunk either as a single vessel that divides or individually from the arterial trunk to the lungs.

Clinical Manifestations

Varying degrees of cyanosis depend on the amount of pulmonary blood flow. If not diagnosed at birth, the infant may develop signs of heart failure as pulmonary vascular resistance decreases. The signs then include tachypnea and cough. Peripheral pulses are usually bounding as a result of the diastolic runoff into the pulmonary arteries. A single S_2 is due to the single valve. There may be a systolic ejection click, and there is often a **systolic murmur** at the left sternal border.

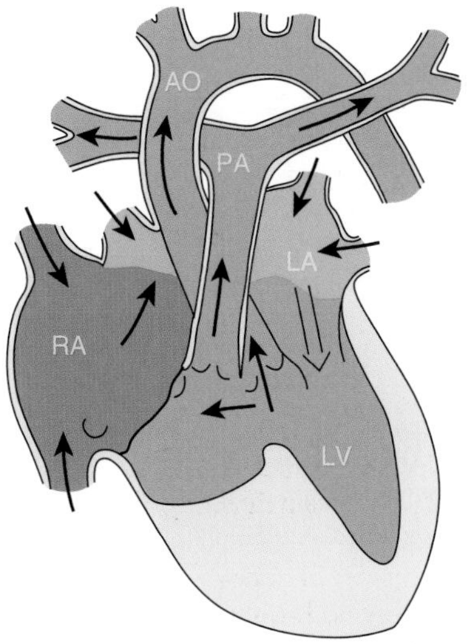

FIGURE 144.3 Tricuspid atresia with ventricular septal defect. *AO*, Aorta; *LA*, left atrium; *LV*, left ventricle; *PA*, pulmonary artery; *RA*, right atrium.

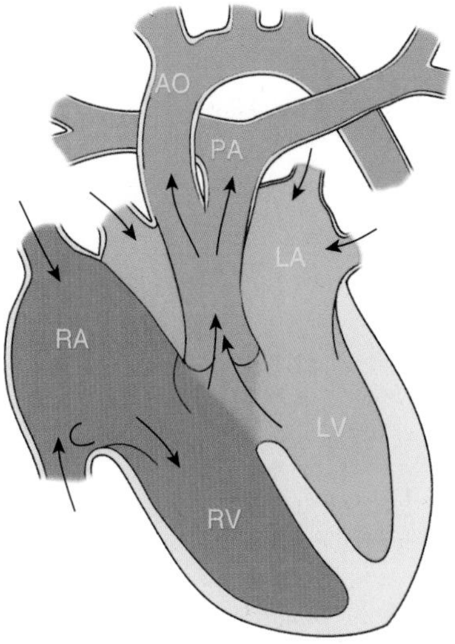

FIGURE 144.4 Truncus arteriosus. *AO*, Aorta; *LA*, left atrium; *LV*, left ventricle; *PA*, pulmonary artery; *RA*, right atrium; *RV*, right ventricle.

Imaging Studies

ECG findings include **combined ventricular hypertrophy** and **cardiomegaly**. A chest x-ray usually reveals **increased pulmonary blood** and may show displaced pulmonary arteries. Echocardiography defines the anatomy, including the VSD, truncal valve function, and origin of the pulmonary arteries.

Treatment

Medical management is usually needed and includes **anticongestive medications**. **Surgical repair** includes VSD closure and placement of a conduit between the right ventricle and pulmonary arteries.

TOTAL ANOMALOUS PULMONARY VENOUS RETURN

Etiology and Epidemiology

Total anomalous pulmonary venous return accounts for about 1% of congenital heart disease (Fig. 144.5). Disruption of the development of normal pulmonary venous drainage during the third week of gestation results in one of four abnormalities. All of the pulmonary veins fail to connect to the left atrium and return abnormally via the right side of the heart. They may have **supracardiac, infracardiac, cardiac,** or **mixed drainage.** An atrial-level communication is required for systemic cardiac output and survival.

Clinical Manifestations

The most important determinant of presentation is the presence or absence of **obstruction** to the pulmonary venous drainage. Infants without obstruction have minimal cyanosis and may be asymptomatic. There is a hyperactive **right ventricular impulse** with a **widely split S_2** (owing to increased right ventricular volume) and a **systolic ejection murmur** at the left upper sternal border. There is usually a mid-diastolic murmur at the lower left sternal border from the increased flow across the tricuspid valve. Growth is relatively poor. Infants with **obstruction** present with cyanosis, marked tachypnea and dyspnea, and signs of right-sided heart failure including hepatomegaly. The obstruction results in little, if any, increase in right ventricular volume, so there may be no murmur or changes in S_2.

Imaging Studies

For infants without obstruction, the ECG is consistent with right ventricular volume overload. Cardiomegaly with increased pulmonary blood flow is seen on chest x-ray. Infants with obstructed veins have right axis deviation and right ventricular hypertrophy on ECG. On chest x-ray, the heart is normal or mildly enlarged with varying degrees of pulmonary edema that can appear similar to hyaline membrane disease or pneumonia. Echocardiography shows the volume-overloaded right side of the heart, right-to-left atrial level shunting, and common pulmonary vein site of drainage and degree of obstruction.

Treatment

At **surgery**, the common pulmonary vein is opened into the left atrium, and there is ligation of any vein or channel that had been draining the common vein.

HYPOPLASTIC LEFT HEART SYNDROME

Etiology and Epidemiology

Hypoplastic left heart syndrome accounts for 1% of all congenital heart defects (Fig. 144.6) but is the most common cause of death from cardiac defects in the first month of life. Hypoplastic left heart syndrome occurs when there is failure of development of the mitral or aortic valve or the aortic arch. A small left ventricle that is unable to support normal systemic circulation is a central finding, regardless of etiology. Associated degrees of hypoplasia of the ascending aorta and aortic arch are present. Left-to-right shunting occurs at the atrial level.

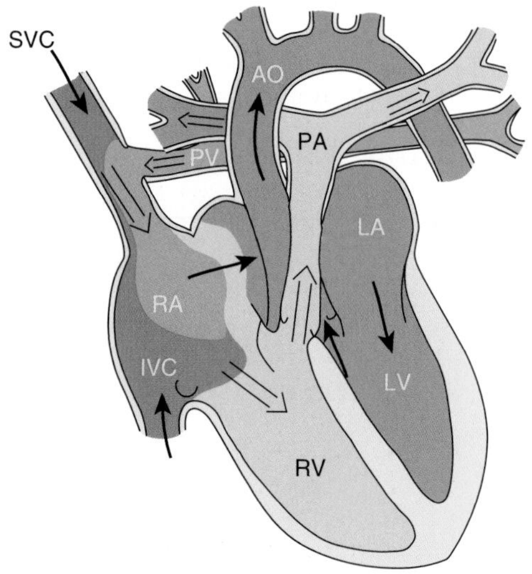

FIGURE 144.5 Total anomalous pulmonary venous return. *AO*, Aorta; *IVC*, inferior vena cava; *LA*, left atrium; *LV*, left ventricle; *PA*, pulmonary artery; *PV*, pulmonary vein; *RA*, right atrium; *RV*, right ventricle; *SVC*, superior vena cava.

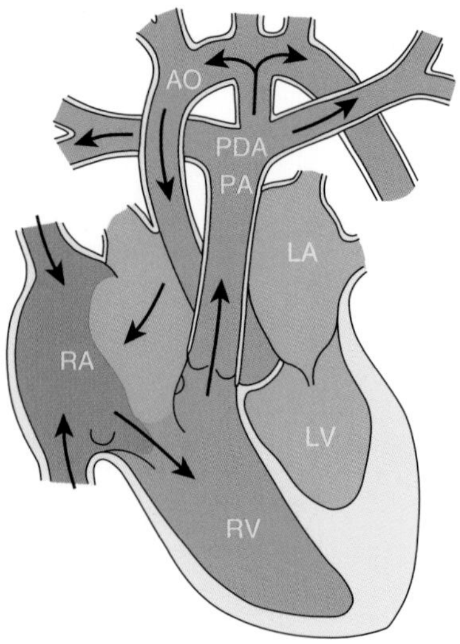

FIGURE 144.6 Hypoplastic left side of the heart. *AO*, Aorta; *LA*, left atrium; *LV*, left ventricle; *PA*, pulmonary artery; *PDA*, patent ductus arteriosus; *RA*, right atrium; *RV*, right ventricle.

TABLE 144.2 Extracardiac Complications of Cyanotic Congenital Heart Disease

PROBLEM	ETIOLOGY	THERAPY
Polycythemia	Persistent hypoxia	Phlebotomy
Relative anemia	Nutritional deficiency	Iron replacement
CNS abscess	Right-to-left shunting	Antibiotics, drainage
CNS thromboembolic stroke	Right-to-left shunting or polycythemia	Phlebotomy
Gingival disease	Polycythemia, gingivitis, bleeding	Dental hygiene
Gout	Polycythemia, diuretic agents	Allopurinol
Arthritis, clubbing	Hypoxic arthropathy	None
Pregnancy	Poor placental perfusion, poor ability to increase cardiac output	Bed rest
Infectious disease	Associated asplenia, DiGeorge syndrome	Antibiotics
	Fatal RSV pneumonia with pulmonary hypertension	Ribavirin, RSV immune globulin
Growth	Failure to thrive, increased oxygen consumption, decreased nutrient intake	Treat heart failure; correct defect early
Psychosocial adjustment	Limited activity, peer pressure; chronic disease, multiple hospitalizations, cardiac surgical techniques	Counseling

CNS, Central nervous system; *RSV*, respiratory syncytial virus.

Clinical Manifestations

The newborn is dependent on right-to-left shunting at the ductus arteriosus for systemic blood flow. As the ductus arteriosus constricts, the infant becomes critically ill with signs and symptoms of heart failure from excessive pulmonary blood flow and obstruction of systemic blood flow. Pulses are diffusely weak or absent. S_2 is single and loud. There is usually no heart murmur. Cyanosis may be minimal, but **low cardiac output** gives a grayish color to the cool, mottled skin.

Imaging Studies

ECG findings include **right ventricular hypertrophy** with **decreased left ventricular forces**. The chest x-ray reveals **cardiomegaly** (with right-sided enlargement) and pulmonary venous congestion or pulmonary edema. Echocardiography shows the small left side of the heart, the degree of stenosis of the aortic and mitral valves, the hypoplastic ascending aorta, and the adequacy of left-to-right atrial flow and right-to-left ductal flow.

Treatment

Medical management includes **prostaglandin E_1** to open the ductus arteriosus, correction of acidosis, and ventilatory and blood pressure support as needed. **Surgical repair** is staged with the first surgery (Norwood or Sano procedure) done during the newborn period. Subsequent procedures create a systemic source for the pulmonary circulation (bidirectional Glenn and Fontan procedures), leaving the right ventricle to supply systemic circulation. There have been many modifications to all three stages of the repair. Prognosis for survival has improved significantly over the past two decades.

COMPLICATIONS OF CONGENITAL HEART DISEASE

Extracardiac complications are summarized in Table 144.2.

CHAPTER 145

Heart Failure

ETIOLOGY AND EPIDEMIOLOGY

The force generated by the cardiac muscle fiber depends on its contractile status and basal length, which is equivalent to the preload. As the preload (fiber length, left ventricular filling pressure, or volume) increases, myocardial performance (stroke volume and wall tension) increases up to a point (the normal Starling curve). The relationship is the **ventricular function curve** (Fig. 145.1). Alterations in the contractile state of the muscle lower the relative position of the curve but retain the relationship of fiber length to muscle work. The cardiac output equals stroke volume times the heart rate; thus heart rate is another important determinant of cardiac work. Additional factors also affect cardiac performance (Table 145.1).

Heart failure occurs when the heart is unable to pump blood at a rate commensurate with metabolic needs (inadequate oxygen delivery). It may be due to a change in **myocardial contractility** that results in low cardiac output or to **abnormal loading conditions** being placed on the myocardium. The abnormal loading conditions may be **afterload** (pressure overload, such as with aortic stenosis, pulmonary stenosis, or coarctation of the aorta) or **preload** (volume overload, such as in ventricular septal defect [VSD], patent ductus arteriosus (PDA), or valvular insufficiency). Volume overload is the most common cause of heart failure in children.

The age of presentation is helpful in creating the differential diagnosis (Table 145.2). In the first weeks of life, excessive afterload being placed on the myocardium is most common. Heart failure presenting around 2 months of age is usually due to increasing left-to-right shunts that become apparent as the pulmonary vascular resistance decreases. Acquired heart disease, such as myocarditis and cardiomyopathy, can present at any age.

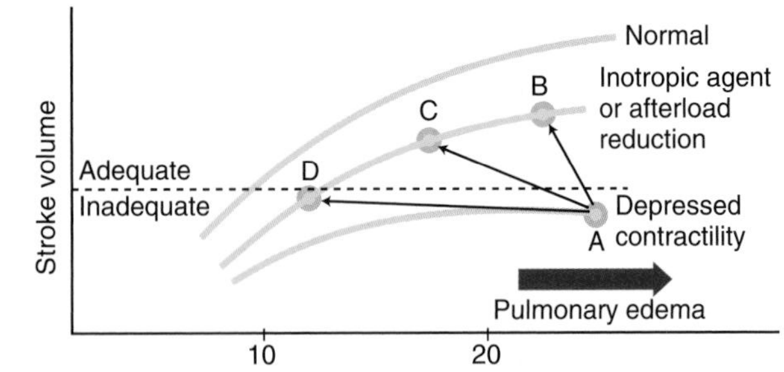

FIGURE 145.1 Ventricular function curve illustrating the effect of inotropic agents or arterial vasodilators. In contrast to diuretics, the effect of digitalis or arterial vasodilator therapy in a patient with heart failure is movement onto another ventricular function curve, which is intermediate between the normal and the depressed curves. When the patient's ventricular function moves from *A* to *B* by the administration of one of these agents, the left ventricular end-diastolic pressure may also decrease because of improved cardiac function; further administration of diuretics or venodilators may shift the function further to the left along the same curve from *B* to *C* and eliminate the risk of pulmonary edema. A vasodilating agent that has arteriolar and venous dilating properties (e.g., nitroprusside) would shift this function directly from *A* to *C*. If this agent shifts the function from *A* to *D* because of excessive venodilation or the administration of diuretics, the cardiac output may decrease too much, even though the left ventricular end-diastolic pressure would be normal (10 mm Hg) for a normal heart. Left ventricular end-diastolic pressures of 15-18 mm Hg are usually optimal in the failing heart to maximize cardiac output, but to avoid pulmonary edema. (From Andreoli TE, Carpenter CCJ, Griggs RC, Loscalzo J, eds. *Cecil Essentials of Medicine*. 5th ed. Philadelphia: Saunders; 2001.)

CLINICAL MANIFESTATIONS

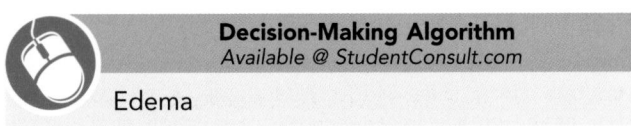

Decision-Making Algorithm
Available @ StudentConsult.com

Edema

Heart failure presents in infants as poor feeding, failure to thrive, tachypnea, and diaphoresis with feeding. Older children may present with shortness of breath, easy fatigability, and edema. The physical examination findings depend on whether pulmonary venous congestion, systemic venous congestion, or both are present. Tachycardia, a gallop rhythm, and thready pulses may be present with either cause. If left-sided failure is predominant, tachypnea, orthopnea, wheezing, and pulmonary edema are seen. Hepatomegaly, edema, and distended neck veins are signs of right-sided failure.

IMAGING STUDIES

The absence of cardiomegaly on a chest x-ray usually rules out the diagnosis of heart failure. An echocardiogram assesses the heart chamber sizes, measures myocardial function, and diagnoses congenital heart defects when present.

TABLE 145.1 Factors Affecting Cardiac Performance

PRELOAD (LEFT VENTRICULAR DIASTOLIC VOLUME)
Total blood volume
Venous tone (sympathetic tone)
Body position
Intrathoracic and intrapericardial pressure
Atrial contraction
Pumping action of skeletal muscle
AFTERLOAD (IMPEDANCE AGAINST WHICH THE LEFT VENTRICLE MUST EJECT BLOOD)
Peripheral vascular resistance
Left ventricular volume (preload, wall tension)
Physical characteristics of the arterial tree (elasticity of vessels or presence of outflow obstruction)
CONTRACTILITY (CARDIAC PERFORMANCE INDEPENDENT OF PRELOAD OR AFTERLOAD)
Sympathetic nerve impulses*
Circulating catecholamines*
Digitalis, calcium, other inotropic agents*
Increased heart rate or postextrasystolic augmentation*
Anoxia, acidosis†
Pharmacological depression†
Loss of myocardium†
Intrinsic depression†
HEART RATE
Autonomic nervous system
Temperature, metabolic rate

*Increases contractility.
†Decreases contractility.
From Andreoli TE, Carpenter CCJ, Griggs RC, Loscalzo J. Cecil Essentials of Medicine. 5th ed. Philadelphia: Saunders; 2001.

TREATMENT

Initial treatment is directed at improving myocardial function and optimizing preload and afterload. Diuretics, inotropic support, and, often, **afterload reduction** are employed (Table 145.3). Long-term therapy usually consists of diuretics followed by afterload reduction. Long-term therapy with **β-blockers** also may be beneficial, although this remains somewhat controversial in pediatric patients. Spironolactone is usually added to the medical regimen because of its effect on cardiac remodeling.

TABLE 145.2 Etiology of Heart Failure by Age Group

FETUS
Severe anemia (hemolysis, fetal-maternal transfusion, hypoplastic anemia)
Supraventricular tachycardia
Ventricular tachycardia
Complete heart block
Atrioventricular valve insufficiency
High-output cardiac failure (arteriovenous malformation, teratoma)
PREMATURE NEONATE
Fluid overload
PDA
VSD
Cor pulmonale (BPD)
FULL-TERM NEONATE
Asphyxial cardiomyopathy
Arteriovenous malformation (vein of Galen, hepatic)
Left-sided obstructive lesions (coarctation of aorta, hypoplastic left heart, critical aortic stenosis)
Transposition of great arteries
Large mixing cardiac defects (single ventricle, truncus arteriosus)
Viral myocarditis
Anemia
Supraventricular tachycardia
Complete heart block
INFANT/TODDLER
Left-to-right cardiac shunts (VSD)
Hemangioma (arteriovenous malformation)
Anomalous left coronary artery
Metabolic cardiomyopathy
Acute hypertension (hemolytic uremic syndrome)
Supraventricular tachycardia
Kawasaki disease
Postoperative repair of congenital heart disease
CHILD/ADOLESCENT
Rheumatic fever
Acute hypertension (glomerulonephritis)
Viral myocarditis
Thyrotoxicosis
Hemochromatosis/hemosiderosis
Cancer therapy (radiation, doxorubicin)
Sickle cell anemia
Endocarditis
Cor pulmonale (cystic fibrosis)
Arrhythmias
Chronic upper airway obstruction (cor pulmonale)
Unrepaired or palliated congenital heart disease
Cardiomyopathy

BPD, Bronchopulmonary dysplasia; *PDA*, patent ductus arteriosus; *VSD*, ventricular septal defect.

TABLE 145.3 Treatment of Heart Failure

THERAPY	MECHANISM
GENERAL CARE	
Rest	Reduces cardiac output
Oxygen	Improves oxygenation in the presence of pulmonary edema
Sodium, fluid restrictions	Decreases vascular congestion; decreases preload
DIURETICS	
Furosemide	Salt excretion at ascending loop of Henle; reduces preload; afterload reduces with control of hypertension; may also cause venodilation
Combination of distal tubule and loop diuretics	Greater sodium excretion
INOTROPIC AGENTS	
Digitalis	Inhibits membrane Na^+, K^+-ATPase and increases intracellular Ca^{2+}, improves cardiac contractility, increases myocardial oxygen consumption
Dopamine	Releases myocardial norepinephrine plus a direct effect on β-receptor, may increase systemic blood pressure; at low infusion rates, dilates renal artery, facilitating diuresis
Dobutamine	β_1-Receptor agent; often combined with dopamine
Milrinone	Phosphodiesterase 3 inhibitor with positive inotropic properties and decreases vascular resistance/afterload
AFTERLOAD REDUCTION	
Hydralazine	Arteriolar vasodilator
Nitroprusside	Arterial and venous relaxation; venodilation reduces preload
Captopril/enalapril	Inhibition of angiotensin-converting enzyme; reduces angiotensin II production
OTHER MEASURES	
Mechanical counterpulsation	Improves coronary flow, afterload
Transplantation	Removes diseased heart
Extracorporeal membrane oxygenation	Bypasses heart
Carvedilol	β-Blocking agent

CHAPTER 146

Rheumatic Fever

ETIOLOGY AND EPIDEMIOLOGY

Although uncommon in the United States, *acute* rheumatic fever remains an important preventable cause of cardiac disease. It is most common in children 6-15 years of age. It is due to an immunological reaction that is a delayed sequela of group A beta-hemolytic streptococcal infections of the pharynx. A family history of rheumatic fever and lower socioeconomic status are additional factors.

CLINICAL MANIFESTATIONS

Decision-Making Algorithms
Available @ StudentConsult.com

Heart Murmurs
Arthritis
Involuntary Movements
Fever and Rash

Acute rheumatic fever is diagnosed using the clinical and laboratory findings of the **revised Jones criteria** (Table 146.1). The presence of either two **major criteria** or one major and two **minor criteria**, along with evidence of an antecedent **streptococcal infection**, confirm a diagnosis of acute rheumatic fever. The infection often precedes the presentation of rheumatic fever by 2-6 weeks. Streptococcal antibody tests, such as the antistreptolysin O titer, are the most reliable laboratory evidence of prior infection.

Arthritis is the most common major manifestation. It usually involves the large joints and is migratory. Arthralgia cannot be used as a minor manifestation if arthritis is used as a major manifestation. **Carditis** occurs in about 50% of patients. Tachycardia, a new murmur (mitral or aortic regurgitation), pericarditis, cardiomegaly, and signs of heart failure are evidence of carditis. **Erythema marginatum**, a serpiginous, nonpruritic, and evanescent rash, is uncommon, occurs on the trunk, and is brought out by warmth. **Subcutaneous nodules** are seen predominantly with chronic or recurrent disease. They are firm, painless, nonpruritic, mobile nodules found on the extensor surfaces of the large and small joints, the scalp, and the spine. **Chorea** (Sydenham chorea or St. Vitus dance) consists of neurological and psychiatric signs. It also is uncommon and often presents long after the infection.

TABLE 146.1 Major Jones Criteria for Diagnosis of Acute Rheumatic Fever*,†

SIGN	COMMENTS
Polyarthritis	Common; swelling, limited motion, tender, erythema Migratory; involves large joints but rarely small or unusual joints, such as vertebrae
Carditis	Common; pancarditis, valves, pericardium, myocardium Tachycardia greater than explained by fever; new murmur of mitral or aortic insufficiency; Carey-Coombs mid-diastolic murmur; heart failure
Chorea (Sydenham disease)	Uncommon; manifests long after infection has resolved; more common in females; antineuronal antibody positive
Erythema marginatum	Uncommon; pink macules on trunk and proximal extremities, evolving to serpiginous border with central clearing; evanescent, elicited by application of local heat; nonpruritic
Subcutaneous nodules	Uncommon; associated with repeated episodes and severe carditis; located over extensor surface of elbows, knees, knuckles, and ankles, or scalp and spine; firm, nontender

Minor criteria include fever (temperatures of 101-102°F [38.2-38.9°C]), arthralgias, previous rheumatic fever, leukocytosis, elevated erythrocyte sedimentation rate/C-reactive protein, and prolonged PR interval.

†One major and two minor, or two major, criteria with evidence of recent group A streptococcal disease (e.g., scarlet fever, positive throat culture, or elevated antistreptolysin O or other antistreptococcal antibodies) strongly suggest the diagnosis of acute rheumatic fever.

TREATMENT AND PREVENTION

Management of acute rheumatic fever consists of **benzathine penicillin** to eradicate the beta-hemolytic streptococcus, antiinflammatory therapy with **salicylates**, and **bed rest.** Additional supportive therapy for heart failure or chorea may be necessary. **Long-term penicillin prophylaxis**, preferably with intramuscular benzathine penicillin G, 1.2 million U every 28 days, is required. Oral regimens for prophylaxis generally are not as effective. The prognosis of acute rheumatic fever depends on the degree of permanent cardiac damage. Cardiac involvement may resolve completely, especially if it is the first episode and the prophylactic regimen is followed. The severity of cardiac involvement worsens with each recurrence of rheumatic fever.

CHAPTER 147

Cardiomyopathies

ETIOLOGY

A cardiomyopathy is an intrinsic disease of the heart muscle and is not associated with other forms of heart disease (Table 147.1). There are three types of cardiomyopathy based on anatomical and functional features:

1. Dilated
2. Hypertrophic
3. Restrictive

Dilated cardiomyopathies are the most common. They are often idiopathic, but they may be due to infection (echovirus or Coxsackie B virus) or be postinfectious, familial, or secondary to systemic disease or to cardiotoxic drugs. Hypertrophic cardiomyopathies are usually familial with autosomal dominant inheritance but may occur sporadically. Restrictive cardiomyopathies are rare; they may be idiopathic or associated with systemic disease (Table 147.2).

TABLE 147.1 Etiology of Myocardial Disease

FAMILIAL/HEREDITARY	**CONNECTIVE TISSUE/GRANULOMATOUS DISEASE**
Duchenne muscular dystrophy	Systemic lupus erythematosus
Other muscular dystrophies (Becker, limb-girdle)	Scleroderma
Myotonic dystrophy	Amyloidosis
Kearns-Sayre syndrome (progressive external ophthalmoplegia)	Rheumatic fever
Carnitine deficiency syndromes	Sarcoidosis
Endocardial fibroelastosis	Dermatomyositis
Mitochondrial myopathy syndromes	**DRUGS/TOXINS**
Familial dilated cardiomyopathy (dominant, recessive, X-linked)	Doxorubicin (Adriamycin)
Familial hypertrophic cardiomyopathy	Ipecac
Familial restrictive cardiomyopathy	Iron overload (hemosiderosis)
Pompe disease (glycogen storage)	Irradiation
INFECTIOUS (MYOCARDITIS)	Cocaine
Viral (e.g., coxsackievirus infection, mumps, Epstein-Barr virus infection, influenza, parainfluenza infection, measles, varicella, HIV infection)	Amphetamines
	CORONARY ARTERIES
Bacterial (e.g., diphtheria, *Mycoplasma* infection, meningococcal disease, leptospirosis, Lyme disease, psittacosis, *Coxiella* infection, Rocky Mountain spotted fever)	Anomalous left coronary artery
	Kawasaki disease
	OTHER DISORDERS/CONDITIONS
Parasitic (e.g., Chagas disease, toxoplasmosis)	Idiopathic
METABOLIC/NUTRITIONAL/ENDOCRINE	Sickle cell anemia
Hypothyroidism	Endomyocardial fibrosis
Hyperthyroidism	Right ventricular dysplasia
Pheochromocytoma	
Mitochondrial myopathies and oxidative respiratory chain defects	
Type II, X-linked 3-methylglutaconic aciduria	

HIV, Human immunodeficiency virus.

TABLE 147.2 Anatomical and Functional Features of Cardiomyopathies

FEATURE	DILATED	HYPERTROPHIC	RESTRICTIVE
Etiology	Infectious Metabolic Toxic Idiopathic	Sporadic Inherited (autosomal dominant)	Infiltrative (amyloidosis, sarcoidosis) Noninfiltrative (idiopathic, familial) Storage disease (hemochromatosis, Fabry disease) Endomyocardial disease
Hemodynamics	Decreased systolic function	Diastolic dysfunction (impaired ventricular filling)	Diastolic dysfunction (impaired ventricular filling)
Treatment	Positive inotropes Diuretics Afterload reduction β-Blockers Antiarrhythmics Anticoagulants Cardiac transplantation	β-Blockers Calcium channel blockers	Diuretics Anticoagulants Cardiac transplantation

CLINICAL MANIFESTATIONS

Decision-Making Algorithms
Available @ StudentConsult.com

Chest Pain
Palpitations
Edema

Dilated cardiomyopathies result in enlargement of the left ventricle only or of both ventricles. Myocardial contractility is variably decreased. Children with dilated cardiomyopathy present with signs and symptoms of inadequate cardiac output and **heart failure**. Tachypnea and tachycardia are present on examination. Peripheral pulses are often weak because of a **narrow pulse pressure**. Rales may be audible on auscultation. The heart sounds may be muffled, and an S_3 is often present. Concurrent infectious illness may result in circulatory collapse and shock in children with dilated cardiomyopathies.

Hypertrophic cardiomyopathy is initially difficult to diagnose. Infants, but not older children, frequently present with signs of heart failure. Sudden death may be the initial presentation in older children. Dyspnea, fatigue, chest pain, syncope or near-syncope, and palpitations may be present. A murmur is heard in more than 50% of children referred after identification of an affected family member. Restrictive cardiomyopathies are relatively rare in pediatrics. Presenting symptoms usually include dyspnea exacerbated by a respiratory illness, syncope, hepatomegaly, and an S_4 heart sound on examination.

IMAGING STUDIES

Decision-Making Algorithm
Available @ StudentConsult.com

Edema

Cardiomegaly usually is seen on chest radiographs for all three types of cardiomyopathies. The electrocardiogram (ECG) in dilated cardiomyopathy may have nonspecific ST-T wave changes and left ventricular hypertrophy. ECG evidence of right ventricular hypertrophy is present in 25% of children with cardiomyopathy. The ECG with hypertrophic cardiomyopathy is universally abnormal, but changes are nonspecific. Primary hypertrophic cardiomyopathy is associated with a prolonged QT interval. Children with restrictive cardiomyopathies may show atrial enlargement on the ECG. Echocardiography features vary by type of cardiomyopathy. Dilated cardiomyopathies result in left atrial and ventricular dilation, a decreased shortening fraction, and globally depressed contractility. Asymmetric septal hypertrophy and left ventricular outflow tract obstruction are seen in hypertrophic cardiomyopathies. Massive atrial dilation is seen in restrictive cardiomyopathies. Endomyocardial biopsy specimens, obtained while the patient is hemodynamically stable, identify histological type and allow tests for mitochondrial or infiltrative diseases.

TREATMENT

Supportive therapy, including **diuretics**, **inotropic medications**, and **afterload reduction**, is provided for all three types of cardiomyopathy. If a specific etiology can be identified, treatment is directed at the etiology. Symptomatic therapy with close monitoring and follow-up is crucial. Because of the high mortality rate associated with all forms of cardiomyopathy, **cardiac transplantation** must be considered.

CHAPTER 148
Pericarditis

ETIOLOGY AND EPIDEMIOLOGY

Pericarditis is inflammation of the parietal and visceral surfaces of the pericardium. It is most often viral in origin, with many viruses identified as causative agents. A bacterial etiology is rare but causes a much more serious and symptomatic pericarditis. *Staphylococcus aureus* and *Streptococcus pneumoniae* are the most likely bacterial causes. Pericarditis is associated with collagen vascular diseases, such as rheumatoid arthritis, and is seen with uremia (Table 148.1). **Postpericardiotomy syndrome** is a relatively common form of pericarditis that follows heart surgery.

CLINICAL MANIFESTATIONS

Decision-Making Algorithm
Available @ StudentConsult.com

Chest Pain

The symptoms of pericarditis (Table 148.2) depend on the amount of fluid in the pericardial space and how fast it accumulates. A small effusion usually is well tolerated. A large effusion may be well tolerated if it accumulates slowly. The faster the fluid accumulates, the sooner the patient is hemodynamically compromised and develops symptoms.

IMAGING AND LABORATORY STUDIES

Echocardiography is the most specific and useful diagnostic test for detection of pericardial effusions. A chest x-ray may reveal cardiomegaly. A large effusion creates a rounded, globular cardiac silhouette. The electrocardiogram (ECG) may show tachycardia, elevated ST segments, reduced QRS voltage, or electrical alternans (variable QRS amplitude). The causative organism may be identified through viral titers, antistreptolysin O (ASO) titers, or diagnostic testing of the pericardial fluid.

TREATMENT

Pericardiocentesis is indicated for the treatment of hemodynamically significant effusions and to determine the etiology of the pericarditis. Additional treatment is directed at the specific etiology. There is no specific treatment for viral pericarditis other than **antiinflammatory medications**.

TABLE 148.1 Etiology of Pericarditis and Pericardial Effusion

IDIOPATHIC (PRESUMED VIRAL) INFECTIOUS AGENTS	Sarcoidosis
Bacterial	Vasculitis
Group A streptococci	**TRAUMATIC**
Staphylococcus aureus	Cardiac contusion (blunt trauma)
Pneumococcus, meningococcus*	Penetrating trauma
*Haemophilus influenzae**	Postpericardiotomy syndrome
Mycobacterium tuberculosis	Radiation
Viral†	**CONTIGUOUS SPREAD**
Coxsackievirus (group A, B)	Pleural disease
Echovirus	Pneumonia
Mumps	Aortic aneurysm (dissecting)
Influenza	**METABOLIC**
Epstein-Barr	Hypothyroidism
Cytomegalovirus	Uremia
Fungal	Chylopericardium
Histoplasma capsulatum	**NEOPLASTIC**
Coccidioides immitis	Primary
Blastomyces dermatitidis	Contiguous (lymphoma)
Candida	Metastatic
COLLAGEN VASCULAR-INFLAMMATORY AND GRANULOMATOUS DISEASES	Infiltrative (leukemia)
Rheumatic fever	**OTHER ETIOLOGICAL DISORDERS/FACTORS**
Systemic lupus erythematosus (idiopathic and drug-induced)	Drug reaction
Rheumatoid arthritis	Pancreatitis
Kawasaki disease	After myocardial infarction
Scleroderma	Thalassemia
Mixed connective tissue disease	Central venous catheter perforation
Inflammatory bowel disease	Heart failure
	Hemorrhage (coagulopathy)

Infectious or immune complex.
†*Common (viral pericarditis or myopericarditis is probably the most common cause of acute pericarditis in a previously normal host).*
From Sigman G. Chest pain. In: Kliegman RM, Greenbaum LA, Lye PS, eds. Practical Strategies in Pediatric Diagnosis and Therapy. *2nd ed. Philadelphia: Saunders;, 2004. Tab 9-9.*

TABLE 148.2 Manifestations of Pericarditis

SYMPTOMS	Hepatomegaly
Chest pain (worsened if lying down or with inspiration)	Pulsus paradoxus (>10 mm Hg with inspiration)
Dyspnea	Narrow pulse pressure
Malaise	Weak pulse, poor peripheral perfusion
Patient assumes sitting position	**Constrictive**
SIGNS	Distended neck veins
Nonconstrictive	Kussmaul sign (inspiratory increase in jugular venous pressure)
Fever	Distant heart sounds
Tachycardia	Pericardial knock
Friction rub (accentuated by inspiration, body position)	Hepatomegaly
Enlarged heart by percussion and x-ray examination	Ascites
Distant heart sounds	Edema
Tamponade	Tachycardia
As above, plus:	
Distended neck veins	

Suggested Readings

Allen HD, Shaddy RE, Penny DJ, et al. *Heart Disease in Infants, Children, and Adolescent*. 9th ed. Philadelphia: Lippincott Williams & Wilkins; 2016.

Eidem BW, Cetta F, O'Leary PW. *Echocardiography in Pediatric and Adult Congenital Heart Disease*. Philadelphia: Lippincott Williams & Wilkins; 2010.

Kliegman RM, Stanton BMD, St. Geme J, et al, eds. *Nelson Textbook of Pediatrics*. 20th ed. Philadelphia: Saunders; 2015.

Park M. *Pediatric Cardiology for Practitioners*. 6th ed. Elsevier Health Sciences; 2014.

Shaddy RE. *Heart Failure in Congenital Heart Disease*. London: Springer; 2014.

PEARLS FOR PRACTITIONERS

CHAPTER 139

Cardiovascular System Assessment

- Rate of growth is one of the most valuable and objective signs of cardiovascular health.
  - In infants with heart failure, weight gain is more significantly affected than height and head circumference.
- Cardiovascular vital signs vary with age, and one needs to know or have a resource for "normal" for all age groups to be able to recognize/diagnose abnormal.
- Blood pressure should be routinely taken in the right arm and, if elevated, then taken in all four extremities.
  - The presence of a normal right arm blood pressure and normal pedal pulses effectively rules out coarctation of the aorta.
- Peripheral cyanosis (hands, feet, perioral), also known as acrocyanosis, is common in infants and needs to be differentiated from central cyanosis (tongue, lips).
- Murmurs are the noises made by turbulent blood flow and are very common in pediatric patients.
  - The timing of the murmur is most important in determining the significance of the murmur and developing a differential diagnosis.
  - Diastolic murmurs, holosystolic murmurs, continuous murmurs (with the exception of the venous hum), and murmurs with a palpable thrill are abnormal murmurs.
  - To be a normal (innocent) murmur, the cardiovascular history and remainder of the cardiovascular exam must be normal.
- A normal heart size on chest radiograph virtually rules out heart failure; however, a large heart is not diagnostic of heart failure.

CHAPTER 140

Syncope

- Syncope is the transient loss of consciousness and muscle tone and is typically associated with an upright position, prodromal symptoms, pale appearance, and brief loss of consciousness with rapid return to normal state of consciousness.
  - Syncope occurring during exercise or with associated cardiac symptoms should be considered atypical until more extensively evaluated.

CHAPTER 141

Chest Pain

- Chest pain is common in Pediatrics but is rarely cardiac in origin. Up to one third of all Pediatric chest pain is idiopathic, with musculoskeletal chest pain being the most common cause of diagnosable chest pain.

CHAPTER 142

Dysrhythmias

- The most common symptomatic dysrhythmia in Pediatrics is supraventricular tachycardia.
- Sinus arrhythmia is common in children and represents a normal variation in heart rate with respiration.

CHAPTER 143

Acyanotic Congenital Heart Disease

- Congenital heart defects occur in about 1% of births and includes a wide spectrum of defects from asymptomatic to fatal lesions.
- Ventricular septal defect (VSD) is the most common congenital heart defect.
  - The amount of shunting at a VSD depends on the size of the defect and the pulmonary vascular resistance.
  - Large shunts are the result of excessive pulmonary blood flow (congestive heart failure), typically presenting with tachypnea, fatigue, and diaphoresis with feeding and poor weight gain.
- Atrial septal defects (ASDs) rarely cause symptoms in childhood.
  - The amount of shunting at an ASD depends on the size of the defect and the relative compliance of the ventricles.
  - In addition to a systolic ejection murmur from increased flow across the pulmonary valve, a widely split second heart sound that does not vary with respiration is the classic exam finding associated with an ASD.
- A patent ductus arteriosus (PDA) results in volume overload of the left heart and shunting, which is dependent on the size of the PDA and the pulmonary vascular resistance.

- The most common congenital heart defect in children with Trisomy 21 is the endocardial cushion defect, which is also called atrioventricular canal defect or atrioventricular septal defect.
- Symptoms and management of pulmonary stenosis and aortic stenosis depend on the severity of the stenosis.
  - Pulmonary valve stenosis is rarely progressive; aortic valve stenosis is usually progressive.
- Coarctation of the aorta usually occurs in the juxtaductal region.
  - Symptoms and presentation depend on the severity of the obstruction and associated congenital heart defects.

CHAPTER 144

Cyanotic Congenital Heart Disease

- Clinical cyanosis occurs when >5 g/100 mL of reduced hemoglobin is present in the systemic blood.
- The most common cyanotic congenital heart defects are the five Ts: Tetralogy of Fallot, Transposition of the great arteries, Tricuspid atresia, Truncus arteriosus, and Total anomalous pulmonary venous return.
- Tetralogy of Fallot is the most common cyanotic congenital heart defect. The degree of cyanosis and the murmur depend on the amount of pulmonary stenosis.
- Transposition of the great arteries is the most common cyanotic lesion to present in the newborn period.
- Congenital heart defects with a functionally single ventricle, such as tricuspid atresia and hypoplastic left heart syndrome (HLHS) require a staged surgical repair.
  - Survival of patients with HLHS—the most common cause of death from a cardiac defect in the first month of life—has improved dramatically with staged surgical and aggressive medical management.

CHAPTER 145

Heart Failure

- The most common cause, as well as the clinical manifestations of congestive heart failure, vary with age of presentation.
- Diseases/issues that impact preload, afterload, and contractility can all result in worsening cardiac performance and heart failure.
- Treatment of heart failure often includes diuresis, inotropic support, and afterload reduction.

CHAPTER 146

Rheumatic Fever

- Rheumatic fever remains an important, preventable cause of cardiac disease worldwide. Diagnosis of Rheumatic Fever is made using the clinical and laboratory findings of the revised Jones criteria.

CHAPTER 147

Cardiomyopathies

- There are three types of cardiomyopathy: (1) dilated (most common); (2) hypertrophic; and (3) restrictive.
- Supportive therapy, including diuretics, inotropic medications, and afterload reduction, are used in all three types.
- Cardiac transplantation must be considered due to the high mortality rate seen in all forms of cardiomyopathy.

CHAPTER 148

Pericarditis

- Pericarditis is inflammation of the parietal and visceral surfaces of the pericardium and is most often viral in origin.
  - The severity of symptoms depends on the amount of fluid present in the pericardial space and the rapidity with which the fluid accumulated.

SECTION 20

HEMATOLOGY

Amanda Brandow | J. Paul Scott

CHAPTER 149

Hematology Assessment

HISTORY

A detailed history of the onset, severity, progression, associated symptoms, presence of systemic complaints, and exacerbating factors is crucial to the diagnosis of a blood disorder. In many blood disorders, a **detailed pedigree** identifying a pattern of inheritance can point to the diagnosis.

PHYSICAL EXAMINATION AND COMMON MANIFESTATIONS

Decision-Making Algorithms
Available @ StudentConsult.com

Jaundice
Anemia
Bleeding
Petechiae/Purpura
Pancytopenia
Failure to Thrive

The physical examination of patients with blood disorders first focuses on hemodynamic stability. Acute episodes of anemia may be life threatening, presenting with impairment of perfusion and cognitive status. The two most common findings of anemia include **pallor** and **jaundice.** The presence of **petechiae, purpura,** or deeper sites of **bleeding,** including generalized hemorrhage, indicates abnormalities of platelets, coagulation factors, or both. **Growth parameters** point to whether anemia is an acute or chronic process. Severe types of anemia, thrombocytopenia, and pancytopenia often are associated with congenital anomalies and a pattern of growth delay. Organ system involvement (especially **hepatosplenomegaly** and **lymphadenopathy**) or systemic illness points to a generalized illness as the cause for hematological abnormalities (Table 149.1).

INITIAL DIAGNOSTIC EVALUATION

Diagnosis of pediatric blood disorders requires a detailed knowledge of normal hematological values that vary according to age and, after puberty, according to sex (Table 149.2). Directed by the history, physical examination, and screening laboratory studies, specific diagnostic testing can confirm the diagnosis.

DEVELOPMENTAL HEMATOLOGY

Hematopoiesis begins by 3 weeks of gestation with **erythropoiesis** in the yolk sac. By 2 months' gestation, the primary site of hematopoiesis migrates to the liver. By 5-6 months' gestation, the process shifts from the liver to the bone marrow. An extremely premature infant may have significant **extramedullary hematopoiesis** due to limited bone marrow hematopoiesis. During infancy, virtually all marrow cavities are actively hematopoietic and the proportion of hematopoietic to stromal elements is quite high. As the child grows, hematopoiesis moves to the central bones of the body (vertebrae, sternum, ribs, and pelvis), and the marrow is gradually replaced with fat. Hemolysis or marrow damage may lead to marrow repopulation of cavities where hematopoiesis previously had ceased or may delay the shift of hematopoiesis. Hepatosplenomegaly in patients with chronic hemolysis may signify extramedullary hematopoiesis. When a patient with cytopenia is being evaluated, a **bone marrow examination** provides valuable information about processes that lead to underproduction of circulating cells. In addition, bone marrow infiltration by neoplastic elements or storage cells often occurs in concert with infiltration in the spleen, liver, and lymph nodes.

The hematopoietic cells consist of the following:

1. Small compartment of **pluripotent progenitor stem cells** that resemble small lymphocytes and are capable of forming all myeloid elements
2. Large compartment of committed, proliferating cells of myeloid, erythroid, and megakaryocytic lineage
3. Large compartment of postmitotic maturing cells (Fig. 149.1)

The bone marrow is the major storage organ for mature neutrophils and contains about seven times the intravascular pool of neutrophils. It contains 2.5-5 times as many cells of myeloid lineage as cells of erythroid lineage. Smaller numbers of megakaryocytes, plasma cells, histiocytes, lymphocytes, and stromal cells are also stored in the marrow.

Erythropoiesis (red blood cell [RBC] production) is controlled by erythropoietin, a glycoprotein that stimulates primitive pluripotential stem cells to differentiate along the erythroid line. It is made by the juxtaglomerular apparatus of the kidney in response to local tissue hypoxia. The normally high hemoglobin level of the fetus is a result of fetal erythropoietin

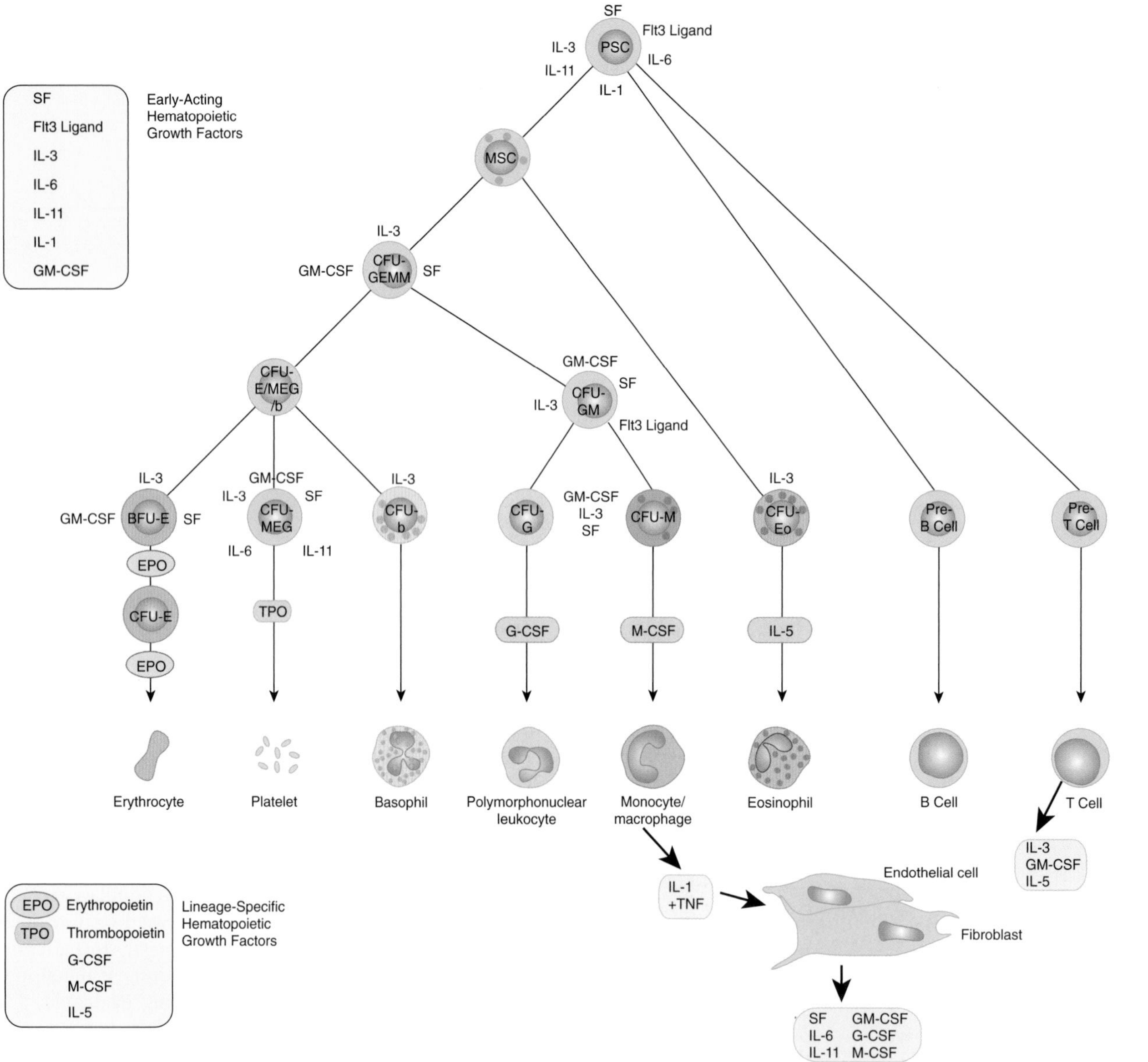

FIGURE 149.1 Major cytokine sources and actions that promote hematopoiesis. Cells of the bone marrow microenvironment, such as macrophages, endothelial cells, and reticular fibroblasts, produce macrophage colony-stimulating factor *(M-CSF)*, granulocyte-macrophage colony-stimulating factor *(GM-CSF)*, and granulocyte colony-stimulating factor *(G-CSF)* after stimulation. For all lineages, optimal development requires a combination of early and late acting factors. *BFU*, Burst-forming unit; *CFU*, colony-forming unit; *EPO*, erythropoietin; *IL*, interleukin; *MSC*, myeloid stem cell; *PSC*, pluripotent stem cell; *TNF*, tumor necrosis factor; *TPO*, thrombopoietin. (From Sieff CA, Nathan DG, Clark SC. The anatomy and physiology of hematopoiesis. In: Orkin SH, Nathan DG, eds. *Hematology of Infancy and Childhood*. 5th ed. Philadelphia: WB Saunders; 1998:168.)

TABLE **149.1** Presentation of Hematological Disorders

CONDITION	SYMPTOMS AND SIGNS	COMMON EXAMPLES
Anemia	Pallor, fatigue, heart failure, jaundice	Iron deficiency, hemolytic anemia
Polycythemia	Irritability, cyanosis, seizures, jaundice, stroke, headache	Cyanotic heart disease, infant of diabetic mother, cystic fibrosis
Neutropenia	Fever, pharyngitis, oral ulceration, cellulitis, lymphadenopathy, bacteremia, gingivitis, perirectal infections	Congenital or drug-induced agranulocytosis, leukemia
Thrombocytopenia	Petechiae, ecchymosis, gastrointestinal hemorrhage, epistaxis	ITP, leukemia
Coagulopathy	Bruising, hemarthrosis, mucosal bleeding	von Willebrand disease, hemophilia, DIC
Thrombosis	Pulmonary embolism, deep vein thrombosis	Lupus anticoagulant; protein C, protein S, or antithrombin III deficiency; factor V Leiden, prothrombin 20210

DIC, Disseminated intravascular coagulation; *ITP*, idiopathic thrombocytopenic purpura.

TABLE 149.2 Hematological Values During Infancy and Childhood

	HEMOGLOBIN (g/dL)		HEMATOCRIT (%)			LEUKOCYTES (per mm³)		NEUTROPHILS (%)		DIFFERENTIAL COUNTS			
AGE	MEAN	RANGE	MEAN	RANGE	RETICULOCYTES (%) MEAN	MEAN	RANGE	MEAN	RANGE	LYMPHOCYTES (%) MEAN	EOSINOPHILS (%) MEAN	MONOCYTES (%) MEAN	NUCLEATED RED CELLS/100 WBCs
Cord blood	16.8	13.7-20.1	55	45-65	5	18,000	9,000-30,000	61	40-80	31	2	6	7
2 wk	16.5	13-20	50	42-66	1	12,000	5,000-21,000	40		48	3	9	3-10
3 mo	12.0	9.5-14.5	36	31-41	1	12,000	6,000-18,000	30		63	2	5	0
6 mo-6 yr	12.0	10.5-14	37	33-42	1	10,000	6,000-15,000	45		48	2	5	0
7-12 yr	13.0	11-16	38	34-40	1	8,000	4,500-13,500	55		38	2	5	0
ADULT													
Female	14.0	12-16	42	37-47	1.6	7,500	5,000-10,000	55	35-70	35	3	7	0
Male	16.0	14-18	47	42-52									

WBCs, White blood cells.
From Behrman RE, ed. Nelson Textbook of Pediatrics. *14th ed. Philadelphia: WB Saunders; 1992.*

production in the liver in response to low partial pressure of oxygen (Po_2) in utero. Erythropoietin leads to production of the **erythroid colony-forming unit**. The earliest recognizable erythroid cell is the erythroblast, which forms eight or more daughter cells. The RBC nucleus becomes gradually pyknotic and eventually is extruded. The cell is then released from the marrow as a **reticulocyte** that maintains residual mitochondrial and protein synthetic capacity. These highly specialized RBC precursors are engaged primarily in the production of **globin chains, glycolytic enzymes,** and **heme.** Iron is taken up via transferrin receptors and incorporated into the heme ring, which combines with globin chains synthesized within the immature RBC. When the messenger RNA and mitochondria are gone from the RBC, heme or protein synthesis is no longer possible; however, the RBC continues to function for its normal life span of about 120 days.

Embryonic hemoglobins are produced during yolk sac erythropoiesis, then replaced by **fetal hemoglobin** (hemoglobin F, $\alpha_2\gamma_2$) during the hepatic phase. During the third trimester, gamma chain production gradually diminishes, replaced by beta chains, resulting in **hemoglobin A** ($\alpha_2\beta_2$). Some fetal factors (e.g., infant of a diabetic mother) delay onset of beta chain production, but premature birth does not. Just after birth, with rapid increases in oxygen saturation, erythropoietin production stops and thus erythropoiesis ceases. Fetal RBCs have a shorter survival time (60 days).

During the first few months of postnatal life, rapid growth, shortened RBC survival, and cessation of erythropoiesis cause a gradual decline in hemoglobin levels, with a nadir at 8-10 weeks of life. This so-called **physiological nadir** is accentuated in premature infants. Erythropoietin is produced in response to the decline in hemoglobin and decreased oxygen delivery. Erythropoiesis subsequently resumes with an increase in the reticulocyte count. The hemoglobin level gradually increases, accompanied by synthesis of increasing amounts of hemoglobin A. By 6 months of age in healthy infants, only trace gamma chain synthesis occurs.

Production of **neutrophil precursors** is controlled predominantly by two different colony-stimulating factors (see Fig. 149.1). The most immature neutrophil precursors are controlled by **granulocyte-macrophage colony-stimulating factor** (GM-CSF), produced by monocytes and lymphocytes. GM-CSF increases the entry of primitive precursor cells into the myeloid line of differentiation. **Granulocyte colony-stimulating factor** (G-CSF) augments the production of more mature granulocyte precursors. GM-CSF and G-CSF, working in concert, can augment production of neutrophils, shorten the usual 10- to 14-day production time from stem cell to mature neutrophil, and stimulate functional activity. The rapid increase in neutrophil count that occurs with infection is caused by release of stored neutrophils from the bone marrow, under the control of GM-CSF. During maturation, a mitotic pool of neutrophil precursors exists—myeloblasts, promyelocytes, and myelocytes possessing primary granules. The postmitotic pool consists of metamyelocytes, bands, and mature polymorphonuclear leukocytes containing secondary or specific granules that define the cell type. Only bands and mature neutrophils are fully functional with regard to phagocytosis, chemotaxis, and bacterial killing. Neutrophils migrate from the bone marrow, circulate for 6-7 hours, and enter the tissues, where they become end-stage cells that do not recirculate. Eosinophil production is under the control of a related glycoprotein hormone, interleukin 3. Eosinophils, which play a role in host defense against parasites, also are capable of living in tissues for prolonged periods.

Megakaryocytes are giant, multinucleated cells derived from the primitive stem cell and are polyploid (16-32 times the normal DNA content) because of nuclear, but not cytoplasmic, cell division. Platelets form by invagination of the megakaryocytic cell membrane and bud off from the periphery. **Thrombopoietin** is the primary regulator of platelet production. Platelets adhere to damaged endothelium and subendothelial surfaces via specific receptors for the adhesive proteins, von Willebrand factor (VWF), and fibrinogen. Platelets also have specific granules that readily release their contents after stimulation and trigger the process of platelet aggregation. Platelets circulate for 7-10 days and have no nucleus.

Lymphocytes are particularly abundant in the bone marrow of young children. These are primarily B lymphocytes arising in the spleen and lymph nodes, but T lymphocytes also are present.

CHAPTER 150

Anemia

ETIOLOGY

The diagnosis of anemia is determined by comparison of the patient's **hemoglobin level** with age-specific and sex-specific normal values (see Table 149.2). The production of androgens at the onset of puberty in boys causes males to maintain a normal hemoglobin value approximately 1.5-2 g/dL higher than girls. The easiest quantitative definition of anemia is any hemoglobin or hematocrit value that is 2 standard deviations (SDs; 95% confidence limits) below the mean for age and gender. However, in certain pathological states, anemia may be present with a normal hemoglobin level (e.g., cyanotic cardiac or pulmonary disease or abnormally high hemoglobin affinity for oxygen). This is a physiological definition of anemia. Anemia is often a manifestation of another other primary process and may accentuate other organ dysfunction.

Anemias are classified based on the size and hemoglobin content of the cells (Fig. 150.1). **Hypochromic, microcytic anemia** is caused by an inadequate production of hemoglobin. The most common causes of this type of anemia are iron deficiency and thalassemia. Most **normocytic anemias** are associated with a systemic illness that impairs adequate marrow synthesis of red blood cells (RBCs). Vitamin B_{12} and folic acid deficiencies lead to **macrocytic anemia**. **Hemolytic diseases** are mediated either by disorders intrinsic or extrinsic to the RBC that increase cell destruction. The most common RBC membrane disorders are **hereditary spherocytosis** and **hereditary elliptocytosis**. In both of these disorders, abnormalities of proteins within the cytoskeleton lead to abnormal RBC shape and function. Numerous RBC enzyme deficiencies may lead to hemolysis, but only two are common: **glucose-6-phosphate dehydrogenase (G6PD) deficiency** and **pyruvate kinase deficiency**. Immune-mediated hemolysis may be extravascular when RBCs coated with antibodies or complement are phagocytosed by the reticuloendothelial system. The hemolysis may be intravascular when antibody binding leads to complement fixation and lysis of RBCs.

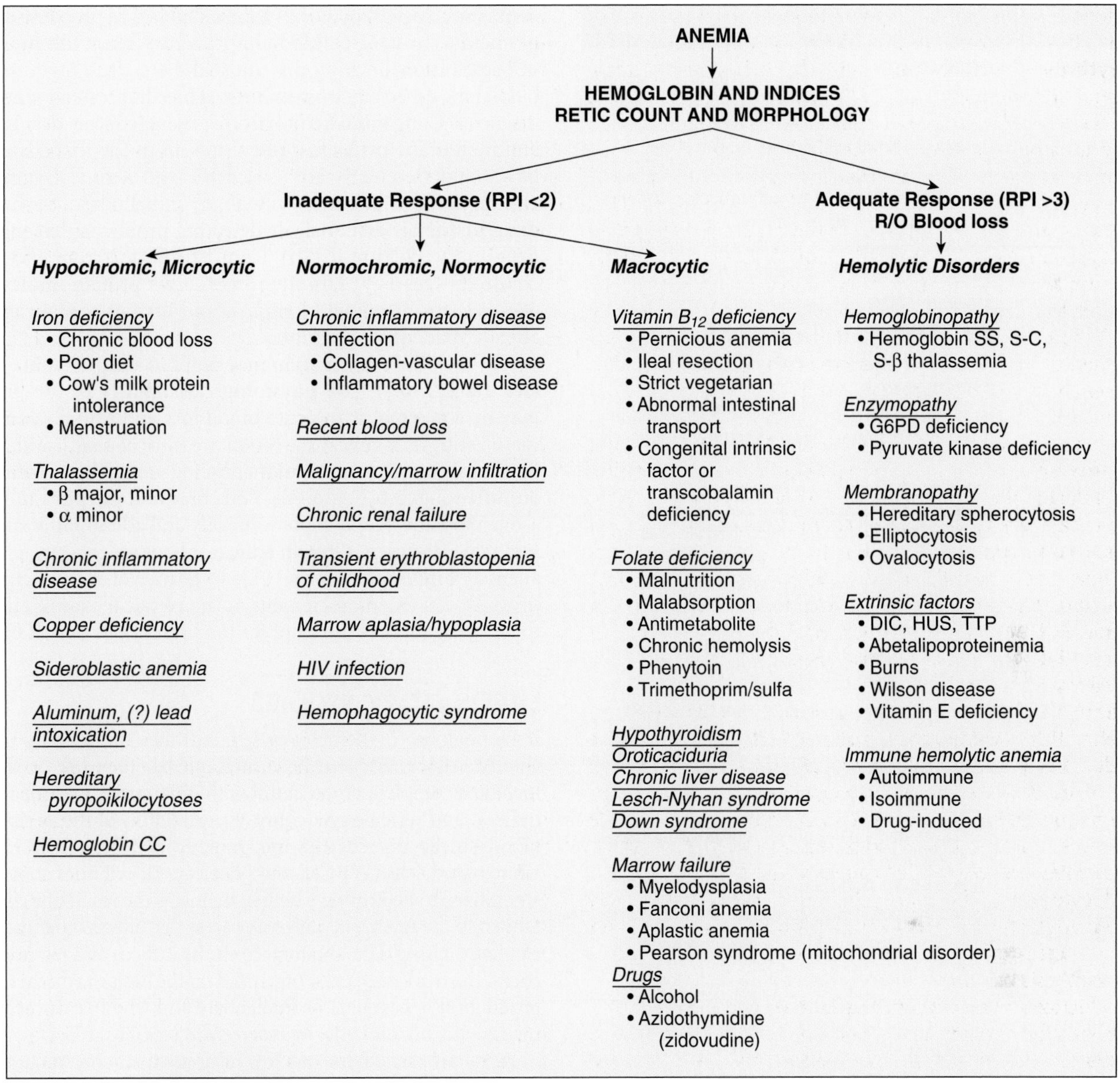

FIGURE 150.1 Use of the complete blood count, reticulocyte count, and blood smear in the diagnosis of anemia. *DIC,* Disseminated intravascular coagulation; *G6PD,* glucose-6-phosphate dehydrogenase; *HUS,* hemolytic uremic syndrome; *R/O,* rule out; *RPI,* reticulocyte production index; *TTP,* thrombotic thrombocytopenic purpura.

CLINICAL MANIFESTATIONS

Decision-Making Algorithms
Available @ StudentConsult.com

Heart Murmurs
Jaundice
Splenomegaly
Edema
Anemia

Acute onset of anemia can result in a poorly compensated state, manifested as an elevated heart rate, a systolic flow murmur, poor exercise tolerance, headache, excessive sleeping (especially in infants) or fatigue, irritability, poor feeding, and syncope. In contrast, chronic anemia often is exceptionally well tolerated in children because of their cardiovascular reserve. Usually, children with chronic anemia will have minimal tachycardia and a systolic flow murmur on examination. The urgency of diagnostic and therapeutic intervention, especially the use of packed RBC transfusion, should be dictated by the extent of cardiovascular or functional impairment more than the absolute level of hemoglobin.

The causes of anemia often can be suspected from a careful history adjusted for the patient's age (Tables 150.1 and 150.2). Anemia at any age demands a search for **blood loss**. A history of jaundice, pallor, previously affected siblings, drug ingestion by the mother, or excessive blood loss at the time of birth provides important clues to the diagnosis in newborns. A careful **dietary history** is crucial. A history of **jaundice**, **pallor**, and/or **splenomegaly** are often present with hemolytic anemia. Because of increased bilirubin production, **gallstones** (bilirubinate) are a common complication of chronic hemolysis. Systemic

TABLE 150.1 Historical Clues in Evaluation of Anemia

VARIABLE	COMMENTS
Age	Iron deficiency rare in the absence of blood loss before 6 mo or in term infants or before doubling of birth weight in preterm infants
	Neonatal anemia with reticulocytosis suggests hemolysis or blood loss; with reticulocytopenia, suggests bone marrow failure
	Sickle cell anemia and β-thalassemia appear as fetal hemoglobin disappears (4-8 mo of age)
Family history and genetic considerations	X-linked: G6PD deficiency
	Autosomal dominant: spherocytosis
	Autosomal recessive: sickle cell anemia, Fanconi anemia
	Family member with history of cholecystectomy (for bilirubin stones) or splenectomy at an early age
	Ethnicity (thalassemia in persons of Mediterranean origin; G6PD deficiency in blacks, Greeks, and people of Middle Eastern origin)
	Race (β-thalassemia in persons of Mediterranean, African, or Asian descent; α-thalassemia in those of African and Asian descent; SC and SS in those of African descent)
Nutrition	Cow's milk diet: iron deficiency
	Strict vegetarian: vitamin B_{12} deficiency
	Goat's milk diet: folate deficiency
	Pica: plumbism, iron deficiency
	Cholestasis, malabsorption: vitamin E deficiency
Drugs	G6PD: oxidants (e.g., nitrofurantoin, antimalarials)
	Immune-mediated hemolysis (e.g., penicillin)
	Bone marrow suppression (e.g., chemotherapy)
	Phenytoin, increasing folate requirements
Diarrhea	Malabsorption of vitamin B_{12} or E or iron
	Inflammatory bowel disease and anemia of inflammation (chronic disease) with or without blood loss
	Milk protein intolerance–induced blood loss
	Intestinal resection: vitamin B_{12} deficiency
Infection	*Giardia lamblia* infection: iron malabsorption
	Intestinal bacterial overgrowth (blind loop): vitamin B_{12} deficiency
	Fish tapeworm: vitamin B_{12} deficiency
	Epstein-Barr virus, cytomegalovirus infection: bone marrow suppression, hemophagocytic syndromes
	Mycoplasma infection: hemolysis
	Parvovirus infection: bone marrow suppression
	HIV infection
	Chronic infection
	Endocarditis
	Malaria: hemolysis
	Hepatitis: aplastic anemia

G6PD, Glucose-6-phosphate dehydrogenase.

complaints suggest acute or chronic illnesses as probable causes of anemia. In later childhood and adolescence, the presence of constitutional symptoms, unusual diets, drug ingestion, or blood loss, especially from menstrual bleeding, often points to a diagnosis. **Congenital hemolytic disorders** (enzyme deficiencies and membrane problems) often present in the first 6 months of life and frequently are associated with neonatal jaundice, although these disorders often go undiagnosed. A careful **drug history** is essential for detecting problems that may be drug induced. Pure dietary iron deficiency is rare except in children's ages 1-3 years when cow's milk protein intolerance causes gastrointestinal blood loss and further complicates an already inadequate iron intake.

The physical examination may point to the potential causes (see Table 150.2). The **physiological stability** of the patient may be abnormal with acute blood loss and acute hemolysis, manifesting as tachycardia, blood pressure changes, and, most ominously, an altered state of consciousness. The presence of **jaundice** suggests hemolysis. **Petechiae** and **purpura** indicate a coagulopathy. **Hepatosplenomegaly** and **adenopathy** suggest infiltrative disorders. **Growth failure** or poor weight gain suggests anemia of inflammation (previously termed anemia of chronic disease). An essential element of the physical examination is the investigation of the stool for the presence of **occult blood.**

LABORATORY STUDIES

A hemoglobin or hematocrit test indicates the severity of the anemia. After anemia has been substantiated, the work-up should include a complete blood count with differential, platelet count, indices, and reticulocyte count. Examination of the peripheral blood smear assesses the morphology of RBCs (Fig. 150.2), white blood cells (WBCs), and platelets. All cell lines should be scrutinized to determine whether anemia is the result of a process limited to the erythroid line or a process that affects other marrow elements. Using data obtained from the indices and reticulocyte count, the work-up can be organized on the basis of whether RBC production is adequate or inadequate and whether the cells are microcytic, normocytic, or macrocytic (see Fig. 150.1).

An appropriate bone marrow response to anemia includes an elevated absolute reticulocyte number, suggesting increased RBC production. This implies either hemolysis or blood loss. Anemia with a normal reticulocyte number suggests decreased or ineffective production for the degree of anemia. Reticulocytopenia signifies either an acute onset of anemia such that the marrow has not had adequate time to respond; that reticulocytes are being destroyed in the marrow (antibody mediated); or that intrinsic bone marrow disease is present. The best indicators of the severity of hemolysis are the hemoglobin level and the elevation of the **reticulocyte count**. Biochemical evidence of hemolysis includes an increase in levels of bilirubin and lactate dehydrogenase and a decrease in haptoglobin.

DIFFERENTIAL DIAGNOSIS

Hypochromic, Microcytic Anemia

Iron Deficiency Anemia

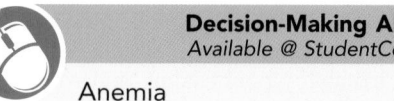

Decision-Making Algorithm
Available @ StudentConsult.com

Anemia

TABLE 150.2 Physical Findings in the Evaluation of Anemia

SYSTEM/STRUCTURE	OBSERVATION	SIGNIFICANCE
Skin	Hyperpigmentation	Fanconi anemia, dyskeratosis congenita
	Café-au-lait spots	Fanconi anemia
	Vitiligo	Vitamin B_{12} deficiency
	Partial oculocutaneous albinism	Chediak-Higashi syndrome
	Jaundice	Hemolysis
	Petechiae, purpura	Bone marrow infiltration, autoimmune hemolysis with autoimmune thrombocytopenia, hemolytic uremic syndrome, hemophagocytic syndromes
	Erythematous rash	Parvovirus or Epstein-Barr virus infection
	Butterfly rash	SLE antibodies
	Bruising	Bleeding disorder, nonaccidental trauma, scurvy
Head	Frontal bossing	Thalassemia major, severe iron deficiency, chronic subdural hematoma
	Microcephaly	Fanconi anemia
Eyes	Microphthalmia	Fanconi anemia
	Retinopathy	Hemoglobin SS, SC disease (see Table 150.7)
	Optic atrophy	Osteopetrosis
	Blocked lacrimal gland	Dyskeratosis congenita
	Kayser-Fleischer ring	Wilson disease
	Blue sclera	Iron deficiency, osteopetrosis
Ears	Deafness	
Mouth	Glossitis	Vitamin B_{12} deficiency, iron deficiency
	Angular stomatitis	Iron deficiency
	Cleft lip	Diamond-Blackfan syndrome
	Pigmentation	Peutz-Jeghers syndrome (intestinal blood loss)
	Telangiectasia	Osler-Weber-Rendu syndrome (blood loss)
	Leukoplakia	Dyskeratosis congenita
Chest	Shield chest or widespread nipples	Diamond-Blackfan syndrome
	Murmur	Endocarditis: prosthetic valve hemolysis; severe anemia
Abdomen	Hepatomegaly	Hemolysis, infiltrative tumor, chronic disease, hemangioma, cholecystitis, extramedullary hematopoiesis
	Splenomegaly	Hemolysis, sickle cell disease, (early) thalassemia, malaria, leukemia/lymphoma, Epstein-Barr virus, portal hypertension
	Nephromegaly	Fanconi anemia
	Absent kidney	Fanconi anemia
Extremities	Absent thumbs	Fanconi anemia
	Triphalangeal thumb	Diamond-Blackfan syndrome
	Spoon nails	Iron deficiency
	Beau line (nails)	Heavy metal intoxication, severe illness
	Mees line (nails)	Heavy metals, severe illness, sickle cell anemia
	Dystrophic nails	Dyskeratosis congenita
Rectal	Hemorrhoids	Portal hypertension
	Heme-positive stool	Gastrointestinal bleeding
Nerves	Irritable, apathy	Iron deficiency
	Peripheral neuropathy	Deficiency of vitamins B_1, B_{12}, and E; lead poisoning
	Dementia	Deficiency of vitamins B_{12} and E
	Ataxia, posterior column signs	Vitamin B_{12} deficiency
	Stroke	Sickle cell anemia, paroxysmal nocturnal hemoglobinuria
General	Small stature	Fanconi anemia, HIV infection, malnutrition

SLE, Systemic lupus erythematosus.

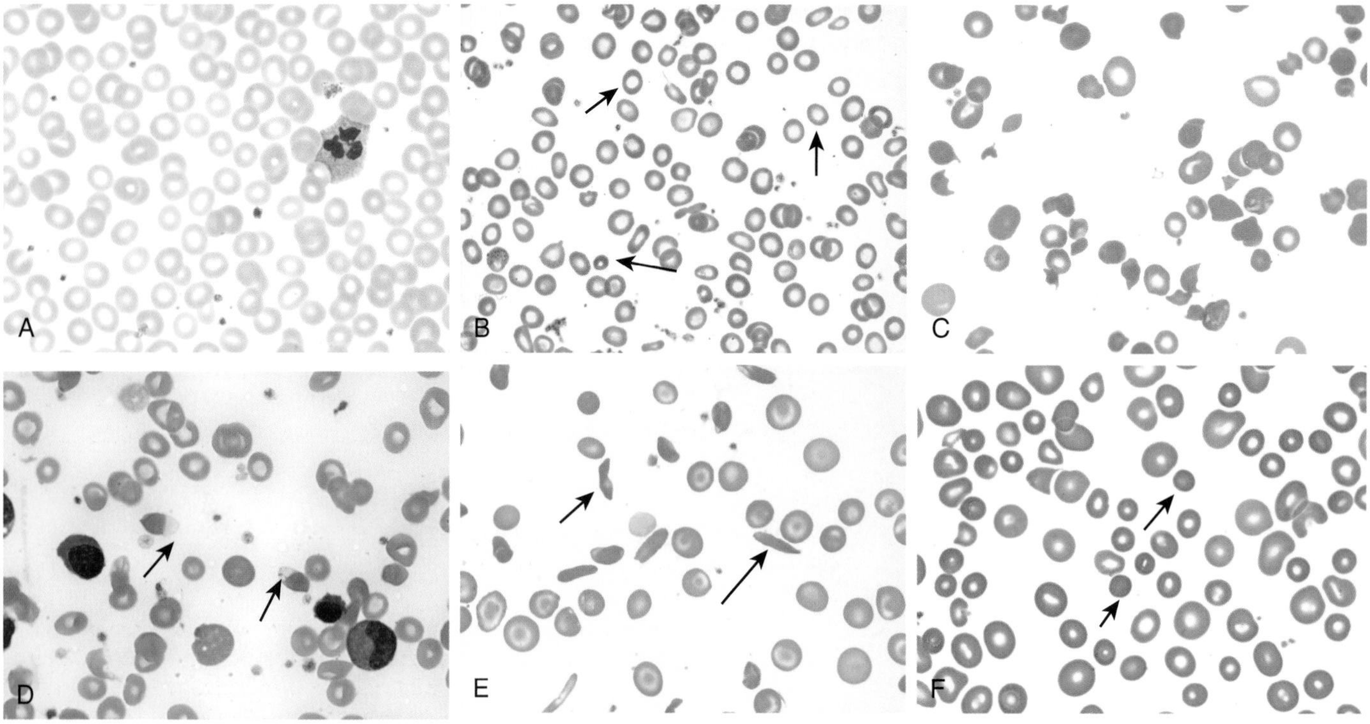

FIGURE 150.2 Morphological abnormalities of the red blood cell. **A,** Normal. **B,** Hypochromic microcytes (iron deficiency). **C,** Schistocytes (hemolytic uremic syndrome. **D,** Blister cells (glucose-6-phosphate dehydrogenase deficiency). **E,** Sickle cells (hemoglobin SS disease). **F,** Spherocytes (autoimmune hemolytic anemia). *Arrows* represent the cell discussed. (Courtesy B. Trost and J.P. Scott.)

TABLE **150.3** Stages in Development of Iron Deficiency Anemia

HEMOGLOBIN (g/dL)	PERIPHERAL SMEAR	SERUM IRON (μg/dL)	BONE MARROW IRON	SERUM FERRITIN (ng/mL)
13+ (normal)	nc/nc	50-150	Fe^{2+}	*Male:* 40-340 *Female:* 40-150
10-12	nc/nc	↓	Fe^{2+} absent, erythroid hyperplasia	<12
8-10	hypo/nc	↓	Fe^{2+} absent, erythroid hyperplasia	<12
<8	hypo/micro*	↓	Fe^{2+} absent, erythroid hyperplasia	<12

**Microcytosis, determined by a mean corpuscular volume (in fL) <2 standard deviations (SD) below the mean, must be adjusted for age (e.g., −2 SD at 3-6 months = 74; at 0.5-2 years = 70; at 2-6 years = 75; at 6-12 years = 77; and at 12-18 years = 78).*
hypo/micro, Hypochromic, microcytic; *hypo/nc,* hypochromic, normocytic; *nc/nc,* normochromic, normocytic.
From Andreoli TE, Bennett JC, Carpenter CC, et al. Cecil Essentials of Medicine. *4th ed. Philadelphia: WB Saunders; 1997.*

Etiology

Infants fed cow's milk when younger than 1 year of age, toddlers fed large volumes of cow's milk, and menstruating adolescent females who are not receiving supplemental iron are at high risk for iron deficiency. **Dietary** iron deficiency anemia is most common in bottle-fed toddlers who are receiving large volumes of cow's milk and eat minimal amounts of food high in iron content (see Chapters 28 and 31). Iron deficiency anemia also may be found in children with chronic inflammatory diseases, even without **chronic blood loss**.

Epidemiology

The prevalence of iron deficiency, the most common cause of anemia in the world, is approximately 9% in toddlers, 9-11% in adolescent females, and less than 1% in adolescent males. Iron deficiency anemia occurs in approximately one third of children who are iron deficient (Table 150.3). Children from low socioeconomic status in the United States may be at increased risk for iron deficiency because of poor dietary intake (see Chapter 31). Breast-fed infants are less likely to have iron deficiency than bottle-fed infants because, although there is less iron in breast milk, this iron is more efficiently absorbed. However, infants who continue to be exclusively breast fed in the second half of the first year of life are at risk for iron deficiency.

Clinical Manifestations

In addition to cardiovascular manifestations of anemia, central nervous system (CNS) abnormalities **(apathy, irritability, poor concentration)** have been linked to iron deficiency, presumably resulting from alterations of iron-containing enzymes (monoamine oxidase) and cytochromes. Poor muscle endurance, gastrointestinal dysfunction, and impaired WBC and T-cell function have been associated with iron deficiency. Iron deficiency in infancy may be associated with later **cognitive deficits** and poor school performance.

TABLE 150.4 Differentiating Features of Microcytic Anemias*

TEST	IRON DEFICIENCY ANEMIA	THALASSEMIA MINOR†	ANEMIA OF INFLAMMATION‡
Serum iron	Low	Normal	Low
Serum iron-binding capacity	High	Normal	Low or normal
Serum ferritin	Low	Normal or high	Normal or high
Marrow iron stores	Low or absent	Normal or high	Normal or high
Marrow sideroblasts	Decreased or absent	Normal or increased	Normal or increased
Free erythrocyte protoporphyrin	High	Normal or slightly increased	High
Hemoglobin A_2 or F	Normal	High β-thalassemia; normal α-thalassemia	Normal
Red blood cell distribution width§	High	Normal	Normal/↑

*See Table 150.3 for definition of microcytosis.
†α-Thalassemia minor can be diagnosed by the presence of Bart hemoglobin on newborn screening.
‡Usually normochromic; 25% of cases are microcytic.
§Red blood cell distribution width quantitates the degree of anisocytosis (different sizes) of red blood cells.

Treatment

In an otherwise healthy child, a **therapeutic trial of oral iron** is the best diagnostic study for iron deficiency as long as the child is re-examined and a response is documented. The response to oral iron includes rapid subjective improvement, especially in neurological function (within 24-48 hours) and reticulocytosis (48-72 hours); increase in hemoglobin levels (4-30 days); and repletion of iron stores (in 1-3 months). The usual therapeutic dose of 4-6 mg/day of elemental iron induces an increase in hemoglobin of 0.25-0.4 g/dL per day (a 1%/day increase in hematocrit). If the hemoglobin level fails to increase within 2 weeks after institution of iron treatment, careful re-evaluation for ongoing blood loss, development of infection, poor compliance, malabsorption, or other causes of microcytic anemia is required (Table 150.4; see Fig. 150.1).

Prevention

Bottle-fed infants should receive an iron-containing formula until 12 months of age. Exclusively breast-fed infants older than 6 months of age should receive an iron supplement. The introduction of iron-enriched solid foods at 6 months of age, followed by a transition to a limited amount of cow's milk and increased solid foods at 1 year, can help prevent iron deficiency anemia. Adolescent females who are menstruating should have a diet enriched with iron-containing foods. A vitamin with iron may also be used.

Thalassemia Minor

Etiology and Epidemiology

α-Thalassemia and **β-thalassemia minor** are common causes of microcytosis, either with or without a mild hypochromic, microcytic anemia. They are prevalent in certain ethnic groups (Mediterranean, Southeast Asian, African Americans). Individuals of Asian descent are at risk of having three or four α genes deleted, resulting in hemoglobin disease (β_4 tetramers) or hydrops fetalis, which is largely Bart (γ_4 tetramers) hemoglobin (Table 150.5 and Fig. 150.3).

Laboratory Testing

The thalassemia minor syndromes (i.e., α-thalassemia trait, β-thalassemia trait) are characterized by a mild hypochromic, microcytic anemia with a low absolute reticulocyte count (see Table 150.5). The RBC count is usually elevated. As a result, if the mean corpuscular volume (MCV) divided by the RBC count is less than 12.5 (Mentzer index), the diagnosis is suggestive of thalassemia trait. The blood smear reveals only microcytosis with α-thalassemia minor. Outside the neonatal period, when Bart hemoglobin is no longer detectable, the hemoglobin electrophoresis is usually normal in α-thalassemia minor (see Fig. 150.3). Blood smears of patients with β-thalassemia minor also reveal microcytic RBCs. In addition, target cells and basophilic stippled RBCs, caused by precipitation of alpha-chain tetramers, may also be present. The diagnosis of β-thalassemia minor is based on an elevation of hemoglobin A_2 and F levels. Molecular testing is indicated for identification of more severe or unusual variants.

Treatment

No treatment is required for children with **thalassemia minor**. However, children with more severe forms of thalassemia, such as β-thalassemia intermedia or major or children with hemoglobin H disease (β_4 tetramers), especially the Constant Spring variant, require chronic transfusion therapy (see Table 150.5).

Lead Poisoning

Lead poisoning may be associated with a hypochromic, microcytic anemia because most patients have concomitant iron deficiency. The history of living in an older home (built before 1980) with chipped paint or lead dust should raise suspicion of lead poisoning, especially in a child with **pica**. The lead content of water should also be assessed due to the potential for lead containing pipes. **Basophilic stippling** on the blood smear is common. Lead intoxication rarely causes hemolytic anemia. Detection by routine screening, removal from exposure, chelation therapy, and correction of iron deficiency are crucial to the potential development of affected children.

Normocytic Anemia

Etiology and Treatment

Anemia is a common component of chronic inflammatory disease. Hepcidin, a protein made in the liver, plays a key role in iron homeostasis. Inflammation causes an increase in the

TABLE 150.5 Thalassemia Syndromes

DISORDER	GENOTYPIC ABNORMALITY	CLINICAL PHENOTYPE
β-THALASSEMIA		
Thalassemia major (Cooley anemia)	Homozygous β^0-thalassemia	Severe hemolysis, ineffective erythropoiesis, transfusion dependency, hepatosplenomegaly, iron overload
Thalassemia intermedia	Compound heterozygous β^0- and β^+-thalassemia	Moderate hemolysis, splenomegaly, moderately severe anemia, but not transfusion dependent; main life-threatening complication is iron overload
Thalassemia minor	Heterozygous β^0- and β^+-thalassemia	Microcytosis, mild anemia
α-THALASSEMIA		
Silent carrier	α-/αα	Normal complete blood count
α-Thalassemia trait	αα/- - (α-thalassemia 1, *cis* deletion) *or* α -/α - (α-thalassemia 2, *trans* deletion)	Mild microcytic anemia
Hemoglobin H	α -/- -	Microcytic anemia and mild hemolysis; not transfusion dependent*
Hydrops fetalis	- -/- -	Severe anemia, intrauterine anasarca from congestive heart failure; death in utero or at birth

**The Constant Spring variant may require chronic transfusion.*
From Andreoli T, Carpenter C, Griggs R, et al. Cecil Essentials of Medicine. *7th ed. Philadelphia: Saunders: 2007.*

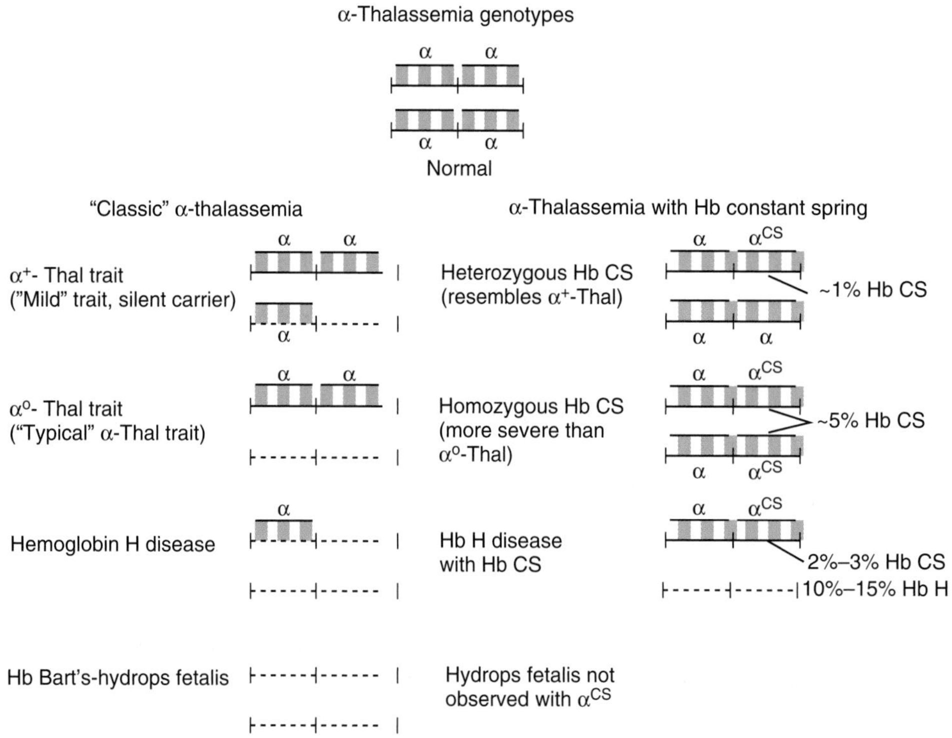

FIGURE 150.3 Genetic origins of the classic α-thalassemia syndromes due to gene deletions in the α-globin gene cluster. Hb Constant Spring (Hb CS) is an α-globin chain variant synthesized in such small amounts (1-2% of normal) that it has the phenotypic impact of a severe nondeletion α-thalassemia allele; however, the α^{CS} allele is always linked to a functioning α-globin gene, so it has never been associated with hydrops fetalis. (From Hoffman R, Benz EJ, Shattil SS, et al, eds. *Hematology: Basic Principles and Practice.* 5th ed. Philadelphia: Churchill Livingstone; 2008.)

production of hepcidin, interrupting the process of iron release by macrophages and the absorption of iron from the intestines leading to anemia. The **anemia of inflammation** may be normocytic or, less often, microcytic. This may pose a clinical challenge, when children with inflammatory disorders associated with blood loss (i.e., inflammatory bowel disease) exhibit a microcytic anemia. In these circumstances, only a bone marrow aspiration with staining of the sample for iron can differentiate the two entities clearly (see Table 150.4). Low ferritin levels indicate concurrent iron deficiency. A trial of iron therapy is

TABLE 150.6 Differentiation of Red Blood Cell Aplasias and Pancytopenia

DISORDER	AGE AT ONSET	CHARACTERISTICS	TREATMENT
CONGENITAL			
Diamond-Blackfan syndrome (congenital hypoplastic anemia)	Newborn-1 mo; 90% of patients are <1 yr of age	Pure red blood cell aplasia, autosomal recessive trait, elevated fetal hemoglobin, fetal i antigen present, macrocytic, short stature, webbed neck, cleft lip, triphalangeal thumb; late-onset leukemia, mutation analysis	Prednisone, transfusion, hematopoietic stem cell transplant
ACQUIRED			
Transient erythroblastopenia	6 mo-5 yr of age; 85% of patients are >1 yr of age	Pure red blood cell defect; no anomalies, fetal hemoglobin, or i antigen; spontaneous recovery, normal MCV	Expectant transfusion for symptomatic anemia
Idiopathic aplastic anemia (status post hepatitis, drugs, unknown)	All ages	All cell lines involved; exposure to felbamate, chloramphenicol, radiation	Hematopoietic stem cell transplantation, antithymocyte globulin, cyclosporine, androgens
FAMILIAL			
Fanconi anemia	Usually before 10 yr of age; mean is 8 yr	All cell lines; microcephaly, absent thumbs, café-au-lait spots, cutaneous hyperpigmentation, short stature; chromosomal breaks, high MCV and hemoglobin F; horseshoe or absent kidney; leukemic transformation; autosomal recessive trait	Androgens, corticosteroids, hematopoietic stem cell transplantation
Paroxysmal nocturnal hemoglobinuria	After 5 yr	Initial hemolysis followed by aplastic anemia; increased complement-mediated hemolysis; thrombosis; iron deficiency; CD59 low	Iron, hematopoietic stem cell transplantation, androgens, steroids, eculizumab
Dyskeratosis congenita	Mean is 10 yr for skin; mean is 17 yr for anemia	Pancytopenia; hyperpigmentation, dystrophic nails, leukoplakia; X-linked recessive; lacrimal duct stenosis; high MCV and fetal hemoglobin	Androgens, splenectomy, hematopoietic stem cell transplantation
Familial hemophagocytic lymphohistiocytosis	Before 2 yr	Pancytopenia; fever, hepatosplenomegaly, hypertriglyceridemia, CSF pleocytosis	Transfusion; often lethal; VP-16, hematopoietic stem cell transplantation, IVIG, cyclosporine
INFECTIOUS			
Parvovirus	Any age	Any chronic hemolytic anemia, typically sickle cell; new-onset reticulocytopenia and severe anemia	Red blood cell transfusion
Epstein-Barr virus (EBV)	Any age; usually <5 yr of age	X-linked immunodeficiency syndrome, pancytopenia	Transfusion, bone marrow transplantation
Virus-associated hemophagocytic syndrome (CMV, HHV-6, EBV)	Any age	Pancytopenia; hemophagocytosis in marrow, fever, hepatosplenomegaly	Transfusion, antiviral therapy, IVIG

CMV, Cytomegalovirus; *CSF,* cerebrospinal fluid; *HHV-6,* human herpesvirus 6; *IVIG,* intravenous immunoglobulin; *MCV,* mean corpuscular volume; *VP-16,* etoposide.

not indicated without a specific diagnosis in children who appear to be systemically ill.

Bone marrow **infiltration by malignant cells** commonly leads to a normochromic, normocytic anemia. The mechanism by which neoplastic cells interfere with RBC and other marrow cell synthesis is multifactorial. The reticulocyte count is often low. Immature myeloid elements may be released into the peripheral blood because of the presence of the infiltrating tumor cells. An examination of the peripheral blood may reveal lymphoblasts; when solid tumors metastasize to the marrow, these cells are seldom seen in the peripheral blood. Teardrop cells may be seen in the peripheral blood. A bone marrow examination is frequently necessary in the face of normochromic, normocytic anemia.

Congenital hypoplastic anemia (Diamond-Blackfan syndrome), a lifelong disorder, usually presents in the first few months of life or at birth with severe anemia and mild macrocytosis or normocytic anemia. This RBC disorder is due to a deficiency of bone marrow RBC precursors (Table 150.6). More than a third of patients have short stature. Many patients (50-66%) respond to corticosteroid treatment but must receive therapy indefinitely. Patients who do not respond to corticosteroid treatment are transfusion dependent and are at risk of the multiple complications of long-term transfusion therapy, especially iron overload. These patients have a higher rate of developing leukemia or other hematological malignancies than the general population.

In contrast to the congenital hypoplastic anemias, **transient erythroblastopenia of childhood**, a normocytic anemia caused by suppression of RBC synthesis, usually appears between 6 months and 5 years of age in an otherwise normal child (see Table 150.6). Viral infections are thought to be the trigger, although the mechanism leading to RBC aplasia is poorly understood. The onset is gradual, but anemia may become severe. Recovery is usually spontaneous. Differentiation from Diamond-Blackfan syndrome, in which erythroid precursors also are absent or diminished in the bone marrow, may be challenging. Transfusion of packed RBCs may be necessary if the anemia becomes symptomatic before recovery.

Aplastic crises may complicate any chronic hemolytic anemia. Human parvovirus B19 (the cause of fifth disease) infects erythroid precursors and shuts down erythropoiesis. In children with chronic hemolytic anemia, these periods of severe reticulocytopenia can lead to an acute exacerbation of the anemia that may precipitate cardiovascular decompensation. Transient erythroid aplasia is without consequence in individuals with normal RBC survival. Recovery from parvovirus infection in hemolytic disease is spontaneous, but patients may need transfusion if the anemia is severe.

Macrocytic Anemia

See Fig. 150.1.

Marrow Failure/Pancytopenia

Decision-Making Algorithm
Available @ StudentConsult.com

Anemia

Etiology

Pancytopenia is a simultaneous quantitative decrease in formed elements of the blood—erythrocytes, leukocytes, and platelets. Patients more often exhibit symptoms of infection or bleeding than anemia because of the relatively short life span of WBCs and platelets compared with the life span of RBCs. Causes of pancytopenia include failure of production (implying intrinsic bone marrow disease), sequestration (hypersplenism), and increased peripheral destruction.

Differential Diagnosis

Features that suggest **bone marrow failure** and mandate an examination of bone marrow include a low reticulocyte count, teardrop forms of RBCs (implying marrow replacement, not just failure), presence of abnormal forms of leukocytes or myeloid elements less mature than band forms, small platelets, and an elevated MCV in the face of a low reticulocyte count. Pancytopenia resulting from bone marrow failure is usually a gradual process, starting with one or two cell lines but later involving all three cell lines. Features suggesting **increased destruction** include reticulocytosis, jaundice, immature erythroid or myeloid elements on the blood smear, large platelets, and increased serum bilirubin and lactic dehydrogenase.

Aplastic Anemia

Decision-Making Algorithm
Available @ StudentConsult.com

Anemia

Etiology and Epidemiology

In a child with aplastic anemia, pancytopenia evolves as the hematopoietic elements of the bone marrow disappear and the marrow is replaced by fat. In developed countries, aplastic anemia is most often idiopathic. The disorder may be induced by drugs such as chloramphenicol and felbamate or by toxins such as benzene. Aplastic anemia also may follow infections, particularly hepatitis and infectious mononucleosis (see Table 150.6). Immunosuppression of hematopoiesis is postulated to be an important mechanism in patients with postinfectious and idiopathic aplastic anemia.

Laboratory Studies

A **bone marrow biopsy** is crucial to determine cellularity or the extent of depletion of the hematopoietic elements.

Treatment

Survival rate is approximately 20% in severe aplastic anemia with supportive care alone, although the duration of survival may be years when vigorous blood product and antibiotic support is provided. For children with severe aplastic anemia—defined by an absolute reticulocyte count less than 50,000/μL, absolute neutrophil count less than 500/mm^3, platelet count less than 20,000/mm^3, and bone marrow cellularity on biopsy specimen less than 25% of normal—the treatment of choice is **hematopoietic stem cell transplantation (HSCT)** from a sibling with identical human leukocyte antigen (HLA) and compatible mixed lymphocytes. When HSCT occurs before the recipient is sensitized to blood products, survival rate is greater than 80%. The treatment of aplastic anemia without an HLA-matched donor for HSCT is evolving, with two major options: potent immunosuppressive therapy or unrelated or partially matched HSCT. Results of trials using immunosuppressive therapy with antithymocyte globulin, cyclosporine, and corticosteroids in combination with hematopoietic growth factors have been encouraging. Such therapy is often toxic, and relapses often occur when therapy is stopped.

Fanconi Anemia

Decision-Making Algorithms
Available @ StudentConsult.com

Anemia
Petechiae/Purpura
Pancytopenia

Etiology and Epidemiology

Fanconi anemia is a constitutional form of aplastic anemia that usually presents in the latter half of the first decade of life and may evolve over years. A group of genetic defects in proteins involved in **DNA repair** have been identified in Fanconi anemia, which is inherited in an autosomal recessive manner. The diagnosis is based on demonstration of increased chromosomal breakage after exposure to agents that damage DNA. The repair mechanism for DNA damage is abnormal in all cells in Fanconi anemia, which may contribute to the increased risk of malignancies. Acute leukemia develops in 10% of cases. Other malignancies that can occur include solid tumors of the head and neck, gastrointestinal tumors, and gynecological tumors.

Clinical Manifestations

Patients with Fanconi anemia have numerous characteristic clinical findings (see Table 150.6).

Treatment

HSCT can cure the pancytopenia caused by bone marrow aplasia. Many patients with Fanconi anemia and approximately 20% of children with aplastic anemia seem to respond for a time to **androgenic therapy**, which induces masculinization and may cause liver injury and liver tumors. Androgenic therapy increases RBC synthesis and may diminish transfusion requirements. The effect on granulocytes, and especially the platelet count, is less impressive.

Other less common etiologies of familial bone marrow failure resulting in pancytopenia are outlined in Table 150.6. These include dyskeratosis congenita and familial hemophagocytic lymphohistiocytosis.

Marrow Replacement

Marrow replacement may occur as a result of **leukemia**, **solid tumors** (especially neuroblastoma), **storage diseases**, **osteopetrosis** in infants, and **myelofibrosis**, which is rare in childhood. The mechanisms by which malignant cells impair marrow synthesis of normal hematopoietic elements are complex and incompletely understood. Bone marrow aspirate and biopsy are needed for precise diagnosis of the etiology of marrow synthetic failure.

Pancytopenia Resulting From Destruction of Cells

Pancytopenia resulting from destruction of cells may be caused by **intramedullary destruction** of hematopoietic elements (myeloproliferative disorders, deficiencies of folic acid and vitamin B_{12}) or by the **peripheral destruction** of mature cells. The usual site of peripheral destruction of blood cells is the spleen, although the liver and other parts of the reticuloendothelial system may contribute. **Hypersplenism** may be the result of anatomical causes (portal hypertension or splenic hypertrophy from thalassemia); infections (including malaria); storage diseases (Gaucher disease); or malignancy (lymphomas, histiocytosis). Splenectomy is indicated only when the pancytopenia is of clinical significance.

Hemolytic Anemias

Major Hemoglobinopathies

Decision-Making Algorithms
Available @ StudentConsult.com

Jaundice
Splenomegaly
Red Urine and Hematuria
Anemia

Alpha-Chain Hemoglobinopathies

Etiology. Because alpha chains are needed for fetal erythropoiesis and production of hemoglobin F ($\alpha_2\gamma_2$), **alpha-chain hemoglobinopathies** are present in utero. Four alpha genes are present on the two number 16 chromosomes (see Fig. 150.3 and Table 150.5). Single gene deletions produce no disorder (silent carrier state) but can be detected by measuring the rates of α and β synthesis or by using molecular biological techniques. Deletion of two genes produces **α-thalassemia minor** with mild or no anemia and microcytosis. In individuals of African origin, the gene deletions occur on different chromosomes *(trans)*. Thus infants born to parents that both have α-thalassemia gene deletions in *trans* have a benign disorder. In the Asian population, deletions may occur on the same chromosome *(cis)*. Thus infants born to parents who both have α-thalassemia gene deletions in *cis* may inherit two number 16 chromosomes lacking three or even four genes resulting in severe disease. Deletion of all four α genes leads to hydrops fetalis, severe intrauterine anemia, and death, unless intrauterine transfusions are administered. Deletion of three genes produces moderate hemolytic anemia with γ_4 tetramers **(Bart hemoglobin)** in the fetus and β_4 tetramers (hemoglobin H) in older children and adults (see Table 150.5).

Beta-Chain Hemoglobinopathies

Beta-chain hemoglobinopathies in the United States are more prevalent than alpha-chain disorders, possibly because these abnormalities are not symptomatic in utero. The major beta hemoglobinopathies include those that alter hemoglobin function, including **hemoglobins S, C, E, and D,** and those that alter beta-chain production, the **β-thalassemias**. Because each RBC has two copies of chromosome 11 and they express both β-globin genes, most disorders of beta chains are not clinically severe, unless both beta chains are abnormal. By convention, when describing β-thalassemia genes, β^0 indicates a thalassemic gene resulting in absent beta-chain synthesis, whereas β^+ indicates a thalassemic gene that permits reduced but not absent synthesis of normal β chains. Disorders of the beta chain usually manifest themselves clinically between 4 and 12 months of age when fetal hemoglobin nadirs, unless they have been detected prenatally or by cord blood screening.

β-Thalassemia Major (Cooley Anemia)

Etiology and Epidemiology

β-Thalassemia major is caused by mutations that impair **beta-chain synthesis**. Because of unbalanced synthesis of alpha and beta chains, alpha chains precipitate within the cells, resulting in RBC destruction either in the bone marrow or in the spleen. β-Thalassemia major is seen most commonly in individuals of Mediterranean or Asian descent. The clinical severity of the illness varies on the basis of the molecular defect (Table 150.5).

Clinical Manifestations

Signs and symptoms of β-thalassemia major result from the combination of chronic hemolytic disease, decreased or absent production of normal hemoglobin A, and ineffective erythropoiesis. The anemia is severe and leads to growth failure and high-output heart failure. **Ineffective erythropoiesis** causes increased expenditure of energy and expansion of the bone marrow cavities of all bones, leading to osteopenia, pathological fractures, extramedullary erythropoiesis with resultant hepatosplenomegaly, and an increase in the rate of iron absorption.

Treatment

Treatment of β-thalassemia major is based on a **hypertransfusion program** that corrects the anemia and suppresses the patient's own ineffective erythropoiesis, limiting the stimulus for increased iron absorption. This suppression permits the bones to heal, decreases metabolic expenditures, increases growth, and limits dietary iron absorption. Splenectomy may reduce the transfusion volume, but it adds to the risk of serious infection. Chelation therapy with deferoxamine or deferasirox should start when laboratory evidence of iron overload **(hemochromatosis)** is present and before there are clinical signs of

TABLE 150.7 Comparison of Sickle Cell Syndromes

GENOTYPE	CLINICAL CONDITION	PERCENT HEMOGLOBIN Hb A	Hb S	Hb A_2	Hb F	Hb C	OTHER FINDING(S)
SA	Sickle cell trait	55-60	40-45	2-3	–	–	Usually asymptomatic
SS	Sickle cell anemia	0	85-95	2-3	5-15	–	Clinically severe anemia; Hb F heterogeneous in distribution
S-β^0 thalassemia	Sickle cell–β^0 thalassemia	0	70-80	3-5	10-20	–	Moderately severe anemia; splenomegaly in 50%; smear: hypochromic, microcytic anemia
S-β+ thalassemia	Sickle cell-β^+ thalassemia	10-20	60-75	3-5	10-20	–	Hb F distributed heterogeneously; mild microcytic anemia
SC	Hb SC disease	0	45-50	–	–	45-50	Moderately severe anemia; splenomegaly; retinopathy; target cells
S-HPFH	Sickle-hereditary persistence of Hb F	0	70-80	1-2	20-30	–	Often asymptomatic; Hb F is uniformly distributed

From Andreoli T, Carpenter C, Griggs R, et al. Cecil Essentials of Medicine. *7th ed. Philadelphia: Saunders; 2007.*

iron overload (nonimmune diabetes mellitus, cirrhosis, heart failure, bronzing of the skin, and multiple endocrine abnormalities). HSCT in childhood, before organ dysfunction induced by iron overload, has had a high success rate in β-thalassemia major and is the treatment of choice.

Sickle Cell Disease

Decision-Making Algorithms
Available @ StudentConsult.com

- Abdominal Pain
- Jaundice
- Hepatomegaly
- Splenomegaly
- Anemia
- Pancytopenia
- Fever Without a Source
- Irritable Infant

Etiology and Epidemiology

The common sickle cell syndromes are **hemoglobin SS disease, hemoglobin S-C disease, hemoglobin S-β^0-thalassemia, hemoglobin S-β^+-thalassemia,** and rare variants (Table 150.7). The specific hemoglobin phenotype must be identified because the clinical complications differ in frequency, type, and severity. As a result of a single **amino acid substitution** (valine for glutamic acid at the β6 position), sickle hemoglobin crystallizes and forms a gel in the deoxygenated state. When reoxygenated, the sickle hemoglobin is normally soluble. The so-called reversible sickle cell is capable of entering the microcirculation. As the oxygen is extracted and saturation declines, sickling may occur, occluding the microvasculature. The surrounding tissue undergoes infarction, inducing pain and dysfunction. This sickling phenomenon is exacerbated by hypoxia, acidosis, fever, hypothermia, and dehydration.

Clinical Manifestations and Treatment

A child with sickle cell disease is vulnerable to **life-threatening infection** by 4 months of age due to splenic dysfunction. **Splenic dysfunction** is caused by sickling of the RBCs within the spleen, resulting in an inability to filter microorganisms from the bloodstream in most patients. Splenic dysfunction is followed, eventually, by **splenic infarction**, usually by 2-4 years of age. The loss of normal splenic function makes the patient susceptible to overwhelming infection by encapsulated organisms, especially *Streptococcus pneumoniae* and other pathogens (Table 150.8). The hallmark of infection is fever. A febrile patient with a sickle cell disease (temperature >38.5°C) must be evaluated immediately (see Chapter 96). Current precautions to prevent infections include prophylactic daily oral penicillin begun at diagnosis and vaccinations against pneumococcus, *Haemophilus influenzae* type b, meningococcus, hepatitis B virus, and influenza virus.

The anemia of hemoglobin SS disease is usually a chronic, moderately severe, hemolytic anemia that is not routinely transfusion dependent. The severity depends in part on the patient's phenotype. Manifestations of chronic anemia include jaundice, pallor, variable splenomegaly in infancy, a cardiac flow murmur, and delayed growth and sexual maturation. Decisions about transfusion should be made on the basis of the patient's clinical condition, the hemoglobin level, and the reticulocyte count.

Sickle cell disease is complicated by sudden, occasionally severe and life-threatening events caused by the acute intravascular sickling of the RBCs, with resultant pain or organ dysfunction (i.e., **crisis**). In two different clinical situations, an acute, potentially life-threatening decline in the hemoglobin level may be superimposed on the chronic compensated anemia. **Splenic sequestration crisis** is a life-threatening, hyperacute drop in the hemoglobin level (blood volume) secondary to splenic pooling of the patient's RBCs and sickling within the spleen. The spleen is moderately to markedly enlarged, and the reticulocyte count is elevated. In an **aplastic crisis**, parvovirus B19 infects RBC precursors in the bone marrow and induces transient RBC aplasia with reticulocytopenia and a rapid worsening of anemia because of the very short life span of sickle RBCs. Simple transfusion therapy is indicated for sequestration and aplastic crises when the anemia is symptomatic.

Vasoocclusive painful events may occur in any organ of the body and manifest as pain and/or significant dysfunction (see Table 150.8). The **acute chest syndrome** is a vasoocclusive

TABLE 150.8 Clinical Manifestations of Sickle Cell Anemia*

MANIFESTATION	COMMENTS
Anemia	Chronic, onset 3-4 mo of age; may require folate therapy for chronic hemolysis; hemoglobin usually 6-10 g/dL
Aplastic crisis	Parvovirus infection, reticulocytopenia; acute and reversible; may need transfusion
Sequestration crisis	Massive splenomegaly (may involve liver), shock; treat with transfusion
Hemolytic crisis	May be associated with G6PD deficiency
Dactylitis	Hand-foot swelling in early infancy
Pain	Microvascular painful vasoocclusive infarcts of muscle, bone, bone marrow, lung, intestines; chronic pain (nervous system sensitization)
Cerebrovascular accidents (overt and silent)	Large and small vessel occlusion → thrombosis/bleeding (stroke); requires chronic transfusion
Acute chest syndrome	Infection, asthma, atelectasis, infarction, fat emboli, severe hypoxemia, infiltrate, dyspnea, absent breath sounds; treated with transfusions, antibiotics, oxygen, bronchodilators
Chronic lung disease	Pulmonary fibrosis, restrictive lung disease, cor pulmonale, pulmonary hypertension
Priapism	Causes eventual impotence; treated with transfusion, oxygen, or corpora cavernosa-to-spongiosa shunt
Ocular	Retinopathy
Gallbladder disease	Bilirubin stones; cholecystitis
Renal	Hematuria, papillary necrosis, renal concentrating defect; nephropathy
Cardiomyopathy	Heart failure
Skeletal	Osteonecrosis (avascular) of femoral or humeral head
Leg ulceration	Seen in older patients
Infections	Functional asplenia, defects in properdin system; pneumococcal bacteremia, meningitis, and arthritis; deafness from meningitis; *Salmonella* and *Staphylococcus aureus* osteomyelitis; severe *Mycoplasma* pneumonia
Growth failure, delayed puberty	May respond to nutritional supplements
Psychological problems	Narcotic addiction (rare), dependence unusual; chronic illness, chronic pain syndrome

**Clinical manifestations with sickle cell trait are unusual but include renal papillary necrosis (hematuria), sudden death on exertion, intraocular hyphema extension, and sickling in unpressurized airplanes.*
G6PD, Glucose-6-phosphate dehydrogenase.

crisis within the lungs with evidence of a new infiltrate on chest radiograph. It is often associated with infection and infarction. The patient may first complain of chest pain but within a few hours develops cough, increasing respiratory and heart rates, hypoxia, and progressive respiratory distress. Physical examination reveals areas of decreased breath sounds and dullness on chest percussion. Treatment involves early recognition and prevention of arterial hypoxemia. Oxygen, fluids, judicious use of analgesic medications, antibiotics, bronchodilators, and RBC transfusion (rarely exchange transfusion) are indicated as therapy for acute chest syndrome. *Incentive spirometry* may help reduce the incidence of acute chest crisis in patients presenting with pain in the chest or abdomen.

Acute painful events are the most common type of vasoocclusive events. Pain usually localizes to the long bones of the arms or legs but may occur in smaller bones of the hands or feet in infancy (dactylitis) or in the abdomen. Painful events usually last 2-7 days. Repeated painful events within the femur may lead to avascular necrosis of the femoral head and chronic hip disease. Treatment of painful events includes administration of fluids, analgesia (usually opioids and nonsteroidal antiinflammatory drugs), and oxygen if the patient is hypoxic. Appropriate use of analgesics is imperative to control pain. Patients with sickle cell disease often require high doses of opioids due to tolerance to provide adequate pain control. The frequency of acute painful events increases with age. In addition, chronic daily pain irrespective of an acute vasoocclusive event is associated with increasing age, occurring in 30% of adults and 23-40% of children. Chronic nervous system sensitization is likely a key driver of the chronic pain seen in patients with sickle cell disease.

Priapism occurs in males, usually between 6 and 20 years old. The child experiences a sudden, painful onset of a tumescent penis that will not relax. Therapeutic steps for priapism include the administration of oxygen, fluids, analgesia, and transfusion when appropriate to achieve a hemoglobin S less than 30%. Urgent partial exchange transfusion is often required to lower the hemoglobin S.

Overt **stroke** occurs in approximately 8-10% of patients with SS disease. These events may present as the sudden onset of an altered state of consciousness, seizures, or focal paralysis. **Silent stroke**, which is defined as evidence of cerebral infarction on imaging studies but a normal neurological examination, is more common and occurs in approximately 20% of patients with SS disease. A significant change in school performance or behavior has been associated with silent stroke. Children with Hg SS disease older than 3 years should be screened for increased risk of stroke using transcranial Doppler (TCD). Chronic monthly transfusions are indicated in those with overt stroke and abnormal TCDs and should be considered for those with silent strokes.

Laboratory Diagnosis

The diagnosis of hemoglobinopathies is made by identifying the precise amount and type of hemoglobin using **hemoglobin electrophoresis**, **isoelectric focusing**, or **high-performance liquid chromatography**. Every member of an at-risk population should have a precise hemoglobin phenotype performed at birth (preferably) or during early infancy. All U.S. states perform newborn screening for sickle cell disease.

Treatment

Direct therapy of sickle cell disease is evolving. The mainstay of care is supportive measures. The use of chronic RBC transfusions to treat patients who have had a stroke has been very successful. Chronic RBC transfusions have also been used successfully for short time periods to prevent recurrent vasoocclusive events, including pain, acute chest syndrome, and priapism. **Hydroxyurea**, which increases hemoglobin F, decreases the number and severity of painful events, frequency of acute chest syndrome and need for transfusions in children as early as 1 year of age. Current published clinical care guidelines from the National Institutes of Health (NIH)/National Heart, Lung, and Blood Institute (NHLBI) for patients with sickle cell disease recommend hydroxyurea should be initiated in asymptomatic children with severe sickle cell disease (HbSS or $HbS\beta^0$-thalassemia). **HSCT** using a matched sibling donor has cured many children with sickle cell disease. HSCT using alternative donors for children, without a suitable sibling match, is being studied.

Enzymopathies

Decision-Making Algorithms
Available @ StudentConsult.com

Splenomegaly
Anemia

Etiology

G6PD deficiency is an abnormality in the **hexose monophosphate shunt pathway** of glycolysis that results in the depletion of reduced nicotinamide adenine dinucleotide phosphate (NADPH) and the inability to regenerate reduced glutathione. When a patient with G6PD is exposed to significant oxidant stress, hemoglobin is oxidized, forming precipitates of sulfhemoglobin **(Heinz bodies)**, which are visible on specially stained preparations. The gene for G6PD deficiency is on the X chromosome.

The severity of hemolysis depends on the enzyme variant. In many G6PD variants the enzymes become unstable with aging of the RBC and cannot be replaced because the cell is anucleated. Older cells are most susceptible to oxidant-induced hemolysis. In other variants the enzyme is kinetically abnormal.

Epidemiology

The most common variants of G6PD deficiency have been found in areas where malaria is endemic. G6PD deficiency protects against parasitism of the erythrocyte. The most common variant with normal activity is termed **type B** and is defined by its electrophoretic mobility. The approximate gene frequencies in African Americans are 70% type B, 20% type A, and 10% type A–. Only the **A– variant**, termed the *African variant,* is unstable. Ten percent of black males are affected. A group of variants found in Sardinians, Sicilians, Greeks, Sephardic and Oriental Jews, and Arabs is termed the **Mediterranean variant** and is associated with chronic hemolysis and potentially life-threatening hemolytic disease. Because the gene for G6PD deficiency is carried on the X chromosome, clinical hemolysis is most common in males. Heterozygous females who have randomly inactivated a higher percentage of the normal gene may become symptomatic, as may homozygous females with the A– variant (0.5-1% of females of African descent).

Clinical Manifestations

G6PD deficiency has two common presentations. Individuals with the A– variant have normal hemoglobin values when well but develop an **acute episode of hemolysis** triggered by serious (bacterial) infection or ingestion of an oxidant drug. The RBC morphology during episodes of acute hemolysis is striking, appearing to have "bites" taken out of them (cookie cells). These are areas of absent hemoglobin that are produced by phagocytosis of Heinz bodies by splenic macrophages; as a result, the RBCs appear blistered. Clinically evident jaundice, dark urine resulting from bilirubin pigments, hemoglobinuria when hemolysis is intravascular, and decreased haptoglobin levels are common during hemolytic episodes. Early on, the hemolysis usually exceeds the ability of the bone marrow to compensate, so the reticulocyte count may be low for 3-4 days.

Laboratory Studies

The diagnosis of G6PD deficiency is based on decreased NADPH formation. However, G6PD levels during an acute, severe hemolytic episode may be normal because the most deficient cells have been destroyed and reticulocytes are enriched with G6PD. Repeating the test at a later time when the patient is in a steady-state condition, testing the mothers of boys with suspected G6PD deficiency, or performing electrophoresis to identify the precise variant present aids in diagnosis.

Treatment and Prevention

The treatment of G6PD deficiency is supportive. Transfusions are indicated when significant cardiovascular compromise is present. Maintaining hydration and urine alkalization protects the kidneys against damage from precipitated free hemoglobin. Hemolysis is prevented by avoidance of known oxidants, particularly long-acting sulfonamides, nitrofurantoin, primaquine, dimercaprol, and moth balls (naphthalene). Fava beans (favism) have triggered hemolysis, particularly in patients with the Mediterranean variant. Serious infection also is a potential precipitant of hemolysis in G6PD-deficient young children.

Pyruvate kinase deficiency is much less common than G6PD deficiency and represents a clinical spectrum of disorders caused by the functional deficiency of pyruvate kinase. Some individuals have a true deficiency state, and others have abnormal enzyme kinetics. The metabolic consequence of pyruvate kinase deficiency is adenosine triphosphate (ATP) depletion, impairing RBC survival. Pyruvate kinase deficiency is usually an autosomal disorder, and most children who are affected (and are not products of consanguinity) are double heterozygotes for two abnormal enzymes. Hemolysis is not aggravated by oxidant stress due to the profound reticulocytosis in this condition. Aplastic crises are potentially life threatening. The spleen is the site for RBC removal in pyruvate kinase deficiency. Most patients have amelioration of the anemia and a reduction of transfusion requirements after splenectomy.

Membrane Disorders

Decision-Making Algorithms
Available @ StudentConsult.com

Anemia
Pancytopenia

Etiology

The biochemical basis of **hereditary spherocytosis** and **hereditary elliptocytosis** are similar. Both conditions appear to have a defect in the protein lattice (spectrin, ankyrin, protein 4.2, band 3) that underlies the RBC lipid bilayer and provides stability of the membrane shape. In hereditary spherocytosis, pieces of membrane bud off as microvesicles because of abnormal vertical interaction of the cytoskeletal proteins and uncoupling of the lipid bilayer from the cytoskeleton. When the RBC loses membrane, cell shape changes from a biconcave disk to a spherocyte. The RBC is less deformable when passing through narrow passages in the spleen. Hereditary elliptocytosis is a disorder of spectrin dimer interactions that occurs primarily in individuals of African descent. The transmission of the two variants is usually autosomal dominant, but spontaneous mutations causing hereditary spherocytosis are common. **Hereditary pyropoikilocytosis** (unusual instability of the erythrocytes when they are exposed to heat at 45°C) is the result of a structural abnormality of spectrin.

Clinical Manifestations

Hereditary spherocytosis varies greatly in clinical severity, ranging from an asymptomatic, well-compensated, mild hemolytic anemia that may be discovered incidentally to a severe hemolytic anemia with growth failure, splenomegaly, and chronic transfusion requirements in infancy necessitating early splenectomy. The most common variant of hereditary elliptocytosis is a clinically insignificant morphological abnormality without shortened RBC survival. The less common variant is associated with spherocytes, ovalocytes, and elliptocytes with a moderate, usually compensated, hemolysis. Far more significant hemolysis occurs in hereditary pyropoikilocytosis. The peripheral blood smear in hereditary pyropoikilocytosis often includes elliptocytes, spherocytes, fragmented RBCs, and striking microcytosis. Such patients may have bizarre blood smears in the newborn period with small, fragmented RBCs.

Laboratory Diagnosis

The clinical diagnosis of hereditary spherocytosis should be suspected in patients with even a few spherocytes found on the blood smear because the spleen preferentially removes spherocytes. An incubated **osmotic fragility test** confirms the presence of spherocytes and increases the likelihood of the diagnosis. The osmotic fragility test result is abnormal in any hemolytic disease in which spherocytes are present (e.g., in antibody-mediated hemolysis). Genetic studies (band 3 gene mutation) can also be done to confirm the diagnosis of hereditary spherocytosis.

Treatment

Splenectomy corrects the anemia and normalizes the RBC survival in patients with hereditary spherocytosis, but the morphological abnormalities persist. Splenectomy should be reserved for any child with severe hereditary spherocytosis and symptoms referable to chronic anemia or growth failure. Splenectomy should be deferred until age 5 years, if possible, to minimize the risk of overwhelming postsplenectomy sepsis and to maximize the antibody response to the polyvalent pneumococcal and meningococcal vaccine. In several reports, partial splenectomy seems to improve the hemolytic anemia and maintain splenic function in host defense.

Hemolytic Anemia Caused by Disorders Extrinsic to the Red Blood Cell

Etiology and Clinical Manifestations

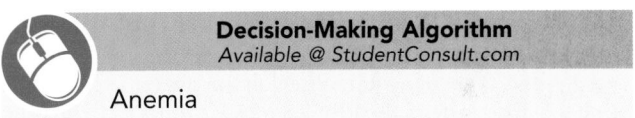

Decision-Making Algorithm
Available @ StudentConsult.com
Anemia

Isoimmune hemolysis is caused by active maternal immunization against fetal antigens that the mother's erythrocytes do not express (see Chapter 62). Examples are antibodies to the A, B, and Rh D antigens; other Rh antigens; and the Kell, Duffy, and other blood groups. Anti-A and anti-B hemolysis is caused by the placental transfer of naturally occurring maternal antibodies from mothers who lack A or B antigen (usually blood type O). Positive results of the direct antiglobulin **(Coombs)** test on the infant's RBCs (Fig. 150.4), the indirect antiglobulin test on the mother's serum, and the presence of spherocytes and

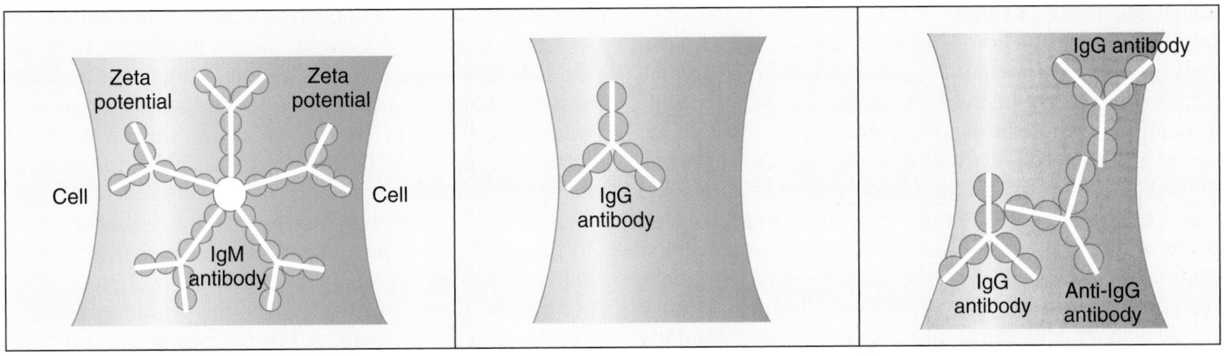

A B C

FIGURE 150.4 Coombs or direct antiglobulin test (DAT). In the DAT, so-called Coombs serum that recognizes human immunoglobulin (Ig) or complement (C) is used to detect the presence of antibody or C on the surface of the red blood cells (RBCs) by agglutination. **A,** An IgM antibody can bind two RBCs simultaneously because of its multiple antigen-binding sites. The great size of the IgM allows it to bridge the surface repulsive forces (zeta potential) between RBCs and cause agglutination. **B,** An IgG antibody is too small to bridge the zeta potential and cause agglutination. **C,** On the addition of Coombs serum, the zeta potential is bridged successfully, and RBCs agglutinate. (Modified from Ware RE, Rosse WF. Autoimmune hemolytic anemia. In: Orkin SH, Nathan DG, Look AT, Ginsburg D, eds. *Hematology of Infancy and Childhood.* 6th ed. Philadelphia: Saunders; 2003:530.)

immature erythroid precursors (erythroblastosis) on the infant's blood smear confirm this diagnosis. Isoimmune hemolytic disease varies in clinical severity. There may be no clinical manifestations or the infant may exhibit jaundice, severe anemia, and hydrops fetalis.

Autoimmune hemolytic anemia is usually an acute, self-limited Coombs-positive process that develops after an infection (*Mycoplasma,* Epstein-Barr, or other viral infections) due to the production of autoantibodies that cause red cell destruction. Autoimmune hemolytic anemia may also be the presenting symptom of a chronic autoimmune disease (systemic lupus erythematosus, lymphoproliferative disorders, or immunodeficiency). Drugs may induce a Coombs-positive hemolytic anemia by forming a hapten on the RBC membrane (penicillin) or by forming immune complexes (quinidine) that attach to the RBC membrane. Antibodies then activate complement-induced intravascular hemolysis. The third type of drug-induced immune hemolysis occurs during treatment with α-methyldopa and a few other drugs. In this type, prolonged drug exposure alters the RBC membrane, inducing neoantigen formation. Antibodies are produced that bind to the neoantigen; this produces a positive antiglobulin test result far more commonly than it actually induces hemolysis. In each of these conditions, the erythrocyte is an *innocent bystander.*

A second form of acquired hemolytic disease is caused by mechanical damage to the RBC membrane during circulation. In **thrombotic microangiopathy** the RBCs are trapped by fibrin strands in the circulation and physically broken by shear stress as they pass through these strands. Hemolytic uremic syndrome, disseminated intravascular coagulation (DIC), thrombotic thrombocytopenic purpura, malignant hypertension, toxemia, and hyperacute renal graft rejection can produce thrombotic microangiopathy. The platelets are usually large, indicating that they are young, but have a decreased survival even if the numbers are normal. Consumption of clotting factors is more prominent in DIC than in the other forms of thrombotic microangiopathy. The smear shows RBC fragments (schistocytes), microspherocytes, teardrop forms, and polychromasia. Other examples of mechanical injury to RBCs include damage by exposure to nonendothelialized surfaces (as in artificial heart valves) or as a result of high flow and shear rates in giant hemangiomas **(Kasabach-Merritt syndrome)**.

Alterations in plasma lipids, especially cholesterol, may lead to damage to the RBC membrane and shorten RBC survival. Lipids in the plasma are in equilibrium with lipids in the RBC membrane. High cholesterol levels increase the membrane cholesterol and the total membrane surface without affecting the volume of the cell. This condition produces **spur cells** that may be seen in abetalipoproteinemia and liver diseases. Hemolysis occurs in the spleen, where poor RBC deformability results in erythrocyte destruction. **Circulating toxins** (e.g., snake venoms and heavy metals) that bind sulfhydryl groups may damage the RBC membrane and induce hemolysis. Irregularly spiculated RBCs (burr cells) are seen in renal failure. **Vitamin E deficiency** can also cause an acquired hemolytic anemia as a result of abnormal sensitivity of membrane lipids to oxidant stress. Vitamin E deficiency may occur in premature infants who are not being supplemented with vitamin E or who have insufficient nutrition, in infants with severe malabsorption syndromes (including cystic fibrosis), and in infants with transfusional iron overload, which can lead to severe oxidant exposure.

Laboratory Diagnosis

The peripheral blood smear in autoimmune hemolytic anemia usually reveals spherocytes and occasionally nucleated RBCs. The reticulocyte count varies because some patients have relatively low reticulocyte counts as a result of autoantibodies that cross react with RBC precursors.

Treatment and Prognosis

Transfusion for the treatment of autoimmune hemolysis is challenging because crossmatching is difficult because the autoantibodies react with virtually all RBCs. In addition to **transfusion**, which may be lifesaving, management of autoimmune hemolytic anemia depends on antibody type. Management may involve administration of **corticosteroids** and, at times, **intravenous immunoglobulin**. Corticosteroids reduce the clearance of sensitized RBCs in the spleen. In drug-induced hemolysis, withdrawal of the drug usually leads to resolution of the hemolytic process. More than 80% of children with autoimmune hemolytic anemia recover spontaneously.

CHAPTER 151

Hemostatic Disorders

NORMAL HEMOSTASIS

Hemostasis is the dynamic process of **coagulation** as it occurs in areas of vascular injury, involving the carefully modulated interaction of platelets, vascular wall, and procoagulant and anticoagulant proteins. After an injury to the vascular endothelium, subendothelial collagen induces a conformational change in von Willebrand factor **(VWF),** an adhesive protein to which platelets bind via their glycoprotein Ib receptor. After adhesion, platelets undergo activation and release numerous intracellular contents, including adenosine diphosphate (ADP). These **activated platelets** subsequently induce aggregation of additional platelets. Simultaneously, tissue factor, collagen, and other matrix proteins in tissue activate the coagulation cascade, leading to the formation of the enzyme **thrombin** (Fig. 151.1). Thrombin causes further aggregation of platelets, a positive feedback activation of factors 5 and 8, the conversion of fibrinogen to fibrin, and the activation of factor 11. A **platelet plug** forms, and bleeding ceases, usually within 3-7 minutes. The generation of thrombin leads to formation of a permanent clot by the activation of factor 13, which cross links fibrin, forming a stable thrombus. Finally, contractile elements within the platelet mediate **clot retraction.** Thrombin also contributes to the eventual limitation of clot size by binding to the protein thrombomodulin on intact endothelial cells, converting protein C into activated protein C. Thrombin contributes to the eventual lysis of the thrombus by activating plasminogen to plasmin. All of the hemostatic processes are closely interwoven and occur on biological surfaces that mediate coagulation by bringing the critical players—platelets, endothelial cells, and subendothelium—into close proximity with pro- and anticoagulant proteins.

Many think of coagulation as having **intrinsic and extrinsic pathways,** but the reality is that these pathways are closely interactive and do not react independently (Fig. 151.2). For ease of use, all coagulation factors are denoted using Arabic rather than Roman numerals to prevent misreading factor VII (7) as

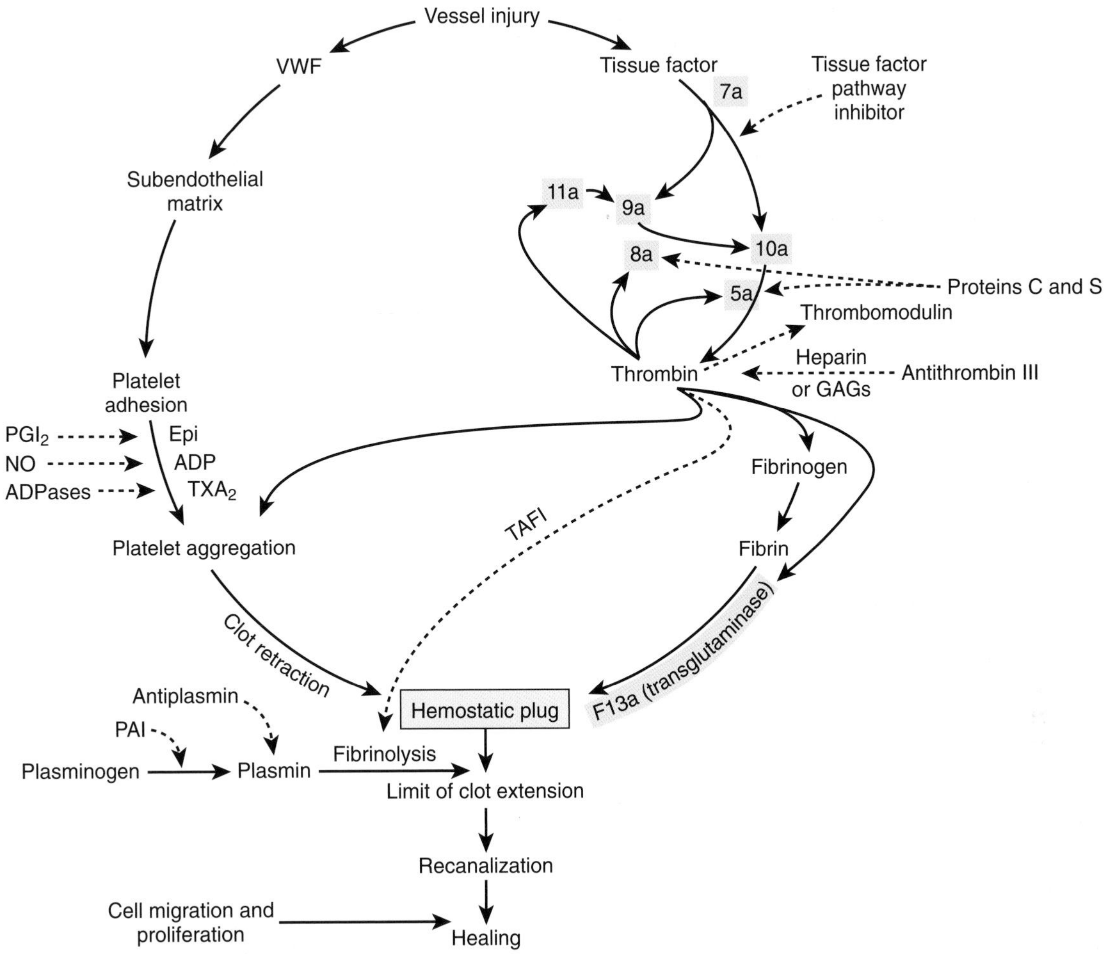

FIGURE 151.1 Diagram of the multiple interactions of the hemostatic mechanism. *Solid lines* indicate reactions that favor coagulation, and *dashed lines* indicate reactions that inhibit clotting. *Epi*, Epinephrine; *GAGs*, glycosaminoglycans; *NO*, nitric oxide; *PAI*, plasminogen activator inhibitor; *PGI_2*, prostaglandin I_2 (prostacyclin); *TAFI*, thrombin-activated fibrinolytic inhibitor; *TXA_2*, thromboxane A_2; *VWF*, von Willebrand factor. (Modified from Scott JP, Montgomery RR. Hemorrhagic and thrombotic diseases. In: Kliegman RM, Behrman RE, Jenson HB, Stanton BF, eds. *Nelson Textbook of Pediatrics*. 18th ed. Philadelphia: Saunders; 2007:2062.)

factor VIII (8). In vivo, factor 7 autocatalyzes to form small amounts of factor 7a. When tissue is injured, **tissue factor** is released and causes a burst of factor 7a generation. Tissue factor, in combination with calcium and factor 7a, activates factor 9 and factor 10. The activation of factor 9 by factor 7a results in eventual generation of thrombin, which feeds back on factor 11, generating factor 11a and accelerating thrombin formation. This process explains why deficiency of factor 8 or factor 9 leads to severe bleeding disorders, whereas deficiency of factor 11 is usually mild, and deficiency of factor 12 is asymptomatic.

A series of **inhibitory factors** serve to tightly regulate the activation of coagulation. **Antithrombin III** inactivates thrombin and factors 10a, 9a, and 11a. The **protein C and protein S** system inactivates activated factors 5 and 8, which are cofactors localized in the "tenase" and "prothrombinase" complexes. The **tissue factor pathway inhibitor**, an anticoagulant protein, limits activation of the coagulation cascade by factor 7a and factor 10a. **Fibrinolysis** is initiated by the action of tissue plasminogen activator on plasminogen, producing plasmin, the active enzyme that degrades fibrin into split products. Fibrinolysis eventually dissolves the clot and allows normal flow to resume. Deficiencies of anticoagulant proteins may predispose to thrombosis.

DEVELOPMENTAL HEMOSTASIS

In the fetus, fibrinogen, factor 5, factor 8, and platelets approach normal levels during the second trimester. Levels of other clotting factors and anticoagulant proteins increase gradually throughout gestation. The premature infant is simultaneously at increased risk of bleeding or clotting complications that are exacerbated by many of the medical interventions needed for care and monitoring, especially indwelling arterial or venous catheters. Most children attain normal levels of procoagulant and anticoagulant proteins by 1 year of age, although levels of protein C lag and normalize in adolescence.

HEMOSTATIC DISORDERS

Etiology and Epidemiology

A detailed **family history** is crucial to the diagnosis of bleeding and thrombotic disorders. **Hemophilia** is X-linked, and almost

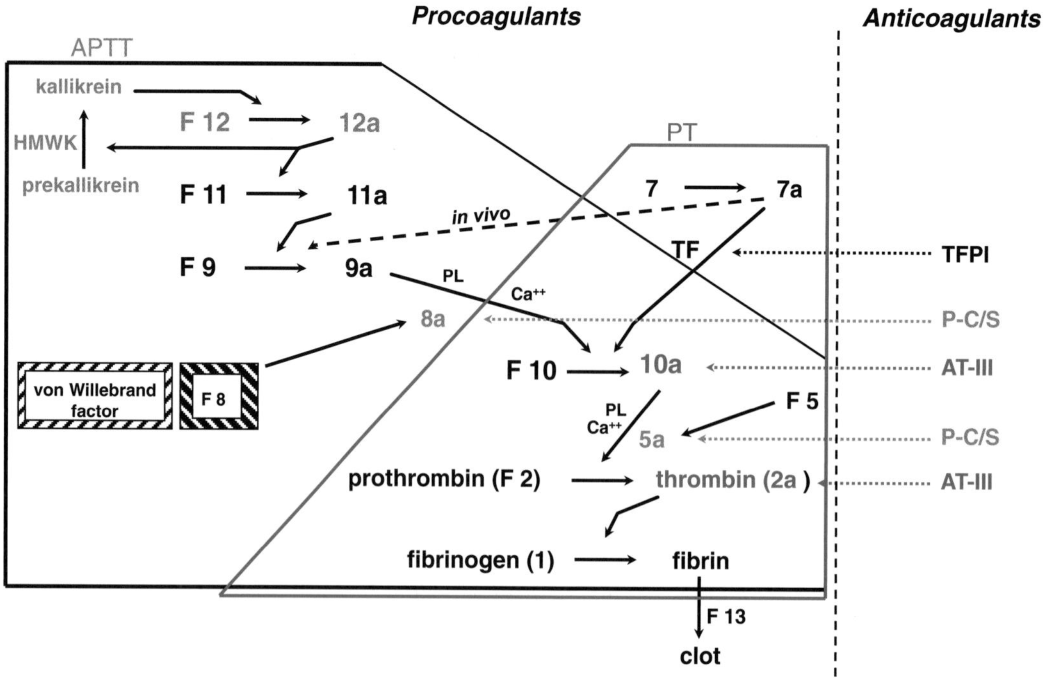

FIGURE 151.2 Simplified pathways of blood coagulation. The area inside the solid black line is the intrinsic pathway measured by the activated partial thromboplastin time (aPTT). The area inside the green line is the extrinsic pathway, measured by the prothrombin time (PT). The area encompassed by both lines is the common pathway. *AT-III*, Antithrombin III; *F*, factor; *HMWK*, high molecular weight kininogen; *P-C/S*, protein C/S; *PL*, phospholipid; *TFPI*, tissue factor pathway inhibitor. (Modified from Scott JP, Montgomery RR. Hemorrhagic and thrombotic diseases. In: Kliegman RM, Behrman RE, Jenson HB, Stanton BF, eds. *Nelson Textbook of Pediatrics*. 18th ed. Philadelphia: Saunders; 2007:2061.)

all affected children are boys. **von Willebrand disease** usually is inherited in an autosomal dominant fashion. In the investigation of thrombotic disorders, a personal or family history of blood clots in the legs or lungs, early-onset stroke, or heart attack suggests a hereditary predisposition to thrombosis. The causes of bleeding may be hematological in origin or due to vascular, nonhematological causes (Fig. 151.3). Thrombotic disorders can be congenital or acquired (Table 151.1) and frequently present after an initial event (central catheter, trauma, malignancy, infection, pregnancy, or treatment with estrogens) provides a nidus for clot formation or a procoagulant stimulus.

Clinical Manifestations

Decision-Making Algorithms
Available @ StudentConsult.com

Gastrointestinal Bleeding
Bleeding
Petechiae/Purpura

Patients with hemostatic disorders may have complaints of either bleeding or clotting. Age at onset of bleeding indicates whether the problem is congenital or acquired. The **sites of bleeding** (mucocutaneous or deep) and **degree of trauma** (spontaneous or significant) required to induce injury suggest the type and severity of the disorder. Certain medications (aspirin and valproic acid) are known to exacerbate preexisting bleeding disorders by interfering with platelet function.

TABLE 151.1 Common Hypercoagulable States

CONGENITAL DISORDERS
Factor V Leiden (activated protein C resistance)
Prothrombin 20210
Protein C deficiency
Protein S deficiency
Antithrombin III deficiency
Plasminogen deficiency
Dysfibrinogenemia
Homocystinuria
ACQUIRED DISORDERS
Indwelling catheters
Lupus anticoagulant/antiphospholipid syndrome
Nephrotic syndrome
Malignancy
Pregnancy
Birth control pills
Autoimmune disease
Immobilization/surgery
Trauma
Infection
Inflammatory bowel disease

From Scott JP. Bleeding and thrombosis. In: Kliegman RM, ed. Practical Strategies in Pediatric Diagnosis and Therapy. *Philadelphia: WB Saunders; 1996.*

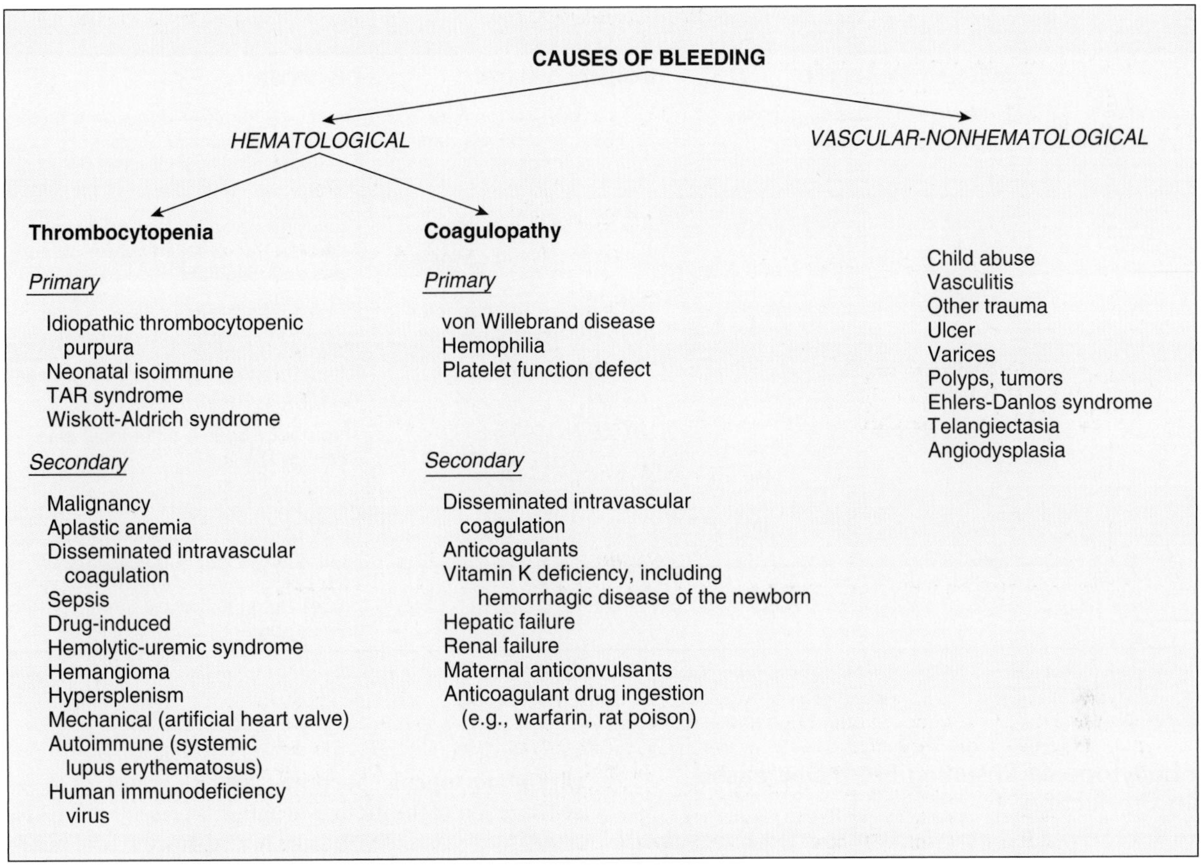

CAUSES OF BLEEDING
HEMATOLOGICAL
VASCULAR-NONHEMATOLOGICAL
Thrombocytopenia
Primary
Idiopathic thrombocytopenic purpura
Neonatal isoimmune
TAR syndrome
Wiskott-Aldrich syndrome
Secondary
Malignancy
Aplastic anemia
Disseminated intravascular coagulation
Sepsis
Drug-induced
Hemolytic-uremic syndrome
Hemangioma
Hypersplenism
Mechanical (artificial heart valve)
Autoimmune (systemic lupus erythematosus)
Human immunodeficiency virus
Coagulopathy
Primary
von Willebrand disease
Hemophilia
Platelet function defect
Secondary
Disseminated intravascular coagulation
Anticoagulants
Vitamin K deficiency, including hemorrhagic disease of the newborn
Hepatic failure
Renal failure
Maternal anticonvulsants
Anticoagulant drug ingestion (e.g., warfarin, rat poison)
Child abuse
Vasculitis
Other trauma
Ulcer
Varices
Polyps, tumors
Ehlers-Danlos syndrome
Telangiectasia
Angiodysplasia

FIGURE 151.3 Common causes of bleeding. *TAR,* Thrombocytopenia with absence of radius (syndrome).

The **physical examination** should characterize the presence of skin or mucous membrane bleeding and deeper sites of hemorrhage into the muscles and joints or internal bleeding sites. The term **petechia** refers to a nonblanching lesion less than 2 mm in size. **Purpura** is a group of adjoining petechiae, **ecchymoses** (bruises) are isolated lesions larger than petechiae, and **hematomas** are raised, palpable ecchymoses.

The physical examination should also search for manifestations of an underlying disease, lymphadenopathy, hepatosplenomegaly, vasculitic rash, or chronic hepatic or renal disease. **Deep venous thrombi** may cause warm, swollen (distended), tender, purplish discolored extremities or organs or no findings. **Arterial clots** cause acute, painful, pale, and poorly perfused extremities. Arterial thrombi of the internal organs present with signs and symptoms of infarction.

Laboratory Testing

Screening laboratory studies for bleeding patients include a **platelet count, prothrombin time, partial thromboplastin time, fibrinogen,** and **bleeding time** or other screening test of platelet function. Many laboratories have adopted the platelet function analyzer (PFA) to replace the bleeding time as a screening test for platelet function abnormalities and von Willebrand disease. The PFA has variable sensitivity and specificity for common bleeding disorders. No single laboratory test can screen for all bleeding disorders. The findings on screening tests for bleeding vary with the specific disorder (Table 151.2).

Differential Diagnosis

Disorders of Platelets

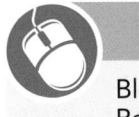

Decision-Making Algorithms
Available @ StudentConsult.com

Bleeding
Petechiae/Purpura

Platelet counts less than $150,000/mm^3$ constitute **thrombocytopenia.** Mucocutaneous bleeding is the hallmark of platelet disorders, including thrombocytopenia. The risk of bleeding correlates imperfectly with the platelet count. Children with platelet counts greater than $80,000/mm^3$ are able to withstand all but the most extreme hemostatic challenges, such as surgery or major trauma. Children with platelet counts less than $20,000/mm^3$ are at risk for spontaneous bleeding. These generalizations are modified by factors such as the age of the platelets (young, large platelets usually function better than old ones) and the presence of inhibitors of platelet function, such as antibodies, drugs (especially aspirin), fibrin degradation products, and toxins formed in the presence of hepatic or renal disease. The size of platelets is routinely measured as the mean platelet volume (MPV). The etiology of thrombocytopenia (Fig. 151.4) may be organized into three mechanisms:

1. Decreased platelet production
2. Increased destruction
3. Sequestration

TABLE 151.2 Screening Tests for Bleeding Disorders

TEST	MECHANISM TESTED	NORMAL VALUES	DISORDER
Prothrombin time	Extrinsic and common pathway	<12 sec beyond neonate; 12-18 sec in term neonate	Defect in vitamin K–dependent factors; hemorrhagic disease of newborn, malabsorption, liver disease, DIC, oral anticoagulants, ingestion of rat poison
Activated partial thromboplastin time	Intrinsic and common pathway	70 sec in term neonate 25-40 sec beyond neonate	Hemophilia; von Willebrand disease, heparin; DIC; deficient factors 12 and 11; lupus anticoagulant
Thrombin time	Fibrinogen to fibrin conversion	12-17 sec in term neonate; 10-15 sec beyond neonate	Fibrin split products, DIC, hypofibrinogenemia, heparin, uremia
Bleeding time	Hemostasis, capillary and platelet function	3-7 min beyond neonate	Platelet dysfunction, thrombocytopenia, von Willebrand disease, aspirin
Platelet count	Platelet number	150,000-450,000/mL	Thrombocytopenia differential diagnosis (see Fig. 151.4)
PFA	Closure time		
Blood smear	Platelet number and size; RBC morphology	–	Large platelets suggest peripheral destruction; fragmented, bizarre RBC morphology suggests microangiopathic process (e.g., hemolytic uremic syndrome, hemangioma, DIC)

DIC, Disseminated intravascular coagulation; *PFA*, platelet function analyzer-100; *RBC*, red blood cell.

Thrombocytopenia Resulting From Decreased Platelet Production

Primary disorders of megakaryopoiesis (platelet production) are rare in childhood, other than as part of an aplastic syndrome. **Thrombocytopenia with absent radii syndrome** is characterized by severe thrombocytopenia in association with orthopedic abnormalities, especially of the upper extremity. The thrombocytopenia usually improves over time. **Amegakaryocytic thrombocytopenia** presents at birth or shortly thereafter with findings of severe thrombocytopenia, but no other congenital anomalies. The marrow is devoid of megakaryocytes and usually progresses to aplasia of all hematopoietic cell lines.

Acquired thrombocytopenia as a result of decreased production is rarely an isolated finding. It is seen more often in the context of **pancytopenia resulting from bone marrow failure** caused by infiltrative or aplastic processes. Certain chemotherapeutic agents may affect megakaryocytes selectively more than other marrow elements. **Cyanotic congenital heart disease with polycythemia** often is associated with thrombocytopenia, but this is rarely severe or associated with significant clinical bleeding. Congenital (TORCH [toxoplasmosis, other agents, rubella, cytomegalovirus, herpes simplex]) and acquired **viral infections** (human immunodeficiency virus [HIV], Epstein-Barr virus, and measles) and some **drugs** (anticonvulsants, antibiotics, cytotoxic agents, heparin, and quinidine) may induce thrombocytopenia. Postnatal infections and drug reactions usually cause transient thrombocytopenia, whereas congenital infections may produce prolonged suppression of bone marrow function.

Thrombocytopenia Resulting From Peripheral Destruction

Etiology

In a child who appears well, **immune-mediated mechanisms** are the most common cause of thrombocytopenia resulting from rapid peripheral destruction of antibody-coated platelets by reticuloendothelial cells. **Neonatal alloimmune thrombocytopenic purpura** (NATP) occurs as a result of sensitization of the mother to antigens present on fetal platelets. Antibodies cross the placenta and attack the fetal platelet (see Chapter 59). Many platelet alloantigens have been identified and sequenced, permitting prenatal diagnosis of the condition in an at-risk fetus. Mothers with idiopathic thrombocytopenic purpura (**maternal ITP**) or with a history of ITP may have passive transfer of antiplatelet antibodies, with resultant neonatal thrombocytopenia (see Chapter 59). The maternal platelet count is sometimes a useful indicator of the probability that the infant will be affected.

Clinical Manifestations

The infant with NATP is at risk for **intracranial hemorrhage** in utero and during the immediate delivery process. In ITP, the greatest risk seems to be present during passage through the birth canal, during which molding of the head may induce intracranial hemorrhage. Fetal scalp sampling or percutaneous umbilical blood sampling may be performed to measure the fetal platelet count.

Treatment

Administration of intravenous immunoglobulin (IVIG) before delivery increases fetal platelet counts and may alleviate thrombocytopenia in infants with NATP and ITP. Delivery by cesarean section is recommended to prevent central nervous system (CNS) bleeding (see Chapter 59). Neonates with severe thrombocytopenia (platelet counts <20,000/mm^3) may be treated with IVIG or corticosteroids or both until thrombocytopenia remits. If necessary, infants with NATP may receive washed maternal platelets.

Idiopathic Thrombocytopenic Purpura

Etiology

Autoimmune thrombocytopenic purpura of childhood (childhood ITP) is a common disorder that usually follows an

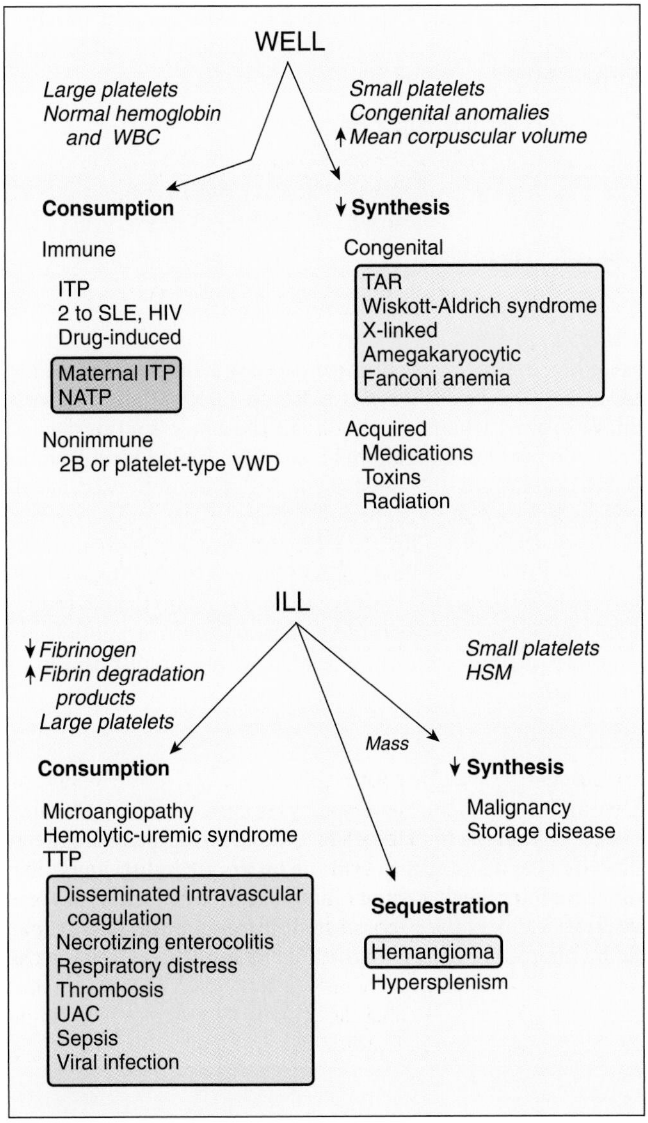

FIGURE 151.4 Differential diagnosis of childhood thrombocytopenic syndromes. The syndromes initially are separated by their clinical appearances. Clues leading to the diagnosis are presented in *italics*. The mechanisms and common disorders leading to these findings are shown in the *lower part of the figure*. Disorders that commonly affect neonates are listed in the *shaded boxes*. *HSM*, Hepatosplenomegaly; *ITP*, idiopathic immune thrombocytopenic purpura; *NATP*, neonatal alloimmune thrombocytopenic purpura; *SLE*, systemic lupus erythematosus; *TAR*, thrombocytopenia with absence of radius (syndrome); *TTP*, thrombotic thrombocytopenic purpura; *UAC*, umbilical artery catheter; *VWD*, von Willebrand disease; *WBC*, white blood cell. (From Scott JP. Bleeding and thrombosis. In: Kliegman RM, Greenbaum LA, Lye PS, eds. *Practical Strategies in Pediatric Diagnosis and Therapy*. Philadelphia: Saunders; 2004:920.)

acute viral infection. Childhood ITP is caused by an antibody (IgG or IgM) that binds to the platelet membrane. The condition results in Fc receptor–mediated splenic destruction of antibody-coated platelets. Rarely, ITP may be the presenting symptom of an autoimmune disease, such as systemic lupus erythematosus (SLE).

Clinical Manifestations

Young children typically exhibit ITP 1-4 weeks after viral illness, with abrupt onset of petechiae, purpura, and epistaxis. The thrombocytopenia usually is severe. Significant adenopathy or hepatosplenomegaly is unusual, and the red blood cell (RBC) and white blood cell (WBC) counts are normal.

Diagnosis

The diagnosis of ITP usually is based on clinical presentation and the platelet count and does not often require a bone marrow examination. If atypical findings are noted, however, marrow examination is indicated to rule out an infiltrative disorder (leukemia) or an aplastic process (aplastic anemia). In ITP, an examination of the bone marrow reveals increased megakaryocytes and normal erythroid and myeloid elements.

Treatment and Prognosis

Therapy is seldom indicated for platelet counts greater than 30,000/mm^3. Therapy does not affect the long-term outcome of ITP but is intended to increase the platelet count acutely. For moderate and severe clinical bleeding with severe thrombocytopenia (platelet count <10,000/mm^3), therapeutic options include **prednisone**, starting dose of 2 mg/kg per 24 hours for 2 weeks or IVIG, 1 g/kg per 24 hours for 1-2 days. All of these approaches seem to decrease the rate of clearance of sensitized platelets, rather than decreasing production of antibody. The optimal choice for therapy (if any) is controversial. Splenectomy is indicated in acute ITP only for life-threatening bleeding. Approximately 80% of children have a spontaneous resolution of ITP within 6 months after diagnosis. Serious bleeding, especially intracranial bleeding, occurs in fewer than 1% of patients with ITP. There is no evidence that early treatment prevents intracranial bleeding.

ITP that persists for 6-12 months is classified as **chronic ITP**. Repeated treatments with IVIG, IV anti-D, or high-dose pulse steroids are effective in delaying the need for splenectomy. Secondary causes of chronic ITP, especially SLE and HIV infection, should be ruled out. Splenectomy induces a remission in 70-80% of childhood chronic ITP cases. The risks of splenectomy (surgery, sepsis from encapsulated bacteria, pulmonary hypertension) must be weighed against the risk of severe bleeding.

Other Disorders

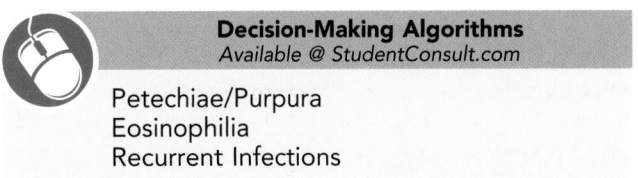

Decision-Making Algorithms
Available @ StudentConsult.com

Petechiae/Purpura
Eosinophilia
Recurrent Infections

Wiskott-Aldrich syndrome is an X-linked disorder characterized by hypogammaglobinemia, eczema, and thrombocytopenia caused by a molecular defect in a cytoskeletal protein common to lymphocytes and platelets (see Chapter 74). Small platelets are seen on a peripheral blood smear. Nevertheless, thrombocytopenia often is improved by splenectomy. Hematopoietic stem cell transplantation cures the immunodeficiency and thrombocytopenia. Familial X-linked thrombocytopenia can be seen as a variant of Wiskott-Aldrich syndrome or a mutation in the *GATA1* gene. Autosomal macrothrombocytopenia is due to deletions in chromosomes 22q11 or mutations in 22q12.

Thrombotic microangiopathy causes thrombocytopenia, anemia secondary to intravascular RBC destruction, and, in some cases, depletion of clotting factors. Children with thrombotic microangiopathy usually are quite ill. In a child with disseminated intravascular coagulation **(DIC),** the deposition of fibrin strands within the vasculature and activation of thrombin and plasmin result in a wide-ranging hemostatic disorder with activation and clearance of platelets. **Hemolytic uremic syndrome** occurs as a result of exposure to a toxin that induces endothelial injury, fibrin deposition, and platelet activation and clearance (see Chapter 164). In **thrombotic thrombocytopenic purpura**, platelet consumption, precipitated by a congenital or acquired deficiency of a metalloproteinase that cleaves VWF, seems to be the primary process, with a modest deposition of fibrin and RBC destruction.

Disorders of Platelet Function

Etiology

Primary disorders of platelet function may involve receptors on platelet membranes for adhesive proteins. Deficiency of glycoprotein Ib complex (VWF receptor) causes **Bernard-Soulier syndrome.** A deficiency of glycoprotein IIb-IIIa (the fibrinogen receptor) causes **Glanzmann thrombasthenia.** Mild abnormalities of platelet aggregation and release, detectable by platelet aggregometry, are far more common. Secondary disorders caused by toxins and drugs (uremia, valproic acid, aspirin, nonsteroidal antiinflammatory drugs, and infections) may cause a broad spectrum of platelet dysfunction.

Clinical Manifestations

Disorders of platelet function present with mucocutaneous bleeding and a prolonged bleeding time or long PFA closure time and may be primary or secondary. The bleeding time is an insensitive screen for mild and moderate platelet function disorders but is usually prolonged in severe platelet function disorders, such as Bernard-Soulier syndrome or Glanzmann thrombasthenia.

Disorders of Clotting Factors

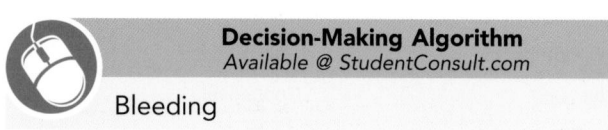

Decision-Making Algorithm
Available @ StudentConsult.com

Bleeding

Etiology

Hereditary deficiencies of most procoagulant proteins lead to bleeding. The genes for factor 8 and factor 9 are on the X chromosome, whereas virtually all the other clotting factors are coded on autosomal chromosomes. **Factor 8 and factor 9 deficiencies** are the most common severe inherited bleeding disorders. **von Willebrand disease** is the most common congenital bleeding disorder. Of the procoagulant proteins, low levels of the so-called contact factors (prekallikrein, high molecular weight kininogen, and Hageman factor [factor 12]) cause a prolonged activated partial thromboplastin time (aPTT) but are not associated with a predisposition to bleeding.

Hemophilia

Etiology

Hemophilia A (factor 8 deficiency) occurs in 1 in 5,000 males. **Hemophilia B** (factor 9 deficiency) occurs in approximately 1 in 25,000 males. Clinically the two disorders are indistinguishable other than by their therapy (Table 151.3). The lack of factor 8 or factor 9 delays the generation of thrombin, which is crucial to forming a normal, functional fibrin clot and solidifying the

TABLE 151.3 Comparison of Hemophilia A, Hemophilia B, and von Willebrand Disease

FEATURE	HEMOPHILIA A	HEMOPHILIA B	VON WILLEBRAND DISEASE
Inheritance	X-linked	X-linked	Autosomal dominant
Factor deficiency	Factor 8	Factor 9	VWF, factor 8
Bleeding site(s)	Muscle, joint, surgical	Muscle, joint, surgical	Mucous membranes, skin, surgical, menstrual
Prothrombin time	Normal	Normal	Normal
Activated partial thromboplastin time	Prolonged	Prolonged	Prolonged or normal
Bleeding time/PFA-100	Normal	Normal	Prolonged or normal
Factor 8 coagulant activity	Low	Normal	Low or normal
VWF antigen	Normal	Normal	Low
VWF activity	Normal	Normal	Low
Factor 9	Normal	Low	Normal
Ristocetin-induced platelet agglutination	Normal	Normal	Normal, low, or increased at low-dose ristocetin
Platelet aggregation	Normal	Normal	Normal
Treatment	DDAVP* or recombinant factor 8	Recombinant factor 9	DDAVP* or VWF concentrate

**Desmopressin (DDAVP) for mild to moderate hemophilia A or type 1 von Willebrand disease.*
PFA, Platelet function analyzer-100; *VWF*, von Willebrand factor.

platelet plug that has formed in areas of vascular injury. The severity of the disorder is determined by the degree of clotting factor deficiency.

Clinical Manifestations

Patients with less than 1% (severe hemophilia) factor 8 or factor 9 may have **spontaneous bleeding** or bleeding with minor trauma. Patients with 1-5% (moderate hemophilia) factor 8 or factor 9 usually require moderate trauma to induce bleeding episodes. In mild hemophilia (>5% factor 8 or factor 9), significant trauma is necessary to induce bleeding; spontaneous bleeding does not occur. Mild hemophilia may go undiagnosed for many years, whereas severe hemophilia manifests in infancy when the child reaches the toddler stage. In severe hemophilia, spontaneous bleeding occurs, usually in the muscles or joints **(hemarthroses).**

Laboratory Studies

The diagnosis of hemophilia is based on a **prolonged aPTT.** In the aPTT, a surface-active agent activates the intrinsic system of coagulation, of which factors 8 and 9 are crucial components. In factor 8 or factor 9 deficiency, the aPTT is quite prolonged but should correct to normal when the patient's plasma is mixed 1:1 with normal plasma. When an abnormal aPTT is obtained, **specific factor assays** are needed to make a precise diagnosis (see Table 151.2) to determine the appropriate factor replacement therapy. Prenatal diagnosis and carrier diagnosis are possible using molecular techniques.

Treatment

Early, appropriate **replacement therapy** is the hallmark of excellent hemophilia care. Acute bleeding episodes are best treated in the home when the patient has attained the appropriate age and the parents have learned home treatment. Bleeding associated with surgery, trauma, or dental extraction often can be anticipated, and excessive bleeding can be prevented with appropriate replacement therapy. Prophylactic therapy starting in infancy has greatly diminished the likelihood of chronic arthropathy in children with hemophilia. For life-threatening bleeding, levels of 80-100% of normal factor 8 or factor 9 are necessary. For mild to moderate bleeding episodes (hemarthroses), a 40% level for factor 8 or a 30-40% level for factor 9 is appropriate. The dose can be calculated using the knowledge that 1 U/kg body weight of factor 8 increases the plasma level 2%, whereas 1.5 U/kg of recombinant factor 9 increases the plasma level 1%:

$$\text{Dose for factor 8} = \text{desired level (\%)} \times \text{weight (kg)} \times 0.5$$

or

$$\text{Dose for recombinant factor 9} = \text{desired level (\%)} \times \text{weight (kg)} \times 1.5$$

Desmopressin acetate is a synthetic vasopressin analog with minimal vasopressor effect. Desmopressin triples or quadruples the initial factor 8 level of a patient with mild or moderate (not severe) hemophilia A, but has no effect on factor 9 levels. When adequate hemostatic levels can be attained, desmopressin is the treatment of choice for individuals with mild and moderate hemophilia A. Aminocaproic acid is an inhibitor of fibrinolysis that may be useful for oral bleeding.

Patients treated with older factor 8 or 9 concentrates derived from large pools of plasma donors were at high risk for **hepatitis B, C, and D** and **HIV**. Recombinant factor 8 and factor 9 concentrates are safe from virally transmitted illnesses. Acquired immunodeficiency syndrome (AIDS) is the most common cause of death in older hemophilia patients (who received plasma-derived factors). Many older patients also have chronic hepatitis C.

Inhibitors are IgG antibodies directed against transfused factor 8 or factor 9 in congenitally deficient patients. Inhibitors arise in 15% of patients with severe factor 8 deficiency but are less common in patients with severe factor 9 deficiency. They may be high or low titer and show an anamnestic response to treatment. The treatment of bleeding patients with an inhibitor is difficult. For low titer inhibitors, options include continuous factor 8 infusions. For high titer inhibitors, it is usually necessary to administer a product that bypasses the inhibitor, preferably recombinant factor 7a. Activated prothrombin complex concentrates, used in the past to treat inhibitor patients, paradoxically increased the risks of thrombosis, resulting in fatal complications, such as myocardial infarction. For long-term treatment of inhibitor patients, induction of immune tolerance by repeated infusion of the deficient factor with or without immunosuppression may be beneficial.

Early institution of factor replacement and continuous prophylaxis beginning in early childhood should prevent the chronic joint disease associated with hemophilia.

von Willebrand Disease

Etiology

von Willebrand disease is a common disorder (1% of the population) caused by a deficiency of **VWF**, an adhesive protein that serves two functions: acting as a bridge between subendothelial collagen and platelets and binding and protecting circulating factor 8 from rapid clearance from circulation. von Willebrand disease usually is inherited as an autosomal dominant trait and, rarely, as an autosomal recessive trait. VWF may be either quantitatively deficient (partial = type 1 or absolute = type 3) or qualitatively abnormal (type 2 = dysproteinemia). Approximately 80% of patients with von Willebrand disease have classic (type 1) disease (i.e., a mild to moderate deficiency of VWF). Several other subtypes are clinically important, each requiring different therapy.

Clinical Manifestations

Mucocutaneous bleeding, epistaxis, gingival bleeding, cutaneous bruising, and menorrhagia occur in patients with von Willebrand disease. In severe disease, factor 8 deficiency may be profound, and the patient may also have manifestations similar to hemophilia A (hemarthrosis). Findings in classic von Willebrand disease differ from findings in hemophilia A and B (see Table 151.3).

Laboratory Testing

VWF testing involves measurement of the amount of protein, usually measured immunologically as the **VWF antigen** (VWF:Ag). VWF activity (VWF:Act) is measured functionally in the **ristocetin cofactor assay** (VWFR:Co), which uses the antibiotic ristocetin to induce VWF to bind to platelets. VWF multimer testing is done to assess the protein structure and assists in the diagnosis of the qualitative disorders (type 2 = dysproteinemia).

Treatment

The treatment of von Willebrand disease depends on the severity of bleeding. **Desmopressin** is the treatment of choice for most bleeding episodes in patients with type 1 disease and some patients with type 2 disease. When high levels of VWF are needed but cannot be achieved satisfactorily with desmopressin, treatment with a virally attenuated, **VWF-containing concentrate** (Humate P) may be appropriate. The dosage can be calculated as for factor 8 in hemophilia. Cryoprecipitate should not be used because it is not virally attenuated. Hepatitis B vaccine should be given before the patient is exposed to plasma-derived products. As in all bleeding disorders, aspirin and nonsteroidal antiinflammatory drugs should be avoided.

Vitamin K Deficiency

For discussion of vitamin K deficiency, see Chapters 27 and 31.

Disseminated Intravascular Coagulation

Decision-Making Algorithms
Available @ StudentConsult.com

Bleeding
Petechiae/Purpura

Etiology

DIC is a disorder in which widespread activation of the coagulation mechanism is usually associated with shock. Normal hemostasis is a balance between hemorrhage and thrombosis. In DIC, this balance is altered by the severe illness, so the patient has activation of coagulation (thrombosis) mediated by thrombin and fibrinolysis mediated by plasmin (bleeding). Coagulation factors—especially platelets, fibrinogen, and factors 2, 5, and 8—are consumed, as are the anticoagulant proteins, especially antithrombin, protein C, and plasminogen. Endothelial injury, tissue release of thromboplastic procoagulant factors, or, rarely, exogenous factors (snake venoms) directly activate the coagulation mechanism (Table 151.4).

Clinical Manifestations

The diagnosis of DIC usually is suspected clinically and is confirmed by laboratory findings of a **decline in platelets and fibrinogen** associated with elevated prothrombin time, partial thromboplastin time, and elevated levels of D-dimer, formed when fibrinogen is clotted and then degraded by plasmin (Table 151.5). In some patients, DIC may evolve more slowly and there may be a degree of compensation. In a severely ill patient, the sudden occurrence of bleeding from a venipuncture or incision site, gastrointestinal or pulmonary hemorrhage, petechiae, or ecchymosis or evidence of peripheral gangrene or thrombosis suggests the diagnosis of DIC.

Treatment

The treatment of DIC is challenging. General guidelines include the following: treat the disorder inducing the DIC first; **support** the patient by correcting hypoxia, acidosis, and poor perfusion; and replace depleted blood-clotting factors, platelets, and anticoagulant proteins by transfusion.

Heparin may be used to treat significant arterial or venous thrombotic disease unless sites of life-threatening bleeding coexist.

TABLE 151.4 Causes of Disseminated Intravascular Coagulation

INFECTIOUS
Meningococcemia (purpura fulminans)
Other gram-negative bacteria (*Haemophilus, Salmonella, Escherichia coli)*
Rickettsiae (Rocky Mountain spotted fever)
Virus (cytomegalovirus, herpes, hemorrhagic fevers)
Malaria
Fungus
TISSUE INJURY
Central nervous system trauma (massive head injury)
Multiple fractures with fat emboli
Crush injury
Profound shock or asphyxia
Hypothermia or hyperthermia
Massive burns
MALIGNANCY
Acute promyelocytic leukemia
Acute monoblastic or myelocytic leukemia
Widespread malignancies (neuroblastoma)
VENOM OR TOXIN
Snake bites
Insect bites
MICROANGIOPATHIC DISORDERS
"Severe" thrombotic thrombocytopenic purpura
Hemolytic uremic syndrome
Giant hemangioma (Kasabach-Merritt syndrome)
GASTROINTESTINAL DISORDERS
Fulminant hepatitis
Severe inflammatory bowel disease
Reye syndrome
HEREDITARY THROMBOTIC DISORDERS
Antithrombin III deficiency
Homozygous protein C deficiency
NEONATAL PERIOD
Maternal toxemia
Group B streptococcal infections
Abruptio placentae
Severe respiratory distress syndrome
Necrotizing enterocolitis
Congenital viral disease (e.g., cytomegalovirus infection or herpes)
Erythroblastosis fetalis
MISCELLANEOUS CONDITIONS/DISORDERS
Severe acute graft rejection
Acute hemolytic transfusion reaction
Severe collagen vascular disease
Kawasaki disease
Heparin-induced thrombosis
Infusion of "activated" prothrombin complex concentrates
Hyperpyrexia/encephalopathy, hemorrhagic shock syndrome

From Scott JP. Bleeding and thrombosis. In: Kliegman RM, ed. Practical Strategies in Pediatric Diagnosis and Therapy. *Philadelphia: WB Saunders; 1996.*

TABLE 151.5 Differential Diagnosis of Coagulopathies That Can Be Confused With Disseminated Intravascular Coagulation

	PROTHROMBIN TIME	PARTIAL THROMBOPLASTIN TIME	FIBRINOGEN	PLATELETS	D-DIMER	CLINICAL KEY(S)
DIC	↑	↑	↓	↓	↑	Shock
Liver failure	↑	↑	↓	Normal or ↓	↑	Jaundice
Vitamin K deficiency	↑	↑	Normal	Normal	Normal	Malabsorption, liver disease
Sepsis without shock	↑	↑	Normal	Normal	↑ or normal	Fever

DIC, Disseminated intravascular coagulation.
From Scott JP. Bleeding and thrombosis. In: Kliegman RM, edr. Practical Strategies in Pediatric Diagnosis and Therapy. *Philadelphia: WB Saunders; 1996.*

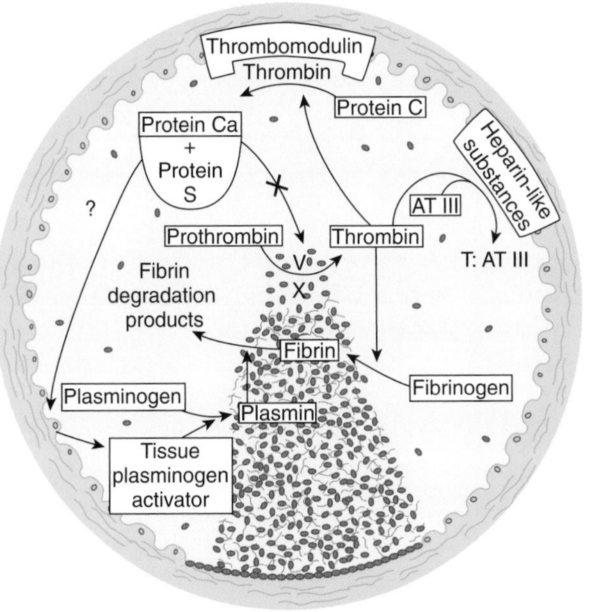

FIGURE 151.5 Formation of the hemostatic plug at the site of vascular injury. Three major physiological anticoagulant mechanisms—antithrombin III (AT III), protein C, and the fibrinolytic system—are activated to limit clot formation to the site of damage and to prevent generalized thrombosis. *T*, Thrombin. (From Schafer A. The hypercoagulable state. *Ann Intern Med.* 1985;102:814–828.)

Thrombosis

Etiology

A hereditary predisposition to **thrombosis** (see Table 151.1) may be caused by a deficiency of an anticoagulant protein (**protein C or S, antithrombin,** or **plasminogen**) (Fig. 151.5), by an abnormality of a procoagulant protein making it resistant to proteolysis by its respective inhibitor **(factor 5 Leiden),** by a mutation resulting in an increased level of a procoagulant protein (prothrombin 20210), or by damage to endothelial cells **(homocysteinemia).** Neonates with deficiency syndromes may be particularly vulnerable to thrombosis. Neonates with homozygous protein C deficiency present with purpura fulminans or thrombosis of the major arteries and veins or both. Many individuals with an inherited predisposition to thrombosis exhibit symptoms in adolescence or early adulthood. Protein C deficiency presenting in adulthood usually is inherited as an autosomal dominant trait, whereas the homozygous form usually is autosomal recessive. Protein S and antithrombin III deficiencies are inherited as autosomal dominant traits. Factor 5 Leiden is the most common hereditary cause of a predisposition to thrombosis, appearing in 3-5% of whites. **Acquired antiphospholipid antibodies** (anticardiolipin and lupus anticoagulant) also predispose to thrombosis.

Clinical Manifestations

Neonates and adolescents are the most likely pediatric patients to present with thromboembolic disease. Indwelling catheters, vasculitis, sepsis, immobilization, nephrotic syndrome, coagulopathy, trauma, infection, surgery, inflammatory bowel disease, oral contraceptive agents, pregnancy, and abortion all predispose to thrombosis. The manifestations of pulmonary emboli vary from no findings to chest pain, diminished breath sounds, a loud S_2, cyanosis, tachypnea, and hypoxemia.

Diagnostic and Imaging Studies

Venous thrombosis can be detected noninvasively by ultrasound Doppler flow compression studies. The gold standard for diagnosis is the venogram. An abnormal *(high probability)* ventilation-perfusion scan or detection of an intravascular thrombus on helical computed tomography is diagnostic of pulmonary emboli. There are no appropriate screening studies for thrombotic disorders. Diagnosis of a congenital or acquired predisposition to thrombosis requires a battery of specific assays.

Treatment

Therapy of thrombotic disorders depends on the underlying condition and usually involves standard or low molecular weight **heparin** followed by longer term anticoagulation with **warfarin.** New agents, including the direct thrombin inhibitors, are currently under active investigation in the pediatric population. Major vessel thrombosis, life-threatening thrombosis, or arterial thrombosis may necessitate treatment with **fibrinolytic agents** (recombinant tissue plasminogen activator). In newborns, inherited deficiency syndromes may present as emergencies and necessitate **replacement** with plasma, antithrombin III concentrates, or protein C concentrates.

CHAPTER 152

Blood Component Therapy

Transfusion of red blood cells (RBCs), platelets, plasma, cryoprecipitate, and granulocytes can be lifesaving or life-maintaining (Table 152.1). **Whole blood** is rarely indicated and is most useful to provide both oxygen-carrying capacity

TABLE 152.1 Commonly Used Transfusion Products

COMPONENT	CONTENT	INDICATION	DOSE	EXPECTED OUTCOME
Packed RBCs	250-300 mL/unit	↓ Oxygen-carrying RBCs	10-15 mL/kg	↑ Hb by 2-3 g/dL
Platelet concentrate from whole blood donation	5-7 × 10^{10} platelets/unit	Severe thrombocytopenia ± bleeding	1 unit/10 kg	↑ Platelet count by 50,000/μL
Platelet concentrate	3 × 10^{11} platelets/unit	Severe thrombocytopenia ± bleeding	1 unit/70 kg	↑ Platelet count by 30,000-50,000/μL
Fresh frozen plasma	1 unit of each clotting factor /mL	Multiple clotting factor deficiency	10-20 mL/kg	Improvement in significantly prolonged prothrombin and partial thromboplastin times
Cryoprecipitate	Fibrinogen, factor 8, VWF, factor 13	Hypofibrinogenemia, factor 13 deficiency	1 unit/5-10 kg	↑ Fibrinogen by 50-100 mg/dL
Recombinant factor concentrates	Units as labeled	Hemophilic bleeding or prophylaxis	F8: 20-50 units/kg F9: 40-120 units/kg	F8: ↑ 2%/unit/kg F9: ↑ 0.7 unit/kg
Recombinant factor VIIa (NovoSeven)	Micrograms (μg)	Hemophilic bleeding in patient with inhibitor; also used for uncontrolled postoperative hemorrhage	30-90 μg/kg/dose	Cessation of bleeding

Hgb, Hemoglobin; *RBCs*, red blood cells; *VWF*, von Willebrand factor.

TABLE 152.2 Evaluation of Transfusion Reactions

TYPE OF REACTION	CLINICAL SIGNS	MANAGEMENT
Acute hemolytic transfusion reaction (incidence of 1:250,000 to 1:1,000,000)	Acute shock, back pain, flushing, early fever, intravascular hemolysis, hemoglobinemia, hemoglobinuria (may be delayed 5-10 days and less severe if anamnestic response is present)	1. Stop transfusion; return blood to bank with fresh sample of patient's blood 2. Hydrate intravenously*; support blood pressure, maintain high urine flow, alkalinize urine 3. Check for and correct electrolyte abnormalities (hyperkalemia)
Delayed hemolytic transfusion reaction (incidence of 1:100,000)	Onset 7-14 days after transfusion: pain, fever, jaundice, hemoglobinuria; fall in hemoglobin; reticulocytopenia	Transfuse only antigen-negative RBCs if needed;
Febrile nonhemolytic transfusion reaction (incidence of 1:100)	Fever during or within 4 hr after end of transfusion, chills, usually from passively transfused cytokines or recipient reaction to leukocytes	Antipyretics for symptomatic treatment or pretreatment for future transfusions; leukocyte reduction has decreased incidence of febrile reactions
	Bacterial contamination can occur in 1:100,000 platelet transfusions	Blood culture if high suspicion for bacterial infection
Allergic transfusion reaction (incidence of 1:100)	Urticaria, pruritus, maculopapular rash, edema, respiratory distress, hypotension during or within 4 hr of transfusion; often because recipient has preformed antibodies against donor antigens, occasionally from passive infusion of antibodies from atopic donor	Diphenhydramine ± hydrocortisone for acute management For future transfusions consider: 1. Pretreatment with diphenhydramine ± hydrocortisone 2. Volume reduction to reduce donor plasma 3. Washing cellular products to remove all donor plasma (for severe reactions)

**Normal saline is the compatible intravenous fluid.*
HLA, Human leukocyte antigen; *RBCs*, red blood cells; *WBC*, white blood cell.
Modified from Andreoli TE, Bennett JC, Carpenter CC, Plum F, et al. Cecil Essentials of Medicine. 4th ed. Philadelphia: WB Saunders; 1997.

and functional procoagulant and anticoagulant factors. Otherwise, **packed RBCs** are used to treat anemia to increase oxygen-carrying capacity. RBC transfusions should not be used to treat asymptomatic nutritional deficiencies that can be corrected by administering the appropriate deficient nutrient (iron or folic acid).

Blood component therapy requires proper anticoagulation of the component unit, screening for infectious agents and blood group compatibility testing before administration. Typical **transfusion reactions** are listed in Table 152.2. Transfusion may also result in circulatory overload, especially in the presence of cardiopulmonary deficiency. Filtering of blood products to remove white blood cells (WBCs) may prevent febrile reactions. Long-term complications of transfusions include graft-versus-host disease and **infectious diseases** such as **hepatitis B** (<1:250,000 units) **and C** (1:1,600,000 units), **human immunodeficiency virus** (<1:1,800,000 units), malaria, syphilis, babesiosis, brucellosis, and Chagas disease. Patients who are chronically transfused are more prone to iron overload and alloimmunization to RBCs and platelets.

Suggested Readings

Alter BP. Bone marrow failure syndromes in children. *Pediatr Clin North Am.* 2002;49:973.

Hartung HD, Olson TS, Bessler M. Acquired aplastic anemia in children. *Pediatr Clin North Am.* 2013;60(6):1311–1336.

Key NS, Negrier C, Klein HG, et al. Transfusion medicine 1, 2, 3. *Lancet.* 2007;370(9585):415–426, 427–438, 439–448.

Lavin M, O'Donnell JS. New treatment approaches to von Willebrand disease. *Hematology Am Soc Hematol Educ Program.* 2016;2016(1):683–689.

Meeks SL, Batsuli G. Hemophilia and inhibitors: current treatment options and potential new therapeutic approaches. *Hematology Am Soc Hematol Educ Program.* 2016;2016(1):657–662.

Monagle P, Chan A, Goldenberg NA, et al. Antithrombotic therapy in neonates and children: antithrombotic therapy and prevention of thrombosis. 9th ed: American College of Chest Physicians evidence-based clinical practice guidelines. *Chest.* 2012;141(suppl 2):3737S.

Nathan DG, Orkin SH, Ginsburg D, et al. *Nathan and Oski's Hematology of Infancy and Childhood.* 6th ed. Philadelphia: Saunders; 2003.

Neunert C, Lim W, Crowther M, et al. American society of hematology: the American Society of Hematology 2011 evidence-based practice guideline for immune thrombocytopenia. *Blood.* 2011;117(16):4190–4207.

NHLBI Expert Panel Report on the Management of Sickle Cell Disease, 2014. http://www.nhlbi.nih.gov/sites/www.nhlbi.nih.gov/files/sickle-cell-disease-report.pdf.

Sackey K. Hemolytic anemia: part 1. *Pediatr Rev.* 1999;20:152.

Sackey K. Hemolytic anemia: part 2. *Pediatr Rev.* 1999;20:204.

Scheinberg P. Aplastic anemia: therapeutic updates in immunosuppression and transplantation. *Hematology Am Soc Hematol Educ Program.* 2012;2012:292–300.

Tolar J, Mehta PA, Walters MC. Hematopoietic cell transplantation for nonmalignant disorders. *Biol Blood Marrow Transplant.* 2012;18(suppl 1):S166–S171.

Tsai SF, Chen SJ, Yen HJ, et al. Iron deficiency anemia in predominantly breastfed young children. *Pediatr Neonatol.* 2014;55:466–469.

Wang W, Bourgeois T, Klima J, et al. Iron deficiency and fatigue in adolescent females with heavy menstrual bleeding. *Haemophilia.* 2013;19:225–230.

Wharton BA. Iron deficiency in children: detection and prevention. *Br J Haematol.* 1999;106:270.

PEARLS FOR PRACTITIONERS

CHAPTER 149

Hematology Assessment

- Normal hematological values vary according to age.
- The physiological nadir occurs at 8-10 weeks of life; this nadir is accentuated in premature infants.
- The presence of petechiae, purpura, or deeper sites of bleeding, including generalized hemorrhage, indicates abnormalities of platelets, coagulation factors, or both.
- Organ system involvement or systemic illness point to a generalized illness as the cause for hematological abnormalities.

CHAPTER 150

Anemia

- Anemia is any hemoglobin or hematocrit value that is 2 standard deviations (SDs) below the mean for age and sex.
- Androgens at the onset of puberty results in male hemoglobin values about 1.5-2 g/dL higher than females.
- Anemias are classified based on red blood cell (RBC) size: microcytic, normocytic, or macrocytic.
- Key clinical findings in patients with hemolytic anemias are jaundice, pallor, and splenomegaly.
- An elevated reticulocyte count suggests increased red blood cell production.
- Anemia with a normal reticulocyte count suggests decreased or ineffective production.

Iron Deficiency Anemia

- Pure dietary iron deficiency is rare except in children 1-3 years of age; it is most common in bottle-fed toddlers receiving large amounts of cow's milk and lacking food high in iron.
- Menstruating adolescent females who are not receiving supplemental iron are at high risk for iron deficiency.
- In an otherwise healthy child, a therapeutic trial of oral iron is the best diagnostic study for iron deficiency as long as the child is re-examined and a response is documented reticulocytosis (48-72 hours); increase in hemoglobin levels (4-30 days); and repletion of iron stores (in 1-3 months).

Thalassemias

- α-thalassemia minor and β-thalassemia minor are common causes of microcytic anemia in otherwise healthy children of Mediterranean, Southeast Asian, or African American descent.

Lead Poisoning

- Lead poisoning may be associated with hypochromic, microcytic anemia since most patients have concomitant iron deficiency.

Normocytic Anemia

- Chronic inflammation can lead to normocytic anemia that is likely mediated through hepcidin.
- Malignancy can result in normocytic anemia; red blood cell aplasias (congenital and acquired) result in normocytic anemia.

Macrocytic Anemia

- Vitamin B_{12} and folate deficiency should be evaluated for in the setting of macrocytic anemia.

Pancytopenia

- Pancytopenia is a simultaneous quantitative decrease in all formed elements of the blood.
- A low reticulocyte count, presence of abnormal forms of leukocytes or myeloid elements less mature than band forms, small platelets, and an elevated mean corpuscular volume in the face of a low reticulocyte count suggest bone marrow failure and require bone marrow examination.
- The etiology of aplastic anemia can be idiopathic, drug-induced, or postinfectious.
- Fanconi anemia, an autosomal recessive defect in DNA repair, leads to bone marrow failure, presents with multiple congenital anomalies, and can evolve into acute leukemia.

Hemoglobinopathies

- α-chain hemoglobinopathies present in utero since alpha chains are needed for fetal erythropoiesis.
- Four alpha genes are present on chromosome 16. A single gene deletion is a silent carrier, 2 gene deletions result in α-thalassemia minor (trait), 3 gene deletion results in hemoglobin H disease (moderate hemolytic anemia), 4 gene deletion results in hydrops fetalis with severe intrauterine anemia.
- β-chain hemoglobinopathies present between 4 and 12 months of age when fetal hemoglobin nadirs.

Sickle Cell Disease

- The common sickle cell syndromes are hemoglobin SS disease, hemoglobin SC disease, hemoglobin S-β°-thalassemia, and hemoglobin S-β⁺-thalassemia.
- A child with sickle cell disease is vulnerable to:
  - Life-threatening infection by 4 months of age due to splenic dysfunction (a febrile patient with sickle cell disease must be evaluated immediately and empirically treated with antibiotics).
  - Sudden, occasionally severe and life-threatening events caused by the acute intravascular sickling of the RBCs, with resultant pain or organ dysfunction.
  - Acute painful events usually localized to the long bones of the arms or legs, but may occur in smaller bones of the hands or feet in infancy (dactylitis) or in the abdomen.
  - Overt stroke occurs in approximately 8-10% of patients with hemoglobin SS or hemoglobin S-β°-thalassemia and is an indication for chronic transfusion.
- Hydroxyurea should be initiated in asymptomatic children with severe sickle cell disease (HbSS or HbSβ°-thalassemia).

Enzymopathies

- The most common red blood cell enzyme disorders are glucose-6-phosphate dehydrogenase (G6PD) deficiency and pyruvate kinase deficiency.
- The gene for G6PD is on the X-chromosome.
- Patients with pyruvate kinase deficiency have depletion of adenosine triphosphate which impairs red blood cell survival.

Membrane Disorders

- The most common red blood cell membrane hemolytic disorders are hereditary spherocytosis and hereditary elliptocytosis.
- A positive osmotic fragility test supports the diagnosis of hereditary spherocytosis.

Hemolytic Anemia Caused by Disorders Extrinsic to the Red Blood Cell

- Isoimmune hemolysis is caused by active maternal immunization against fetal antigens (i.e., A, B, and Rh D antigens).
- Autoimmune hemolytic anemia is Coombs-positive due to the production of autoantibodies that cause red blood cell destruction, often following an infection.
- Treatment often requires red blood cell transfusion in addition to corticosteroids for some types.

CHAPTER 151

Hemostatic Disorders

Normal Hemostasis

- All of the hemostatic processes are closely interwoven and occur on biological surfaces that mediate coagulation by bringing platelets, endothelial cells, and subendothelium into close proximity with pro- and anticoagulant proteins.
- Deficiency of factor 8 or factor 9 leads to severe bleeding disorders, deficiency of factor 11 can be associated with mild bleeding, and deficiency of factor 12 is asymptomatic.
- Fibrinolysis is initiated by the action of tissue plasminogen activator on plasminogen, producing plasmin, the active enzyme that degrades fibrin into split products.

Developmental Hemostasis

- Most children attain normal levels of procoagulant and anticoagulant proteins by 1 year of age; levels of protein C lag and normalize in adolescence.

Hemostatic Disorders

- A detailed family history is crucial to the diagnosis of bleeding and thrombotic disorders.
- No single laboratory test can screen for all bleeding disorders.

Platelet Disorders

- Platelet counts less than 150,000 /mm^3 constitute thrombocytopenia. Mucocutaneous bleeding is the hallmark of platelet disorders. The risk of bleeding correlates imperfectly with the platelet count.
- The etiology of thrombocytopenia is organized into three mechanisms:
  - Decreased platelet production.
  - Increased platelet destruction: neonatal autoimmune thrombocytopenia, acute idiopathic thrombocytopenia purpura, and thrombotic microangiopathy.
  - Platelet sequestration.
- Disorders of platelet function present with mucocutaneous bleeding, prolonged bleeding time, or long PFA closure time and can be primary or secondary disorders.

Disorders of Clotting Factors

- Hemophilia A (factor 8 deficiency) and hemophilia B (factor 9 deficiency) are X-linked, severe bleeding disorders.
  - Clinical bleeding often occurs in the muscles and joints; the severity of bleeding is proportional to the patient's baseline level of factor 8 or 9.
  - Factor 8 or factor 9 recombinant replacement therapy is used to treat acute bleeds, for hemostasis for surgical procedures, and as prophylaxis in patients with severe hemophilia.
- von Willebrand disease is a congenital bleeding disorder that affects about 1% of the population.
  - Associated with mucocutaneous bleeding such as epistaxis, gingival bleeding, cutaneous bruising, and menorrhagia.
  - The treatment depends on the type and the severity of bleeding; it commonly includes desmopressin (DDAVP).

Disseminated Intravascular Coagulation

- Disseminated intravascular coagulation (DIC) is a disorder with widespread activation of coagulation (thrombosis) and fibrinolysis (bleeding).
  - Diagnosis usually is suspected clinically and is confirmed by laboratory findings.
  - General treatment guidelines include:
    - Treat the disorder inducing DIC first.
    - Support the patient by correcting hypoxia, acidosis, and poor perfusion.
    - Replace depleted blood-clotting factors, platelets, and anticoagulant proteins by transfusion.

Thrombosis

- Hereditary predisposition to thrombosis:
  - Protein C or S, antithrombin, or plasminogen deficiency.
  - Abnormality of a procoagulant protein (factor 5 Leiden).
  - Increased level of a procoagulant protein (prothrombin 20210).
  - Damage to endothelial cells (homocysteinemia).
- Acquired thrombosis due to indwelling catheters, vasculitis, sepsis, immobilization, nephrotic syndrome, coagulopathy, trauma, infection, surgery, inflammatory bowel disease, oral contraceptive agents, and pregnancy.
- Venous thromboses cause warm, swollen, tender, or purplish discolored extremities; arterial thromboses cause painful, pale and poorly perfused extremities.
  - Venous thrombosis can be detected noninvasively by ultrasound Doppler flow compression studies. The gold standard for diagnosis is the venogram.
- Therapy of thrombotic disorders usually involves standard or low molecular weight heparin followed by longer-term anticoagulation with warfarin.

CHAPTER 152

Blood Component Therapy

- Transfusion of red blood cells (RBCs), platelets, plasma, cryoprecipitate, and granulocytes can be lifesaving or life-maintaining.
- Packed red blood cells are used to treat anemia to increase oxygen-carrying capacity.
- Long-term complications of transfusions include:
  - Graft-versus-host disease.
  - Infectious diseases such as hepatitis B (<1:250,000 units) and C (1:1,600,000 units), human immunodeficiency virus (<1:1,800,000 units), malaria, syphilis, babesiosis, brucellosis, and Chagas disease.
- Patients who are chronically transfused are more prone to iron overload and alloimmunization to red blood cells and platelets.

SECTION **21**

ONCOLOGY

Thomas B. Russell | Thomas W. McLean

CHAPTER **153**

Oncology Assessment

Childhood cancer is rare. Although only about 1% of new cancer cases in the United States occur among children younger than 19 years of age, cancer is the leading cause of disease-related death in children age 1-14 years. Hematopoietic tumors (leukemia, lymphoma) are the most common childhood cancers, followed by brain/central nervous system (CNS) tumors and sarcomas of soft tissue and bone (Fig. 153.1). There is wide variability in the age-specific incidence of childhood cancers. Embryonal tumors, such as neuroblastoma and retinoblastoma, peak during the first 2 years of life; acute lymphoblastic leukemia (ALL) peaks during early childhood (ages 2-5 years); osteosarcoma peaks during adolescence; and Hodgkin disease peaks during late adolescence (Fig. 153.2). The overall incidence of cancer among white children is higher than that among other ethnic groups and is twice that of African American children in the United States.

HISTORY

Many signs and symptoms of childhood cancer are nonspecific. Although most children with fever, fatigue, weight loss, or limp do not have cancer, each of these symptoms may be a manifestation of an underlying malignancy. Uncommonly, a child with cancer will have no symptoms at all. An abdominal mass may be palpated on routine examination, or a complete blood count (CBC) may be unexpectedly abnormal. Some children have a genetic susceptibility to cancer and should be screened appropriately (Table 153.1).

It is important to explore quality, duration, location, severity, and precipitating events of the chief complaint. A prominent lymph node that does not resolve (with or without antibiotics) may warrant a biopsy. A limp that does not improve within weeks should prompt a CBC and a radiograph. Fever, night sweats, or weight loss should raise the concern for lymphoma. In addition, it is important to obtain the birth history, medical and surgical history, growth history, developmental history, family history, and social history. Even though family history in most patients does not predict an underlying predisposition syndrome, cancer-predisposing genes (such as *TP53*) are mutated in approximately 9% of children and adolescents with cancer.

PHYSICAL EXAMINATION

Growth parameters and vital signs are important to obtain in all patients. Pulse oximetry should be obtained if respiratory symptoms are present. The overall appearance of the patient should be noted, particularly general appearance, pain, cachexia, pallor, and respiratory distress. Palpable masses should be measured. Lymphadenopathy and organomegaly should be quantified, if present. A thorough examination of the skin may reveal rashes, bruises, and petechiae. Careful neurological and ophthalmological examinations are crucial if headache or vomiting is present because the vast majority of patients with CNS tumors have abnormal neurological examinations.

COMMON MANIFESTATIONS

Decision-Making Algorithms
Available @ StudentConsult.com

Visual Impairment and Leukocoria
Vomiting
Hepatomegaly
Splenomegaly
Headaches
Lymphadenopathy
Anemia
Petechiae/Purpura
Pancytopenia
Fever of Unknown Origin

The most common manifestations of childhood cancer are fatigue, anorexia, malaise, pain, fever, abnormal lump or mass, pallor, bruising, petechiae, bleeding, headache, vomiting, visual changes, weight loss, and night sweats (Table 153.2). Lymphadenopathy and organomegaly are common in leukemia, particularly with T-cell ALL or non-Hodgkin lymphoma. Patients with solid tumors usually have a palpable or measurable mass. Other signs and symptoms may include limp, cough, dyspnea, cranial nerve palsies, and papilledema. In general, malignant masses are firm, fixed, and nontender, whereas masses that are infectious or inflammatory in nature are relatively softer, mobile, and tender to palpation.

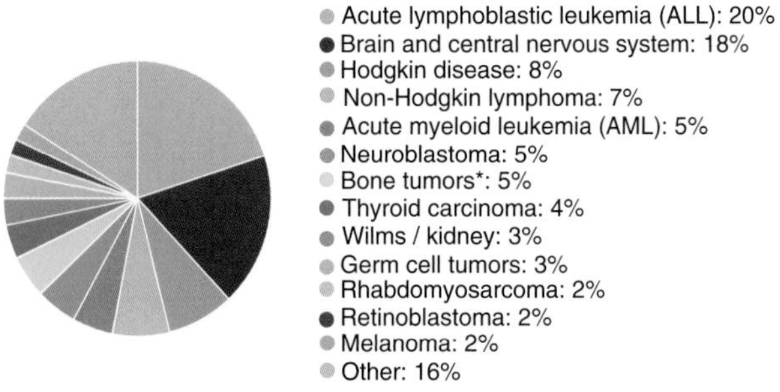

FIGURE 153.1 Number of Childhood Cancer Diagnoses per Year. Total = 15,780, Age 0-19 years. (Courtesy CureSearch for Children's Cancer, *http://curesearch.org/Number-of-Diagnoses;* Source of data: American Cancer Society, Cancer Facts and Figures, 2014.)

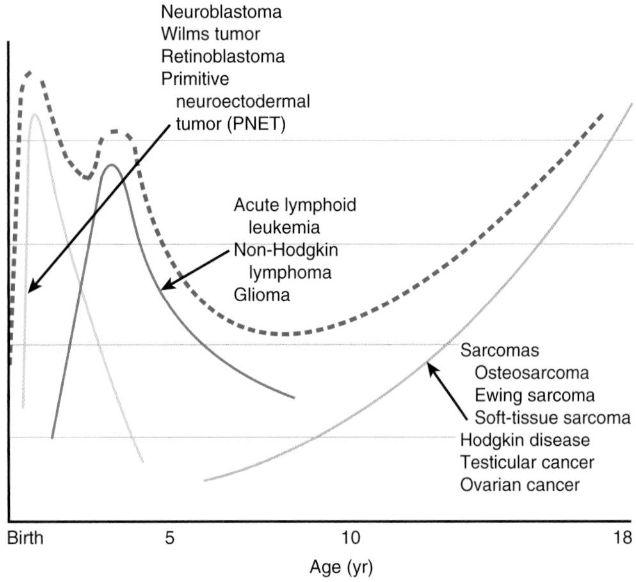

FIGURE 153.2 Incidence of the most common types of cancer in children by age. The cumulative incidence is shown as a *dashed line.* (Courtesy Archie Bleyer, MD.)

DIFFERENTIAL DIAGNOSIS

Distinguishing a malignant process from another disease can be difficult. Ultimately, a tissue diagnosis (from bone marrow or solid tumor biopsy) with pathological confirmation is required to confirm a diagnosis of cancer. Infection commonly masquerades as a potential malignancy. In particular Epstein-Barr virus, cytomegalovirus, and mycobacterial infections can mimic leukemia or lymphoma by causing fever, lymphadenopathy, organomegaly, weight loss, and abnormal blood counts. Trauma may produce swelling that can mimic solid tumors. Idiopathic thrombocytopenic purpura and iron deficiency can produce thrombocytopenia and anemia, respectively. Immune deficiencies or irregularities (autoimmune hemolytic anemia or neutropenia) can also produce cytopenias. Juvenile idiopathic arthritis and other collagen vascular disease can cause musculoskeletal pain and anemia, mimicking leukemia. Benign tumors are relatively common in children, including mature germ cell tumors/hamartomas, hemangiomas or other vascular tumors, mesoblastic nephromas, and bone cysts.

INITIAL DIAGNOSTIC EVALUATION

Screening Tests

A CBC with differential and review of the peripheral blood smear is the best screening test for many pediatric malignancies. Leukopenia (with or without neutropenia), anemia, or thrombocytopenia may be present in leukemia or any cancer that invades the bone marrow (e.g., neuroblastoma, rhabdomyosarcoma, and Ewing sarcoma). Leukemia may also produce leukocytosis, usually with blasts present on the peripheral blood smear. An isolated cytopenia (neutropenia, anemia, or thrombocytopenia) widens the differential diagnosis but still may be the only abnormal laboratory finding. Of note, a patient with leukemia may also have a normal CBC. Lactate dehydrogenase and uric acid are often elevated in fast-growing tumors (leukemia or lymphoma) and occasionally in sarcomas or neuroblastoma. In many cases, it is appropriate to assess electrolytes and renal and hepatic function in the screening process. Elevated blood pressure, if confirmed by repeat measurements, should prompt a urinalysis, as should the palpation of an abdominal mass. Serum (and/or cerebrospinal fluid) alpha-fetoprotein (AFP) and beta-human chorionic gonadotropin (β-HCG) are screening tests (and tumor markers) for germ cell tumors. Serum AFP is also a tumor marker for hepatoblastoma. Urine homovanillic acid (HVA) and vanillylmandelic acid (VMA) are tumor markers for neuroblastoma.

Diagnostic Imaging

A chest x-ray (CXR; posteroanterior and lateral) is the best screening radiographic study for a patient with suspicious cervical lymphadenopathy, fever, and weight loss. Mediastinal masses and pleural effusions can often be detected on CXR. Abdominal signs or symptoms warrant an ultrasound or computed tomography (CT) scan. Persistent headaches or morning vomiting should prompt a CT or magnetic resonance imaging (MRI) scan of the head. If bone tumors are suspected, plain radiographs are indicated and will usually reveal the lesion(s), if present. Radiographs may be normal when a bony pelvic lesion is suspected; thus a CT or MRI should be obtained. Other imaging studies to delineate a mass and to search for suspected metastases are often indicated, but these decisions are usually best left to the pediatric oncology team with input from radiologists. Table 153.3 shows the general use of diagnostic imaging following confirmation of a diagnosis of cancer to assess the primary tumor and metastases. Positron emission tomography (PET), with or without CT, has proved useful for staging and assessing response for lymphomas and sarcomas. Metaiodobenzylguanidine (mIBG) scans are useful for neuroblastoma.

TABLE 153.1 Known Risk Factors for Selected Childhood Cancers

CANCER TYPE	RISK FACTOR	COMMENTS
Acute lymphoid leukemia	Ionizing radiation	Prenatal diagnostic x-ray exposure and therapeutic irradiation for cancer treatment increases risk.
	Race	White children have a twofold higher rate than black children in the United States.
	Genetic conditions	Down syndrome is associated with an estimated 10- to 20-fold increased risk. Neurofibromatosis 1, Bloom syndrome, and ataxia-telangiectasia, among others, are associated with an elevated risk.
Acute myeloid leukemias	Chemotherapy and radiation therapy	Alkylating agents and epipodophyllotoxins increase risk, as does receiving radiation therapy for other cancers.
	Genetic factors	Down syndrome and neurofibromatosis 1 are strongly associated. Familial monosomy 7 and several other genetic syndromes are also associated with increased risk.
Brain cancers	Ionizing radiation to the head	Radiation therapy for one brain tumor can lead to a secondary brain tumor.
	Genetic factors	Neurofibromatosis 1 is strongly associated with optic gliomas and, to a lesser extent, with other CNS tumors. Tuberous sclerosis and several other genetic syndromes are associated with increased risk.
Hodgkin disease	Family history	Monozygotic twins and siblings are at increased risk.
	Infections	Epstein-Barr virus is associated with increased risk.
Non-Hodgkin lymphoma	Immunodeficiency	Acquired and congenital immunodeficiency disorders and immunosuppressive therapy increase risk.
	Infections	Epstein-Barr virus is associated with increased risk in African countries.
Osteosarcoma	Ionizing radiation	Cancer radiation therapy and high radium exposure increase risk.
	Chemotherapy	Alkylating agents increase risk.
	Genetic factors	Increased risk is apparent with Li-Fraumeni syndrome and hereditary retinoblastoma.
Ewing sarcoma	Race	Incidence is about nine times higher in white children than in black children in the United States.
Neuroblastoma	Genetic factors	Chromosome 6p22 variants and mutations in the *ALK* and *PHOX* genes are associated with increased risk.
Retinoblastoma	Genetic factors	Mutations in the Rb gene on chromosome 14
Wilms tumor	Congenital anomalies	Aniridia, Beckwith-Wiedemann syndrome, and other congenital and genetic conditions are associated with increased risk.
Renal medullary carcinoma	Sickle cell trait	Etiology is unknown.
Rhabdomyosarcoma	Congenital anomalies and genetic conditions	Li-Fraumeni syndrome and neurofibromatosis 1 are associated with increased risk.
Hepatoblastoma	Prematurity	Etiology is unknown.
	Genetic factors	Beckwith-Wiedemann syndrome, hemihypertrophy, Gardner syndrome, and familial adenomatous polyposis are associated with increased risk.
Hepatocellular carcinoma	Infections	Hepatitis B virus infection increases risk.
Malignant germ cell tumors	Cryptorchidism	Cryptorchidism is a risk factor for testicular germ cell tumors.

CNS, Central nervous system.
Modified from Scheurer ME, Lupo PL, and Bondy ML. Epidemiology of childhood cancer. In: Pizzo PA, Poplack DG, eds. Principles and Practice of Pediatric Oncology. *7th ed. Philadelphia: Wolters Kluwer; 2016:10.*

TABLE 153.2 Common Manifestations of Childhood Malignancies

SIGN/SYMPTOM	SIGNIFICANCE	EXAMPLE
HEMATOLOGICAL		
Pallor, anemia	Bone marrow infiltration	Leukemia, neuroblastoma
Petechiae, thrombocytopenia	Bone marrow infiltration	Leukemia, neuroblastoma
Fever, neutropenia	Bone marrow infiltration	Leukemia, neuroblastoma
SYSTEMIC		
Bone pain, limp, arthralgia	Primary bone tumor, metastasis to bone	Osteosarcoma, Ewing sarcoma, leukemia, neuroblastoma
Fever of unknown origin, weight loss, night sweats	Lymphoreticular malignancy	Hodgkin disease, non-Hodgkin lymphoma
Painless lymphadenopathy	Lymphoreticular malignancy, metastatic solid tumor	Leukemia, Hodgkin disease, non-Hodgkin lymphoma, Burkitt lymphoma, thyroid carcinoma
Cutaneous lesion	Primary or metastatic disease	Neuroblastoma, leukemia, Langerhans cell histiocytosis, melanoma
Abdominal mass	Abdominal/pelvic organ	Neuroblastoma, Wilms tumor, lymphoma, hepatoblastoma, germ cell tumor
Hypertension	Sympathetic nervous system tumor	Wilms tumor, neuroblastoma, pheochromocytoma
Diarrhea	Vasoactive intestinal polypeptide	Neuroblastoma
Soft tissue mass	Local or metastatic tumor	Ewing sarcoma, osteosarcoma, neuroblastoma, rhabdomyosarcoma, germ cell tumor, thyroid carcinoma
Diabetes insipidus, galactorrhea, poor growth	Neuroendocrine involvement of hypothalamus or pituitary gland	Germ cell tumor, adenoma, craniopharyngioma, prolactinoma, Langerhans cell histiocytosis
Emesis, visual disturbances, ataxia, headache, papilledema, cranial nerve palsies	Increased intrathecal pressure	Primary brain tumor; metastasis to the brain
OPHTHALMOLOGICAL		
Leukocoria	White pupil	Retinoblastoma
Periorbital ecchymosis	Metastasis	Neuroblastoma
Miosis, ptosis, heterochromia	Horner syndrome: compression of cervical sympathetic nerves	Neuroblastoma
Opsomyoclonus, ataxia	Neurotransmitters (?) Autoimmunity (?)	Neuroblastoma
Exophthalmos, proptosis	Orbital tumor	Rhabdomyosarcoma, neuroblastoma, lymphoma
THORACIC		
Anterior mediastinal mass	Cough, stridor, pneumonia, tracheal-bronchial compression	Germ cell tumor, T-cell lymphoma/leukemia, Hodgkin disease, primary mediastinal large B-cell lymphoma
Posterior mediastinal mass	Vertebral or nerve root compression; dysphagia	Neuroblastoma, ganglioneuroblastoma, ganglioneuroma

TABLE 153.3 Minimum Work-Up Required for Common Pediatric Malignancies to Assess Primary Tumor and Potential Metastases*

MALIGNANCY	BMA/bx	CXR	CT Scan	MRI	BONE SCAN, PET SCAN, or PET-CT SCAN	CSF ANALYSIS	MARKER(S)	OTHER
Leukemia	Yes	Yes	—	—	—	Yes	—	—
Non-Hodgkin lymphoma	Yes	Yes	Yes	—	Yes	Yes	—	—
Hodgkin lymphoma	Yes	Yes	Yes	—	Yes	—	—	—
CNS tumors	—	—	—	Yes	—	Yes	—	—
Neuroblastoma	Yes	—	Yes	—	Yes	—	VMA, HVA	mIBG scan
Wilms tumor	—	Yes	Yes	—	—	—	—	—
Rhabdomyosarcoma	Yes	Yes	Yes	—	Yes	Yes, for parameningeal tumors only	—	—
Osteosarcoma	—	Yes	Yes (chest)	Yes (primary)	Yes	—	—	—
Ewing sarcoma	Yes	Yes	Yes (chest)	Yes (primary)	Yes	—	—	—
Germ cell tumors	—	Yes	Yes	—	—	—	AFP, β-hCG	Consider brain MRI
Liver tumors	—	Yes	Yes	—	—	—	AFP	—
Retinoblastoma	±	—	Yes, if MRI not available	Yes (brain)	±	Yes	—	Rb gene analysis

Individual cases may require additional studies.
AFP, Alpha-fetoprotein; *β-hCG*, beta-human chorionic gonadotropin; *BMA/bx*, bone marrow aspirate/biopsy; *CNS*, central nervous system; *CSF*, cerebrospinal fluid; *CT*, computed tomography; *CXR*, chest x-ray; *HVA*, homovanillic acid; *mIBG*, metaiodobenzylguanidine; *MRI*, magnetic resonance imaging; *PET*, positron emission tomography; *Rb*, retinoblastoma; *VMA*, vanillylmandelic acid.

CHAPTER 154

Principles of Cancer Treatment

The overall goal of pediatric oncology is to cure all patients with minimal toxicity. Treatment for children with cancer is often multimodal and may involve surgery, radiation therapy, chemotherapy, and immunotherapy. Surgery and radiation are generally local treatment modalities (an exception is total body irradiation as part of a bone marrow or stem cell transplant), whereas chemotherapy and immunotherapy have both local and systemic effects.

Primary prevention strategies for most pediatric malignancies are unknown. Two exceptions are the use of hepatitis B vaccine to lower the rates of hepatocellular carcinoma and the use of human papillomavirus vaccine to reduce the risk of genitourinary and oropharyngeal cancers. Childhood malignancies are not associated with tobacco or alcohol use, dietary factors, or sun exposure. Treatment with certain chemotherapy agents and radiation therapy increases the rate of second malignancies. Secondary prevention may be accomplished by screening the at-risk child (e.g., a child with Beckwith-Wiedemann syndrome or twin of a leukemia patient), but these opportunities are rare.

ONCOLOGICAL EMERGENCIES

Adverse effects of tumors and treatments may result in oncological emergencies in children and adolescents (Table 154.1). Mediastinal masses from lymphoma can cause life-threatening airway obstruction. Tumors with a large tumor burden (e.g., lymphoma, leukemia) may affect renal function adversely from tubular deposition of uric acid crystals. Allopurinol or rasburicase can be administered before chemotherapy to minimize this effect.

A common metabolic emergency is **tumor lysis syndrome,** often seen in treatment of leukemia and lymphoma. Large amounts of phosphate, potassium, and uric acid are released into the circulation from lysed cells. Overwhelming infection and spinal cord compression with neurological compromise are other oncological emergencies.

SURGERY

Appropriate imaging (usually with computed tomography [CT] or magnetic resonance imaging [MRI]) for solid tumors presenting as a palpable mass or mass-related symptoms (pain, respiratory distress, intestinal obstruction) should be obtained and followed by resection (when possible) or biopsy (if complete resection is not feasible or indicated). Pediatric lymphomas are chemosensitive and rarely require complete surgical resection.

It is crucial to determine the amount of tissue required and the appropriate distribution of the tissue for testing so that all necessary studies are performed. A general oncological surgery principle is to resect not just the tumor but also, in most cases, a surrounding margin of normal tissue to ensure the entire tumor has been resected.

TABLE 154.1 Oncological Emergencies

CONDITION	MANIFESTATIONS	ETIOLOGY	MALIGNANCY	TREATMENT
METABOLIC				
Hyperuricemia	Uric acid nephropathy, renal insufficiency or failure	Tumor lysis syndrome	Lymphoma, leukemia	Allopurinol; hydration; rasburicase
Hyperkalemia	Arrhythmias	Tumor lysis syndrome	Lymphoma, leukemia	Kayexalate; sodium bicarbonate; glucose plus insulin
Hyperphosphatemia	Hypocalcemic tetany; metastatic calcification, photophobia, pruritus	Tumor lysis syndrome	Lymphoma, leukemia	Hydration, diuresis; oral aluminum hydroxide to bind phosphate
Hypercalcemia	Anorexia, nausea, polyuria, pancreatitis, gastric ulcers; prolonged PR/shortened QT interval	Bone resorption; ectopic parathormone, vitamin D, or prostaglandins	Metastasis to bone, rhabdomyosarcoma	Hydration and furosemide diuresis; corticosteroids; mithramycin; calcitonin, diphosphonates
HEMATOLOGICAL				
Anemia	Pallor, weakness, heart failure	Bone marrow suppression or infiltration; blood loss	Any with chemotherapy	Packed red blood cell transfusion
Thrombocytopenia	Petechiae, hemorrhage	Bone marrow suppression or infiltration	Any with chemotherapy	Platelet transfusion
Disseminated intravascular coagulation	Shock, hemorrhage	Sepsis, hypotension, tumor factors	Promyelocytic leukemia, others	Fresh frozen plasma; platelets, treat infection
Neutropenia	Infection	Bone marrow suppression or infiltration	Any with chemotherapy	If patient is febrile, administer broad-spectrum antibiotics, consider filgrastim (G-CSF)
Hyperleukocytosis (WBC $\geq$50,000/mm^3)	Hemorrhage, thrombosis; pulmonary infiltrates, hypoxia; tumor lysis syndrome	Leukostasis; vascular occlusion	Leukemia	Hydration; chemotherapy; leukapheresis?
Graft-versus-host disease	Dermatitis, diarrhea, hepatitis	Immunosuppression and nonirradiated blood products; bone marrow transplantation	Any with immunosuppression	Corticosteroids; cyclosporine; methotrexate; tacrolimus; mycophenolate mofetil; antithymocyte globulin
SPACE-OCCUPYING LESIONS				
Spinal cord compression	Back pain, motor and sensory deficits	Invasion of spinal canal by primary tumor or metastases	Neuroblastoma, medulloblastoma	MRI for diagnosis; corticosteroids; radiation therapy; laminectomy; chemotherapy
Increased intracranial pressure	Headache, confusion, coma, emesis, headache, hypertension, bradycardia, seizures, papilledema, hydrocephalus; cranial nerve III and VI palsies	Primary or metastatic brain tumor	Astrocytoma, medulloblastoma, others; neuroblastoma	CT or MRI for diagnosis; corticosteroids; ventriculoperitoneal shunt; radiation therapy; chemotherapy
Superior vena cava syndrome	Distended neck veins, plethora, edema of head and neck, cyanosis, proptosis; Horner syndrome	Superior mediastinal mass	Lymphoma	Chemotherapy; radiation therapy
Tracheal compression	Respiratory distress	Mediastinal mass compressing trachea	Lymphoma	Radiation therapy, corticosteroids

CNS, Central nervous system; *CT*, computed tomography; *G-CSF*, granulocyte colony-stimulating factor; *MRI*, magnetic resonance imaging; *WBC*, white blood cell.

CHEMOTHERAPY

Because most pediatric solid tumors have a high risk for micrometastatic disease at the time of diagnosis, chemotherapy is used in almost all cases (Table 154.2). Exceptions include low-stage neuroblastoma and Wilms tumor (particularly in infants) and low-grade central nervous system (CNS) tumors. For patients with localized solid tumors, chemotherapy administered after removal of the primary tumor is referred to as **adjuvant therapy.** Chemotherapy administered while the primary tumor is still present is referred to as **neoadjuvant chemotherapy.** Neoadjuvant chemotherapy has a number of potential benefits, including an early attack on presumed micrometastatic disease, shrinkage of the primary tumor to facilitate local control, and additional time to plan for definitive surgery.

Resistance to particular chemotherapeutic agents can develop relatively quickly. Thus combinations of chemotherapy drugs are used, as opposed to sequential single agents, to treat childhood cancer. The blood-brain barrier prevents the penetration of chemotherapeutic drugs into the CNS. Thus administration of the chemotherapeutic agent directly into the cerebrospinal fluid (by lumbar puncture) is used for leukemia and lymphoma. Radiation therapy also circumvents the blood-brain barrier.

RADIATION THERAPY

Radiation therapy is the process of delivering ionizing radiation to malignant cells to kill them directly or, more commonly, prevent them from dividing by interfering with DNA replication. Conventional radiation therapy uses photons, but atomic particles such as electrons, protons, and neutrons can also be used. Not all tumors are radiosensitive, and radiation therapy is not necessary in all tumors that are radiosensitive.

OTHER THERAPIES

Certain cancers have been treated with biological response modifiers, tyrosine kinase inhibitors, or monoclonal antibodies in addition to standard treatments. **Targeted therapies** specifically target the tumor cells, sparing normal host cells. Imatinib and dasatinib are tyrosine kinase inhibitors that target the effects of the t(9;22) translocation *(BCR-ABL)* of chronic myeloid leukemia and acute lymphoblastic leukemia. Rituximab is a monoclonal antibody directed against the cell surface antigen CD20 expressed in some lymphomas. Dinutuximab is an anti-G_{D2} monoclonal antibody used for neuroblastoma. Chimeric antigen receptor T-cell therapy and bi-specific T-cell engager therapy are immunotherapies that leverage the patient's own T cells to kill cancer cells.

Supportive care also plays an important role in pediatric oncology, including the use of appropriate antimicrobial agents, blood products, nutritional support, intensive care, and integrative therapies.

ADVERSE EFFECTS

Because chemotherapy agents are cellular toxins, numerous adverse effects are associated with their use. Bone marrow suppression, immunosuppression, nausea, vomiting, and alopecia are general adverse effects of commonly used chemotherapy drugs. Each chemotherapy drug also has specific toxicities. Doxorubicin can cause cardiac damage; cisplatin can cause renal damage and ototoxicity; cyclophosphamide and ifosfamide can cause hemorrhagic cystitis; and vincristine can cause peripheral neuropathy. Radiation therapy produces many adverse effects such as mucositis, growth retardation, organ dysfunction, and the later development of secondary cancers. Significant therapy-related **late effects** may develop in pediatric cancer patients (Table 154.3).

TABLE 154.2 Cancer Chemotherapy

DRUG	ACTION	INDICATION	ACUTE TOXICITY*
ANTIMETABOLITES			
Methotrexate	Folic acid antagonist; inhibits dihydrofolate reductase	ALL, lymphoma, medulloblastoma, osteosarcoma	Myelosuppression (nadir 7-10 days), mucositis, dermatitis, hepatitis, renal and CNS effects with high-dose administration; prevent with hydration and leucovorin, monitor levels
6-Mercaptopurine	Purine analog	ALL	Myelosuppression; hepatitis; mucositis; allopurinol increases toxicity
Cytosine arabinoside (Ara-C)	Pyrimidine analog; inhibits DNA polymerase	ALL, AML, lymphoma	Myelosuppression, conjunctivitis, mucositis, neurotoxicity
ALKYLATING AGENTS			
Cyclophosphamide	Alkylates guanine; inhibits DNA synthesis	ALL, lymphoma, sarcoma, brain tumors	Myelosuppression; hemorrhagic cystitis
Ifosfamide	Similar to cyclophosphamide	Lymphoma, Wilms tumor, sarcoma, germ cell and testicular tumors	Similar to cyclophosphamide; neurotoxicity, cardiac toxicity
Carmustine (BCNU), lomustine (CCNU)	Carbamylation of DNA; inhibits DNA synthesis	CNS tumors, lymphoma, Hodgkin disease	Delayed myelosuppression (4-6 wk); pulmonary fibrosis, carcinogenic, stomatitis

Continued

TABLE 154.2 Cancer Chemotherapy—cont'd

DRUG	ACTION	INDICATION	ACUTE TOXICITY*
Cisplatin	Inhibits DNA synthesis	Osteosarcoma, neuroblastoma, CNS tumors, germ cell tumors	Nephrotoxic; myelosuppression, ototoxicity, neurotoxicity, hemolytic uremic syndrome
Carboplatin	Inhibits DNA synthesis	Same as for cisplatin	Myelosuppression
TOPOISOMERASE INHIBITORS			
Doxorubicin and daunorubicin	Intercalation, DNA strand breaks	ALL, AML, osteosarcoma, Ewing sarcoma, lymphoma, neuroblastoma	Cardiomyopathy, red urine, tissue necrosis on extravasation, myelosuppression, conjunctivitis, radiation dermatitis, arrhythmia
Dactinomycin	Intercalation, DNA strand breaks	Wilms tumor, rhabdomyosarcoma, Ewing sarcoma	Tissue necrosis on extravasation, myelosuppression, hepatopathy with thrombocytopenia, stomatitis
Etoposide (VP-16)	DNA strand breaks	ALL, AML, lymphoma, germ cell tumor, sarcoma	Myelosuppression, secondary leukemia, allergic reaction
Topotecan	DNA strand breaks	Neuroblastoma, rhabdomyosarcoma	Myelosuppression, diarrhea, mucositis
TUBULIN INHIBITORS			
Vincristine	Inhibits microtubule formation	ALL, lymphoma, Wilms tumor, Hodgkin disease, Ewing sarcoma, neuroblastoma, rhabdomyosarcoma, brain tumors	Local cellulitis, peripheral neuropathy, constipation, ileus, jaw pain, inappropriate ADH secretion, seizures, ptosis, minimal myelosuppression
Vinblastine	Inhibits microtubule formation	Hodgkin disease, Langerhans cell histiocytosis	Local cellulitis, myelosuppression
ENZYME			
Asparaginase	Depletion of asparagine	ALL, AML	Allergic reaction; pancreatitis, hyperglycemia, platelet dysfunction and coagulopathy, encephalopathy, stroke, thrombosis
HORMONES			
Prednisone, dexamethasone	Direct lymphocyte cytotoxicity	ALL; Hodgkin disease, lymphoma	Cushing syndrome, cataracts, diabetes, hypertension, myopathy, osteoporosis, infection, peptic ulceration, irritability, psychosis, hunger, fluid retention
MONOCLONAL ANTIBODIES			
Rituximab	Anti-CD20	CD20+ B-cell leukemia, lymphoma	Fever, chills, allergy
Brentuximab	Anti-CD30	CD30+ lymphomas	Myelosuppression, peripheral neuropathy, fatigue, fever
Blinatumomab	Anti-CD19 and anti-CD3	CD19+ refractory B-lymphoblastic leukemia	Cytokine release syndrome, neurotoxicity
Dinutuximab	Anti-G_{D2}	High-risk neuroblastoma	Neuropathic pain, hypotension, hypoxia, fever, capillary leak syndrome, hypersensitivity reactions
SMALL MOLECULE PATHWAY INHIBITORS			
Imatinib	Inhibits BCR-ABL, VEGF, c-KIT kinases	Ph+ CML, ALL	Nausea, vomiting, fatigue, headache
Dasatinib	Inhibits BCR-ABL, c-KIT, and other kinases	Ph+ CML, ALL	Fluid retention, rash, nausea
MISCELLANEOUS			
Tretinoin (all-trans retinoic acid) and isotretinoin (cis-retinoic acid)	Promotes differentiation	Acute promyelocytic leukemia (ATRA); neuroblastoma (CRA)	Fever, respiratory distress, leukocytosis (ATRA); dry mouth, hair loss, pseudotumor cerebri (CRA)
Arsenic	Promotes differentiation, apoptosis	Acute promyelocytic leukemia	Transaminitis, nausea, vomiting, abdominal pain, QTc prolongation

Many drugs produce nausea and vomiting during administration; many cause alopecia with repeated doses.

ADH, Antidiuretic hormone; *ALL*, acute lymphoblastic leukemia; *AML*, acute myeloid leukemia; *ATRA*, all-trans retinoic acid; *CML*, chronic myeloid leukemia; *CNS*, central nervous system; *VEGF*, vascular endothelial growth factor.

TABLE 154.3 Long-Term Sequelae of Cancer Therapy

PROBLEM	ETIOLOGICAL AGENT(S)
Infertility	Alkylating agents; radiation
Second cancers	Genetic predisposition; radiation; alkylating agents, etoposide, topoisomerase II inhibitors
Sepsis	Splenectomy
Hepatotoxicity	Methotrexate, 6-mercaptopurine; radiation
Hepatic venoocclusive disease	High-dose, intensive chemotherapy (busulfan, cyclophosphamide) ± bone marrow transplant
Scoliosis	Radiation
Pulmonary (fibrosis)	Radiation; bleomycin, busulfan
Cardiomyopathy	Doxorubicin, daunorubicin; radiation
Leukoencephalopathy	Cranial radiation, methotrexate
Cognition/intelligence	Cranial radiation, methotrexate
Pituitary dysfunction (growth hormone deficiency, panhypopituitarism)	Cranial radiation
Psychosocial	Stress, anxiety, death of peers; conditioned responses to chemotherapy
Thyroid dysfunction	Radiation
Osteonecrosis	Corticosteroids

CHAPTER 155

Leukemia

ETIOLOGY

The etiology of childhood leukemia is unknown and is thought to be multifactorial with both genetics and environmental factors contributing to malignant transformation. In **chronic myeloid leukemia (CML)** and, less commonly, in **acute lymphoblastic leukemia (ALL)**, a translocation involving chromosomes 9 and 22 (Philadelphia [Ph] chromosome) creates a novel fusion gene called *BCR-ABL*. This results in the production of a constitutively activated tyrosine kinase that drives the development of CML and Ph-positive ALL. In addition, a number of genetic syndromes/diseases including Down syndrome (Trisomy 21), Fanconi anemia, Bloom syndrome, ataxia-telangiectasia, Wiskott-Aldrich syndrome, neurofibromatosis type 1, and rare familial leukemia syndromes can predispose children to the development of acute leukemia. Siblings of children with leukemia are at an increased risk of developing leukemia with an approximately two- to fourfold risk above the general pediatric population (approximately 25% risk for monozygotic twins). Environmental factors that may increase the risk of leukemia include ionizing radiation and chemical exposures including certain chemotherapy agents (particularly the topoisomerase II inhibitors).

EPIDEMIOLOGY

ALL accounts for approximately 75%, acute myeloid leukemia (AML) accounts for approximately 20%, and CML accounts for less than 5% of leukemia cases in the pediatric population. Other chronic leukemias, including juvenile myelomonocytic leukemia, chronic myelomonocytic leukemia, and chronic lymphocytic leukemia, are rare in childhood. ALL is the most common childhood cancer, comprising 25% of cancer prior to the age of 15 years (40 per 1 million children under the age of 15 years) and 19% of cancer prior to the age of 20 years.

ALL is classified according to lymphoid lineage as either B cell or T cell. The incidence of B-lineage ALL peaks at 2-5 years of age and is slightly more common in boys than in girls. T-cell ALL is associated with male predominance and an older age of onset. In the United States, ALL is more common in whites than in African American children. The incidence of AML is relatively higher in the neonatal period, then drops and stabilizes until adolescence when there is a slight increase, which continues into adulthood (especially beyond 55 years of age). Males and females are equally affected by AML. Hispanic and African American children have a slightly higher incidence of AML than white children.

CLINICAL MANIFESTATIONS

Decision-Making Algorithms
Available @ StudentConsult.com

Arthritis
Extremity Pain
Lymphadenopathy
Anemia
Bleeding

Signs and symptoms of acute leukemia are related to the infiltration of leukemic cells into normal tissues, resulting in either bone marrow failure (anemia, neutropenia, thrombocytopenia) and/or specific tissue infiltration (lymph nodes, liver, spleen, brain, bone, skin, gingiva, testes). Common presenting symptoms are fever, pallor, petechiae and/or ecchymoses, lethargy, malaise, anorexia, and bone/joint pain. Physical examination frequently reveals lymphadenopathy and hepatosplenomegaly. The testes and central nervous system (CNS) are common extramedullary sites for ALL involvement; neurological symptoms or a painless enlargement of one or both testes may be seen. Patients with T-cell ALL often have high white blood cell (WBC) counts, an anterior mediastinal mass (mediastinal adenopathy and/or thymic infiltration), cervical lymphadenopathy, hepatosplenomegaly, and CNS involvement. In patients with AML, extramedullary soft tissue tumors may be found in various sites.

LABORATORY AND IMAGING STUDIES

The diagnosis of acute leukemia is confirmed by findings of immature blast cells on the peripheral blood smear, bone marrow aspirate, or both. Most patients have abnormal blood counts; anemia and thrombocytopenia are common. The WBC count may be low, normal, or high; 15-20% of patients have a

WBC count of 50,000/mm^3 or higher (hyperleukocytosis) at presentation. Definitive diagnosis requires the evaluation of cell surface markers (immunophenotype) by flow cytometry. Cytogenetic analysis should be undertaken in all cases of acute leukemia because many reoccurring cytogenetic abnormalities have prognostic implications and are used, in combination with other risk factors, to assign therapy to optimize outcome. In B-lineage ALL, the t(12;21) translocation (previously called *TEL/AML;* now referred to as *ETV6/RUNX1*) is the most common (approximately 20% of all cases) and is associated with a favorable prognosis when combined with other low-risk features. The t(9;22) translocation occurs in 3% of cases and, historically, has a poor prognosis. However, much like in CML, the use of tyrosine kinase inhibitors in Ph-positive ALL has resulted in dramatic improvements in outcomes. The t(4;11) translocation (and other translocations involving the MLL gene on chromosome 11) often occurs in infant ALL and patients with secondary AML (often in patients that have been exposed to topoisomerase II inhibitors). It is associated with a poor prognosis. Fluorescent in situ hybridization or polymerase chain reaction techniques are now used in most cases of leukemia because many chromosomal abnormalities are not apparent on routine karyotypes. DNA microarray techniques are becoming an important diagnostic and prognostic tool. Recently, a new high-risk subgroup called Philadelphia-like ALL has been identified using this technique. A lumbar puncture should always be performed at the time of diagnosis to evaluate the possibility of CNS involvement. A chest x-ray should be obtained in all patients to assess for an anterior mediastinal mass. Electrolytes (particularly potassium, phosphorous, and calcium), uric acid, and renal and hepatic function should be monitored in all patients to assess and treat patients at risk for tumor lysis syndrome.

DIFFERENTIAL DIAGNOSIS

The differential diagnosis of acute leukemia includes nonmalignant and malignant diseases. Infection is probably the most common mimicker of acute leukemia, particularly Epstein-Barr virus. Other infections (cytomegalovirus, other viruses, mycobacteria) may also produce signs and symptoms common to leukemia. Noninfectious considerations include aplastic anemia, histiocytosis, juvenile idiopathic arthritis, immune thrombocytopenic purpura, and congenital or acquired conditions that result in neutropenia or anemia. Several malignant diagnoses including neuroblastoma, rhabdomyosarcoma, and Ewing sarcoma can also mimic leukemia. Newborns with trisomy 21 may have a condition known as transient myeloproliferative disorder, which produces elevated WBC counts with peripheral blasts, anemia, and thrombocytopenia. It usually resolves with supportive care only, but these children have a significantly increased risk (30%) of developing acute leukemia (ALL or AML) within the next few months to years of life.

TREATMENT

Patients with B-lineage ALL generally receive three- or four-agent induction chemotherapy (patients with T-cell ALL receive a four-agent induction) based on their initial risk group assignment. Standard-risk patients receive vincristine, corticosteroids, and pegylated asparaginase over 4 weeks; high-risk patients also receive an anthracycline (typically daunorubicin). Intrathecal therapy with cytarabine or methotrexate is given to treat existing or subclinical CNS leukemia. Following induction therapy, patients undergo an end-of-induction bone marrow evaluation to assess for remission (nearly all patients with ALL achieve a remission). The intensity of postinduction therapy relies on risk adaptation using a variety of prognostic tools (cytogenetics, rapidity and depth of remission using tests for minimal residual disease [MRD], etc.). ALL patients with CNS involvement detected at diagnosis often require more intensive treatment that can include an escalation in their intrathecal therapy as well as the use of cranial radiation therapy. Recently, the omission of cranial radiation therapy for all pediatric leukemia patients holds great promise. Patients with ALL receive chemotherapy for a total of 2-3 years. The treatment of AML is divided into three general types including (1) acute promyelocytic leukemia with a t(15;17) translocation *(PML-RARA)* that relies heavily on all-trans retinoic acid and arsenic trioxide; (2) myeloid leukemias of Down syndrome in which less intensive therapy is administered, and (3) AML that parallels the risk and biological features most commonly seen in adult AML. The latter results in the need for intensive therapy and, in select high-risk patients, the use of stem cell transplantation after completing upfront intensive chemotherapy. The majority of pediatric patients with AML require four cycles of intensive cytarabine-based chemotherapy for low- and intermediate-risk patients and stem cell transplant for high-risk patients. Much like ALL, risk adaptive therapy is based on cytogenetics and response to therapy. Additionally, the availability of a human leukocyte antigen (HLA)-matched donor (ideally an HLA-matched sibling) determines the use of stem cell transplantation in first remission. Unlike ALL, there is little evidence that low-dose continuation therapy is helpful in AML (with the exception of acute promyelocytic leukemia).

COMPLICATIONS

Major short-term complications associated with the treatment of leukemia result from bone marrow suppression caused by chemotherapy. Patients may have bleeding and significant anemia that necessitates transfusion of platelets and red blood cells. The development of neutropenia predisposes patients to a significant risk of both bacterial and fungal infections. Cell-mediated immunosuppression increases the risk of *Pneumocystis jiroveci (carinii)* pneumonia; hence, prophylaxis, most commonly with oral trimethoprim-sulfamethoxazole, is recommended. Prophylaxis with antibiotics and antifungal agents is becoming more commonplace, particularly in patients with AML who are at high risk for treatment-related mortality (obese patients and adolescent/young adult patients). Long-term sequelae of therapy are less common than in previous treatment eras but continue to be a priority for prevention, recognition, and treatment. These sequelae include neurocognitive impairment, short stature, obesity, cardiac dysfunction, infertility, second malignant neoplasms, and psychosocial problems (Table 154.3).

PROGNOSIS

Patients with ALL are classified into prognostic risk groups (B-lineage ALL currently separates patients into low, average, high, and very high risk) based on age, initial WBC count, genetic characteristics (cytogenetics), extramedullary involvement at diagnosis (testicular and/or CNS involvement), and response to induction therapy using MRD techniques. Risk

TABLE 155.1 General Prognostic Factors in Acute Lymphoblastic Leukemia

FACTOR	FAVORABLE (LOWER RISK)	UNFAVORABLE (HIGHER RISK)
Age	1-9.99 years	<1 or ≥10 years
Gender	Female	Male
Race and ethnicity	Caucasian, Asian/Pacific Islanders	African American, Hispanic, Native American
Initial WBC count	<50,000/mm^3	≥50,000/mm^3
CNS disease at diagnosis	Absent	Present
Immunophenotype	B-lineage	T cell
Ploidy	Hyperdiploidy	Hypodiploidy
Genetics	t(12;21), trisomies of chromosomes 4 and 10	t(4;11), t(9;22), Ph-like, iamp21
Minimal residual disease after remission induction	Negative	Positive

CNS, Central nervous system; *WBC*, white blood cell.

stratification factors are evolving (Table 155.1). The overall cure rate for childhood B-lineage ALL is approaching 90%. Relapse of ALL occurs most commonly in the bone marrow but can involve other extramedullary sites, such as the CNS or testicles. Relapse therapy relies on several treatment options based on the timing and location of relapse as well as the patient's response to initial reinduction with chemotherapy. Thereafter a number of treatment options are employed including chemotherapy only, combination of chemotherapy with immunotherapy, immunotherapy alone, and stem cell transplantation. The current overall cure rate for childhood AML is approximately 65%. The prognosis for relapsed AML is poor, particularly in patients who have received a stem cell transplant.

CHAPTER 156

Lymphoma

ETIOLOGY

Lymphomas are malignancies of lymphoid tissues and are the third most common malignancy in childhood, behind leukemias and central nervous system (CNS) tumors. There are two major types of lymphoma: **Hodgkin lymphoma (HL)** and **non-Hodgkin lymphoma (NHL)**. The etiologies are multifactorial. Both congenital and acquired immunodeficiencies are more commonly associated with NHL, whereas the Epstein-Barr virus (EBV) has been associated with both HL and NHL.

Almost all cases of NHL in childhood are diffuse, highly malignant, and show little differentiation. NHL has three histological subtypes: small noncleaved cell (Burkitt lymphoma), lymphoblastic, and large cell. For simplicity, these may be regarded as B cell, T cell, and large cell (which may be of B-cell or T-cell origin; Table 156.1). Chromosomal translocations can result in unregulated/increased expression of an oncogene that drives malignant transformation. In Burkitt lymphoma, translocations occurring between chromosome 8 (*c-myc* oncogene) and the immunoglobulin gene locus (found on chromosomes 2, 14, or 22) lead to overexpression of *c-myc*, causing malignant transformation.

EPIDEMIOLOGY

The incidence of HL has a bimodal distribution with peaks in the adolescent/young adult years and again after age 50; it is rarely seen in children younger than 5 years of age. In children, boys are affected more commonly than girls; in adolescents, the gender ratio is approximately equal. The incidence of NHL increases with age. It is twice as common in whites as in African Americans and has a male predominance. NHL has been described in association with congenital or acquired immunodeficiency states and after organ or stem cell transplantation. Burkitt lymphoma is commonly divided into two forms: a sporadic form, commonly seen in North America, and an endemic form, with a strong association with EBV and commonly seen in Africa.

CLINICAL MANIFESTATIONS

Decision-Making Algorithms
Available @ StudentConsult.com

Lymphadenopathy
Neck Masses
Abdominal Pain
Fever

The most common clinical presentation of HL is painless, firm lymphadenopathy often confined to one or two contiguous lymph node areas (most commonly the supraclavicular and cervical nodes). Mediastinal lymphadenopathy, which produces cough or shortness of breath, is a frequent presenting symptom. The presence of one of three B symptoms has prognostic value: fever (>38°C for 3 consecutive days), drenching night sweats, and unintentional weight loss of 10% or more within 6 months of diagnosis.

The sporadic (North American) form of Burkitt lymphoma more commonly has an abdominal presentation (typically with pain), whereas the endemic (African) form frequently presents with tumors of the jaw. The anterior mediastinum and cervical nodes are the usual primary sites for T-cell lymphomas. These lymphomas may cause airway or superior vena cava obstruction, pleural effusion, or both.

The diagnosis of lymphoma is established by biopsy of an involved lymph node. Systemic symptoms such as fever and weight loss may be present, particularly in patients with anaplastic large cell lymphoma (ALCL), which can be insidious in onset. If the bone marrow contains 25% or greater blasts, the disease is classified as acute leukemia (either B-lineage acute lymphoblastic leukemia [ALL], T-cell ALL, or Burkitt leukemia). This distinction makes little prognostic or therapeutic difference as they all require aggressive, systemic therapy in addition to CNS-directed therapy.

TABLE 156.1 Subtypes of Non-Hodgkin Lymphoma in Children

HISTOLOGICAL CATEGORY	IMMUNOPHENOTYPE	USUAL PRIMARY SITE	MOST COMMON TRANSLOCATION(S)
Small noncleaved (Burkitt lymphoma)	Mature B-cell (surface immunoglobulin present)	Abdomen (sporadic form) Head and neck (endemic form)	t(8;14)(q24;q32) t(2;8)(p11;q24) t(8;22)(q24;q11)
Lymphoblastic	T-cell (rarely pre-B-cell)	Neck and/or anterior mediastinum	Many
Large cell	T-cell, B-cell, or indeterminate	Lymph nodes, skin, soft tissue, bone	t(2;5)(p23;q35)

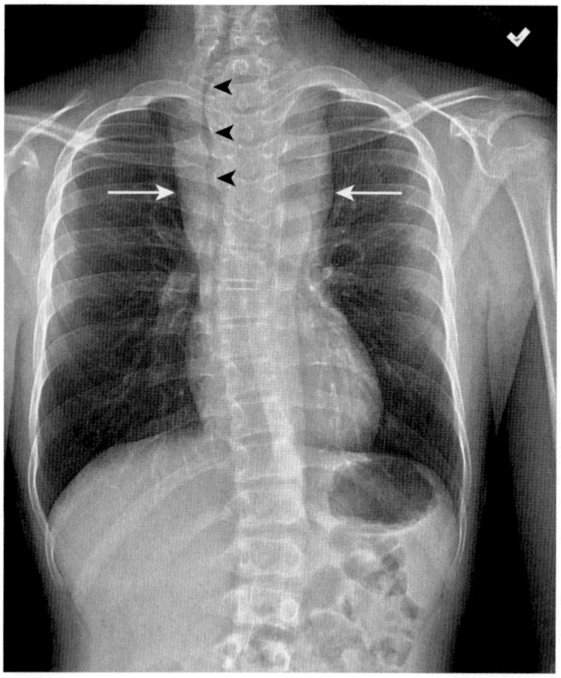

FIGURE 156.1 Chest x-ray of a 15-year-old boy demonstrating a large superior anterior mediastinal mass *(large arrows)* compressing the trachea and deviating it to the right *(arrowheads)*. Biopsy revealed non-Hodgkin lymphoma.

LABORATORY/IMAGING STUDIES

Patients suspected of having lymphoma should have a complete blood count, erythrocyte sedimentation rate, and measurement of serum electrolytes (particularly potassium, phosphorous, and calcium), lactate dehydrogenase, and uric acid as well as a chest x-ray to assess for a mediastinal mass (Fig. 156.1). The diagnosis ultimately requires a pathological confirmation from tissue or fluid sampling (pleural or peritoneal fluid). For staging purposes, a bone marrow evaluation, positron emission tomography (PET) and, less commonly, a bone scan are indicated to assess extent of disease (staging). The pathological hallmark of HL is the identification of Reed-Sternberg cells. Histopathological subtypes in childhood HL are the same as those reported in adults. Nodular sclerosis (NS) is the most common subtype in adolescents/young adults, whereas mixed cellularity subtypes and nodular lymphocyte predominant are more common in younger children. Staging of HL is according to the Ann Arbor system. About half of pediatric patients will have Stage II involvement at presentation (I 19%, II 49%, III 19%, IV 13%), and about 39% will have B symptoms.

DIFFERENTIAL DIAGNOSIS

The differential diagnosis for lymphomas in children includes leukemia, rhabdomyosarcoma, nasopharyngeal carcinoma, germ cell tumors, and thymomas. Nonmalignant diagnoses include infectious mononucleosis (EBV infection), branchial cleft and thyroglossal duct cysts, cat scratch disease *(Bartonella henselae)*, bacterial or viral lymphadenitis, mycobacterial infection, toxoplasmosis, and even tinea capitis, all of which can produce significant lymphadenopathy that can mimic lymphoma. Patients with acute abdominal pain from Burkitt lymphoma may be misdiagnosed as having appendicitis.

TREATMENT

Pediatric HL is highly curable even with advanced disease; overall survival rates now exceed 90%. Risk-adaptive therapy using stage, the presence of bulky disease, the presence or absence of B symptoms, serum albumin, and the response to upfront chemotherapy has been employed to reduce the need for radiation therapy and excess chemotherapy. Multiagent chemotherapy usually consists of drugs such as doxorubicin, vincristine, bleomycin, vinblastine, etoposide, prednisone, and cyclophosphamide. In general, four to six courses of chemotherapy are given. The use of anti-CD30 monoclonal therapy (Brentuximab vedotin) and the elimination of bleomycin are currently under investigation in pediatric HL. Response to therapy is often assessed after two cycles of upfront chemotherapy, relying on PET (to assess metabolic response) and computed tomography (CT; to assess bulk reduction) to determine the need for subsequent chemotherapy (slow response obligates more aggressive chemotherapy) and the need for radiation therapy. Of interest, patients with Stage I (single-node with complete resection) nodular lymphocyte predominant HL are cured with surgery alone 80% of the time.

Distant, noncontiguous metastases are common in childhood NHL. Systemic chemotherapy is mandatory and should be administered to all children with NHL, even those with clinically localized disease at diagnosis. B- and T-cell lymphoblastic lymphoma and ALCL are generally treated with aggressive multidrug regimens similar to the regimens used in ALL. Surgery and radiation therapy are not commonly used because the disease is rarely localized and is highly sensitive to chemotherapy. Burkitt lymphoma and diffuse large B-cell lymphomas are highly curable with cyclophosphamide, vincristine, prednisolone, and doxorubicin. Much like HL treatment, monoclonal antibody therapy is being added to the traditional chemotherapy backbone in Burkitt lymphoma (anti-CD20) and in ALCL (anti-CD30).

COMPLICATIONS

The short-term complications from the treatment of lymphoma are similar to other pediatric malignancies and commonly include immunosuppression, related sequelae from myelosuppression, nausea, vomiting, and alopecia. Late adverse effects include second malignant neoplasms (acute myeloid leukemia or myelodysplasia, thyroid malignancies, and breast cancer), hypothyroidism, impaired soft tissue and bone growth, cardiac dysfunction, and pulmonary fibrosis.

PROGNOSIS

Children and adolescents with HL are classified as low, intermediate, or high risk according to stage, nodal bulk, the presence of B symptoms, and the serum albumin at presentation. The prognosis is generally excellent with overall survival exceeding 90% for most patients (approaching 100% for low-risk patients). The overall 3-year survival rates for B-cell, T-cell, and large cell NHL are 70-90%.

CHAPTER 157

Central Nervous System Tumors

ETIOLOGY

Most central nervous system (CNS) tumors in children and adolescents are **primary tumors** that originate in the CNS and include gliomas (especially low-grade gliomas) and embryonic neoplasms (such as medulloblastoma and CNS primitive neuroectodermal tumors). In contrast, CNS tumors in adults are often high-grade astrocytomas or **secondary tumors** that are metastatic from other carcinomas. CNS tumors also may arise in patients previously treated with radiation therapy. CNS tumors are likely multifactorial in etiology. The classification of CNS tumors is complex and evolving, with the World Health Organization classification being the most complete and accurate system.

EPIDEMIOLOGY

CNS tumors are the most common solid tumors in children, second to leukemia in overall cancer incidence during childhood. However, due primarily to improved outcomes for leukemia, CNS tumors are now the leading cause of childhood cancer deaths. About 1,700 new cases occur each year in the United States; the rate is approximately 33 cases per 1 million children under 15 years of age. The incidence peaks before age 10 years and then decreases until a second peak after age 70. For medulloblastoma and ependymoma, males are more affected than females; for other tumor types, no gender differences exist. In the first 2-3 years of life, whites are affected more than nonwhite children; otherwise incidence rates are essentially equal for whites and nonwhite children.

Children with certain inherited syndromes, such as neurofibromatosis (types 1 and 2), Li-Fraumeni syndrome, tuberous sclerosis, Turcot syndrome, and von Hippel-Lindau syndrome, have an increased risk for developing a CNS tumor. However, most CNS tumors arise in children with no known underlying disorder or risk factor.

CLINICAL MANIFESTATIONS

Decision-Making Algorithms
Available @ StudentConsult.com

Abnormal Head Size, Shape, and Fontanels
Visual Impairment and Leukocoria
Strabismus
Vomiting
Headaches
Ataxia

Brain tumors can cause symptoms by impingement on normal tissue (usually cranial nerves) or by an increase in intracranial pressure caused either by obstruction of cerebrospinal fluid (CSF) flow or by a direct mass effect. Tumors that obstruct the flow of CSF quickly become symptomatic. Symptoms of **increased intracranial pressure** are lethargy, headache, and vomiting (particularly in the morning on awakening). Irritability, anorexia, poor school performance, and loss of developmental milestones all may be signs of slow-growing CNS tumors. In young children with open cranial sutures, an increase in head circumference may occur. Optic pathway tumors may lead to loss of visual acuity or visual field defects. Inability to abduct the eye as the result of sixth cranial nerve palsy is a common sign of increased intracranial pressure. Other cranial nerve deficits suggest involvement of the brainstem. Seizures occur in 20-50% of patients with supratentorial tumors; focal weakness or sensory changes also may be seen. Pituitary involvement can produce neuroendocrine effects such as precocious puberty or diabetes insipidus. Cerebellar tumors are associated with ataxia and diminished coordination. A history and physical examination are fundamental for evaluation and should include a careful neurological assessment, including visual fields and a funduscopic examination.

LABORATORY/IMAGING STUDIES

If an intracranial lesion is suspected, **magnetic resonance imaging (MRI)** is currently the examination of choice (Fig. 157.1). Examination of CSF by cytocentrifuge histological testing is indicated to determine the presence of metastatic disease in primitive neuroectodermal tumors, germ cell tumors, and pineal region tumors. A lumbar puncture should not be performed before imaging has been obtained to evaluate for evidence of increased intracranial pressure. If a tumor is suspected to have metastatic potential (medulloblastoma), MRI of the entire spine should be obtained before surgery to assess for neuraxial dissemination. A postoperative MRI study of the brain should be obtained within 24-48 hours of surgery to assess the extent of resection. During follow-up, magnetic resonance spectroscopy can help distinguish recurrent tumor from radiation necrosis.

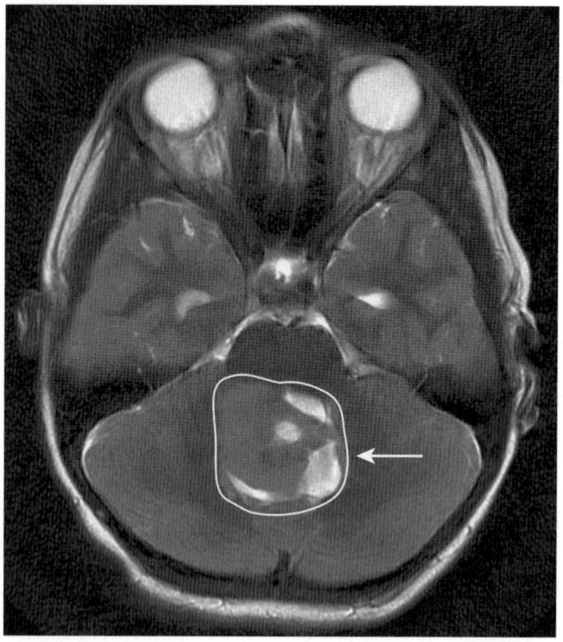

FIGURE 157.1 Magnetic resonance imaging scan of a 9-year-old boy showing a heterogeneously enhancing fourth ventricular mass *(arrow)*. It was resected, and pathology revealed medulloblastoma.

TABLE 157.1 Location, Incidence, and Prognosis of Central Nervous System Tumors in Children

LOCATION	INCIDENCE (%)	5-YEAR SURVIVAL (%)
Infratentorial (posterior fossa)	50-60	
Astrocytoma (cerebellum)	15	90
Medulloblastoma	15	50-80
Glioma (brainstem)	15	High grade: 0-5; low grade: 30
Ependymoma	5	50-60
Supratentorial (cerebral hemispheres)	35-45	
Astrocytoma	20	50-75
Glioblastoma multiforme	10	0-5
Ependymoma	5	50-75
Choroid plexus papilloma	2	95
Midline	10-15	
Craniopharyngioma	6	70-90
Germ cell tumors	3	65-95
Pineal	1	65-75
Optic nerve glioma	3	90

DIFFERENTIAL DIAGNOSIS

The differential diagnosis of a CNS mass lesion includes malignant tumor, benign tumor, arteriovenous malformation, aneurysm, brain abscess, cysticercosis, granulomatous disease (tuberculosis, sarcoid), intracranial hemorrhage, pseudotumor cerebri, vasculitis, and, rarely, metastatic tumor.

TREATMENT

The therapy for children with CNS tumors is individualized and depends on the tumor type, location, size, and associated symptoms. High-dose **dexamethasone** is often administered immediately to reduce tumor-associated edema. Surgical objectives are complete excision, if possible, and maximal debulking if a complete excision is not possible. In children, radiation therapy is often combined with chemotherapy; in young children, radiation therapy may be delayed or avoided altogether. Proton radiation therapy is an emerging therapy that holds promise for decreased toxicity. Primitive neuroectodermal tumors (including medulloblastoma) and germ cell tumors are sensitive to chemotherapy; gliomas are less sensitive to chemotherapy. Chemotherapy plays an especially important role in infants in whom the effects of high-dose CNS radiation may have devastating effects on growth and neurocognitive development.

COMPLICATIONS

Short-term adverse effects of therapy include nausea, vomiting, anorexia, fatigue, immunosuppression, and cushingoid features. Long-term adverse effects include neurocognitive deficits, endocrinological sequelae, decreased bone growth, ototoxicity, renal insufficiency, cataracts, infertility, and second malignant neoplasms. The neurocognitive deficits can be significant, particularly in infants and young children, and are the primary reason for the continued search for the lowest efficacious radiation therapy dose and the most conformal delivery methods for the radiation therapy boosts. **Posterior fossa syndrome** (also known as "cerebellar mutism") occurs in up to 25% of patients after resection of a posterior fossa tumor and is characterized by an acute decrease in speech, behavioral changes (e.g., irritability, apathy, or both), diffuse cerebellar dysfunction, and other neurological abnormalities. It may begin within hours to days of surgery and is usually self-resolving within weeks to months, although some neurological complications may persist. **Somnolence syndrome,** which is characterized by excessive fatigue and sleepiness, may occur in the months after completion of radiation therapy and is self-limited.

PROGNOSIS

Improvements in neurodiagnosis, neurosurgical techniques, chemotherapy regimens, and radiation therapy techniques have improved overall outcome. The 5-year overall survival rate associated with all childhood CNS tumors is approximately 50-60%, resulting in large measure from the high curability of cerebellar astrocytomas and the increasing cure rate for patients with medulloblastoma (Table 157.1). Intrinsic brainstem gliomas and glioblastoma multiforme have extremely poor prognoses.

CHAPTER 158

Neuroblastoma

ETIOLOGY

Neuroblastoma is derived from **neural crest cells** that form the adrenal medulla and the sympathetic nervous system. The cause is unknown. Most cases occur in young children. Neuroblastoma may rarely (1-2% of cases) be hereditary. Mutations in the *ALK*, *PHOX2B*, and *TP53* genes have been associated with familial cases. In sporadic cases, several somatic genetic mutations have been identified, with *MYCN* amplification being the most common.

EPIDEMIOLOGY

Neuroblastoma is the most common extracranial solid tumor of childhood and the most common malignancy in infancy. The median age at diagnosis is 17 months. There are approximately 800 new cases of neuroblastoma in the United States each year. The prevalence is estimated to be 1 in 7,000 live births.

CLINICAL MANIFESTATIONS

Decision-Making Algorithms
Available @ StudentConsult.com

Abdominal Masses
Neck Masses
Abnormal Eye Movements
Limp
Pancytopenia

Neuroblastoma is remarkable for its broad spectrum of clinical behavior ranging from spontaneous regression to rapid progression with metastases resulting in death. Children with localized disease are often asymptomatic at diagnosis, whereas children with metastases often appear ill and have systemic complaints such as fever, weight loss, and pain. The most common presentation is abdominal pain or mass. The mass is often palpated in the abdomen or flank and is hard and nontender. Approximately 45% of tumors arise in the adrenal gland, and 25% arise in the retroperitoneal sympathetic ganglia. Other sites of origin are the paravertebral ganglia of the chest and neck. Paraspinal tumors may invade through the neural foramina and cause spinal cord compression. Horner syndrome is sometimes seen with neck or apical masses. Several **paraneoplastic syndromes,** including secretory diarrhea, profuse sweating, and **opsomyoclonus**, are associated with neuroblastoma.

Neuroblastoma may metastasize to multiple organs, including the liver, bone, bone marrow, and lymph nodes. Periorbital ecchymoses are a sign of orbital bone metastases. A unique category of neuroblastoma, **stage MS**, is defined in infants (<18 months old) with metastases limited to skin, liver, or bone marrow. It is associated with a favorable outcome.

LABORATORY/IMAGING STUDIES

A complete blood count and plain radiographs may help identify patients with neuroblastoma. Calcification within abdominal neuroblastoma tumors is often observed on plain radiographs of the abdomen. About 90% of neuroblastomas produce **catecholamines (vanillylmandelic acid; homovanillic acid)** that can be detected in the urine. Definitive diagnosis of neuroblastoma requires tissue biopsy for microscopic examination and genetic testing. A computed tomography (CT) scan of the chest, abdomen, and pelvis; a bone scan and/or metaiodobenzylguanidine scan; bilateral bone marrow aspiration and biopsies; and urinary catecholamines complete the evaluation.

DIFFERENTIAL DIAGNOSIS

The abdominal presentation of neuroblastoma must be differentiated from Wilms tumor, which also presents as an abdominal or flank mass. Ultrasound or CT examination usually differentiates the tumors prior to surgery. Periorbital ecchymoses from orbital metastases can be mistaken for child abuse. Because children with bone marrow involvement may have anemia, thrombocytopenia, or neutropenia, leukemia is often considered in the differential.

TREATMENT

Treatment of neuroblastoma is based on risk classification (Table 158.1), an evolving scheme based on emerging genetic discoveries, and treatment advances. Complete surgical excision is the initial treatment of choice for localized neuroblastoma. Children with very low– or low-risk tumors who undergo a gross total resection require no further therapy. Patients with intermediate-risk disease are usually treated with surgery and 4-8 cycles of chemotherapy. In patients with high-risk disease, combination chemotherapy is given after confirmation of the diagnosis. The most commonly used agents are vincristine, cyclophosphamide, topotecan, doxorubicin, cisplatin, and etoposide. Resection of the primary tumor is undertaken after several courses of chemotherapy. Patients then undergo **high-dose chemotherapy with autologous stem cell rescue**; recent data suggest two courses of high-dose therapy are better than one. Radiation therapy is then administered to the primary tumor bed and areas of metastatic disease. Finally, **cis-retinoic acid** (isotretinoin) and **Dinutuximab** (a form of immunotherapy directed against the G_{D2} antigen) are administered to treat minimal residual disease.

COMPLICATIONS

Spinal cord compression from neuroblastoma may cause an irreversible neurological deficit and is an oncological emergency. Children with opsomyoclonus syndrome may suffer from developmental delay. The aggressive chemotherapy and radiation therapies currently used to treat high-risk neuroblastoma may result in complications such as ototoxicity, nephrotoxicity, growth problems, and second malignancies.

PROGNOSIS

The prognosis is affected by age at diagnosis, stage (based on presence or absence of metastasis and image-defined risk factors), DNA ploidy, *MYCN* status, 11q aberration, and histopathology (grade of tumor differentiation). Currently, children with neuroblastoma can be divided into four groups: very low, low, intermediate, and high risk. Patients with favorable biology tend to be younger and often have localized disease. Older patients with metastatic disease most commonly have unfavorable biology; approximately 50% will ultimately relapse due to drug-resistant residual disease. Although neuroblastoma represents only 8% of cases of childhood cancer, it is responsible for 15% of cancer deaths in children.

TABLE 158.1 International Neuroblastoma Risk Group Pretreatment Classification Schema

INRG STAGE	AGE (MONTHS)	HISTOLOGICAL CATEGORY	GRADE OF TUMOR DIFFERENTIATION	*MYCN*	11q ABERRATION	PLOIDY	PRETREATMENT RISK GROUP
L1/L2		GN maturing, GNB intermixed					A (very low)
L1		Any, except GN maturing or		NA			B (very low)
		GNB intermixed		Amplified			K (high)
L2	<18	Any, except GN maturing or		NA	No		D (low)
		GNB intermixed			Yes		G (intermediate)
	≥18	GNB nodular neuroblastoma	Differentiating	NA	No		E (low)
					Yes		H (intermediate)
			Poorly differentiated or undifferentiated	NA			H (intermediate)
				Amplified			N (high)
M	<18			NA		Hyperdiploid	F (low)
	<12			NA		Diploid	I (intermediate)
	12-<18			NA		Diploid	J (intermediate)
	<18			Amplified			O (high)
	≥18						P (high)
MS	<18			NA	No		C (very low)
					Yes		Q (high)
				Amplified			R (high)

GN, Ganglioneuroma; *GNB*, ganglioneuroblastoma; *INRG*, International Neuroblastoma Risk Group; *NA*, not amplified.

CHAPTER **159**

Wilms Tumor

ETIOLOGY AND EPIDEMIOLOGY

Wilms tumor is thought to arise from primitive, metanephric blastema, the precursor of a normal kidney. Nephrogenic rests are foci of embryonal cells that are rarely (<1%) found in normal infant kidneys but commonly (25-40%) found in Wilms tumor–bearing kidneys. Although the cause of Wilms tumor is unknown, approximately 15-20% of sporadic tumors have *WT1* mutations or deletions. Over 70% of Wilms tumors demonstrate loss of imprinting or loss of heterozygosity at 11p15, leading to overexpression of *IGF2*, thought to play a key role in tumorigenesis. Certain syndromes including Beckwith-Wiedemann and WAGR (Wilms tumor, aniridia, genitourinary anomalies, and retardation; mutation involving 11p13 region) are at increased risk of developing the disease.

Wilms tumor is the most common malignant renal tumor of childhood, with approximately 500 new cases per year in the United States. Unilateral tumors have a median age of diagnosis of 44 months versus bilateral tumors, which have a median age of diagnosis of 31 months. Bilateral presentations are commonly associated with hereditary forms of the disease.

CLINICAL MANIFESTATIONS

Decision-Making Algorithms
Available @ StudentConsult.com

Abdominal Pain
Abdominal Masses
Hematuria

Most children with Wilms tumor are brought to medical attention because they have an abdominal mass that is discovered by their parents. Although many children do not have complaints at the time that the mass is first noted, associated symptoms may include abdominal pain (often mistaken for constipation), fever, hypertension, and hematuria.

LABORATORY/IMAGING STUDIES

An abdominal ultrasound or computed tomography (CT) scan can usually distinguish an intrarenal mass from a mass arising from the adrenal gland (most commonly neuroblastoma) or other surrounding structures. Evaluation of the inferior vena cava is crucial because the tumor may extend from the kidney into the vena cava. The diagnostic work-up includes a complete blood count, urinalysis, liver and renal function studies, as well as a CT scan of the chest, abdomen, and pelvis to assess for metastatic involvement (pulmonary involvement is the most common metastatic site). The diagnosis is confirmed by histological examination of the tumor.

DIFFERENTIAL DIAGNOSIS

The differential diagnosis of Wilms tumor includes hydronephrosis and polycystic disease of the kidney; benign renal tumors, such as mesoblastic nephroma and hamartoma; and other malignant tumors, such as neuroblastoma, renal cell carcinoma, lymphoma, and retroperitoneal rhabdomyosarcoma.

TREATMENT

The timing of nephrectomy for unilateral, resectable Wilms tumor remains divided between the North American approach and the European approach. Both approaches have a similar overall survival. The North American approach recommends an upfront nephrectomy (confirming tissue diagnosis) followed by adjuvant chemotherapy with or without radiation therapy, whereas the European approach is to make a diagnosis relying predominantly on imaging (sometimes a biopsy), provide upfront (neoadjuvant) chemotherapy, then nephrectomy of the involved kidney followed by adjuvant chemotherapy with or without radiation therapy. The Children's Oncology Group (North American approach) relies on stage, histology (favorable versus anaplastic/unfavorable), patient age, tumor weight, loss of heterozygosity of 1p and 16q, and imaging response of pulmonary nodules after initial chemotherapy to risk stratify patients. Most patients will receive a 2-3 drug chemotherapy regimen (vincristine, actinomycin, with or without doxorubicin) as well as radiation therapy for those with high-risk features. Patients designated with very-low-risk unilateral Wilms tumor can often be cured with nephrectomy only.

Bilateral Wilms tumor is present in about 5% of children on initial presentation. The treatment goal for patients with bilateral Wilms tumor is to balance the need to achieve a cure while retaining as much normal kidney function as possible.

PROGNOSIS AND COMPLICATIONS

The overall survival rate for Wilms tumor is 90%. Unfortunately, 25% of survivors will experience serious chronic health conditions. Survivors of Wilms tumor are at risk for cardiomyopathy, scoliosis, hypertension and prehypertension, renal and bladder insufficiency, pulmonary dysfunction, hepatic dysfunction, infertility, and second malignancies. Patients with bilateral Wilms tumor are sometimes left with renal insufficiency or failure. Female survivors may have complicated pregnancies and deliveries most commonly associated with flank radiation.

CHAPTER 160

Sarcomas

Sarcomas are divided into soft tissue sarcomas and bone cancers. Soft tissue sarcomas arise primarily from the connective tissues of the body, such as muscle tissue, fibrous tissue, and adipose tissue. **Rhabdomyosarcoma (RMS)**, the most common soft tissue sarcoma in children, is derived from mesenchymal cells of muscle lineage. Less common soft tissue sarcomas include fibrosarcoma, synovial sarcoma, and extraosseous Ewing sarcoma. The most common malignant bone cancers in children are **osteosarcoma** and **Ewing sarcoma**. Osteosarcomas derive from primitive bone-forming mesenchymal stem cells. Ewing sarcomas are thought to be of neural crest cell origin.

ETIOLOGY

The cause is unknown for most children diagnosed with sarcoma, although a few observations have been made regarding risks. Individuals with Li-Fraumeni syndrome (associated with a germline p53 mutation) and neurofibromatosis (associated with *NF1* mutations) have an increased risk of soft tissue sarcomas. There is a 500-fold increased risk for osteosarcoma for individuals with hereditary retinoblastoma. Prior treatment for childhood cancer with radiation therapy or chemotherapy (specifically alkylating agents), or both, increases the risk for osteosarcoma as a second malignancy.

EPIDEMIOLOGY

In the United States, 850-900 children and adolescents under 20 years of age are diagnosed with soft tissue sarcomas each year; approximately 350 are RMS. The incidence of RMS peaks in children 2-6 years old and again in adolescents. The early peak is associated with tumors in the genitourinary region, head, and neck; the later peak is associated with tumors in the extremities, trunk, and male genitourinary tract. Boys are affected 1.5 times more often than girls. Of the 650-700 U.S. children and adolescents under 20 years of age diagnosed with bone tumors each year, approximately two thirds have osteosarcoma and one third have Ewing sarcoma. Osteosarcoma most commonly affects adolescents; the peak incidence occurs during the period of maximum growth velocity. The incidence of Ewing sarcoma peaks between ages 10 and 20 years but may occur at any age. Ewing sarcoma primarily affects whites; it rarely occurs in African American children or Asian children.

CLINICAL MANIFESTATIONS

Decision-Making Algorithms
Available @ StudentConsult.com

Extremity Pain
Limp
Neck Masses
Scrotal Swelling (Painless)
Vaginal Discharge
Lymphadenopathy

The clinical presentation of RMS varies, depending on the site of origin, subsequent mass effect, and presence of metastatic disease. Periorbital swelling, proptosis, and limitation of extraocular motion may be seen with an orbital tumor. Nasal mass, chronic otitis media, ear discharge, dysphagia, neck mass, and cranial nerve involvement may be noted with tumors in other head and neck sites. Urethral or vaginal masses, paratesticular swelling, hematuria, and urinary frequency or retention may be noted with tumors in the genitourinary tract. Trunk or extremity lesions tend to present as rapidly growing masses that may or may not be painful. If there is metastatic disease to bone or bone marrow, limb pain and evidence of marrow failure may be present.

Osteosarcoma is often located at the epiphysis or metaphysis of long bones that are associated with maximum growth velocity (distal femur, proximal tibia, proximal humerus), but any bone may be involved. It presents with pain and may be associated with a palpable mass. Because the pain and swelling often are initially thought to be related to trauma, radiographs of the affected region are frequently obtained; the radiographs usually reveal a lytic lesion, sometimes associated with calcification in the soft tissue surrounding the lesion. Although 75-80% of patients with osteosarcoma have apparently localized disease at diagnosis, most patients are believed to have micrometastatic disease as well.

Although Ewing sarcoma can occur in almost any bone in the body, the femur and pelvis are the most common sites. In addition to local pain and swelling, clinical manifestations may include constitutional symptoms such as fever, fatigue, and weight loss.

LABORATORY/IMAGING STUDIES

Tissue biopsy is needed for a definitive diagnosis of sarcoma. Selection of the biopsy site is important and has implications for future surgical resection and radiation therapy. Under light microscopy, RMS and Ewing sarcoma appear as small, round, blue cell tumors. Osteosarcomas are distinguishable by the presence of osteoid.

Immunohistochemical staining for muscle-specific proteins, such as actin and myosin, helps confirm the diagnosis of RMS. Two major histological variants exist for RMS: embryonal and alveolar. The **embryonal (ERMS; embryonal RMS)** histological variant is most common in younger children with head, neck, and genitourinary primary tumors. The **alveolar (ARMS; alveolar RMS)** histological variant occurs in older patients and is seen most commonly in trunk and extremity tumors. Alveolar RMS is often characterized by specific translocations: t(2;13) or t(1;13). Although histology is still used to determine risk group assignment/treatment, *FOXO1* fusion status is more predictive of outcome. The vast majority of ARMS are *PAX3-FOXO1* or *PAX7-FOXO1* translocation positive. Metastatic evaluation for patients with RMS should include positron emission tomography (PET) scan (when available), chest computed tomography (CT), and bilateral bone marrow aspiration/biopsy. A lumbar puncture is required in patients with a parameningeal primary site due to the risk of direct extension into the central nervous system (CNS).

The diagnosis of osteosarcoma is established with the presence of osteoid and immunohistochemical analysis of the biopsy material. The extent of the primary tumor should be delineated carefully with magnetic resonance imaging (MRI) before starting chemotherapy to determine surgical resection options. Osteosarcoma tends to metastasize to the lungs, most commonly, and rarely to other bones. Metastatic evaluation includes a chest CT scan and a bone scan (or PET scan).

The diagnosis of Ewing sarcoma is established with immunohistochemical analysis along with cytogenetic and molecular diagnostic studies of the biopsy material. Ewing sarcoma is characterized by a specific chromosomal translocation, t(11;22), which is seen in 95% of tumors. MRI of the primary lesion should be performed to delineate extent of the lesion and any associated soft tissue mass. Metastatic evaluation involves a PET scan (when available), chest CT scan, and bilateral bone marrow aspiration/biopsy.

DIFFERENTIAL DIAGNOSIS

Patients with Ewing sarcoma may be misdiagnosed as having osteomyelitis; children with osteogenic sarcoma are often initially believed to have pain and swelling related to trauma. The differential diagnosis for RMS depends on the location of the tumor. Tumors of the trunk and extremities often present as a painless mass and may initially be thought to be benign tumors. Head and neck RMS may be misdiagnosed as allergies, orbital cellulitis, or chronic infection of ears or sinuses. The differential diagnosis for intraabdominal RMS includes other abdominal malignancies, such as Wilms tumor and neuroblastoma.

TREATMENT

Treatment of RMS is currently based on a staging system that incorporates a number of diagnostic features including primary site, histological subtype, *FOXO1* fusion status, stage (local, regional or metastatic involvement), and surgical grouping (the ability or inability to achieve a gross total resection prior to chemotherapy/radiation). The most common chemotherapy agents used in RMS are vincristine, dactinomycin, and cyclophosphamide. Other active agents include irinotecan, ifosfamide, and etoposide. The use of temsirolimus, temozolomide, and ganitumab (anti-IGF-1R monoclonal antibody) is currently under investigation. Radiation is administered to the primary tumor when surgical resection is incomplete or would be morbid. It may also be administered to involved regional nodal sites, and sometimes to distant metastatic sites.

The current treatment of osteosarcoma involves neoadjuvant chemotherapy, surgical resection of the primary tumor, followed by adjuvant chemotherapy. The most common chemotherapy agents used for osteosarcoma are high-dose methotrexate, doxorubicin, and cisplatin. Radiation therapy is ineffective for osteosarcoma, although it is sometimes used for palliative intent to treat pain. The treatment for Ewing sarcoma is similar to osteosarcoma and requires neoadjuvant chemotherapy, local control measures, followed by adjuvant chemotherapy. The most common chemotherapy agents used for Ewing sarcoma are vincristine, doxorubicin, and cyclophosphamide in combination with ifosfamide and etoposide. The addition of topotecan in nonmetastatic patients and ganitumab in metastatic patients is currently under investigation. In contrast to osteosarcoma, Ewing sarcoma is radiation sensitive, and radiation therapy is administered to patients where the primary tumor cannot be safely resected as well as for metastatic sites.

COMPLICATIONS

In addition to potential late effects from the chemotherapy, children with sarcomas may have complications related to local control of the tumor. If the local disease is controlled with surgery, the long-term sequelae may include loss of limb or limitation of function. If local control is accomplished with radiation therapy, the late effects depend on the dose of radiation given, the extent of the radiated site, and the development of the child at the time of radiation therapy. Irradiating tissues interferes with growth and development, causes organ damage, and increases the risk of second malignant neoplasms.

PROGNOSIS

For all children with sarcoma, presence or absence of metastatic disease at presentation is the most important prognostic factor. The outlook remains poor for patients who have distant metastases from Ewing sarcoma, RMS, or osteosarcoma. Patients with localized RMSs in favorable sites have an excellent prognosis when treated with surgery followed by chemotherapy. In patients with osteosarcoma, the amount of tumor necrosis after preoperative chemotherapy is prognostic. Patients who achieve >90% tumor necrosis after neoadjuvant chemotherapy have an overall survival rate of approximately 80% versus approximately 50% for patients who have <90% tumor necrosis. The overall cure rate for patients with localized osteosarcoma and Ewing sarcoma is approximately 60-70%. Patients who have lung metastasis at diagnosis have a cure rate of approximately 30%. Patients with metastases to other bones have a very poor prognosis (less than 20%).

Suggested Readings

Adamson PC. Improving the outcome for children with cancer: development of targeted new agents. *CA Cancer J Clin.* 2015;65: 212–220.

Allen CE, Kelly KM, Bollard CM. Pediatric lymphomas and histiocytic disorders of childhood. *Pediatr Clin North Am.* 2015;62:139–165.

Chintagumpala M, Gajjar A. Brain tumors. *Pediatr Clin North Am.* 2015;62:167–178.

Cooper SL, Brown PA. Treatment of pediatric acute lymphoblastic leukemia. *Pediatr Clin North Am.* 2015;62:61–73.

HaDuong JH, Martin AA, Skapek SX, et al. Sarcomas. *Pediatr Clin North Am.* 2015;62:179–200.

Malkan AD, Loh A, Bahrami A, et al. An approach to renal masses in pediatrics. *Pediatrics.* 2015;135:142–158.

Pinto NR, Applebaum MA, Volchenboum SL, et al. Advances in risk classification and treatment strategies for neuroblastoma. *J Clin Oncol.* 2015;33:3008–3017.

PEARLS FOR PRACTITIONERS

CHAPTER 153

Oncology Assessment

- The most common cancers in children and adolescents are leukemia, brain tumors, and lymphoma followed by sarcomas of soft tissue and bone.
  - Cancers that are seen almost exclusively in children, as opposed to adolescents and adults, include neuroblastoma, Wilms tumor, retinoblastoma, and hepatoblastoma.
- Many signs and symptoms of childhood cancer are nonspecific. Pain, fatigue, pallor, bruising/petechiae/bleeding, and a growing mass are all common on presentation.
- In general, malignant lymph nodes tend to be large, firm, fixed, and nontender; reactive lymph nodes tend to be small, soft, mobile, and tender.
- Almost all cancers require a biopsy of some type to make a definitive diagnosis.
- A child with an abdominal mass should prompt consideration for neuroblastoma, Wilms tumor, and hepatoblastoma.
  - In general, toddlers and older children with neuroblastoma are ill, whereas children with Wilms tumor have few associated symptoms.
- Serum (and/or cerebrospinal fluid) alpha-fetoprotein (AFP) and beta-human chorionic gonadotropin (β-HCG) are tumor markers for germ cell tumors. AFP is a tumor marker for hepatoblastoma.
- Urine homovanillic acid (HVA) and vanillylmandelic acid (VMA) are tumor markers for neuroblastoma.
- The prognosis for children with cancer has improved dramatically in the past 60 years, with long-term survival improving from about 20% to 80%.
- Prognostic factors include age, histology, and the presence or absence of metastases. However, genetic factors (of both the cancer and the patient) and response to initial therapy are becoming more powerful determinants of survival.

CHAPTER 154

Principles of Cancer Treatment

- Treatment for children with cancer is usually multimodal and may involve surgery, radiation therapy, chemotherapy, and immunotherapy. Targeted therapies and immunotherapies are more commonly being used to treat pediatric cancers, often with dramatic results and manageable toxicities.
- Current primary prevention strategies for pediatric malignancy are uncommon but include use of the hepatitis B vaccine (hepatocellular carcinoma) and human papillomavirus vaccine (GU/oropharyngeal cancers).
- Adverse effects of treatment may lead to oncological emergencies.
  - Tumor lysis syndrome may be seen in patients with leukemia and lymphoma. It is best treated with hydration, allopurinol and/or rasburicase (to treat hyperuricemia), and treating the underlying cancer.

  - Airway compression, spinal cord compression, and infection are other oncological emergencies.
- Many survivors of childhood cancer suffer from long-term side effects from the treatment.
  - As the prognosis for childhood cancer improves, clinical trials are shifting focus from improving survival to decreasing long-term side effects.

CHAPTER 155

Leukemia

- Children with cytopenias and/or leukocytosis should be considered for bone marrow aspiration to assess for acute leukemia.
- Acute lymphoblastic leukemia (ALL) accounts for approximately 75% of pediatric leukemia; acute myeloid leukemia (AML) accounts for approximately 20% and chronic myeloid leukemia (CML) accounts for less than 5%.
  - ALL is more common in whites, whereas AML has a slightly higher incidence in Hispanic and African American children.
- ALL is classified as B-cell or T-cell.
  - The incidence of B-cell ALL peaks at 2-5 years of age with a slight male predominance. T-cell ALL has a male predominance and presents at an older age.
- The diagnosis of acute leukemia is confirmed by findings of immature blast cells on a peripheral blood smear or bone marrow aspirate.
- Cytogenetic analysis should be undertaken because cytogenetic abnormalities have prognostic indications and can be used to tailor treatment.
- Unlike adults, children with acute lymphoblastic leukemia generally have an excellent prognosis (90% survival). Children with acute myeloid leukemia have a more guarded prognosis (65% survival).

CHAPTER 156

Lymphoma

- Lymphomas are the third most common pediatric malignancy (following leukemia and central nervous system tumors).
- Hodgkin lymphoma peaks in the adolescent/young adult years (and again after age 50). It most commonly presents as painless, firm lymphadenopathy. Diagnosis is established by biopsy of an involved lymph node. It is highly curable, even with advanced disease.
- Non-Hodgkin lymphoma (NHL) incidence increases with age, is more common in whites, and has a male predominance. Distant, noncontiguous metastases are common in childhood NHL. Systemic chemotherapy is mandatory.

CHAPTER 157

Central Nervous System Tumors

- Most central nervous system (CNS) tumors in children and adolescents are primary tumors that originate in the CNS and include low-grade astrocytomas or embryonic neoplasms (such as medulloblastoma and CNS primitive neuroectodermal tumors).
- CNS tumors are the most common solid tumor in childhood and are now the leading cause of childhood cancer deaths.
- Lethargy, headache, ataxia, and morning vomiting are common presenting symptoms of brain tumors; these symptoms should prompt consideration for imaging the brain (computed tomography [CT] and/or magnetic resonance imaging [MRI]).
- Treatment is individualized and may include surgery, chemotherapy, and/or radiation therapy. Radiation therapy is often delayed or avoided in young children.
- The 5-year survival is improving. It is now 50-60%, resulting, in large part, because of the curability of cerebellar astrocytomas and the increasing cure rate for medulloblastoma.

CHAPTER 158

Neuroblastoma

- Neuroblastoma is the most common malignancy in infancy.
  - Compared with toddlers and older children, infants with neuroblastoma are generally well, have less aggressive disease, and an excellent prognosis.
- The most common presentation of neuroblastoma is an abdominal mass or pain.
- Children with high-risk neuroblastoma have a guarded prognosis, even with aggressive treatment including chemotherapy, surgery, radiation therapy, retinoid acid, and immunotherapy.

CHAPTER 159

Wilms Tumor

- Wilms tumor is thought to arise from primitive, metanephric blastema.
  - Over 70% of Wilms tumors demonstrate loss of imprinting or loss of heterozygosity at 11p15.
- The most common presentation is an abdominal mass.
- Treatment of Wilms tumor is nephrectomy and chemotherapy with or without radiation therapy.
- The overall survival rate is 90%, although 25% of survivors experience chronic health problems.

CHAPTER 160

Sarcomas

- There are two types of sarcomas: soft tissue sarcomas (rhabdomyosarcoma) or bone cancers (osteosarcoma, Ewing sarcoma).
- Sarcomas originating in the bone, such as osteosarcoma and Ewing sarcoma, usually present with a mass and/or pain.
- Prognostic factors for patients with sarcomas include the presence or absence of metastases, the extent of surgical resection, and the response to chemotherapy (usually measured by the amount of tumor necrosis).
- Survival in patients with localized rhabdomyosarcoma is excellent following surgery and chemotherapy.
- Patients with osteosarcoma with >90% tumor necrosis following chemotherapy have a >80% survival rate (50% survival if <90% tumor necrosis).
- Overall survival for localized osteosarcoma or Ewing sarcoma is 60-70%.
  - Survival with lung metastases is ~30%.
  - Survival with metastases to other bones is <20%.

NEPHROLOGY AND UROLOGY

Hiren P. Patel | John D. Mahan

CHAPTER 161

Nephrology and Urology Assessment

The kidneys preserve homeostasis through (1) maintaining fluid and electrolyte balance; (2) excreting metabolic waste products through glomerular filtration and tubular secretion; (3) generating energy (gluconeogenesis); and (4) producing important endocrine hormones (renin, vitamin D metabolites, erythropoietin). Renal disorders, by disturbing homeostasis, can affect growth and development and cause a variety of clinical manifestations (Table 161.1). Renal disorders in children may be intrinsic renal diseases or derive from systemic conditions (Table 161.2).

HISTORY

Fetal urine production contributes to amniotic fluid volume, lung maturation, and somatic development. Congenital renal disorders may be associated with reduced (oligohydramnios) or increased amniotic fluid volume (polyhydramnios). Pulmonary hypoplasia and fetal maldevelopment of the face and extremities may result from insufficient amniotic fluid (Potter syndrome; see Chapters 58 and 60).

Risk factors for renal disease (e.g., perinatal hypoxia-ischemia, acute tubular necrosis, renal vein thrombosis) can often be detected by a careful history. A detailed family history may identify hereditary renal conditions. Poor growth and/or feeding and abnormal fluid intake and/or output may indicate underlying renal dysfunction. Common manifestations of renal and urinary tract disorders are listed in Table 161.1.

PHYSICAL EXAMINATION

Renal diseases in children may be initially asymptomatic and detected during routine visits. Abnormal growth, hypertension (HTN), dehydration, or edema may suggest underlying renal disease (see Chapter 33). Abnormal facial features may suggest syndromes associated with renal disorders (fetal alcohol syndrome, Down syndrome). Preauricular tags, external ear deformities, or ophthalmological abnormalities (keratoconus, aniridia, iridocyclitis, cataracts) can be associated with congenital renal defects. Abdominal examination may reveal renal masses or bladder distention due to urine-concentrating defect or urinary tract obstruction.

RENAL PHYSIOLOGY

Normal renal function depends on intact **glomerular filtration** and **tubular function** (**proximal tubule** [PT], **loop of Henle**, and **distal tubule** [DT]) to produce **urine** (Fig. 161.1). Net glomerular pressure favors movement of fluid out of glomerular capillaries into Bowman's space. Intraglomerular pressure is regulated by afferent and, particularly, efferent arteriolar tone. **Renin** is generated by cells in the juxtaglomerular apparatus, located at the base of each glomerulus near the afferent/efferent arterioles and DT of that nephron. Renin is released in response to glomerular flow and perfusion.

The PT conducts isosmotic reabsorption (see Fig. 161.1) to reclaim two thirds of filtered volume, sodium, and chloride. Glucose, amino acids, potassium, and phosphate are almost completely reabsorbed. Approximately 75% of filtered bicarbonate is reabsorbed in the PT. When filtered bicarbonate exceeds the PT threshold, it is spilled into the urine. The PT also secretes compounds such as organic acids, penicillins, and other drugs. The most potent vitamin D analog—1,25$(OH)_2$-cholecalciferol (**calcitriol**)—is produced by PT cells in response to parathyroid hormone and intracellular calcium/phosphorus concentrations.

The loop of Henle is the site of reabsorption of 25% of filtered sodium chloride (see Fig. 161.1). Active chloride transport drives the countercurrent multiplier and constructs the medullary interstitial hypertonic gradient required for urinary concentration.

The DT is composed of the **distal convoluted tubule** (DCT) and **collecting ducts (CD).** The DCT is water impermeable and contributes to urine dilution by active sodium chloride absorption. The CD is the primary site of **antidiuretic hormone** (vasopressin) response, which leads to urine concentration. Sodium-potassium and sodium-hydrogen exchange in the CD is regulated by aldosterone. Active hydrogen ion secretion, responsible for final acidification of the urine, also occurs in the CD.

Renal **ammonia** production and intraluminal generation of ammonium (NH_4^+) facilitate urine hydrogen ion excretion. Urinary NH_4^+ is not easily measured but can be inferred by calculation of the **urinary anion gap.** The *gap* between measured anions and cations largely consists of NH_4^+. Problems with renal acid excretion or ammonia production decrease the urinary anion gap. A urinary gap of approximately 1 mEq/kg body weight is typical in normal children.

Maximum **urinary concentrating capacity** in a preterm newborn (~400 mOsm/L) is less than in a full-term newborn (600-800 mOsm/L), which is less than in older children and

TABLE 161.1 Common Manifestations of Renal Disease by Age

FINDING	SIGNIFICANCE
NEONATE	
Flank mass	Multicystic dysplasia, UT obstruction (hydronephrosis), polycystic disease, tumor
Hematuria	UTI, acute tubular/cortical necrosis, UT malformation, trauma, renal vein thrombosis
Anuria and oliguria	Renal agenesis, obstruction, acute tubular necrosis, vascular thrombosis
CHILD/ADOLESCENT	
Cola red-colored urine	Hemoglobinuria (hemolysis), myoglobinuria (rhabdomyolysis), pigmenturia (porphyria, urate, beets, drugs), hematuria (UTI, GN, Henoch-Schönlein purpura, hypercalciuria, stones)
Gross hematuria	UTI, GN, trauma, benign hematuria, nephrolithiasis, tumor
Edema	Nephrotic syndrome, GN, acute/chronic renal failure, cardiac/liver disease
Hypertension	Acute GN, acute/chronic renal failure, obstruction, cysts, dysplasia, coarctation of the aorta, renal artery stenosis
Polyuria	Diabetes mellitus, central and nephrogenic diabetes insipidus, obstruction, dysplasia, hypokalemia, hypercalcemia, psychogenic polydipsia, sickle disease/trait, polyuric renal failure, diuretic abuse
Oliguria	Dehydration, acute tubular necrosis, acute GN, interstitial nephritis, hemolytic uremic syndrome
Dysfunctional voiding/urgency	Neurogenic bladder, UTI, vaginitis, hypercalciuria, foreign body

GN, Glomerulonephritis; *UT*, Urinary tract; *UTI*, urinary tract infection.

TABLE 161.2 Primary and Systemic Causes of Renal Disease in Children

PRIMARY	SECONDARY (SYSTEMIC)
Minimal change nephrotic syndrome	Postinfectious glomerulonephritis
Focal segmental glomerulosclerosis	IgA nephropathy
Membranoproliferative glomerulonephritis	Henoch-Schönlein purpura-related nephritis
	Membranoproliferative glomerulonephritis (related to chronic infection, liver disease)
Membranous nephropathy	Hemolytic uremic syndrome
	Systemic lupus erythematosus
	Granulomatosis with polyangiitis and other vasculitides
Congenital nephrotic syndrome	Tubular toxins
Alport syndrome	Antibiotics
Intrinsic tubular disorders	Chemotherapeutic agents
Structural renal disorders	Hemoglobin/myoglobin
Congenital urinary tract abnormalities	Tubular disorders
Polycystic kidney disease	Cystinosis, oxalosis
Renal/urinary tract tumor	Galactosemia, hereditary fructose intolerance
	Stones
	Sickle disease/trait
	Trauma
	Extrarenal malignancy (leukemia, lymphoma)

Ig, Immunoglobulin.

adults (~1,200 mOsm/L). Neonates can dilute urine similar to adults (75-90 mOsm/L), but because **glomerular filtration rate** (GFR) is lower, the capacity to excrete a water load is less in infants. GFR reaches adult levels by 1-2 years of age. Tubular reabsorption of sodium, potassium, bicarbonate, and phosphate and excretion of hydrogen are all reduced in infants relative to adults. These functions mature independently and at different ages, so a neonate rapidly develops the ability to reabsorb sodium efficiently, but it takes 2 years for bicarbonate reabsorption to mature. **Erythropoietin** is secreted by interstitial cells in the renal medulla in response to low oxygen delivery and helps regulate bone marrow red blood cell production.

COMMON MANIFESTATIONS

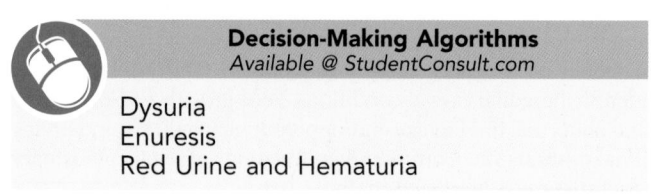

Decision-Making Algorithms
Available @ StudentConsult.com

Dysuria
Enuresis
Red Urine and Hematuria

Renal disorders can be classified as **primary** or **secondary** (due to systemic illnesses; see Table 161.2). Renal diseases may present with obvious signs (hematuria or edema), or with subtle signs detected on screening examinations (abdominal or flank mass, HTN, proteinuria). Fever, irritability, and vomiting may be presenting symptoms in neonates and infants with **urinary tract infections** (UTIs), whereas frequency and dysuria suggest UTI in older children. Chronic kidney disease is often associated with poor growth and feeding, but may be initially detected on screening examinations (HTN, hematuria). An abnormal urine stream may indicate posterior urethral valves other obstructive lesions or bladder disorders.

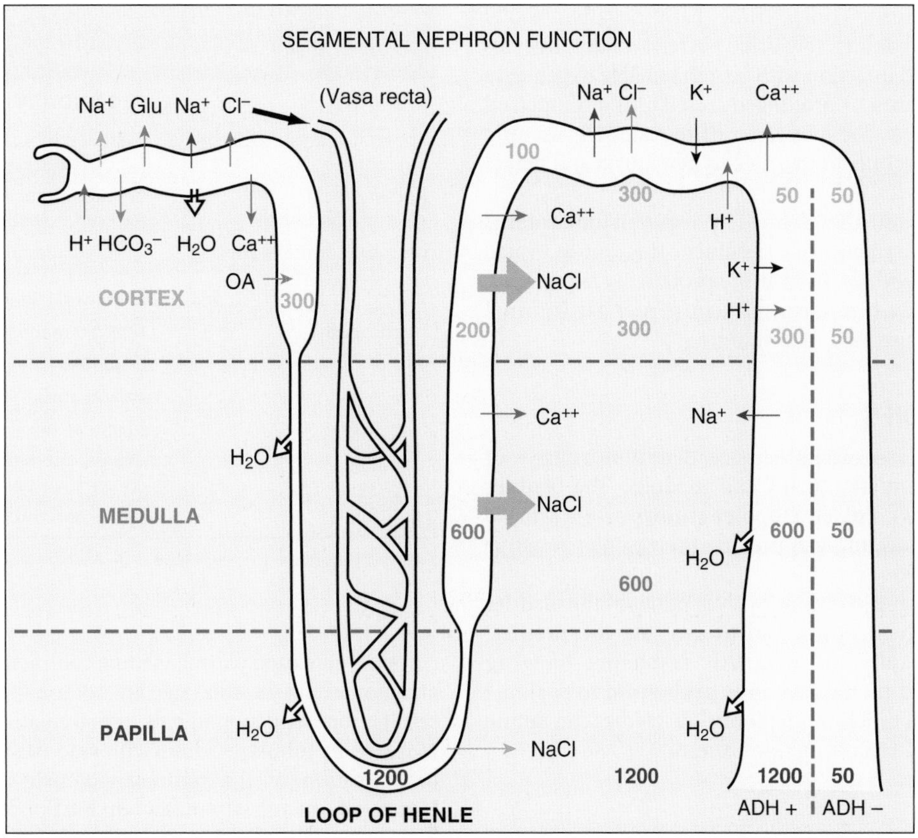

FIGURE 161.1 Major transport functions of each nephron segment, including representative osmolalities in vasa recta, interstitium, and tubule at different levels within the kidney. *ADH*, Antidiuretic hormone; *Glu*, glucose; *OA*, organic acid. (From Andreoli TE, Carpenter CCJ, Plum F, et al., ed. *Cecil Essentials of Medicine*. Philadelphia: WB Saunders;1986.)

DIAGNOSTIC STUDIES

Laboratory Studies

GFR is measured most *accurately* by infusion of a substance that is *freely* filtered by the glomerulus but not metabolized, reabsorbed, or secreted in or by the tubules. GFR is calculated as follows:

$$GFR = [U]V/[P]$$

where *[U]* is urine concentration, *[P]* is serum concentration of a substance (mg/dL) used to measure clearance, and *V* is urine flow rate (mL/min).

By convention, GFR is corrected to body surface area of 1.73 m^2 to allow comparison between different-sized individuals. In a full-term newborn, an uncorrected GFR of 4-5 mL/min corrects to approximately 40 mL/min per 1.73 m^2. GFR increases rapidly during the first 2 years of life until it achieves adult values (100-120 mL/min per 1.73 m^2). After that, GFR and body size increase proportionately, so GFR/1.73 m^2 remains stable.

Plasma creatinine reflects muscle mass, increases with age, and is used to approximate GFR. Creatinine is also secreted by the PT, resulting in less accurate measurement of GFR with immature kidneys or with decreased renal function. **Blood urea nitrogen** is affected by renal function, but is also affected by hydration, nutrition, catabolism, and tissue breakdown. The correlation between creatinine and GFR can be used to estimate GFR. The revised Schwartz formula is the following:

$$GFR = \frac{0.413 \times Ht}{Cr_{serum}}$$

(height in cm; serum creatinine in mg/dL). This formula is most useful when body habitus and muscle mass are reasonably normal and when renal function is relatively stable. This formula is most accurate in GFR range of 15-75 mL/min per 1.73 m^2. Values greater than 75 are typically reported as greater than 75 rather than as a specific number. **Creatinine clearance** ($[U_{Cr}]V/[P_{Cr}]$) estimates GFR, but overestimates GFR when renal function is decreased.

Urinalysis is a useful screen for renal abnormalities. In addition to urine color and turbidity, **macroscopic urinalysis** uses a **urine dipstick** for pH and the presence of protein, glucose, ketones, blood, and leukocytes. Dilute urine may result in a false-negative result for protein; false-positive results may occur with extremely alkaline or concentrated urine or if there is a delay in reading the test. Dipsticks are exquisitely sensitive to presence of hemoglobin (or myoglobin); there are few false-negative test results but many false-positive results. **Glucose** is detected via glucose oxidase-peroxidase reaction, and leukocytes are detected via **leukocyte esterase** reaction. The **nitrite test** may detect bacteriuria if the bacteria can reduce nitrate to nitrite and have sufficient urine contact time. False-negative results occur with frequent voiding, low urine bacterial count, urinary tract obstruction, and infection with bacteria unable to generate nitrite. Gross hematuria or prolonged contact (uncircumcised boys) may result in a false-positive nitrite test. **Microscopic urinalysis** is used to confirm pyuria and hematuria and detect casts and crystals.

Proteinuria can be further defined by a **spot urine protein/creatinine** ($U_{Pr}/_{Cr}$) in a single urine specimen. This unit-less value correlates very well with 24-hour urine protein excretion: spot $U_{Pr}/_{Cr}$ approximates 24-hour urine protein/m^2 per day (normal <0.20; nephrotic range >2.0 in children).

IMAGING STUDIES

Ultrasound reliably assesses kidney size, determines degree of dilation, and differentiates cortex and medulla. The bladder also can be visualized. **Pulsed Doppler studies** assess arterial and venous blood flow and can provide the vascular resistive index in each kidney.

A **voiding cystourethrogram** involves filling of the bladder to detect vesicoureteral reflux and to evaluate the urethra. **Computed tomography** and **magnetic resonance imaging** have mostly replaced the **intravenous pyelogram** to evaluate kidney structure and function. Radionuclide studies can define renal size, scars, and renal function/excretion.

CHAPTER 162

Nephrotic Syndrome and Proteinuria

ETIOLOGY AND EPIDEMIOLOGY

Small amounts of protein are found in urine of healthy children (<4 mg/m^2 per hour or $U_{Pr}/_{Cr}$ <0.2). **Nephrotic proteinuria** in children is defined as protein >40 mg/m^2 per hour or $U_{Pr/Cr}$ >2.0. Proteinuria between these levels is mildly to moderately elevated but not nephrotic.

Proteinuria may be **transient** or **persistent, asymptomatic** or **symptomatic,** and **orthostatic** (present in the upright position but not in the recumbent position) or **fixed** (present in all positions). Proteinuria may be **glomerular** (disruptions of the normal glomerular barrier to protein filtration) or **tubular** (increased filtration, impaired reabsorption, or secretion of proteins).

Nephrotic syndrome (NS) is characterized by persistent heavy **proteinuria** (mainly albuminuria; >2 g/m^2 per 24 hour); **hypoproteinemia** (serum albumin <3.0 g/dL); **hypercholesterolemia** (>250 mg/dL); and **edema**. Age, race, and geography affect the incidence of NS. Certain human leukocyte antigen (HLA) types (HLA-DR7, HLA-B8, and HLA-B12) are associated with increased incidence of NS. Increased glomerular permeability is due to alterations in the normal glomerular cellular and basement membrane barrier that restrict serum protein filtration. The resultant massive proteinuria leads to decreased serum proteins, especially albumin. Plasma oncotic pressure is diminished, leading to fluid shifts from vascular to interstitial compartments and plasma volume contraction. Renal blood flow and glomerular filtration rate are not usually diminished. Edema results from reduction in effective circulating blood volume and increase in tubular sodium chloride reabsorption secondary to activation of the renin-angiotensin-aldosterone system. Hypoproteinemia stimulates hepatic lipoprotein synthesis and diminishes lipoprotein metabolism, leading to elevated serum lipids (cholesterol, triglycerides) and lipoproteins.

TABLE 162.1 Primary and Secondary Forms of Nephrotic Syndrome

PRIMARY	SECONDARY
Minimal change nephrotic syndrome	Systemic lupus erythematosus
Primary focal glomerulosclerosis	Henoch-Schönlein purpura, Granulomatosis with polyangiitis and other vasculitides
Membranoproliferative glomerulonephritis	Chronic infections (hepatitis B, hepatitis C, malaria, human immunodeficiency virus)
Idiopathic membranous nephropathy	Allergic reactions
	Diabetes
	Amyloidosis
	Malignancies
	Congestive heart failure, constrictive pericarditis
	Renal vein thrombosis

NS may be **primary** or **secondary** (Table 162.1). A child with apparent primary NS, prior to renal biopsy, is considered to have **idiopathic nephrotic syndrome. Minimal change nephrotic syndrome** (MCNS) is the most common histological form of primary NS in children. More than 80% of children less than 7 years of age with NS have MCNS. Children 7-16 years old with NS have a ~50% chance of having MCNS. Males are affected more frequently than females (2:1).

Focal segmental glomerulosclerosis (FSGS) accounts for ~10-20% of children with primary NS. It may present like MCNS or with less impressive proteinuria. FSGS may develop from MCNS or represent a separate entity. A circulating factor that increases glomerular permeability is found in some patients with FSGS. More than 35% of children with FSGS progress to renal failure.

Membranoproliferative glomerulonephritis (MPGN) is characterized by hypocomplementemia with signs of glomerular renal disease. MPGN represents 5-15% of children with primary NS, is typically persistent, and has a high likelihood of progression to renal failure over time.

Membranous nephropathy represents <5% of children with primary NS. It is seen most commonly in adolescents and children with systemic infections (hepatitis B, syphilis, malaria, and toxoplasmosis) or specific medications (gold, penicillamine).

Congenital NS presents during the first 2 months of life. There are two common types. The Finnish type is an autosomal recessive disorder most common in persons of Scandinavian descent and is due to a mutation in the nephrin protein component in the glomerular filtration slit. The second type is a heterogeneous group of abnormalities, including diffuse mesangial sclerosis and conditions associated with drugs or infections. Prenatal onset is supported by elevated levels of maternal alpha-fetoprotein.

Secondary NS may result from many different causes in children and are listed in Table 162.1.

CLINICAL MANIFESTATIONS

Decision-Making Algorithms
Available @ StudentConsult.com

Abdominal Pain
Red Urine and Hematuria
Proteinuria
Edema

The sudden onset of dependent pitting edema or ascites is the most common presentation for children with NS. Anorexia, malaise, and abdominal pain are often present. Blood pressure may be elevated in up to 25% of children on presentation; acute tubular necrosis and significant hypotension may occur with sudden decline in serum albumin and significant volume depletion. Diarrhea (intestinal edema) and respiratory distress (pulmonary edema or pleural effusion) may be present. Typical MCNS is characterized by *absence* of gross hematuria, renal insufficiency, hypertension (HTN), and hypocomplementemia.

DIAGNOSTIC STUDIES

Proteinuria of 1+ or higher on 2-3 random urine specimens suggests persistent proteinuria that should be further quantified. A $U_{Pr}/_{Cr} > 0.2$ on a first morning specimen excludes orthostatic proteinuria. $U_{Pr}/_{Cr} > 2.0$ indicates nephrotic range proteinuria.

In addition to a demonstration of proteinuria, hypercholesterolemia, and hypoalbuminemia, routine testing typically includes a serum C3 complement. A low serum C3 implies a lesion other than MCNS, and a renal biopsy is indicated before trial of corticosteroid therapy. Microscopic hematuria may be present in up to 25% of cases of MCNS but does not predict response to steroids. Additional laboratory tests, including electrolytes, blood urea nitrogen, creatinine, total protein, and serum albumin level, are performed based on history and physical examination features. Renal ultrasound is often useful. Biopsy is performed when MCNS is not suspected.

DIFFERENTIAL DIAGNOSIS

Transient proteinuria can be seen after vigorous exercise, fever, dehydration, seizures, and adrenergic agonist therapy. Proteinuria usually is mild ($U_{Pr}/_{Cr} < 1$), glomerular in origin, and always resolves within a few days. It does not indicate renal disease.

Postural (orthostatic) proteinuria is a benign condition defined by normal protein excretion while recumbent but significant proteinuria when upright. It is glomerular in origin, more common in adolescents and tall, thin individuals, and not associated with progressive renal disease. Many children with orthostatic proteinuria continue this process into adulthood.

Tubular proteinuria is characterized by preponderance of urine low molecular weight proteins and is seen with acute tubular necrosis, pyelonephritis, structural renal disorders, polycystic kidney disease, and tubular toxins such as antibiotics or chemotherapeutic agents. The combination of tubular proteinuria with tubular electrolyte wasting and glycosuria is termed **Fanconi syndrome.**

Glomerular proteinuria is characterized by a combination of urine large and small molecular weight proteins, variable levels of proteinuria, and often other evidence of glomerular disease (hematuria, red blood cell casts, HTN, and renal insufficiency). Causes of glomerular proteinuria include glomerular capillary disruption (hemolytic uremic syndrome, crescentic glomerulonephritis); glomerular capillary immune complex deposition (poststreptococcal glomerulonephritis and lupus nephritis); and altered glomerular capillary permeability (MCNS, congenital NS).

TREATMENT

Because greater than 80% of children less than 13 years of age with primary NS have steroid-responsive forms (chiefly MCNS), steroid therapy may be initiated without a renal biopsy if a child has typical features of NS. Typical therapy for MCNS is prednisone, 2 mg/kg per day (60 mg/m^2 per 24 hour, maximum 60 mg/day), provided once a day or split into multiple doses. Over 90% of children who respond to steroids do so within 4 weeks. Responders should receive steroids for 12 weeks for best long-term results. A renal biopsy is indicated for nonresponders because steroid resistance decreases the chance that MCNS is the underlying disease. Frequent relapses or steroid resistance may necessitate additional immunosuppressive therapy.

Treatment responses in FSGS are highly variable. Approximately 35% respond to steroid therapy; others may respond to immunosuppressive therapy. MPGN and membranous glomerulonephritis often improve with chronic steroid or immunosuppressive therapy but do not reliably remit with standard NS steroid therapy. Aggressive medical therapy of familial congenital NS, with early nephrectomy, dialysis, and transplantation, is the only effective approach to this syndrome.

NS edema is treated by restricting salt intake. Severe edema may require use of loop diuretics. When these therapies do not alleviate severe edema, cautious parenteral administration of 25% albumin (0.5-1.0 g/kg intravenously over 1-2 hours) with an intravenous loop diuretic usually results in diuresis. The administered albumin is excreted rapidly, and thus salt restriction and diuretics must be continued. Significant pleural effusions may require drainage. Acute HTN is treated with β-blockers or calcium channel blockers. Persistent HTN usually responds to angiotensin-converting enzyme inhibitors.

COMPLICATIONS

An increased incidence of serious infections, particularly **bacteremia** and **peritonitis** (particularly *Streptococcus pneumoniae, Escherichia coli,* or *Klebsiella),* is due to urinary loss of immunoglobulins and complement. Side effects of steroids are most common in steroid-dependent and frequently relapsing patients. Hypovolemia may result from diarrhea or diuretic use. Loss of coagulation factors, antithrombin, and plasminogen may lead to a hypercoagulable state with a risk of **thromboembolism** (TE). Warfarin, Lovenox, low-dose aspirin, or dipyridamole may minimize risk of thrombosis in NS patients with a history of TE or high risk for TE. Hyperlipidemia promotes increased atherosclerotic vascular disease.

PROGNOSIS

Most children with NS eventually go into remission. Nearly 80% of children with MCNS experience NS relapse, defined as heavy proteinuria that persists for 3 or more consecutive days. Transient proteinuria (up to 3 days) may occur with intercurrent infection in children with MCNS and is not considered a relapse. Steroid therapy is typically effective for true relapse. Steroid-responsive patients have little risk of chronic renal failure. Patients with FSGS may initially respond to steroids but later develop resistance. Many children with FSGS progress to end-stage kidney failure (see Chapter 165). Recurrence of FSGS occurs in ~30% of children who undergo renal transplantation.

CHAPTER 163

Glomerulonephritis and Hematuria

ETIOLOGY AND EPIDEMIOLOGY

A child with **gross hematuria** may have a serious disease and requires prompt evaluation. **Microscopic hematuria,** defined as >3-5 red blood cells (RBCs) per high-power field on freshly voided and centrifuged urine, can be benign. Isolated asymptomatic microscopic hematuria is found in up to 4% of healthy children. In most cases this is a transient finding. Hematuria may originate from glomerular, tubulointerstitial, or lower urinary tract disorders (Table 163.1).

TABLE 163.1 Differential Diagnosis of Red Urine/Hematuria
FACTITIOUS HEMATURIA
Nonpathological (urate crystals in infants, ingested foods, medications, dyes)
Pathological (hemoglobinuria from hemolytic anemia, myoglobinuria from rhabdomyolysis)
GLOMERULAR
Immunological injury (GN—e.g., PSGN, IgA nephropathy, MPGN, systemic diseases)
Structural disorder (Alport syndrome, thin basement membrane disease)
Toxin-mediated injury (HUS)
TUBULOINTERSTITIAL/PARENCHYMAL
Inflammation (interstitial nephritis, pyelonephritis)
Vascular (sickle cell trait/disease, Nutcracker syndrome)
Structural (cyst rupture, Wilms tumor, urinary tract obstruction, renal trauma)
LOWER URINARY TRACT
Inflammation (cystitis, hemorrhagic cystitis, urethritis)
Injury (trauma, kidney stone)
Hypercalciuria

GN, Glomerulonephritis; *HUS*, hemolytic uremic syndrome; *Ig*, immunoglobulin; *MPGN*, membranoproliferative glomerulonephritis; *PSGN*, poststreptococcal glomerulonephritis.

Immune-mediated inflammation causes most **glomerulonephritis** (GN). Poststreptococcal glomerulonephritis (PSGN) is the most common form of acute GN, and immunoglobulin (Ig)A nephropathy is the most common chronic GN, but many other types of GN can occur. The most common identifiable lower urinary tract causes of hematuria include urinary tract infection (UTI), kidney stones, and hypercalciuria.

CLINICAL MANIFESTATIONS

Decision-Making Algorithms
Available @ StudentConsult.com

Red Urine and Hematuria
Proteinuria
Edema
Hypertension

Children with **acute GN** commonly present with hematuria (gross or microscopic) and other cardinal features of glomerular injury (proteinuria, hypertension, edema, oliguria, renal insufficiency). **PSGN** occurs most frequently in children 2-12 years of age and is more common in boys. Manifestations of PSGN are typical of acute GN and develop 5-21 days (average 10 days) after streptococcal pharyngitis infections and 4-6 weeks after impetigo. **Acute postinfectious GN** presents similar to PSGN following infections with other bacterial and viral pathogens. PSGN can develop even in the child treated with antibiotics for the infection. Special attention must be paid to the blood pressure as hypertension may be severe enough to cause heart failure, seizures, and/or encephalopathy.

The presentation of **IgA nephropathy** is more variable and may take the form of acute GN, asymptomatic microscopic hematuria, or recurrent gross hematuria concurrent with an upper respiratory infection (rather than several days later, as with PSGN). Children with hematuria secondary to systemic disorders such as Henoch-Schönlein purpura nephritis, lupus nephritis, and vasculitis-associated GN typically present with other systemic features of the respective disease.

A special form of GN is **rapidly progressive glomerulonephritis (RPGN)** that presents with typical features of acute GN where renal insufficiency progresses more quickly and severely. Renal biopsy shows glomerular epithelial cell proliferation with crescents. RPGN may be idiopathic or secondary to any type of GN. Early recognition of RPGN is crucial to prevent progression to end-stage renal disease (ESRD) that occurs without prompt treatment.

Alport syndrome is typically caused by X-linked chromosome mutations, but has also been associated with mutations of genes for type IV collagen, both leading to abnormal glomerular basement membrane (GBM). The disease may present with either asymptomatic microscopic or gross hematuria. Males typically develop progressive renal failure and sensorineural hearing loss during adolescence and young adulthood. Females typically have a more benign course but usually have at least microscopic hematuria. **Thin basement membrane disease** (benign familial hematuria) is caused by mutations leading to isolated GBM thinning; these mutations are often autosomal dominant with hematuria frequently noted in first-degree relatives. As opposed to Alport syndrome, thin basement

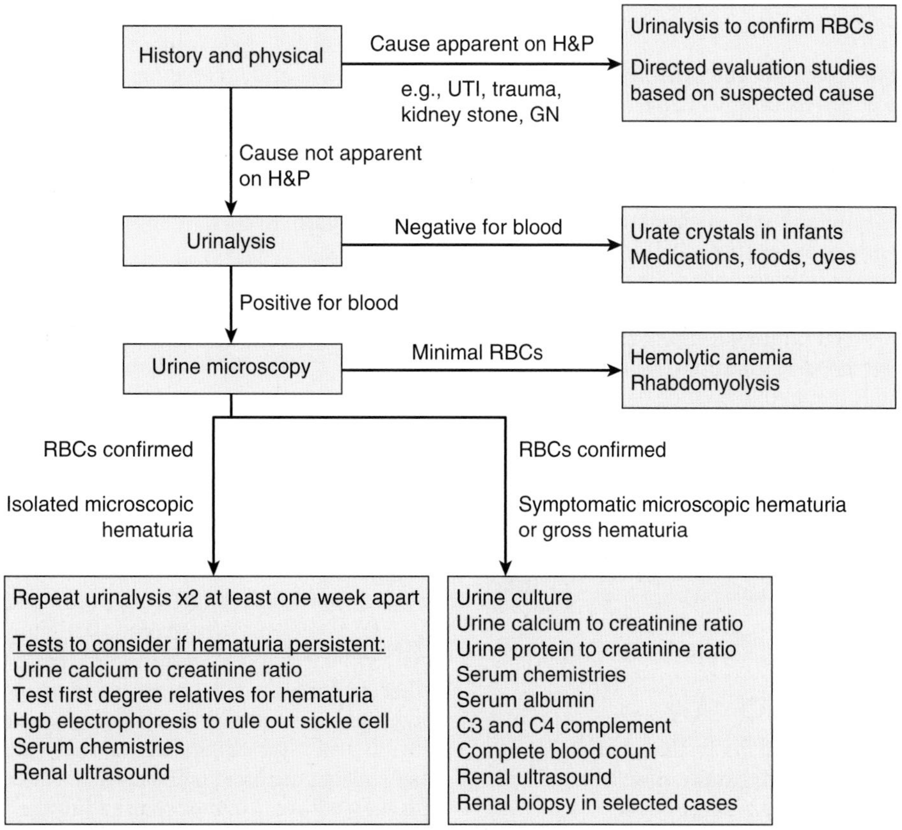

FIGURE 163.1 Suggested algorithm for evaluation of red urine/hematuria. *GN*, Glomerulonephritis; *Hgb*, hemoglobin; *H&P*, history and physical; *RBCs*, red blood cells; *UTI*, urinary tract infection.

membrane disease is typically not progressive and usually has an excellent prognosis.

The presentation of nonglomerular causes of hematuria is more variable and related to the underlying etiology. Hematuria due to tubular disorders is usually microscopic and may be associated with proteinuria, glycosuria, and polyuria. These children typically do not have hypertension and develop renal insufficiency only with more severe disease. Painless gross hematuria may be seen with strenuous exercise, sickle cell trait/disease, or Wilms tumor. Hematuria may be associated with pain when due to bleeding from renal cysts or Nutcracker syndrome (renal vein compression). Gross hematuria following trauma may signify more severe renal or lower urinary tract injury. **UTI** is typically associated with dysuria and urinary frequency. **Urolithiasis** may be associated with asymptomatic hematuria or with flank or abdominal pain. **Hypercalciuria** can cause both gross and microscopic hematuria and may be associated with urinary tract symptoms such as dysuria and urinary frequency or may be asymptomatic.

DIAGNOSTIC STUDIES

All patients with hematuria should have a careful history and physical (including blood pressure) along with urinalysis including microscopic examination to identify RBCs. Glomerular hematuria is suggested by brownish (tea- or cola-colored) urine and presence of RBC casts and/or dysmorphic RBCs on urine microscopy. A urine color that is more bright red without RBC casts or dysmorphic RBCs is more suggestive of lower urinary tract source. However, there may be overlap of these findings.

A suggested algorithm for the evaluation of hematuria is given in Fig. 163.1. Gross hematuria and microscopic hematuria with associated concerning findings should have additional laboratory evaluation. Presence of low C3 complement narrows the differential diagnosis to PSGN, membranoproliferative GN, and lupus nephritis. Children with isolated, asymptomatic microscopic hematuria may be observed with repeat urinalyses. If hematuria is persistent, additional evaluation may then be appropriate.

THERAPY

Therapy for PSGN is supportive and involves dietary sodium restriction, diuretics, and antihypertensive agents as needed. Although treating the streptococcal infection does not prevent PSGN, antibiotic treatment is still warranted with active streptococcal infection. Therapies for children with other forms of GN depend on underlying cause and severity. In some cases, antiinflammatory therapy involving corticosteroids and/or other immunosuppressive agents may be warranted. Treatment with angiotensin-converting enzyme inhibitors may reduce proteinuria and glomerular hyperperfusion, but should be used with caution in the setting of acute kidney injury.

PROGNOSIS AND PREVENTION

PSGN usually has a benign outcome. In typical cases, the gross hematuria, proteinuria, and edema decline quickly (5-10 days). Microscopic hematuria may persist for months or even years;

greater than 95% of children recover completely with no long-term sequelae.

Children with IgA nephropathy and other forms of chronic GN have greater risk of progression to ESRD. The prognosis for renal recovery in chronic GN and in RPGN is variable and related to the underlying disorder and disease severity. The presence of persistent, heavy proteinuria, hypertension, decreased kidney function, and severe glomerular lesions on biopsy is associated with poor outcomes.

Children with idiopathic isolated, asymptomatic microscopic hematuria or suspected thin basement membrane disease typically have an excellent renal prognosis. Long-term follow-up, including yearly urinalysis (to rule out proteinuria) and blood pressure measurement, is required to exclude progressive forms of renal disease.

CHAPTER 164

Hemolytic Uremic Syndrome

ETIOLOGY AND EPIDEMIOLOGY

Hemolytic uremic syndrome (HUS) is characterized by the triad of **microangiopathic hemolytic anemia, thrombocytopenia,** and **renal injury** and is an important cause of acute kidney injury in children. HUS typically occurs in children less than 5 years of age, but can occur in older children. The most common type of HUS is associated with a prodromal diarrheal illness (**D + HUS**). Contamination of meat, fruit, vegetables, or water with verotoxin (VT)-producing *Escherichia coli* (most commonly ***E. coli*** **O157:H7**) is responsible for many outbreaks. VT may be produced by other *E. coli* strains as well as other bacteria such as *Shigella*. VT causes hemorrhagic enterocolitis of variable severity and results in HUS in ~5-15% of affected children.

HUS presenting without a prodrome of diarrhea **(atypical HUS)** may occur at any age. The clinical course is usually more severe than D + HUS. Atypical HUS can be secondary to infection (*Streptococcus pneumonia*, human immunodeficiency virus), genetic and acquired defects in complement regulation, medications, malignancy, systemic lupus erythematosus, and pregnancy.

CLINICAL MANIFESTATIONS

Decision-Making Algorithms
Available @ StudentConsult.com

Diarrhea
Petechiae/Purpura

Classic D + HUS begins with enterocolitis, often with bloody stools, followed in 7-10 days by weakness, lethargy, and oliguria/anuria. Physical examination reveals irritability, pallor, and petechiae. Dehydration is frequent; however, some children have volume overload. Hypertension may be due to volume overload and/or renal injury. Central nervous system (CNS) involvement, including seizures, occurs in up to 25% of cases. Other potential organ involvement includes pancreatitis, cardiac dysfunction, and colonic perforation.

Children without evidence of diarrheal prodrome may have a similar microangiopathic syndrome, identified as **thrombotic thrombocytopenic purpura** (TTP). Children with TTP typically have predominant CNS symptoms but may also have significant renal disease. Recurrent episodes are common. Because CNS involvement is also seen in HUS, TTP can be difficult to distinguish from HUS in some cases. Deficiencies of ADAMTS13, a von Willebrand factor-cleaving protease, have been identified in children affected with TTP.

DIAGNOSTIC STUDIES

Common laboratory findings in HUS are listed in Table 164.1. Peripheral blood smear reveals evidence of microangiopathic hemolysis. Coombs test is negative. Diarrhea and presence of toxin-producing *E. coli* may have resolved by the time HUS is diagnosed.

TREATMENT AND PROGNOSIS

Therapy for HUS is supportive and includes volume repletion, hypertension control, and managing complications of renal insufficiency, including dialysis when indicated. Red blood cell transfusions are provided as needed. Platelet transfusions should be avoided because they may add to the thrombotic microangiopathy and are indicated only by active hemorrhage or prior to a procedure. Antibiotics and antidiarrheal agents may increase risk of developing HUS. Early hydration during the diarrheal phase may lessen the severity of renal insufficiency. Most children (>95%) with D + HUS survive the acute phase and recover normal renal function, although some may have evidence of long-term renal and other morbidity.

TABLE 164.1 Common Laboratory Findings With Hemolytic Uremic Syndrome

EVIDENCE OF MICROANGIOPATHIC HEMOLYTIC ANEMIA
Anemia
Thrombocytopenia
Presence of schistocytes, helmet cells, and burr cells on peripheral blood smear
Increased LDH
Decreased haptoglobin
Increased indirect bilirubin
Increased AST
Elevated reticulocyte count
EVIDENCE OF RENAL INJURY
Elevated creatinine
Presence of hematuria, proteinuria, pyuria, casts on urinalysis
OTHER POTENTIAL FINDINGS
Leukocytosis
Positive stool culture for *E. coli* O157:H7
Positive stool test for shiga-toxin
Elevated amylase/lipase

AST, Aspartate aminotransferase; *E. coli*, *Escherichia coli*; *LDH*, lactate dehydrogenase.

CHAPTER 165

Acute and Chronic Renal Failure

ACUTE KIDNEY INJURY

Etiology

Acute kidney injury (AKI), formerly termed *acute renal failure,* refers to an abrupt decrease in glomerular filtration rate (GFR) and tubular function. This may lead to decreased excretion of waste products (e.g., urea) and disturbance in fluid and electrolyte homeostasis. Early recognition and management of AKI are crucial.

AKI may be **oliguric** (<1 mL/kg/hr in neonates and infants, <0.5 mL/kg/hr in children) or **nonoliguric**, which is more difficult to recognize. Although urine output in nonoliguric AKI is normal or polyuric, electrolyte disturbances and uremia may become significant. Major causes of AKI may be divided into **prerenal** (renal hypoperfusion), **intrinsic renal** (tubular, glomerular, or vascular injury), and **postrenal** (urinary tract obstruction) categories (Table 165.1). In many cases, the cause of AKI is multifactorial.

Prerenal azotemia is most commonly due to **dehydration,** but may be secondary to other mechanisms of glomerular hypoperfusion. Tubular injury encompasses the most common causes of intrinsic AKI in children. Tubular injury may occur from hypoxia-ischemia **(acute tubular necrosis),** infection **(sepsis), nephrotoxic agents** (medications, contrast, myoglobin), and inflammation **(interstitial nephritis).** Postrenal AKI may be due to either structural or functional **urinary tract obstruction**.

Clinical Manifestations

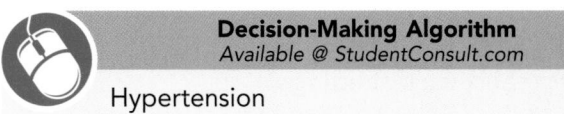

Decision-Making Algorithm
Available @ StudentConsult.com
Hypertension

History, physical examination, and basic studies usually allow proper classification of the child with AKI (Table 165.2). Prerenal azotemia is characterized by history of precipitating factors and oliguria. Intrinsic tubular injury is associated with precipitating factors, but urine output may be low, normal, or high, depending on the severity of the injury. Glomerular and vascular disorders may present with hematuria, edema, hypertension, and oliguria. The urine output with postrenal AKI may be low or normal and may be associated with flank masses or a distended bladder on examination. Depending on the underlying cause and severity of illness, AKI can be associated with signs of dehydration or volume overload.

Diagnostic Studies

A **urinalysis** (UA) should be obtained in all children with AKI. In prerenal azotemia, UA is unremarkable with high specific gravity reflecting appropriate renal retention of water associated with renal hypoperfusion. However, neonates are not able to

TABLE 165.1 Causes of Acute Kidney Injury

PRERENAL
Dehydration
Hemorrhage
Septic shock
Burns
Heart failure
Cirrhosis
POSTRENAL (OBSTRUCTION)
Urethral obstruction (stricture, posterior urethral valves)
Ureteral obstruction
Ureterocele
Extrinsic tumor compressing bladder outlet
Neurogenic bladder (myelomeningocele, spinal cord injury)
INTRINSIC
Acute tubular necrosis
Nephrotoxins (medications, contrast, myoglobin)
Infection (sepsis)
Interstitial nephritis
Glomerular injury (primary glomerulonephritis, vasculitis, hemolytic uremic syndrome)
Vascular (renal vein thrombosis, arterial emboli, malignant hypertension)

TABLE 165.2 Laboratory and Clinical Evaluation of Acute Kidney Injury

LABORATORY/CLINICAL FEATURE	PRERENAL		RENAL		
	CHILD	**NEONATE**	**CHILD**	**NEONATE**	**POSTRENAL**
Urine output	Low		Low, normal, or high		Low or normal
Urinalysis	Normal		RBCs, WBCs, protein, casts		Variable
Urine Na^+ (mEq/L)	<15	<20-30	>40	>50	Variable, may be >40
FE_{Na}* (%)	<1	<2.5	>2	>2.5	Variable, may be >2
Urine osmolality (mOsm/L)	>500	>350	~300	~300	Variable, may be <300
Renal ultrasound	Normal		Increased echogenicity, decreased corticomedullary differentiation		Hydronephrosis

*FE_{Na} (%) = [(urine sodium/plasma sodium) ÷ (urine creatinine/plasma creatinine)] × 100.
FE_{Na}, Fractional excretion of sodium; *RBCs,* red blood cells; *WBCs,* white blood cells.

concentrate urine as well. With intrinsic tubular injury and postrenal AKI, UA may show mild hematuria and/or proteinuria with specific gravity 1.015 or less. With glomerular and vascular injury, hematuria and proteinuria are usually moderate to severe. In oliguric states, differentiation between prerenal azotemia and acute tubular necrosis may be aided by determining urine osmolality and fractional excretion of sodium (see Table 165.2). **Renal ultrasound** is often helpful in defining AKI category (see Table 165.2). Renal biopsy is indicated only in select cases.

Common electrolyte abnormalities seen with AKI include hyperkalemia, metabolic acidosis, hypocalcemia, and hyperphosphatemia. These labs may need to be monitored frequently, depending on initial results and clinical course. A complete blood count should be obtained as anemia is frequently observed. Other studies may be obtained as clinically indicated.

Treatment

In some cases the underlying disorder can be treated. Examples include volume repletion in dehydration, stopping an offending nephrotoxic medication, and relieving urinary tract obstruction. In all cases efforts should be made to limit additional renal injury (e.g., ensuring adequate renal perfusion and avoiding nephrotoxic medications). Medication dosages should be adjusted for decreased renal function as appropriate.

Fluid therapy depends on volume status and urine output. If hypovolemia is present, intravascular volume should be expanded by intravenous saline administration. If hypervolemia is present, 1-2 mg/kg of furosemide and fluid restriction may be attempted. If euvolemia is present, total fluid input should be adjusted to meet the urine output, which may be higher or lower than normal. Assessment of intake and output should be augmented with serial body weight measurements.

AKI treatment particularly involves management of potential complications. Electrolyte disorders are treated as appropriate. Potassium intake and medications that increase potassium should be restricted. If hyperkalemia is present, intravenous calcium will lower the risk of arrhythmia while measures are initiated to shift potassium into cells (bicarbonate, β-agonists, insulin/dextrose) and hasten removal (diuretics, sodium-potassium exchange resins, dialysis). Preferred treatment of hypocalcemia involves oral calcium supplementation and calcitriol; intravenous (IV) calcium is reserved for severe cases. Hypertension may be treated with diuretics, calcium channel blockers, and vasodilators. Angiotensin-converting enzyme (ACE) inhibitors are usually avoided in the setting of AKI.

Major indications for **acute dialysis** are listed in Table 165.3. Medical therapy may be attempted before initiating renal replacement therapy. There is no set blood urea nitrogen or creatinine level at which dialysis is started in AKI. Renal replacement options in children include peritoneal dialysis, hemodialysis, and continuous renal replacement therapy. The mode is selected based on individual factors.

Prognosis

Recovery from AKI depends on etiology, severity, availability of specific treatments, and other patient aspects. Nonoliguric AKI usually recovers well, whereas outcomes with oliguric AKI are more variable. Even with seemingly good recovery, a history of AKI places the child at increased risk for future renal complications, including chronic kidney disease (CKD).

TABLE 165.3 Indications for Renal Replacement Therapy

ACUTE AND/OR CHRONIC DIALYSIS
Volume overload
Metabolic acidosis
Electrolyte abnormalities
Uremia
ACUTE DIALYSIS
Certain ingestions
Hyperammonemia
CHRONIC DIALYSIS
Poor growth
Stage 5 chronic kidney disease (end-stage renal disease)

TABLE 165.4 Classification of the Stages of Chronic Kidney Disease

STAGE	GFR (mL/min/1.73 m^2)*	DESCRIPTION
1	>90	Minimal kidney damage
2	60-89	Kidney damage with mild reduction of GFR
3	30-59	Moderate reduction of GFR
4	15-29	Severe reduction of GFR
5	<15 (or dialysis)	End-stage renal disease

**GFR ranges apply for children 2 years of age and older.*
GFR, Glomerular filtration rate.
From National Kidney Foundation Kidney Disease Outcomes Quality Initiative.

CHRONIC KIDNEY DISEASE

Etiology and Epidemiology

Congenital anomalies of the kidney and urinary tract (CAKUT) are the most common causes of CKD that present between birth and 10 years of age. After age 10, acquired renal diseases, such as focal segmental glomerulosclerosis and glomerulonephritis (GN), are more common causes of CKD. Risk of progression to end-stage renal disease (ESRD) is related to the underlying cause and severity of CKD. During puberty, renal function may deteriorate if the damaged kidneys are not able to grow and adapt to increased demands. CKD is staged to facilitate appropriate evaluation and monitoring (Table 165.4). GFR can be estimated in children using the Schwartz formula (see Chapter 161). Most complications of CKD do not manifest until at least stage 3 CKD. In stage 4 CKD, complications become more numerous and severe. Children with stage 5 CKD (ESRD) are typically treated with either dialysis or renal transplantation.

Clinical Manifestations

The clinical presentation of a child with CKD is related to both underlying cause and complications of CKD. A child with CAKUT may have polyuria, polydipsia, and recurrent urinary tract infections. A child with glomerular disease may have hematuria, proteinuria, edema, and hypertension. Common complications of CKD in children are listed in Table 165.5.

TABLE 165.5 Common Complications and Treatments of Chronic Kidney Disease

COMPLICATION	TREATMENT
1. Poor growth	Increased caloric intake, treat acidosis, treat CKD-MBD, recombinant GH
2. Anemia	Erythropoietin, iron supplementation
3. CKD-Mineral Bone Disorder/secondary hyperparathyroidism	1,25-Dihydroxyvitamin D supplementation, calcium supplementation, dietary phosphorous restriction, phosphate binders
4. Cardiovascular	
4a. Hypertension	Antihypertensive medications
4b. Left ventricular hypertrophy	Volume control
5. Electrolyte abnormalities	
5a. Hyperkalemia	Low K diet, furosemide, sodium polystyrene sulfonate
5b. Hyponatremia	Sodium supplementation
5c. Metabolic acidosis	Alkali replacement

CKD, Chronic kidney disease; *CKD-MBD*, chronic kidney disease—mineral bone disorder; *GH*, growth hormone; *K*, potassium.

Most of these complications are multifactorial in etiology. For example, factors associated with **growth failure** include poor nutrition, **CKD-mineral bone disorder (CKD-MBD)**, metabolic acidosis, hormonal abnormalities, and resistance to growth hormone. **Anemia** results primarily from a failure to produce adequate **erythropoietin** and iron deficiency. CKD-MBD is usually due to **secondary hyperparathyroidism** as a result of diminished renal 1,25-dihydroxyvitamin D production, hypocalcemia, and hyperphosphatemia (from decreased renal excretion). If prolonged and/or severe, CKD-MBD may lead to rickets and bone deformities. **Hypertension** and **left ventricular hypertrophy** are common cardiovascular complications. Delayed puberty results from altered gonadotropin secretion and regulation. Learning and school performance may also be impaired in CKD.

Treatment

The management of children with advanced CKD requires a multidisciplinary team of pediatric practitioners. Adequate nutrition should be provided even if this requires dietary supplements and tube feedings. In infants, a low-solute formula may be indicated. Unless a child is oliguric, fluid restriction is not necessary. Many children with CAKUT require supplemental salt due to urine sodium wasting. Conversely, children with GN tend to retain sodium and may become hypertensive or edematous if given excess salt. Common treatment considerations for other CKD complications are given in Table 165.5.

Measures can be taken to preserve kidney function or slow progression of CKD. Hypertension and proteinuria can be treated with ACE inhibitors or angiotensin receptor blockers. Potentially nephrotoxic medications should be avoided when feasible. Medication adjustment for reduced kidney function is important. Protein intake is typically not restricted in pediatric CKD.

The optimal treatment of ESRD is **renal transplantation.** Both deceased and living donors can be used for renal transplantation. Living donors are preferred when available. **Maintenance dialysis** is effective for a child awaiting renal transplantation or when renal transplantation is not possible. Indications for chronic dialysis are given in Table 165.3. **Peritoneal dialysis** is done at home by the family. **Hemodialysis** is typically done three times a week at a dialysis facility.

Prognosis

Children with mild CKD (stages 1 and 2) may do well but need to be monitored for progressive loss of kidney function. Children with stages 3 and 4 CKD have a high likelihood of progressing to ESRD at some point, although the timing can vary. Children with kidney transplants generally do well, but have to take immunosuppressive medications associated with a variety of side effects, including infections, nephrotoxicity, cardiovascular complications, and increased risk for certain malignancies. Unfortunately, most transplanted kidneys fail over time but can last for >10-20 years. Children on maintenance dialysis have the highest morbidity and mortality, especially with longer time spent on dialysis. Thus the primary goal is to provide a kidney transplant for children with ESRD.

CHAPTER 166 Hypertension

DEFINITION

In children, hypertension (HTN) is defined as blood pressure (BP) greater than 95th percentile for age, gender, and height measured on at least three different occasions. The context of BP measurement (e.g., cuff size, pain, anxiety) is important. Staging of HTN is listed in Table 166.1. Hypertensive emergency is defined as severe BP elevation associated with target organ damage (encephalopathy, heart failure).

ETIOLOGY

Pediatric HTN has many causes (Table 166.2) that are either **primary** (essential) *or* **secondary. Essential HTN** is the most common cause of HTN in younger children and adolescents. Obese children are more likely to develop essential HTN. Secondary HTN should be suspected with younger age and more severely elevated BP. **Renal disease** is the most common cause of secondary HTN in children.

TABLE 166.1 Classification of Blood Pressure

BLOOD PRESSURE CATEGORY	BLOOD PRESSURE PERCENTILE (%)
Normal	<90th
Prehypertension	90th-95th*
Stage 1 hypertension	95th to (99th + 5 mm Hg)
Stage 2 hypertension	>99th + 5 mm Hg

If 90th % is greater than 120/80, use 120/80 as the lower limit.

TABLE 166.2 Causes of Hypertension

PRIMARY HYPERTENSION
Essential hypertension
Metabolic syndrome
RENAL CAUSES
Congenital anomalies (renal dysplasia, obstructive uropathy)
Structural disorders (Wilms tumor, polycystic kidney disease)
Glomerulonephritis
Acquired injury (renal scarring, acute tubular necrosis)
ENDOCRINE CAUSES
Catecholamine-secreting tumors (pheochromocytoma, neuroblastoma)
Hypercortisolism (Cushing syndrome)
Hyperaldosteronism
Hyperthyroidism
NEUROLOGICAL CAUSES
Increased sympathetic activity (stress, anxiety, pain)
Dysautonomia
Increased intracranial pressure
VASCULAR CAUSES
Coarctation of the aorta
Renal artery embolism (from umbilical artery catheter)
Renal vein thrombosis
Renal artery stenosis
Vasculitis
OTHER CAUSES
Obstructive sleep apnea
Medications, illicit drugs

CLINICAL MANIFESTATIONS

Decision-Making Algorithms
Available @ StudentConsult.com

Red Urine and Hematuria
Hypertension
Headaches
Obesity
Alkalemia

Most children with HTN have no symptoms. Signs and symptoms associated with severe HTN include encephalopathy (headache, vomiting, seizures), heart failure, stroke, and retinopathy (blurred vision, flame hemorrhage, and cotton wool spots on retinal exam). Neonatal history (low birth weight or use of umbilical artery catheter); family history of HTN, stroke, or heart disease; and dietary history (excessive salt or caffeine, drugs) are important. Additional findings that may suggest specific causes include abdominal bruit (renal artery stenosis); diminished leg pressure and weak femoral pulse (coarctation of aorta); café-au-lait spots (neurofibromatosis-associated renal artery stenosis); flank mass (hydronephrosis, Wilms tumor); tachycardia with flushing and diaphoresis (pheochromocytoma); and truncal obesity, acne, striae, and buffalo hump (Cushing syndrome). Signs of underlying kidney disease may be present.

DIAGNOSTIC STUDIES

In addition to history and physical examination, evaluation of children with confirmed HTN includes:

1. Baseline etiological assessment (urinalysis, electrolytes, blood urea nitrogen, creatinine, and renal ultrasound)
2. Focused studies based on clinical suspicion (e.g., plasma metanephrines, thyroid studies, vascular imaging)
3. Assessment for target organ damage (echocardiogram for left ventricular hypertrophy)
4. Assessment of other cardiovascular risk factors (lipids, fasting glucose, uric acid)

TREATMENT

Therapeutic lifestyle changes (diet, exercise) should be initiated for asymptomatic stage 1 HTN without target organ damage or systemic disease. Medication should be started for stage 2 or symptomatic HTN and stage 1 HTN that fails to respond to lifestyle changes over 6-12 months. Calcium channel blockers or angiotensin-converting enzyme inhibitors are the most frequently chosen first-line options in children. Angiotensin receptor blockers, β-blockers, or diuretics are also effective first-line antihypertensive agents. More than one agent may be needed. Hypertensive emergency requires prompt hospitalization and may require parenteral antihypertensive treatment with nicardipine, labetalol, esmolol, or sodium nitroprusside.

PROGNOSIS

Prognosis depends on underlying etiology and BP control. Essential HTN is usually not associated with morbidity at presentation. Left untreated, however, even asymptomatic stage 1 HTN may increase risk for cardiovascular, central nervous system, and renal morbidity in adults.

CHAPTER 167

Vesicoureteral Reflux

ETIOLOGY AND EPIDEMIOLOGY

Vesicoureteral reflux (VUR) is retrograde flow of urine from the bladder up the ureter or even into the kidney. Most VUR results from congenital incompetence of the ureterovesical (UV) junction, a structure that matures through early childhood. In a significant minority of children, structural UV abnormalities exist that never resolve. VUR may be familial; 30-40% of siblings of a child with VUR also have VUR. VUR may also be secondary to distal bladder obstruction or other urinary tract anomalies.

VUR exposes the kidney to increased hydrodynamic pressure during voiding and increases likelihood of renal infection due to incomplete emptying of the ureter and bladder (see Chapter 114). **Reflux nephropathy** refers to development and progression of renal scarring. This is a particular risk if VUR is associated with urinary tract infection (UTI) or obstruction. Although a single UTI may result in renal scarring, the incidence is higher in children with recurrent UTIs. Renal dysplasia is associated with congenital VUR. Because of increasing use of maternal-fetal ultrasonography, a number of newborns are now identified with VUR before UTI has occurred, creating opportunities for early intervention and prevention strategies. **Duplication of the ureters,** with or without associated ureterocele, may obstruct the upper collecting system. Often, the ureter draining the lower pole of a duplicated renal unit has VUR. **Neurogenic bladder** is accompanied by VUR in up to 50% of affected children. VUR may also be due to increased intravesicular pressure when the bladder outlet is obstructed from inflammation of the bladder (cystitis) or by acquired bladder obstruction.

CLINICAL MANIFESTATIONS

VUR is most often identified during radiological evaluation following a UTI (see Chapter 114). The younger the patient with UTI, the more likely VUR is present. No clinical signs reliably differentiate children with UTI with and without VUR.

DIAGNOSTIC STUDIES

An imaging study can be performed after initiation of UTI treatment with no need to wait days or weeks before performing the test. **Renal ultrasound** (RUS) is the best study to evaluate the urinary tract in children. A **voiding cystourethrogram** (VCUG) or **radionuclide cystogram** (NCG) is performed to detect urethral/bladder abnormalities and/or VUR. Recent American Academy of Pediatrics guidelines for infants with a first UTI between 2 and 24 months of age recommend a VCUG if a RUS reveals hydronephrosis, scarring, or other findings suggestive of either high-grade VUR or obstructive uropathy and in other atypical or complex clinical circumstances. VCUG should also be performed if there is a recurrence of a febrile UTI. Although VCUG provides additional anatomical detail, a NCG may detect more children with mild VUR and involves less radiation. An international grading system is useful to describe reflux (Fig. 167.1). Incidence of renal scarring in patients with low-grade VUR is low (15%) and increases with grade IV or V reflux (65%). Grade I or II VUR is likely to resolve without surgical intervention, but VUR resolves in <50% grade IV or V. **Nuclear renal scanning** best identifies renal scars.

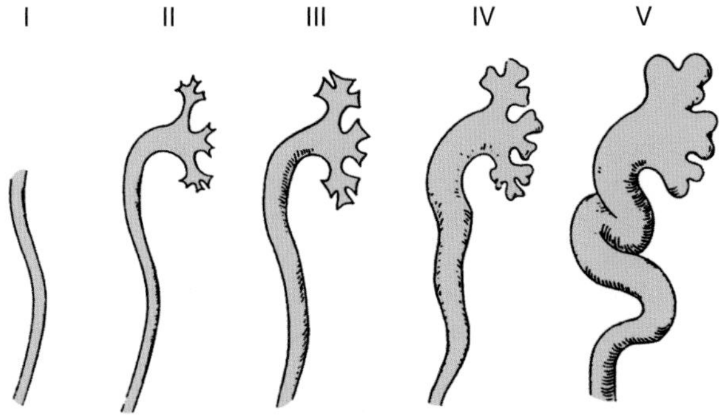

FIGURE 167.1 International classification of vesicoureteral reflux. Grade I: into a nondilated ureter; grade II: into the pelvis and calyces without dilation; grade III: mild to moderate dilation of the ureter, renal pelvis, and calyces with minimal blunting of the fornices; grade IV: moderate ureteral tortuosity and dilation of the pelvis and calyces; grade V: gross dilation of the ureter, pelvis, and calyces; loss of papillary impressions; and ureteral tortuosity. (From Wein A, Kavoussi L, Novick A, et al. *Campbell-Walsh Urology*. 9th ed. Philadelphia: Saunders; 2007.)

TREATMENT

Controversy remains about whether long-term prophylactic antibiotic therapy (trimethoprim-sulfamethoxazole or nitrofurantoin) is indicated in mild to moderate VUR. It is optional in this population and may be particularly useful in children with high-grade VUR and/or recurrent symptomatic UTI. **Complications** of reflux nephropathy are hypertension and chronic kidney disease (CKD). CKD is typically heralded by mild proteinuria and involves development of focal and segmental glomerulosclerosis as well as interstitial scarring. Indications for surgical repair of VUR are controversial, and options now include instillation of dextranomer/hyaluronic acid copolymer into the bladder wall (Deflux procedure), which appears to be a very successful, minimally invasive correction of mild to moderate VUR.

CHAPTER 168

Congenital and Developmental Abnormalities of the Urinary Tract

ETIOLOGY AND EPIDEMIOLOGY

Anomalies of the urinary tract (UT) occur in up to 4% of infants. **Bilateral renal agenesis** occurs in 1 in 4,000 births. Renal agenesis is a component of **Potter syndrome** (flat facies, clubfoot, and pulmonary hypoplasia). Any intrauterine UT disorder that results in little fetal urine and therefore little amniotic fluid can lead to Potter syndrome. **Unilateral renal agenesis** occurs in 1 in 3,000 births and is more common in infants of diabetic mothers and African Americans. It is accompanied by normal or minimally reduced renal function. This condition can also be found with vesicoureteral reflux (VUR) and other anomalies of the genital tract, ear, skeletal system, and cardiovascular system. Unilateral renal agenesis can be a component of Turner syndrome, Poland syndrome, or VACTERL association (vertebral abnormalities, anal atresia, cardiac abnormalities, tracheoesophageal fistula, renal agenesis and dysplasia, and limb defects).

Renal hypoplasia/dysplasia refers to kidneys that are congenitally small, malformed, or both. Many affected children progress to chronic kidney disease (CKD) over time because of reduced nephron number. The kidneys are often unable to fully reabsorb sodium and water, and these children often require salt and water supplementation to optimize growth.

Multicystic renal dysplasia (MCD) is due to abnormal nephron development and occurs in 1 in 4,000 births. There is minimal or no functioning renal tissue in the affected kidney; bilateral disease is lethal. There is an association with VUR in the contralateral kidney. MCD often spontaneously involutes over the first few years of life and is rarely associated with hypertension (HTN) or recurrent urinary tract infection (UTI).

Polycystic kidney diseases (PKDs) are a group of genetic disorders affecting the kidneys and other tissues. PKD may

TABLE 168.1 Site and Etiology of Urinary Tract Obstruction

SITE	ETIOLOGICAL CONDITION/DISORDER
Infundibula/pelvis	Congenital, calculi, infection, trauma/hemorrhage, tumor
Ureteropelvic junction	Congenital stenosis,* calculi, trauma/hemorrhage
Ureter	Obstructive megaureter,* ectopic ureter, ureterocele, calculi,* inflammatory bowel disease
	Retroperitoneal tumor (lymphoma), retroperitoneal fibrosis, chronic granulomatous disease
Bladder	Neurogenic dysfunction,* tumor (rhabdomyosarcoma), diverticula, ectopic ureter
Urethra	Posterior valves,* diverticula, strictures, atresia, ectopic ureter, foreign body, phimosis,* priapism

**Relatively common.*

be primary (autosomal recessive or autosomal dominant) or associated with other syndromes. Autosomal recessive PKD occurs in 1 in 10,000-40,000 children and is due to genetic defects in fibrocystin. Autosomal dominant PKD, due to defects in polycystin 1 or 2, occurs in 1 in 1,000 individuals, making it the most common inherited kidney disease. Although there is some overlap clinically, the two conditions differ morphologically. Both may appear in infancy or in older children. Renal cysts also are observed in other inherited disorders, such as von Hippel–Lindau syndrome, tuberous sclerosis, and Bardet-Biedl syndrome.

Urinary tract obstruction can occur at any anatomical level of the genitourinary system (Table 168.1). Early in gestation, severe obstruction results in renal dysplasia. Ureteral obstruction later in fetal life or after birth results in dilation of the ureter and collecting system, often with subsequent renal parenchymal alterations. An obstructed UT is susceptible to infections, which may worsen renal injury. **Posterior urethral valves** are the most common cause of **bladder outlet obstruction** in males, present in 1 in 50,000 boys. Parents may note a poor urine stream in affected children. The valves are sail-shaped membranes that arise from the verumontanum and attach to the urethral wall. The prostatic urethra becomes dilated, VUR may be present, and hypertrophied detrusor muscle develops. Renal dilation varies in severity. Renal dysplasia is often present. Severe obstruction may be associated with oligohydramnios, resulting in lethal pulmonary hypoplasia. Intrauterine renal pelvis rupture produces **urinary ascites,** a common cause of ascites in the newborn period.

CLINICAL MANIFESTATIONS

Decision-Making Algorithms
Available @ StudentConsult.com

Red Urine and Hematuria
Hyponatremia

Bilateral renal agenesis results in insufficient lung development and Potter syndrome. Respiratory distress is severe, pneumothoraces can occur, and severe pulmonary hypoplasia is fatal. Unilateral renal agenesis may be asymptomatic because the nonaffected kidney undergoes compensatory growth and provides normal renal function.

Autosomal recessive PKD is characterized by marked bilateral renal enlargement. Interstitial fibrosis and tubular atrophy progress over time. Kidney failure usually occurs in early childhood. **Hepatic fibrosis** is present and may lead to portal HTN. Bile duct ectasia and biliary dysgenesis occur. Many affected infants display flank masses, hepatomegaly, pneumothorax, proteinuria, and/or hematuria.

Autosomal dominant PKD typically presents in middle adulthood but may present in infancy or childhood. Infants may have a clinical picture similar to autosomal recessive PKD, but older children typically show a pattern similar to that of adults, with large isolated cysts developing over time. The defect may occur anywhere along the nephron unit. Hepatic cysts are often present, and pancreatic, splenic, and ovarian cysts can also develop. **Cerebral aneurysms** may develop, and risk of cerebral hemorrhage depends on size, blood pressure, and family history of intracranial hemorrhage.

UT obstruction may be silent but is usually discovered during prenatal ultrasound or with UTI or flank mass in early childhood. In a newborn, the most common type of abdominal mass is renal (most commonly **ureteropelvic junction obstruction**).

DIAGNOSTIC IMAGING

Renal ultrasound (RUS) and **radionuclide renography** (usually with diuretic administered) are the standard tests for diagnosis of UT obstruction. RUS can identify renal agenesis, hypoplasia, dysplasia, cysts, and/or UT dilation. Obstruction may be suggested, but a dilated UT may also result from VUR, ureteral hypoplasia, or neurogenic bladder. A **voiding cystourethrogram** (VCUG) is usually part of the evaluation. Many boys with posterior urethral valves are identified by prenatal ultrasound. Postnatally, the diagnosis and extent of renal damage are established by RUS and VCUG.

TREATMENT

Infants and children with bilateral dysplasia often require additional sodium and water due to renal wasting. With MCD, surgical kidney removal is rarely indicated unless severe HTN or recurrent UTI occurs.

Treatment of HTN can prolong maintenance of renal function. General therapy of CKD (see Chapter 165) can improve growth and development.

UT obstruction often requires drainage or surgical correction. Treatment of posterior urethral valve consists of either primary valve ablation or diversion (usually via vesicostomy) if ablation is not possible. Ectopic ureters are frequently obstructed; when this happens, surgical intervention is required.

Children with neurogenic bladder are prone to UTI and renal impairment from poor urine emptying. Clean intermittent catheterization or a urinary diversion can minimize these complications.

CHAPTER 169

Other Urinary Tract and Genital Disorders*

URINARY TRACT STONES

Etiology

Urinary tract calculi are called **nephrolithiasis** or **urolithiasis.** Primary bladder stones can be seen with recurrent urinary tract infections (UTIs), neurogenic bladder or bladder surgery (sutures serve as a nidus), and intestinal bladder augmentation. Renal stones can result from obstructive abnormalities or an underlying metabolic predisposition. In industrialized societies, most stones (>90%) in children arise in the urinary tract (UT) and become symptomatic with passage or if lodged (commonly at the ureteropelvic junction or the ureterovesical junction). Metabolic causes include idiopathic familial hypercalciuria (IHC), hyperoxaluria, uric acid disorders, distal renal tubular acidosis, cystinuria, hypercalcemic hypercalciuria, and primary hyperparathyroidism. Some children with UT abnormalities and stones have a concomitant metabolic predisposition.

Clinical Manifestations

Decision-Making Algorithm
Available @ StudentConsult.com
Red Urine and Hematuria

Acute obstruction of urine flow is the cause of renal colic, a severe sharp intermittent pain in the flank or lower abdomen often radiating to the groin. Vomiting, distress, and inability to relieve pain with position changes are characteristic. In younger children, fussiness and vomiting may be the only symptoms. Hematuria may be gross or microscopic and typically clears rapidly with passage of gravel or stone material.

Diagnostic Studies

Renal ultrasound may identify stones in the kidney but can easily miss UT stones. Computed tomography (CT), particularly a helical CT, can identify stones throughout the UT, but stones can be obscured by oral or intravenous contrast material. Etiological diagnosis is facilitated when stone material can be obtained and sent for analysis. Spot or 24-hour urine studies for mineral and electrolyte determinations, obtained on a typical diet for the child, are important to characterize any underlying metabolic predisposition and are valuable even when a stone is available for analysis.

Treatment

Acute treatment of urinary calculi consists of hydration and analgesia. Chronic treatment for all types of metabolic stones involves vigorous fluid intake, usually twice the maintenance volume. Infection-related stones require treatment of infection and, often, removal of the stone as well as correction of any predisposing anatomical abnormality. Specific metabolic conditions require specific treatments; for IHC, normal calcium intake with low sodium and low oxalate intake is prescribed. For some children with IHC, potassium citrate or thiazides are required to minimize stone recurrence. Tamsulosin has been increasingly used with success in older children with distal ureteral stones to promote passage. Lithotripsy or surgery by a pediatric urologist may be required for children with large, infected, or obstructing stones.

VOIDING DYSFUNCTION

Etiology

Voiding difficulties are frequent in preschool age children due to delay in maturation of bladder and micturition pathways. Normal micturition and continence rely on structural UT integrity, neurological maturation, and coordination between somatic and autonomic nervous system units, including central nervous system, spinal cord pathways, bladder/urinary sphincter pathways, and the autonomic system. Daytime continence is usually achieved before nighttime continence. Most children are dry, day and night, by 4-5 years of age. Nocturnal enuresis is the involuntary loss of urine during sleep. Children with primary enuresis have never had a prolonged (usually >3 months) span of nighttime continence. Up to 10% of 5-year-old children have primary enuresis with 15% spontaneous resolution per year. Boys are affected more than girls with increased incidence in families (40% at 6 years of age if one affected parent, 70% if two affected parents). Secondary enuresis involves loss of nighttime control after an extended period of dryness and generally requires evaluation to uncover the cause.

Clinical Manifestations

Dysfunctional voiding (DV) may manifest as incontinence, frequency, urgency, hesitancy, dysuria, lower abdominal pain, or recurrent UTI. Symptoms may vary over time and be associated with obvious neurological problems (spinal cord injury, encephalitis), constipation, and/or behavioral problems. DV symptoms may vary, depending on recent UTI or changes in family or school life/stressors. The majority of children with DV are anatomically, neurologically, and psychologically normal.

Diagnostic Studies

Evaluation for DV may be performed at any age, but isolated urinary incontinence in an otherwise normal child is not usually evaluated until 5 years of age. Urinalysis and urine culture should be done to exclude occult infection and renal disease. Children with daytime incontinence should undergo renal/bladder ultrasound to exclude structural abnormalities. Urodynamic evaluation is typically reserved for children with suspicion of neurogenic bladder or known neurological etiology.

Treatment

For children with recurrent UTI, prophylactic antibiotics may be useful. Timed voiding and anticholinergic medications are

*We gratefully acknowledge the invaluable contributions of Rama Jayanthi, MD, Pediatric Urology, Nationwide Children's Hospital, Columbus, Ohio.

used to treat bladder hyperactivity and sensory defects. More complicated treatment regimens include biofeedback, α-blockers, and intermittent catheterization. For children with simple primary enuresis, the bed-wetting alarm provides safe and effective resolution of the problem for greater than 70% of affected children; medical therapy with anticholinergics, imipramine, or desmopressin may also be useful in selected children.

DISORDERS OF THE PENIS

Etiology

Hypospadias occurs in ~1 in 500 newborn infants. In this condition, the urethral folds fail to fuse completely over the urethral groove, leaving the urethral meatus located ventrally and proximally to its normal position. The ventral foreskin is also lacking, and the dorsal portion gives the appearance of a hood. Severe hypospadias with undescended testes is a form of ambiguous genitalia. Etiologies include congenital adrenal hyperplasia with masculinization of females or androgen insensitivity. UT anomalies are uncommon in association with hypospadias. Hypospadias may occur alone, but in severe cases can be associated with a **chordee** (a fixed ventral curvature of the penile shaft). Rarely, when the urethra opens onto the perineum, the chordee is extreme, and the scrotum is bifid and sometimes extends to the dorsal base of the penis.

In 90% of uncircumcised males, the foreskin should be retractable by adolescence. Before this age, the prepuce may normally be tight and does not need treatment. After this age, the inability to retract the prepuce is termed **phimosis.** The condition may be congenital or the result of inflammation. **Paraphimosis** occurs when the prepuce has been retracted behind the coronal sulcus, cannot resume its normal position, and causes swelling of the glans or pain.

Clinical Manifestations and Treatment

The meatal opening in **hypospadias** may be located anteriorly (on the glans, coronal, or distal third of the shaft); on the middle third of the shaft; or posteriorly (near the scrotum). Testes are undescended in 10% of boys with hypospadias. Inguinal hernias are common. Males with hypospadias should not be circumcised, particularly if the meatus is proximal to the glans, as the foreskin may be necessary for later repair. Most pediatric urologists repair hypospadias before the patient is 18 months old.

Phimosis is rarely symptomatic. Parents should be reassured that loosening of the prepuce usually occurs during puberty. Treatment, if needed, is topical steroids. If the narrowing is severe, gentle stretching may be useful. Circumcision is reserved for the most severe cases. **Paraphimosis** with venous stasis and edema leads to severe pain. When paraphimosis is discovered early, reduction of the foreskin may be possible with lubrication. In some cases, emergent circumcision is needed.

DISORDERS AND ABNORMALITIES OF THE SCROTUM AND ITS CONTENTS

Etiology

Undescended testes (cryptorchidism) are found in ~1% of boys after 1 year of age. It is more common in full-term newborns (3.4%) than in older children. In neonates, cryptorchidism is more common with shorter gestation (20% in 2,000-2,500-g infants and 100% in <900-g infants). Cryptorchidism is bilateral in 30% of cases. Spontaneous testicular descent does not tend to occur after 1 year of age, but failure to find one or both testes in the scrotum does not indicate undescended testicles. **Retractile testes, absent testes**, and **ectopic testes** may resemble cryptorchidism in presentation.

Clinical Manifestations

Decision-Making Algorithms
Available @ StudentConsult.com

Scrotal Pain
Scrotal Swelling (Painless)

A history of maternal drug use (steroids) and family history are important in the evaluation of a child for apparent cryptorchidism. Whether the testis was ever noted in the scrotum should be asked. The true undescended testis is found along the normal embryological path of descent, usually in the presence of a patent processus vaginalis. An undescended testis is often associated with an inguinal hernia; it is also subject to **torsion.** There is a high incidence of infertility in adulthood. When bilateral and untreated, infertility is uniform. There is increased malignancy risk (five times the normal rate) with undescended testis, usually presenting between the ages of 20 and 30. The risk is greater in untreated males or those with surgical correction during or after puberty.

Retractile testes are normal testes that retract into the inguinal canal from an exaggerated cremasteric reflex. The diagnosis of retractile testes is likely if testes are palpable in the newborn period but not at later examination. Frequently parents describe seeing their son's testes in his scrotum when he is in the bath and seeing one or both "disappear" when he gets cold.

Complications

Decision-Making Algorithm
Available @ StudentConsult.com

Scrotal Pain

Torsion of the testis is an emergency requiring prompt diagnosis and treatment to save the affected testis. Torsion accounts for 40% of cases of acute scrotal pain and swelling and is the major cause of the acute scrotum in boys less than 6 years of age. It is thought to arise from abnormal fixation of the testis to the scrotum. On examination, the testicle is swollen and tender, and the cremasteric reflex is absent. The absence of blood flow on nuclear scan or Doppler ultrasound is consistent with torsion.

The differential diagnosis of testicular pain includes trauma, an incarcerated hernia, and torsion of the testicular epididymal appendix. Torsion of the appendix testis is associated with point tenderness over the lesion and minimal swelling. In adolescents, the differential diagnosis of testicular torsion also must include **epididymitis,** the most common cause of acute scrotal pain and swelling in older adolescents. Diagnosis is aided by an antecedent history of sexual activity or UTI. Testicular torsion must be considered as the principal diagnosis when severe acute testicular pain is present.

Treatment

The undescended testis is usually histologically normal at birth. Atrophy and dysplasia are found after the first year of life. Some boys have congenital dysplasia in the contralateral descended testis. Surgical correction at an early age results in greater chance of adult fertility. Administration of human chorionic gonadotropin causes testosterone release from functioning testes and may result in descent of retractile testes.

Orchidopexy is usually done in the second year of life. Most extraabdominal testes can be brought into the scrotum with correction of the associated hernia. If the testis is not palpable, ultrasound or magnetic resonance imaging may determine its location. The closer the testis is to the internal inguinal ring, the better the chance of successful orchidopexy.

Surgical correction of testicular torsion is called *detorsion and fixation of the testis.* If performed within 6 hours of torsion, there is >90% chance of testicular salvage. The contralateral testis usually is fixed to the scrotum to prevent possible torsion. If torsion of the appendix is found, the necrotic tissue is removed.

Suggested Readings

Andreoli SP. Acute kidney injury in children. *Pediatr Nephrol.* 2009;24:253–263.

Ariceta G. Clinical practice: proteinuria. *Eur J Pediatr.* 2011;170:15–20.

Brady TM. Hypertension. *Pediatr Rev.* 2012;33:541–552.

Greenbaum LA, Benndorf R, Smoyer WE. Childhood nephrotic syndrome—current and future therapies. *Nat Rev Nephrol.* 2012;8:445–458.

Kaspar CD, Bholah R, Bunchman TE. A review of pediatric chronic kidney disease. *Blood Purif.* 2016;41:211–217.

Massengill SF. Hematuria. *Pediatr Rev.* 2008;29:342–348.

Schwartz GJ, Munoz A, Schneider MF, et al. New equation to estimate GFR in children with CKD. *J Am Soc Nephrol.* 2009;20:629–637.

Subcommittee on Urinary Tract Infection, Steering Committee on Quality Improvement and Management, Roberts KB. Urinary tract infection: clinical practice guideline for the diagnosis and management of the initial UTI in febrile infants and children 2 to 24 months. *Pediatrics.* 2011;128:595–610.

Valentini RP, Lakshmanan Y. Nephrolithiasis in children. *Adv Chronic Kidney Dis.* 2011;18:370–375.

PEARLS FOR PRACTITIONERS

CHAPTER 161

Nephrology and Urology Assessment

- Fetal urine production contributes to amniotic fluid volume, lung maturation, and somatic development; reduced (oligohydramnios) or increased amniotic fluid volume (polyhydramnios) may be a sign of a congenital renal disorder.
- Glomerular filtration rate (GFR) is normally low in newborns infants (~25 mL/min/1.73 m^2), and it takes up to 2 years of age to develop adult levels of GFR (100-120 mL/min/1.73 m^2).
- The proximal tubule (PT) is responsible for most water and electrolyte reabsorption; this nephron portion consumes >90 % of renal O_2 and suffers most severe injury with anoxic-ischemic kidney injury (acute tubular necrosis); the inability of PT to maximally reabsorb bicarbonate leads to proximal renal tubular acidosis.
- The distal tubule collecting duct (CD) is the primary site of antidiuretic hormone (vasopressin) response, which leads to urine concentration; CD sodium-potassium and sodium-hydrogen exchange CD is regulated by aldosterone; abnormalities in CD active hydrogen ion secretion lead to distal and/or hyperkalemic renal tubular acidosis.
- The revised Schwartz formula [GFR = 0.413 × Ht (cm)/serum Cr (mg/dL)] is used to estimate GFR in children.

CHAPTER 162

Nephrotic Syndrome and Proteinuria

- Urine protein is best quantified by a spot urine Pr/Cr, with normal <0.2 and heavy (nephrotic range) proteinuria >2.0; U Pr/Cr 0.2-2.0 indicates mild to moderate proteinuria.
- Nephrotic syndrome (NS) is characterized by persistent heavy proteinuria (mainly albuminuria; >2 g/m^2/24 hr); hypoproteinemia (serum albumin <3.0 g/dL); hypercholesterolemia (>250 mg/dL); and edema.
- Primary forms of NS include minimal change nephrotic syndrome (MCNS—most common form of childhood NS; >80% of those with NS <7 years old having MCNS), focal glomerulosclerosis (FSGS), membranoproliferative glomerulonephritis (MPGN), and membranous glomerulonephritis.
- For the child with likely MCNS (presentation between 2 and 12 years of age, no signs of systemic disorder, minimal hematuria, normal GFR, and normal C_3), a corticosteroid trial is warranted.
- Complications of childhood NS include poor growth, hypertension, episodes of acute kidney injury (AKI), serious bacterial infections, episodes of thrombi and thromboemboli, and accelerated atherosclerotic disease.

CHAPTER 163

Glomerulonephritis and Hematuria

- Glomerulonephritis (GN) in children presents with some, but not necessarily all, of the cardinal features of GN: hematuria, proteinuria, decreased renal function, hypertension, oliguria and/or edema; poststreptococcal GN is most common form of acute GN while immunoglobulin (Ig)A nephropathy is most common form of chronic GN in children.
- Hypocomplementemia (low C_3) characterizes acute poststreptococcal, postinfectious GN, MPGN, and lupus nephritis; all other causes of GN have normal C_3.

CHAPTER 164

Hemolytic Uremic Syndrome

- Hemolytic uremic syndrome (HUS) is characterized by triad of microangiopathic hemolytic anemia, thrombocytopenia, and renal injury and is an important cause of AKI in children, typically occurring in children <5 years of age; the most common type of HUS is associated with a prodromal diarrheal illness (D + HUS) due to contamination of meat, fruit, vegetables, or water with verotoxin (VT)-producing *Escherichia coli* (most commonly *E. coli* O157:H7).
- HUS is a self-limited disorder that can be asymptomatic or involve full renal failure requiring dialysis; 95% of patients recover, although 20% of these patients have chronic sequelae such as hypertension or chronic kidney disease; atypical HUS secondary to certain pneumococcal infections or complement abnormalities can be recurrent and more severe than D + HUS.

CHAPTER 165

Acute and Chronic Renal Failure

- AKI is an abrupt decrease in GFR and tubular function that may lead to decreased excretion of waste products and disturbance in fluid and electrolyte homeostasis; AKI may be oliguric (<1 mL/kg/hr in neonates and infants, <0.5 mL/kg/hr in children) or nonoliguric, and can be classified as prerenal (renal hypoperfusion), intrinsic renal (tubular, glomerular, or vascular injury), or postrenal (urinary tract obstruction).
- Indications for acute dialysis in children include volume overload, metabolic acidosis, electrolyte abnormalities, severe uremia, certain ingestions and metabolic disorders (e.g., hyperammonemia); indications for chronic dialysis include all of the above as well as poor growth due to CKD and CKD Stage 5 due to its significant risks of serious complications.
- Complications of CKD in children include poor growth, anemia, CKD-mineral bone disorder (bone deformities, fractures), cardiovascular issues (hypertension, left ventricular hypertrophy), and electrolyte disturbances (Na, K, HCO_3, Ca, P).

CHAPTER 166

Hypertension

- Hypertension in children (preadolescent and adolescent) is most frequently essential (primary) with secondary forms less common; the most common secondary cause in children is due to renal disease.
- In addition to history and physical examination, evaluation of children with confirmed HTN includes (1) baseline studies (urinalysis, electrolytes, blood urea nitrogen, creatinine, and renal ultrasound); (2) focused studies based on clinical suspicion (e.g., plasma metanephrines, thyroid studies, vascular imaging); (3) assessment for target organ damage (echocardiogram); and assessment of cardiovascular risk factors (lipids, fasting glucose, uric acid).

CHAPTER 167

Vesicoureteral Reflux

- Vesicoureteral reflux (VUR) results from congenital incompetence of the ureterovesical (UV) junction, a structure that often, but not always, matures through early childhood; VUR may be familial (seen in 30-40% of siblings of child) or may be secondary to distal bladder obstruction or other urinary tract anomalies.
- Reflux nephropathy refers to development and progression of renal scarring with VUR; it is more common when VUR is associated with UTI or obstruction; although a single UTI may result in renal scarring, the incidence is higher in children with recurrent UTIs; renal dysplasia is also associated with congenital VUR.

CHAPTER 168

Congenital and Developmental Abnormalities of the Urinary Tract

- Anomalies of the urinary tract (UT) occur in up to 4% of infants and include bilateral and unilateral renal agenesis, renal hypoplasia/dysplasia, multicystic renal dysplasia, polycystic kidney diseases (PKD—autosomal recessive PKD, autosomal dominant PKD and PKD associated with syndromes), and UT obstruction disorders (posterior urethral valves, ureterocele), which vary greatly in severity and are often diagnosed through prenatal ultrasound examinations.

CHAPTER 169

Other Urinary Tract and Genital Disorders

- In childhood nephrolithiasis, primary bladder stones are seen with recurrent urinary tract infections (UTIs), neurogenic bladder or bladder surgery (sutures as nidus), and intestinal bladder augmentation while renal stones result from obstruction or an underlying metabolic predisposition; metabolic causes include idiopathic familial hypercalciuria (IHC), hyperoxaluria, uric acid disorders, distal renal tubular acidosis, cystinuria, hypercalcemic hypercalciuria, and primary hyperparathyroidism.
- In children daytime continence is usually achieved before nighttime; most children are dry, day and night, by 4-5 years of age; nocturnal enuresis is involuntary loss of urine during sleep; primary enuresis = never had >3 month span of nighttime continence (up to 10% of 5-year-olds; 15% spontaneous resolution/year; boys > girls; increased incidence in families); secondary enuresis involves loss of nighttime control after period of dryness and requires evaluation for cause.

- Dysfunctional voiding (DV) may manifest as incontinence, frequency, urgency, hesitancy, dysuria, lower abdominal pain, or recurrent UTI; most children with DV are anatomically, neurologically, and psychologically normal; for children with recurrent UTI, prophylactic antibiotics may be useful; for children with simple primary enuresis, the bed-wetting alarm provides safe and effective resolution for >70% of affected children; medical therapy with anticholinergics, imipramine, or desmopressin may also be useful in selected children.

ENDOCRINOLOGY

Paola Palma Sisto | MaryKathleen Heneghan

CHAPTER 170

Endocrinology Assessment

The endocrine system regulates vital body functions by means of hormonal messengers. **Hormones** are defined as circulating messengers, with action at a distance from the organ **(gland)** of origin of the hormone. Hormones can be regulated by nerve cells; endocrine agents can serve as neural messengers. There is also a relationship between the endocrine system and the immune system; autoantibodies may cause an organ to produce an excess or deficiency of a hormone. Manifestations of an endocrine disorder are related to the response of the peripheral tissue to a hormone excess or deficiency.

Hormone action also may be **paracrine** (acting on adjacent neighboring cells to the cell of origin of the hormone) or **autocrine** (acting on the cell of origin of the hormone itself); agents acting in these ways are called *factors* rather than hormones (Fig. 170.1). Hormones generally are regulated in a feedback loop so that the production of a hormone is linked to its effect or its circulating concentration. Endocrine disorders generally manifest from one of four ways:

1. By **excess hormone:** In Cushing syndrome, there is an excess of glucocorticoid present; if the excess is secondary to autonomous glucocorticoid secretion by the adrenal gland, the trophic hormone adrenocorticotropic hormone (ACTH) is suppressed.
2. By **deficient hormone:** In glucocorticoid deficiency, the level of cortisol is inadequate; if the deficiency is at the adrenal gland, the trophic hormone is elevated (ACTH).
3. By an abnormal **response of end-organ** to hormone: In pseudohypoparathyroidism, defects in the gene *(GNAS1)* encoding the alpha subunit of the stimulatory G protein (Gsa) is manifested by elevated parathyroid hormone (PTH) levels in the face of deficient PTH function (PTH resistance).
4. By **gland enlargement** that may have effects as a result of size rather than function: With a large nonfunctioning pituitary adenoma, abnormal visual fields and other neurological signs and symptoms result even though no hormone is produced by the tumor.

Peptide hormones act through specific cell membrane receptors; when the hormone is attached to the receptor, the complex triggers various intracellular second messengers that cause the biological effects. Peptide hormone receptor number and avidity may be regulated by hormones. **Steroid hormones** exert their effects by attachment to intranuclear receptors, and the hormone-receptor complex translocates to the nucleus, where it binds with DNA and leads to further gene activation.

The interpretation of serum hormone levels must be related to their controlling factors. For example, a given value of parathyroid hormone may be normal in a eucalcemic patient but inadequate in a hypocalcemic patient with partial hypoparathyroidism or excessive in a hypercalcemic patient with hyperparathyroidism.

HYPOTHALAMIC-PITUITARY AXIS

The **hypothalamus** controls many endocrine systems, either directly or through the pituitary gland. Higher central nervous system (CNS) centers control the hypothalamus. Hypothalamic releasing or inhibiting factors travel through capillaries of the pituitary portal system to control the anterior pituitary gland, regulating the hormones specific for the factor (Fig. 170.2). The pituitary hormones enter the peripheral circulation and exert their effects on target glands, which produce other hormones that feed back to suppress their controlling hypothalamic and pituitary hormones. Insulin-like growth factor-1 (IGF-1), growth hormone (GH), cortisol, sex steroids, and thyroxine (T_4) all feedback on the hypothalamic-pituitary system. Prolactin is the only pituitary hormone that is suppressed by a hypothalamic factor, dopamine. The hypothalamus is also the location of vasopressin-secreting axons that either terminate in the posterior pituitary gland and exert their effect via vasopressin secretion from this area or terminate in the

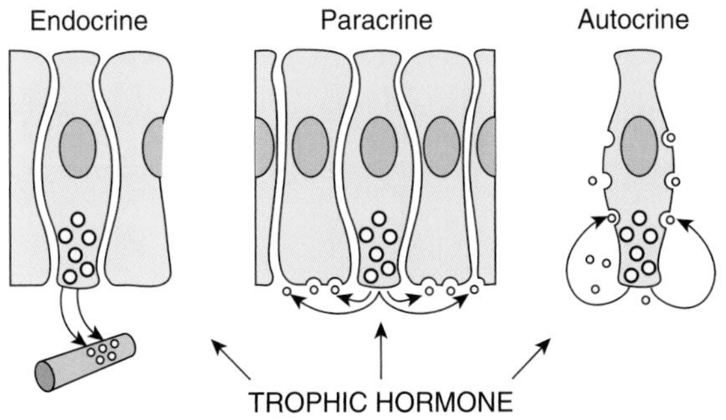

FIGURE 170.1 Schematic representation of mechanisms of action of hormones and growth factors. Although traditional hormones are formed in endocrine glands and transported to distant sites of action through the bloodstream (endocrine mechanism), peptide growth factors may be produced locally by the target cells themselves (autocrine modality of action) or by neighboring cells (paracrine action). (From Wilson JD, Foster DW, eds. *Williams Textbook of Endocrinology*. 8th ed. Philadelphia: WB Saunders; 1992:1007.)

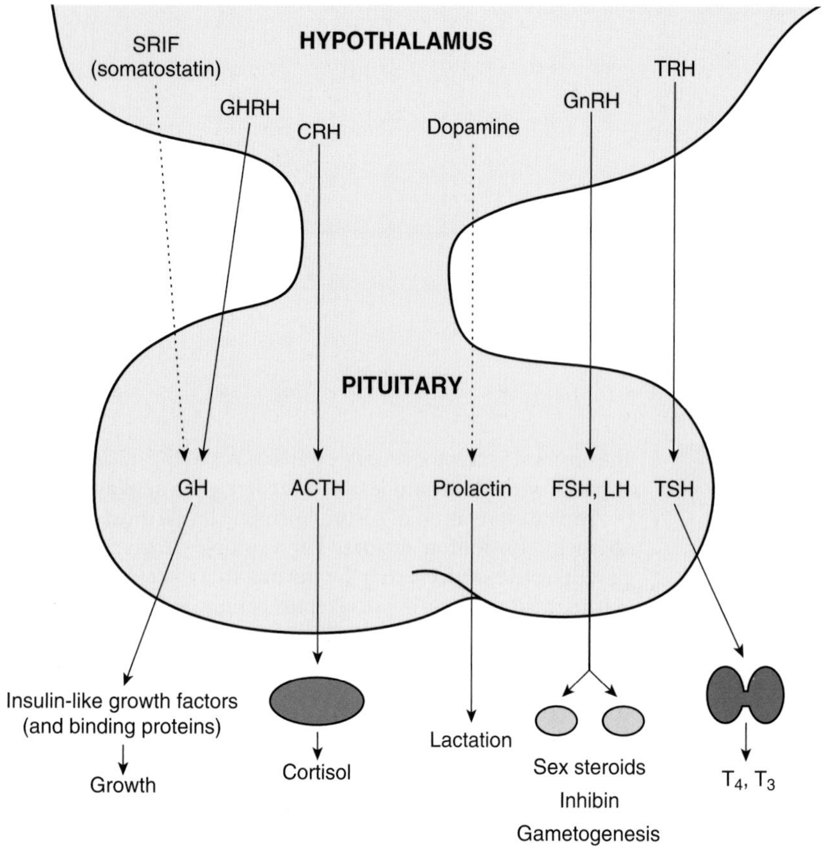

FIGURE 170.2 Hormonal influences of the hypothalamus and pituitary gland. Solid line represents stimulatory influence; dotted line represents inhibitory influence. *ACTH*, Adrenocorticotropic hormone; *CRH*, corticotropin-releasing hormone or CRF; *FSH*, follicle-stimulating hormone; *GH*, growth hormone; *GHRH*, GH-releasing hormone or GRF; *GnRH*, gonadotropin-releasing hormone or luteinizing hormone releasing factor, LRF or LHRH; *LH*, luteinizing hormone; *SRIF*, somatotropin release-inhibiting factor, somatostatin or SS; *TRH*, thyrotropin-releasing hormone or TRF; *TSH*, thyroid-stimulating hormone; *T3*, triiodothyronine; *T4*, thyroxine.

TABLE **170.1** Diagnostic Evaluation for Hypopituitarism

MANIFESTATION	CAUSE	TESTS*
Growth failure, hypothyroidism, or both	GH deficiency, TRH/TSH deficiency, or both	Provocative GH tests, free T_4, bone age, IGF-1, IGF-BP3
Hypoglycemia	GH deficiency, ACTH insufficiency, or both	Provocative GH tests, test of ACTH secretion, IGF-1, IGFBP3
Micropenis, pubertal delay or arrest	Hypogonadotropic hypogonadism with or without GH deficiency	Sex steroids (E_2, testosterone), basal LH and FSH (analyzed by ultrasensitive assays) or after LHRH administration, provocative GH tests, IGF-1, IGFBP3
Polyuria, polydipsia	ADH deficiency	Urine analysis (specific gravity), serum electrolytes, urine and serum osmolality, water deprivation test

**Each patient with hypopituitarism should have CNS MRI as part of evaluation to determine the etiology of the condition.*
ACTH, Adrenocorticotropic hormone; *ADH*, Antidiuretic hormone; *CNS*, central nervous system; E_2, estradiol; *FSH*, follicle-stimulating hormone; *GH*, growth hormone; *GnRH*, gonadotropin-releasing hormone; *IGF-1*, insulin-like growth factor-1; *IGF-BP3*, insulin-like growth factor-binding protein 3; *LH*, luteinizing hormone; *LHRH*, luteinizing hormone releasing hormone; *MRI*, magnetic resonance imaging; *TRH*, thyrotropin-releasing hormone; *TSH*, thyroid-stimulating hormone; T_4, thyroxine.

mediobasal hypothalamus, from which they can exert effects on water balance, even in the absence of the posterior pituitary gland.

The **assessment** of pituitary function may be determined by measuring some of the specific pituitary hormone in the basal state; other assessments require the measurement after stimulation. Indirect assessment of pituitary function can be obtained by measuring serum concentrations of the target gland hormones (Table 170.1). Several tests of pituitary function are listed in Table 170.2.

DISORDERS OF THE HYPOTHALAMIC-PITUITARY AXIS

Decision-Making Algorithms
Available @ StudentConsult.com

Visual Impairment and Leukocoria
Amenorrhea
Pubertal Delay
Polyuria

TABLE 170.2 Anterior Pituitary Hormone Function Testing

RANDOM HORMONE MEASUREMENTS	PROVOCATIVE OR OTHER TESTS	TARGET HORMONE MEASUREMENT
GH (not useful as a random determination except in newborns, and in GH resistance or in pituitary gigantism)	Arginine (a weak stimulus) L-Dopa (useful clinically) Insulin-induced hypoglycemia (a dangerous but accurate test) Clonidine (useful clinically) GHRH 12- to 24-hr integrated GH levels (of questionable utility)	IGF-1, IGF-BP3 (affected by malnutrition as well as GH excess)
ACTH (early morning sample useful only if in high-normal range)	Cortisol after insulin-induced hypoglycemia (a dangerous but accurate test)	8 A.M. cortisol
		24-hr urinary free cortisol
	ACTH stimulation test (may differentiate ACTH deficiency from primary adrenal insufficiency)	
TSH*	TRH (not commonly performed)	FT_4
LH, FSH*	GnRH (difficult to interpret in prepubertal subjects)	Testosterone/estradiol
Prolactin (elevated in hypothalamic disease and decreased in pituitary disease)	TRH (not commonly performed)	None

New supersensitive assays allow determination of abnormally low values found in hypopituitarism.
ACTH, Adrenocorticotropic hormone; *CRH,* corticotropin-releasing hormone; *FSH,* follicle-stimulating hormone; *FT_4,* free thyroxine; *GH,* growth hormone; *GnRH,* gonadotropin-releasing hormone; *GHRH,* growth hormone-releasing hormone; *IGF-1,* insulin-like growth factor-1; *IGF-BP3,* insulin-like growth factor-binding protein 3; *L-dopa,* L-dihydroxyphenylalanine; *LH,* luteinizing hormone; *TRH,* thyrotropin-releasing hormone; *TSH,* thyroid-stimulating hormone.

Hypothalamic deficiency leads to a decrease in most pituitary hormone secretions but may lead to an increase in prolactin secretion. Destructive lesions of the pituitary gland or hypothalamus are more common in childhood than increased pituitary secretion of various hormones. A **craniopharyngioma,** a tumor of the Rathke pouch, may descend into the sella turcica, causing erosion of the bone and destruction of pituitary and hypothalamic tissue. **Acquired hypopituitarism** also may result from pituitary infections; from infiltration (Langerhans cell histiocytosis [histiocytosis X], lymphoma, and sarcoidosis); after radiation therapy or trauma to the CNS; and as a consequence of autoimmunity against the pituitary gland.

Congenital hypopituitarism can be caused by the absence of hypothalamic-releasing factors. Without hypothalamic stimulation, the pituitary gland does not release its hormones. Congenital defects associated with hypopituitarism range from **holoprosencephaly** (cyclopia, cebocephaly, orbital hypotelorism) to cleft palate (6% of cases of cleft palate are associated with GH deficiency). **Optic nerve hypoplasia,** formerly known as septooptic dysplasia, may result in significant visual impairment with pendular ("roving") nystagmus (inability to focus on a target) in addition to varying degrees of hypopituitarism. The magnetic resonance imaging (MRI) findings of congenital hypopituitarism may include an ectopic posterior pituitary gland *bright spot,* the appearance of a *pituitary stalk transection,* and/or small pituitary gland.

CHAPTER 171
Diabetes Mellitus

Diabetes mellitus (DM) is characterized by hyperglycemia and glycosuria and is an end-point of a few disease processes (Table 171.1). The most common type occurring in childhood is type 1 DM (T1D), which is caused by autoimmune destruction of the insulin-producing β cells (islets) of the pancreas, leading to permanent insulin deficiency. Type 2 DM (T2D) results from insulin resistance and relative insulin deficiency usually in the context of exogenous obesity. The incidence of T1D and T2D in the United States is increasing. Less common types of diabetes result from genetic defects of the insulin receptor or inherited abnormalities in sensing of ambient glucose concentration by pancreatic β cells (see Table 171.1).

DEFINITION

A **diagnosis** of DM is made based on four glucose abnormalities that may need to be confirmed by repeat testing: (1) Fasting serum glucose concentration ≥126 mg/dL, (2) a random venous plasma glucose ≥200 mg/dL with symptoms of hyperglycemia, (3) an abnormal oral glucose tolerance test (OGTT) with a 2-hour postprandial serum glucose concentration ≥200 mg/dL, and (4) a HgbA1c ≥6.5%.

A patient is considered to have **impaired fasting glucose** if fasting serum glucose concentration is 100-125 mg/dL or **impaired glucose tolerance** if 2-hour plasma glucose following an OGTT is 140-199 mg/dL. Sporadic hyperglycemia can occur in children, usually in the setting of an intercurrent illness. When the hyperglycemic episode is clearly related to an illness or other physiological stress, the probability of incipient diabetes is small (<5%).

TYPE 1 DIABETES MELLITUS

Etiology

T1D results from the autoimmune destruction of insulin-producing β cells (islets) of the pancreas. In addition to the presence of diabetes susceptibility genes, an unknown environmental insult presumably triggers the autoimmune process. A variety of studies have produced conflicting data regarding a host of environmental factors. These include cow's milk feeding at an early age, viral infectious agents (coxsackie virus, cytomegalovirus, mumps, rubella), vitamin D deficiency, and perinatal factors. T1D is thought to be primarily a T cell–mediated disease.

Antibodies to islet cell antigens may be seen months to years before the onset of β cell dysfunction (Fig. 171.1). These include islet cell antibodies, insulin autoantibodies, antibodies to tyrosine phosphatase IA-2, antibodies to glutamic acid decarboxylase, and others. The risk for diabetes increases with the number of antibodies detected in the serum. In individuals with only one detectable antibody, the risk is only 10-15% while in individuals with three or more antibodies the risk is 55-90%. When 80-90% of the β cell mass has been destroyed, the remaining β cell mass is insufficient to maintain euglycemia and clinical manifestations of diabetes result (see Fig. 171.1).

TABLE 171.1 Classification of Diabetes Mellitus in Children and Adolescents

TYPE	COMMENT
TYPE 1 (INSULIN-DEPENDENT)	
Transient neonatal	Manifests immediately after birth; lasts 1-3 mo
Permanent neonatal	Other pancreatic defects possible
Classic type 1	Glycosuria, ketonuria, hyperglycemia, islet cell positive; genetic component
TYPE 2 (NON-INSULIN-DEPENDENT)	
Secondary	Cystic fibrosis, hemochromatosis, drugs (L-asparaginase, tacrolimus)
Adult type (classic)	Associated with obesity, insulin resistance; genetic component
OTHER	
Gestational diabetes	Abnormal glucose tolerance during pregnancy only, which reverts to normal postpartum; increased risk for later onset of diabetes
Maturity-onset diabetes of youth	Autosomal dominant, onset before age of 25 years; not associated with obesity or autoimmunity
Mitochondrial diabetes	Single-gene mutations include hepatocyte nuclear factors 1β,1α, 4α; glucokinase; insulin promoter factor 1
	Associated with deafness and other neurological defects, maternal transmission—mtDNA point mutations

Epidemiology

The annual incidence of T1D is increasing steadily but with significant geographic differences. In the United States, the annual incidence is approximately 20 in 100,000. The annual incidence in children ranges from a high of 40 in 100,000 among Scandinavian populations to less than 1 in 100,000 in China. The prevalence of T1D in the United States is highest in non-Hispanic whites followed by African Americans, Hispanics, and American Indians.

Genetic determinants play a role in the susceptibility to T1D, although the mode of inheritance is complex and multigenic. Siblings or offspring of patients with diabetes have a risk of 2-8% for the development of diabetes; an identical twin has a 30-50% risk. The human leukocyte antigen (HLA) region on chromosome 6 provides the strongest determinant of susceptibility, accounting for approximately 40% of familial inheritance of T1D. Specific class II DR and DQ HLA alleles (HLA DR3

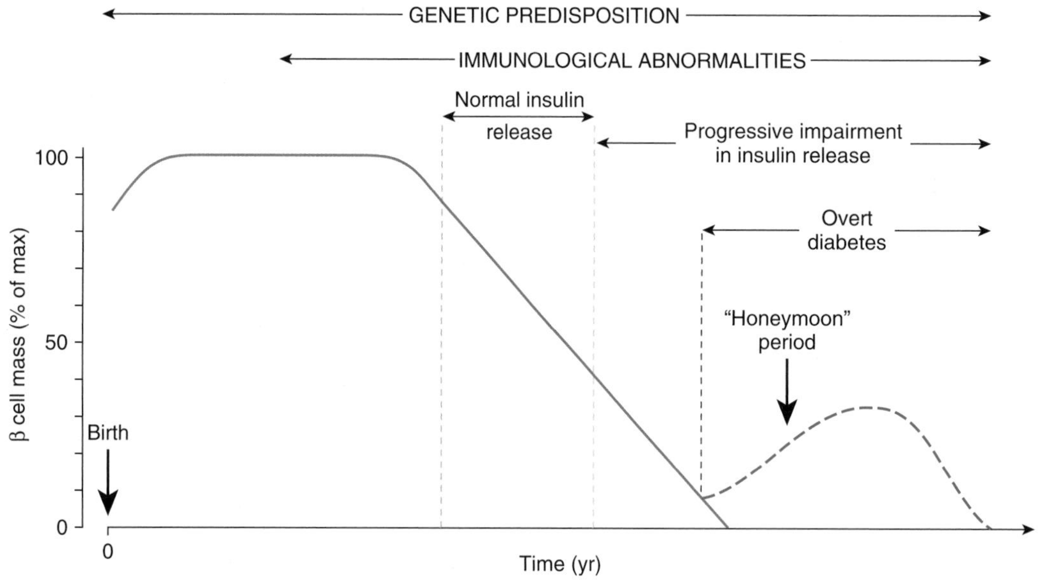

FIGURE 171.1 Schematic representation of the autoimmune evolution of diabetes in genetically predisposed individuals.

and HLA DR4) increase the risk of developing T1D, whereas other specific HLA alleles exert a protective effect. More than 90% of children with T1D possess HLA DR3 alleles, HLA DR4 alleles, or both. The insulin gene region variable number tandem repeat on chromosome 11 is also linked to T1D susceptibility. There is evidence for association, beyond HLA, of more than 100 other loci with T1D. Genetic factors do not fully account for susceptibility to T1D; environmental factors also play a role.

Clinical Manifestations

Decision-Making Algorithms
Available @ StudentConsult.com

Polyuria
Failure to Thrive

Hyperglycemia results when insulin secretory capacity becomes inadequate to enhance peripheral glucose uptake and to suppress hepatic and renal glucose production. Insulin deficiency usually first causes postprandial hyperglycemia and then fasting hyperglycemia. Ketogenesis is a sign of more complete insulin deficiency. Lack of suppression of gluconeogenesis and glycogenolysis further exacerbates hyperglycemia, while fatty acid oxidation generates the ketone bodies: β-hydroxybutyrate, acetoacetate, and acetone. Protein stores in muscle and fat stores in adipose tissue are metabolized to provide substrates for gluconeogenesis and fatty acid oxidation.

Glycosuria occurs when the serum glucose concentration exceeds the renal threshold for glucose reabsorption (from 160 to 190 mg/dL). Glycosuria causes an osmotic diuresis (including obligate loss of sodium, potassium, and other electrolytes) leading to dehydration. Polydipsia occurs as the patient attempts to compensate for the excess fluid losses. Weight loss results from the persistent catabolic state and the loss of calories through glycosuria and ketonuria. The classic presentation of T1D includes polyuria, polydipsia, polyphagia, and weight loss.

DIABETIC KETOACIDOSIS

If the clinical features of new-onset T1D are not detected, **diabetic ketoacidosis (DKA)** will occur. DKA may also occur in patients with known T1D if insulin injections are omitted or during an intercurrent illness when greater insulin requirements are unmet in the presence of elevated concentrations of the counter-regulatory and stress hormones (glucagon, growth hormone [GH], cortisol, and catecholamines). DKA can be considered to be present if (1) the arterial pH is below 7.3, (2) the serum bicarbonate level is below 15 mEq/L, and (3) ketones are elevated in serum or urine.

Pathophysiology

In the absence of adequate insulin secretion, persistent partial hepatic oxidation of fatty acids to ketone bodies occurs. Two of these three ketone bodies are organic acids and lead to metabolic acidosis with an elevated anion gap. Lactic acid may contribute to the acidosis when severe dehydration results in decreased tissue perfusion. Hyperglycemia causes an osmotic diuresis that is initially compensated for by increased fluid intake. As the hyperglycemia and diuresis worsen, most patients are unable to maintain the large fluid intake and dehydration occurs. Vomiting and increased insensible water losses caused by tachypnea can worsen the dehydration. Electrolyte abnormalities occur through a loss of electrolytes in the urine and transmembrane alterations resulting from acidosis. As hydrogen ions accumulate as a result of ketoacidosis, intracellular potassium is exchanged for hydrogen ions. Serum concentrations of potassium increase initially with acidosis then decrease as serum potassium is cleared by the kidney. Depending on the duration of ketoacidosis, serum potassium concentrations at diagnosis may be increased, normal, or decreased, but intracellular potassium concentrations are depleted. A decreased serum potassium concentration is an ominous sign of total body potassium depletion. Phosphate depletion also can occur as a result of the increased renal phosphate excretion required for elimination of excess hydrogen ions. Sodium depletion is also common in ketoacidosis resulting from renal losses of sodium caused by osmotic diuresis and from gastrointestinal losses from vomiting (Fig. 171.2).

Clinical Presentation

Decision-Making Algorithms
Available @ StudentConsult.com

Abdominal Pain
Polyuria
Acidemia
Hypernatremia

Patients with DKA present initially with polyuria, polydipsia, nausea, and vomiting. Abdominal pain occurs frequently and can mimic an acute abdomen. The abdomen may be tender from vomiting or distended secondary to a paralytic ileus. The presence of polyuria, despite a state of clinical dehydration, indicates osmotic diuresis and differentiates patients with DKA from patients with gastroenteritis or other gastrointestinal disorders. Respiratory compensation for acidosis results in tachypnea with deep **(Küssmaul)** respirations. The *fruity* odor of acetone frequently can be detected on the patient's breath. An altered mental status can occur, ranging from disorientation to coma.

Laboratory studies reveal hyperglycemia (serum glucose concentrations ranging from 200 mg/dL to >1,000 mg/dL). Arterial pH is below 7.30, and the serum bicarbonate concentration is less than 15 mEq/L. Serum sodium concentrations may be elevated, normal, or low, depending on the balance of sodium and free water losses. The measured serum sodium concentration is artificially low, however, because of hyperglycemia. Hyperlipidemia also contributes to the decrease in measured serum sodium. The level of blood urea nitrogen (BUN) can be elevated with prerenal azotemia secondary to dehydration. The white blood cell count is usually elevated and can be left-shifted without implying the presence of infection. Fever is unusual and should prompt a search for infectious sources that may have triggered the episode of DKA.

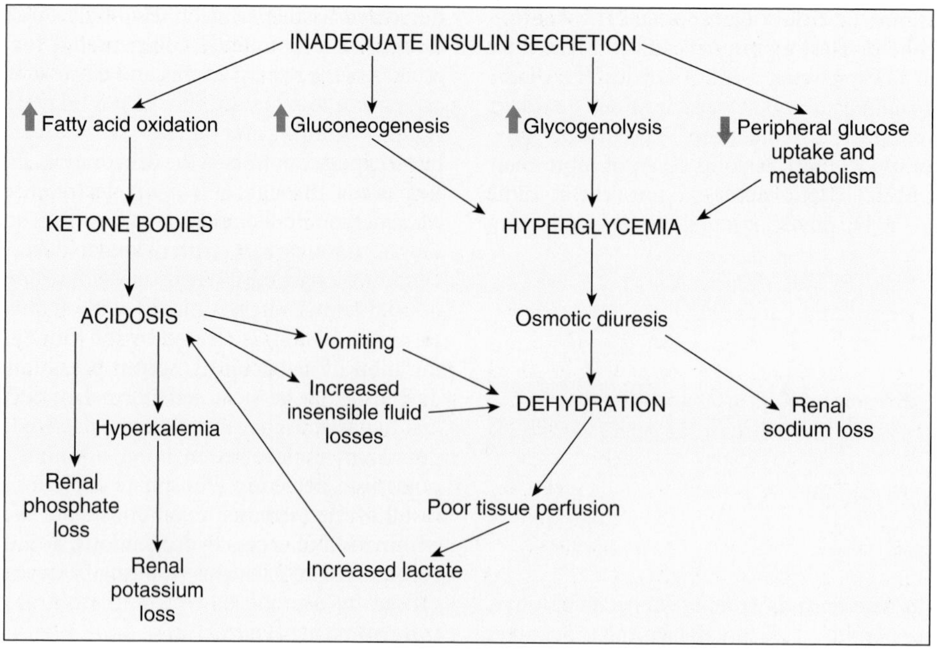

FIGURE 171.2 Pathophysiology of diabetic ketoacidosis.

Treatment

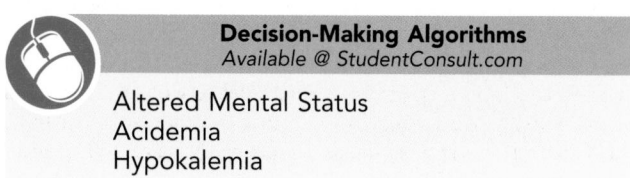

Decision-Making Algorithms
Available @ StudentConsult.com

Altered Mental Status
Acidemia
Hypokalemia

Therapy for patients with DKA involves careful replacement of fluid deficits, correction of acidosis and hyperglycemia via insulin administration, correction of electrolyte imbalances, and monitoring for complications of treatment. The optimal approach to management of DKA must strike a balance between adequate correction of fluid losses and avoidance of rapid shifts in osmolality and fluid balance. The most serious complication of DKA and its treatment is **cerebral edema** and cerebral herniation.

A patient with severe DKA is assumed to be approximately 10% dehydrated. If a recent weight measurement is available, the precise extent of dehydration can be calculated. An initial intravenous (IV) fluid bolus of a glucose-free isotonic solution (normal saline, lactated Ringer solution) at 10-20 mL/kg should be given to restore intravascular volume and renal perfusion. The remaining fluid deficit after the initial bolus should be added to maintenance fluid requirements, and the total should be replaced slowly over 36-48 hours. Ongoing losses resulting from osmotic diuresis usually do not need to be replaced unless urine output is large or signs of poor perfusion are present. Osmotic diuresis is usually minimal when the serum glucose concentration decreases to less than 300 mg/dL. To avoid rapid shifts in serum osmolality, 0.9% sodium chloride can be used as the replacement fluid for the initial 4-6 hours, followed by 0.45% sodium chloride.

Hyperglycemia

Fast-acting soluble insulin should be administered as a continuous IV infusion (0.1 U/kg/hr). Serum glucose concentrations should decrease at a rate no faster than 100 mg/dL/hr. When serum glucose concentrations decrease to less than 250-300 mg/dL, glucose should be added to the IV fluids. If serum glucose concentrations decrease to less than 200 mg/dL before correction of acidosis, the glucose concentration of the IV fluids should be increased, but the insulin infusion should not be decreased by more than half, and it should never be discontinued before resolution of acidosis.

Acidosis

Insulin therapy decreases the production of free fatty acids and protein catabolism and enhances glucose usage in target tissues. These processes correct acidosis. Bicarbonate therapy should be avoided. Potential adverse effects of bicarbonate administration include paradoxical increases in central nervous system (CNS) acidosis caused by increased diffusion of carbon dioxide across the blood-brain barrier, potential tissue hypoxia caused by shifts in the oxyhemoglobin dissociation curve, abrupt osmotic changes, and increased risk of the development of cerebral edema.

As acidosis is corrected, urine ketone concentrations may appear to rise. β-Hydroxybutyrate, which is not detected in urine ketone assays, is converted with treatment to what the assay most detects, acetoacetate. Hence minute-to-minute urine ketone concentrations are not a required index of the adequacy of therapy.

Electrolyte Imbalances

Regardless of the serum potassium concentration at presentation, total body potassium depletion is likely. Serum potassium concentrations can decrease rapidly as insulin and then glucose therapy improves acidosis, and potassium is exchanged for intracellular hydrogen ions. When adequate urine output is shown, potassium should be added to the IV fluids. Potassium replacement should be given as 50% potassium chloride and 50% potassium phosphate at a concentration of 20-40 mEq/L. This combination provides phosphate for replacement of deficits, but avoids excess phosphate administration, which may precipitate hypocalcemia. If the serum potassium level is greater than 6 mEq/L, potassium should not be added to IV fluids until the potassium level decreases.

Monitoring

Initial laboratory measurements should include serum glucose, sodium, potassium, chloride, bicarbonate, BUN, creatinine, calcium, phosphate, and magnesium concentrations; arterial or venous pH; and a urinalysis. Serum glucose measurement should be repeated every hour during therapy; electrolyte concentrations should be repeated every 2-3 hours. Calcium, phosphate, and magnesium concentrations should be measured every 4-6 hours during therapy. Neurological and mental status should be assessed at frequent intervals. Any complaints of headache or deterioration of mental status should prompt rapid evaluation for possible **cerebral edema.** Indicative symptoms include a decreased sensorium, sudden severe headache, vomiting, change in vital signs (bradycardia, hypertension, apnea), a dilated pupil, ophthalmoplegia, or seizure.

Complications

Clinically apparent **cerebral edema** occurs in 1-5% of cases of DKA. Cerebral edema is the most serious complication of DKA, with a mortality rate of 20-80%. The pathogenesis of cerebral edema likely involves osmolar shift resulting in fluid accumulation in the intracellular compartment and cell swelling. Subclinical cerebral edema is common in patients with DKA, but the factors that exacerbate this process leading to symptomatic brain swelling and possible cerebral herniation are not clearly defined. Cerebral edema typically occurs 6-12 hours after therapy for DKA is begun, often following a period of apparent clinical improvement. Factors that correlate with increased risk for cerebral edema include higher initial BUN concentration, lower initial P_{CO_2}, failure of the serum sodium concentration to increase as glucose concentration decreases during treatment, and treatment with bicarbonate.

Signs of advanced cerebral edema include obtundation, papilledema, pupillary dilation or inequality, hypertension, bradycardia, and apnea. **Treatment** involves the rapid use of IV mannitol, endotracheal intubation, and ventilation and may require the use of a subdural bolt. Other complications of DKA are intracranial thrombosis or infarction, acute kidney injury with acute renal failure caused by severe dehydration, pancreatitis, arrhythmias caused by electrolyte abnormalities, pulmonary edema, and bowel ischemia. Peripheral edema occurs commonly 24-48 hours after therapy is initiated and may be related to residual elevations in antidiuretic hormone and aldosterone.

Transition to Outpatient Management

When the acidosis has been corrected and the patient tolerates oral feedings, the IV insulin infusion can be discontinued and a regimen of subcutaneous (SC) insulin injections can be initiated. The first SC insulin dose should be given 30-45 minutes before discontinuation of the IV insulin infusion. Further adjustment of the insulin dose should be made over the following 2-3 days. A patient already diagnosed with T1D may be restarted on the prior doses if they were adequate. For a patient with new-onset T1D, typical starting total daily doses are approximately 0.5-0.7 U/kg/24 hr for prepubertal patients and approximately 0.7-1 U/kg/24 hr for adolescents, using any number of the available insulin combinations. The best and most common choice for making the transition to SC insulin is to begin by giving injections of fast-acting (bolus) insulin (lispro, aspart, or glulisine insulin) with each meal and long-acting (basal) insulin (glargine or detemir) at bedtime. This regimen of multiple daily injections provides the most flexibility but requires the patient to administer many injections per day and to count carbohydrates in food. An alternative is a fixed mixed split dosing regimen (neutral protamine Hagedorn [NPH] and fasting-acting insulin) with two daily injections.

Externally worn pumps that provide a continuous SC infusion of fast-acting insulin are available, although not usually used at the very onset of T1D. Insulin pumps provide fast-acting insulin in small basal amounts continuously every hour and will provide bolus insulin when instructed. Insulin pumps may be used by all age groups who are highly motivated to achieve tight control. The absence of SC depot insulin (glargine or detemir) can increase the risk of DKA.

Serum glucose concentrations should be assessed before each meal, at bedtime, and periodically at 2-3 A.M. to provide information for adjustment of the regimen. Patients and their families should begin learning the principles of diabetes care as soon as possible. Demonstration of the ability to administer insulin injections and test glucose concentrations using a glucose meter is necessary before discharge, as is knowledge of hypoglycemia management. Meal planning is crucial to control glucose in T1D. Nutrition services must be part of the care delivered to the families from diagnosis.

Honeymoon Period

In some patients with new onset of T1D, the β cell mass has not been completely destroyed. The remaining functional β cells seem to recover function with insulin treatment. When this occurs, exogenous insulin requirements decrease. This is a period of stable blood glucose control, often with nearly normal glucose concentrations. This phase of the disease, known as the honeymoon period, usually starts in the first weeks of therapy, often continues for 3-6 months, and can last 2 years.

Outpatient Type 1 Diabetes Mellitus Management

Management of T1D in children requires a comprehensive approach with attention to medical, nutritional, and psychosocial issues. Therapeutic strategies should be flexible with the individual needs of each patient and the family taken into account. Optimal care involves a team of diabetes professionals, including a physician, a diabetes nurse educator, a dietitian, and a social worker or psychologist.

Goals

The Diabetes Control and Complications Trial established that intensive insulin therapy, with the goal of maintaining blood glucose concentrations as close to normal as possible, can delay the onset and slow the progression of complications of diabetes (retinopathy, nephropathy, neuropathy). Attaining this goal using intensive insulin therapy can increase the risk of hypoglycemia. The adverse effects of hypoglycemia in young children may be significant because the immature CNS may be more susceptible to glycopenia. Although the risk for diabetic complications increases with duration of diabetes, there is controversy as to whether the increase of risk is slower in the prepubertal years than in adolescence and adulthood.

Given the benefits of stable, near normal blood glucose concentrations, a goal of HgbA1c <7.5% is set for children of all ages. Preprandial blood glucose target concentrations are 90-130 mg/dL and concentrations before bedtime and overnight of 90-150 mg/dL. Goals of therapy need to take into account other individual characteristics, such as a past history of severe hypoglycemia and the abilities of the patient and family.

Insulin Regimens

Many types of insulin differ in duration of action and time to peak effect (Table 171.2). These insulins can be used in various combinations, depending on the needs and goals of the individual patient. The most commonly used regimen is that of multiple injections of fast-acting insulin given with meals in combination with long-acting basal insulin given at bedtime. This regimen provides flexibility but requires administration of many injections per day and will require assistance for young children. After the total daily dose of insulin is determined, 30-50% is given as long-acting insulin, and the remainder is given as fast-acting insulin, divided according to the need for corrections of high glucose levels and for meals. To correct for hyperglycemia, one can determine the insulin sensitivity using the 1,800/1,500 rule: dividing 1,800 (or 1,500) by the total daily dose of insulin to determine how many milligrams per deciliter of glucose will decrease with one unit of insulin. The insulin:carbohydrate ratio is used to calculate insulin for the carbohydrate content of food; 500 divided by the total daily dose determines the number of grams of carbohydrate that requires one unit of insulin.

Insulin pumps that provide a continuous SC infusion of short-acting insulin also are available and are being used by children and adolescents who are highly motivated to achieve tight control.

Lispro, aspart, and glulisine insulin are synthetic human insulin analogs in which amino acid alterations result in fast absorption and onset of action (see Table 171.2). Because of the short duration of action, these are used in combination with long-acting insulin. Glargine and detemir are insulin analogs with increased solubility at acidic pH and decreased solubility at physiological pH. They have a duration of greater than 24 hours and act as a basal insulin.

Newly diagnosed patients in the honeymoon period may require 0.4-0.6 U/kg/24 hr. Prepubertal patients with diabetes longer than 1-2 years typically require 0.5-1 U/kg/24 hr. During middle adolescence when elevated GH concentrations produce relative insulin resistance, insulin requirements increase by 40-50%, and doses of 1-2 U/kg/24 hr are typical.

Nutrition

Balancing the daily meal plan with the dosages of insulin is crucial for maintaining serum glucose concentrations within the target range and avoiding hypoglycemia or hyperglycemia. The content and schedule of meals vary according to the type of insulin regimen used. It is recommended that carbohydrates contribute 50-65% of the total calories, protein 12-20%, and fat <30%. Saturated fat should contribute <10% of the total caloric intake, and cholesterol intake should be less than 300 mg/24 hr. High-fiber content is recommended.

Patients using multiple daily injections or the insulin pump can maintain a more flexible meal schedule with regard to the timing of meals and the carbohydrate content. These patients give an injection of insulin before or immediately after each meal with the total dose calculated according to the carbohydrate content of the meal. Further adjustments in the dose can be made based on the measured serum glucose concentration and plans for activity during the day. Children using a twice-a-day combination of intermediate-acting and fast-acting insulins need to maintain a relatively consistent meal schedule so that carbohydrate absorption and insulin action peaks correspond. A typical meal schedule for a patient using this type of regimen involves three meals and three snacks daily. The total carbohydrate content of the meals and snacks should be kept constant.

TABLE 171.2 Representative Profiles of Insulin

INSULIN	ONSET	PEAK ACTION	DURATION
VERY SHORT ACTING			
Lispro, aspart, glulisine	5-15 min	30-90 min	3-5 hr
SHORT ACTING			
Regular	30-60 min	2-3 hr	5-8 hr
INTERMEDIATE ACTING			
Neutral protamine Hagedorn (NPH) (isophane)	2-4 hr	4-10 hr	10-16 hr
LONG ACTING			
Glargine	2-4 hr	None	20-24 hr
Detemir	2-4 hr	6-14 hr	16-20 hr
Degludec	2-4 hr	None	24+ hr

Data from Wolfsdorf JI, ed. Intensive Diabetes Management. *4th ed. Alexandria, VA: American Diabetes Associations; 2009.*

Blood Glucose Testing

Blood glucose should be routinely monitored before each meal and at bedtime. Hypoglycemia during the night or excessive variability in the morning glucose concentrations should prompt additional testing at 2 or 3 A.M. to ensure that there is no consistent hypoglycemia or hyperglycemia. During periods of illness or when blood glucose concentrations are higher than 300 mg/dL, urine ketones also should be tested. Continuous glucose monitors, which provide minute-to-minute blood glucose concentration information, can be useful in following trends of blood glucose concentrations, but should not be used in calculations of mealtime insulin doses.

Long-Term Glycemic Control

Measurements of **glycohemoglobin** or **hemoglobin A_{1c} (HgbA1c)** reflect the average blood glucose concentration over the preceding 3 months and provide a means for assessing long-term glycemic control. HgbA1c should be measured four times a year, and the results should be used for counseling of patients. The American Diabetes Association has set HgbA1c targets for children at <7.5%. Measurements of HgbA1c are inaccurate in patients with hemoglobinopathies. Glycosylated albumin or fructosamine can be used in these cases.

Complications

Patients with T1D for more than 3-5 years should receive an annual ophthalmological examination for retinopathy. Urine should be collected annually for assessment of microalbuminuria, which suggests early renal dysfunction and indicates a high risk of progression to nephropathy. Treatment with angiotensin-converting enzyme inhibitors may halt the progression of microalbuminuria. In children with T1D, annual cholesterol measurements and periodic assessment of blood pressure are recommended. Early detection of hypertension and hypercholesterolemia with appropriate intervention can help limit future risk of coronary disease.

Other Disorders

Chronic autoimmune lymphocytic thyroiditis is particularly common and can result in hypothyroidism. Because symptoms can be subtle, thyroid function tests should be performed annually. Other disorders that occur with increased frequency in children with T1D include celiac disease, immunoglobulin A deficiency, Addison disease, and peptic ulcer disease.

Special Problems: Hypoglycemia

Hypoglycemia occurs commonly in patients with T1D. For patients in adequate or better control, it is expected to occur on average once or twice a week. Severe episodes of hypoglycemia, resulting in seizures or coma or requiring assistance from another person, occur in 10-25% of these patients per year.

Hypoglycemia in patients with T1D results from a relative excess of insulin in relation to the serum glucose concentration. This excess can be caused by alterations in the dose, timing, or absorption of insulin; alterations of carbohydrate intake; or changes in insulin sensitivity resulting from activity. Defective counter-regulatory responses also contribute to hypoglycemia. Abnormal glucagon responses to falling serum glucose concentrations develop within the first few years of the disease, and abnormalities in epinephrine release occur after a longer duration.

Lack of awareness of hypoglycemia occurs in approximately 25% of patients with diabetes. Recent episodes of hypoglycemia may play a role in the pathophysiology of *hypoglycemia unawareness*; after an episode of hypoglycemia, autonomic responses to subsequent episodes are reduced. A return of symptoms of hypoglycemia can be exhibited in these patients after 2-3 weeks of strict avoidance of hypoglycemic episodes.

Symptoms of hypoglycemia include symptoms resulting from neuroglycopenia (headache, visual changes, confusion, irritability, or seizures) and symptoms resulting from the catecholamine response (tremors, tachycardia, diaphoresis, or anxiety). Mild episodes can be treated with administration of rapidly absorbed oral glucose (glucose gel or tablets or fruit juices). More severe episodes that result in seizures or loss of consciousness at home should be treated with glucagon injections. IV glucose should be given in hospital settings.

Prognosis

Long-term complications of T1D include retinopathy, nephropathy, neuropathy, and macrovascular disease. Evidence of organ damage caused by hyperglycemia is rare in patients with diabetes of less than 5-10 years' duration; clinically apparent disease rarely occurs before 10-15 years' duration. Diabetic retinopathy is the leading cause of blindness in the United States. Nephropathy eventually occurs in 30-40% and accounts for approximately 30% of all new adult cases of end-stage renal disease. Neuropathy occurs in 30-40% of postpubertal patients with T1D and leads to sensory, motor, or autonomic deficits. Macrovascular disease results in an increased risk of myocardial infarction and stroke among individuals with diabetes.

Intensive control of diabetes, using frequent blood glucose testing, continuous glucose monitoring, and multiple daily injections of insulin or an insulin pump, can reduce the development or progression of diabetic complications, including a 76% reduction of risk for retinopathy, a 39% reduction in microalbuminuria, and a 60% reduction in clinical neuropathy. For pubertal and adult patients, the benefits of intensive therapy likely outweigh the increased risk for hypoglycemia. For younger patients, in whom the risks for hypoglycemia are greater and the benefits of tight glucose control may be lower, a less intensive regimen may be appropriate.

TYPE 2 DIABETES MELLITUS

Pathophysiology

T2D can occur as the result of various pathophysiological processes; however, the most common form results from peripheral insulin resistance and compensatory hyperinsulinemia, followed by failure of the pancreas to maintain adequate insulin secretion (see Table 171.1).

Epidemiology

The prevalence of T2D in children is increasing in parallel with childhood obesity and is highest in children of ethnic groups with a high prevalence of T2D in adults, including Native

Americans, Hispanic Americans, and African Americans. Obesity, the metabolic syndrome, ethnicity, and a family history of T2D are risk factors. Autoantibodies to the pancreas are present among some clinically assumed to have T2D, compounding the difficulty in differentiating T1D from T2D at the time of diagnosis.

Clinical Manifestations and Differential Diagnosis

Fasting and postprandial glucose levels for diagnosis of T2D are the same as those for T1D. The diagnosis of T2D may be suspected on the basis of polyuria and polydipsia in a background of the metabolic syndrome. Differentiating T2D from T1D in children on only clinical grounds can be challenging. The possibility of T2D should be considered in patients who are obese, have a strong family history of T2D, have other characteristics of the metabolic syndrome, or have absence of antibodies to β cell antigens at the time of diagnosis of diabetes. **Acanthosis nigricans,** a dermatological manifestation of hyperinsulinism and insulin resistance, presents as hyperkeratotic pigmentation in the nape of the neck and in flexural areas and is noted as a sign in the metabolic syndrome. Although ketoacidosis occurs far more commonly in T1D, it also can occur in patients with T2D under conditions of physiological stress and cannot be used as an absolute differentiating factor. T2D can be confirmed by the evaluation of insulin or C-peptide responses to stimulation with oral carbohydrate and in the absence of islet cell autoreactivity.

Therapy

T2D is the result of a combination of insulin resistance, relative insulin deficiency, and a secretory β cell defect. Asymptomatic patients with mildly elevated glucose values (slightly >126 mg/dL for fasting or slightly >200 mg/dL for random glucose) may be managed initially with lifestyle modifications, including nutrition therapy (dietary adjustments) and increased exercise. Exercise has been shown to decrease insulin resistance. In most children with new-onset, uncomplicated T2D, oral agents are usually the first line of therapy. Only metformin, an insulin secretagogue, is approved by the U.S. Food and Drug Administration for use in children. A rare side effect of metformin is lactic acidosis, occurring mainly in patients with compromised renal function. The most common side effect is gastrointestinal upset. If ketonuria or ketoacidosis occurs, insulin treatment is necessary to first achieve adequate glycemic control, but may be discontinued within weeks with continuation of oral medications. Insulin therapy may be required if adequate glycemic control is not achieved with lifestyle modifications and metformin.

Because T2D may have a long preclinical course, early diagnosis is possible in subjects at risk who have the **metabolic syndrome.** Significant lifestyle modifications, such as improved eating habits and increased exercise, have a role in preventing or decreasing the morbidity of T2D. Finally, it is critical to monitor and manage the other components of metabolic syndrome, such as advanced pubertal development, hypertension, hyperlipidemia, and polycystic ovary syndrome in females.

MATURITY-ONSET DIABETES OF YOUTH (MODY)

MODY comprises a group of dominantly inherited forms of relatively mild diabetes. Insulin resistance does not occur in these patients; instead, the primary abnormality is an insufficient insulin secretory response to glycemic stimulation. Treatment depends on the type and can include the use of sulfonylureas.

CHAPTER 172

Hypoglycemia

Hypoglycemia in infancy and childhood can result from a large variety of hormonal and metabolic defects (Table 172.1). Hypoglycemia occurs most frequently in the early neonatal period, often as a result of transient neonatal hyperinsulinemia in infants of diabetic mothers or as a result of inadequate energy stores to meet the disproportionately large metabolic needs of premature or small for gestational age newborns. Hypoglycemia during the first few days of life in an otherwise normal newborn is less frequent and warrants concern (see Chapter 6). After the initial 2-3 days of life, hypoglycemia is far less common and is more frequently the result of endocrine or metabolic disorders (although sepsis must always be ruled out).

DEFINITION

Clinical hypoglycemia is defined as a plasma glucose (PG) concentration low enough to cause symptoms and/or signs of impaired brain function. Brain glucose utilization is reduced at a PG concentration of approximately 55-65 mg/dL. **Autonomic system** (neurogenic) symptoms are perceived at a PG concentration <55 mg/dL. Cognitive function is impaired **(neuroglycopenia)** at a PG concentration <50 mg/dL (Table 172.2).

CLINICAL MANIFESTATIONS

Decision-Making Algorithms
Available @ StudentConsult.com

Hypotonia and Weakness
Altered Mental Status
Irritable Infant

The symptoms and signs of hypoglycemia result from direct depression of the central nervous system owing to lack of energy substrate and the counter-regulatory adrenergic response to low glucose via catecholamine secretion designed to correct hypoglycemia (see Table 172.2). Compared with older children, infants do not usually show adrenergic symptoms. The signs and symptoms of hypoglycemia in infants are relatively nonspecific and include jitteriness, feeding difficulties, pallor, hypotonia, hypothermia, episodes of apnea and bradycardia, depressed levels of consciousness, and seizures. In older children, signs and symptoms include confusion, irritability, headaches,

TABLE 172.1 Classification of Hypoglycemia in Infants and Children

ABNORMALITIES IN THE HORMONAL SIGNAL INDICATING HYPOGLYCEMIA	Fatty Acid Oxidation (incomplete list)
Counter-Regulatory Hormone Deficiency	Long-, medium-, or short-chain fatty acid acyl-CoA dehydrogenase deficiency
MPHD	Carnitine deficiency (primary or secondary)
Isolated growth hormone deficiency	Carnitine palmitoyltransferase deficiency
ACTH deficiency	*Other*
Addison disease	Enzymatic defects
Glucagon deficiency	Galactosemia
Epinephrine deficiency	Hereditary fructose intolerance
Hyperinsulinism	Propionic acidemia
Infant of a diabetic mother	Methylmalonic acidemia
Infant with erythroblastosis fetalis	Tyrosinosis
β cell adenoma (insulinoma)	Glutaric aciduria
Congenital hyperinsulinemic hypoglycemia	Global hepatic dysfunction
Beckwith-Wiedemann syndrome	Reye syndrome
Anti-insulin receptor antibodies	Hepatitis
Inadequate Substrate	Heart failure
Prematurity/small for gestational age infant	Sepsis, shock
Ketotic hypoglycemia	Carcinoma/sarcoma (IGF-2 secretion)
Maple syrup urine disease	Malnutrition/starvation
Disorders of Metabolic Response Pathways	Hyperviscosity syndrome
Glycogenolysis	Drugs/Intoxications
Glucose-6-phosphatase deficiency	Oral hypoglycemic agents or insulin
Amylo-1,6-glucosidase deficiency	Alcohol
Liver glycogen phosphorylase deficiency	Salicylates
Glycogen synthase deficiency	Propranolol
Glycogen debranching enzyme deficiency	Valproic acid
Phosphorylase kinase deficiency	Pentamidine
GLUT2 transporter mutations	Ackee fruit (unripe)
Gluconeogenesis	Quinine
Fructose-1,6-diphosphatase deficiency	Trimethoprim-sulfamethoxazole (with renal failure)
Pyruvate carboxylase deficiency	
Phosphoenolpyruvate carboxykinase deficiency	

ACTH, Adrenocorticotropic hormone; *acyl-CoA*, acyl coenzyme A; *IGF-2*, insulin-like growth factor-2; *MPHD*, multiple pituitary hormone deficiency.

visual changes, tremors, pallor, sweating, tachycardia, weakness, seizures, and coma.

Failure to recognize and treat severe, prolonged hypoglycemia can result in serious long-term morbidity, including intellectual disability and nonhypoglycemic seizures. Younger infants and patients with more severe or prolonged hypoglycemia are at greatest risk for adverse outcomes.

PATHOPHYSIOLOGY

Hormonal Signal

Normal regulation of serum glucose concentrations requires appropriate interaction of a number of hormonal signals and metabolic pathways (Fig. 172.1). In a normal individual, a decrease in serum glucose concentrations leads to a suppression of insulin secretion and increased secretion of the counter-regulatory hormones (growth hormone [GH], cortisol, glucagon, and epinephrine; see Fig. 172.1). This hormonal signal promotes the release of amino acids (particularly alanine) from muscle to fuel gluconeogenesis and the release of triglyceride from adipose tissue stores to provide free fatty acids (FFAs) for hepatic ketogenesis. FFAs and ketones serve as alternate fuels for muscle. This hormonal signal also stimulates the breakdown of hepatic glycogen and promotes gluconeogenesis. Failure of any of the components of this hormonal signal can lead to hypoglycemia.

Hyperinsulinemia

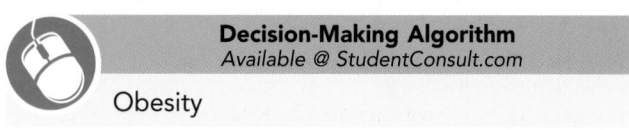

Decision-Making Algorithm
Available @ StudentConsult.com

Obesity

A lack of suppression of insulin secretion in response to low serum glucose concentrations can occur in infants but is uncommon beyond the neonatal period. This situation arises most frequently in infants of diabetic mothers who were exposed to high concentrations of maternally derived glucose in utero, resulting in fetal islet cell hyperplasia. The hyperinsulinemic state is transient, usually lasting hours to days.

TABLE 172.2 Symptoms and Signs of Hypoglycemia

FEATURES ASSOCIATED WITH EPINEPHRINE RELEASE*	FEATURES ASSOCIATED WITH CEREBRAL GLYCOPENIA
Perspiration	Headache
Palpitation (tachycardia)	Mental confusion
Pallor	Somnolence
Paresthesia	Dysarthria
Trembling	Personality changes
Anxiety	Inability to concentrate
Weakness	Staring
Nausea	Hunger
Vomiting	Convulsions
	Ataxia
	Coma
	Diplopia
	Stroke

**These features and perceptions of the features may be blunted if the patient is receiving β-blocking agents.*

Hyperinsulinism that persists beyond a few days of age can result from distinct genetic disorders affecting glucose-regulated insulin release, or **congenital hyperinsulinism.** In these infants, hyperplasia of the pancreatic islet cells develops in the absence of excess stimulation by maternal diabetes. There are currently 11 genes associated with monogenic forms of hyperinsulinism *(ABCC8, KCNJ11, GLUD1, GCK, HADH1, UCP2, MCT1, HNF4A, HNF1A, HK1, PGM1)*, as well as several syndromic genetic forms of HI (e.g., Beckwith-Wiedemann, Kabuki, and Turner syndromes). The most common causes for congenital hyperinsulinism involve inactivating K_{ATP} channel mutations and account for approximately 60% of all identifiable mutations. Hyperinsulinism also can occur in **Beckwith-Wiedemann syndrome** (a condition characterized by neonatal somatic gigantism, macrosomia, macroglossia, omphalocele, visceromegaly, and earlobe creases).

Regardless of the cause, neonates with hyperinsulinism are characteristically large for gestational age (see Chapter 60). Hypoglycemia is severe and frequently occurs within 1-3 hours of a feeding. Glucose requirements are increased, often two to three times the normal basal glucose requirement of 6-8 mg/kg/min. The *diagnosis* of hyperinsulinism in children is determined by evaluating markers of inappropriate insulin effects (e.g., suppressed ketogenesis) because plasma insulin concentrations are frequently not clearly elevated. Diagnosis is most reliably based on a closely monitored provocative fasting test that includes (1) frequent sampling of plasma concentrations of glucose, insulin, β-hydroxybutyrate, and FFAs and (2) terminating the test when glucose concentrations decline toward 50 mg/dL with a determination of the glycemic response to glucagon. The absence of serum and urine ketones at the time of hypoglycemia is an important diagnostic feature, distinguishing hyperinsulinism from defects in counter-regulatory hormone secretion.

Treatment initially involves the infusion of intravenous (IV) glucose at high rates and of diazoxide to suppress insulin secretion. If diazoxide therapy is unsuccessful, long-acting somatostatin analogs can be tried. Often medical therapy for persistent hyperinsulinemic hypoglycemia of the newborn is unsuccessful, and subtotal (90%) pancreatectomy is required to prevent long-term neurological sequelae of hypoglycemia.

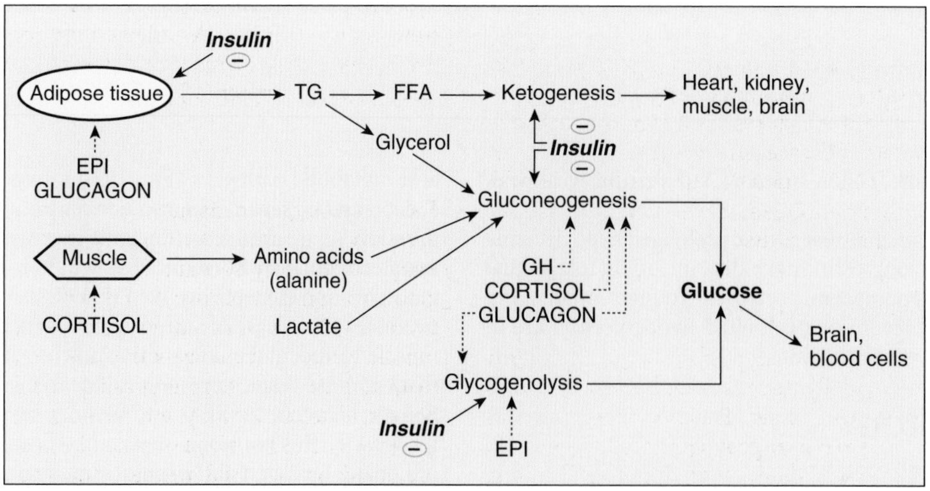

FIGURE 172.1 Regulation of serum glucose. ⊖ represents inhibitions. *EPI*, Epinephrine; *FFA*, free fatty acid; *GH*, growth hormone; *TG*, triglyceride.

Factitious Hyperinsulinemia

In rare cases, insulin or a hypoglycemic medication is administered by a parent or caregiver to a child as a form of child abuse, which is a condition referred to as **Munchausen syndrome by proxy.** This *diagnosis* should be suspected if extremely high insulin concentrations are detected (>100 μU/mL). C-peptide concentrations are low or undetectable, which confirms that the insulin is from an exogenous source.

Defects in Counter-Regulatory Hormones

Abnormalities in the secretion of counter-regulatory hormones that produce hypoglycemia usually involve GH, cortisol, or both. Deficiencies in glucagon and epinephrine secretion are rare. GH and cortisol deficiency occur as a result of hypopituitarism. Hypopituitarism results from congenital hypoplasia or aplasia of the pituitary or, more commonly, from deficiency of hypothalamic releasing factors (see Chapter 173). Clues to this diagnosis in infants include the presence of hypoglycemia in association with midline facial or neurological defects (e.g., cleft lip and palate or absence of the corpus callosum), pendular (roving) nystagmus (indicating visual impairment from possible abnormalities in the development of the optic nerves, which can occur in optic nerve hypoplasia), and the presence of microphallus and cryptorchidism in boys (indicating abnormalities in gonadotropin secretion). Jaundice and hepatomegaly also can occur, simulating neonatal hepatitis. Despite the presence of GH deficiency, these infants are usually of normal size at birth.

Deficient cortisol secretion also can occur in primary adrenal insufficiency, resulting from a variety of causes. In infants it often results from congenital adrenal hyperplasia, most frequently as a result of 21-hydroxylase deficiency (see Chapters 177 and 178). In older children, primary adrenal insufficiency is seen most frequently in **Addison disease** and other disorders (see Chapter 178).

Confirmation of GH or cortisol deficiency as the cause of hypoglycemia requires the detection of low serum GH and cortisol concentrations during an episode of hypoglycemia or after other stimulatory testing. In contrast to hyperinsulinism, serum and urine ketones are positive at the time of hypoglycemia and FFAs are elevated. Treatment involves supplementation of the deficient hormones in physiological doses.

ENERGY STORES

Sufficient energy stores in the form of glycogen, adipose tissue, and muscle are necessary to respond appropriately to hypoglycemia. Deficiencies in these stores are a common cause of hypoglycemia in neonates who are small for gestational age or premature (see Chapter 60). Beyond the early neonatal period, energy stores are usually sufficient to meet the metabolic requirements except in malnourished children.

IDIOPATHIC KETOTIC HYPOGLYCEMIA

A common cause of new-onset hypoglycemia is idiopathic ketotic hypoglycemia, usually seen in children between 18 months and remits by 8 years of age. Patients have symptoms of hypoglycemia after a period of prolonged fasting, often in the setting of an intercurrent illness with decreased feeding. Children with this disorder are often thin and small and may have a history of being small for gestational age. Defective mobilization of alanine from muscle to fuel gluconeogenesis is thought to be the cause, although the condition may derive mostly from having lower fuel reserves. Because there are no specific diagnostic tests for this disorder, ketotic hypoglycemia is a *diagnosis of exclusion.*

Treatment involves avoidance of fasting and frequent feedings of a high-protein, high-carbohydrate diet. Patients may require hospitalization for IV glucose infusion if they cannot maintain adequate oral intake during a period of illness.

DISRUPTED METABOLIC RESPONSE PATHWAYS

Maintenance of normal serum glucose concentrations in the fasting state requires glucose production via glycogenolysis and gluconeogenesis and the production of alternative energy sources (FFAs and ketones) via lipolysis and fatty acid oxidation.

Glycogenolysis

Some glycogen storage diseases (GSDs) occur in a variety of subtypes that differ in severity (see Chapter 52). Among the subtypes that result in hypoglycemia, the most severe form is glucose-6-phosphatase deficiency, which is characterized by severe hypoglycemia, massive hepatomegaly, growth retardation, and lactic acidosis. In contrast, deficiencies in the glycogen phosphorylase enzymes may cause isolated hepatomegaly with or without hypoglycemia.

The *diagnosis* of GSD is suggested by a finding of hepatomegaly without splenomegaly (although GSD type 0 is not associated with hepatomegaly). Confirmation of the diagnosis requires specific biochemical studies of leukocytes or liver biopsy specimens. *Treatment* for the most common types involves frequent high-carbohydrate feedings during the day and continuous feedings at night via nasogastric tube. Feedings of uncooked cornstarch overnight are sufficient to maintain serum glucose concentrations in some patients.

Gluconeogenesis

Defects in gluconeogenesis are uncommon and include fructose-1,6-diphosphatase deficiency and phosphoenolpyruvate carboxykinase deficiency. Affected patients exhibit fasting hypoglycemia, hepatomegaly, lactic acidosis, and hyperuricemia. Ketosis occurs, and FFA and alanine concentrations are high. *Treatment* involves frequent high-carbohydrate, low-protein feedings (see Chapter 52).

Fatty Acid Oxidation

Fatty acid oxidation disorders of ketogenesis include the fatty acid acyl-coenzyme A (CoA) dehydrogenase deficiencies; long-chain, medium-chain, and short-chain acyl-CoA dehydrogenase deficiencies; and hereditary carnitine deficiency (see Chapter 55). Of these disorders, medium-chain acyl-CoA dehydrogenase deficiency is the most common; it occurs in 1 in 4,000-17,000 live births, depending on the population. Patients often are well in infancy and have the first episode of hypoglycemia at 2 years of age or older. Mild hepatomegaly may be present along with mild hyperammonemia, hyperuricemia, and mild elevations in hepatic transaminases. Episodes of nonketotic hypoglycemia usually occur with prolonged fasting or during episodes of intercurrent illness. *Treatment* involves avoidance of fasting.

OTHER METABOLIC DISORDERS

Many metabolic disorders can lead to hypoglycemia, including galactosemia, hereditary fructose intolerance, and disorders of organic acid metabolism (see Table 172.1). Hypoglycemia in these disorders is usually a reflection of global hepatic dysfunction secondary to the buildup of hepatotoxic intermediates. Many of these disorders present with low concentrations of ketone bodies because ketogenesis also is affected. The finding of non-glucose-reducing substances in the urine after ingestion of offending substances suggests a diagnosis of galactosemia or hereditary fructose intolerance. *Treatment* requires dietary restriction of the specific offending substances.

MEDICATIONS AND INTOXICATION

Hypoglycemia can occur as an adverse effect of numerous medications (see Table 172.1). Ethanol ingestion also can cause hypoglycemia, especially in younger children, because the metabolism of ethanol results in the depletion of cofactors necessary for gluconeogenesis.

DIAGNOSIS

Although the list of causes of hypoglycemia is long and complex, establishing the *etiology* in a particular patient is important. Frequently it is difficult to make an accurate diagnosis until one can obtain a *critical sample* of blood and urine at the time of the hypoglycemic episode. In a child with unexplained hypoglycemia, a serum sample should be obtained before treatment for the measurement of glucose and insulin, GH, cortisol, FFAs, and β-hydroxybutyrate and acetoacetate. Measurement of serum lactate levels also should be considered. A urine specimen should be obtained for measuring ketones and reducing substances. *Hypoglycemia without ketonuria suggests hyperinsulinism or a defect in fatty acid oxidation.* The results of this initial testing can establish whether endocrine causes are responsible and, if not, provide initial information regarding which types of metabolic disorders are most likely.

EMERGENCY MANAGEMENT

Acute care of a patient with hypoglycemia consists of rapid administration of IV glucose (2 mL/kg of 10% dextrose in water). After the initial bolus, an infusion of IV glucose should provide approximately 1.5 times the normal hepatic glucose production rate (8-12 mg/kg/min in infants, 6-8 mg/kg/min in children). This infusion allows for suppression of the catabolic state and prevents further decompensation in patients with certain metabolic disorders. If adrenal insufficiency is suspected, stress doses of glucocorticoids should be administered.

CHAPTER 173

Short Stature

GROWTH

Normal growth is the final common pathway of many factors, including endocrine, environmental, nutritional, and genetic influences (see Chapter 5). A normal linear growth pattern is good evidence of overall health and can be considered a *bioassay* for the well-being of the whole child. The effects of certain hormones on growth and ultimate height are listed in Table 173.1. Just as various factors influence stature, stature itself influences psychological, social, and potentially economic well-being. Parental concern about the psychosocial consequences of abnormal stature often causes a family to seek medical attention.

Growth Hormone Physiology

Growth hormone (GH) secretion is pulsatile, stimulated by hypothalamic GH-releasing factor (GRF), and inhibited by GH release inhibitory factor (somatostatin, somatotropin release-inhibiting factor [SRIF]), which interact with their individual receptors on the pituitary somatotrope in a noncompetitive manner. GH is also stimulated by a number of factors (e.g., ghrelin, sex steroid hormones, clonidine, hypoglycemia,

TABLE 173.1 Hormonal Effects on Growth

HORMONE	BONE AGE	GROWTH RATE	ADULT HEIGHT*
Androgen excess	Advanced	Increased	Diminished
Androgen deficiency	Normal or delayed	Normal or decreased	Increased slightly or normal
Thyroxine excess	Advanced	Increased	Normal or diminished
Thyroxine deficiency	Retarded	Decreased	Diminished
Growth hormone excess	Normal or advanced	Increased	Excessive
Growth hormone deficiency	Retarded	Decreased	Diminished
Cortisol excess	Retarded	Decreased	Diminished
Cortisol deficiency	Normal	Normal	Normal

*Effect in most patients with treatment.
Modified from Underwood LE, Van Wyk JJ. Normal and aberrant growth. In: Wilson JD, Foster DW, eds. Textbook of Endocrinology. *8th ed. Philadelphia: WB Saunders; 1992.*

etc.). GH circulates bound to a GH-binding protein (GHBP); GHBP abundance reflects the abundance of GH receptors. GH has direct effects on tissue and also causes production and secretion of insulin-like growth factor-1 (IGF-1) in many tissues. GH stimulates IGF-1 production in the liver along with production of the acid-labile subunit and the IGF-binding protein (IGF-BP3); this forms the complex that delivers IGF-1 to tissue.

IGF-1 acts primarily as a paracrine and autocrine agent and is most closely associated with postnatal growth. When IGF-1 attaches to its membrane-bound receptor, second messengers are stimulated to change the physiology of the cell and produce growth effects. IGF-1 production is influenced by disease states such as malnutrition, chronic renal and liver disease, hypothyroidism, or obesity.

IGF-BP3 is measurable in clinical assays and is less influenced by nutrition and age than is IGF-1; measuring IGF-1 and IGF-BP3 is useful in evaluating GH adequacy, particularly in infancy and early childhood.

Measurement of Growth

The correct measurement of an infant's length requires one adult to hold the infant's head still and another adult to extend the feet with the soles perpendicular to the lower legs. A caliper-like device, such as an infantometer, or the movable plates on an infant scale are used so that the exact distance between the two calipers or plates can be determined. Marking the position of the head and feet of an infant lying on a sheet of paper on the examining table leads to inaccuracies and may miss true disorders of growth or create false concerns about a disorder of growth in a normal child. Accurate measurements of height (standing), or length (lying down), and weight should be plotted on the Centers for Disease Control and Prevention growth charts for the timely diagnosis of growth disorders (http://www.cdc.gov/growthcharts/).

After 2 years of age, the height of a child should be measured in the standing position. Children measured in the standing position should be barefoot against a hard surface. A Harpenden stadiometer or equivalent device is optimal for the measurement of stature. A decrease of roughly 1.25 cm in height measurement may occur when the child is measured in the standing position rather than in the lying position, leading to the inappropriate referral of many children who appear to be *not growing* to a subspecialist.

Measurement of the **arm span** is essential when the diagnoses of Marfan or Klinefelter syndrome, short-limbed dwarfism, or other dysmorphic conditions are considered. Arm span is measured as the distance between the tips of the fingers when the patient holds both arms outstretched horizontally while standing against a solid surface. The **upper-to-lower segment ratio** is the ratio of the upper segment (determined by subtraction of the measurement from the symphysis pubis to the floor [known as the lower segment] from the total height) to the lower segment. This ratio changes with age. A normal term infant has an upper-to-lower ratio of 1.7:1, a 1-year-old has a ratio of 1.4:1, and a 10-year-old has a ratio of 1:1. Conditions of hypogonadism, not commonly discerned or suspected until after the normal age for onset of puberty, lead to greatly decreased upper-to-lower ratio in an adult, whereas long-lasting and untreated hypothyroidism leads to a high upper-to-lower ratio in the child.

Endocrine Evaluation of Growth Hormone Secretion

Decision-Making Algorithm
Available @ StudentConsult.com
Short Stature

GH is a 191–amino acid protein secreted by the pituitary gland under the control of GRF and SRIF (see Fig. 170.2). GH secretion is enhanced by α-adrenergic stimulation, hypoglycemia, starvation, exercise, early stages of sleep, and stress and inhibited by β-adrenergic stimulation and hyperglycemia. Because concentrations of GH are low throughout the day, except for brief secretory peaks in the middle of the night or early morning, the daytime ascertainment of GH deficiency or sufficiency on the basis of a single determination of a random GH concentration is impossible. Adequacy of GH secretion may be determined by a stimulation test to measure peak GH secretion. A normal response is a vigorous secretory peak after stimulation; the lack of such a peak is consistent with GH deficiency. However, there is a high false-positive rate (on any day, about 10% or more of normal children may not reach the normal GH peak after even two stimulatory tests). Indirect measurements of GH secretion, such as serum concentrations of IGF-1 and IGF-BP3, are considered better screens for GH deficiency.

The factors responsible for postnatal growth are not the same as the factors that mediate fetal growth. **Thyroid hormone** is essential for normal postnatal growth, although a thyroid hormone-deficient fetus achieves a normal birth length; similarly, a GH-deficient fetus has a normal birth length, although in IGF-1 deficiency resulting from GH resistance **(Laron dwarfism),** fetuses are shorter than control subjects. Adequate thyroid hormone is necessary to allow the secretion of GH. Hypothyroid patients may appear falsely to be GH deficient; with thyroid hormone repletion, GH secretion normalizes. Gonadal steroids are important in the pubertal growth spurt. The effects of other hormones on growth are noted in Table 173.1.

ABNORMALITIES OF GROWTH

Short Stature of Nonendocrine Causes

Decision-Making Algorithm
Available @ StudentConsult.com
Short Stature

Short stature is defined as subnormal height relative to other children of the same gender and age, taking family heights into consideration. It can be caused by numerous conditions (Table 173.2). The Centers for Disease Control and Prevention growth charts use the 3rd percentile of the growth curve as the demarcation of the lower limit. **Growth failure** denotes a slow growth rate regardless of stature. Ultimately a slow growth rate leads to short stature, but a disease process is detected sooner if the decreased growth rate is noted before the stature becomes short. Plotted on a growth chart, growth failure appears as a curve that crosses percentiles downward and is associated with a height velocity below the 5th percentile of height velocity for

TABLE 173.2 Causes of Short Stature

VARIATIONS OF NORMAL	**SYNDROMES OF SHORT STATURE**
Constitutional (delayed bone age)	Turner syndrome (syndrome of gonadal dysgenesis)
Genetic (short familial height)	Noonan syndrome
ENDOCRINE DISORDERS	Autosomal trisomy 13, 18, 21
GH deficiency	Laurence-Moon-Bardet-Biedl syndrome
Congenital	Prader-Willi syndrome
• Isolated GH deficiency	Autosomal abnormalities
• With other pituitary hormone deficiencies	Dysmorphic syndromes (e.g., Russell-Silver or Cornelia de Lange syndrome)
• With midline defects	Pseudohypoparathyroidism
• Pituitary agenesis	**CHRONIC DISEASE**
• With gene deficiency	Cardiac disorders
Acquired	Left-to-right shunt
• Hypothalamic/pituitary tumors	Heart failure
• Langerhans cell histiocytosis	Pulmonary disorders
• CNS infections and granulomas	Cystic fibrosis
• Head trauma (birth and later)	Asthma (severe steroid dependent)
• Hypothalamic/pituitary irradiation	Gastrointestinal disorders
• CNS vascular accidents	Malabsorption (e.g., celiac disease)
• Hydrocephalus	Disorders of swallowing
• Autoimmune	Inflammatory bowel disease
• Psychosocial dwarfism (functional GH deficiency)	Hepatic disorders
• Amphetamine treatment for hyperactivity*	Hematological disorders
Laron dwarfism (increased GH and decreased IGF-1)	Sickle cell anemia
Pygmies (normal GH and IGF-2 but decreased IGF-1)	Thalassemia
Hypothyroidism	Renal disorders
Glucocorticoid excess	Renal tubular acidosis
Endogenous	Chronic uremia
Exogenous	Immunological disorders
Diabetes mellitus under poor control	Connective tissue disease
Diabetes insipidus (untreated)	Juvenile idiopathic arthritis
Hypophosphatemic vitamin D-resistant rickets	Chronic infection
Virilizing congenital adrenal hyperplasia (tall child, short adult) $P\text{-}450_{c21}$, $P\text{-}450_{c11}$ deficiencies	AIDS
SKELETAL DYSPLASIAS	Hereditary fructose intolerance
Osteogenesis imperfecta	Malnutrition
Osteochondrodysplasias	Kwashiorkor, marasmus
LYSOSOMAL STORAGE DISEASES	Iron deficiency
Mucopolysaccharidoses	Zinc deficiency
Mucolipidoses	Anorexia caused by chemotherapy for neoplasms
	Cerebral palsy

Only if caloric intake is severely diminished.
AIDS, Acquired immunodeficiency syndrome; *CNS*, central nervous system; *GH*, growth hormone; *IGF*, insulin-like growth factor.
Modified from Styne DM. Growth disorder. In: Fitzgerald PA, ed. Handbook of Clinical Endocrinology. *Norwalk, CT: Appleton & Lange; 1986.*

age (Fig. 173.1). A corrected midparental, or genetic target, height helps determine whether the child is growing well for the family (see Chapter 6). To determine a range of normal height for the family under consideration, the corrected midparental height is bracketed by 2 standard deviations (SDs), which, for the United States, is approximately 10 cm (4 in.). The presence of a height 3.5 SDs below the mean, a height velocity below the 5th percentile for age, or a height below the target height corrected for midparental height requires a diagnostic evaluation.

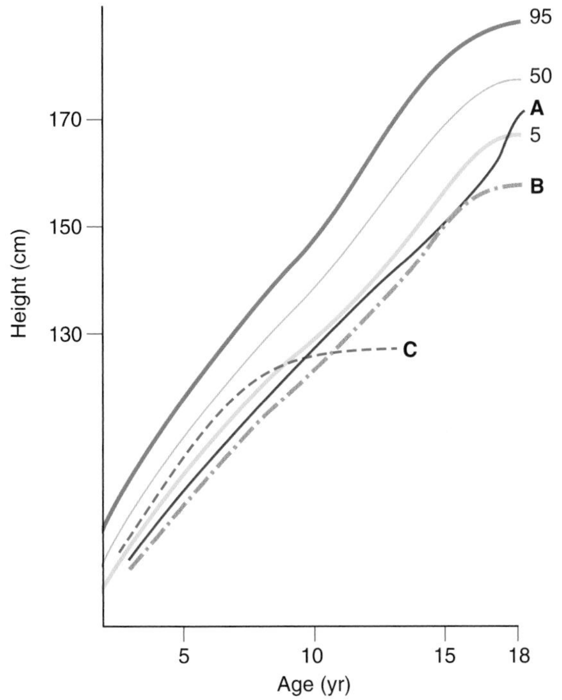

FIGURE 173.1 Patterns of linear growth. Normal growth percentiles (5th, 50th, and 95th) are shown along with typical growth curves for *(A)* constitutional delay of growth and adolescence (short stature with normal growth rate for bone age, delayed pubertal growth spurt, and eventual achievement of normal adult stature); *(B)* familial short stature (short stature in childhood and as an adult); and *(C)* acquired pathological growth failure (e.g., acquired untreated primary hypothyroidism) (see Chapter 5).

Nutrition is the most important factor affecting growth on a worldwide basis (see Chapter 28). Failure to thrive may develop in the infant as a result of **maternal deprivation** (nutritional deficiency or aberrant psychosocial interaction) or as a result of organic illness (anorexia, nutrient losses through a form of malabsorption, or hypermetabolism caused by hyperthyroidism or other causes; see Chapter 21). Psychological difficulties also can affect growth, as in **psychosocial** or **deprivation dwarfism,** in which the child develops functional temporary GH deficiency and poor growth as a result of psychological abuse; when placed in a different, healthier psychosocial environment, GH physiology normalizes, and growth occurs.

The common condition known as **constitutional delay** in growth or puberty or both is considered a variation of normal growth, caused by a reduced tempo, or cadence, of physiological development (see Fig. 173.1). Usually a family member had delayed growth or puberty but achieved a normal final height. The bone age is delayed, but the growth rate remains mostly within the lower limits of normal. Constitutional delay usually leads to a delay in secondary sexual development. **Genetic or familial short stature** (Table 173.3) refers to the stature of a child of short parents, who is expected to reach a lower than average height and yet normal for these parents. If the parents were malnourished as children, grew up in a zone of war, or suffered famine, the heights of the parents are less predictive.

Phenotypic features suggesting an underlying chromosomal disorder can occur in many syndromes. These syndromes can be suspected by attending to arm spans and upper-to-lower segment ratios. Genetic syndromes often combine obesity and decreased height, whereas otherwise normal obese children are usually taller than average and have advanced skeletal development and physical maturation (see Table 173.2). The **Prader-Willi syndrome** includes fetal and infantile hypotonia, small hands and feet, postnatal acquired obesity with an insatiable appetite, developmental delay, hypogonadism, almond-shaped eyes, and abnormalities on the snRNP (small nuclear ribonucleic particle) portion of the 15th chromosome at 15q11-q13. Most cases have deletion of the paternal sequence, but about 20-25% have uniparental disomy, in which both chromosomes 15 derive from the mother. **Laurence-Moon-Bardet-Biedl syndrome** is characterized by retinitis pigmentosa, hypogonadism, and developmental delay with an autosomal dominant inheritance pattern. Laurence-Moon syndrome is associated with spastic paraplegia; Bardet-Biedl syndrome is associated with obesity and polydactyly. **Pseudohypoparathyroidism** leads to short stature and developmental delay with short fourth and fifth digits (Albright hereditary osteodystrophy phenotype), resistance to parathyroid hormone and resultant hypocalcemia, and elevated levels of serum phosphorus. **Turner syndrome** is characterized by a karyotype of 45,XO or by a mosaic karyotype and clinically presents with short stature, shield chest, wide-spaced nipples, wide-carrying angle of the upper extremities, high-arched palate, gonadal failure, kidney dysplasias with normal function, and aortic arch abnormalities. Affected girls are often susceptible to autoimmune disorders.

Decision-Making Algorithms
Available @ StudentConsult.com

Hypotonia and Weakness
Short Stature
Pubertal Delay
Obesity
Hypocalcemia

Short Stature Caused by Growth Hormone Deficiency

Etiology and Epidemiology

Decision-Making Algorithm
Available @ StudentConsult.com

Short Stature

Classic congenital or **idiopathic GH deficiency** occurs in about 1 in 4,000 children. Idiopathic GH deficiency, of unidentified specific etiology, is the most common cause of both congenital and acquired GH deficiency. Less often, GH deficiency is caused by anatomical defects of the pituitary gland, such as pituitary aplasia or other midline defects, with variable degrees of deficiency of other pituitary functions. Hereditary forms of GH deficiency that affect pituitary differentiation are the result of heterogeneous defects of the gene for GH, GRF, or GH receptor. *Classic GH deficiency* refers to very reduced to absent secretion of GH; numerous short children may have intermediate forms of decreased GH secretion. Acquired GH deficiency causing late-onset growth failure suggests the possibility of a **tumor** of the hypothalamus or pituitary causing compression of the area (see Tables 173.2 and 173.3).

TABLE 173.3 Differential Diagnosis and Therapy of Short Stature

DIAGNOSTIC FEATURE	HYPOPITUITARISM GH DEFICIENCY*	CONSTITUTIONAL DELAY	FAMILIAL SHORT STATURE	DEPRIVATIONAL DWARFISM	TURNER SYNDROME	HYPOTHYROIDISM	CHRONIC DISEASE
Family history positive	Rare	Frequent	Always	No	No	Variable	Variable
Gender	Both	Males more often affected than females	Both	Both	Female	Both	Both
Facies	Immature or with midline defect (e.g., cleft palate or optic hypoplasias)	Immature	Normal	Normal	Turner facies or normal	Coarse (cretin if congenital)	Normal
Sexual development	Delayed	Delayed	Normal	May be delayed	Female prepubertal	Usually delayed, may be precocious if hypothyroidism is severe	Delayed
Bone age	Delayed	Delayed	Normal	Usually delayed; growth arrest lines present	Delayed	Delayed	Delayed
Dentition	Delayed	Normal; delay usual	Normal	Variable	Normal	Delayed	Normal or delayed
Hypoglycemia	Variable	No	No	No	No	No	No
Karyotype	Normal	Normal	Normal	Normal	45,X or partial deletion of X chromosome or mosaic	Normal	Normal
Free T_4	Low (with TRH deficiency) or normal	Normal	Normal	Normal or low	Normal: hypothyroidism may be acquired	Low	Normal
Stimulated GH	Low	Normal for bone age	Normal	Possibly low, or high if patient malnourished	Usually normal	Low	Usually normal
Insulin-like growth factor-1	Low	Normal or low for chronological age	Normal	Low	Normal	Low	Low or normal (depending on nutritional status)
Therapy	Replace deficiencies	Reassurance; sex steroids to initiate secondary sexual development in selected patients	None	Change or improve environment	Sex hormone replacement, GH; oxandrolone may be useful	T_4	Treat malnutrition, organ failure (e.g., dialysis, transplant, cardiotonic drugs, insulin)

**Possibly with GnRH, CRH, or TRH deficiency.*
CRH, Corticotropin-releasing hormone; *GH,* growth hormone; *GnRH,* gonadotropin-releasing hormone; *TRH,* thyrotropin-releasing hormone; *T_4,* thyroxine.

Clinical Manifestations

Infants with congenital GH deficiency achieve a normal or near-normal birth length and weight at term, but the growth rate slows after birth, most noticeably after age 2-3 years. These children become progressively shorter for age and tend to have an elevated weight-to-height ratio. Careful measurements in the first year of life may suggest the diagnosis, but most patients elude diagnosis until several years of age. A patient with classic GH deficiency has the appearance of a **cherub (a chubby, immature appearance),** with a high-pitched voice resulting from an immature larynx. Unless severe hypoglycemia occurs or dysraphism (midline defects) of the head includes a central nervous system (CNS) defect that affects mentation, the patient has normal intellectual growth and age-appropriate speech. Male neonates with isolated GH deficiency with or without gonadotropin deficiency may have a microphallus (a stretched penile length of <2 cm [normal is 3-5 cm]) and fasting hypoglycemia. Patients who lack the adrenocorticotropic hormone (ACTH, stimulates cortisol) in addition to GH may have more profound hypoglycemia because cortisol also stimulates gluconeogenesis.

A very rare cause of growth failure is GH resistance or GH insensitivity, caused by abnormal number or function of GH receptors or by a postreceptor defect. Patients with the autosomal recessive **Laron syndrome,** involving mutations of the GH receptor, have a prominent forehead, hypoplastic nasal bridge, delayed dentition, sparse hair, blue sclerae, delayed bone maturation and osteoporosis, progressive adiposity, hypercholesterolemia, and low blood glucose. They have elevated serum GH concentrations, although serum IGF-1 and IGF-BP3 concentrations are low. Malnutrition, medications (corticosteroids), or severe liver disease may cause **acquired GH resistance** because serum GH is elevated and IGF-1 is decreased.

Diagnosis

If family or other medical history does not provide a likely diagnosis, screening tests should include a metabolic panel to evaluate kidney and liver function, a complete blood count (CBC) to rule out anemia, a celiac panel to rule out celiac disease, erythrocyte sedimentation rate (ESR), thyroid function testing, and IGF-1, IGFBP-3 for children under age 3 years. A urine study should be performed to assess renal function and evaluate for renal tubular acidosis. In a girl, a karyotype to rule out **Turner syndrome** should be considered. A bone age will establish skeletal maturation.

If chronic disease or familial short stature are ruled out and routine laboratory testing is normal (Table 173.4), two GH stimulatory tests are commonly performed (see Table 170.2). GH testing should be offered to a patient who is short (<5th percentile and usually >3.5 SDs below the mean), growing poorly (<5th percentile growth rate for age), or whose height projection, based on bone age, is considerably below the target height when corrected for family height.

Classic GH-deficient patients do not show an increase in serum GH levels after stimulation. Some patients release GH in response to secretagogue testing but cannot release GH spontaneously during the day or night. Tests for GH secretion are insensitive, not very specific, and fairly variable. In equivocal cases, an operational definition of GH deficiency might be that patients grow significantly faster when administered a normal dose of GH than before treatment.

TABLE 173.4 Growth Failure: Screening Tests

TEST	RATIONALE
CBC	*Anemia:* nutritional, chronic disease, malignancy *Leukopenia:* bone marrow failure syndromes *Thrombocytopenia:* malignancy, infection
ESR, CRP	Inflammation of infection, inflammatory diseases, malignancy
Metabolic panel (electrolytes, liver enzymes, BUN)	Signs of acute or chronic hepatic, renal, adrenal dysfunction; hydration and acid-base status
Carotene, folate, and prothrombin time; celiac antibody panel	Assess malabsorption; detect celiac disease
Urinalysis with pH	Signs of renal dysfunction, hydration, water and salt homeostasis; renal tubular acidosis
Karyotype	Determines Turner (XO) or other syndromes
Cranial imaging (MRI)	Assesses hypothalamic-pituitary tumors (craniopharyngioma, glioma, germinoma) or congenital midline defects
Bone age	Compare with height age and evaluate height potential
IGF-1, IGF-BP3	Reflects growth hormone status or nutrition
Free thyroxine	Detects MPHD or isolated hypothyroidism
Prolactin	Elevated in hypothalamic dysfunction or destruction, suppressed in pituitary disease

BUN, Blood urea nitrogen; *CBC,* complete blood count; *CRP,* C-reactive protein; *ESR,* erythrocyte sedimentation rate; *IGF-1,* insulin-like growth factor-1; *IGF-BP3,* insulin-like growth factor-binding protein 3; *MRI,* magnetic resonance imaging; *MPHD,* multiple pituitary hormone deficiency.

Treatment

GH deficiency is treated with biosynthetic recombinant DNA-derived GH. Dosage is titrated to the growth rate, weight of the patient, and IGF-1 levels. Treatment with GH carries the low risk of an increased incidence of slipped capital femoral epiphysis, especially in rapidly growing adolescents, and of pseudotumor cerebri. Patients who have GH deficiency due to treatment for malignancy may be at higher risk for a secondary malignancy with GH therapy. Risks and benefits must be weighed with the family and treatment team.

Administration of GH to patients with normal GH responsiveness to secretagogues is controversial, but, as noted earlier, diagnostic tests are imperfect; if the patient is growing extremely slowly without alternative explanation, GH therapy is sometimes used. GH is effective in increasing the growth rate and final height in Turner syndrome and in chronic renal failure; GH also is used for treatment of short stature and muscle weakness of Prader-Willi syndrome. Other indications include children born small for gestational age who have not exhibited catch-up growth by 2 years of age and the long-term treatment of idiopathic short stature with height 2.25 SDs or less below the mean. Psychological support of children with severe short stature is important. Although there is controversy, marital status, satisfaction with life, and vocational achievement may be decreased in children of short stature who are not given supportive measures.

CHAPTER 174

Disorders of Puberty

PHYSIOLOGY

The staging of pubertal changes and the sequence of events are discussed in Chapter 67. The onset of puberty is marked by pubarche and gonadarche. **Pubarche** results from adrenal maturation or adrenarche and is marked with the appearance of pubic hair; other features include oiliness of hair and skin, acne, axillary hair, and body odor. **Gonadarche** is characterized by increasing secretion of gonadal sex steroids as a result of the maturation of the hypothalamic-pituitary-gonadal axis. These sex steroids differ by gender, consisting of testosterone from the testes and estradiol and progesterone from the ovaries. In males physical signs are pubic hair, axillary hair, facial hair, increased muscularity, deeper voice, increased penile size, and increased testicular volume. In females the physical signs are breast development, development of the female body habitus, increased size of the uterus, and menarche with regular menstrual cycles. The third component is the growth spurt of puberty.

Hypothalamic gonadotropin-releasing hormone (GnRH), produced by cells in the arcuate nucleus, is secreted from the median eminence of the hypothalamus into the pituitary portal system and reaches the membrane receptors on the pituitary gonadotropes to cause the production and release of luteinizing hormone (LH) and follicle-stimulating hormone (FSH) into the circulation. Mutations in genes encoding neurokinin B and neurokinin B receptor can alter the timing of puberty. Neurokinin B might play a role in regulating the secretion of kisspeptin, a compound responsible for the release of GnRH and, indirectly, release of LH and FSH. The hypothalamic-pituitary-gonadal axis is active in the fetus and newborn but is suppressed in the childhood years until activity increases again at the onset of puberty.

In females FSH stimulates the ovarian production of estrogen and, later in puberty, causes the formation and support of corpus luteum. In males LH stimulates the production of testosterone from the Leydig cells; later in puberty, FSH stimulates the development and support of the seminiferous tubules. The gonads also produce the protein inhibin. Both sex steroids and inhibin suppress the secretion of gonadotropins. The interplay of the products of the gonads and GnRH modulates the serum concentrations of gonadotropins. GnRH is released in episodic pulses that vary during development and during the menstrual period. These pulses ensure that gonadotropins are released in a pulsatile manner. With the onset of puberty, the amplitude of the pulses of gonadotropins and, in turn, the sex steroids increases, first at night and then throughout the day. Adrenarche generally occurs several years earlier than gonadarche and is heralded by increasing circulating dehydroepiandrosterone (DHEA) or androstenedione. Serum DHEA increases years before the appearance of its effects.

The typical developmental sequence in girls is **thelarche** (due to gonadarche), followed closely by **pubarche** (due to adrenarche), and finally **menarche** 2-3 years later. In boys the first typical event is scrotal thinning followed by the enlargement of testes and by the appearance of pubic hair (long diameter of the testis >2.5 cm, volume >4 mL). Most of the enlargement of testes during puberty is the result of seminiferous tubule maturation.

DELAYED PUBERTY

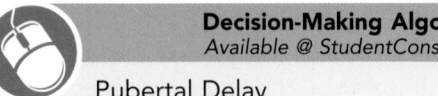

Decision-Making Algorithm
Available @ StudentConsult.com
Pubertal Delay

Puberty is delayed when there is no sign of pubertal development by age 13 years in girls and 14 years in boys living in the United States (Tables 174.1 and 174.2).

Constitutional Delay in Growth and Adolescence

Patients with constitutional delay have delayed onset of pubertal development and significant bone age delay (2 standard deviations below the mean, which is equal to a 1.5- to 2-year delay as a teenager). Usually height gain is below, although fairly parallel to, the normal percentiles on the growth curve. The prepubertal nadir, or deceleration before their pubertal growth spurt, is prolonged or protracted. A family history of delayed puberty in a parent or sibling is reassuring. Spontaneous puberty usually begins in these patients by the time the bone age reaches 12 years in boys and 11 years in girls. Other causes of delayed puberty must be eliminated before a diagnosis of constitutional delay in puberty is made. Observation and reassurance are appropriate. Adult height normal for the genetic potential is generally attained. In some cases, boys may be treated with low-dose testosterone for a few months if the bone age is at least 11-12 years. Treatment is not required for longer than 4-8 months because endogenous hormone production usually ensues. Boys who do not initiate endogenous hormone production should be evaluated for other causes of hypogonadism. Estrogen treatment has been used in girls with constitutional delay, but there are no clear studies showing the added benefits. Young women with delayed puberty may need to be evaluated for primary amenorrhea.

Hypogonadotropic Hypogonadism

As a cause of delayed or absent puberty, hypogonadotropic hypogonadism may be difficult to distinguish from constitutional delay (see Tables 174.1 and 174.2). Hypogonadotropic hypogonadism precludes spontaneous entry into gonadarche; adrenarche usually occurs to some degree. Throughout childhood and in early puberty, patients with hypogonadotropic hypogonadism have normal proportions and growth. When these patients reach adulthood, *eunuchoid* proportions may ensue because their long bones grow for longer than normal, producing an upper-to-lower ratio below the lower limit of normal of 0.9 and an arm span greater than their height.

TABLE 174.1 Classification of Delayed Puberty and Sexual Infantilism

CONSTITUTIONAL DELAY IN GROWTH AND PUBERTY
HYPOGONADOTROPIC HYPOGONADISM
CNS disorders
Tumors (craniopharyngioma, germinoma, glioma, prolactinoma)
Congenital malformations
Radiation therapy
Other causes
Isolated gonadotropin deficiency
Kallmann syndrome (anosmia-hyposmia)
Other disorders
Idiopathic and genetic forms of multiple pituitary hormone deficiencies
Miscellaneous disorders
Prader-Willi syndrome
Laurence-Moon-Bardet-Biedl syndrome
Functional gonadotropin deficiency
• Chronic systemic disease and malnutrition
• Hypothyroidism
• Cushing disease
• Diabetes mellitus
• Hyperprolactinemia
• Anorexia nervosa
• Psychogenic amenorrhea
Impaired puberty and delayed menarche in female athletes and ballet dancers (exercise amenorrhea)
HYPERGONADOTROPIC HYPOGONADISM
Klinefelter syndrome (syndrome of seminiferous tubular dysgenesis) and its variants
Other forms of primary testicular failure
Anorchia and cryptorchidism
Syndrome of gonadal dysgenesis and its variants (Turner syndrome)
Other forms of primary ovarian failure
XX and XY gonadal dysgenesis
Familial and sporadic XX gonadal dysgenesis and its variants
Familial and sporadic XY gonadal dysgenesis and its variants
Noonan syndrome
Galactosemia

CNS, Central nervous system.
Modified from Grumbach MM, Styne DM. Puberty. In: Wilson JD, Foster DW, eds. Williams Textbook of Endocrinology. *9th ed. Philadelphia: WB Saunders; 1998.*

Isolated Gonadotropin Deficiency

Decision-Making Algorithms
Available @ StudentConsult.com

Pubertal Delay
Obesity

Disorders that can cause hypogonadism include congenital hypopituitarism, such as midline defects, tumors, infiltrative disease (hemochromatosis), and many syndromes, including Laurence-Moon-Bardet-Biedl, Prader-Willi, and Kallmann syndromes. If there is an inability to release gonadotropins but no other pituitary abnormality, the patient has isolated gonadotropin deficiency (almost universally a result of absent GnRH). Patients grow normally until the time of the pubertal growth spurt, when they fail to experience the accelerated growth characteristic of the normal growth spurt. There are a number of additional genetic mutations associated with hypogonadism that are very rare (*GnRH1, DAX1, TAC3, FGF8,* and others).

Kallmann syndrome combines isolated gonadotropin deficiency with disorders of olfaction. There is genetic heterogeneity; some patients have a decreased sense of smell, others have abnormal reproduction, and some have both. Most cases are sporadic, but a number of patients may have mutations in the *KAL1* gene at Xp 22.3 (X chromosome), *KAL2* gene (8p11.2), or *KAL3* gene (20p13). The mutation causes the GnRH neurons to remain ineffectually located in the primitive nasal area, rather than migrating to the correct location at the medial basal hypothalamus. Olfactory bulbs and olfactory sulci are often absent on magnetic resonance imaging (MRI). Other symptoms include disorders of the hand, with one hand copying the movements of the other hand, shortened fourth metacarpal bone, and an absent kidney.

Abnormalities of the Central Nervous System

Decision-Making Algorithms
Available @ StudentConsult.com

Amenorrhea
Pubertal Delay

Central nervous system (CNS) tumors, including pituitary adenoma, glioma, prolactinoma, or craniopharyngioma, are important causes of gonadotropin deficiency. Craniopharyngiomas have a peak incidence in the teenage years and may cause any type of anterior or posterior hormone deficiency. Craniopharyngiomas usually calcify, eroding the sella turcica when they expand. They may impinge on the optic chiasm, leading to bitemporal hemianopsia and optic atrophy. Other tumors that may affect pubertal development include astrocytomas and gliomas.

Idiopathic hypopituitarism is the congenital absence of various combinations of pituitary hormones. Genes associated with this include *HESX1, PROP1, POU1F1(PIT1), LHX3, LHX4, TBX19, SOX2,* and *SOX3*. Although this disorder may occur in family constellations, in X-linked or autosomal recessive patterns, sporadic types of congenital idiopathic hypopituitarism are more common. Congenital hypopituitarism may manifest in a male with growth hormone (GH) deficiency and associated gonadotropin deficiency with a microphallus or with hypoglycemia with seizures, especially if adrenocorticotropic hormone and GH deficiency occurs as well.

TABLE 174.2 Differential Diagnostic Features of Delayed Puberty and Sexual Infantilism

CAUSATIVE CONDITION/ DISORDER	STATURE	PLASMA GONADOTROPINS	GNRH TEST: LH RESPONSE	PLASMA GONADAL STEROIDS	PLASMA DHEAS	KARYOTYPE	OLFACTION
Constitutional delay in growth and adolescence	Short for chronological age, usually appropriate for bone age	Prepubertal, later pubertal	Prepubertal, later pubertal	Prepubertal, later normal	Low for chronological age, appropriate for bone age	Normal	Normal
HYPOGONADOTROPIC HYPOGONADISM							
Isolated gonadotropin deficiency	Normal, absent pubertal growth spurt	Low	Prepubertal or no response	Low	Appropriate for chronological age	Normal	Normal
Kallmann syndrome	Normal, absent pubertal growth spurt	Low	Prepubertal or no response	Low	Appropriate for chronological age	Normal	Anosmia or hyposmia
Idiopathic multiple pituitary hormone deficiencies	Short stature and poor growth since early childhood	Low	Prepubertal or no response	Low	Usually low	Normal	Normal
Hypothalamic-pituitary tumors	Decrease in growth velocity of late onset	Low	Prepubertal or no response	Low	Normal or low for chronological age	Normal	Normal
PRIMARY GONADAL FAILURE							
Syndrome of gonadal dysgenesis and variants	Short stature since early childhood	High	Hyperresponsive for age	Low	Normal for chronological age	XO or variant	Normal
Klinefelter syndrome and variants	Normal to tall	High	Hyperresponsive at puberty	Low or normal	Normal for chronological age	XXY or variant	Normal
Familial XX or XY gonadal dysgenesis	Normal	High	Hyperresponsive for age	Low	Normal for chronological age	XX or XY	Normal

DHEAS, Dehydroepiandrosterone sulfate; *GnRH*, gonadotropin-releasing hormone; *LH*, luteinizing hormone.
From Grumbach MM, Styne DM. Puberty. In: Wilson JD, Foster DW, eds. Williams Textbook of Endocrinology. *9th ed. Philadelphia: WB Saunders; 1997.*

Syndromes of Hypogonadotropic Hypogonadism

Decision-Making Algorithms
Available @ StudentConsult.com

Amenorrhea
Pubertal Delay

Decreased gonadotropin function occurs when voluntary dieting, malnutrition, or chronic disease results in weight loss to less than 80% of ideal weight. **Anorexia nervosa** is characterized by striking weight loss and psychiatric disorders (see Chapter 70). Primary or secondary amenorrhea frequently is found in affected girls, and pubertal development is absent or minimal, depending on the level of weight loss and the age at onset. Regaining weight to the ideal level may not immediately reverse the condition. Increased physical activity, even without weight loss, can lead to decreased menstrual frequency and gonadotropin deficiency in **athletic amenorrhea;** when physical activity is interrupted, menstrual function may return. Chronic or systemic illness (e.g., cystic fibrosis, diabetes mellitus, inflammatory bowel disease, or hematological diseases) can lead to pubertal delay or to amenorrhea from hypothalamic dysfunction. **Hypothyroidism** inhibits the onset of puberty and delays menstrual periods. Conversely, severe primary hypothyroidism may lead to precocious puberty.

Hypergonadotropic Hypogonadism

Decision-Making Algorithms
Available @ StudentConsult.com

Pubertal Delay
Gynecomastia

Hypergonadotropic hypogonadism is characterized by elevated gonadotropins and low sex steroid levels resulting from primary gonadal failure. This permanent condition is almost always diagnosed following the lack of entry into gonadarche and is not suspected throughout childhood. Gonadotropins do not increase to greater than normal until shortly before or around the normal time of puberty.

Ovarian failure is diagnosed by elevated gonadotropins. **Turner syndrome** is a common cause of ovarian failure and short stature. The karyotype is classically 45,XO, but other abnormalities of the X chromosome, or mosaicism, are possible. The incidence of Turner syndrome is 1 in 2,000-1 in 3,000 births. The features of a girl with Turner syndrome need not be evident on physical examination or by history. The diagnosis must be considered in any girl who is short without a contributory history. Patients with other types of gonadal dysgenesis, or galactosemia, as well as patients who have undergone radiation therapy or chemotherapy for malignancy may develop ovarian failure.

Klinefelter syndrome (seminiferous tubular dysgenesis) is the most common cause of **testicular failure**. The karyotype is 47,XXY, but variants with more X chromosomes are possible. The incidence is approximately 1 in 500-1 in 1,000 in males. Testosterone levels may be close to normal, at least until mid-puberty, because Leydig cell function may be spared; however, seminiferous tubular function characteristically is lost, causing infertility. Commonly LH levels may be normal to elevated, whereas FSH levels are usually more unequivocally elevated. The age of onset of puberty is usually normal, but secondary sexual changes may not progress because of inadequate Leydig cell function.

Primary Amenorrhea

Decision-Making Algorithms
Available @ StudentConsult.com

Amenorrhea
Pubertal Delay

In addition to other diagnoses mentioned, other conditions need to be considered when evaluating girls with lack of menses. The Mayer-Rokitansky-Kuster-Hauser (MRKH) syndrome of congenital absence of the uterus occurs in 1 in 4,000-5,000 female births. Anatomical obstruction by imperforate hymen or vaginal septum also presents with normal secondary sexual development without menstruation. The complete syndrome of **androgen insensitivity** includes normal feminization, absence of pubic or axillary hair, and primary amenorrhea. In this syndrome, all müllerian structures, including ovaries, uterus, fallopian tubes, and upper third of the vagina, are lacking; the karyotype is 46,XY, and patients have intraabdominal testes.

Evaluation

When no secondary sexual development is present after the upper age limits of normal pubertal development, serum gonadotropin levels should be obtained to determine whether the patient has a hypogonadotropic or hypergonadotropic hypogonadism (see Table 174.2). Based on gonadotropin measurements only, the differentiation between constitutional delay in growth and hypogonadotropic hypogonadism is difficult; the gonadotropin levels are low in both conditions. Sometimes observation for months or years is necessary before the diagnosis is confirmed. Ultrasound of the pelvic structures in females would be helpful in the work-up of delayed puberty.

Treatment

If a permanent condition is apparent, replacement with sex steroids is indicated. Females are given titrated doses of transdermal estradiol, low-dose oral ethinyl estradiol, or conjugated estrogens until breakthrough bleeding occurs, at which time cycling is started with a dose for 25 days; on days 20-25, a progestational agent, such as medroxyprogesterone acetate (5 mg), is added to mimic the normal increases in gonadal hormones and to induce a normal menstrual period. Alternatively, combined estrogen and progesterone agents (oral contraceptives) may be used after breakthrough bleeding occurs. In males, testosterone enanthate or cypionate (50-100 mg monthly with a progressive increase to 100-200 mg) is given intramuscularly once every 4 weeks. This starting regimen is appropriate for patients with hypogonadotropic or hypergonadotropic hypogonadism, and doses are increased gradually to adult levels, often increasing the frequency of injections as needed. Alternatively, patients are transitioned to daily topical testosterone agents to keep levels more consistent. Oral agents are not used for fear of hepatotoxicity. Patients with apparent constitutional delay in puberty who have, by definition, passed the upper limits of normal onset of puberty may be given a 3- to 6-month course of low-dose, sex-appropriate gonadal steroids to see whether spontaneous puberty occurs. This course of therapy might be repeated once without undue advancement of bone age.

All patients with any form of delayed puberty are at risk for decreased bone density; adequate calcium intake is essential. Patients with hypogonadotropic hypogonadism may be able to achieve fertility by the administration of gonadotropin therapy or pulsatile hypothalamic-releasing hormone therapy administered by a programmable pump on an appropriate schedule.

In subjects with **Turner syndrome**, the goals of therapy include promoting growth with exogenous human GH supplementation and induction of the secondary sexual characteristics and of menses with low-dose cyclic estrogen/progesterone replacement therapy. Patients with Turner syndrome have had successful pregnancies after in vitro fertilization with a donor ovum and endocrine support.

SEXUAL PRECOCITY

Decision-Making Algorithms
Available @ StudentConsult.com

Precocious Puberty in the Male
Precocious Puberty in the Female

Classification

Sexual precocity **(precocious puberty)** is classically defined as secondary sexual development occurring before the age of 9 years in boys or 8 years in girls (Tables 174.3 and 174.4). During the past 15-20 years, studies from the United States and Europe reported earlier breast development in girls, as compared to historical data. Studies clearly suggest an earlier age at puberty onset in American girls in the 1980s to 1990s compared to the 1930s and 1940s. However, age at menarche occurred at the same time or slightly earlier. Thus the time span from breast development to menarche seemed to have increased. The findings

TABLE 174.3 Classification of Sexual Precocity

TRUE PRECOCIOUS PUBERTY OR COMPLETE ISOSEXUAL PRECOCITY
Idiopathic true precocious puberty
CNS tumors
Hamartomas (ectopic GnRH pulse generator)
Other tumors
Other CNS disorders
True precocious puberty after late treatment of congenital virilizing adrenal hyperplasia
INCOMPLETE ISOSEXUAL PRECOCITY (GnRH-INDEPENDENT SEXUAL PRECOCITY)
Males
Chorionic gonadotropin-secreting tumors (hCG-dependent sexual precocity)
CNS tumors (e.g., germinoma, chorioepithelioma, teratoma)
Tumors in locations outside of the CNS (hepatoblastoma)
LH-secreting pituitary adenoma
Increased androgen secretion by adrenal or testis
Congenital adrenal hyperplasia (21-hydroxylase deficiency, 11-hydroxylase deficiency)
Virilizing adrenal neoplasm
Leydig cell adenoma
Familial male-limited precocious puberty
Females
Estrogen-secreting ovarian or adrenal neoplasms
Ovarian cysts
Males and females
McCune-Albright syndrome
Primary hypothyroidism
Peutz-Jeghers syndrome
Iatrogenic sexual precocity
VARIATIONS OF PUBERTAL DEVELOPMENT
Premature thelarche
Premature menarche
Premature adrenarche
Adolescent gynecomastia
CONTRASEXUAL PRECOCITY
Males (feminization)
Adrenal neoplasm
Increased extraglandular conversion of circulating steroids to estrogen
Females (virilization)
(Congenital adrenal hyperplasia, $P\text{-}450_{c21}$ deficiency, $P\text{-}450_{c11}$ deficiency, 3β-Hydroxysteroid dehydrogenase deficiency)
Virilizing adrenal neoplasms
Virilizing ovarian neoplasms (e.g., arrhenoblastomas)

CNS, Central nervous system; *GnRH,* gonadotropin-releasing hormone; *hCG,* human chorionic gonadotropin; *LH,* luteinizing hormone.
From Grumbach MM, Styne DM. Puberty. In: Wilson JD, Foster DW, eds. Williams Textbook of Endocrinology. *9th ed. Philadelphia: WB Saunders; 1998.*

could reflect that exogenous or lifestyle factors may influence the typical sequence of pubertal events.

Central precocious puberty, resulting in gonadarche, emanates from premature activation of the hypothalamic-pituitary-gonadal axis (GnRH-dependent). **Peripheral precocious puberty,** gonadarche or adrenarche, does not involve the hypothalamic-pituitary-gonadal axis (GnRH-independent).

Central Precocious Puberty (GnRH-Dependent Precocious Puberty)

In central precocious puberty, every endocrine and physical aspect of pubertal development is normal but too early; this includes tall stature, advanced bone age consistent with somatic age, increased sex steroid and pulsatile gonadotropin secretion, and increased response of LH to GnRH. The clinical course of central precocious puberty may wax and wane. Benign precocious puberty is the presumptive diagnosis in individuals who begin puberty early on a **constitutional** or **familial** basis. If no cause can be determined, the diagnosis is idiopathic precocious puberty, which occurs much more often in girls than in boys. Obese girls have earlier adrenarche, and sometimes menarche as well, than appropriate-weight girls. Compared with girls, boys with precocious puberty have a higher incidence of CNS disorders, such as tumors and hamartomas, precipitating the precocious puberty.

Almost any condition that affects the CNS, including hydrocephalus, meningitis, encephalitis, suprasellar cysts, head trauma, epilepsy, mental retardation, and irradiation, can precipitate central precocious puberty and must be considered before central precocious puberty is diagnosed. **Hamartomas** are nonmalignant tumors of the tuber cinereum with a characteristic appearance on computed tomography (CT) or MRI; biopsy is rarely required. The mass of GnRH neurons secrete GnRH and cause precocious puberty. Although hamartomas are not true neoplasms, they may require neurosurgical attention. The resulting precocious puberty is responsive to medical therapy with GnRH agonists, and surgery is rarely indicated.

GnRH-Independent Precocious Puberty

Decision-Making Algorithm
Available @ StudentConsult.com

Precocious Puberty in the Female

The most common cause of GnRH-independent precocious puberty, **McCune-Albright syndrome,** is more frequent in girls than boys and includes precocious gonadarche, a bone disorder with polyostotic fibrous dysplasia and hyperpigmented cutaneous macules (café-au-lait spots). The precocious gonadarche results from ovarian hyperfunction and sometimes cyst formation, leading to episodic estrogen secretion. This disorder results from a postconception somatic mutation in the G protein intracellular signaling system (specifically G_{sa}, which leads to unregulated constitutive activation of adenylate cyclase, and of cAMP in the absence of trophic hormone stimulation), in the affected cells in ovary, bone, and skin; other endocrine organs may also autonomously hyperfunction for the same reason. Hyperthyroidism, hyperadrenalism, or acromegaly may

TABLE 174.4 Differential Diagnosis of Sexual Precocity

CAUSATIVE DISORDER	SERUM GONADOTROPIN CONCENTRATION*	LH RESPONSE TO GNRH	SERUM SEX STEROID CONCENTRATIONS	GONADAL SIZE	MISCELLANEOUS
True precocious puberty	Pubertal values	Pubertal	Pubertal values of testosterone or estradiol	Normal pubertal testicular enlargement or ovarian and uterine enlargement (by sonography)	MRI scan of brain to rule out CNS tumor or other abnormality; bone scan for McCune-Albright syndrome
Incomplete sexual precocity (pituitary gonadotropin-independent)					
MALES					
Chorionic gonadotropin-secreting tumor in males	High hCG (low LH)	Prepubertal (suppressed)	Pubertal values of testosterone	Slight to moderate uniform enlargement of testes	Hepatomegaly suggests hepatoblastoma; MRI scan of brain if chorionic gonadotropin-secreting CNS tumor suspected
Leydig cell tumor in males	Suppressed	Suppressed	Very high testosterone	Irregular asymmetric enlargement of testes	
Familial male-limited precocious puberty	Suppressed	Suppressed	Pubertal values of testosterone	Testes symmetric and >2.5 cm but smaller than expected for pubertal development; spermatogenesis may occur	Familial; probably sex-linked, autosomal dominant trait
Premature adrenarche	Prepubertal	Prepubertal	Prepubertal testosterone; DHEAS values appropriate for pubic hair stage 2	Testes prepubertal	Onset usually after 6 yr of age; more frequent in brain-injured children
FEMALES					
Granulosa cell tumor (presentation may be similar to that with follicular cysts)	Suppressed	Suppressed	Very high estradiol	Ovarian enlargement on physical examination, MRI, CT, or sonography	Tumor often palpable on abdominal examination
Follicular cyst	Suppressed	Suppressed	Prepubertal to very high estradiol values	Ovarian enlargement on physical examination, MRI, CT, or sonography	Single or repetitive episodes; exclude McCune-Albright syndrome (e.g., perform skeletal survey and inspect skin)
Feminizing adrenal tumor	Suppressed	Suppressed	High estradiol and DHEAS values	Ovaries prepubertal	Unilateral adrenal mass
Premature thelarche	Prepubertal	Prepubertal	Prepubertal or early pubertal estradiol	Ovaries prepubertal	Onset usually before 3 yr of age
Premature adrenarche	Prepubertal	Prepubertal	Prepubertal estradiol; DHEAS values appropriate for pubic hair Tanner stage 2	Ovaries prepubertal	Onset usually after 6 yr of age; more frequent in brain-injured children

**In supersensitive assays.*

CNS, Central nervous system; *CT*, computed tomography; *DHEAS*, dehydroepiandrosterone sulfate; *GnRH*, gonadotropin-releasing hormone; *hCG*, human chorionic gonadotropin; *LH*, luteinizing hormone; *MRI*, magnetic resonance imaging.

Modified from Grumbach MM, Styne DM. Puberty. In: Wilson JD, Foster DW, eds. Williams Textbook of Endocrinology. *9th ed. Philadelphia: WB Saunders; 1997.*

occur. **Adrenal carcinomas** usually secrete adrenal androgens, such as DHEA; **adrenal adenomas** may virilize a child as a result of the production of androgen or may feminize a child as a result of the production of estrogen.

Boys may have precocious gonadarche on the basis of a rare entity called **familial male-limited precocious puberty.** This condition, with germ cell maturation caused by an X-limited dominant defect, produces constitutive activation of the LH receptor that leads to continuous production and secretion of testosterone without requiring LH or human chorionic gonadotropin (hCG).

hCG-secreting tumors stimulate LH receptors and increase testosterone secretion. These tumors may be found in various places, including the pineal gland (dysgerminomas) or the liver (hepatoblastoma).

Germinomas are noncalcifying hypothalamic or pineal tumors that frequently produce hCG, which may cause sexual precocity in prepubertal boys (hCG cross reacts with the LH receptor because of the similarity of structure between LH and hCG). **Optic** or **hypothalamic gliomas** (with or without neurofibromatosis), astrocytomas, and ependymomas may cause precocious puberty by disrupting the negative restraint of the areas of the CNS that normally inhibit pubertal development throughout childhood. These tumors may require radiotherapy, which contributes to a significant risk for hypopituitarism.

Ovarian cysts may occur once or may be recurrent. High serum estrogen values may mimic ovarian tumors. **Congenital adrenal hyperplasia (CAH)** is a cause of virilization in girls (see Chapter 177).

Evaluation of Sexual Precocity

The first step in evaluating sexual precocity is to determine which characteristics of normal puberty are apparent (see Chapter 67) and whether estrogen effects, androgen effects, or both are present (see Table 174.4). In girls the estrogen effect manifests as breast development, uterine increase, and, eventually, menarche. Both boys and girls manifest the androgen effect as adult body odor, pubic and axillary hair, and facial skin oiliness and acne. In boys it is also important to note whether the testes are enlarged more than 2.5 cm in length (4 mL volume), which implies gonadarche. If the testes are not enlarged but virilization is progressing, the source of the androgens may be the adrenal glands or exogenous sources.

Laboratory evaluation includes determination of adrenal androgen and sex steroid levels (testosterone, estradiol, DHEAS [dehydroepiandrosterone sulfate]) and baseline gonadotropin concentrations. The inherent nature of gonadotropin secretion is characterized by low secretory rates throughout childhood and pulsatile secretion in adolescents and adults. If baseline gonadotropin values are elevated into the normal pubertal range, central precocious puberty is likely. If baseline gonadotropins are low, however, no immediate conclusion may be drawn as to GnRH-dependent versus GnRH-independent precocious puberty. This distinction often requires the assessment of gonadotropin responsiveness to GnRH stimulation. A prepubertal GnRH response is FSH predominant, whereas a pubertal response is more LH predominant. Thyroid hormone determination also is useful because severe primary hypothyroidism can cause incomplete precocious puberty. If there is a suggestion of a CNS anomaly or a tumor (CNS, hepatic, adrenal, ovarian, or testicular), MRI of the brain and pituitary with and without contrast is indicated. MRI of the is recommended in patients with the diagnosis of central precocious puberty; however, the yield is generally low in girls over age 6. Boys as well as young girls have a higher risk of CNS lesions as a cause of precocious puberty.

Treatment

Long-acting, superactive analogs of GnRH (leuprolide depot, histrelin depot) are the treatment of choice for central precocious puberty. They suppress gonadotropin secretion by downregulating GnRH receptors in the pituitary gonadotropes (Table 174.5), causing gonadal secretion to revert to the prepubertal state. Boys with GnRH-independent premature Leydig cell and

TABLE 174.5 Pharmacological Therapy of Sexual Precocity

DISORDER	TREATMENT	ACTION AND RATIONALE
GnRH-dependent true or central precocious puberty	GnRH agonists	Desensitization of gonadotropes; blocks action of endogenous GnRH
GnRH-independent incomplete sexual precocity		
Girls		
Autonomous ovarian cysts	Medroxyprogesterone acetate	Inhibition of ovarian steroidogenesis; regression of cyst (inhibition of FSH release)
McCune-Albright syndrome	Medroxyprogesterone acetate*	Inhibition of ovarian steroidogenesis; regression of cyst (inhibition of FSH release)
Boys	Testolactone*	Inhibition of P-450 aromatase; blocks estrogen synthesis
Familial GnRH-independent sexual precocity with premature Leydig cell maturation	Ketoconazole*	Inhibition of P-450_{c17} (mainly 17,20-lyase activity)
	Spironolactone* or flutamide *and* testolactone	Antiandrogen inhibition of aromatase; blocks estrogen synthesis
	Medroxyprogesterone acetate*	Inhibition of testicular steroidogenesis

**If true precocious puberty develops, a GnRH agonist can be added.*
FSH, Follicle-stimulating hormone; *GnRH*, gonadotropin-releasing hormone.
Modified from Grumbach MM, Kaplan SL. Recent advances in the diagnosis and management of sexual precocity. Acta Paediatr Jpn. *1988;30(Suppl):155.*

germ cell maturation do not respond to GnRH analogs but require treatment with an inhibitor of testosterone synthesis (e.g., ketoconazole), an antiandrogen (e.g., spironolactone), or an aromatase inhibitor (e.g., testolactone or letrozole). Patients with precocious puberty from a hormone-secreting tumor require surgical removal, if possible. The precocious puberty of the McCune-Albright syndrome is GnRH independent and unresponsive to therapy with GnRH analog. Therapy is provided with testolactone and antiandrogens or antiestrogen, such as tamoxifen or aromatase inhibitor such as letrozole.

VARIATIONS IN PUBERTAL DEVELOPMENT

Isolated Premature Thelarche (Premature Breast Development)

Decision-Making Algorithm
Available @ StudentConsult.com

Precocious Puberty in the Female

Benign **premature thelarche** is the isolated appearance of unilateral or bilateral breast tissue in girls, usually at ages 6 months to 3 years. There are no other signs of puberty and no evidence of excessive estrogen effect (vaginal bleeding, thickening of the vaginal secretions, increased height velocity, or bone age acceleration). Ingestion or dermal application of estrogen-containing compounds must be excluded. Laboratory investigations are not usually necessary, but a pelvic ultrasound study rarely may be indicated to exclude ovarian disease. Girls with this condition should be re-evaluated at intervals of 6-12 months to ensure that apparent premature thelarche is not the beginning of progression into precocious puberty. The prognosis is excellent; if no progression occurs, no treatment other than reassurance is necessary.

Gynecomastia

Decision-Making Algorithm
Available @ StudentConsult.com

Gynecomastia

In males breast tissue is termed *gynecomastia,* and it may occur to some degree in 45-75% of normal pubertal boys (see Chapter 67). Androgens normally are converted to estrogen by aromatization; in early puberty, only modest amounts of androgens are produced, and the estrogen effect can overwhelm the androgen effects at this stage. Later in pubertal development, the androgen production is so great that there is little effect from the estrogen produced by aromatization. Gynecomastia also can suggest the possibility of **Klinefelter syndrome** as puberty progresses. Prepubertal gynecomastia suggests an unusual source of estrogen either from exogenous sources (oral or dermal estrogen administration is possible from contamination of food or ointments) or from endogenous sources (from abnormal function of adrenal gland or ovary or from increased peripheral aromatization).

Isolated Premature Adrenarche (Pubarche)

Decision-Making Algorithms
Available @ StudentConsult.com

Amenorrhea
Precocious Puberty in the Male
Precocious Puberty in the Female

The isolated appearance of pubic hair before age 6-7 years in girls or before age 9 years in boys is termed **premature pubarche,** usually resulting from adrenarche. It is relatively common. If the pubic hair is associated with any other feature of virilization (clitoral or penile enlargement or advanced bone age) or other signs (acne, rapid growth, or voice change), a detailed investigation for a pathological cause of virilization is indicated. Measurements of serum testosterone, 17-hydroxyprogesterone, and DHEAS are indicated to investigate the possibility of CAH. Ultrasound studies may reveal a hyperplastic adrenal gland or a virilizing adrenal or ovarian tumor. Most patients with isolated pubic hair do not have progressive virilization and simply have premature adrenarche *(pubarche)* resulting from premature activation of DHEA secretion from the adrenal gland. The skeletal maturation, as assessed by bone age, may be slightly advanced and the height slightly increased, but testosterone concentrations are normal. DHEA levels usually are high for prepubertal age but are consistent with Tanner (sexuality maturity rating) stages II and III. In girls, there have been studies linking premature adrenarche to the development of irregular menses or polycystic ovarian syndrome (PCOS) later in adolescence.

CHAPTER 175

Thyroid Disease

THYROID PHYSIOLOGY AND DEVELOPMENT

Thyrotropin-releasing hormone (TRH), a tripeptide synthesized in the hypothalamus, stimulates the release of pituitary thyroid-stimulating hormone (TSH). Pituitary TSH is a glycoprotein that stimulates the synthesis and release of thyroid hormones by the thyroid gland. Thyroid function develops in three stages. At the end of the first trimester, the gland descends from the floor of the primitive oral cavity to its definitive position in the anterior lower neck. The hypothalamic-pituitary-thyroid axis becomes functional in the second trimester. Peripheral metabolism of thyroid hormones matures in the third trimester.

Thyroxine (T_4), triiodothyronine (T_3), and TSH do not cross the placenta in significant amounts. Concentrations in fetal serum reflect primarily fetal secretion and metabolism. Maternal thyroid antibodies, iodides (including radioactive iodides), and medications given to mothers to treat hyperthyroidism (methimazole and propylthiouracil) cross the placenta and affect fetal thyroid function. An infant born prematurely or with intrauterine growth restriction may have an interruption of the normal maturational process and appear to have hypothyroidism by standard tests (and newborn screen).

The thyroid gland concentrates iodine and binds it to tyrosine molecules to produce either monoiodotyrosine or diiodotyrosine, with subsequent coupling of two tyrosines, T_4 or T_3. The major fraction of circulating T_3 (approximately 2/3) is derived from peripheral deiodination of T_4 to T_3, but some is produced by the gland itself. The conversion of T_4 to T_3 requires the removal of one iodine from the outer ring of tyrosine; removing an iodine from the inner ring results in reverse T_3, which has little biological effect. Preferential conversion of T_4 to reverse T_3 rather than T_3 occurs in utero and in all forms of severe illness, including respiratory distress syndrome, fevers, anorexia, and starvation. Conversion from T_4 to T_3 increases immediately after birth and throughout life. T_4 and T_3 are noncovalently bound to a specific serum carrier protein, **thyroxine-binding globulin,** and to a lesser extent, albumin. Only small (<0.02%) fractions of T_4 and T_3 are not bound; free T_4 (as it is converted to free T_3) and free T_3 are biologically active. Free T_3 exerts metabolic effects and negative feedback on TSH release (Fig. 175.1).

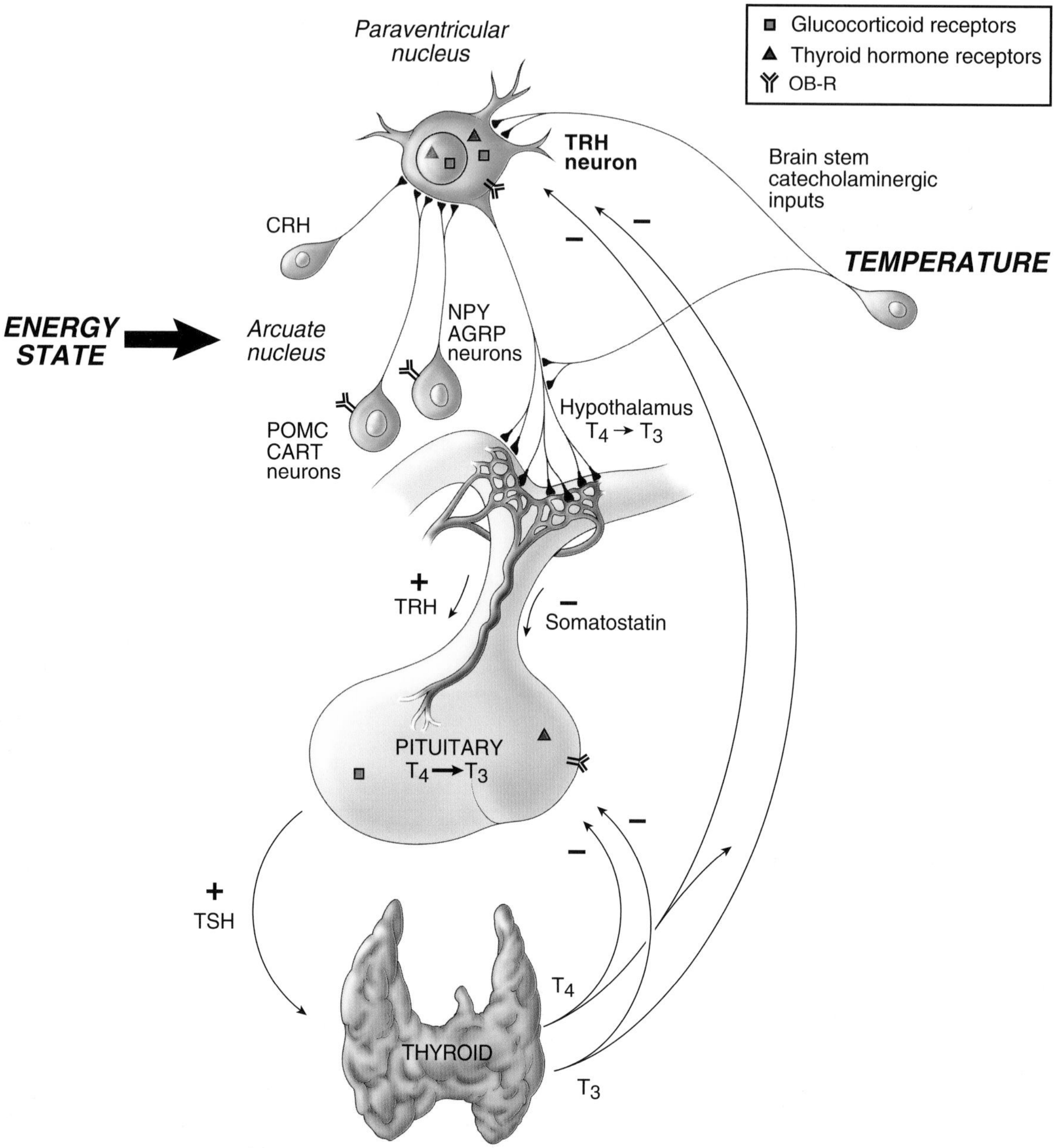

FIGURE 175.1 Interrelationships of the hypothalamic-pituitary-thyroid axis. Thyroid-stimulating hormone *(TSH)* from the pituitary gland stimulates the secretion of thyroxine *(T_4)* and triiodothyronine *(T_3)* from the thyroid gland. These act at the pituitary gland level to control secretion of TSH by a negative feedback mechanism. In addition, T_4 is metabolized to the potent T_3 within the pituitary gland by a deiodinase. Secretion of TSH is stimulated by thyrotropin-releasing hormone *(TRH)* from the hypothalamus and inhibited by somatostatin. Thyroid hormone acts at the hypothalamus to stimulate secretion of somatostatin (somatostatin acts as a negative signal to the pituitary secretion of TSH). *CRH,* Corticotropin-releasing hormone; *OB-R,* leptin receptor. (From Melmed S, Polonsky K, Kronenberg H, Larsen R, eds. *Williams Textbook of Endocrinology.* 10th ed. Philadelphia: Saunders; 2003:101.)

TABLE 175.1 Laboratory Test Results in Various Types of Thyroid Function Abnormalities in Children*

	SERUM			
ABNORMALITY	**TOTAL T_4**	**FREE T_4**	**SERUM TSH**	**SERUM TBG**
Primary hypothyroidism	↓	↓	↑	N
Hypothalamic (TRH) tertiary hypothyroidism	↓	↓	↓	N
Pituitary (TSH) secondary hypothyroidism	↓	↓	↓	N
TBG deficiency	↓	N	N	↓
TBG excess	↑	N	N	↑

**TSH may be slightly elevated.*
↓, Decreased; ↑, increased; *N*, Normal; *T_4*, thyroxine; *TBG*, thyroxine-binding globulin; *TRH*, thyrotropin-releasing hormone; *TSH*, thyroid-stimulating hormone.

Serum TSH increases just after birth but soon decreases to lower values considered normal for later life. T_4 secretion increases after birth as a result of the peak in TSH and because of maturation of thyroid metabolism. It is important to refer to age-adjusted normative data to interpret thyroid function tests properly, whether relative to making diagnoses of hyperthyroidism or hypothyroidism or when adjusting therapy. Free T_4 is the test of choice because it eliminates the effects of variation in protein binding, which can be substantial.

Table 175.1 summarizes laboratory test results in various types of thyroid abnormalities. In usual circumstances, plasma concentrations of TSH above the normal range indicate primary hypothyroidism and concentrations below the normal range most often indicate the presence of hyperthyroidism. Thyroid scans with 99m-pertechnetate or 123-I-iodine are occasionally indicated in the evaluation of pediatric thyroid disease. They can be useful in identifying thyroid agenesis or ectopic thyroid tissue.

THYROID DISORDERS

Hypothyroidism

Decision-Making Algorithms
Available @ StudentConsult.com

Short Stature
Pubertal Delay
Precocious Puberty in the Male
Precocious Puberty in the Female

Hypothyroidism is diagnosed by a decreased serum free T_4 and may be the result of diseases of the thyroid gland (primary hypothyroidism), abnormalities of the pituitary gland (secondary), or abnormalities of the hypothalamus (tertiary). Hypothyroidism is congenital or acquired and may or may not be associated with a goiter (Table 175.2).

TABLE 175.2 Causes of Hypothyroidism in Infancy and Childhood

AGE GROUP	MANIFESTATION	CAUSE
Newborn	No goiter	Thyroid gland dysgenesis or ectopic location
		Exposure to iodides
		TSH deficiency
		TRH deficiency
	± Goiter	Inborn defect in hormone synthesis* or effect
		Maternal goitrogen ingestion, including propylthiouracil, methimazole, iodides
		Severe iodide deficiency (endemic)
Child	No goiter	Thyroid gland dysgenesis
		Cystinosis
		Hypothalamic-pituitary insufficiency
		Surgical after thyrotoxicosis or other thyroid surgery
	Goiter	Hashimoto thyroiditis: chronic lymphocytic thyroiditis
		Inborn defect in hormone synthesis or effect
		Goitrogenic drugs, infiltrative (sarcoid, lymphoma)

**Impaired iodide transport, defective thyroglobulin iodination, defective iodotyrosine dehalogenase, or defective thyroglobulin or its coupling to iodotyrosine.*
TRH, Thyrotropin-releasing hormone; *TSH*, thyroid-stimulating hormone.

Congenital Hypothyroidism

Congenital hypothyroidism occurs in approximately 1 in 2,000-4,000 live births and is caused by dysgenesis (agenesis, aplasia, ectopia) or, less often, dyshormonogenesis (e.g., enzyme defects). Thyroid tissue usually is not palpable in these sporadic nongoitrous conditions. Dyshormonogenesis, disorders of intrathyroid metabolism, or goitrous congenital hypothyroidism occurs in about 1 in 30,000 live births. A goiter reflects an inborn error of metabolism in the pathway of iodide incorporation or thyroid hormone biosynthesis or reflects the transplacental passage of antithyroid drugs given to the mother. Routine neonatal screening programs to measure cord blood or heel-stick TSH values occur in every state in the United States. An immediate confirmatory serum sample should be obtained from any infant having a positive result on a **screening test**. A low free T_4 and high TSH confirm the finding.

Isolated secondary or tertiary hypothyroidism occurs in 1 in 100,000 live births; the free T_4 is normal to low, as is the TSH. When tertiary or secondary hypothyroidism is detected, assessment of other pituitary hormones and investigation of pituitary-hypothalamic anatomy via magnetic resonance imaging are indicated. Although not a hypothyroid condition, **congenital thyroxine-binding globulin deficiency** occurs in about 1 in 10,000 live births and is associated with low serum total T_4 concentration, normal TSH, and normal serum free T_4. This is a euthyroid condition and does not require treatment with thyroid hormone because it is merely a binding protein abnormality. It is commonly X-linked dominant.

Clinical manifestations of congenital hypothyroidism in the immediate newborn period usually are subtle but become more evident weeks or months after birth. By then it is too late to ensure that there is not a detriment to the infant's cognitive development. Newborn screening is crucial to make an early diagnosis and initiate thyroid replacement therapy by younger than 1 month of age. Findings at various stages after birth include hypothermia, acrocyanosis, respiratory distress, large fontanels, abdominal distention, lethargy and poor feeding, prolonged jaundice, edema, umbilical hernia, mottled skin, constipation, large tongue, dry skin, and hoarse cry. Thyroid hormones are crucial for maturation and differentiation of tissues, such as bone and brain (most thyroid-dependent brain maturation occurs in the first 2-3 years after birth; Table 175.3).

When **treatment** (with levothyroxine) is initiated within 1 month or less after birth, the prognosis for normal intellectual development is excellent. State screening programs usually allow for therapy within 1-2 weeks of birth. If therapy is instituted after 6 months when the signs of severe hypothyroidism are present, the likelihood of normal intellectual function is markedly decreased. Growth improves after thyroid replacement even in late diagnosed cases. The dose of levothyroxine changes with age; 10-15 µg/kg of levothyroxine is used for a newborn, but about 3 µg/kg is used later in childhood. In neonatal hypothyroidism, the goal is to bring the serum free T_4 rapidly into the upper half of the range of normal. Suppression of TSH is not seen and not necessary in all cases because such suppression may lead to excessive doses of levothyroxine.

Acquired Hypothyroidism

The **etiology** of acquired hypothyroidism is presented in Table 175.2. The clinical manifestations may be subtle. Hypothyroidism should be suspected in any child who has a decline in growth velocity, especially if **not** associated with weight loss (see Table 175.3). The most common cause of acquired hypothyroidism in older children in the United States is lymphocytic autoimmune thyroiditis **(Hashimoto thyroiditis).** In many areas of the world, iodine deficiency is the etiology of endemic goiter **(endemic cretinism).** The failure of the thyroid gland may be heralded by an increase of TSH before T_4 levels decrease. In contrast to untreated congenital hypothyroidism, acquired hypothyroidism is not a cause of permanent developmental delay.

Hashimoto Thyroiditis

Also known as autoimmune or *lymphocytic thyroiditis,* Hashimoto thyroiditis is a common cause of goiter and acquired thyroid disease in older children and adolescents. A family history of thyroid disease is present in 25-35% of patients. The *etiology* is an autoimmune process targeted against the thyroid gland with lymphocytic infiltration and lymphoid follicle and germinal center formation preceding fibrosis and atrophy.

Clinical manifestations include a firm, nontender euthyroid, hypothyroid, or, rarely, hyperthyroid (hashitoxicosis) diffuse goiter with a pebble-like surface. See Table 175.3 for signs and symptoms, which can be diverse. Onset typically occurs after

TABLE 175.3 Symptoms and Signs of Hypothyroidism
ECTODERMAL
Poor growth
Dull facies: thick lips, large tongue, depressed nasal bridge, periorbital edema
Dry scaly skin
Sparse brittle hair
Diminished sweating
Carotenemia
Vitiligo
CIRCULATORY
Sinus bradycardia/heart block
Cold extremities
Cold intolerance
Pallor
ECG changes: low-voltage QRS complex
NEUROMUSCULAR
Muscle weakness
Hypotonia: constipation, potbelly
Umbilical hernia
Myxedema coma (carbon dioxide narcosis, hypothermia)
Pseudohypertrophy of muscles
Myalgia
Physical and mental lethargy
Developmental delay
Delayed relaxation of reflexes
Paresthesias (nerve entrapment: carpal tunnel syndrome)
Cerebellar ataxia
SKELETAL
Delayed bone age
Epiphyseal dysgenesis, increased upper-to-lower segment ratio
METABOLIC
Myxedema
Serous effusions (pleural, pericardial, ascites)
Hoarse voice (cry)
Weight gain
Menstrual irregularity
Arthralgia
Elevated CK
Macrocytosis (anemia)
Hypercholesterolemia
Hyperprolactinemia
Precocious puberty in severe cases

CK, Creatine kinase; *ECG,* electrocardiographic.

6 years of age with a peak incidence in adolescence with a female predominance. Associated autoimmune diseases include celiac disease, type 1 diabetes mellitus, adrenal insufficiency, and hypoparathyroidism. **Autoimmune polyglandular syndrome type I** consists of hypoparathyroidism, Addison disease, mucocutaneous candidiasis, and hypothyroidism. **Autoimmune polyglandular syndrome type II** consists of Addison disease, type 1 diabetes mellitus, and frequently hypothyroidism. Trisomy 21 and Turner syndrome are predisposed to the development of autoimmune thyroiditis.

The **diagnosis** may be confirmed by serum antithyroid peroxidase (previously antimicrosomal) and antithyroglobulin antibodies. Neither biopsy nor thyroid scan is indicated in Hashimoto thyroiditis, although a thyroid scan with reduced uptake may differentiate hashitoxicosis from Graves disease.

Treatment with thyroid hormone sufficient to normalize TSH and free T_4 is indicated for hypothyroidism in Hashimoto thyroiditis. Patients without manifestation of hypothyroidism require thyroid function testing (serum TSH and free T_4) every 6-12 months to detect the later development of hypothyroidism. Goiter with a normal TSH usually is not an indication for treatment.

Hyperthyroidism

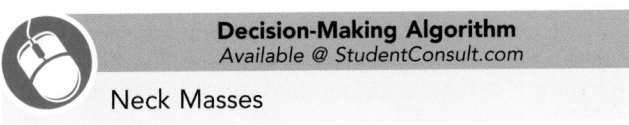

Decision-Making Algorithm
Available @ StudentConsult.com

Neck Masses

Graves Disease

Most children with hyperthyroidism have Graves disease, the autonomous functioning of the thyroid caused by autoantibodies (thyroid-stimulating immunoglobulins [TSIs]) stimulating the thyroid. The resulting excessive synthesis, release, and peripheral metabolism of thyroid hormones produce the clinical features. Hashimoto thyroiditis and thyrotoxicosis are on a continuum of autoimmune diseases; there is overlap in their immunological findings.

Antithyroid peroxidase and antithyroglobulin antibodies may be present in thyrotoxicosis, although the values are usually lower than in Hashimoto thyroiditis. Exceptionally high titers of antibodies may indicate the thyrotoxic phase of Hashimoto thyroiditis with the subsequent evolution toward permanent hypothyroidism. In Graves disease, serum free T_4, free T_3, or both levels are elevated, whereas TSH is suppressed. Rare causes of hyperthyroidism include McCune-Albright syndrome, thyroid nodule (often an adenoma), TSH hypersecretion, subacute thyroiditis, and iodine or thyroid hormone ingestion.

Clinical Manifestations

Graves disease presents as hyperthyroidism (Table 175.4) and is about five times more common in girls than in boys with a peak incidence in adolescence. Personality changes, mood instability, and poor school performance are common initial problems. Tremor, anxiety, inability to concentrate, and weight loss may be insidious and confused with a psychological disorder until thyroid function tests reveal the elevated serum free T_4 level. In rare cases, serum free T_4 may be near-normal, whereas serum T_3 is selectively elevated (T_3 toxicosis). A firm homogeneous goiter is usually present. Many patients complain of neck fullness. Thyroid gland enlargement is best visualized with the neck only slightly extended and with the examiner lateral to the patient. Palpation of the thyroid gland is best performed with the examiner's hands around the neck from the back. The patient swallows so that the examiner can feel and examine the size, consistency, nodularity, and motion of the gland. The examiner should watch the patient swallow to note any discernible enlargement or asymmetry of the thyroid lobes. Auscultation may reveal a bruit over the gland that needs to be differentiated from a carotid bruit.

TABLE 175.4 Clinical Manifestations of Hyperthyroidism

ASSOCIATED CHANGE	SIGN/SYMPTOM
Increased catecholamine effects	Nervousness
	Palpitations
	Tachycardia
	Atrial arrhythmias
	Systolic hypertension
	Tremor
	Brisk reflexes
Hypermetabolism	Increased sweating
	Shiny, smooth skin
	Heat intolerance
	Fatigue
	Weight loss—increased appetite
	Increased bowel movement (loose stools)
	Hyperkinesis
Myopathy	Weakness
	Periodic paralysis
	Cardiac failure—dyspnea
Miscellaneous	Proptosis, stare, exophthalmos, lid lag, ophthalmopathy
	Hair loss
	Inability to concentrate
	Personality change (emotional lability)
	Goiter
	Thyroid bruit
	Onycholysis
	Painful gland*
	Acute thyroid storm (hyperpyrexia, tachycardia, coma, high-output heart failure, shock)

**Unusual except in subacute thyroiditis with hyperthyroid phase.*

Treatment

Three treatment choices are available: pharmacological, radioactive iodine, and surgical.

Drugs

Medical therapy to block thyroid hormone synthesis consists of methimazole (0.4-0.6 mg/kg/day once or twice daily) or propylthiouracil (5-7 mg/kg/day divided every 8 hours). Both medications are equally effective; however, propylthiouracil is no longer a first-line therapy secondary to concerns of severe liver injury and acute liver failure. A β blocker, such as propranolol or atenolol, is started if symptoms are severe to control cardiac manifestations and is tapered as the methimazole takes effect. Antithyroid medication is usually continued for 1-2 years because the remission rate is approximately 25% per year. In patients complying with the treatment regimen, the 2-year course of treatment can be repeated. Medication should suppress thyroid function to normal without the need to add thyroid hormone replacement to normalize serum free T_4. Complications of methimazole are muscle pain, rash, granulocytopenia, and jaundice. The granulocytopenia is an idiosyncratic complication of rapid onset, which is observed only in the early months after institution of antithyroid medication and requires monitoring the complete blood count. If a suppressed white blood cell count is observed, antithyroid therapy must be discontinued. This potentially lethal rare complication affects 3 in 10,000 users a year. After resolution, the other of the two antithyroid medications can be started because there is usually less than a 50% chance of a similar reaction from the other medication. Iodine administration, which may suppress thyroid function but becomes ineffective in a few weeks, is sometimes used as a preparation for surgery, but never for long-term therapy.

Radioiodine

Radioiodine (^{131}I) is slower in exerting therapeutic effects, may require repeated dosing, and is likely to cause permanent hypothyroidism. Hypothyroidism is the desired outcome because it is easier and safer to treat than continued hyperthyroidism. Although studies reveal no long-term consequences, concern remains about possible sequelae in children. This method of treatment is entering the mainstream for children and adolescents. Radioiodine given to a pregnant teenager renders the fetus hypothyroid and is contraindicated.

Surgery

Surgical treatment consists of partial or complete thyroidectomy. Risks associated with thyroidectomy include the use of anesthesia and the possibility that the thyroid removal will be excessive, causing hypothyroidism, or that it will be inadequate, resulting in persistent hyperthyroidism. In addition, keloid formation, recurrent laryngeal nerve palsy, and hypoparathyroidism (transient postoperative or permanent) may occur. Thyroid storm caused by the release of large amounts of preformed hormone is a serious but rare complication. Even with optimal immediate postoperative results, patients may become hypothyroid within 10 years.

Thyroid Storm

Thyroid storm (see Table 175.4) is a rare medical emergency consisting of tachycardia, disorientation, elevated blood pressure, and hyperthermia. Treatment includes reducing the hyperthermia with a cooling blanket and administering a β blocker to control the tachycardia, hypertension, and autonomic hyperfunction symptoms. Iodine may be given to block thyroid hormone release after an antithyroid medication is started. Hydrocortisone may be indicated for relative adrenal insufficiency and therapy for heart failure includes diuretics and digoxin.

Congenital Hyperthyroidism

This disorder results from transplacental passage of maternal TSIs and may be masked for several days until the short-lived effects of transplacental maternal antithyroid medication wear off (assuming the mother was receiving such medication), at which time the effects of TSIs are observed. Irritability, tachycardia (often with signs of cardiac failure simulating *cardiomyopathy*), polycythemia, craniosynostosis, bone age advancement, poor feeding, and failure to thrive are the clinical hallmarks. This condition may be anticipated if the mother is known to be thyrotoxic or has an elevated TSI during third trimester of pregnancy. Cure of hyperthyroidism before pregnancy (surgery or radioiodine treatment) limits or curtails T_4 production but not the underlying immune disturbance producing TSIs; thus the infant still may be affected, at least transiently.

Treatment for a severely affected neonate includes methimazole and, as needed, a β blocker to help decrease symptoms. Because the half-life of the immunoglobulin is several weeks, spontaneous resolution of neonatal thyrotoxicosis resulting from transplacental passage of TSIs usually occurs by 2-3 months of age. Observation without treatment is indicated in patients who are minimally affected.

NODULES/TUMORS OF THE THYROID

About 2% of children develop solitary thyroid nodules, most of which are benign. Evaluation of a nodule includes thyroid function tests, neck ultrasound, and, if needed, fine-needle aspiration (FNA). Ultrasound guidance may be needed for aspiration of small nodules or those not palpable. Nodules found to be benign on FNA may be monitored through clinical exam and ultrasound.

Carcinoma of the thyroid is rare in children (1% of all pediatric cancers in the 5- to 9-year-old age group and up to 7% of cancers in the 15- to 19-year-old age group). Papillary and follicular carcinomas represent 90% of childhood thyroid cancers. A history of therapeutic head or neck irradiation or radiation exposure from nuclear accidents predisposes a child to thyroid cancer. Carcinoma usually presents as a firm to hard, painless, nonfunctional solitary nodule and may spread to adjacent lymph nodes. Rapid growth, hoarseness (recurrent laryngeal nerve involvement), and lung metastasis may be present. If the nodule is solid on ultrasound, is *cold* on radioiodine scanning, and feels hard, the likelihood of a carcinoma is high. Excisional biopsy usually is performed, but FNA biopsy also may be diagnostic.

Treatment includes total thyroidectomy, selective regional node dissection, and radioablation with ^{131}I for residual or recurrent disease. The **prognosis** is usually good if the disease is diagnosed early.

Medullary carcinoma of the thyroid may be asymptomatic except for a mass. Diagnosis is based on the presence of elevated calcitonin levels, either in the basal state or after pentagastrin stimulation (difficult to obtain) and histological examination. This tumor most often occurs with multiple endocrine neoplasia 2a or 2b (MEN), possibly in a familial pattern. In some families, the presence of mutations of the *RET* protooncogene is predictive of the development of medullary carcinoma of the thyroid. The location of the mutation can help determine when removal of the thyroid is warranted. Genetic screening of other members of the family is indicated after a proband is recognized. Prophylactic thyroidectomy is indicated for the family members with the same allele.

CHAPTER 176

Disorders of Parathyroid Bone and Mineral Endocrinology

PARATHYROID HORMONE AND VITAMIN D

Calcium and phosphate are regulated mainly by diet and three hormones: parathyroid hormone (PTH), vitamin D, and calcitonin. PTH is secreted in response to a decrease in serum ionized calcium level. PTH attaches to its membrane receptor then acts via adenylate cyclase to mobilize calcium from bone into the serum and to enhance fractional reabsorption of calcium by the kidney while inducing phosphate excretion; all increase the serum calcium concentration and decrease serum phosphate. Lack of PTH effect is heralded by low serum calcium in the presence of elevated phosphate for age. PTH stimulates vitamin D secretion by increasing renal 1α-hydroxylase activity and acts indirectly to elevate serum calcium concentration by stimulating the production of 1,25-dihydroxyvitamin D from 25-hydroxyvitamin D. Calcitonin increases the deposition of calcium into bone; in normal states the effect is subtle, but calcitonin may be used temporarily to suppress extremely elevated serum calcium values.

1,25-Dihydroxyvitamin D enhances calcium absorption from the gastrointestinal tract, increasing serum calcium levels and bone mineralization. Vitamin D is derived from exposure of the skin to ultraviolet rays (usually via the sun) or from oral ingestion. It is modified first to 25-hydroxyvitamin D in the liver and then 1α-hydroxylated to the metabolically active form (1,25-dihydroxyvitamin D) in the kidney. The serum concentration of 25-hydroxyvitamin D is a better reflection of vitamin D sufficiency than the measurement of 1,25-hydroxyvitamin D (see Chapter 31).

HYPOCALCEMIA

Decision-Making Algorithm
Available @ StudentConsult.com
Hypocalcemia

The **clinical manifestations** of hypocalcemia result from increased neuromuscular irritability and include muscle cramps, carpopedal spasm (tetany), weakness, paresthesia, laryngospasm, and seizure-like activity. Tetany can be detected by the *Chvostek sign* (facial spasms produced by lightly tapping over the facial nerve just in front of the ear) or by the *Trousseau sign* (carpal spasms exhibited when arterial blood flow to the hand is occluded for 3-5 minutes with a blood pressure cuff inflated to 15 mm Hg above systolic blood pressure). Total serum calcium concentration is usually measured, although a determination of serum ionized calcium, the biologically active form, is preferable. Albumin is the major reservoir of protein-bound calcium. Disorders that alter plasma pH or serum albumin concentration must be considered when circulating calcium concentrations are being evaluated. The fraction of ionized calcium is inversely related to plasma pH; **alkalosis** can precipitate hypocalcemia by lowering ionized calcium without changing total serum calcium. Alkalosis may result from hyperpnea caused by anxiety or from hyperventilation related to physical exertion. Hypoproteinemia may lead to a false suggestion of hypocalcemia because the serum total calcium level is low even though the ionized Ca^{2+} remains normal. It is best to measure serum ionized calcium if hypocalcemia or hypercalcemia is suspected.

Primary hypoparathyroidism causes hypocalcemia but does not cause rickets. The etiology of primary hypoparathyroidism includes the following:

1. Congenital malformation (e.g., DiGeorge syndrome or other complex syndromes) resulting from developmental abnormalities of the third and fourth branchial arches (see Chapters 143 and 144)
2. Surgical procedures, such as thyroidectomy or parathyroidectomy, in which parathyroid tissue is removed either deliberately or as a complication of surgery for another goal
3. Autoimmunity, which may destroy the parathyroid gland

Pseudohypoparathyroidism (all with hypocalcemia and hyperphosphatemia) may occur in one of four forms as follows:

1. *Type Ia:* an abnormality of the G_{sa} protein linking the PTH receptor to adenylate cyclase; biologically active PTH is secreted in great quantities, but does not stimulate its receptor
2. *Type Ib:* normal phenotype, normal G_{sa} with abnormalities in the production of adenylate cyclase
3. *Type Ic:* abnormal phenotype, normal production of adenylate cyclase, but a distal defect eliminates the effects of PTH
4. *Type II:* normal phenotype, normal production of adenylate cyclase, with a postreceptor defect, close to type Ib

Pseudohypoparathyroidism is an autosomal dominant condition that may present at birth or later. Pseudohypoparathyroidism is associated with **Albright hereditary osteodystrophy**, whose clinical manifestations include short stature, stocky body habitus, round facies, short fourth and fifth metacarpals, calcification of the basal ganglia, subcutaneous calcification, and developmental delay. Albright hereditary osteodystrophy may be inherited separately so that a patient may have a normal appearance with hypocalcemia or may have the Albright hereditary osteodystrophy phenotype with normal serum calcium, phosphate, PTH, and response to PTH.

Transient neonatal hypocalcemia. During the first 3 days after birth, serum calcium concentrations normally decline in response to withdrawal of the maternal calcium supply via the placenta. Sluggish PTH response in a neonate may result in a transient hypocalcemia. Hypocalcemia caused by decreased PTH release is found in infants of mothers with hyperparathyroidism and hypercalcemia; the latter suppresses fetal PTH release, causing **transient hypoparathyroidism** in the neonatal period.

Normal serum magnesium concentrations are required for normal parathyroid gland function and action. **Hypomagnesemia** may cause a secondary hypoparathyroidism, which responds poorly to therapies other than magnesium replacement.

The **etiology** of hypocalcemia usually can be discerned by combining features of the clinical presentation with determinations of serum ionized calcium, phosphate, alkaline phosphatase, PTH (preferably at a time when the calcium is low), magnesium, and albumin. If the PTH concentration is not appropriately elevated in relation to the low serum calcium, hypoparathyroidism (transient, primary, or caused by hypomagnesemia) is present. Vitamin D stores can be estimated by measuring

TABLE 176.1 Important Physiological Changes in Bone and Mineral Diseases

CONDITION	CALCIUM	PHOSPHATE	PARATHYROID HORMONE	25(OH)D
Primary hypoparathyroidism	↓	↑	↓	Nl
Pseudohypoparathyroidism	↓	↑	↑	Nl
Vitamin D deficiency	Nl(↓)	↓	↑	↓
Familial hypophosphatemic rickets	Nl	↓	Nl (sl↑)	Nl
Hyperparathyroidism	↑	↓	↑	Nl
Immobilization	↑	↑	↓	Nl

25(OH)D, 25-Hydroxyvitamin D; *Nl*, normal; *sl*, slight; *↑*, high; *↓*, low.

serum 25-hydroxyvitamin D. Renal function is assessed by a serum creatinine measurement or determination of creatinine clearance (Table 176.1).

Treatment of severe tetany or seizures resulting from hypocalcemia consists of intravenous calcium gluconate (1-2 mL/kg of a 10% solution) given slowly over 10 minutes while cardiac status is monitored by electrocardiogram for bradycardia, which can be fatal. Long-term treatment of hypoparathyroidism involves administering vitamin D, preferably as 1,25-dihydroxyvitamin D and calcium. Therapy is adjusted to keep the serum calcium in the lower half of the normal range to avoid episodes of hypercalcemia that might produce nephrocalcinosis and to avoid pancreatitis.

RICKETS

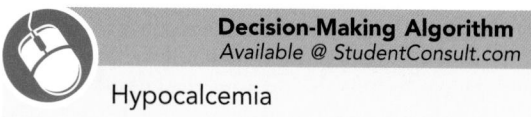

Decision-Making Algorithm
Available @ StudentConsult.com

Hypocalcemia

Rickets is defined as decreased or defective bone mineralization in growing children; **osteomalacia** is the same condition in adults. The proportion of osteoid (the organic portion of bone) is excessive. As a result, the bone becomes soft and the metaphyses of the long bones widen. In older infants, poor linear growth, bowing of the legs on weight bearing (which can be painful), thickening at the wrists and knees, and prominence of the costochondral junctions (rachitic rosary) of the rib cage occur. At this stage, x-ray findings are diagnostic.

In **nutritional vitamin D deficiency** calcium is not absorbed adequately from the intestine (see Chapter 31). Poor vitamin D intake or avoidance of sunlight in infants (exacerbated by those exclusively breastfed) may contribute to the development of rickets. Fat malabsorption resulting from hepatobiliary disease (biliary atresia, neonatal hepatitis) or other causes (cystic fibrosis) also may produce vitamin D deficiency because vitamin D is a fat-soluble vitamin. Defects in vitamin D metabolism by the kidney (renal failure, autosomal recessive deficiency of 1α-hydroxylation, **vitamin D-dependent rickets**) or liver (defect in 25-hydroxylation) also can cause rickets.

In **familial hypophosphatemic rickets,** the major defect is failure of the kidney to adequately reabsorb filtered phosphate so that serum phosphate decreases and urinary phosphate is high. The *diagnosis* of this X-linked disease usually is made within the first few years of life and is typically more severe in males.

The **etiology** of rickets usually can be determined by an assessment of the mineral and vitamin D status (25-hydroxyvitamin D <8 ng/mL suggests nutritional vitamin D deficiency) (see Table 176.1). Further testing of mineral balance or measurement of other vitamin D metabolites may be required.

Several forms of vitamin D can be used for **treatment** of the different rachitic conditions, but their potencies vary widely. Required dosages depend on the condition being treated (see Chapter 31). Rickets may also be treated with 1,25-hydroxyvitamin D and supplemental calcium. In hypophosphatemic rickets, phosphate supplementation (not calcium) must accompany vitamin D therapy, which is given to suppress secondary hyperparathyroidism. Adequate therapy restores normal skeletal growth and produces resolution of the radiographic signs of rickets. Nutritional rickets is treated with vitamin D given as a single large weekly dose or multiple smaller replacement doses. Surgery may be required to straighten legs in untreated patients with long-standing disease.

CHAPTER 177

Disorders of Sexual Development

NORMAL SEXUAL DEVELOPMENT

The successive sequence of chromosomal sex, gonadal sex, and phenotypic sex leads to gender identity of the individual. Genes usually determine the morphology of internal organs and of gonads (gonadal sex); this directs the appearance of the external genitalia that form the secondary sex characteristics (phenotypic sex); self-perception of the individual (gender identity) and the perception of the individual by others (gender role) follow. In most children, these features blend and conform, but, in some patients, one or more features may not follow this sequence, leading to the disorder of sexual development (DSD; see Chapter 23).

The internal and external genitalia are formed between 6 and 13 weeks of gestation. Fetal gonad and external genitalia are bipotential and have the capacity to support development of a normal male or female phenotype (Fig. 177.1). In the presence of a gene called *SRY* for sex-determining region on the Y chromosome, the primitive fetal gonad differentiates into a testis (Fig. 177.2). The Leydig cells of the testis secrete

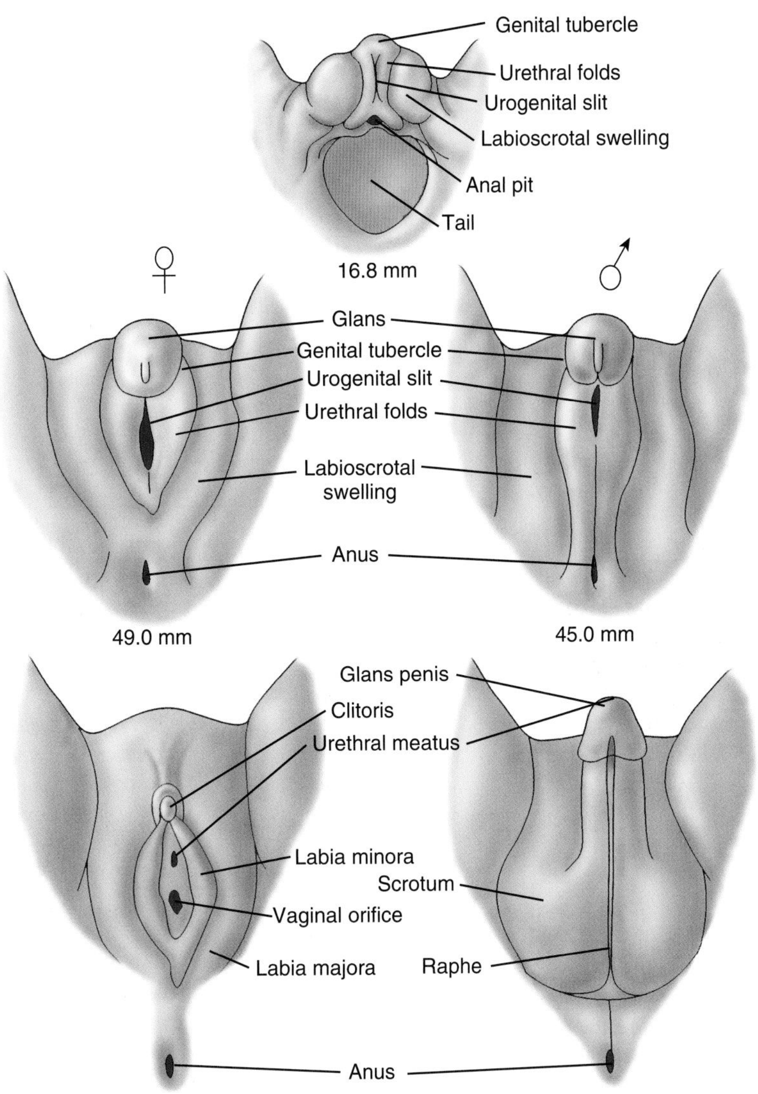

FIGURE 177.1 Differentiation of male and female external genitalia as proceeding from a common embryonic anlage. Testosterone acts at 9-13 weeks of gestation to virilize the bipotential anlage. In the absence of testosterone action, the female phenotype develops. (From Grumbach MM, Conte FA. Disorders of sexual differentiation. In: Wilson JD, Foster DW, eds. *Textbook of Endocrinology*. 8th ed. Philadelphia: WB Saunders; 1990:873; modified from Spaulding MH, *Contrib Embryol Instit.* 1921;13:69–88.)

testosterone, which has direct effects (stimulating development of the wolffian ducts) but also is locally converted to dihydrotestosterone (DHT) by the 5α-reductase enzyme. DHT causes enlargement, rugation, and fusion of the labioscrotal folds into a scrotum; fusion of the ventral surface of the penis to enclose a penile urethra; and enlargement of the phallus with ultimate development of male external genitalia. Testicular production and secretion of müllerian-inhibitory substance by Sertoli cells cause the regression and disappearance of the müllerian ducts and their derivatives, such as the fallopian tubes and uterus. In the presence of testosterone, the wolffian ducts develop into the vas deferens, seminiferous tubules, and prostate.

The female phenotype develops unless specific *male* influences alter development, although recent studies find there are female determining genes necessary for development as well. In the absence of *SRY*, an ovary spontaneously develops from the bipotential, primitive gonad. In the absence of fetal testicular secretion of müllerian-inhibitory substance, a normal uterus, fallopian tubes, and posterior third of the vagina develop out of the müllerian ducts, and the wolffian ducts degenerate. In the total absence of androgens, the external genitalia appear female.

Classification

The terminology for conditions associated with variations in sexual development is evolving. Sometimes referred to as intersex, disorders of sex differentiation, or differences of sex development, DSDs are categorized under three main subgroups according to karyotype (XX, XY, and sex chromosome for mosaic karyotypes).

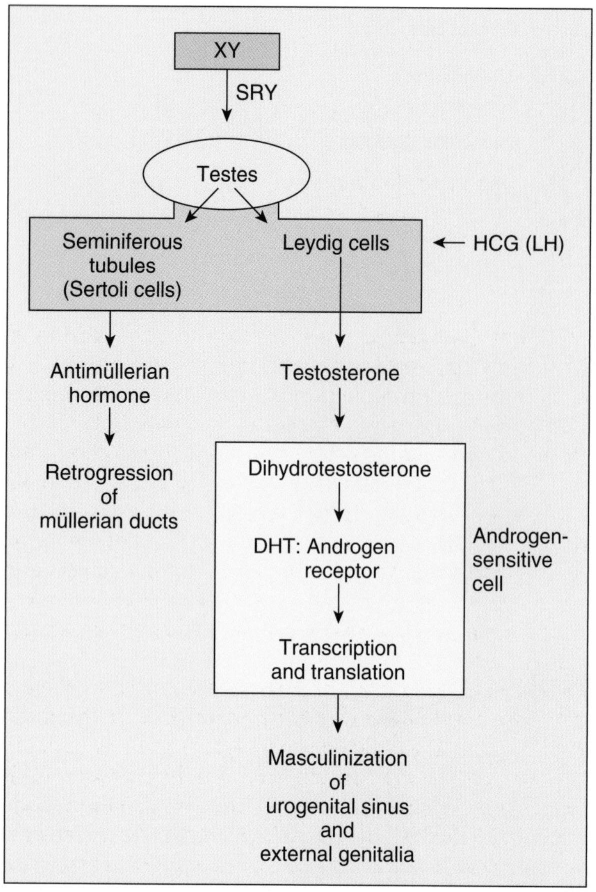

FIGURE 177.2 A diagrammatic scheme of male sex determination and differentiation. *SRY* is the master gene controlling male sex differentiation, but there are many other genes and their products that control male and female sexual differentiation. *DHT,* Dihydrotestosterone; *HCG,* human chorionic gonadotropin; *LH,* luteinizing hormone; *SRY,* the gene for the testis-determining factor. (From Wilson JD, Foster DW, eds. *Williams Textbook of Endocrinology.* 8th ed. Philadelphia: WB Saunders; 1992:918.)

ABNORMAL SEXUAL DEVELOPMENT

46,XX Disorders of Sexual Development

Decision-Making Algorithms
Available @ StudentConsult.com

Hypertension
Amenorrhea
Precocious Puberty in the Male
Precocious Puberty in the Female
Ambiguous Genitalia
Alkalemia

Masculinization of the external genitalia of genotypic females (except for isolated enlargement of the clitoris, which can occur from later androgen exposure) is always caused by the presence of excessive androgens during the critical period of development (8-13 weeks of gestation) (Table 177.1). The degree of virilization can range from mild clitoral enlargement to the appearance of a *male* phallus with a penile urethra and fused scrotum with raphe. Congenital virilizing adrenal hyperplasia is the most common cause of female ambiguous genitalia; it is most commonly the result of an enzyme deficiency that impairs synthesis of glucocorticoids, but does not affect androgen production. The impaired cortisol secretion leads to adrenocorticotropic hormone (ACTH) hypersecretion, which stimulates hyperplasia of the adrenal cortex and excessive adrenal production of androgens (see Chapter 178).

TABLE 177.1 Causes of Virilization in the Female

CONDITION	ADDITIONAL FEATURE(S)
P-450_{c21} deficiency (21 hydroxylase)	Salt loss in some
3β-Hydroxysteroid dehydrogenase deficiency	Salt loss
P-450_{c11} deficiency (11 hydroxylase)	Salt retention/hypertension
Androgenic drug exposure (e.g., progestins)	Exposure between 9 and 12 weeks of gestation
Mixed gonadal dysgenesis or mosaic Turner syndrome	Karyotype = 46,XY/45,X
Ovotesticular DSD	Testicular and ovarian tissue present
Maternal virilizing adrenal or ovarian tumor	Rare, positive history

DSD, Disorder of sexual development.

46,XY Disorders of Sexual Development

Decision-Making Algorithms
Available @ StudentConsult.com

Amenorrhea
Pubertal Delay
Ambiguous Genitalia
Gynecomastia

Underdevelopment of the male external genitalia occurs because of a relative deficiency of testosterone production or action (Table 177.2). The penis is small, with various degrees of hypospadias (penile or perineal) and associated chordee or ventral binding of the phallus; unilateral, but more often bilateral, cryptorchidism may be present. The testes should be sought carefully in the inguinal canal or labioscrotal folds by palpation or ultrasound. Rarely a palpable gonad in the inguinal canal or labioscrotal fold represents a herniated ovary or an ovotestis. The latter patients have ovarian and testicular tissue and usually ambiguous external genitalia. Production of testosterone by a gonad implies that testicular tissue is present and that at least some cells carry the *SRY* gene.

Testosterone production can be reduced by specific deficiencies of the enzymes needed for androgen biosynthesis or by dysplasia of the gonads. In the latter, if müllerian-inhibiting substance production also is reduced, a rudimentary uterus and fallopian tubes are present.

The complete form of **androgen resistance** or **androgen insensitivity syndrome** is the most dramatic example of resistance to hormone action by defects in the androgen receptor. Affected patients have a **46,XY** karyotype, normally formed testes

TABLE 177.2 Causes of Inadequate Masculinization in the Male

CONDITION	ADDITIONAL FEATURE(S)
P-450scc (StAR) deficiency	Salt loss
3β-Hydroxysteroid dehydrogenase deficiency	Salt loss
P-450_{c17} deficiency	Salt retention/hypokalemia/hypertension
Isolated P-450_{c17} deficiency with 17,20-desmolase deficiency	Adrenal function normal
17β-Hydroxysteroid oxidoreductase deficiency	Adrenal function normal
Dysgenetic testes	Possible abnormal karyotype; possible mutations in DAX1, SOX9, GATA4, WT1
Leydig cell hypoplasia	Rare
Complete androgen insensitivity	Female external genitalia, absence of müllerian structures
Partial androgen insensitivity	As previous with ambiguous external genitalia
5α-Reductase deficiency	Autosomal recessive, virilization at puberty

StAR, Steroid acute regulatory protein.

(usually located in the inguinal canal or labia majora), and female external genitalia with a short vagina and no internal müllerian structures. At the time of puberty, testosterone concentrations increase to normal or above normal male range. Because a portion of the testosterone is normally converted to estradiol in peripheral tissues and the estrogen cannot be opposed by the androgen, breast development ensues at the normal age of puberty without growth of pubic, facial, or axillary hair or the occurrence of menstruation.

5α-Reductase deficiency presents at birth with predominantly female phenotype or with ambiguous genitalia, including perineoscrotal hypospadias. The defect is in 5α reduction of testosterone to its metabolite DHT. At puberty, spontaneous secondary male sexual development occurs.

Sex Chromosome and Ovotesticular Disorders of Sexual Development

Decision-Making Algorithms
Available @ StudentConsult.com

Short Stature
Pubertal Delay
Gynecomastia

Turner syndrome and **Klinefelter syndrome** and their mosaic variants are classified as sex chromosome DSD. Mixed gonadal dysgenesis (45,X; 46,XY) often may present with genital ambiguity, asymmetric external genitalia, and inguinal hernias. There may be virilization on one side and none on the other. Similar findings may be seen with **ovotesticular DSD**, another classification of DSD.

APPROACH TO THE INFANT WITH GENITAL AMBIGUITY

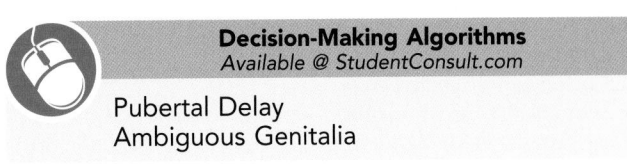

Decision-Making Algorithms
Available @ StudentConsult.com

Pubertal Delay
Ambiguous Genitalia

Ambiguous genitalia in a newborn must be attended to with as little delay as possible and with informed sensitivity to the psychosocial context as required. The laboratory evaluations required might take days or weeks to complete, delaying a sex assignment and naming of the infant, such that choice often precedes diagnosis. Beyond infancy and childhood, and to offset any gender uncertainty in the patient and confusion in the parents, health care providers must help families come to an appropriate closure and gender choice. With that, most centers caring for patients with ambiguous genitalia include a behavioral health specialist with a focus on patients and families encountering these issues.

On physical examination, it is essential to note where the urethral opening lies and whether there is fusion of the anterior portion of the labioscrotal folds. Endogenous excessive production of androgen (as in congenital adrenal hyperplasia [CAH]) in a female fetus between 9 and 13 weeks of gestation leads to ambiguous genitalia. If the vaginal opening is normal, and there is no fusion, but the clitoris is enlarged without ventral fusion of the ventral urethra, the patient likely had later exposure to androgens. In a patient with a fully formed scrotum, even if small, and a normally formed but small penis, termed a *microphallus,* the patient likely had normal exposure to and action of androgen during 9-13 weeks of gestation.

The major goal is a rapid identification of any life-threatening disorders (salt loss and shock caused by the salt-losing form of CAH). Although the classic approach to sex assignment has been based on the feasibility of genital reconstruction and potential fertility rather than on karyotype or gonadal histology, the effects of prenatal androgen must be considered. Experts recommend waiting until the child is able to be part of the dialogue regarding gender identity and reconstruction when appropriate. Present management of ambiguous genitalia involves extensive open discussion with parents involving the biology of the infant and the likely prognosis. Treatment should be individualized and managed by a team, including an experienced pediatric endocrinologist, urologist or gynecologist, psychologist, geneticist, and the primary care physician.

Diagnosis

The first step toward diagnosis is to determine whether the findings represent virilization of a genetic female (androgen excess) or underdevelopment of a genetic male (androgen deficiency; see Fig. 177.2). Inguinal gonads that are evident on palpation usually are testes and indicate that incomplete development of a male phenotype has occurred; this pattern is not consistent, and ovaries and ovotestes may feel similar. Similarly, absence of female internal genitalia (detected by ultrasound) implies that müllerian-inhibiting substance was present and secreted by fetal testes. Karyotype determination is only one of many factors needed to assist the family in the decision of sex of rearing; the *SRY* gene may be found on chromosomes other than the Y chromosome, and, conversely, a Y chromosome may lack an *SRY* gene (it may have been translocated to an X chromosome, leading to the development of a 46,XX male-XX sex reversal, testicular DSD).

Statistically, most virilized females have CAH; 90% of these females have 21-hydroxylase deficiency. The diagnosis is established by measuring the plasma concentration of 17-hydroxyprogesterone and androstenedione (see Chapter 178), which typically is hundreds of times above the normal range. Other enzymatic defects also may be diagnosed by quantifying circulating levels of the adrenal steroid precursor proximal to the defective enzyme block.

Establishing an accurate diagnosis is more difficult in underdeveloped males. When certain types of adrenal hyperplasia coexist with defects in androgen production of the testes, excessive ACTH secretion elevates substantially levels of specific adrenal steroid precursors, allowing a diagnosis. If the defect is restricted to testosterone biosynthesis, the measurement of testosterone and its precursors in the basal state and after stimulation by HCG may be required. Patients with normal levels of testosterone either have persistent androgen resistance or have had an interruption of normal morphogenesis of the genitalia. Abnormalities of the sex chromosomes may be associated with dysgenetic gonads, which may be associated with persistence of müllerian structures.

Treatment

Treatment consists of replacing deficient hormones (cortisol in adrenal hyperplasia or testosterone in a child with androgen biosynthetic defects who will be raised as male), surgical restoration to make the individual look more appropriate for the gender of rearing, and psychological support of the whole family. Gonads and internal organs discordant for the gender of rearing may be removed. Dysgenetic gonads with Y-genetic material always should be removed because **gonadoblastomas** or **dysgerminomas** may develop in the organ. Age at which reconstructive surgery is recommended is controversial; some advocate that surgery not be performed in infancy or early childhood so that the child or young adolescent can be involved in the decision. A decision for gender of rearing is recommended from birth; however, the knowledge that the person with a DSD may change gender later on is shared with parents from the outset.

CHAPTER 178

Adrenal Gland Dysfunction

PHYSIOLOGY

The adrenal gland consists of an outer cortex, which is responsible for the synthesis of steroids, and an inner medulla derived from neuroectodermal tissue, which synthesizes catecholamines. The *adrenal cortex* consists of three zones: an outer glomerulosa (end product is the mineralocorticoid aldosterone, which regulates sodium and potassium balance), a middle fasciculata (end product is cortisol), and an inner reticularis (synthesizes sex steroids). The general scheme of these synthetic steps is shown in Fig. 178.1.

Hypothalamic corticotropin-releasing hormone (CRH) stimulates the release of pituitary adrenocorticotropic hormone (ACTH or corticotropin), derived by selective processing from pro-opiomelanocortin. ACTH governs the synthesis and release of cortisol and adrenal androgens. Primary adrenal insufficiency or cortisol deficiency from any defect in the adrenal gland results in an oversecretion of ACTH; adrenal insufficiency may also occur from ACTH (secondary) or CRH (tertiary) deficiency, resulting in low serum ACTH concentrations and low cortisol. Endogenous (or exogenous) glucocorticoids feedback to inhibit ACTH and CRH secretion. The renin-angiotensin system and potassium regulate aldosterone secretion; ACTH has little effect on aldosterone production except in excess, when it may increase aldosterone secretion.

Steroids that circulate in the free form (not bound to cortisol-binding protein [transcortin]) may cross the placenta from mother to fetus, but ACTH does not. The placenta plays an important role in steroid biosynthesis in utero by acting as a metabolic mediator between mother and child. As the fetal CRH-ACTH-adrenal axis is operational in utero, any deficiencies in cortisol synthesis lead to excessive ACTH secretion. If a virilizing adrenal enzyme defect is present, such as 21-hydroxylase deficiency, the fetal adrenal gland secretes excess androgens, resulting in a virilized fetus. Normal variation of serum cortisol and ACTH levels leads to values that are high early in the morning and lower at night. This normal diurnal variation may take months to years to fully develop in neonates.

ADRENAL INSUFFICIENCY

Decision-Making Algorithms
Available @ StudentConsult.com

Ambiguous Genitalia
Hyponatremia
Hyperkalemia

The **clinical manifestations** of inadequate adrenal function result from inadequate secretion or action of glucocorticoids, mineralocorticoids, or both (Table 178.1). In the case of enzyme defects that affect the gonad and the adrenal gland, overproduction or underproduction of potent androgens can occur depending on the site of enzyme blockade (see Fig. 178.1). Progressive prenatal virilization of the external genitalia may occur in females while incomplete virilization may occur in males. Ambiguity of the external genitalia is a common manifestation of disordered fetal adrenal enzyme function. Precise *diagnosis* is essential for the prescription of appropriate therapy, long-term outlook, and genetic counseling. In patients with enzyme defects, an elevation in the precursor steroid is present proximal to the enzyme block and is metabolized through remaining normal alternate enzyme pathways, whereas a deficiency of steroids is present subsequent to the block.

The dominant clinical features of **congenital adrenal mineralocorticoid deficiency** are hyponatremia and hyperkalemia, usually developing by 5-7 days after birth but not immediately after birth. Vomiting, dehydration, and acidosis soon follow as

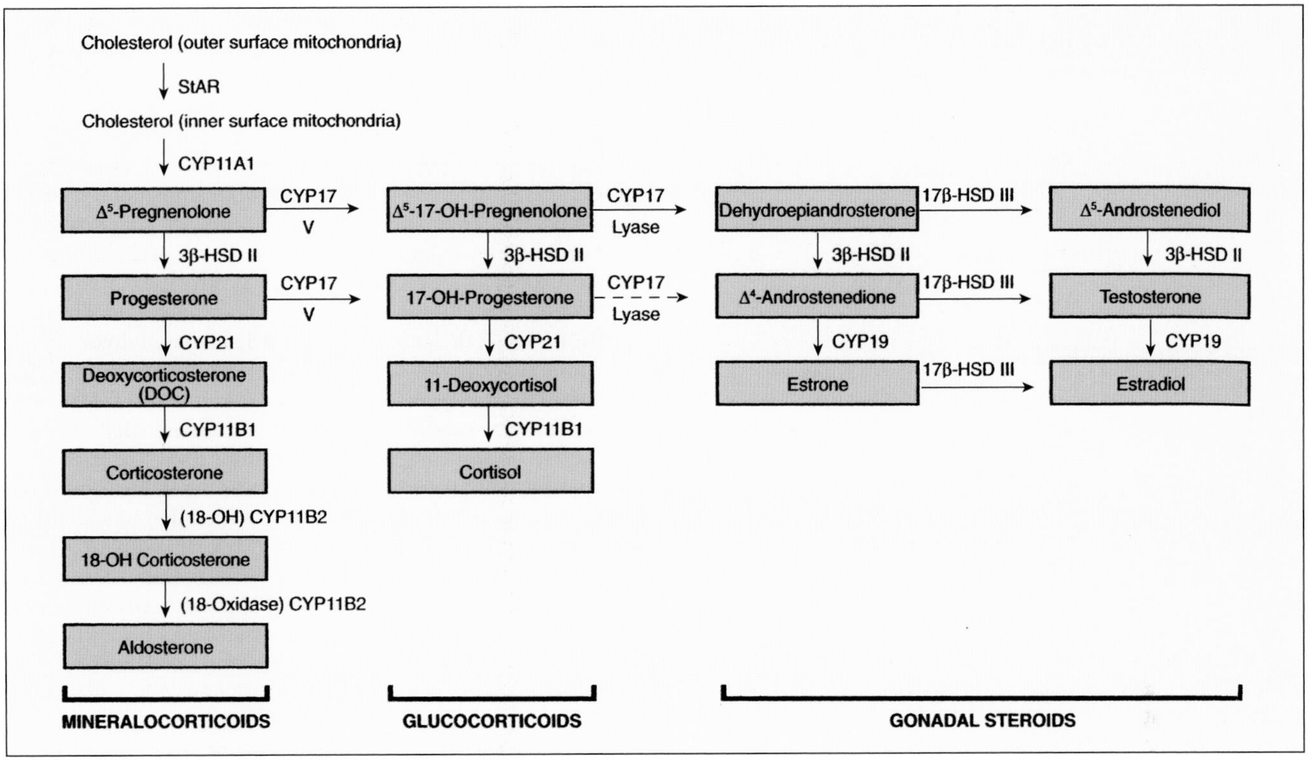

FIGURE 178.1 Diagram of the steroid biosynthetic pathways and the biosynthetic defects that result in congenital hyperplasia. The defect in patients with lipoid adrenal hyperplasia is not (except for one reported case) in the CYP11A1 (cholesterol side-chain cleavage) enzyme, but in StAR, the steroidogenic acute regulatory protein. This protein is involved in the transport of cholesterol from the outer mitochondrial membrane to the inner membrane, where the CYP11A1 enzyme is located. CYP11B1 (11β-hydroxylase) catalyzes 11β-hydroxylation of deoxycorticosterone and 11β-deoxycortisol primarily. CYP17 (17α-hydroxylase/17,20-lyase) catalyzes 17α-hydroxylation and splitting of the 17,20 bond, but for the latter it has preferential D^5-17,20-lyase activity. CYP19 (aromatase) catalyzes the conversion of corticosterone to aldosterone. 3β-HSD I and 3β-HSD II, 3β-hydroxysteroid dehydrogenase/$\Delta^{4,5}$-isomerase types I and II; CYP21 (P450c21), 21-hydroxylase; 17β-HSD 3, 17β-hydroxysteroid dehydrogenase type 3. In the human, deletion of a homozygous null mutation of CYP11A ($P450_{ccc}$) is probably lethal in utero, but a heterogeneous mutation caused congenital lipoid adrenal hyperplasia. (From Melmed S, Polonsky K, Kronenberg H, et al, eds. *Williams Textbook of Endocrinology. 10th ed.* Philadelphia: Saunders; 2003:917.)

does hypotensive shock from glucocorticoid deficiency. Death may occur if the disorder remains undiagnosed and untreated. In females, the ambiguity of the external genitalia is an obvious clue that salt-losing congenital adrenal hyperplasia (CAH) or simple virilizing CAH must be ruled out. Because these forms cannot be distinguished clinically, all presentations of ambiguous genitalia should involve evaluation for mineralocorticoid deficiency. In males, 21-hydroxylase deficiency (the most common form of CAH) does not cause abnormal genitalia; although there may be hyperpigmentation of the scrotal skin, this is a subtle sign and can result in delayed diagnosis. In all infants, the diagnosis of adrenal insufficiency may be overlooked or confused with pyloric stenosis. In pyloric stenosis, vomiting of stomach contents results in hypochloremia, low or normal serum potassium, and alkalosis in contrast to CAH, which has hyponatremia, hyperkalemia, and acidosis. This distinction may be lifesaving in preventing unnecessary investigations or inappropriate therapy.

Not all forms of adrenal hyperplasia present at birth; the spectrum of disorder ranges from severe (classic) to mild (late-onset) or nonclassic. Milder forms may manifest in childhood, adolescence, or even young adulthood (not as glucocorticoid or mineralocorticoid deficiencies, but as androgen excess).

In patients with **congenital adrenal hypoplasia** or **adrenal hemorrhage**, the secretion of all adrenal steroids is low. In contrast, CAH leads to a diagnostic steroid pattern in blood and urine (see Fig. 178.1). Deficiency of 21-hydroxylase is the most common form (95%) and serves as a paradigm for these disorders.

21-HYDROXYLASE DEFICIENCY

Decision-Making Algorithms
Available @ StudentConsult.com

Hypertension
Precocious Puberty in the Male
Precocious Puberty in the Female
Ambiguous Genitalia
Hirsutism

TABLE 178.1 Clinical Manifestations of Adrenal Insufficiency

Cortisol deficiency
Hypoglycemia
Inability to withstand stress
Vasomotor collapse
Hyperpigmentation (in primary adrenal insufficiency with excess of adrenocorticotropic hormone)
Apneic spells
Muscle weakness, fatigue
Aldosterone deficiency
Hyponatremia
Hyperkalemia
Vomiting
Urinary sodium wasting
Salt craving
Acidosis
Failure to thrive
Volume depletion
Hypotension
Dehydration
Shock
Diarrhea
Muscle weakness
Androgen excess or deficiency (caused by adrenal enzyme defect)
Ambiguous genitalia in certain conditions

The incidence of classic 21-hydroxylase deficiency is about 1 in 15,000 among various white populations. Nonclassic CAH may occur with an incidence of 1 in 50 in certain populations. The gene for 21-hydroxylase lies on the short arm of chromosome 6; the genotype may be determined in a proband, permitting prenatal diagnosis in a subsequent pregnancy.

Deficient 21-hydroxylase activity ($P\text{-}450_{c21}$ deficiency) impairs the conversion of 17-hydroxyprogesterone (17-OHP) to 11-deoxycortisol and in the salt-losing form, of progesterone to deoxycorticosterone, a mineralocorticoid proximal in the pathway to the production of aldosterone. The decreased production of cortisol causes hypersecretion of ACTH, which stimulates the synthesis of steroids immediately proximal to the block and shunting of these to overproduction of androgens. The primary clinical manifestation is the virilization of the external genitalia of the affected female fetus. The development of the uterus, ovaries, and fallopian tubes are unaffected by the androgens. The degree of virilization varies, ranging from mild clitoromegaly to complete fusion of labioscrotal folds, with severe clitoromegaly simulating a phallus (see Chapter 177). A male infant with this defect appears normal at birth, although penile enlargement may be apparent thereafter. The deficiency in aldosterone, found in about 75% of patients, causes salt wasting with shock and dehydration until the diagnosis is established and appropriate treatment is given.

The treatment of 21-hydroxylase deficiency requires hydrocortisone and fludrocortisone in the case of the salt-losing form. Therapy must be adjusted throughout childhood at regular intervals. Overtreatment will cause growth stunting and weight gain (cushingoid features), whereas undertreatment will cause excessive height gain, skeletal advance, and early appearance puberty, ultimately jeopardizing adult height potential.

Late-onset CAH is typically noted years after birth. Affected subjects have milder manifestations without ambiguous genitalia, but they may have acne, hirsutism, and, in girls, irregular menstrual cycles or amenorrhea. Late-onset CAH in girls may be confused with **polycystic ovarian syndrome**.

Biochemical diagnostic studies show elevated levels of serum 17-OHP, the substrate for the defective 21-hydroxylase enzyme activity. In newborns with CAH, the values are elevated a 100-fold to a 1,000-fold. In late-onset CAH, an ACTH stimulation test may be necessary to show an abnormally high response of 17-OHP. Serum cortisol and aldosterone levels (in salt losers) are low and renin levels are high, whereas the testosterone level is elevated because it is derived from 17-OHP.

The goals of **treatment** are to achieve normal linear growth and bone age advancement. Long-term therapy consists of providing glucocorticoids at a dose of approximately 10-15 mg/m^2/24 hr in three divided doses of oral hydrocortisone or its equivalent. Mineralocorticoid therapy for salt losers consists of fludrocortisone at a dose of 0.1-0.2 mg/24 hr, often with sodium chloride supplementation in infancy and early childhood. Surgical correction of ambiguous external genitalia may be considered. The adequacy of glucocorticoid replacement therapy is monitored by determining serum concentrations of adrenal precursors, including androstenedione and 17-OHP for 21-hydroxylase deficiency. In addition, the assessment of linear growth and skeletal age, by bone age determination, is required as a reflection of appropriate therapy. To avoid adrenal insufficiency, threefold higher doses of glucocorticoids are given during **stressful states**, such as febrile illnesses and surgery. Intramuscular hydrocortisone is used in severe emergencies or with illnesses involving emesis. Mineralocorticoid therapy is monitored with serum sodium, potassium, and plasma renin activity levels. Prenatal treatment with dexamethasone to suppress fetal ACTH-induced androgen production can reduce or eliminate the ambiguity of the external genitalia in affected female fetuses, if begun at approximately 7 weeks of gestation; however, this remains controversial.

OTHER ENZYME DEFECTS

Other enzyme defects are rare in contrast to 21-hydroxylase deficiency. In **11-hydroxylase deficiency,** the next most common cause of CAH, virilization occurs with salt retention and hypokalemia as a result of the buildup of deoxycorticosterone (see Fig. 178.1), a potent mineralocorticoid. Hypertension develops as a result of excessive mineralocorticoid production. Table 178.2 summarizes the clinical and biochemical features of adrenal insufficiency in infancy.

ADDISON DISEASE

Decision-Making Algorithms
Available @ StudentConsult.com

Hyponatremia
Hyperkalemia

TABLE 178.2 Clinical and Biochemical Features in Newborn Adrenal Insufficiency

FEATURE	ELECTROLYTE DISTURBANCE*	AMBIGUOUS GENITALIA: VIRILIZED FEMALE	AMBIGUOUS GENITALIA: UNDERVIRILIZED MALE	SERUM CORTISOL	URINE 11-DEOXYCORTISOL	17-OHP	DHEA	ALDOSTERONE	17-OHCS	17-KS	PREGNANETRIOL
Hypoplasia	Severe	No	No	D	D	D	D	D	D	D	D
Hemorrhage	Moderate to severe	No	No	D	D	D	D	D	D	D	D
StAR deficiency	Severe	No	Yes	D	D	D	D	D	D	D	D
3β-HSD	Severe	Yes	Yes	D	D	D	I	D	D	I	D
P-450_{c21} deficiency	Absent to severe	Yes	No	D	D	I	I	D	D	I	I
Aldosterone synthesis block	Severe	No	No	Nl	Nl	Nl	Nl	D	Nl	Nl	Nl
Pseudohypo-aldosteronism	Severe	No	No	Nl	Nl	Nl	Nl	I	Nl	Nl	Nl
P-450_{c11} deficiency	None	Yes	No	D	I	Nl or I	Nl	D	I	I	Nl-sl I
P-450_{c17} deficiency	†	No	Yes	D	Nl-D	D	D	Nl-D	D	D	D
Unresponsiveness to ACTH	†	No	No	D	Nl-D	Nl-D	Nl-D	Nl-D	D	D	Nl-D

Usually manifested after 5 days of age.
†*High normal Na^+ and low normal to low K^+.*
17-KS, 17-Ketosteroid; *17-OHCS,* 17-hydroxycorticosteroid; *ACTH,* adrenocorticotropic hormone; *D,* decrease; *HSD,* hydroxysteroid dehydrogenase; *I,* increase; *Nl,* normal; *StAR,* steroid acute regulatory protein.

Addison disease is a rare acquired disorder of childhood, usually associated with autoimmune destruction of the adrenal cortex. It is a form of primary adrenal insufficiency with absence of glucocorticoid and mineralocorticoid.

Clinical manifestations are hyperpigmentation, salt craving, postural hypotension, fasting hypoglycemia, anorexia, weakness, and episodes of shock during severe illness. Subnormal baseline and ACTH-stimulated cortisol values confirm the diagnosis. The presence of hyponatremia, hyperkalemia, and elevated plasma renin activity indicate mineralocorticoid deficiency. Addison disease may occur within the context of autoimmune polyglandular syndromes (APS I and APS II). Other rare causes of adrenal insufficiency include adrenal leukodystrophy and conditions that affect the hypothalamus-pituitary, whether acquired, such as in craniopharyngioma, or iatrogenic, such as in irradiation for treatment of malignancy.

Replacement **treatment** with 10-15 $mg/m^2/24$ hr of hydrocortisone is indicated, with supplementation during stress at three times the maintenance dosage or the use of intramuscular hydrocortisone. The dose is titrated to allow a normal growth rate. Mineralocorticoid replacement with fludrocortisone is monitored by plasma renin activity along with serum sodium and potassium determinations.

CUSHING SYNDROME

Decision-Making Algorithms
Available @ StudentConsult.com

Short Stature
Hirsutism
Obesity
Alkalemia
Hyponatremia
Hypokalemia

Classic **clinical manifestations** of Cushing syndrome in children include progressive central or generalized obesity, marked failure of longitudinal growth, hirsutism, weakness, a nuchal fat pad, acne, striae, hypertension, and often hyperpigmentation when ACTH is elevated. The most frequent cause is long-term administration of exogenous glucocorticoids due to chronic medical conditions. Endogenous causes include adrenal adenoma, carcinoma, nodular adrenal hyperplasia, an ACTH-secreting pituitary microadenoma resulting in bilateral adrenal hyperplasia **(Cushing disease),** or an extremely rare ACTH-secreting tumor. **Diagnostic tests** include 24-hour urinary cortisol excretion, low-dose dexamethasone suppression test, high-dose dexamethasone suppression test (helps distinguish Cushing syndrome from Cushing disease), and late evening salivary cortisol sampling.

Treatment of Cushing syndrome is directed to the etiology and may include excision of adrenal, pituitary, or ectopic ACTH-secreting tumors. Rarely, adrenalectomy is needed to control the symptoms. Parenteral glucocorticoid therapy is necessary during and immediately after surgical treatment to avoid acute adrenal insufficiency.

Suggested Readings

Backeljauw PF, Chernausek SD. The insulin-like growth factors and growth disorders of childhood. *Endocrinol Metab Clin North Am.* 2012;41(2):265–282.
Kliegman RM, Stanton B, St Geme J III, et al, eds. *Nelson Textbook of Pediatrics.* 19th ed. Philadelphia: Elsevier; 2011.
Nimkarn S, Lin-Su K, New MI. Steroid 21 hydroxylase deficiency congenital adrenal hyperplasia. *Pediatr Clin North Am.* 2011;58(5):1281–1300.
Palmert MR, Dunkel L. Clinical practice: delayed puberty. *N Engl J Med.* 2012;366(5):443–453.
Péter F, Muzsnai A. Congenital disorders of the thyroid: hypo/hyper. *Pediatr Clin North Am.* 2011;58(5):1099–1115.
Romero CJ, Nesi-França S, Radovick S. The molecular basis of hypopituitarism. *Trends Endocrinol Metab.* 2009;20(10):506–516.
Schatz DA, Haller MJ, Atkinson MA. Type 1 diabetes. Preface. *Endocrinol Metab Clin North Am.* 2010;39(3):481–667.
Williams RM, Ward CE, Hughes IA. Premature adrenarche. *Arch Dis Child.* 2012;97(3):250–254.

PEARLS FOR PRACTITIONERS

CHAPTER 170

Endocrinology Assessment

- Hormones are defined as circulating messengers, with action at a distance from the organ (gland) of origin of the hormone.
- Endocrine disorders generally manifest from one of four ways: excess hormone, deficient hormone, abnormal response of end-organ, gland enlargement.
- The assessment of pituitary function may be determined by measuring some of the specific pituitary hormone in the basal state; other assessments require the measurement after stimulation.

CHAPTER 171

Diabetes Mellitus

- Type 1 diabetes mellitus is typically treated with multiple daily injections of a short-acting (bolus) insulin and a single dose of long acting (basal) insulin.
- Type 1 diabetes is an autoimmune disease and most often presents with hyperglycemia, ketoacidosis, polyuria, and polydipsia.
- Type 1 diabetes mellitus is a complex chronic illness that requires a team of providers, including endocrinologist, diabetes educator, nutritionist, social worker/psychologist, and close interactions for the family for success.

- Type 2 diabetes is associated with obesity and insulin resistance.

CHAPTER 172

Hypoglycemia

- After the initial 2-3 days of life, hypoglycemia is far less common and is more frequently the result of endocrine or metabolic disorders (although sepsis must always be ruled out).
- Clinical hypoglycemia is defined as a plasma glucose (PG) concentration low enough to cause symptoms and/or signs of impaired brain function.
- The most common causes for congenital hyperinsulinism involve inactivating K_{ATP} channel mutations and account for approximately 60% of all identifiable mutations.
- The *diagnosis* of hyperinsulinism in children is determined by evaluating markers of inappropriate insulin effects (e.g., suppressed ketogenesis) because plasma insulin concentrations are frequently not clearly elevated.
- Idiopathic ketotic hypoglycemia, usually begins at about 18 months of age in thin children and remits by 8 years of age, presents with symptoms of hypoglycemia after a period of prolonged fasting, often in the setting of an intercurrent illness with decreased feeding.
- The *diagnosis* of glycogen storage disease (GSD) is suggested by a hypoglycemia in the setting of hepatomegaly without splenomegaly (although GSD type 0 is not associated with hepatomegaly).
- A *critical sample* of blood and urine at the time of the hypoglycemic episode should be obtained before treatment for the measurement of glucose and insulin, growth hormone (GH), cortisol, free fatty acids (FFAs), and β-hydroxybutyrate and acetoacetate.

CHAPTER 173

Short Stature

- A normal linear growth pattern is good evidence of overall health and can be considered a *bioassay* for the well-being of the whole child.
- Insulin-like growth factor-1 (IGF-1) acts primarily as a paracrine and autocrine agent and is most closely associated with postnatal growth.
- Accurate measurements of height (standing), or length (lying down), and weight should be plotted on the Centers for Disease Control and Prevention growth charts for the timely diagnosis of growth disorders.
- Short stature is defined as subnormal height relative to other children of the same gender and age, taking family heights into consideration.
- Nutrition is the most important factor affecting growth on a worldwide basis.
- Adequacy of GH secretion may be determined by a stimulation test to measure peak GH secretion.
- A patient with classic GH deficiency has the appearance of a **cherub (a chubby, immature appearance),** with a high-pitched voice resulting from an immature larynx.
- GH deficiency is treated with biosynthetic recombinant DNA-derived GH. Dosage is titrated to the growth rate, weight of the patient, and IGF-1 levels.
- The common condition known as **constitutional delay** in growth or puberty or both is considered a variation of normal growth, caused by a reduced tempo, or cadence, of physiological development.

CHAPTER 174

Disorders of Puberty

- Pubarche results from adrenal maturation or adrenarche and is marked with the appearance of pubic hair, oiliness of hair and skin, acne, axillary hair, and body odor; gonadarche is characterized by increasing secretion of gonadal sex steroids as a result of the maturation of the hypothalamic-pituitary-gonadal axis.
- Puberty is delayed when there is no sign of pubertal development by age 13 years in girls and 14 years in boys living in the United States.
- Disorders that can cause hypogonadotropic hypogonadism include congenital hypopituitarism, such as midline defects, tumors, infiltrative disease, and many syndromes, including Laurence-Moon-Bardet-Biedl, Prader-Willi, and Kallmann syndromes.
- Decreased gonadotropin function occurs when voluntary dieting, malnutrition, or chronic disease results in weight loss to less than 80% of ideal weight.
- Hypergonadotropic hypogonadism is characterized by elevated gonadotropins and low sex steroid levels resulting from primary gonadal failure.
- Turner syndrome is a common cause of ovarian failure and short stature; Klinefelter syndrome (seminiferous tubular dysgenesis) is the most common cause of testicular failure.
- When no secondary sexual development is present after the upper age limits of normal pubertal development, serum gonadotropin levels should be obtained to determine whether the patient has a hypogonadotropic or hypergonadotropic hypogonadism.
- Central precocious puberty, resulting in gonadarche, emanates from premature activation of the hypothalamic-pituitary-gonadal axis (gonadotropin-releasing hormone [GnRH]-dependent); peripheral precocious puberty, gonadarche or adrenarche, does not involve the hypothalamic-pituitary-gonadal axis (GnRH-independent).
- Compared with girls, boys with precocious puberty have a higher incidence of CNS disorders, such as tumors and hamartomas, precipitating the precocious puberty.
- The most common cause of GnRH-independent precocious puberty, McCune-Albright syndrome, is more frequent in girls than boys and includes precocious gonadarche, a bone disorder with polyostotic fibrous dysplasia, and hyperpigmented cutaneous macules (café-au-lait spots).
- The first step in evaluating sexual precocity is to determine which characteristics of normal puberty are apparent and whether estrogen effects, androgen effects, or both are present; laboratory evaluation includes determination of adrenal androgen and sex steroid levels (testosterone, estradiol, DHEAS [dehydroepiandrosterone sulfate]) and baseline gonadotropin concentrations.

- A prepubertal GnRH response is follicle-stimulating hormone (FSH) predominant, whereas a pubertal response is more luteinizing hormone (LH) predominant.
- Long-acting, superactive analogs of GnRH (leuprolide depot, histrelin depot) are the treatment of choice for central precocious puberty; antiandrogens, antiestrogens, and aromatase inhibitors are used for peripheral precocious puberty.
- Most patients with isolated pubic hair do not have progressive virilization and simply have premature adrenarche *(pubarche)* resulting from premature activation of DHEA secretion from the adrenal gland; no treatment is needed.

CHAPTER 175

Thyroid Disease

- Early treatment in congenital hypothyroidism is essential to prevent delayed development.
- Hypothyroidism is common in children, and treatment with levothyroxine is typically initiated when a thyroid-stimulating hormone (TSH) is >10 mIU/L.
- Hypothyroidism must be considered in evaluation of short stature, especially if not associated with weight gain.
- Acquired hypothyroidism is an autoimmune disease and may be associated with type 1 diabetes, Addison disease, hypoparathyroidism, and celiac disease.
- Hyperthyroidism is initially treated with pharmacological therapy, and if remission does not occur, ablation or surgical removal is initiated.
- Most thyroid nodules in children and adolescents are benign.

CHAPTER 176

Disorders of Parathyroid Bone and Mineral Endocrinology

- Calcium and phosphate are regulated mainly by diet and three hormones: parathyroid hormone (PTH), vitamin D, and calcitonin.
- Neonatal hypocalcemia has multiple causes depending on timing of onset and may require treatment with intravenous (IV) and/or oral calcium.
- It is essential to make sure vitamin D is adequate as well as magnesium when replacing calcium.
- Hypocalcemia may be associated with multiple nonendocrine disorders and diseases, thus requiring a complete evaluation.

CHAPTER 177

Disorders of Sexual Development

- Genes usually determine the morphology of internal organs and of gonads (gonadal sex); this directs the appearance of the external genitalia that form the secondary sex characteristics (phenotypic sex). Self-perception of the individual (gender identity) and the perception of the individual by others (gender role) follow.
- Sometimes referred to as intersex, disorders of sex differentiation, or differences of sex development, disorders of sexual development (DSDs) are categorized under three main subgroups according to karyotype (XX, XY, and sex chromosome for mosaic karyotypes).
- Congenital virilizing adrenal hyperplasia is the most common cause of female ambiguous genitalia.
- Testosterone production can be reduced by specific deficiencies of the enzymes needed for androgen biosynthesis or by dysplasia of the gonads.
- Although the classic approach to sex assignment has been based on the feasibility of genital reconstruction and potential fertility rather than on karyotype or gonadal histology, the effects of prenatal androgen must be considered; experts recommend waiting until the child is able to be part of the dialogue regarding gender identity and reconstruction when appropriate.
- The first step toward diagnosis of ambiguous genitalia is to determine whether the findings represent virilization of a genetic female (androgen excess) or under development of a genetic male (androgen deficiency)
- Treatment of DSDs consists of replacing deficient hormones (cortisol in adrenal hyperplasia or testosterone in a child with androgen biosynthetic defects who will be raised as male), surgical restoration to make the individual look more appropriate for the gender of rearing, and psychological support of the whole family.

CHAPTER 178

Adrenal Gland Dysfunction

- Early diagnosis and treatment of salt wasting congenital adrenal hyperplasia involves replacement therapy with hydrocortisone, fludrocortisone, and saline solution.
- Adrenal insufficiency is associated with hyperpigmentation, salt craving, postural hypotension, fasting hypoglycemia, anorexia, weakness, and episodes of shock during severe illness.
- Cushing syndrome is commonly a result of chronic use of high-dose oral steroids.

NEUROLOGY

Jocelyn Huang Schiller | Renée A. Shellhaas

CHAPTER 179

Neurology Assessment

A neurological evaluation, including history, physical examination, and judicious use of ancillary studies, allows the localization and diagnosis of nervous system pathology. The process and interpretation of the neurological examination varies with age; the newborn is unique, with many transient and primitive reflexes, whereas the examinations of adolescents and adults are similar. Careful evaluations of social, cognitive, language, fine motor, and gross motor skills, and their age appropriateness are key.

HISTORY

Gathering neurological history follows the traditional medical model with three additions: the **pace** and **localization** of the problem and the developmental assessment. The symptom evolution provides clues to the underlying process. Symptoms may evolve in a **progressive, static,** or **episodic** fashion. Progressive symptoms may present suddenly (seizures, stroke); acutely over minutes or hours (epidural hemorrhage); subacutely over days or weeks (brain tumor); or slowly over years (hereditary neuropathies). Static neurological abnormalities are observed early in life and do not change in character over time (cerebral palsy). Static lesions are often caused by congenital brain abnormalities or prenatal/perinatal brain injury. Intermittent attacks of recurrent, stereotyped episodes suggest epilepsy or migraine syndromes, among others. Episodic disorders are characterized by periods of symptoms, followed by partial or complete recovery (demyelinating, autoimmune, vascular diseases).

Careful evaluations of social, cognitive, language, fine motor, and gross motor skills are key (Chapter 7) to distinguish normal development from isolated or global delays. Loss of skills over time (regression) is particularly worrisome and may suggest an underlying degenerative disease, emerging autism spectrum disorder, epileptic encephalopathy, or other neurological diagnoses.

PHYSICAL EXAMINATION

Observation of the child's appearance, movement, and behavior begins at the start of the encounter. For example, the child may display an unusual posture, abnormal gait, or lack of awareness of the environment.

The brain and skin have the same embryonic origin (ectoderm), so abnormalities of hair, skin, teeth, and nails are associated with congenital brain disorders (neurocutaneous disorders) such as neurofibromatosis (NF type 1), in which **café-au-lait macules** (flat, light brown macules) are characteristic. **Adenoma sebaceum** (fibrovascular lesions that look like acne on the nose and malar regions), nail fibromas, ash-leaf spots (hypopigmented macules), and Shagreen patches (flesh-colored soft plaques with prominent follicular openings) are commonly seen in older children and adults with tuberous sclerosis.

The **head circumference** is measured in its largest occipitofrontal circumference and plotted against standard growth curves (Chapter 5). **Microcephaly** and **macrocephaly** represent an occipitofrontal circumference 2 standard deviations below or above the mean, respectively. Measurements plotted over time may show an accelerating pattern (hydrocephalus) or decelerating pattern (brain injury, degenerative neurological disorder). The anterior fontanelle is slightly depressed and pulsatile when a calm infant is upright. A tense or bulging fontanelle may indicate increased intracranial pressure (ICP) but may also be seen in a crying or febrile infant. Premature closure of one or more sutures **(craniosynostosis)** results in an unusual shape of the head. Abnormal shape, location, or condition of the face, eyes, nares, philtrum, lips, or ears (dysmorphic features) are found in many genetic syndromes.

A careful **ocular examination** is essential and should include a search for epicanthal folds, coloboma, conjunctival telangiectasias, and cataracts. Direct ophthalmoscopy assesses the optic discs and macula for abnormalities, such as papilledema or a cherry red spot. A complete examination of the retina involves dilating the pupil and use of indirect ophthalmoscopy.

Examination of the hands and feet may reveal abnormal creases or digits (Chapters 50 and 201). The neck and spine should be examined for obvious (myelomeningocele) or subtle (cutaneous dimples, sinus tracts, hair tufts, subcutaneous lipomas) midline defects. Nervous system abnormalities may result in kyphosis or scoliosis (Chapter 202).

NEUROLOGICAL EXAMINATION OF A NEONATE

The neonatal neurological examination primarily assesses the function of the basal ganglia, brainstem, and more caudal structures.

TABLE 179.1 Central Nervous System Reflexes of Infancy

REFLEX	DESCRIPTION	AGE AT APPEARANCE	AGE AT DISAPPEARANCE
Moro	Light drop of head produces sudden extension followed by flexion of the arms and legs	Birth	6 mo
Grasp	Placing finger in palm results in flexing of infant's fingers	Birth	6 mo
Rooting	Tactile stimulus at the side of the mouth results in the mouth pursuing the stimulus	Birth	4-6 mo
Trunk incurvation (Gallant)	Stroking the skin along the edge of vertebrae produces curvature of the spine with concavity on the side of the stimulus	Birth	4 mo
Placing	When dorsum of foot is brought into contact with the edge of a surface, infant places foot on the surface	Birth	4-6 mo
Asymmetrical tonic neck	With infant supine, turning of the head results in ipsilateral extension of the arm and leg with flexion of opposite extremities in a "fencing" posture	Birth	3 mo
Parachute	Infant is suspended face down by the chest. When infant is moved toward a table, the arms extend as if to protect self	8-10 mo	Never
Babinski	Stroking lateral aspect of sole from heel up results in dorsiflexion of the great toe and fanning of the remaining toes	Birth	12-18 mo

Mental Status

A healthy newborn infant should have periods of quiet, sustained wakefulness interspersed with sleep. Irritability, lethargy, or more severely depressed consciousness are nonspecific signs of abnormal brain function.

Reflexes

Examination of the **primitive reflexes** provides assessment of the functional integrity of the brainstem and basal ganglia (Table 179.1). Many of these stereotyped motor responses are present at birth. They are symmetrical and disappear at 4-6 months of age, indicating the normal maturation of descending inhibitory cerebral influences. Asymmetry or persistence of the primitive reflexes may indicate focal brain or peripheral nerve lesions.

Motor Examination and Tone

Posture is the position that a calm infant naturally assumes when placed supine. An infant at 28 weeks of gestation shows an extended posture. By 32 weeks, there is a trend toward increase in tone and flexion of the lower extremities. At 34 weeks, the lower extremities are flexed; the upper extremities are extended. The term infant flexes lower and upper extremities. **Recoil**, the readiness with which an arm or leg springs back to its original position after passive stretching and release, is essentially absent in very premature infants but is brisk at term. Because of the asymmetrical tonic neck reflex, it is essential to maintain the infant's head in a neutral position (not turned to the side) during assessment of posture and tone. Spontaneous movements of premature infants are slow and writhing; those of term infants are more rapid.

NEUROLOGICAL EXAMINATION OF A CHILD

The purpose of the neurological examination is to *localize* or identify the region from which the symptoms arise. The **mental status and developmental examinations** assess cerebral cortex function. The **cranial nerve examination** evaluates the integrity of the brainstem. The **motor examination** evaluates upper and lower motor neuron function. The **sensory examination** assesses the peripheral sensory receptors and their central reflections. **Deep tendon reflexes** assess upper and lower motor connections.

Mental Status and Developmental Evaluation

Alertness is assessed in infants by observing spontaneous activities, feeding behavior, and visual ability to fix and follow objects. Responses to tactile, visual, and auditory stimuli are noted. If consciousness is altered, the response to painful stimuli is noted. Observation of toddlers at play allows a nonthreatening assessment of developmentally appropriate skills. In addition to language function, older children can be tested for reading, writing, numerical skills, fund of knowledge, abstract reasoning, judgment, humor, and memory.

The simplest way to assess intellectual abilities is through language skills. **Language function** is receptive (understanding speech or gestures) and expressive (speech and use of gestures). Abnormalities of language resulting from cerebral hemisphere disorders are referred to as **aphasias**. Anterior, expressive, or *Broca aphasia* is characterized by sparse, nonfluent language. Posterior, receptive, or *Wernicke aphasia* is characterized by an inability to understand language, with speech that is fluent but nonsensical. Global aphasia refers to impaired expressive and receptive language.

CRANIAL NERVE EVALUATION

The cranial nerve evaluation assesses brainstem integrity, but depends on the stage of brain maturation and the ability to cooperate. A colorful toy may capture a young child's attention and permit observation of coordination, movement, and cranial nerve function.

Cranial Nerve I

Smell can be assessed in verbal, cooperative children older than 2 years of age. Aromatic substances (perfumes, vanilla) should be used instead of volatile substances (ammonia), which irritate the nasal mucosa and stimulate the trigeminal nerve.

Cranial Nerve II

Full-term newborns in a quiet awake state follow human faces, lights in a dark room, or large, opticokinetic strips. Visual acuity has been estimated to be 20/200 in newborns and gradually matures throughout childhood. Standard visual charts displaying pictures instead of letters can be used to assess visual acuity in toddlers. Peripheral vision is tested by surreptitiously bringing objects into the visual field from behind. A reduced pupillary reaction to light suggests anterior visual pathway (retina, optic nerves, chiasm) lesions. Unilateral lesions are identified by the *swinging flashlight test.* With an optic nerve abnormality, both pupils constrict when light is directed into the normal eye. When light is swung over to the abnormal eye, both pupils dilate inappropriately; this is called an *afferent pupillary defect* or **Marcus Gunn pupil.** Interruption of the sympathetic innervation to the pupil produces **Horner syndrome** (ptosis, miosis, and unilateral facial anhidrosis). In this instance, anisocoria (unequal pupils) is more pronounced in a dark room because the affected pupil is unable to dilate appropriately. Lesions of the posterior visual pathway, including the lateral geniculate, optic radiations, and occipital cortex, have normal pupillary light reactions but are expressed by loss of visual fields.

Cranial Nerves III, IV, and VI

These three cranial nerves control eye movements and are most easily examined with the use of a colorful toy to capture the child's attention. For infants too young to fix and follow, rotating the infant's head assesses **oculocephalic vestibular reflexes** (doll's eye maneuver). If the brainstem is intact, rotating a newborn or comatose patient's head to the right causes the eyes to move to the left, and vice versa. In awake, older patients, voluntary eye movements mask the reflex.

Abnormalities of these cranial nerves may cause diplopia (double vision). With unilateral third cranial nerve (oculomotor nerve) palsy, the involved eye deviates down and out (infraducted, abducted), with associated ptosis and a dilated (mydriatic) pupil. Injury to cranial nerve IV (trochlear nerve) causes weakness of downward eye movement with consequent vertical diplopia. Cranial nerve VI (abducens nerve) palsy results in the inability to move the eye outward. Cranial nerve VI has a long intracranial route within the subarachnoid space; failure of abduction of one or both eyes is a frequent, but nonspecific, sign of increased intracranial pressure (ICP).

Cranial Nerve V

The muscles of mastication can be observed as an infant sucks and swallows. The **corneal reflex** can test cranial nerves V ophthalmic division and VII at any age. Facial sensation of light touch and pain can be determined with cotton gauze and pinprick. Facial sensation can be functionally assessed in an infant by gently brushing the cheek, which will produce the **rooting reflex** (turns head and neck with mouthing movement, as if seeking to nurse).

Cranial Nerve VII

Facial muscles are assessed by observing the face during rest, crying, and blinking. At older, cooperative ages, children can be asked to smile, blow out their cheeks, blink forcibly, and furrow their foreheads. Weakness of all unilateral muscles of the face, including the forehead, eye, and mouth, indicates a lesion of the ipsilateral peripheral facial nerve **(Bell palsy).** Since the upper third of the face receives bilateral cortical innervation, if the weakness affects only the lower face and mouth, a contralateral lesion of upper motor neurons in the brain (tumor, stroke, abscess) must be considered.

Cranial Nerve VIII

Lesions of cranial nerve VIII cause deafness, tinnitus, and vertigo. Normally, alert neonates blink in response to a bell or other abrupt, loud sound. Four-month-old infants turn their head and eyes to localize a sound. Hearing can be tested in a verbal child by whispering a word in one ear while covering the opposite ear. If there are any concerns about hearing, formal audiologic assessment is indicated. Delayed language development should trigger a referral for a formal hearing assessment.

Lesions of the vestibular component of cranial nerve VIII produce symptoms of vertigo, nausea, vomiting, diaphoresis, and nystagmus. Nystagmus is an involuntary beating eye movement with a rapid phase in one direction and a slow phase in the opposite direction. By convention, the direction of the nystagmus is defined by the fast phase and may be horizontal, vertical, or rotatory.

Cranial Nerves IX and X

The gag reflex is brisk at all ages except the very immature neonate. An absent gag reflex suggests a lesion of the brainstem, cranial nerves IX or X, neuromuscular junction, or pharyngeal muscles. Weak, breathy, or nasal speech, weak sucking, drooling, inability to handle secretions, gagging, and nasal regurgitation of food are additional symptoms of cranial nerve X dysfunction.

Cranial Nerve XI

Observing the infant's posture and spontaneous activity assesses the functions of the trapezius and sternocleidomastoid muscles. Head tilt and drooping of the shoulder suggest lesions involving cranial nerve XI. In later childhood, strength in these muscles can be tested directly.

Cranial Nerve XII

Atrophy and fasciculation of the tongue usually indicate a lesion of the anterior horn cells (spinal muscular atrophy). Assessment is most reliable when an infant is asleep. The tongue deviates toward the weak side in unilateral lesions.

MOTOR EXAMINATION

Strength

In infants, strength is assessed by observation of spontaneous movements and movements against gravity. Extremity movements should be symmetrical and are best seen when the infant is held supine with one hand supporting the buttocks and one supporting the shoulders. Strength is graded as follows:

5 Normal
4 Weak but able to provide resistance
3 Able to move against gravity but not against resistance
2 Unable to move against gravity
1 Minimal movement
0 Complete paralysis

Strength in toddlers is assessed by observing functional abilities, such as walking, stooping to pick up an object, and standing up from the floor. An older child should be able to easily reach high above his or her head, wheelbarrow walk, run, hop, go up and down stairs, and arise from the ground. Cooperative children can undergo individual muscle strength testing. **Gower sign** (child arises from lying on the floor by using his arms to *climb up* his legs and body) is a sign of significant proximal weakness. Subtle upper extremity asymmetry can be detected when the child extends arms out in front with the palms upward and eyes closed. The hand on the weaker side cups and begins to pronate slowly **(pronator drift). Muscle fasciculations** indicate denervation from disease of the anterior horn cell or peripheral nerve.

Tone

Tone represents the dynamic resistance of muscles to passive stretch. Lower motor and cerebellar lesions produce decreased tone **(hypotonia).** Upper motor lesions produce increased tone **(spasticity).** In extrapyramidal disease, an increase in resistance is present throughout passive movement of a joint **(rigidity).**

Bulk

Muscle bulk may be decreased due to disuse or to lower motor neuron or neuromuscular disease. Excessive muscle bulk is seen in rare conditions, such as myotonia congenita; boys with Duchenne muscular dystrophy have *pseudohypertrophy* of their calves.

Coordination

Ataxia is the lack of coordination of movement, which is typically due to a dysfunction of the cerebellar pathways. Observation and functional analysis help assess coordination in infants and toddlers. Watching the child sit or walk assesses truncal stability. Exchanging toys or objects with the child permits assessment of intention tremor and **dysmetria** (errors in judging distance), signs of cerebellar dysfunction. Cooperative children can do repetitive finger or foot tapping to test rapid alternating movements. Cerebellar and corticospinal tract dysfunction produce slow and irregular alternating movements.

Gait

Watching a child creep, crawl, cruise, or walk is the best global assessment for the motor and coordination systems (Chapter 197). Subtle deficits and asymmetries in strength, tone, or balance may be observed. The toddler gait is normally wide-based and unsteady. The base of the gait narrows with age. By 6 years, a typical child is able to walk on their toes or heels and can tandem walk (heel to toe). Cerebellar dysfunction results in a broad-based, unsteady gait accompanied by difficulty in executing turns. Corticospinal tract dysfunction produces a stiff, scissoring gait and toe walking; arm swing is decreased, and the affected arm is flexed across the body. Extrapyramidal dysfunction produces a slow, stiff, shuffling gait with dystonic postures. A waddling gait occurs with hip weakness due to lower motor neuron or neuromuscular disorders. A steppage gait results from weakness of ankle dorsiflexors (common peroneal palsy).

Reflexes

Deep tendon reflexes can be elicited at any age and are reported on a five-point scale:

0 Absent
1 Trace
2 Normal
3 Exaggerated reflex, with spread to contiguous areas (tapping a patellar reflex and observing a bilaterally brisk quadriceps response)
4 Clonus (self-limited or sustained)

These reflexes are decreased in lower motor neuron diseases and increased in upper motor neuron disease. **Babinski response**, or extensor plantar reflex, is an upward movement of the great toe and flaring of the toes on stimulation of the lateral foot and is a sign of corticospinal tract dysfunction. This reflex is unreliable in neonates, except when asymmetrical, because the "normal" response at this age varies. By 12-18 months of age, the plantar response should consistently be flexor (toes flexing down).

SENSORY EXAMINATION

The sensory examination of newborns and infants is limited to observing the behavioral response to light touch or gentle sterile pinprick. Stimulation of a limb should produce a facial grimace. A spinal reflex alone may produce withdrawal movement of a limb. In a cooperative child, the senses of pain, touch, temperature, vibration, and joint position can be tested individually. The cortical areas of sensation must be intact to identify an object placed in the hand **(stereognosis)** or a number written in the hand **(graphesthesia)** or to distinguish between two sharp objects applied simultaneously and closely on the skin **(two-point discrimination).**

SPECIAL DIAGNOSTIC PROCEDURES

Cerebrospinal Fluid Analysis

Analysis of cerebrospinal fluid (CSF) is essential when central nervous system infection is suspected and provides important clues to other diagnoses (Table 179.2). Differentiating hemorrhagic CSF caused by a traumatic lumbar puncture (LP) from a true subarachnoid hemorrhage may be difficult. In most cases of traumatic LP, the fluid clears significantly as the sequence of tubes is collected. If there is clinical evidence of increased ICP (papilledema, depression of consciousness, focal neurological deficits), caution must be exercised before performing an LP to limit risk of cerebral herniation. A computed tomography (CT) scan should be performed and confirmed to be normal

TABLE 179.2 Analysis of Cerebrospinal Fluid

	NORMAL CSF VALUES	
CSF FINDING	**NEWBORN**	**>1 MO OLD**
Cell count*	10-25/mm^3	5/mm^3
Protein	65-150 mg/dL	<40 mg/dL
Glucose	>2/3 blood glucose or >40 mg/dL	>2/3 blood glucose or >60 mg/dL

CSF Change	**Significance**
Increased polymorphonuclear cells and decreased CSF glucose	Bacterial infection
	Partially treated bacterial meningitis
	Brain or parameningeal abscess
	Parasitic infection
	Leak of dermoid contents
Increased lymphocytes and decreased CSF glucose	Mycobacterial infection (tuberculosis)
	Fungal infection
	Carcinomatous meningitis
	Sarcoidosis
Increased lymphocytes and normal CSF glucose	Viral meningitis
	Postinfectious disease (ADEM)
	Vasculitis
Increased CSF protein	Infection
	Guillain-Barré syndrome
	Inflammatory disease (ADEM, multiple sclerosis)
	Leukodystrophy
	Venous thrombosis
	Hypertension
	Spinal block (Froin syndrome)
	Carcinomatous meningitis
Decreased glucose without pleocytosis	GLUT-1 transporter deficiency
Mild CSF pleocytosis	Tumor
	Infarction
	Multiple sclerosis
	Subacute bacterial endocarditis
Bloody CSF	Subarachnoid hemorrhage
	Subdural hemorrhage
	Intraparenchymal hemorrhage
	Hemorrhagic meningoencephalitis (group B streptococci, HSV)
	CNS trauma
	Vascular malformation
	Coagulopathy
	Traumatic lumbar puncture

**In normal children, cells present should be lymphocytes.*
ADEM, Acute disseminated encephalomyelitis; *CNS,* central nervous system; *CSF,* cerebrospinal fluid; *HSV,* herpes simplex virus.

before the LP if increased ICP is suspected. If increased ICP is present, it must be treated before an LP is performed.

Electroencephalography

The electroencephalogram (EEG) records electrical activity generated by the cerebral cortex. EEG rhythms mature throughout childhood. There are three key features present: background patterns, behavioral state modulation, and presence or absence of epileptiform patterns. The background varies with age but in general should be symmetrical and synchronous between the two hemispheres without any localized area of higher amplitude or slower frequencies (focal slowing). Persistent focal slowing suggests an underlying structural abnormality (brain tumor, abscess, stroke). Bilateral disturbances of brain activity (increased ICP, metabolic encephalopathy) must be suspected when there is diffuse slow wave activity. Spikes, polyspikes, and spike-and-wave abnormalities, either in a localized region (focal) or distributed bihemispherically (generalized), suggest an increased risk for seizures.

Electromyography and Nerve Conduction Studies

Electromyography and nerve conduction velocities (NCVs) assess for abnormalities of the neuromuscular apparatus, including anterior horn cells, peripheral nerves, neuromuscular junctions, and muscles. Normal muscle is electrically silent at rest. Spontaneous discharges of motor fibers **(fibrillations)** or groups of muscle fibers **(fasciculation)** indicate denervation, revealing dysfunction of anterior horn cells or peripheral nerves. Abnormal muscle responses to repetitive nerve stimulation are seen with neuromuscular junction disorders, such as myasthenia gravis and botulism. The amplitude and duration of the muscle compound action potentials are decreased in primary diseases of muscle. NCVs assess the action potential transmission along peripheral nerves. NCVs are slowed in demyelinating neuropathies (Guillain-Barré syndrome). The amplitude of the signal is diminished in axonal neuropathies.

Neuroimaging

Imaging the brain and spinal cord is accomplished using CT or magnetic resonance imaging (MRI). CT is quick and accessible for emergency purposes. MRI provides finer detail and, with different sequences, permits detection of posterior fossa lesions, subtle cerebral abnormalities, vascular anomalies, low-grade tumors, and ischemic changes. For a child with an acute head injury or sudden headache, cranial CT is the study of choice because it can rapidly reveal intracranial hemorrhage or other large lesions. For a child with new-onset focal seizures, MRI is the study of choice because an area of focal cortical dysplasia or other subtle lesions might not be apparent on CT. MRI also provides excellent views of the spinal cord. Cranial ultrasonography is a noninvasive bedside procedure used to visualize the brain and ventricles of infants with open fontanelles.

CHAPTER 180
Headache and Migraine

ETIOLOGY AND EPIDEMIOLOGY

Headache is a common symptom among children and adolescents. Headaches can be a primary problem (migraines, tension-type headaches) or secondary to another condition.

Secondary headaches are most often associated with minor illnesses such as viral upper respiratory infections or sinusitis but may be the first symptom of serious conditions (meningitis, brain tumors), so a systematic approach is necessary.

CLINICAL MANIFESTATIONS

Decision-Making Algorithm
Available @ StudentConsult.com
Headaches

The temporal pattern of the headache must be clarified. Each pattern (acute, recurrent-episodic, chronic-progressive, chronic-nonprogressive) has its own differential diagnosis (Table 180.1).

Tension-type headaches are the most common type of recurrent primary headaches in children and adolescents. They are generally mild and lack associated symptoms so are not typically disruptive to patients' lifestyle or activities. The pain is global and squeezing or pressing in character and can last for hours or days. There is no associated nausea, vomiting, phonophobia, or photophobia. Headaches can be related to environmental stresses or symptomatic of underlying psychiatric illnesses, such as anxiety or depression.

Migraine headaches are another common type of recurrent headaches and frequently begin in childhood. Headaches are stereotyped attacks of frontal, bitemporal or unilateral, moderate to severe, pounding or throbbing pain that are aggravated by activity and last 1-72 hours. Associated symptoms include nausea, vomiting, pallor, photophobia, phonophobia, and an intense desire to seek a quiet, dark room for rest. Toddlers may be unable to verbalize the source of their discomfort and exhibit episodes of irritability, sleepiness, pallor, and vomiting. An aura can precede or coincide with the headache and typically persists for 15-30 minutes. Visual auras are very common and consist of spots, flashes, or lines of light that flicker in one or both visual fields. Complex, atypical auras (hemiparesis, monocular blindness, ophthalmoplegia, vertigo, confusion), accompanied by a headache, warrant careful diagnostic investigation, including a combination of neuroimaging, electroencephalogram, and appropriate metabolic studies.

Common causes of **secondary headaches** include head trauma, viral illness, and sinusitis. Medication-overuse headaches may complicate primary and secondary headaches. Serious causes of secondary headache include increased intracranial pressure (ICP) caused by a mass (tumor, vascular malformation) or intrinsic increase in pressure (pseudotumor cerebri). Increased ICP should be suspected if the headache and associated vomiting are worse when lying down or on first awakening; awaken the child from sleep; remit on arising; or are exacerbated by coughing, Valsalva maneuver, or bending over. Papilledema (Fig. 180.1) or focal neurological deficits should trigger an intensive etiological investigation.

DIAGNOSTIC STUDIES

For most children, a thorough history and physical examination provide an accurate diagnosis and obviate the need for further testing. Neuroimaging is usually not necessary. Imaging is warranted, however, if the patient has an abnormal neurological examination, symptoms of increased ICP, there are unusual neurological features during the headache (atypical aura), or the headaches are progressively worsening. In these cases, brain magnetic resonance imaging (MRI), with and without gadolinium contrast, is the study of choice, providing the highest sensitivity for detecting posterior fossa lesions and other, more subtle abnormalities. When the headache has a sudden, severe onset, emergent computed tomography (CT) can quickly evaluate

TABLE 180.1 Four Temporal Patterns of Childhood Headache

Acute: Single episode of pain without a history of such episodes. The "first and worst" headache raises concerns for aneurysmal subarachnoid hemorrhage in adults, but is commonly due to *febrile illness* related to upper respiratory tract infection in children. Regardless, more ominous causes of acute headache (hemorrhage, meningitis, tumor) must be considered.
Acute recurrent: Pattern of attacks of pain separated by symptom-free intervals. Primary headache syndromes, such as *migraine or tension-type* headache, usually cause this pattern. Recurrent headaches are occasionally due to specific epilepsy syndromes (benign occipital epilepsy), substance abuse, or recurrent trauma.
Chronic progressive: Implies a gradually increasing frequency and severity of headache. The pathological correlate is *increasing ICP*. Causes of this pattern include pseudotumor cerebri, brain tumor, hydrocephalus, chronic meningitis, brain abscess, and subdural collections.
Chronic nonprogressive or chronic daily: Pattern of frequent or constant headache. Chronic daily headache generally is defined as >3-mo history of >15 headaches/mo, with headaches lasting >4 hr. Affected patients have normal neurological examinations; psychological factors and anxiety about possible underlying organic causes are common.

ICP, Intracranial pressure.

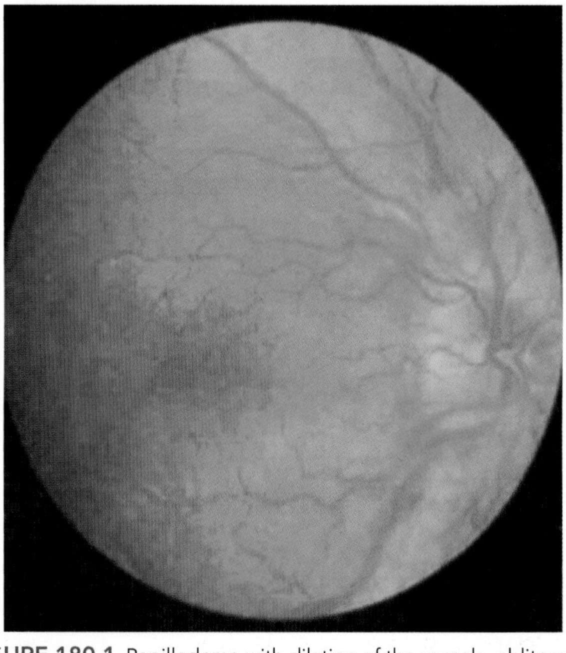

FIGURE 180.1 Papilledema with dilation of the vessels, obliteration of the optic cup, loss of disc margin, and hemorrhages around disc. (From Kliegman RE, Behrman RM, Jenson HB, eds. *Nelson Textbook of Pediatrics.* 18th ed. Philadelphia: Saunders; 2007:2107.)

for intracranial bleeding. If the CT is negative, a lumbar puncture should be performed to measure opening pressure and evaluate for pleocytosis, elevated red blood cells, and xanthochromia.

TREATMENT

Treating migraines requires an individually tailored regimen to address the frequency, severity, and disability produced by the headaches. Intermittent *symptomatic,* or abortive, analgesics are the mainstay for treatment of infrequent episodes of migraine. Symptomatic therapy requires early analgesic administration, often accompanied by rest in a quiet, dark room. Acetaminophen or a nonsteroidal antiinflammatory drug such as ibuprofen or naproxen sodium is often effective. Hydration and antiemetics are useful adjunctive therapies. If these first-line medications are insufficient, *triptan* agents may be considered. Triptans, available in injectable, nasal spray, oral disintegrating, and tablet form, are serotonin receptor agonists that can alleviate migraine symptoms promptly. Triptans are contraindicated for patients with focal neurological deficits associated with their migraines or signs consistent with basilar migraine (syncope) because of the risk of stroke.

Many children suffer with severe and frequent migraines that disrupt their daily lives. Children with more than one disabling headache per week may require **daily preventive agents** to reduce both attack frequency and severity. Preventive medications include tricyclic antidepressants (amitriptyline, nortriptyline), anticonvulsants (topiramate, valproic acid), antihistamines (cyproheptadine), beta-blockers (propranolol), and calcium channel blockers (verapamil).

Before initiating daily medications, lifestyle modifications must be put into place to regulate sleep, daily routines, and exercise and to identify and eliminate any precipitating or aggravating influences (caffeine, certain foods, stress, missed meals, dehydration). Other adjunctive treatment options include psychological support, stress management, and biofeedback.

CHAPTER 181 Seizures

A seizure is a transient occurrence of signs or symptoms resulting from abnormal excessive or synchronous neuronal activity in the brain.

ETIOLOGY AND EPIDEMIOLOGY

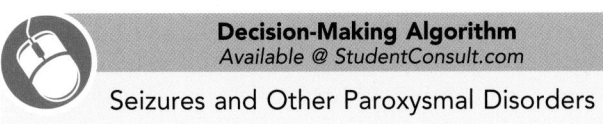

Decision-Making Algorithm
Available @ StudentConsult.com
Seizures and Other Paroxysmal Disorders

The differential diagnosis of paroxysmal disorders includes **seizures** and **nonepileptic events** (Table 181.1). Nonepileptic paroxysmal events are often normal or benign phenomena, although some are clinically significant and consequential. A thorough medical history from the patient and primary witnesses is the most reliable tool for establishing the correct diagnosis.

TABLE 181.1 Paroxysmal Disorders of Childhood

Seizures/epilepsy
Migraine and variants • Paroxysmal torticollis of infancy • Benign paroxysmal vertigo
Syncope • Vasovagal syncope • Breath-holding spells • Cardiac syncope (arrhythmias, long QT syndrome) • Apnea
Transient ischemic attack
Metabolic disorders • Hypoglycemia • Inborn errors of metabolism
Sleep disorders • Narcolepsy, cataplexy • Night terrors
Paroxysmal dyskinesias and other movement disorders • Tics
Shudder attacks
Sandifer syndrome (gastroesophageal reflux causing paroxysmal stiffening and posturing)
Conversion disorder
Malingering
Normal behavior • Neonatal jitteriness • Benign sleep myoclonus
Self-stimulatory behavior

Acute symptomatic seizures are secondary to an acute problem affecting brain excitability, such as electrolyte imbalance or infection (Table 181.2). **Epilepsy** is defined as recurrent, *unprovoked* seizures. Epileptic seizures are generally classified as *focal,* arising from one region of the cortex, or *generalized,* which arise from both hemispheres simultaneously (Table 181.3). Approximately 4-10% of children experience at least one seizure. The incidence of childhood epilepsy is 1-2%.

FOCAL SEIZURES

Focal seizures with retained awareness (previously termed simple partial seizures) arise from a specific anatomical focus and may or may not spread to surrounding brain regions. Clinical symptoms include motor (tonic, clonic, myoclonic), sensory, psychic, or autonomic abnormalities, but consciousness is preserved. The location and extent of spread of the seizure focus determine the clinical symptoms.

Focal seizures with altered awareness (previously termed complex partial seizures) can have similar sensorimotor signs, but also have associated alteration of consciousness. Although the child may not be completely unresponsive, subtle slowing or alteration of mental status (*dyscognitive* features) may occur. Along with altered responsiveness, patients may have automatisms or stare during these seizures. Automatisms are

TABLE 181.2 Causes of Seizures

PERINATAL CONDITIONS
Malformation of cortical development
Intrauterine infection
Hypoxic-ischemic encephalopathy*
Trauma
Hemorrhage*
INFECTIONS
Encephalitis*
Meningitis*
Brain abscess
METABOLIC CONDITIONS
Hypoglycemia*
Hypocalcemia
Hypomagnesemia
Hyponatremia
Hypernatremia
Storage diseases
Reye syndrome
Degenerative disorders
Porphyria
Pyridoxine dependency and deficiency
POISONING
Lead
Drug toxicity
Drug withdrawal
NEUROCUTANEOUS SYNDROMES
Tuberous sclerosis
Neurofibromatosis
Sturge-Weber syndrome
Incontinentia pigmenti
SYSTEMIC DISORDERS
Vasculitis
Systemic lupus erythematosus
Hypertensive encephalopathy
Hepatic encephalopathy
OTHER CAUSATIVE DISORDERS/CONDITIONS
Accidental trauma*
Child abuse*
Increased intracranial pressure
Tumor
Remote brain injury
Febrile illnesses*
Cryptogenic* (no underlying disorder found)
Familial*

*Common.

TABLE 181.3 Classification of Seizures and Epilepsy Syndromes

FOCAL SEIZURES
With retained awareness With observable motor signs (can be tonic, clonic, myoclonic) With sensory phenomena (visual, auditory, olfactory, gustatory, vertiginous, somatosensory) Autonomic
With impaired consciousness (dyscognitive features) Psychic (déjà vu, jamais vu, fear) Impaired consciousness at onset Development of impaired consciousness
Focal seizures with evolution to bilateral convulsions Jacksonian seizures
GENERALIZED SEIZURES
Absence (staring, unresponsiveness)
Convulsive seizures • Tonic (sustained contraction) • Clonic (rhythmic contractions) • Tonic-clonic (tonic phase followed by clonic phase)
Atonic (abrupt loss of tone)
Myoclonic (rapid, shock-like contraction)
Epileptic spasms (flexion or extension of trunk and extremities for <2 sec)

automatic semipurposeful movements of the mouth (lip smacking, chewing) or extremities (rubbing of fingers, shuffling of feet). Focal seizures that manifest only with psychic or autonomic symptoms, such as a feeling of déjà vu during a temporal lobe seizure, can be difficult to recognize.

When focal seizures spread to involve both cerebral hemispheres, they are said to have *evolved to a bilateral convulsive seizure* (previously called a secondarily generalized seizure). It is often difficult to distinguish primary generalized tonic and clonic seizures from those that evolved from focal seizures on purely clinical grounds. This distinction is important, however, because evaluation and treatment for focal or generalized epilepsy syndromes are quite different.

GENERALIZED SEIZURES

Tonic, clonic, and biphasic **tonic-clonic** seizures may occur alone or in association with other seizure types. Typically the seizure begins abruptly but occasionally is preceded by a series of myoclonic jerks. During a tonic-clonic seizure, consciousness and control of posture are lost, followed by tonic stiffening and upward deviation of the eyes. Pooling of secretions, pupillary dilation, diaphoresis, and hypertension are common. Clonic jerks follow the tonic phase. In the post-ictal phase, the child might be hypotonic. Irritability and headache are common as the child awakens.

Absence Seizures

Seizures in which the primary clinical feature is staring can be either absence (generalized) or focal seizures. The clinical

TABLE 181.4 Differentiating Absence Seizures From Focal Seizures With Altered Awareness

FEATURE	ABSENCE SEIZURE	FOCAL SEIZURE WITH ALTERED AWARENESS
Duration	Seconds	Minutes
Provoking maneuver	Hyperventilation Photic stimulation	Variable, but often none
Postictal phase	None (return immediately to baseline)	Confusion, sleepiness
Number of seizures	Many per day	Infrequent (rarely more than one per day)
EEG features	Interictal: normal except bursts of generalized spike wave and sometimes occipital intermittent rhythmic delta activity Ictal: 3-Hz generalized spike-wave	Interictal: focal slowing, sharp waves, or spikes Ictal: focal discharges (with or without spread to contiguous regions or the contralateral hemisphere)
Neurological examination	Normal	Normal, or focal deficits
Neuroimaging	Normal*	Normal, or focal abnormalities (mesial temporal sclerosis, focal cortical dysplasia, neoplasm, encephalomalacia)
First-line treatment	Ethosuximide or valproic acid†	Oxcarbazepine

**In the proper clinical context, and with an appropriate EEG, a diagnosis of absence epilepsy should be made without neuroimaging.*
†Oxcarbazepine and carbamazepine are relatively contraindicated for children with typical absence epilepsy, as their seizures can be exacerbated by these medications.
EEG, Electroencephalographic.

hallmark of absence seizures is a brief (<15 seconds) loss of awareness accompanied by eyelid fluttering or simple automatisms, such as fumbling with the fingers and lip smacking. Absence seizures usually begin between 4 and 6 years of age. Neurological examination and brain imaging are normal. The characteristic electroencephalographic (EEG) patterns consist of **generalized 3-Hz spike-and-wave activity.** An absence seizure can often be provoked by **hyperventilation.** Differentiating absence from focal seizures with altered awareness can be difficult but is essential for appropriate evaluation and treatment (Table 181.4).

Atypical Absence, Myoclonic, and Atonic Seizures

Atypical absence seizures manifest as episodes of impaired consciousness with automatisms, autonomic phenomena, and motor manifestations, such as eye opening, eye deviation, and body stiffening. They are associated with slower EEG discharges (2 Hz) and accompany other seizure types. **Myoclonus** is a sudden jerk of all or part of the body; not all myoclonus is due to epilepsy. Nonepileptic myoclonus may be benign, as in sleep myoclonus, or indicate serious disease. Myoclonic epilepsy usually is associated with multiple seizure types. The underlying disorder producing myoclonic epilepsy may be static (**juvenile myoclonic epilepsy** [JME]) or progressive and associated with neurological deterioration (neuronal ceroid lipofuscinosis). **Myoclonic absence** refers to body jerks that commonly accompany typical or atypical absence seizures. Although **atonic seizures** are typically brief (lasting 1-2 seconds), they are very disabling because of a sudden loss of postural tone that often results in falls and injuries.

Febrile Seizures

Seizures in the setting of fever may be caused by central nervous system infections (meningitis, encephalitis, brain abscess), unrecognized epilepsy triggered by fever, or **febrile seizures.** The latter represents the most common cause of seizures among children between 6 months and 6 years of age, occurring in about 4% of all children. By definition, a febrile seizure occurs in the presence of fever. **Simple febrile seizures** are generalized at onset, last less than 15 minutes, and occur only once in a 24-hour period in a neurologically and developmentally normal child. If the seizure has focal features, lasts longer than 15 minutes, recurs within 24 hours, or the child has preexisting neurological challenges, the seizure is referred to as a **complex febrile seizure.**

The prognosis of children with simple febrile seizures is excellent. Although febrile seizures recur in 30-50% of children, intellectual achievements are normal. The risk of subsequent epilepsy is not substantially greater than that of the general population (approximately 2%). Factors that increase the risk for the development of epilepsy include abnormal neurological examination or development, family history of epilepsy, and complex febrile seizures.

Since simple febrile seizures are brief and the outcome is benign, most children require no treatment. Rectal diazepam can be administered during a seizure to abort a prolonged convulsion; it is appropriate to provide a rescue medication for children with a history of prolonged febrile seizures. Since antiseizure medications have side effects and children with febrile seizures have an excellent prognosis, daily antiseizure medication to prevent febrile seizures is not recommended. Administration of antipyretics during febrile illnesses does not prevent febrile seizures; the seizure can often be the first sign of a child's illness.

Psychogenic Nonepileptic Seizures

Psychogenic nonepileptic seizures (PNES) (previously termed pseudoseizures) may be the manifestation of conversion disorders or malingering. Additionally, children with epilepsy may, consciously or subconsciously, exhibit concurrent PNES. PNES semiology typically differs from epileptic seizures. In PNES, the patient's eyes are often closed (typically eyes are open during epileptic seizures) and the movements are tremulousness or thrashing rather than tonic or clonic. Verbalization and pelvic thrusting are seen more commonly in PNES, urinary and fecal continence is usually preserved, and injury does not usually occur. If the tongue is bitten, more often the tip of the tongue is injured (as opposed to the sides of the tongue in epileptic seizures). PNES can often be initiated or terminated by suggestion. An EEG performed during PNES does not show epileptiform patterns. The diagnosis is critical because appropriate mental health care, and not anticonvulsant medications, is the crux of treatment. Careful assessment and intervention for physical or sexual abuse, as well as other social stressors, is a key component of the care of children with PNES.

EPILEPSY SYNDROMES

Epilepsy syndromes have distinctive EEG and clinical features (age of seizure onset, specific seizure types). Recognition of epilepsy syndromes provides useful information regarding the underlying etiologies that must be considered, treatments that may be helpful (or harmful), and long-term prognostic information.

Benign childhood epilepsy with centrotemporal spikes, also known as **benign Rolandic epilepsy,** is among the most common epilepsy syndromes and usually begins between ages 5 and 10 years. The seizures typically occur only during sleep or on awakening. Affected children usually have focal motor seizures involving the face and arm (abnormal movement or sensation around the face and mouth, drooling, rhythmic guttural sound, impaired speech and swallowing). Seizures sometimes evolve to bilateral convulsions. The interictal EEG demonstrates independent bilateral centrotemporal sharp waves but is otherwise normal. With a classic history and EEG and a normal neurological examination, the diagnosis can be made with confidence and neuroimaging is not required. Seizures usually respond promptly to antiseizure medication. Intellectual outcome is normal, and the epilepsy resolves after puberty. Comorbid learning difficulties (especially language-based learning disabilities) and attention-deficit/hyperactivity disorder (ADHD) are common.

Childhood absence epilepsy is another common syndrome. Absence seizures typically begin in the early school years and usually resolve by late childhood or adolescence. If absence does not remit, 44% will go on to develop JME (see later discussion). Ethosuximide is the first-choice medication. A subset of patients also has generalized tonic-clonic seizures. For these children, valproic acid is the first choice as it can prevent both absence and convulsive seizures. Comorbid learning disabilities and ADHD are common. There is no contraindication to treating these children's ADHD with stimulant medication.

JME is the most common generalized epilepsy among adolescents and young adults. Onset is typically in early adolescence with myoclonic jerks (exacerbated in the morning, often causing the patient to drop objects), generalized tonic-clonic seizures, and absence seizures. Seizures usually resolve promptly with antiseizure medication. JME is classically treated with valproic acid; however, there are concerns about side effects and teratogenicity. Levetiracetam has a much lower risk of teratogenicity and is generally well tolerated. As such, levetiracetam is now favored, particularly for girls and women since treatment of JME is usually lifelong.

Infantile spasms are brief contractions of the neck, trunk, and arm muscles, followed by a phase of sustained muscle contraction lasting less than 2 seconds. Spasms occur most frequently when the child is awakening from or going to sleep. Each jerk is followed by a brief period of relaxation with repeated spasms in clusters of variable duration. When flexion of the thighs and crying are prominent, the syndrome may be mistaken for colic or gastroesophageal reflux. **West syndrome** is the triad of infantile spasms, developmental regression, and a dramatically abnormal EEG pattern (**hypsarrhythmia**—a pattern of chaotic high-voltage slow waves, spikes, and polyspikes). The peak age at onset of infantile spasms is 3-8 months. The underlying etiology of the spasms dictates the prognosis. More than 200 different etiologies have been identified, including tuberous sclerosis, malformations of cortical development (lissencephaly), genetic syndromes (trisomy 21), acquired brain injury (stroke, perinatal hypoxic-ischemic encephalopathy), and metabolic disorders (phenylketonuria). Infants for whom an etiology is determined are classified as having *symptomatic* infantile spasms and are at very high risk for long-term neurodevelopmental difficulties. The etiology is not determined for a small subset of children; these patients have a somewhat better long-term prognosis but remain at high risk for adverse outcomes. With advances in genetic testing, fewer children have infantile spasms of uncertain etiology.

Infantile spasms are a neurological emergency since rapid initiation of effective therapy offers the best chance for favorable neurodevelopmental outcomes. First-line treatment options for infantile spasms include adrenocorticotropic hormone, high-dose oral corticosteroids, and vigabatrin. Other antiseizure medications are much less effective. For infants with underlying tuberous sclerosis, vigabatrin is the treatment of choice. For other patients, treatment determinations are made on a case-by-case basis.

Lennox-Gastaut syndrome is a severe epilepsy syndrome with variable age of onset. Most children present before age 5 years. Frequent, multiple seizure types including atonic, focal, atypical absence, and generalized tonic, clonic, or tonic-clonic semiologies characterize the disorder. Many children have underlying brain injury, malformations, or genetic etiologies. The seizures are typically difficult to control, and most patients have significant intellectual disability.

Benign neonatal convulsions are an autosomal dominant genetic disorder linked to abnormal neuronal potassium channels. Otherwise well newborns present with focal seizures toward the end of the first week of life, leading to the colloquial term *fifth-day fits*. Response to treatment is generally excellent, and the long-term outcome is typically favorable.

Acquired epileptic aphasia (Landau-Kleffner syndrome) is characterized by the abrupt loss of previously acquired language in young children. The language disability is an acquired cortical auditory deficit (auditory agnosia). The EEG is highly epileptiform in sleep, the peak area of abnormality often being in the dominant perisylvian region (language areas). This diagnosis should be considered for young patients with clear autistic regression, as it is a potentially treatable entity.

STATUS EPILEPTICUS

Status epilepticus is a neurological emergency and is defined as (1) ongoing seizure activity or (2) repetitive seizures without recovery of consciousness for greater than 30 minutes. Status epilepticus carries an approximately 14% risk of new neurological deficits and 4-5% mortality, both related to the underlying etiology. Etiologies include new-onset epilepsy, drug intoxication, drug withdrawal (especially missed anticonvulsant doses among children with epilepsy), hypoglycemia, electrolyte imbalance, acute head trauma, infection, ischemic stroke, intracranial hemorrhage, metabolic disorders, and hypoxia.

The first priority of treatment is to ensure an adequate airway, breathing, and circulation (Chapter 38). Vital signs should be obtained and oxygen administered if needed. If respirations are inadequate, positive-pressure ventilation may be required. Intravenous (IV) access should be obtained, and laboratory evaluation should be undertaken (see below).

Several pharmacological options exist for management of status epilepticus (Table 181.5). Initial management is with a benzodiazepine and should begin if the seizure persists longer than 5 minutes. Lorazepam, diazepam, and midazolam are all effective agents and should be given as an adequate single dose (rather than successive smaller doses), which can be repeated one time. IV administration is preferred. However, when IV access is not available, benzodiazepines may be administered via rectal, intranasal, buccal, or intramuscular routes.

If the seizure does not resolve after two doses of benzodiazepine, a second-line agent must be administered. There are few data from clinical trials to guide subsequent management. For newborns and infants, phenobarbital is reasonable. For older children, IV fosphenytoin (preferred over phenytoin due to tolerability), valproic acid, or levetiracetam may be considered. If the seizures persist, options include repeating one of the second-line medications or beginning a continuous infusion of midazolam or pentobarbital (with appropriate airway protection, blood pressure support, and strong consideration of video-EEG monitoring to evaluate for ongoing subclinical seizures; see Table 181.5). If this approach is ineffective, preparations for general anesthesia are undertaken. When status epilepticus stops, maintenance therapy is initiated with the appropriate anticonvulsant.

TABLE 181.5 Management of Status Epilepticus

STABILIZATION
ABCs (airway, breathing, circulation)
Cardiac monitoring
Oxygen and pulse oximetry
Intravenous access
Immediate laboratory tests
Glucose
Basic metabolic panel—sodium, calcium, magnesium
Anticonvulsant drug levels
Toxicology studies as appropriate
Complete blood counts, platelets, and differential
PHARMACOLOGICAL MANAGEMENT
Benzodiazepine (max rate of administration = 1 mg/min)
Lorazepam IV, IN 0.1 mg/kg (maximum 4 mg per dose)
Diazepam IV, PR 0.15-0.2 mg/kg (maximum 10 mg per dose)
Rectal diazepam 0.2-0.5 mg/kg (maximum 20 mg per dose)
Midazolam IV, IM, IN, buccal 0.1-0.2 mg/kg (maximum 10 mg per dose)
Standard anticonvulsant medications
Fosphenytoin IV, IM 20 mg/kg (phenytoin equivalents; maximum 1,500 PE per dose)
Phenobarbital IV 20 mg/kg (maximum 1,000 mg per dose)
Levetiracetam IV 60 mg/kg (maximum 4,500 mg per dose)
Valproic acid IV, PR 20 mg/kg (maximum 3,000 mg per dose)
Continuous infusions
Pentobarbital
Midazolam
General anesthesia

IM, Intramuscularly; *IN*, intranasally; *IV*, intravenous; *PE*, phenytoin; *PR*, per rectum.

LABORATORY AND DIAGNOSTIC EVALUATION

For an otherwise healthy child with a self-resolved, unprovoked seizure and a normal physical and neurological examination, no laboratory evaluation is required. Children with *simple febrile seizures* who have recovered completely require little or no laboratory evaluation other than studies necessary to evaluate the source of the fever. If the clinical presentation does not meet these criteria and acute symptomatic seizures are suspected, evaluation for potentially life-threatening causes such as meningitis, sepsis, head trauma, and toxins must be pursued. A complete laboratory evaluation for new onset of seizures includes a complete blood count and measurement of glucose, calcium, sodium, potassium, chloride, bicarbonate, urea nitrogen, creatinine, magnesium, and phosphorus, as well as blood or urine toxicology screening. Children with clinical signs and symptoms of meningitis (neck stiffness, Kernig sign, Brudzinski sign), or history or physical examination suggestive of intracranial infection, should undergo a lumbar puncture. Cerebrospinal fluid (CSF) should be analyzed for cell counts, culture, protein, and glucose levels. In children less than 18 months old, particularly young infants, the clinical symptoms of meningitis may be subtle. Neonates also may require testing for inborn errors of metabolism; blood ammonia; CSF glycine and lactate; and a clinical trial of pyridoxine. Evaluation for infections, such as urine and stool cultures, and polymerase chain reactions for herpes simplex virus, cytomegalovirus, and enterovirus should be considered.

The **EEG** is the most useful neurodiagnostic test for distinguishing seizures from nonepileptic paroxysmal disorders and for classifying seizures as having focal or generalized onset. The EEG must be interpreted in the context of the clinical history; some normal children have focal or epileptiform EEG patterns. Conversely, children with seizures may have normal interictal EEGs. When the diagnosis is unclear, EEG with prolonged recordings and simultaneous video monitoring in an attempt to capture a typical event may be necessary.

Magnetic resonance imaging (MRI) is superior to computed tomography (CT) in showing most brain pathology, but in the emergency department setting, CT can be performed rapidly and often shows acute intracranial hemorrhage more clearly than MRI. MRI is unnecessary in patients with the primary generalized epilepsies, such as typical childhood absence and JME. Lesions (tumors, arteriovenous malformations, cysts, strokes, gliosis, focal atrophy) may be identified in 25% of patients with other epilepsy types, even when the clinical examination and EEG do not suggest focal features. Identification of some lesions, such as focal cortical dysplasia, hamartoma, and mesial temporal sclerosis, can assist in consideration of surgical treatment of pharmacoresistant epilepsy.

LONG-TERM THERAPY

The decision to institute daily seizure medications for a first unprovoked seizure is based on the likelihood of recurrence balanced against the risk of long-term drug therapy. Determination

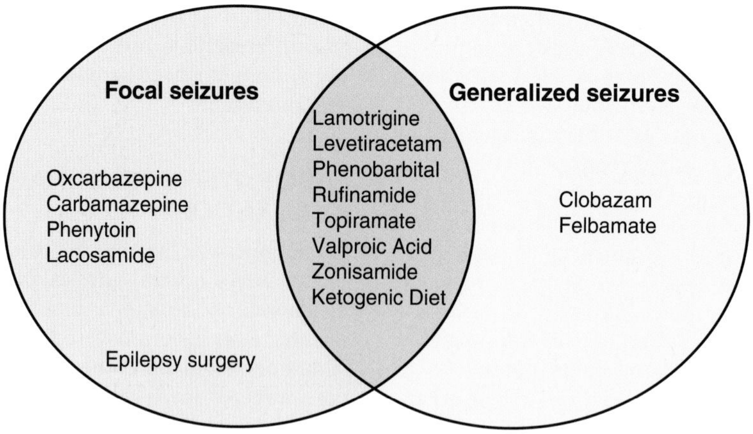

Special circumstances:
1. For absence epilepsy, ethosuximide is the first-line treatment.
2. Adrenocorticotropic hormone, oral corticosteroids, or vigabatrin are used to treat infantile spasms.

FIGURE 181.1 Treatment for epilepsy.

TABLE 181.6 Recurrence Risk After a First Unprovoked Seizure*

SEIZURE TYPE	EEG NORMAL, EXAM NORMAL	EEG EPILEPTIFORM OR EXAM ABNORMAL	BOTH EEG AND EXAM ABNORMAL
Generalized	25%	50%	75%
Focal	50%	75%	>90%

Most recurrences occur within 2 years
EEG, Electroencephalographic.

of the recurrence risk is based on the clinical history and neurodiagnostic testing (Table 181.6). If the recurrence risk is 75% or greater, it is usually suggested that daily medication be prescribed. Absence seizures, infantile spasms, atypical absence seizures, and atonic seizures are universally recurrent at the time of diagnosis, so treatment should be initiated immediately.

The goal of treatment is to maintain an optimal functional state. Medication toxicity should be weighed against the risk of the seizures. Initial drug selection is based on the seizure type (Fig. 181.1). Using a single agent limits toxicity, contains cost, and improves compliance. Approximately 60% of children obtain satisfactory seizure control and minimal side effects with the initial drug. If seizure control is not achieved, despite good compliance, addition of a second drug is considered. Measuring anticonvulsant blood levels can sometimes be helpful in adjusting dosing and monitoring compliance. Levels should be interpreted in light of the patient's clinical state; a patient with a "low" drug level who is seizure free does not necessarily need a higher dose. Anticonvulsant drug levels should be drawn at trough, usually before the morning doses. When hepatic or renal disease is present, especially in critically ill children, protein binding of medications is often altered and measurements of free and total anticonvulsant levels can be helpful.

The duration of antiseizure treatment varies according to seizure type and epilepsy syndrome. For most children, medications can be weaned off after 2 years without seizures. There are some exceptions. For example, children with JME, progressive myoclonic epilepsy, atypical absence seizures, and Lennox-Gastaut syndrome usually require lifelong treatment. Children who have other neurological comorbidities, seizures that were initially difficult to control, or persistently epileptiform EEGs are at highest risk for recurrence when therapy is discontinued.

Although cognitively normal children with epilepsy have the same rates of injury as normal healthy children, there are important safety considerations for people with epilepsy. The risk of drowning is high, so swimming and bathing must only occur under direct adult supervision. Children should use appropriate helmets for sports such as bicycling or ice skating. There is no contraindication to participation in contact sports, but scuba diving, hang gliding, and free climbing are not safe for people with epilepsy. Each country and individual states have specific laws regarding driving for people with epilepsy. Most require a period of seizure freedom before driving.

CHAPTER 182
Weakness and Hypotonia

Weakness is a decreased ability to voluntarily and actively move muscles. This may be generalized or localized to one aspect of the body. Hypotonia is a state of low muscle resistance to movement. Hypotonia can be associated with weakness, but in some cases is present with normal motor strength. The differential diagnosis for weakness is extensive (Table 182.1).

ETIOLOGY

Weakness and hypotonia may be due to disorders of **upper motor neurons** or **lower motor neurons**. Upper motor neurons

TABLE 182.1 Disorders Causing Weakness in Infants and Children

ANATOMICAL REGION	CORRESPONDING DISORDERS
Central nervous system—brain	Brain tumor
	Trauma (accidental, nonaccidental)
	Infection (meningitis, encephalitis, abscess, TORCH)
	Ischemia (arterial or venous)
	Hemorrhage
	Demyelinating disease
	Metabolic disease (leukodystrophy; inborn error of metabolism; mitochondrial encephalomyopathy, lactic acidosis, and stroke-like episodes)
	Degenerative disease
Central nervous system—spinal cord	Transverse myelitis
	Tumor
	Abscess
	Trauma
	Infarction
Anterior horn cell	Spinal muscular atrophy
	Poliomyelitis
Peripheral nerve	Guillain-Barré syndrome
	Hereditary motor sensory neuropathy
	Tick paralysis
	Bell palsy
Neuromuscular junction	Myasthenia gravis (juvenile, transient neonatal, congenital)
	Botulism
Muscle	Muscular dystrophies (Duchenne, Becker, limb-girdle)
	Myotonic dystrophies
	Congenital myopathies
	Metabolic myopathies
	Dermatomyositis
	Polymyositis

TORCH, Toxoplasmosis, other [syphilis, varicella-zoster, parvovirus B19], rubella, cytomegalovirus, and herpes.

originate in the cerebral motor cortex; their axons form the corticospinal tract ending in the spinal cord and control voluntary motor activity. The anterior horn cells, their motor roots, peripheral motor nerves, neuromuscular junctions, and muscles represent the lower motor neurons and muscle units. Maintenance of normal strength, tone, and coordination requires integrated communication throughout this complex system, including the cerebral cortex, cerebellum, brainstem, thalamus, basal ganglia, and spinal cord.

CLINICAL MANIFESTATIONS

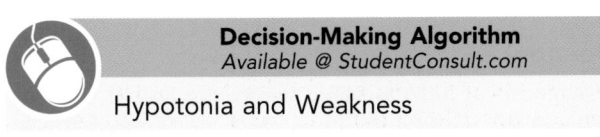

Decision-Making Algorithm
Available @ StudentConsult.com

Hypotonia and Weakness

TABLE 182.2 Clinical Distinction Between Upper Motor Neuron and Lower Motor Neuron Lesions

CLINICAL SIGN	UPPER MOTOR NEURON (CORTICOSPINAL TRACT)	LOWER MOTOR NEURON (NEUROMUSCULAR)
Tone	Increased (spastic)	Decreased
Reflexes	Increased	Decreased
Babinski reflex	Present	Absent
Atrophy	Possible	Possible
Fasciculations	Absent	Possible

Weakness caused by upper motor neuron disease differs from weakness produced by lower motor units (Table 182.2). Dysfunction of the upper motor neuron causes loss of voluntary control, but not total loss of movement because motor nuclei of the basal ganglia, thalamus, and brainstem have tracts that produce simple or complex stereotyped patterns of movement. The corticospinal tract permits fine motor activity and is best tested by rapid alternating movements of the distal extremities. In the acute phase, upper motor neuron disorders cause hypotonia and decreased deep tendon reflexes. Over time, spasticity and hyperreflexia develop. Mild dysfunction produces slowed, stiff motions. More severe dysfunction produces stiff, abnormal involuntary postures and spasticity. A central lesion usually results in weakness that is more pronounced in the flexors of the lower extremities than in the extensors, so affected patients tend to be spastic with legs extended and adducted. In the upper extremities, the extensors are weaker than flexors, so elbows and wrists are flexed.

Damage to the spinal cord leaves residual simple, stereotyped reflex movements coordinated by local spinal reflexes below the level of the lesion.

Destruction of the lower motor neuron, the final common pathway producing muscle activity, leads to hypotonia and total absence of movement. Function is best tested by measuring the strength of individual muscle groups or, in a young child, by observing the ability to perform tasks requiring particular muscle groups (walk up or down stairs, arise from the ground, walk on toes or heels, raise the hands above the head, squeeze a ball). With lower motor neuron disorders, atrophy and fasciculations are common and deep tendon reflexes are typically decreased or absent.

DISEASE OF THE UPPER MOTOR NEURON

Etiology and Epidemiology

Tumors, traumatic brain injury, infections, stroke, demyelinating syndromes, spinal cord trauma or mass, metabolic diseases, and neurodegenerative diseases (see Chapters 100, 101, 157, 184, 185; Section 10) may injure the brain or spinal cord, producing an upper motor neuron pattern of weakness coupled with increased deep tendon reflexes, spasticity, and extensor plantar responses (Babinski sign). In neonates, weakness with upper motor neuron patterns may be caused by TORCH (toxoplasmosis, other [syphilis, varicella-zoster, parvovirus B19], rubella, cytomegalovirus, and herpes) infections (see Chapter 66), developmental brain anomalies, hemorrhage, stroke, hypoxia, genetic syndromes, metabolic/electrolyte disturbances, or toxic exposure.

The distribution of weakness depends on the location of the lesion. A tumor in the left parietal region may produce a right hemiparesis. A brainstem glioma may produce a slowly progressive quadriparesis. A diffuse disorder of myelin synthesis, such as a leukodystrophy, would produce progressive symmetrical quadriparesis.

Decision-Making Algorithm
Available @ StudentConsult.com
Hypotonia and Weakness

Acute disseminated encephalomyelitis (ADEM) is an acute, inflammatory demyelinating disorder that may affect infants and children after a febrile illness. Children may present with a variety of symptoms and signs including acute optic neuritis, hemiparesis, ataxia, seizures, headache, weakness, or dysphagia. The pathophysiology resembles that of multiple sclerosis. An important difference is that children with ADEM have encephalopathy. Although multiple sclerosis is most commonly diagnosed in adulthood, childhood cases have been increasingly recognized. ADEM and multiple sclerosis exacerbations are treated with high-dose steroids and intravenous immunoglobulin (IVIG). Physical and occupational therapies are often helpful.

Acute spinal cord lesions, such as infarction or compression, may produce a **flaccid, areflexic paralysis** that mimics lower motor neuron disease. A child who exhibits an acute or subacute flaccid paraparesis is most likely to have an acute cord syndrome or Guillain-Barré syndrome. The hallmarks of spinal cord disease are a sensory level and a motor level of impairment, disturbance of bowel and bladder function, and local spinal pain or tenderness. Patients may be bradycardic and hypotensive due to neurogenic shock. The acute cord syndrome may be the result of infection, cord tumor, infarction, demyelination, or trauma. **Transverse myelitis**, an acute postinfectious demyelinating disorder of the spinal cord, is treated with high-dose steroids. Symptoms of an epidural abscess include fever, spinal pain, and neurological deficits. Trauma and tumors (neuroblastoma, lymphoma, sarcoma) compressing the spinal cord necessitate immediate neurosurgical management to preserve vital function. Lesions of the spinal cord are best delineated with magnetic resonance imaging (MRI).

DISEASES OF THE LOWER MOTOR NEURON

Neuromuscular disease affects any component of the lower motor neuron unit. The distribution of muscle weakness can point toward specific diseases (Table 182.3).

TABLE 182.3 Topography of Neuromuscular Diseases

LOCATION	CLINICAL SYNDROMES/DISORDERS
Proximal muscle weakness	Muscular dystrophy
	Duchenne/Becker
	Limb-girdle dystrophy
	Dermatomyositis; polymyositis
	Kugelberg-Welander disease (spinal muscular atrophy type 2)
Distal limb weakness	Polyneuropathy (Guillain-Barré syndrome)
	Hereditary motor sensory neuropathy I
	Hereditary motor sensory neuropathy II
	Myotonic dystrophy
	Distal myopathy
Ophthalmoplegia and limb weakness	Myasthenia gravis
	Botulism
	Myotonic dystrophy
	Congenital myotubular myopathy
	Miller Fisher variant of Guillain-Barré syndrome
Facial and bulbar weakness	Myasthenia gravis
	Botulism
	Polio
	Miller Fisher variant of Guillain-Barré syndrome
	Myotonic dystrophy
	Congenital myopathy
	Facioscapulohumeral dystrophy

Spinal Muscular Atrophy

Etiology

Progressive degeneration of anterior horn cells is the key manifestation of spinal muscular atrophy (SMA), a genetic disease with signs and symptoms that may begin in intrauterine life or any time thereafter. About 25% of patients have a severe infantile form (SMA type 1/**Werdnig-Hoffmann disease**), 50% have a late infantile and more slowly progressive form (SMA type 2/**Kugelberg-Welander syndrome**), and 25% have a more chronic, juvenile form (SMA type 3). SMA is one of the most frequent autosomal recessive diseases, with a carrier frequency of 1 in 50.

Clinical Manifestations

Decision-Making Algorithm
Available @ StudentConsult.com
Hypotonia and Weakness

The earlier in life the signs develop, the more severe the progression. Infants with SMA type 1 present in early infancy with severe hypotonia, generalized weakness, and facial involvement. Infants have normal cognitive, social, and language skills and sensation. **Fasciculations** (quivering muscle movements that are typically best seen on the lateral aspect of the tongue) are best identified by inspecting the mouth when the child is asleep. Deep tendon reflexes are absent. With disease progression, breathing becomes rapid, shallow, and predominantly abdominal. In an extremely weak child, respiratory compromise leads to atelectasis, pulmonary infection, and death. Most infants with SMA type 1 die within the first 2 years. Children with SMA type 2 may survive to adulthood. Children with SMA type 3 can initially appear normal with slower progression of weakness and a normal life expectancy.

Laboratory and Diagnostic Studies

The diagnosis of SMA is made by genetic testing. Creatine phosphokinase (CK) may be normal or mildly elevated.

Electromyelogram (EMG) shows fasciculations, fibrillations, and other signs of denervation. Muscle biopsy specimens show grouped atrophy.

Treatment

No specific treatment delays progression of SMA, although a number of promising agents including nusinersen, an antisense oligonucleotide, are being studied. Symptomatic therapy is directed toward minimizing contractures, preventing scoliosis, optimizing nutrition, and avoiding infections. Respiratory infections are managed early and aggressively with pulmonary hygiene, oxygen, and antibiotics. The use or nonuse of artificial ventilation and tube feedings must be individualized for each patient in each stage of the illness.

Peripheral Neuropathy

There are many peripheral nerve diseases in childhood, but the most classic presentations are Guillain-Barré syndrome, chronic inflammatory demyelinating polyneuropathy (CIDP), hereditary motor sensory neuropathy (HMSN), and tick paralysis. Peripheral neuropathies produced by diabetes mellitus, alcoholism, chronic renal failure, exposure to toxins, vasculitis, and the effects of neoplasm are common in adults but are rare in children.

Guillain-Barré Syndrome

Guillain-Barré syndrome (acute inflammatory demyelinating polyradiculoneuropathy) is a postinfectious autoimmune peripheral neuropathy that can occur about 10 days after a respiratory or gastrointestinal infection (classically *Mycoplasma pneumonia* or *Campylobacter jejuni*). It occurs in people of all ages and is the most common cause of acute flaccid paralysis in children.

The characteristic symptoms are *areflexia, flaccidity,* and *symmetrical ascending weakness.* Progression can occur rapidly, in hours, or more indolently over weeks. Typically, symptoms start with numbness or paresthesia in the hands and feet, then a heavy, weak feeling in the legs. Weakness ascends to involve the arms, trunk, and bulbar muscles (tongue, pharynx, larynx). Deep tendon reflexes are absent even when strength is relatively preserved. Objective signs of sensory loss are usually minor compared with the dramatic weakness. Bulbar and respiratory insufficiency may progress rapidly. Dysfunction of autonomic nerves can lead to blood pressure changes, tachycardia and other arrhythmias, urinary retention or incontinence, or stool retention. This polyneuropathy can be difficult to distinguish from an acute spinal cord syndrome. Preservation of bowel and bladder function, loss of arm reflexes, absence of a sensory level, and lack of spinal tenderness point toward Guillain-Barré syndrome. A cranial nerve variant of Guillain-Barré syndrome called the **Miller Fisher variant** manifests with ataxia, partial ophthalmoplegia, and areflexia.

The cerebrospinal fluid in Guillain-Barré syndrome is sometimes normal early in the illness but classically shows elevated protein levels without significant pleocytosis. MRI with gadolinium may reveal enhancement of the spinal nerve roots. EMG and nerve conduction velocity are not always required but can provide corroborative diagnostic evidence and prognostic indicators.

Children in early stages of the disease should be admitted to the hospital. Those with moderate, severe, or rapidly progressive weakness should be treated in an intensive care unit. Pulmonary and cardiac functions are monitored continuously. Endotracheal intubation is required by patients with impending respiratory failure or an inability to clear secretions. Most patients are treated initially with IVIG. Plasma exchange and immunosuppressive drugs are alternatives when IVIG is unsuccessful or in rapidly progressive disease. Physical, occupational, and speech therapies are mainstays of treatment.

The illness usually resolves spontaneously, albeit slowly; 80% of patients recover normal function within 1-12 months. Twenty percent of patients are left with mild to moderate residual weakness. Some children will suffer acute relapse or chronic symptoms.

Chronic Inflammatory Demyelinating Polyneuropathy

CIDP is an immune-mediated peripheral neuropathy and can affect patients of all ages. Patients present with both proximal and distal weakness (usually in an episodic, relapsing-remitting pattern) affecting the extremities. Patients may also experience sensation changes such as numbness, tingling, or pain. The diagnosis is clinical, although EMG or nerve biopsy may confirm the diagnosis. The mainstays of treatment for CIDP are IVIG, glucocorticoids, and plasmapheresis. Prognosis varies; some patients have complete remission, whereas others experience partial remission or severe persistent disability.

Hereditary Motor Sensory Neuropathy

HMSN (also called Charcot-Marie-Tooth disease [CMT]) is a group of progressive peripheral nerve diseases. Motor components generally dominate the clinical picture, with sensation and autonomic functions affected later. Some subtypes present with severe symptoms starting in infancy while other forms may have milder symptoms.

The peroneal and tibial nerves are the earliest and most severely affected. Most often, complaints begin in the preschool to early adolescent years, with weakness of the ankles and frequent tripping. Examination shows **pes cavus deformity of the feet** (high-arched feet), bilateral weakness of foot dorsiflexors, and normal sensation despite occasional complaints of paresthesia. Peripheral nerves can become markedly enlarged and may be palpable on exam. Progression of HMSN is slow, extending over years and decades. Eventually, patients develop weakness and atrophy of the entire lower legs and hands and mild to moderate sensory loss in the hands and feet. Some patients never have more than a mild foot deformity, loss of ankle reflexes, and electrophysiological abnormalities. Others in the same family may be confined to a wheelchair and have difficulties performing everyday tasks with their hands.

HMSN can be characterized by demyelination (CMT1) or axonal (CMT2) damage. Specific genetic testing is available for many subtypes of HMSN. Specific treatment for HMSN is not available, but braces that maintain the feet in dorsiflexion can improve function.

Tick Paralysis

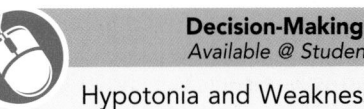

Decision-Making Algorithm
Available @ StudentConsult.com
Hypotonia and Weakness

Tick paralysis produces an acute lower motor neuron pattern of weakness, clinically similar to Guillain-Barré syndrome. An attached female tick releases a toxin, similar to botulism, blocking neuromuscular transmission. Affected patients present with a severe generalized flaccid weakness, including ocular, papillary, and bulbar paralysis. A methodical search for an affixed tick, particularly in hairy areas, must be made in any child with acute weakness. Removal of the tick results in a prompt return of motor function.

Myasthenia Gravis

Decision-Making Algorithm
Available @ StudentConsult.com
Hypotonia and Weakness

Myasthenia gravis is an autoimmune condition. Most commonly, antibodies block the acetylcholine receptors (AChR) at the neuromuscular junction, decreasing the number of effective receptors, which results in rapid fatigability of striated muscle; other types of autoantibodies exist. The three childhood varieties are **juvenile myasthenia gravis** in late infancy and childhood, **transient neonatal myasthenia**, and **congenital myasthenia**.

Juvenile Myasthenia

Variable ptosis, diplopia, ophthalmoplegia, and facial weakness are the presenting symptoms. Dysphagia, poor head control, and extremity weakness may occur. Rapid fatigue of muscles distinguishes myasthenia from other neuromuscular disorders, with progressive worsening over the day or with repetitive activity. In some children, the disease never advances beyond ophthalmoplegia and ptosis (ocular myasthenia). Others have a progressive and potentially life-threatening illness that involves all musculature, including that of respiration and swallowing. Treatment includes pyridostigmine (an acetylcholinesterase inhibitor) and, depending on severity, various forms of immunosuppression.

Transient Neonatal Myasthenia Gravis

A transient myasthenic syndrome develops in the first hours to days after birth in neonates born to mothers with myasthenia gravis. Almost all infants born to mothers with myasthenia have maternal anti-AChR antibodies, but only 10-20% will develop signs. Signs include ptosis, ophthalmoplegia, weak facial movements, poor feeding, hypotonia, respiratory difficulty, and variable extremity weakness. Neonates with transient myasthenia gravis require cholinesterase inhibitors and supportive care for a few days to weeks until the weakness remits.

Congenital Myasthenia Gravis

A variety of rare disorders of the neuromuscular junction have been reported that are not autoimmune mediated. The congenital myasthenic syndromes (CMS) are due to gene mutations in the components of the neuromuscular junction. They typically present in infancy with hypotonia, ophthalmoparesis, facial diplegia, and extremity weakness, although they can present throughout childhood. Respiratory function and feeding may be compromised. Children with CMS usually have lifelong disability. Some children will respond to pyridostigmine or other drugs that improve neuromuscular junction function.

Diagnostic Studies

Autoimmune myasthenia is most commonly diagnosed through the combination of clinical symptoms and antibody testing. The majority of individuals have antibodies to the AChR, although some have antibodies to other components of the neuromuscular junction. Nerve conduction studies classically reveal an electrodecrement with 3-Hz repetitive stimulation. Administration of a cholinesterase inhibitor (edrophonium chloride) can result in transient improvement in strength, particularly of ptosis, and thus can additionally be used for diagnostic verification.

Infant Botulism

Decision-Making Algorithm
Available @ StudentConsult.com
Hypotonia and Weakness

Infant botulism results from intestinal infection by *Clostridium botulinum*, which produces a neurotoxin that blocks presynaptic cholinergic transmission. Young age and the absence of competitive bowel flora predispose infants to this disease. Infants may ingest dust, soil, or food (honey or poorly canned foods) contaminated with spores. The progressive neuromuscular blockade ranges from mild to severe. Infants typically present with constipation and poor feeding. Hypotonia and weakness develop progressively, along with cranial nerve dysfunction manifested by decreased gag reflex, diminished eye movements, decreased pupillary contraction, and ptosis. Heart rate and blood pressure may fluctuate. Affected infants may develop respiratory failure. The diagnosis is made by detecting *C. botulinum* spores and toxin in stool samples. Therapy with botulism IVIG should be administered as soon as the diagnosis is suspected. With prompt treatment and respiratory and supportive care, the prognosis is good.

Duchenne Muscular Dystrophy

Muscular dystrophies are a group of genetic muscle diseases characterized by progressive myofiber degeneration and the gradual replacement of muscle by fibrotic tissue. Duchenne muscular dystrophy is the most common muscular dystrophy and one of the most common genetic disorders of childhood.

Etiology

Duchenne muscular dystrophy is an X-linked disorder (Xp21) that arises from a mutation in the dystrophin gene. Approximately 1 in 3,500 boys is affected. **Becker muscular dystrophy** is an allelic disorder associated with more mild symptoms; its mutations at least partially preserve the function of the resulting gene product.

Clinical Manifestations

Decision-Making Algorithm
Available @ StudentConsult.com
Hypotonia and Weakness

Boys are only rarely symptomatic in early infancy. At about 2-3 years of age, boys develop an awkward gait and an inability to run properly. Some have an antecedent history of mild delay in attaining motor milestones or of poor head control during infancy. Examination shows firm calf hypertrophy and mild to moderate proximal leg weakness with a hyperlordotic, waddling gait. The child typically arises from a lying position on the floor by using his arms to *climb up* his legs and body **(Gower sign).** Arm weakness is evident by age 6 years. Most boys are wheelchair dependent by age 12 years. Other manifestations include cardiomyopathy, scoliosis, respiratory decline, and cognitive and behavioral dysfunction. Many boys with Duchenne live into adulthood. Most die in their 20s or early 30s, usually as a result of progressive respiratory decline or cardiac dysfunction.

Laboratory and Diagnostic Studies

Serum CK levels are always markedly elevated. Diagnosis is established by genetic testing for the dystrophin gene mutation. Approximately one-third of cases represent new mutations. Prenatal genetic testing is possible, and newborn screening for elevated CK is available in some states. Occasionally the diagnosis is not made until a muscle biopsy shows muscle fiber degeneration and regeneration accompanied by increased intrafascicular connective tissue.

Treatment

Chronic oral steroid therapy is now instituted to slow the pace of the disease, delay motor disability, and improve longevity. Supportive care includes physical therapy, bracing, proper wheelchairs, and treatment of cardiac dysfunction or pulmonary infections. A multidisciplinary approach is recommended.

Myotonic Dystrophy

Etiology and Epidemiology

Myotonic dystrophy (DM) is the second most common muscular dystrophy and the most common form to present in adulthood. An autosomal dominant genetic disease, DM is caused by progressive expansion of a triplet repeat, CTG, in the DM protein kinase gene. Presentation is roughly correlated with the number of CTG repeats, and the disease is characterized by genetic anticipation, where each generation presents with earlier and more severe symptoms.

Clinical Manifestations

Although DM most typically presents in adulthood, it can present at any age. Clinical features of childhood-onset "classic" DM include slowly progressive facial and *distal* extremity weakness as well as **myotonia**. Myotonia is a disorder of muscle relaxation after contraction. When patients grasp onto an object, they have difficulty releasing their grasp and may appear to peel their fingers away slowly. The facial appearance is characteristic, with hollowing of muscles around temples, jaw, and neck; ptosis; facial weakness; and drooping of the lower lip. The voice is nasal and mildly dysarthric. Not only is the striated muscle affected, but smooth muscle of the alimentary tract and cardiac muscle are involved. Patients have variable arrhythmias, endocrinopathies, immunological deficiencies, cataracts, and intellectual impairment.

A severe congenital form of DM can appear in infants of mothers with DM because of rapid expansion of the CTG repeat length. Infants are immobile and hypotonic, with ptosis, absence of sucking and Moro reflexes, poor feeding, and respiratory difficulties. Often, weakness and atony of uterine smooth muscle during labor lead to associated hypoxic ischemic encephalopathy and its sequelae, which make the clinical diagnosis more difficult. The presence of congenital contractures, clubfoot, or a history of poor fetal movements indicates intrauterine neuromuscular disease. Those requiring prolonged ventilation have an infant mortality of 25%. Individuals with congenital DM often make significant gains in terms of motor skills, and nearly all children eventually ambulate independently. However, approximately 50% of DM patients have mental retardation. In addition, children with congenital DM experience a second progressive phase of the disease in the teen years, including potentially fatal cardiac arrhythmias. Diagnosis is established by genetic testing.

Other Forms of Childhood Muscle Disease

Congenital muscular dystrophies (CMDs) refer to a group of genetically determined conditions that present in infancy or early childhood. The most common subtypes include merosin-deficient CMD, Ullrich CMD, and the dystroglycanopathies. The characteristic clinical features include hypotonia, extremity weakness, delayed motor development, and congenital contractures. Contractures and scoliosis are often progressive and severely worsen; respiratory status diminishes with age. Diagnosis is established through the combination of elevated serum CK and dystrophic changes detected on muscle biopsy. **Emery-Dreifuss muscular dystrophy** (EDMD), also known as humeroperoneal muscular dystrophy, can be inherited as an X-linked recessive, autosomal dominant, or autosomal recessive disorder. Symptoms typically begin in childhood, although adult onset has been noted. Patients may experience early contractures, slowly progressive humeroperoneal muscle weakness or wasting, and cardiac disease with conduction defects and arrhythmias. EDMD is associated with mild elevations of serum CK levels, abnormal electrocardiograms (ECG), characteristic changes on muscle imaging, and abnormal but nonspecific muscle biopsies. There are no disease-specific modifying therapies for EDMD, although early placement of defibrillators in patients with abnormal ECGs reduces the incidence of sudden death.

Several forms of **limb-girdle muscular dystrophy** (LGMD), usually inherited in an autosomal recessive pattern, have been described. Depending on the subtype of LGMD, presentation can be throughout childhood. A subset of children will have a Duchenne-like presentation. LGMD primarily affects muscles of the hip and shoulder girdles. Distal muscles may later become weak and atrophic; some children have progressive cardiac and respiratory failure.

Facioscapulohumeral dystrophy is an autosomal dominant myopathy. Weakness first appears in the facial and shoulder girdle muscles. Shoulder weakness results in the characteristic observation of scapular winging, which can often be asymmetrical. Patients have mild ptosis, a decrease in facial expression, inability to pucker the lips or close eyes during sleep, neck weakness, difficulty in fully elevating the arms, and thinness of upper arm musculature.

Congenital myopathies (CM) are a group of nondystrophic muscle disorders that, like CMDs, most typically present in infancy with hypotonia and weakness. Additional signs and symptoms include congenital contractures, hip subluxation/

dislocation, small/atrophic muscles, thin body habitus, and characteristic facial appearance (the "myopathic facies"). Symptoms are often nonprogressive or only slowly progressive, although children often have severe lifelong disabilities including wheelchair dependence, severe scoliosis, and respiratory failure. Clinical findings may distinguish CMDs and other dystrophies (involvement of the facial musculature in CM). Diagnosis is ultimately established based on laboratory studies, biopsy findings, and genetic test results. Histopathological subtypes are distinguished by characteristic features on muscle biopsy, the most common being nemaline myopathy, centronuclear myopathy, and core myopathy. Although no specific therapies currently exist for any CM subtype, several promising therapies have shown efficacy in preclinical models of disease.

Metabolic Myopathies

Glycogen storage disease type II (Pompe disease) and muscle carnitine deficiency are discussed in Chapters 52 and 55. **Several mitochondrial myopathies** may present with hypotonia, ophthalmoplegia, and progressive weakness, but the phenotype of these disorders is broad (see Chapter 57). **Endocrine myopathies**, including hyperthyroidism, hypothyroidism, hyperparathyroidism, and Cushing syndrome, are associated with proximal muscle weakness (see Chapters 175, 176, and 178). **Periodic paralysis** due to familial forms of hypokalemia or hyperkalemia produces episodic weakness.

Laboratory and Diagnostic Studies

The diagnostic evaluation should be guided by the clinical history and physical examination (see Chapter 179).

Malignant Hyperthermia

Malignant hyperthermia is a life-threatening syndrome manifested by a rapid increase of body temperature, muscle rigidity, metabolic and respiratory acidosis, hypotension, arrhythmias, and convulsions. Acute episodes are precipitated by exposure to anesthetic agents in patients with a genetic predisposition. Patients with Duchenne muscular dystrophy, central core myopathy, and other myopathies are susceptible, although malignant hyperpyrexia can also occur in children without muscle disease as an autosomal dominant genetic disorder. A family history of unexplained death during anesthesia is often noted. Serum CK levels rise and myoglobinuria can result in tubular necrosis and acute renal failure. Diagnosis of idiopathic malignant hyperthermia is possible with genetic testing or an in vitro muscle contraction test that reveals excessive tonic contracture on exposure to halothane and caffeine. Treatment consists of dantrolene, sodium bicarbonate, and cooling.

NEONATAL AND INFANTILE HYPOTONIA

The clinical distinction between upper and lower motor neuron disorders in infants is blurred because incomplete myelinization of the developing nervous system limits expression of many of the cardinal signs, such as spasticity. The two critical clinical points are whether the child is weak and the presence

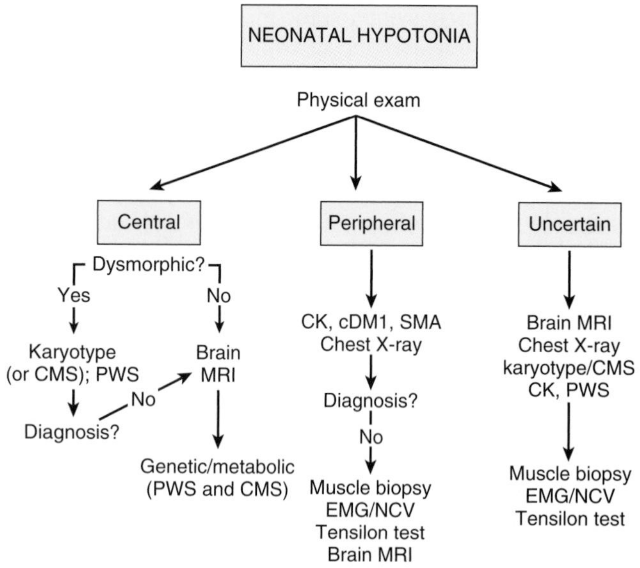

FIGURE 182.1 Evaluation of an infant with hypotonia. *cDM1*, Congenital myotonic dystrophy; *CK*, creatine kinase; *CMS*, chromosomal microarray analysis; *EMG*, electromyelogram; *MRI*, magnetic resonance imaging; *NCV*, nerve conduction velocity; *PWS*, Prader-Willi syndrome; *SMA*, spinal muscular atrophy. (Courtesy James Dowling, MD, PhD.)

or absence of deep tendon reflexes. Hypotonia and weakness coupled with depressed or absent deep tendon reflexes suggest a neuromuscular disorder. A stronger child with brisk reflexes suggests an upper motor neuron source for the hypotonia. Causes of neonatal weakness are outlined earlier. A diagnostic algorithm for infants with hypotonia or weakness is presented in Fig. 182.1.

Hypotonia Without Significant Weakness (Central Hypotonia)

Decision-Making Algorithm
Available @ StudentConsult.com
Hypotonia and Weakness

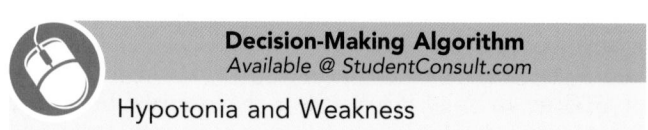

Some infants who appear to move well when supine in their cribs are *floppy* when handled or moved. When lifted, their heads flop, they *slip through* at the shoulders, do not support weight on their legs, and form an *inverted* U in prone suspension **(Landau posture).** When placed prone as neonates, they may lie flat instead of keeping their arms and legs flexed. Passive tone is decreased, but reflexes are normal. Hypotonia may be associated with significant cerebral disease or may be a benign phenomenon that is outgrown. The most common cause of hypotonia is hypoxic-ischemic encephalopathy.

Prader-Willi syndrome (PWS) presents with severe neonatal hypotonia; severe feeding problems leading to failure to thrive; small hands and feet; and, in boys, a small penis, small testicles, and cryptorchidism. Severe hyperphagia and obesity develop in early childhood. Approximately 60-70% of affected individuals have an interstitial deletion of *paternal* chromosome 15q11q13.

PWS and trisomy 21 are the most common genetic causes of neonatal hypotonia.

Infants who have a connective tissue disorder, such as **Ehlers-Danlos syndrome, Marfan syndrome,** or familial laxity of the ligaments, may exhibit marked passive hypotonia, ligamentous laxity, and increased skin elasticity. They have normal strength and cognition and achieve motor and mental milestones normally. They may have peculiar postures of their feet or unusual gaits.

Infants with **benign congenital hypotonia** typically present at 6-12 months old with delayed gross motor skills. They are unable to sit, creep, or crawl but have good verbal, social, and manipulative skills. Strength appears normal, and the infants can kick arms and legs briskly and bring their toes to their mouths. The children often display head lag, slip-through in vertical suspension, and floppiness of passive tone. The infant seems floppy from birth. The differential diagnosis includes upper and motor neuron disorders and connective tissue diseases. Extensive laboratory investigation is often unrevealing. Most of these children catch up to peers and appear normal by 3 years of age. Often, other family members have exhibited a similar developmental pattern.

STROKE IN CHILDHOOD

Etiology

The incidence of pediatric stroke is 2.5-10 per 100,000 children and is higher among neonates, approaching that of elderly patients. A wide spectrum of conditions can produce stroke in childhood (Table 182.4). Pediatric strokes may be due to ischemia (**arterial ischemic stroke** [AIS], **cerebral sinovenous thrombosis** [CSVT]) or hemorrhage. AIS is focal brain infarction that results from occlusion of the arteries in the brain. The most common causes are vasculitis resulting in abnormal cerebral arteries (either autoimmune or infectious, such as vasculitis associated with meningitis) and cardioembolic infarcts due to congenital heart disease, sickle cell anemia, or coagulation disorders. Coagulation disorders also increase the risk of CSVT, the occlusion of venous structures in the brain, which can result in ischemia as the cerebral venous pressure rises. CSVT can also be caused by infections or dehydration. **Hemorrhagic strokes** (HS) may be intraparenchymal (primary or secondary bleeding after AIS) or associated with intraventricular, subarachnoid, subdural, or epidural bleeds. The most common causes of HS are vascular malformations, head trauma, and vasculitis.

TABLE 182.4 Causes of Stroke in Childhood

ARTERIAL ISCHEMIC STROKE
Arteriopathic • Idiopathic arterial stenosis • Vasculitis (autoimmune or infectious; may be focal or diffuse) • Arterial dissection (traumatic or spontaneous) • Moyamoya disease Cardiac • Cyanotic congenital heart disease • Valvular disease • Patent foramen ovale • Arrhythmias • Cardiomyopathy • Infective endocarditis Hematological • Sickle cell anemia • Iron-deficiency anemia • Hypercoagulable state • Hereditary prothrombotic states (factor V Leiden) • Acquired prothrombotic states (antiphospholipid antibodies) • Prothrombotic medications (oral contraception)
CEREBRAL SINOVENOUS THROMBOSIS
Hematological • Hypercoagulable states (see above) • Iron-deficiency anemia • Severe dehydration Infections • Meningitis • Otitis media • Mastoiditis Systemic disease • Leukemia • Inflammatory bowel disease • Nephrotic syndrome Trauma
HEMORRHAGIC STROKE
Head trauma (accidental or abusive) Vascular malformations • Arteriovenous malformations • Cerebral aneurysms Brain tumor Vasculitis Moyamoya disease

Clinical Manifestations

The acute onset of focal neurological deficits in a child is stroke until proven otherwise. Symptoms may be subtle and nonspecific, which can lead to a delay in diagnosis. AIS typically presents with acute, focal neurological deficits. Hemiparesis is most common, but visual, speech, sensory, or balance deficits may be present. Unlike AIS in adults, focal seizures are quite common in childhood presentation of AIS. Similarly, neonatal AIS most often presents with acute symptomatic focal seizures (typically in the first day of life) or encephalopathy.

Symptoms of CSVT may progress more gradually and be more variable and nonspecific than AIS. In CSVT, acute focal deficits may be present or the child may have progressive signs of elevated intracranial pressure, including headache, papilledema, diplopia (most often from cranial nerve VI palsy), seizures, lethargy, or confusion.

HS tends to present acutely, with a sudden "thunderclap" headache. HS may also present with loss of consciousness, nuchal rigidity, focal deficits, or seizures and can be rapidly fatal.

Some early-life strokes are not recognized until later in life, when an infant or child presents with hemiplegia. Such congenital hemiplegia becomes increasingly apparent as infants develop; they have decreased use of one side of the body, early handedness, or may seem to ignore one side of their body or of their environment. Neuroimaging reveals an area of encephalomalacia in the contralateral cerebral hemisphere that is the residual effect of a prior stroke. The area of encephalomalacia may predispose the child to epilepsy. The details of the child's intrauterine, labor, delivery, and postnatal history are often unremarkable, so the timing of the stroke typically remains uncertain.

Differential Diagnosis

There are many conditions that mimic pediatric stroke, most of which are more common than AIS, HS, or CSVT. Some of these mimics are benign (migraine, psychogenic weakness, musculoskeletal abnormalities), but others require specific, prompt diagnosis and treatment (transient postictal weakness, intracranial infection, inflammatory disease of the central nervous system, tumor, posterior reversible leukoencephalopathy syndrome).

Diagnostic Tests and Imaging

On initial presentation, acute neuroimaging is necessary. A noncontrast head computed tomography (CT) scan is highly sensitive to acute HS and can reveal larger, mature AIS; acute, nonhemorrhagic stroke may not be seen on routine CT. Therefore MRI with diffusion-weighted imaging is required for most presentations. Angiography by magnetic resonance angiography (MRA) or CT angiography is used to confirm arterial occlusion in AIS and can identify underlying arteriopathy, vascular malformations, and aneurysms. Diagnosis of CSVT requires a high clinical suspicion and purposeful imaging of the cerebral venous system by MRI or CT. If clinical assessment does not reveal the cause of the stroke, a complete laboratory investigation should be undertaken promptly based on suspected etiologies (see Table 182.4). Many children with AIS have more than one predisposing factor, so identifying one risk factor does not obviate the need for a complete evaluation.

Treatment

Treatment must focus on limiting secondary neuronal injury and prevention of future strokes. Neuroprotection by maintaining control of temperature, blood pressure, glucose, and seizures is essential. Emergency thrombolysis with medications or catheterization is not yet established for children; it is an area of active clinical research. Anticoagulants (IV heparin, subcutaneous low molecular weight heparin, oral warfarin) and platelet antiaggregants (aspirin) are used for secondary stroke prevention in some instances. For those with acute, progressive CSVT, anticoagulation is the mainstay of therapy. Long-term rehabilitation programs are required for most survivors.

CHAPTER 183

Ataxia and Movement Disorders

ATAXIA

Ataxia is the inability to make accurate, smooth, and coordinated movements. **Truncal ataxia** reflects disturbances of the midline cerebellar vermis (medulloblastoma, acute postinfectious cerebellar ataxia, ethanol intoxication). **Appendicular ataxia** reflects disturbances of the ipsilateral cerebellar hemisphere (cystic cerebellar astrocytoma). Ataxias may be acute or chronic. The most common causes of acute ataxia in childhood are postinfectious acute cerebellar ataxia and drug intoxications. Discrete lesions within the posterior fossa, tumors (medulloblastoma, ependymoma, cerebellar astrocytoma), cerebellar abscess, demyelinating diseases, acute labyrinthitis, strokes, and hemorrhages may cause ataxia. Other causes include benign paroxysmal vertigo, head trauma, seizures, postictal states, migraine, paraneoplastic opsoclonus-myoclonus syndrome associated with neuroblastoma, and inborn errors of metabolism. Congenital disorders also may produce chronic, nonprogressive ataxia. There are a number of inherited ataxia syndromes (Table 183.1).

Clinical Manifestations

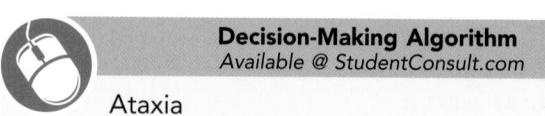

Decision-Making Algorithm
Available @ StudentConsult.com

Ataxia

Signs of ataxia include a broad-based, unsteady gait, difficulty sitting (truncal ataxia), and **dysmetria** (over- or undershooting of the target due to abnormal distance perception). An intention tremor worsens as the arm/hand approaches the target. Some children may be perceived as clumsy. Classically, these signs stem from disorders of the cerebellar pathways, but peripheral nerve lesions causing loss of proprioceptive inputs to the cerebellum (Guillain-Barré syndrome) may present with similar findings. In addition, weakness may intensify or mimic ataxia, so strength must be assessed, along with coordination.

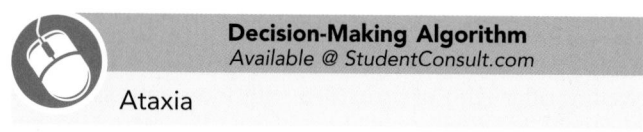

Etiologies

Decision-Making Algorithm
Available @ StudentConsult.com

Ataxia

Drug intoxication is the most common cause of acute ataxia among children. Overdosage of any sedative-hypnotic agent can produce acute ataxia and lethargy, but ataxia without lethargy usually results from intoxication with ethanol or anticonvulsant drugs. Over-the-counter cough syrups (dextromethorphan), essential oils (tea tree), and other toxins (e.g., pesticides) may also cause ataxia. It is important to ask about any medications, drugs of abuse, or other toxins to which the child may have access. Treatment is supportive.

Postinfectious acute cerebellar ataxia may occur 1-3 weeks following varicella, infectious mononucleosis, mild respiratory or gastrointestinal viral illnesses, or other infections. The pathogenesis is uncertain and may represent a direct viral infection of the cerebellum or, more likely, an autoimmune response precipitated by the viral infection and directed at

TABLE 183.1 Causes of Ataxia

BRAIN TUMORS	**VASCULAR DISORDERS**
Medulloblastoma*	Cerebellar hemorrhage or infarction
Ependymoma	Vertebral artery dissection
Cerebellar astrocytoma*	**DEMYELINATING DISORDERS**
Brainstem glioma	Multiple sclerosis
PARANEOPLASTIC DISEASE	Acute disseminated encephalomyelitis
Neuroblastoma (opsoclonus-myoclonus-ataxia)	**STRUCTURAL OR CONGENITAL DISORDERS**
INFECTIOUS DISORDERS	Cerebellar hypoplasia
Encephalitis*	Vermal aplasia
Brainstem encephalitis	Dandy-Walker malformation
Meningitis	Arnold-Chiari malformation
Labyrinthitis*	Hydrocephalus
Cerebellar abscess	**HEREDITARY ATAXIC DISORDERS**
POSTINFECTIOUS DISORDERS	Episodic ataxia
Acute cerebellar ataxia (acute postinfectious cerebellitis)*	Friedreich ataxia
Guillain-Barré syndrome	Ramsay Hunt syndrome
MIGRAINOUS DISORDERS	Spinocerebellar ataxia 1 and 2
Basilar migraine*	Ataxia-telangiectasia
Benign paroxysmal vertigo	Marinesco-Sjögren syndrome
TRAUMA	**GENETIC AND METABOLIC DISORDERS**
Cerebellar hemorrhage	Metachromatic leukodystrophy
Cerebellar contusion	Adrenoleukodystrophy
Concussion	Maple syrup urine disease
Postconcussive syndrome*	Hartnup disease
Vertebrobasilar occlusion	GM_2 gangliosidosis (juvenile)
TOXIC INGESTIONS*	Refsum disease
Ethanol	Vitamin E deficiency
Anticonvulsants	Leigh disease
Antihistamines	Wilson disease
Benzodiazepines	Abetalipoproteinemia
Carbon monoxide	
Inhalants	
Drugs of abuse	

**Common.*

the cerebellar white matter. Symptoms begin abruptly, causing truncal ataxia, staggering, and frequent falling. Dysmetria of the arms, dysarthria, nystagmus, vomiting, irritability, and lethargy may be prominent. Symptoms, which may be severe enough to prevent standing or sitting, usually peak within 2 days, then stabilize and resolve over several weeks. Cerebrospinal fluid (CSF) examination sometimes shows a mild lymphocytic pleocytosis or mild elevation of protein content. Brain magnetic resonance imaging may reveal cerebellar enhancement. No specific therapy is available except to prevent injury during the ataxic phase.

Brain tumors are the second most common neoplasm in children. About 50% arise from within the posterior fossa. Tumors that arise in the posterior fossa or brainstem produce progressive ataxia with headache that may be acute or gradual in onset. There is a progressive worsening over days, weeks, or months, typically with associated signs and symptoms of elevated intracranial pressure. The ataxia and dysmetria may result from primary cerebellar invasion or from obstruction of the CSF pathways (aqueduct of Sylvius fourth ventricle) with resultant hydrocephalus. The most common tumors in this region include medulloblastoma, ependymoma, cerebellar astrocytoma, and brainstem glioma.

Rarely, a **neuroblastoma,** located in the adrenal medulla or anywhere along the paraspinal sympathetic chain in the thorax or abdomen, is associated with degeneration of Purkinje cells and the development of severe ataxia, dysmetria, irritability, myoclonus, and opsoclonus. An immunological reaction directed toward the tumor may be misdirected to attack Purkinje cells and other neuronal elements. The myoclonic movements are irregular, lightning-like movements of a limb or the head. Opsoclonus is a rapid, multidirectional, conjugate movement of the eyes, which suddenly dart in random directions. The presence of **opsoclonus-myoclonus** in a child should prompt a vigorous search for an occult neuroblastoma.

Difficulty walking with a severe staggering gait is one manifestation of **acute labyrinthitis,** but the diagnosis is usually clarified by the associated symptoms of a severe sense of spinning dizziness (vertigo), nausea and vomiting, and associated signs of pallor, sweating, and nystagmus.

Ataxia-telangiectasia, an autosomal recessive genetic disorder of the ATM gene, is the most common of the degenerative ataxias (Chapter 73). Affected patients present with ataxia around age 2 years, progressing to loss of ambulation by adolescence. In mid-childhood, telangiectasias are evident over the sclerae, nose, ears, and extremities. Abnormalities in immune function and greatly increased risk of lymphoreticular tumors result in early death.

Friedreich ataxia is a relentlessly progressive, autosomal recessive disorder. Children present in the late elementary school years with ataxia, dysmetria, dysarthria, diminished proprioception and vibration sense, absent deep tendon reflexes, and nystagmus. Many develop hypertrophic cardiomyopathy and skeletal abnormalities (high-arched feet, hammer toes, kyphoscoliosis).

Several rare **inborn errors of metabolism** can present with intermittent episodes of ataxia and somnolence. These include Hartnup disorder, maple syrup urine disease, mitochondrial disorders, abetalipoproteinemia, and vitamin E deficiency (Chapters 31 and 53).

MOVEMENT DISORDERS

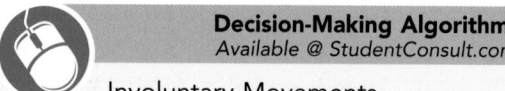

Decision-Making Algorithm
Available @ StudentConsult.com

Involuntary Movements

Movement disorders or **dyskinesias** are a diverse group of entities associated with abnormal excessive, exaggerated, chaotic, or explosive movements of voluntary muscles. They are generally the result of abnormalities of the extrapyramidal system or the basal ganglia. Movement disorders in children are typically **hyperkinetic** (increased movement). The abnormal movements are activated by stress and fatigue and often, but not always, disappear in sleep. They are typically diffuse and migratory (chorea) but may be isolated to specific muscle groups (segmental myoclonus, palatal myoclonus).

Chorea is a hyperkinetic, rapid, unsustained, irregular, purposeless movement that seems to flow from one body part to another. Affected patients demonstrate difficulty keeping the tongue protruded or maintaining grip (milkmaid grip). Patients often attempt to incorporate the involuntary movements into more purposeful movements, which make them appear fidgety. Choreiform movement disorders may be autoimmune/parainfectious, infectious, genetic, structural, metabolic, or toxic in origin (Table 183.2). The movements may occur alone or as part of a more extensive neurological disorder (Sydenham chorea, Huntington chorea, systemic lupus erythematosus, encephalitis).

Athetosis is a hyperkinetic, slow, coarse, writhing movement that is most pronounced in the distal muscle groups. Athetosis is seen frequently in combination with chorea (choreoathetosis) and is usually present in conjunction with other neurological

TABLE 183.2 Causes of Movement Disorders

CHOREA
Autoimmune/parainfectious (acute rheumatic fever,* systemic lupus erythematosus)
Infectious (human immunodeficiency virus, neurosyphilis, scarlet fever, encephalitis)
Genetic (Huntington disease, ataxia-telangiectasia)
Structural (stroke, neoplasm)
Metabolic/toxic (hepatic/renal failure, hyperthyroidism)
Drug induced
ATHETOSIS
Cerebral palsy*
Kernicterus
Hypoxic-ischemic encephalopathy
Drug induced
Pantothenate kinase-associated neurodegeneration
Pelizaeus-Merzbacher disease
DYSTONIA
Inherited primary dystonias
Acute dystonic reaction*
Tardive dyskinesia
Cerebral palsy*
Metabolic disorders (Wilson disease)
TREMOR
Physiological*
Essential tremor*
Hereditary, degenerative (Huntington disease, Wilson disease)
Stroke
Metabolic (hyperthyroidism, hepatic encephalopathy, electrolyte disturbances)
Drugs/toxins* (caffeine, bronchodilators, amphetamines, tricyclic antidepressants)
Psychogenic tremor
MYOCLONUS
Epilepsy
Benign*
Infection
Toxin
Metabolic encephalopathies
TICS*
Transient
Chronic motor tic disorder
Tourette syndrome

**Common*

signs. It may be seen in virtually all the disorders mentioned as causes of chorea. Many children with mixed forms of cerebral palsy have spasticity and choreoathetosis.

Dystonia is characterized by abnormally sustained muscle contraction, causing twisting motions (torsion spasm) and repetitive movements or abnormal postures, usually associated with basal ganglia or thalamic lesions. Cerebral palsy is the most common cause of dystonia among children, but many genetic mutations have been implicated in primary dystonias. Antipsychotics and antiemetics can produce **acute dystonic reactions**, typically involving the face and neck with torticollis, retrocollis, tongue protrusions, and oculogyric crises (eye rotation). **Tardive dyskinesia** is usually associated with chronic antipsychotic drug use and presents with characteristic facial involvement (tongue thrusting, chewing).

Tremor is a hyperkinetic, rhythmic, oscillatory movement caused by simultaneous contractions of antagonistic muscles. The amplitude and frequency are regular. In children, tremor is usually due to a physiological tremor, or essential tremor. Essential tremor is the most common movement disorder in adults, and half report onset in childhood. Other causes of tremor include thyrotoxicosis, hypoglycemia, or drugs (caffeine, bronchodilators, amphetamines, tricyclic antidepressants).

Myoclonus is a hyperkinetic, brief contraction of a muscle group, resulting in a sudden jerk. Myoclonus may be caused by seizures or by other etiologies (see Chapter 181). Nonepileptic myoclonus is distinguished from tremor in that it is a simple contraction of an agonist muscle, whereas tremor is a simultaneous contraction of agonist and antagonist muscles. Myoclonus is seen as a manifestation of various epilepsies and infectious, toxic, and metabolic encephalopathies. Benign myoclonus is commonly observed during sleep and may be particularly pronounced in neonates.

Tics are rapid, purposeless, involuntary, stereotyped movements and typically involve the face, eyes, shoulder, and arm. Examples of simple motor tics include blinking, nose twitching, and extremity jerking. Complex motor tics are more orchestrated movements, including head shaking, gesturing, or jumping. Phonic tics may be simple (grunting, throat clearing) or complex (uttering words, phrases). Approximately 25% of children have transient tics. Most tic disorders in children are transient and not intrusive into the child's life, but may be a source of parental anxiety. Occasionally, tics may be unmasked by stimulant agents. Persistent motor tics (lasting >12 months) in association with vocal tics are characteristic of **Tourette syndrome**, a chronic tic disorder that usually begins before age 7 years. The pathophysiology underlying tics is unknown, but a family history of tics is elicited in more than 50% of cases. Comorbid features, such as obsessive-compulsive disorder and attention-deficit/hyperactivity disorder, are present in half of children with Tourette disorder (see Chapters 13 and 19). Tic disorders are clinical diagnoses, and neurodiagnostic studies have limited value. Many children with tic disorders or Tourette syndrome are unperturbed by their tics and require no therapy. Others may benefit from psychological support, including habit reversal training, and pharmacological therapy with α-adrenergic receptor agonists (clonidine) or neuroleptics (pimozide, haloperidol, risperidone). Chronic tic disorders wax and wane regardless of intervention and most often improve substantially or resolve entirely by late adolescence.

CHAPTER 184

Altered Mental Status

DISORDERS OF CONSCIOUSNESS

Consciousness is a cortical function that allows for awareness of self and environment (place, time). **Arousal** represents the system that initiates and maintains consciousness and is mediated by the ascending reticular activating system (ARAS), which extends from the pons through the midbrain to the hypothalamus and thalamus. **Lethargic** patients have difficulty maintaining an aroused state. Patients who are **obtunded** have decreased arousal but are responsive to stimuli. **Stupor** is a state of responsiveness to pain but not to other stimuli. **Coma** is a state of unresponsive unconsciousness and is caused by dysfunction of the cerebral hemispheres bilaterally, the brainstem, or both.

Acute Disorders of Consciousness

Decision-Making Algorithm
Available @ StudentConsult.com
Altered Mental Status

Acute changes in consciousness vary in degree from mild lethargy and confusion to deep coma. In childhood, the most common causes of coma are toxins, infections, head trauma, hypoxia-ischemia (cardiac arrest, near-drowning), and seizures (postictal state, subclinical status epilepticus; Table 184.1).

Assessment

The most common cause of long-term morbidity in a patient with depressed consciousness is hypoxia; therefore, airway, breathing, and circulation are addressed first. Vital signs, including pulse oximetry, must be assessed. Breathing patterns may provide important clues to the depth, neurological localization, and etiology of the depressed consciousness. A low respiratory rate may be associated with central nervous system (CNS) depressants or increased intracranial pressure (ICP). Tachypnea may be due to hypoxia, metabolic acidosis, or fever, but in more ominous situations may be due to brainstem herniation. Systemic diseases such as sepsis, ingestions, or cardiac failure may lead to shock. Hypotension may also result from severe traumatic brain injury (TBI) or spinal cord injury. Hypertension may be due to increased ICP. The glucose level should also be checked immediately because hypoglycemia is a rapidly treatable cause of altered mental status. Physical examination searches for clues as to the cause of altered consciousness, such as unusual odors, needle tracts, trauma, or signs of dehydration or organ system failure.

The **Glasgow Coma Scale** (see Table 42.1) can be used to assess unresponsive patients regarding their best verbal and motor responses and eye opening to stimulation with scores ranging from 3-15 points.

Diminished levels of consciousness require either bilateral hemispheric or ARAS dysfunction, so testing the structures immediately adjacent to the reticular system is essential. Changes

TABLE 184.1 Causes of Coma and Diagnostic Approach

CAUSES	**Increased Intracranial Pressure**
Infection	Brain tumor
Meningitis	Cerebral edema
Encephalitis (Herpes simplex virus, arboviruses)	Hydrocephalus
Brain abscess or subdural empyema	**Migraine**
Human immunodeficiency virus	**Systemic Disorders**
Tuberculosis meningitis	Gastrointestinal (intussusception)
Toxic shock syndrome	Vasculitis (systemic lupus erythematosus)
Postinfectious (acute disseminated encephalomyelitis)	Hepatic failure
Trauma	Hypertensive encephalopathy
Abusive head trauma	Reye syndrome
Hemorrhage (epidural, subdural, subarachnoid)	Endocrine disorders (adrenal insufficiency, thyroid disorders)
Brain contusion	Renal disorders (uremia)
Concussion	Demyelinating disorders (multiple sclerosis, ADEM)
Diffuse axonal injury	**Metabolic Derangements**
Toxins (Intoxication or Withdrawal)	Hypoglycemia
Ethanol	Hyponatremia or rapid correction
Narcotics	Hypernatremia or rapid correction
Barbiturates	Hyperosmolality or rapid correction
Antihistamines	Hypercapnia
Anticonvulsants	Hyperammonemia
Iron	Inborn errors of metabolism
Acetaminophen	Diabetes mellitus—ketoacidosis or hypoglycemia
Aspirin (Reye syndrome)	**DIAGNOSTIC APPROACH**
Illicit drugs	Routine laboratory testing
Lead poisoning	Glucose
Thiamine deficiency (Wernicke encephalopathy)	Sodium, potassium, calcium, magnesium, chloride, bicarbonate, BUN, creatinine, AST, ALT, blood gases, ammonia
Hypoxia-Ischemia	Blood, urine analyses for toxic substances
Near-drowning	Blood, urine cultures if infection suspected
Post–cardiopulmonary arrest (cardiac arrhythmia, obstructive cardiomyopathy)	Skeletal survey, ophthalmological examination if child abuse suspected
Carbon monoxide intoxication	CSF analysis including opening pressure, white and red blood cell counts, protein, glucose, and culture (± viral PCR testing)
Perinatal asphyxia	Neuroimaging
Strangulation	Head CT
Epilepsy	Brain MRI, MRA, MRV
Subclinical (or nonconvulsive) status epilepticus	Electrodiagnostic studies
Postictal states	EEG
Stroke	Secondary laboratory testing (if cause remains unknown)
Arterial ischemic stroke	Lead level, pyruvate, lactate, serum amino acids, urine organic acids, acylcarnitine profile
Cerebral sinovenous thrombosis	
Hemorrhage	

ADEM, Acute disseminated encephalomyelitis; *ALT*, alanine aminotransferase; *AST*, aspartate aminotransferase; *BUN*, blood urea nitrogen; *CSF*, cerebrospinal fluid; *CT*, computed tomography; *EEG*, electroencephalogram; *MRI/MRA/MRV*, magnetic resonance imaging/angiography/venography; *PCR*, polymerase chain reaction.

in pupillary response suggest midbrain lesions. In comatose patients, eye movements are observed or elicited with the **oculocephalic vestibular reflexes** (doll's eye maneuver) (see Chapter 179). If the oculocephalic responses are not elicited or are unclear, the **oculovestibular response** (cold caloric stimulation) is elicited by flushing cold water into the external ear canal. In a comatose patient, cold water irrigation into the ear canal elicits a tonic eye deviation toward the irrigated ear if the brainstem is functioning.

Body posture at rest and after noxious stimulation can indicate the anatomical level responsible for the alteration of consciousness. Mildly altered mental status may be manifested by a comfortable *sleeping* posture with frequent spontaneous readjustments of position, yawns, and sighs. Patients who lie in a flat, extended, unvarying position with eyes half-open exhibit a deeper coma. An asymmetrical posture suggests motor dysfunction of one side. This asymmetry may be subtle, such as mild external rotation of the affected leg.

Posturing in response to noxious stimulation indicates more serious neurological conditions. **Decorticate posturing** consists of rigid extension of the lower extremities, flexion and supination of the arms, and fisting of the hands. It indicates bilateral cortical or subcortical abnormalities or herniation, with preserved brainstem function. **Decerebrate posturing** (rigid extension and internal rotation of the upper and lower extremities) is associated with herniation with midbrain compression or toxic-metabolic abnormalities. These postures may be symmetrical or asymmetrical. A structural cause is most likely when posturing is asymmetrical, whereas symmetrical posturing may suggest an underlying toxic-metabolic etiology.

Etiology

The evolution of change in consciousness is an important clue to the etiology. A detailed history and physical examination usually provide sufficient clues to differentiate among the three major diagnostic categories producing coma: **metabolic/toxic**, **infectious**, and **structural**. In most clinical situations, the cause of coma is readily identified.

Care must be taken to investigate background medical conditions that may produce a decline in consciousness (diabetes mellitus, leukemia, kidney failure, liver disease). Metabolic derangements are common causes of altered mental status and are suggested by spontaneous fluctuations in the level of consciousness, tremors, myoclonus, asterixis, visual and tactile hallucinations, and deep coma with preservation of pupillary light reflexes. Disturbances of blood chemistries (glucose, sodium, calcium, bicarbonate, blood urea nitrogen, ammonia) may produce depressed mental status, as can hypoxemia (inadequate oxygen delivery to the brain) and cerebral ischemia (inadequate cerebral perfusion). Acute metabolic or toxic disorders usually produce a hypotonic, limp state, but hypertonia, rigidity, and decorticate and decerebrate posturing are sometimes observed in coma caused by hypoglycemia, hepatic encephalopathy, and short-acting barbiturates.

Intoxication and ingestion are common causes of acute alteration of consciousness. A thorough history must be taken to search for the offending agent (see Chapter 45). A history of social or emotional difficulties, drug abuse, or depression raises concern for self-inflicted injury or toxic ingestion. A subacute course of somnolence progressing to difficulty arousing from a deep *sleep* (stupor) over hours suggests drug intoxication or organ system failure (kidney, liver) producing a metabolic encephalopathy. CNS infection, usually causes abrupt alteration of mental status, although viral meningoencephalitis (particularly herpes simplex virus) can present with subacute alterations in mental status. The presence of fever, petechiae, chills, and sweats suggests infection. Prodromal photophobia and pain on movement of the head or eyes are symptoms of meningeal irritation. Premonitory symptoms, such as abdominal pain, diarrhea, sore throat, conjunctivitis, cough, or rash, point toward viral encephalitis or postinfectious syndrome as the cause of the altered consciousness.

Structural processes, such as hemorrhage, acute hydrocephalus, or stroke, can cause sudden depressed consciousness in children. An evolution of headache and morning vomiting suggests increased ICP. A gradual fading of alertness or declining school performance over preceding weeks suggests an expanding intracranial mass, subdural hematoma, or chronic infection (tuberculous meningitis, human immunodeficiency virus).

Clinical Manifestations

Papilledema or paralysis of cranial nerves III or VI in a patient with depressed consciousness is strong evidence of elevated ICP, a medical and neurosurgical emergency. **Herniations** can occur under the falx, through the tentorial notch, or into the foramen magnum (Table 184.2). Recognition of the signs associated with the major herniation syndromes can be lifesaving if emergent neuroimaging and treatment are initiated. **Uncal herniation** implies displacement of the mesial temporal lobe over the tentorial edge, producing a unilateral third nerve palsy ("blown pupil") and hemiparesis (which can be ipsilateral due to compression of the contralateral cerebral peduncle or contralateral if the uncus compresses the ipsilateral peduncle). **Transtentorial (central) herniation** occurs with gradual downward pressure from the diencephalon through the tentorium, resulting in compression of the brainstem (first midbrain, then progressing to pons and medulla). A progressive loss of consciousness accompanied by

TABLE 184.2 Herniation Syndromes

LOCATION	ETIOLOGY	DESCRIPTION	CLINICAL FINDING(S)
Transtentorial Unilateral (uncal) or bilateral	Supratentorial mass lesions, diffuse brain swelling, focal edema, or acute hydrocephalus	Downward displacement of supratentorial brain tissue into infratentorial compartment (below tentorium), compressing the cerebral peduncles, midbrain, third cranial nerve, and posterior circulation	Headache Altered consciousness Dilated ipsilateral pupil Cranial nerve III palsy Hemiparesis Decerebrate posturing Cushing triad Respiratory arrest
Subfalcian	Increased pressure in one hemisphere (mass, focal edema)	Brain tissue displaced under the falx cerebri, compressing the anterior cerebral artery	Weakness, bladder incontinence, coma
Foremen magnum	Cerebellar mass or edema	Downward displacement of cerebellar tonsils, compressing the medulla oblongata and upper spinal cord	Bradycardia, bradypnea, hypertension, death

miosis, decorticate posturing, and Cheyne-Stokes respirations (rhythmic waxing and waning of respiratory amplitude) suggests incipient transtentorial herniation. Late findings include decerebrate posturing and Cushing's triad (bradycardia, irregular respirations, hypertension).

Laboratory and Diagnostic Imaging

Evaluation is guided by the history and physical examination. Clinicians should rapidly consider causes of unresponsiveness that could easily and quickly be reversed (see Table 184.1). If trauma or immersion injuries are suspected, neck manipulation should be avoided until cervical spine imaging excludes vertebral fracture or subluxation.

Computed tomography (CT) remains the preferred imaging technique in emergency situations because it can be performed rapidly and accurately identifies intracranial acute hemorrhages, large space-occupying lesions, edema, and shifts of the midline. The initial head CT scan is done without contrast to identify blood and calcifications. Contrast can be administered to identify inflammatory and neoplastic lesions but is not usually required for identification of major lesions.

Examination of the cerebrospinal fluid (CSF) may establish the cause of the alteration of consciousness. Lumbar puncture (LP) in a patient with elevated ICP can result in transtentorial herniation, so neuroimaging must be performed before LP if elevated ICP is suspected, especially if there are any focal neurological deficits on exam. The presence of red blood cells in the CSF may suggest primary subarachnoid hemorrhage, parenchymal hemorrhage, or hemorrhagic infection (herpes simplex virus), or it may be due to a traumatic procedure. White blood cells in the CSF usually denote infectious meningitis or meningoencephalitis but may also be associated with vasculitis, autoimmune disorders, or parainfectious syndromes. Elevated CSF protein is seen in patients with meningeal inflammation, tumors, or white matter diseases, whereas abnormal CSF glucose levels are also markers of infection and inflammation.

Treatment

Beyond supportive measures, the etiology of altered mental status determines the treatment. Ingestions may necessitate gastric lavage, charcoal administration, forced diuresis, dialysis, or specific antidotes (see Chapter 45). Infections are treated with appropriate antibiotics or antiviral agents (see Chapters 100, 101). If mental status changes are due to increased ICP, acute medical interventions (osmotic agents, steroids, a trial of hyperventilation, elevating the head of the bed to 30 degrees) must be instituted, emergent neuroimaging performed, and urgent neurosurgical consultation obtained. Structural brain lesions may necessitate medical treatment of increased ICP or surgical excision.

Prognosis

The outcome of altered mental status relates to many variables, including etiology. Intoxication typically carries a good prognosis, whereas herniation carries a poor prognosis. Other prognostic factors include the duration of coma and the age of the patient; children have better outcomes than adults. Complete recovery from traumatic coma of several days' duration is possible in children; however, many survivors of prolonged coma are left in a persistent vegetative state or with severe neuropsychiatric disability.

Transient, Recurrent Depression of Consciousness

Episodic alteration or depression of consciousness with full recovery is usually due to seizure, migraine, syncope, or metabolic abnormality (hypoglycemia). Consciousness can be impaired during seizures or in the postictal state. Nonconvulsive (subclinical) status epilepticus (generalized or focal) can directly impair consciousness and is a common complicating factor for infants and children with acute neurological disorders (head trauma, meningitis, stroke, following convulsive status epilepticus). Basilar artery or **confusional migraines** can last hours and be accompanied by agitation, ataxia, cortical blindness, vertigo, or cranial nerve palsies. Headache may precede or follow the neurological signs.

Syncope is one of the most common causes of abrupt, episodic loss of consciousness. Neurocardiogenic syncope, cardiac arrhythmia, or obstructive cardiomyopathy can cause recurrent episodes of loss of consciousness. Two thirds of children with syncope have irregular, myoclonic movements as they lose consciousness (anoxic seizures), which must be distinguished from epilepsy (unprovoked seizures). Children with unexplained syncope require a complete cardiac evaluation (see Chapter 140).

Metabolic derangements, particularly **hypoglycemia**, give rise to episodes of lethargy, confusion, seizures, or coma. Several other metabolic disorders cause recurrent bouts of **hyperammonemia** (see Chapter 53). Symptoms include nausea, vomiting, lethargy, confusion, ataxia, hyperventilation, and coma.

INCREASED INTRACRANIAL PRESSURE

Etiology

When the cranial sutures are fused, the skull becomes a rigid container enclosing a fixed volume, including the brain (80-85%), CSF (10-15%), and blood (5-10%). The exponential relationship between the volume within a closed container and pressure results in a massive increase in ICP as intracranial volume increases. The brain accommodates increased ICP initially by expelling CSF and blood from the intracranial compartment into the spinal subarachnoid space. When the limits of this accommodation are reached, the brain itself begins to shift in response to the continuing elevation of ICP. Brain shifts may cause herniations across the dural extensions or skull barriers (Table 184.2).

The most common causes of increased ICP include mass lesions, hydrocephalus, cerebral edema due to trauma or infection, and idiopathic intracranial hypertension (Tables 184.3 and 184.4).

Mass lesions (brain tumor, abscess, hemorrhage) may produce increased ICP not only by virtue of large size, but by blockage of CSF pathways, blockage of venous outflow, or production of vasogenic cerebral edema. Brain abscesses usually present as mass lesions, producing focal neurological signs and increased ICP. Symptoms of infection, including fever, malaise, anorexia, and stiff neck, may be subtle or absent. Children with chronic cardiac or pulmonary disease may embolize infected material to their brains, predisposing them to brain abscesses. Brain tumors in children are most often located in the posterior fossa and can result in elevated ICP due to obstruction of CSF flow through the cerebral aqueduct and fourth ventricle. Brain

TABLE 184.3 Causes of Increased Intracranial Pressure

MASS EFFECT
Hydrocephalus
Hemorrhage
Tumor
Abscess
Cyst
Inflammatory mass
Arterial ischemic stroke with edema
Intracranial venous sinus thrombosis
DIFFUSE EDEMA
Hypoxic-ischemic injury
Trauma
Infection
Meningitis
Encephalitis
Hypertension
Metabolic derangement or toxin
Hyponatremia
Diabetic ketoacidosis
Dialysis disequilibrium syndrome
Reye syndrome
Fulminant hepatic encephalopathy
Pulmonary insufficiency with hypercarbia
Lead intoxication
Idiopathic intracranial hypertension (pseudotumor cerebri)
Drugs
Withdrawal of long-term steroid administration
Endocrinological disturbance
Obesity

TABLE 184.4 Causes of Hydrocephalus

PATHOGENIC MECHANISM	ETIOLOGICAL DISORDER/CONDITION
Obstruction of CSF pathways	Intraventricular foramina (Monro) obstruction
	Parasellar mass (craniopharyngioma, germinoma, pituitary tumor)
	Intraventricular tumor (ependymoma)
	Tuberous sclerosis with subependymal giant cell astrocytoma
	Aqueduct of Sylvius (cerebral aqueduct) obstruction
	Aqueductal stenosis
	Midbrain or pineal region tumor
	Postinfectious or postinflammatory
	Posthemorrhagic
	Impaired flow from the fourth ventricle foramina of Luschka and Magendie
	Basilar impression
	Platybasia
	Dandy-Walker malformation
	Arnold-Chiari malformation
	Bone lesions of the cranial base (achondroplasia, rickets)
Overproduction of CSF	Choroid plexus papilloma
Defective reabsorption of CSF (extraventricular obstruction or communicating hydrocephalus)	Hypoplasia of the arachnoid villi
	Postinfectious or posthemorrhagic destruction of arachnoid villi or subarachnoid fibrosis
	Extensive cerebral sinovenous thrombosis

CSF, Cerebrospinal fluid.

tumors and abscesses can both result in vasogenic edema, which further increases ICP.

Hydrocephalus from congenital abnormalities or due to an intracranial mass is typically characterized by a slowly evolving syndrome of increased ICP extending over weeks or months. CSF is continuously produced by the choroid plexus within the lateral, third, and fourth ventricles. CSF circulates through the ventricular systems and is then absorbed, predominantly by the arachnoid villi into the large dural sinuses. Hydrocephalus is due to the obstruction of CSF flow anywhere along its course (see Table 184.4). **Obstructive hydrocephalus** is caused by a block before the CSF flows to the subarachnoid space, usually within the fourth ventricle or at the level of the aqueduct. Congenital hydrocephalus can result from CNS malformations, intrauterine infection, intraventricular hemorrhage, genetic defects, trauma, and teratogens. Acquired hydrocephalus may be caused by CNS infections, brain tumors, or hemorrhage. Impairment of CSF flow within the subarachnoid space or impairment of absorption is known by the misnomer *communicating hydrocephalus*, where there is actually extraventricular obstruction of CSF flow *(external hydrocephalus)*. Hydrocephalus caused by overproduction of CSF without true obstruction is seen in choroid plexus papillomas, which account for 2-4% of childhood intracranial tumors.

Bacterial meningitis may produce increased ICP by blockage of CSF pathways, cytotoxic cerebral edema, increase in cerebral blood flow, or multifocal cerebral infarctions (see Chapter 100). Most children with bacterial meningitis can undergo LP safely because the brain swelling is diffuse and distributed evenly throughout the brain and spinal CSF compartments. A few patients with meningitis, however, develop transtentorial herniation within a few hours of LP. Focal neurological signs, poorly reactive pupils, and a tense fontanelle are contraindications to LP in a patient with suspected bacterial meningitis.

Idiopathic intracranial hypertension (pseudotumor cerebri) is a cause of increased ICP with normal brain imaging. Patients exhibit a daily debilitating headache associated with diplopia, abducens palsy, transient visual obscurations, and papilledema. If untreated, permanent visual field loss may develop. The syndrome has been associated with ingestion of medications (tetracycline, vitamin A, oral contraceptive agents) and endocrine disturbances (thyroid disease, Addison disease). Most commonly, this condition is idiopathic and affects children who are otherwise well except for being overweight, with rapid weight gain being a predisposing factor. **Treatment** including acetazolamide or other diuretic, topiramate, or corticosteroids, is generally effective. Weight loss and cessation of triggering medications are also mainstays of treatment. Infrequently, chronic papilledema from persistent idiopathic intracranial hypertension produces visual impairment, and more aggressive management is required (optic nerve fenestration) to preserve visual function.

Clinical Manifestations

Decision-Making Algorithms
Available @ StudentConsult.com

Strabismus
Vomiting
Headaches
Altered Mental Status

The symptoms and signs of increased ICP include headache, vomiting, lethargy, irritability, altered consciousness, sixth nerve palsy, strabismus, diplopia, and papilledema. Headaches suggestive of increased ICP are those associated with nocturnal wakening; worse in the morning; with cough, micturition, defecation, or Valsalva maneuver; or progressively worsening. Specific signs of increased ICP in the infratentorial compartment (posterior fossa) include stiff neck and head tilt. Focal neurological deficits reflect the site of the lesion that is producing the increased ICP and may include hemiparesis from supratentorial lesions, or ataxia and cranial nerve palsies from infratentorial lesions. Critically increased ICP may result in herniation syndromes, as discussed earlier. In addition, the **Cushing triad** of elevated blood pressure, bradycardia, and irregular respirations is a late sign of critically elevated ICP. Infants who have an open fontanelle may present with less specific symptoms such as irritability, lethargy, and poor feeding. Specific signs of increased ICP in infants consist of a bulging fontanelle, suture diastasis, distended scalp veins, a persistent downward deviation of the eyes *(sunsetting)*, and rapid growth of head circumference. Manifestations of increased ICP may evolve slowly when there is slow growth of a mass or incomplete obstruction allowing for transependymal absorption of CSF into the veins. On the other hand, symptoms may develop rapidly in the setting of acute intracranial hemorrhage or abrupt CSF obstruction.

Laboratory and Diagnostic Studies

The cause of increased ICP is determined by brain imaging with either head CT or brain magnetic resonance imaging (MRI). CT is rapid, readily available, and provides clear visualization of an acute hemorrhage, dilated ventricles, or mass lesions. Diffuse brain swelling produced by hypoxic-ischemic injury, meningitis, encephalitis, metabolic abnormalities, or toxins may be better delineated by MRI. MRI is also superior to CT for visualizing the posterior fossa and cortical contusions. In order to avoid radiation from head CT, many centers now use limited sequences to allow for a rapid MRI without sedation as an initial screen for acute causes of elevated ICP. LP is the diagnostic test for infection and for documentation of elevated ICP (essential for patients with idiopathic intracranial hypertension). However, LP is contraindicated in the setting of an intracranial mass lesion or clear hydrocephalus because withdrawal of CSF can change pressures between the intracranial compartments and promote brainstem shifts and herniation. Idiopathic intracranial hypertension is diagnosed when direct measurement of ICP with a manometer during LP reveals elevated ICP in the absence of other CSF or imaging abnormalities.

Treatment of Elevated Intracranial Pressure

The treatment of acute increased ICP should be carried out in an intensive care setting with continuous monitoring and vigilant attention to vital signs. The first goal is stabilization of the cardiopulmonary status. Once the child is stabilized, the head is placed at midline and the head of the bed is elevated to 30 degrees. Indications for endotracheal intubation include refractory hypoxia, hypoventilation, Glasgow coma score of ≤8, loss of airway protective reflexes, and acute herniation requiring controlled hyperventilation. Slight hyperventilation (to a Pa_{CO_2} not lower than 35 mm Hg) produces rapid, but transient, reduction in ICP by cerebral vasoconstriction, leading to decreased cerebral blood volume. More aggressive hyperventilation may cause cerebral ischemia and is only indicated if there are clinical signs of acute herniation. Mannitol or 3% saline may be used acutely to produce an osmotic shift of fluid from the brain to the plasma. A ventricular catheter may be used to monitor the ICP continuously and to remove CSF. In refractory cases, a pentobarbital-induced coma reduces pressure by severely suppressing cerebral metabolism. The antiinflammatory effects of corticosteroids may be helpful in the management of vasogenic edema associated with tumors and abscesses. Acetazolamide and furosemide may transiently decrease CSF production in idiopathic intracranial hypertension. Because acute interventions such as hyperventilation, osmotic therapies, and barbiturates can have negative impacts on systemic and cerebral perfusion and have only transient effects on ICP, they must be used judiciously.

Vasopressor drugs may be necessary to maintain adequate arterial blood pressure and cerebral perfusion pressure. Serum electrolytes and osmolarity should be monitored because of risk of the syndrome of inappropriate antidiuretic hormone or cerebral salt wasting (Chapter 35). Maintaining normoglycemia may have a positive impact on outcomes. Other supportive measures include controlling agitation, fever, and seizures.

The **treatment of hydrocephalus** may be medical or surgical, depending on the etiology. After subarachnoid hemorrhage or meningitis, the flow or absorption of CSF may be transiently impaired. In this circumstance, the use of medication that decreases CSF production, such as acetazolamide, may be beneficial. Surgical management consists of removing the obstructive lesion, placing a shunt, or both. A shunt consists of polyethylene tubing extending usually from a lateral ventricle to the peritoneal cavity **(ventriculoperitoneal shunt).** Shunts carry the hazards of infection or sudden occlusion with signs and symptoms of acute hydrocephalus.

All treatments for increased ICP are temporary measures intended to prevent herniation until the underlying disease process either is treated or resolves spontaneously. Timely intervention can prevent or reverse cerebral herniation. Complete neurological recovery is possible, but rare, after signs of transtentorial or foramen magnum herniation have begun. When these signs are complete, however, with bilaterally dilated, unreactive pupils, absent eye movements, and flaccid quadriplegia, recovery is no longer possible.

TRAUMATIC BRAIN INJURY

Following head injury, children may have immediate depression of consciousness and neurological deficits or may be completely alert without any immediate signs of neurological injury. Most serious trauma results from motor vehicle crashes, sports, recreation-related injuries, and violence. Head trauma may result in concussion, posttraumatic intracranial hemorrhage, skull fractures, or cranial nerve or cervical spine injuries. Head injury, or other injuries, with associated retinal hemorrhages in infants and young children should raise the suspicion of abusive head trauma (see Chapter 22).

Concussion

Concussion is the process in which traumatic forces on the brain result in the rapid onset of short-lived neurological impairment that typically resolves spontaneously. In some cases, however, symptoms and signs may evolve over minutes to hours, so patients should not be left alone following the injury. Patients may have signs or symptoms in one or more domain: somatic (headache), cognitive (slowed reaction times, poor attention), emotional (lability, irritability), sleep disturbance (drowsiness), or physical signs (loss of consciousness, amnesia). A player with any features of a concussion should be evaluated by a licensed health care provider onsite or be referred to a physician. Acute symptoms usually reflect a functional disturbance rather than structural injury, and no abnormalities are seen on standard imaging. If the child appears well after several hours and is discharged home, parents should be instructed to call their physician for any change in alertness, orientation, or neurological functioning. An increase in somnolence, headache, or vomiting is cause for concern and emergent neuroimaging. The majority of concussions resolve within 10 days, although the recovery may be slower in children, and in a small percentage of cases, the symptoms are prolonged. Physical and cognitive rest are the cornerstones of concussion management. Children must not be permitted to resume physical activities until well after the symptoms resolve (Table 184.5). Repeated concussions, especially within a short time frame (days or weeks), carry a significant risk of permanent brain injury **(second impact syndrome).**

TABLE 184.5 Protocol for Return to Sport After Concussion

Return to play protocol follows a stepwise progress with each step taking ≥24 hours. The athlete should continue to the next level if asymptomatic at the current level.

1. No activity, complete physical and mental rest.
2. Light aerobic exercise such as walking or stationary cycling; no resistance training.
3. Sport-specific exercise (skating in hockey, running in soccer).
4. Noncontact, more progressive training drills; resistance training.
5. Full-contact training after medical clearance.
6. Game play.

Modified from McCrory P, Meeuwisse W, Aubry M, et al. Consensus statement on concussion in sport: the 4th International Conference on Concussion in Sport, held in Zurich, November 2012. Br J Sports Med. *2013;47:250–258.*

Traumatic Intracranial Hemorrhage

Head trauma can result in epidural, subdural, parenchymal, and subarachnoid intracranial hemorrhages, as well as brain contusions (Table 184.6). Symptoms include headache, vomiting lethargy, decreased consciousness, and seizures. The classic presentation of **epidural hemorrhages** involves a lucid interval: following the primary brain injury, a child has a decreased level of consciousness, then returns to normal for several hours before developing rapidly progressive neurological symptoms. When associated with neurological decompensation, prompt evacuation of the epidural hematoma is the primary therapy. **Subdural hemorrhages** may result from direct trauma or rotational forces from vigorous shaking (abusive head trauma).

TABLE 184.6 Syndromes of Posttraumatic Intracranial Hemorrhage

SYNDROME	CLINICAL AND RADIOLOGICAL CHARACTERISTICS	TREATMENT
Epidural	Onset over minutes to hours Lucid interval followed by progressive neurological deficits Lens-shaped extracerebral hemorrhage compressing brain	Surgical evacuation or observation Prognosis good with prompt treatment, otherwise poor
Acute subdural	Onset over hours Focal neurological deficits Crescentic extracranial hemorrhage compressing brain	Surgical evacuation Prognosis guarded
Chronic subdural	Onset over weeks to months Anemia, macrocephaly Seizures, vomiting Crescentic, low-density mass on CT	Subdural taps or subdural shunt as necessary Prognosis can be good
Intraparenchymal	Depressed consciousness Focal neurological deficits ± Additional multiple contusions	Supportive care Prognosis guarded
Subarachnoid	Stiff neck Worst headache of life Late hydrocephalus	Supportive care Prognosis variable
Contusion	Focal neurological deficits Brain swelling with transtentorial herniation CT findings: multifocal low-density areas with punctate hemorrhages	Medical treatment of elevated intracranial pressure* Prognosis guarded

Mannitol, elevation of head of bed, diuresis, hyperventilation (pCO_2 32-38 torr unless acutely herniating), steroids.
CT, Computed tomography.

In neonates and infants with open fontanelles, signs and symptoms may be absent or nonspecific. **Subarachnoid hemorrhages** classically present as a sudden, severe headache due to rupture of an intracranial aneurysm. Brain **contusions** are areas of bruising with associated localized ischemia, edema, and mass effect.

Skull Fractures

Skull fractures may present with localized swelling and pain; subcutaneous bleeding over the mastoid process **(Battle sign)** or around the orbit **(raccoon eyes);** blood behind the tympanic membrane **(hemotympanum);** or CSF leak from the nose (rhinorrhea) or ear (otorrhea). Skull fractures may be linear, diastatic (spreading the suture), depressed (an edge displaced inferiorly), or compound (bone fragments breaking the skin surface). Linear, diastatic, and minimally depressed fractures necessitate no specific treatment, but imaging is indicated to evaluate for associated intracranial hemorrhages. If the depression is more than 0.5-1 cm, surgical elevation of bone fragments and repair of associated dural tears are generally recommended. Compound fractures or penetrating injuries necessitate emergent surgical debridement and tetanus prophylaxis. The risk of associated brain contusion and early seizures is high in compound fractures.

Rarely, a few weeks to months after linear skull fractures, a soft, pulsatile scalp mass is palpable; the fracture edges are separated by a soft tissue mass that consists of fibrotic tissue and accumulated brain and meningeal tissue and, possibly, a **leptomeningeal cyst**.

CSF leak occurs when a skull fracture tears adjacent dura, creating communications between the subarachnoid space and the nose, paranasal sinuses, mastoid air cells, or ear. Clear fluid that leaks from the nose or ear after head trauma is presumed to be CSF until proved otherwise. The presence of air within the subdural, subarachnoid, or ventricular space also indicates a dural tear and open communication between the nose or paranasal sinuses and brain. In most cases, the dura heals spontaneously when the patient's head is kept elevated. Patients with CSF leaks are at risk for the development of meningitis or extradural abscesses. If the leak persists or recurs or if meningitis develops, the dura is surgically repaired. **Cranial nerve palsies**, secondary to a laceration or contusion of the cranial nerves, may result from a skull fracture and may be transitory or permanent.

Other Complications of Head Trauma

Cervical spine injuries must be suspected in any unconscious child, especially if bruises are present on the head, neck, or back. In conscious children, findings of neck or back pain, burning or stabbing pains radiating to the arms, paraplegia, quadriplegia, or asymmetrical motor or sensory responses of arms or legs suggest spinal cord injury. Cervical spine injury (displaced or fractured vertebra) may result in complete transection of the cord with spinal shock, loss of sensation, and flaccid paralysis. A contused cord (without vertebral abnormality) may present in a similar manner. Any patient with a clinical or radiological abnormality of the spine requires immediate spine immobilization, cardiopulmonary stabilization, and neurosurgical consultation.

Posttraumatic seizures are divided into one of three patterns: impact seizures, early posttraumatic seizures, and late posttraumatic seizures. Impact seizures occur within seconds of the injury and are presumed to reflect a direct mechanical stimulation to the cortex. The prognosis is excellent and likelihood of later epilepsy is negligible. Early posttraumatic seizures occurring within the first week of the head injury are likely the result of a localized area of cerebral contusion or edema. The long-term prognosis for these seizures is quite favorable. Late posttraumatic seizures arise more than a week after the trauma and most likely indicate an area of cortical gliosis or scarring that will be a source for long-term epilepsy. These patients often require long-term antiepileptic drug therapy.

Transient neurological disturbances may develop a few minutes after head trauma and last for minutes to hours before clearing. The most common symptoms are cortical blindness and confusional states, but hemiparesis, ataxia, or any other neurological deficit may appear. These symptoms may represent a trauma-triggered migraine in susceptible children. Care must be exercised to exclude intracranial pathology.

Drowsiness, headache, and **vomiting** are common after head trauma. They are not, by themselves, of concern if consciousness is preserved, the clinical trend is one of improvement, and results of the neurological examination are normal. Children are especially susceptible to somnolence after head trauma but should be easily arousable. If symptoms worsen or persist for more than 1-2 days, neuroimaging may be indicated to evaluate for intracranial hemorrhage or cerebral edema.

Evaluation and Treatment

Children who have loss of consciousness or amnesia following a head injury should be evaluated in an emergency department. High-risk patients include those with persistent depressed or decreasing level of consciousness, focal neurological signs, penetrating skull injury, depressed skull fractures, or worsening symptoms. Because patients with intracranial hemorrhage may progressively deteriorate and require immediate neurosurgical care, these patients warrant care in a skilled trauma center.

The **Glasgow Coma Scale** is a valuable tool for monitoring the course of patients' after trauma for signs of deterioration (see Chapter 42). Management includes ensuring an appropriate airway, breathing, and circulation. Neuroimaging with CT or MRI, and skull and cervical spine radiographs are obtained emergently. Neuroimaging is not necessary for uncomplicated concussions but should be employed whenever suspicion of structural intracranial lesion exists.

The observation period varies with the severity of the injury and may include hospitalization. Patients with intracranial hemorrhage may require emergent surgical intervention for decompression and drainage of the blood collection. Increased ICP may require monitoring, placement of a ventricular drain, and aggressive medical management, including intubation and ventilation, osmotic therapy, and sedation. ICP may rise abruptly after fluid resuscitation for a child with both head injury and systemic injuries; such children must be monitored intensively so that interventions to maintain cerebral perfusion pressure are immediately available.

Prognosis

Children with TBI without subsequent neurological deficits have a favorable long-term prognosis and late sequelae are rare. Children with moderate TBI usually make good recoveries even when neurological signs persist for weeks. Long-term sequelae may include poor memory, slowing of motor skills, decline in cognitive skills, behavioral alterations, or attention deficits. Language function, especially in a young child, frequently makes a good recovery. Rehabilitation programs with physical therapy, behavioral management, and appropriate education may be necessary.

Coma lasting for weeks after head trauma may be compatible with a good outcome, although the risk of late sequelae is significant. Mortality rates for children with severe TBI range from 10% to 30%. Poor prognostic signs include a Glasgow Coma Scale score <4 on admission without improvement in 24 hours, absent pupillary light reflexes, and persistent extensor plantar reflexes. Extracranial trauma also contributes to the morbidity of these patients (aspiration pneumonia, acute respiratory distress syndrome, sepsis, emboli). Children with TBI who experience acute cerebral swelling may improve gradually or may remain in a vegetative state. Maximal recovery may take weeks or months. Patients who remain in a vegetative state for months after head injury are unlikely to improve.

CHAPTER 185

Neurodegenerative Disorders

Children typically acquire developmental milestones in a variable but predictable sequence (see Chapter 7). Rarely, children present with stagnation of development or frank loss of previously acquired skills. The **neurodegenerative disorders** encompass a large heterogeneous group of diseases that result from specific genetic and biochemical defects and varied unknown causes. Neurodegenerative disorders can present at any age. Clinical phenotypes also vary, but neurological deterioration may be demonstrated as loss of speech, vision, hearing, and intellectual or motor abilities—sometimes in concert with seizures, feeding difficulties, and intellectual disability. Progression may be slow over many years or may lead to death in early childhood.

HEREDITARY AND METABOLIC DEGENERATIVE DISEASES

Degenerative diseases may affect gray matter **(neuronal degenerative disorders),** white matter **(leukodystrophies),** both gray and white matter, or specific, focal regions of the brain. Early seizures and intellectual impairment mark gray matter disorders, whereas upper motor neuron signs and progressive spasticity are the hallmarks of white matter disorders. Many neurodegenerative illnesses result from enzymatic disorders within subcellular organelles, including lysosomes, mitochondria, and peroxisomes (Table 185.1). Therefore any patient with a degenerative neurological condition of unknown cause should have leukocytes or skin fibroblasts harvested for measurement of a standard battery of lysosomal, peroxisomal, and mitochondrial enzymes (see Chapters 56 and 57). Neuroimaging, usually with brain magnetic resonance imaging (MRI), is also typically warranted. The diagnosis of leukodystrophy can usually be made confidently on the basis of extensive cerebral white matter changes on MRI. Histological and biochemical studies may be normal in gray matter encephalopathy, making the diagnosis much less secure. Acquired lesions (infectious, inflammatory, vascular, toxic) are difficult to exclude completely. Brain biopsy is not likely to be helpful.

TABLE 185.1 Selected Clinical Features of Neurodegenerative Disorders and Relevant Diagnostic Tests

SPHINGOLIPIDOSES
Niemann-Pick Disease
Cognitive regression, hepatosplenomegaly, jaundice, seizures
Test: acid sphingomyelinase enzyme activity
Gaucher Disease
Hepatosplenomegaly, cytopenia, spasticity, hyperextension, extraocular palsies, trismus, difficulty swallowing
Test: glucosylceramidase enzyme activity
GM1 Gangliosidoses
Infantile form—early feeding difficulties, global retardation, seizures, coarse facial features, hepatosplenomegaly, cherry red spot
Juvenile form—incoordination, weakness, language regression; later, seizures, spasticity, blindness
Adult form
Test: GM1 ganglioside enzyme activity; *GLB1* gene testing
GM2 Gangliosidoses
Tay-Sachs Disease—progressive weakness, marked startle reaction, blindness, convulsions, spasticity, and cherry red spots
Test: β-hexosaminidase A enzymatic activity
Sandhoff Disease—phenotype similar to Tay-Sachs
Test: β-hexosaminidase A and B enzyme activity (both deficient)
Krabbe Disease/Globoid Cell Leukodystrophy
Irritability, hyperpyrexia, vomiting, seizures, hypertonia, blindness
Test: galactocerebrosidase enzyme activity
Metachromic Leukodystrophy
Late infantile form—stiffening and ataxia of gait, spasticity, optic atrophy, intellectual deterioration, absent reflexes
Juvenile and adult forms
Tests: 1. arylsulfatase A (ARSA) enzyme activity
2. If ARSA activity is <10% of controls, exclude ARSA pseudodeficiency with genetic testing of ARSA and/or abnormal urinary sulfatide excretion
NEURONAL CEROID LIPOFUSCINOSES
Visual loss, progressive dementia, seizures, motor deterioration
Tests: Diagnostic algorithm depends on age of symptom onset, and relies on stepwise testing for palmitoyl-protein thioesterase 1 and tripeptidyl-peptidase 1 enzyme activity
X-LINKED ADRENOLEUKODYSTROPHY
Classic Adrenoleukodystrophy
Academic difficulties, behavioral disturbances, hypoadrenalism, seizures, spasticity, ataxia, and swallowing difficulties.
Adrenomyeloneuropathy
Spastic paraparesis, urinary incontinence, adrenal insufficiency
Test: very long chain fatty acids
MUCOPOLYSACCHARIDOSES (MPS)
Short stature, kyphoscoliosis, coarse facies, hepatosplenomegaly, cardiovascular abnormalities, and corneal clouding

Continued

TABLE 185.1 Selected Clinical Features of Neurodegenerative Disorders and Relevant Diagnostic Tests—cont'd

TYPES
Hurler (MPS type I-H)
Hunter (MPS type II)
Sanfilippo Disease (MPS type III)
Sly Syndrome (MPS type VII)
Tests:
1. lysosomal enzymes
2. urinary glycosaminoglycan excretion
MITOCHONDRIAL DISORDERS
MELAS
Mitochondrial myopathy, encephalopathy, lactic acidosis, and stroke-like episodes
MERRF
Myoclonus, epilepsy, and ragged red fibers, dementia, hearing loss, optic nerve atrophy, ataxia, and loss of deep sensation
NARP
Neuropathy, ataxia, and retinitis pigmentosa
Tests: testing for mitochondrial disorders is complex and must be tailored to the individual clinical scenario; screening for blood and serum lactate and pyruvate is reasonable
SUBACUTE NECROTIZING ENCEPHALOMYELOPATHY (LEIGH DISEASE)
Hypotonia, feeding difficulties, respiratory irregularity, weakness of extraocular movements, and ataxia
Test: depends on clinical phenotype; blood and CSF lactate and pyruvate are elevated
RETT SYNDROME
Loss of purposeful hand movements and communication skills, social withdrawal, gait apraxia, seizures, spasticity, and kyphoscoliosis
Test: *MECP2* gene testing
WILSON DISEASE
Inborn error of copper metabolism resulting in signs of cerebellar and basal ganglia dysfunction
Tests: serum ceruloplasmin levels, urinary copper excretion

CSF, Cerebrospinal fluid; *MECP2*, methyl CpG binding protein 2; *MPS*, mucopolysaccharidoses; *MERRF*, myoclonus, epilepsy, and ragged red fibers; *NARP*, neuropathy, ataxia, and retinitis pigmentosa.

Sphingolipidoses

The sphingolipidoses are characterized by intracellular storage of lipid substrates resulting from defective catabolism of the cell membrane sphingolipids. They are inherited in an autosomal recessive pattern. In most cases, there are several forms of these diseases and the tempo of disease progression reflects the amount of residual enzyme activity. The infantile forms are generally the most severe, usually presenting in the first or second year of life with rapid disease progression; affected individuals have virtually no normal enzyme activity. Juvenile and chronic forms are manifest somewhat later in childhood or even adulthood and have a less fulminant disease course as there is some residual enzyme activity.

Classic **Niemann-Pick disease** is caused by a deficiency of sphingomyelinase and should be suspected in infants who exhibit the combination of hepatosplenomegaly, developmental delay, interstitial lung disease, and **retinal cherry red spots.** The ganglion cells of the retina and macula are distended and appear as a large area of white surrounding a small red fovea that is not covered by ganglion cells. Cognitive regression, myoclonic seizures, hypotonia, and jaundice are also noted within the first year of life. Genetic testing for *SMPD1* mutations is clinically available.

Although the most common form of **Gaucher disease** is an indolent illness of adults, there is a rapidly fatal infantile form featuring severe neurological involvement caused by deficiency of the enzyme glucocerebrosidase. Glucoceramide accumulates in the liver, spleen, and bone marrow. The characteristic neurological signs are opisthotonos (arching of the trunk), trismus (difficulty opening mouth), eye movement abnormalities, and bulbar signs including difficulty swallowing.

Decision-Making Algorithm
Available @ StudentConsult.com
Splenomegaly

Tay-Sachs disease (GM_2 gangliosidosis) is caused by deficiency of hexosaminidase A and results in the accumulation of GM_2 ganglioside in cerebral gray matter and cerebellum. Infants are typically normal, except for a marked startle response, until 6 months of age, when they develop listlessness, irritability, hyperacusis, cognitive regression, and retinal cherry red spots. Within months, blindness, convulsions, spasticity, and opisthotonos develop.

Metachromatic leukodystrophy (MLD) is a lipidosis caused by deficiency of arylsulfatase that results in demyelination of the central nervous system (CNS) and peripheral nervous system. Children with the late-infantile form present between 1 and 2 years of age. After a period of normal development, progressive gait ataxia, spasticity, optic atrophy, intellectual deterioration, and absent reflexes occur. Diagnostic testing reveals increased cerebral spinal fluid protein (a sign of CNS demyelination) and slowing of motor nerve conduction velocity (a sign of peripheral demyelination). Older school-age children with the juvenile form of MLD may present with gradual onset of behavior difficulties and declining academic abilities, followed by gait difficulties, clumsiness, slurred speech, and, sometimes, seizures. Relentless progression is the rule. Bone marrow transplant is a treatment option, particularly if a sibling is diagnosed with MLD before symptom onset.

Krabbe disease (globoid cell leukodystrophy) is caused by a deficiency of galactocerebrosidase. Individuals with the infantile form (85-90% of cases) appear to be normal during the first months of life. Symptoms begin by 6 months of age and include extreme irritability, hyperpyrexia, vomiting, seizures, hypertonia, and blindness. Demyelination of the CNS and peripheral nervous system results in upper and lower motor neuron signs. Bone marrow transplant during infancy may be a treatment option.

Neuronal Ceroid Lipofuscinoses

The neuronal ceroid lipofuscinoses are a group of inherited, neurodegenerative lysosomal storage disorders characterized by progressive vision loss, seizures, declining cognitive abilities, motor deterioration, and early death. Ten different types have been characterized, including infantile, late-infantile, and juvenile types.

Adrenoleukodystrophy

The adrenoleukodystrophies (ALDs) are a group of X-linked neurodegenerative disorders that are often associated with adrenocortical insufficiency. ALD is caused by accumulation of very long chain fatty acids in neuronal and adrenal tissue (see Chapter 178) and is diagnosed by abnormal very long chain fatty acid testing. The most common leukodystrophy is **classic X-linked adrenoleukodystrophy**, caused by a mutation in the *ABCD1* gene. Boys present between ages 5 and 15 years with academic difficulties, behavioral disturbances, and gait abnormalities, progressing to seizures, spasticity, ataxia, and swallowing difficulties. Brain MRI demonstrates a classic pattern of symmetrical abnormal white matter signal in the parietal-occipital regions, with contrast enhancement at the anterior margin. Symptomatic *adrenocortical insufficiency* with fatigue, vomiting, and hypotension develops in 20-40% of patients with X-linked ALD. ALD should be considered in any male with primary adrenocortical insufficiency, even in the absence of clear-cut neurological abnormalities. **Adrenomyeloneuropathy**, a chronic disorder of the spinal cord and peripheral nerves, presents in the third decade of life. Female carriers of the *ABCD1* mutation may also have symptoms similar to adrenomyeloneuropathy, beginning later in life (>35 years of age).

Mucopolysaccharidoses

Mucopolysaccharidoses are caused by defective lysosomal hydrolases resulting in the accumulation of mucopolysaccharides within lysosomes (see Chapter 56). The clinical manifestations include coarse facies, short stature, kyphoscoliosis, hepatosplenomegaly, cardiovascular abnormalities, and corneal clouding. Neurological involvement is seen in mucopolysaccharidosis types I **(Hurler syndrome)**, II **(Hunter syndrome)**, III **(Sanfilippo syndrome)**, and VII **(Sly syndrome)**. Children with Hurler syndrome, the most severe of these illnesses, appear normal during the first 6 months of life, then develop the characteristic skeletal and neurological features. Intellectual disability, spasticity, deafness, and optic atrophy are progressive. Hydrocephalus frequently occurs because of obstruction to cerebrospinal fluid (CSF) flow by thickened leptomeninges.

Mitochondrial Disorders

Mitochondrial diseases represent a clinically heterogeneous group of disorders that fundamentally share a disturbance in oxidative phosphorylation (adenosine triphosphate synthesis; see Chapter 57). Abrupt symptoms are often manifest concurrent with periods of physiological stress such as febrile illness or fasting. Specific genetic diagnoses are often difficult to identify because several different gene mutations can cause the same disease, single mutations can have multiple phenotypes, and analysis of mitochondrial protein function is technically demanding. Specific syndromes include **MELAS** (mitochondrial myopathy, encephalopathy, lactic acidosis, and stroke-like episodes); **MERRF** (myoclonus, epilepsy, and ragged red fibers), which can also manifest as combinations of dementia, sensorineural hearing loss, optic nerve atrophy, peripheral neuropathy, and occasionally cardiomyopathy with Wolff-Parkinson-White syndrome; and **NARP** (neuropathy, ataxia, and retinitis pigmentosa).

Rett Syndrome

Rett syndrome is a neurodevelopmental disorder that classically affects girls. Typically development appears normal during the first 6-18 months of life, but this is followed by developmental *regression*, loss of purposeful hand movements, loss of verbal communication skills, gait apraxia, and stereotypic repetitive hand movements that resemble washing, wringing, or clapping of the hands. Girls also develop *acquired microcephaly*. Episodic apnea and/or hyperpnea, peripheral vasomotor disturbances, growth retardation, abnormal muscle tone, and prolonged QTc interval often occur. The developmental regression plateaus and stabilizes, but seizures, spasticity, and kyphoscoliosis develop. The etiology is a mutation on an X chromosome gene coding for methyl-CpG-binding protein 2 *(MECP2)* transcription factor. Boys with *MECP2* mutations usually do not survive to delivery but can present with severe neonatal encephalopathy, seizures, microcephaly, abnormal tone, and respiratory insufficiency.

Degenerative Diseases With Focal Manifestations

Some neurodegenerative disorders have predilections to target specific regions or systems within the neuraxis and produce symptoms referable to the affected region.

Wilson disease is a treatable degenerative condition that manifests as cerebellar and basal ganglia dysfunction. It is an autosomal recessive inborn error of copper metabolism. Serum ceruloplasmin levels are low. Abnormal copper deposition is found in the liver, producing cirrhosis; in the peripheral cornea, producing a characteristic green-brown (Kayser-Fleischer) ring; and in the CNS, producing neuronal degeneration and protoplasmic astrocytosis. Neurological symptoms characteristically begin in the early teenage years with dysarthria, dysphasia, drooling, fixed smile, tremor, dystonia, and emotional lability. MRI shows abnormalities of the basal ganglia. Treatment is with a copper-chelating agent, such as oral penicillamine.

Decision-Making Algorithms
Available @ StudentConsult.com

Jaundice
Hepatomegaly
Involuntary Movements
Hypocalcemia

Subacute necrotizing encephalomyelopathy, or Leigh disease, is a neuropathologically defined, degenerative, inherited CNS disease primarily involving the periaqueductal region of the brainstem, caudate, and putamen. Symptoms usually begin before 2 years of age and consist of hypotonia, feeding difficulties, respiratory irregularity, weakness of extraocular movements, and ataxia. Blood and CSF lactate and pyruvate levels are elevated. Several alterations of mitochondrial function produce this clinical syndrome.

ACQUIRED ILLNESSES MIMICKING DEGENERATIVE DISEASES

Children with poorly controlled epilepsy may be continuously in either an ictal or a postictal state and may appear stuporous because of their *epileptic encephalopathy*. Antiepileptic drugs that are sedating or affect mood, memory, motivation, or attention may contribute to the lack or loss of developmental abilities and school failure.

Chronic drug use or overuse (sedatives, tranquilizers, anticholinergics) can cause progressive confusion, lethargy, and ataxia. Intoxications with heavy metals, such as lead, may cause chronic learning difficulties or may present acutely with irritability, listlessness, anorexia, and pallor, progressing to fulminant encephalopathy. Vitamin deficiency of thiamine, niacin, vitamin B_{12}, and vitamin E can produce encephalopathy, peripheral neuropathy, and ataxia.

Congenital and acquired hypothyroidism impairs cognition and slows developmental progress. Unrecognized congenital hypothyroidism produces irreversible damage if it is not treated immediately after birth (see Chapter 175).

Structural brain diseases, such as hydrocephalus and slowly growing tumors, may cause slowly progressive cognitive decline and other focal deficits. Certain indolent brain infections, such as rubeola (measles, causing subacute sclerosing panencephalitis), rubella (German measles), syphilis, and some fungal infections, cause neurological deterioration over months and years. Congenital human immunodeficiency virus infection causes failure of normal development and regression of acquired skills.

Psychiatric disorders, such as depression and severe psychosocial deprivation in infancy, can give rise to apathy and failure to attain developmental milestones (see Chapter 21). Children with autism spectrum disorder may go through a phase of developmental stagnation or disintegration at about 12-18 months of age after a period of early normal milestones. Depression in older children can lead to blunting of affect, social withdrawal, and poor school performance, which raise the question of encephalopathy or dementia.

CHAPTER 186
Neurocutaneous Disorders

The skin, teeth, hair, nails, and brain are derived embryologically from ectoderm. Abnormalities of these surface structures may indicate abnormal brain development. Not all of the so-called neurocutaneous disorders have characteristic cutaneous lesions, however, and not all are of ectodermal origin. Neurofibromatosis (types 1 and 2), tuberous sclerosis, Sturge-Weber syndrome, von Hippel-Lindau disease, and ataxia-telangiectasia are the most common of the more than 40 neurocutaneous disorders.

NEUROFIBROMATOSIS TYPE 1

Etiology

Neurofibromatosis type 1 (NF1), also known as von Recklinghausen disease, is an autosomal-dominant disorder with an incidence of approximately 1 in 3,000. It is caused by mutations of the *NF1* gene, which codes for a tumor suppressor gene, neurofibromin. Neurofibromin is a major negative regulator of a key signal transduction pathway, the Ras pathway. Mutations result in increased downstream mitogenic signaling. Somatic mosaicism, in which an abnormality in one copy of the *NF1* gene is present in some cells but not others, indicates a postzygotic mutation and is called **segmental neurofibromatosis**.

Clinical Manifestations

Decision-Making Algorithms
Available @ StudentConsult.com
Hearing Loss
Gynecomastia

The cardinal features of neurofibromatosis are café-au-lait spots, axillary or inguinal freckling, cutaneous neurofibromas, and iris hamartomas (Lisch nodules). **Café-au-lait spots** are present in more than 90% of patients who have NF1 (Fig. 186.1). They typically appear in the first few years of life and increase in number and size over time. The presence of six or more café-au-lait spots larger than 5 mm in a prepubescent child suggests the diagnosis. **Lisch nodules** also increase in frequency with age and are present in more than 90% of adults who have NF1.

Neurofibromas are composed of various combinations of Schwann cells, fibroblasts, mast cells, and vascular elements. Dermal neurofibromas are nearly universal and consist of discrete, small, soft lesions that lie within the dermis and

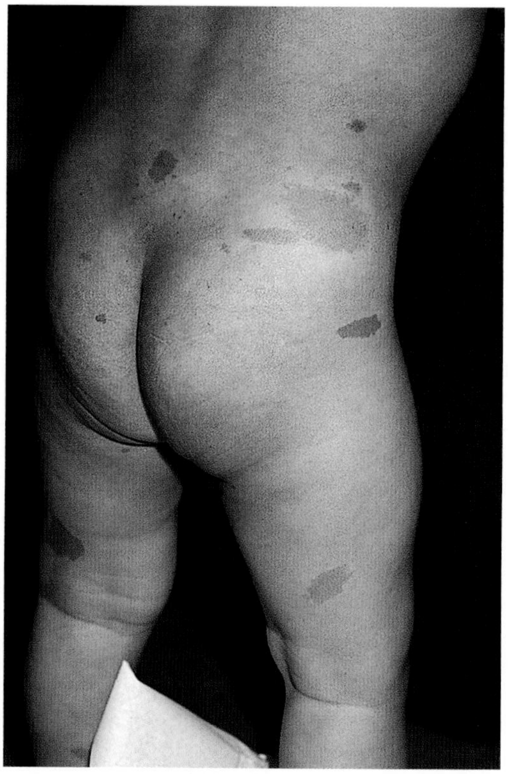

FIGURE 186.1 Café-au-lait macules. (From Kliegman RE, Behrman RE, Jenson HB, eds. *Nelson Textbook of Pediatrics*. 19th ed. Philadelphia: Saunders; 2007:2680.)

epidermis and move passively with the skin. They rarely cause any symptoms but can cause significant cosmetic concerns. Neurofibromas may also be situated within viscera or along blood vessels and peripheral nerves. Plexiform neurofibromas are large, occasionally nodular, subcutaneous lesions that lie along the major peripheral nerve trunks. They often cause symptoms including pain, weakness, and invasion of adjacent viscera, bone, or spinal cord. Sarcomatous degeneration may occur. Surgical treatment may be attempted, but results are often unsatisfactory.

Common complications are learning disability, scoliosis, seizures, and cerebral vasculature abnormalities. Other tumors that occur in NF1 are optic nerve gliomas, astrocytomas of brain and spinal cord, and malignant peripheral nerve tumors. T2-weighted magnetic resonance images (MRIs) reveal hyperintense lesions (hamartomas) in the optic tracts, internal capsule, thalamus, cerebellum, and brainstem that are common and distinctive for the disease. They are benign and disappear in adulthood.

The average life expectancy of patients with NF1 may be reduced by 10-15 years. Malignancy is the most common cause of death. Genetic and psychological counseling are important components of care for this chronic disorder. Although it is an autosomal-dominant disorder, spontaneous mutations account for 30-50% of cases.

Neurofibromatosis Type 2

Neurofibromatosis type 2 (NF2) is an autosomal-dominant disorder with an incidence of 1 in 25,000. Half the cases have no family history. The *NF2* gene is a tumor suppressor gene and disease results in neurological, eye, and skin lesions. NF2 predisposes patients to multiple intracranial and spinal tumors, including bilateral acoustic schwannomas, schwannomas of other cranial and spinal nerves, meningiomas, and gliomas. Posterior capsular or cortical cataracts are common, and skin lesions include plaque-like lesions, subcutaneous nodules, and cutaneous schwannomas. Lisch nodules, café-au-lait spots, and axillary freckling (seen in NF1) are *not* features of NF2.

TUBEROUS SCLEROSIS COMPLEX

Etiology

Tuberous sclerosis complex (TSC), an autosomal-dominant disorder, is characterized by hamartomas in many organs, especially the brain, eyes, skin, kidneys, and heart. The incidence is 1 in 10,000 births. Two thirds of cases are sporadic and thought to represent new mutations. Germline mosaicism is uncommon but explains how parents who apparently do not have the disease can have multiple children with tuberous sclerosis. Mutations affecting either of the presumed tumor suppressor genes, *TSC1* or *TSC2*, cause tuberous sclerosis. The *TSC1* and *TSC2* genes encode distinct proteins, hamartin and tuberin, which are widely expressed in the brain and result in constitutive activation of the protein kinase mTOR (mammalian target of rapamycin), leading to the formation of numerous benign tumors (hamartomas).

Clinical Manifestations

TSC is an extremely heterogeneous disease with variable expression and a wide clinical spectrum varying from normal intelligence without seizures to severe intellectual disability with refractory seizures and autism, often within the same family. People with TSC may have retinal lesions (retinal hamartomas, white depigmented patches) and brain lesions (cortical tubers, subependymal nodules, hydrocephalus). **Tubers** in the cerebral cortex are areas of dysplasia that, in combination with other microscopic areas of abnormal development, are responsible for the symptoms of intellectual disability and epilepsy. TSC is one of the most common causes of infantile spasms; in this context, the infantile spasms often respond to treatment with vigabatrin. **Subependymal nodules** are hamartomas that may mutate into a growth phase and become **subependymal giant cell astrocytomas** (SEGAs), causing obstruction of cerebrospinal fluid outflow and resultant hydrocephalus. SEGAs can be treated with everolimus, a mammalian target of rapamycin inhibitor, and preliminary studies suggest that this medication can also reduce seizure burden for people with TSC.

Extracerebral manifestations include typical skin findings of hypomelanotic macules **(ash leaf spots),** which are easiest to visualize under a Wood ultraviolet lamp and are apparent in infancy. Facial angiofibromas **(adenoma sebaceum)** appear as small red nodules over the nose and cheeks that are sometimes confused with acne. **Shagreen patches** are elevated, rough plaques of skin with a predilection for the lumbar and gluteal regions that develop in late childhood or early adolescence. Cardiac rhabdomyomas are largest during prenatal life and infancy and are rarely symptomatic. Occasionally, they may cause arrhythmias or cardiac outflow obstruction. Renal angiomyolipomas may undergo malignant transformation and are the most common cause of death in adults with TSC. Interstitial pulmonary disease also affects adults with TSC (pulmonary lymphangioleiomyomatosis).

STURGE-WEBER SYNDROME

Sturge-Weber syndrome is sporadic (not inherited) and is caused by a somatic mosaic mutation of the *GNAQ* gene. It is characterized by abnormal blood vessels **(angiomas)** of the leptomeninges overlying the cerebral cortex in association with an ipsilateral facial **port-wine stain** involving the ophthalmic division of the trigeminal nerve (forehead and upper eyelid) and, often, glaucoma. The port-wine stain, also known as nevus flammeus, is due to an ectasia of superficial venules and may have a much more extensive and even bilateral distribution. Not all children with a facial port-wine stain have Sturge-Weber syndrome.

MRI with contrast demonstrates leptomeningeal angioma and white matter abnormalities thought to be due to chronic hypoxia and atrophy. Angiomas produce venous engorgement and, presumably, stasis within the involved areas, which are thought to result in hypoxia. Seizures are the most common associated neurological abnormality, occurring in 75% of patients. Children may also present with hemiparesis, stroke-like episodes, headaches, developmental delay, and learning disabilities. Many children with Sturge-Weber syndrome are intellectually normal, and seizures are well controlled with standard anticonvulsants. However, progressive ischemia of the underlying brain develops in some children with Sturge-Weber syndrome, resulting in hemiparesis, hemianopia, intractable focal seizures, and cognitive impairment. Hemispherectomy has been proposed for individuals with unilateral disease whose seizures are difficult to control, both to control the epilepsy and to preserve cognitive and motor development. Low-dose aspirin may result in improved perfusion and thereby reduce stroke-like events and seizures. Pulse dye laser surgery is the most promising therapeutic option for cosmetic management of the facial nevus flammeus. Expert ophthalmological management of glaucoma is required. Endocrinology evaluations are also necessary, as these patients often have growth hormone deficiency and/or hypothyroidism.

CHAPTER 187

Congenital Malformations of the Central Nervous System

Central nervous system malformations include disorders of spinal cord and neural tube formation, structure specification (neuronal migration, gray matter), brain growth and size, and skull growth and shape.

The precursor of the nervous system is the neural plate of the embryonic ectoderm, which develops at 18 days of gestation. The neural plate gives rise to the neural tube, which forms the brain and spinal cord, and neural crest cells, which form the peripheral nervous system, meninges, melanocytes, and adrenal medulla. The neural tube begins to form on day 22 of gestation. The rostral end forms the brain, and the caudal region forms the spinal cord. The lumen of the neural tube forms the ventricles of the brain and the central canal of the spinal cord. Most brain malformations are produced by a variety of injuries occurring during a vulnerable period of gestation. Precipitating factors include chromosomal, genetic, and metabolic abnormalities; infections (toxoplasmosis, rubella, cytomegalovirus, herpes); and exposure to irradiation, certain drugs, and maternal illness during pregnancy.

CONGENITAL ANOMALIES OF THE SPINAL CORD

Etiology and Clinical Manifestations

Defective closure of the caudal neural tube at the end of week 4 of gestation results in anomalies of the lumbar and sacral vertebrae or spinal cord called **spina bifida**. These anomalies range in severity from clinically insignificant defects of the L5 or S1 vertebral arches to major malformations, leaving the spinal cord uncovered by skin or bone on the infant's back. The latter severe defect, called a **myelomeningocele**, results in flaccid paralysis and loss of sensation in the legs and incontinence of bowel and bladder, with the extent and degree of neurological deficit dependent on the location of the myelomeningocele. In addition, affected children usually have an associated **Chiari type II malformation** (downward displacement of the cerebellar tonsils and medulla), resulting in hydrocephalus and weakness of face and swallowing. In a **meningocele**, the spinal canal and cystic meninges are exposed on the back, but the underlying spinal cord is anatomically and functionally intact. In **spina bifida occulta,** the skin of the back is apparently intact, but defects of the underlying bone or spinal canal are present. Meningoceles and spina bifida occulta may be associated with a lipoma, dermoid cyst, or tethering of the cord to a thick filum terminale. A dimple or tuft of hair may be present over the affected area. Patients may also have an associated dermoid sinus, an epithelial tract extending from the skin surface to the meninges; this increases the risk of meningitis. Patients with spina bifida occulta or meningocele may have weakness and numbness in the feet that can result in recurrent ulcerations, or difficulties controlling bowel or bladder function that may result in recurrent urinary tract infections, reflux nephropathy, and renal insufficiency. In **diastematomyelia,** a bone spicule or fibrous band divides the spinal cord into two longitudinal sections. An associated lipoma that infiltrates the cord and tethers it to the vertebrae may be present. Symptoms include weakness and numbness of the feet and urinary incontinence.

Diagnostic Studies

Myelomeningocele in the fetus is suggested by an elevated **alpha-fetoprotein** in the mother's blood and confirmed by ultrasound and high concentrations of alpha-fetoprotein and acetylcholinesterase in the amniotic fluid. After birth, screening ultrasound may be used with magnetic resonance imaging to confirm less dramatic underlying spinal abnormalities.

Treatment and Prevention

Neonates with myelomeningocele must undergo operative closure of the open spinal defects (fetal or postnatal surgery) and often require treatment of hydrocephalus by placement of a ventriculoperitoneal shunt. Compared to postnatal surgery, fetal surgery prior to 26 weeks' gestation to close the myelomeningocele reduces the need for cerebrospinal fluid (CSF) shunting and improves neurodevelopmental outcomes. Toddlers and children with lower spinal cord dysfunction require physical therapy, bracing of the lower extremities, and intermittent bladder catheterization. In the absence of associated brain anomalies, most survivors have normal intelligence, but learning problems and epilepsy are more common than in the general population.

Spina bifida can be prevented in many cases by **folate** administration to the pregnant mother. Because the defect occurs so early in gestation, all women of childbearing age are advised to take oral folic acid daily.

CONGENITAL MALFORMATIONS OF THE BRAIN

Defective closure of the rostral neural tube produces anencephaly or encephaloceles. Neonates with **anencephaly** have a rudimentary brainstem or midbrain, but no cortex or cranium. This is rapidly fatal after delivery. Patients with **encephalocele** usually have a skull defect and exposure of meninges alone or meninges and brain. The recurrence risk in subsequent pregnancies for either cranial or spinal neural tube defects is 3-4%. Within a family, an anencephalic birth may be followed by the birth of a child affected with a lumbosacral myelomeningocele. The inheritance of neural tube defects is polygenic.

Agenesis of the corpus callosum may be partial or complete and may occur in an isolated fashion or in association with other anomalies of cellular migration. **Dandy-Walker malformation** is diagnosed on the basis of the classic triad: complete or partial agenesis of the cerebellar vermis, cystic dilation of the fourth ventricle, and enlarged posterior fossa. There may be associated hydrocephalus, absence of the corpus callosum, and neuronal migration abnormalities. Intelligence may be normal or impaired, depending on the degree of associated cerebral dysgenesis.

Holoprosencephaly represents varying degrees of failure of the forebrain (prosencephalon) to divide into two distinct cerebral hemispheres. Holoprosencephaly is often associated with midline facial defects (hypotelorism, cleft lip, cleft palate). This anomaly may be isolated or associated with a chromosomal or genetic disorder. The prognosis for infants with severe *(alobar)* holoprosencephaly is uniformly poor, but those with milder forms *(semilobar, lobar)* may have less severe neurological outcomes. Children with trisomy 13 and trisomy 18 characteristically have varying degrees of holoprosencephaly.

Hydranencephaly is a condition in which the brain presumably develops normally, but then is destroyed by an intrauterine, probably vascular, insult. The result is virtual absence of the cerebrum with an intact skull. The thalamus, brainstem, and some occipital cortex are typically present. Children may have a normal external appearance at the time of birth, but do not achieve developmental milestones.

Macrocephaly and Microcephaly

Macrocephaly represents a head circumference above the 97th percentile and may be the result of **macrocrania** (increased skull thickness), **hydrocephalus** (enlargement of the ventricles; see Chapter 184), or **megalencephaly** (enlargement of the brain). Diseases of bone metabolism or hypertrophy of the bone marrow causes macrocrania. Megalencephaly may be the result of a significant disorder of brain development or an accumulation of abnormal metabolic substances (Table 187.1). Most often, however, macrocephaly is a familial trait of no clinical significance. If the child is developmentally normal but has macrocephaly, plotting the parents' head circumference on a growth chart can provide reassurance and help to avoid unnecessary neurodiagnostic testing.

Microcephaly represents a head circumference below the 3rd percentile. A myriad of syndromes and metabolic disorders are associated with microcephaly, some of which are hereditary (Table 187.2). In most instances, a small head circumference is a reflection of a small brain. Brain growth is rapid during the perinatal period, and any insult (infectious, metabolic, toxic, vascular) sustained during this period or during early infancy is likely to impair brain growth and result in microcephaly. Rarely, a small head is the result of premature closure of one or more skull sutures, called **craniosynostosis**. This diagnosis is readily made by the abnormal shape of the skull. As a rule, macrocephaly and microcephaly raise a concern about cognitive ability, but head circumference alone should never be used to establish a prognosis for intellectual development.

Disorders of Neuronal Migration

Many malformations result from the failure of normal migration of neurons from the periventricular germinal matrix zone to the cortical surface at 1-5 months of gestation. Multiple malformations may exist in the same patient. Neurological development with these anomalies varies and depends on the type and extent of the malformation. Many children with disorders of neuronal migration have treatment-resistant epilepsy.

TABLE 187.1 Causes of Macrocephaly
Macrocrania (increased skull thickness)
Achondroplasia
Hypochondroplasia
Fragile X syndrome
Osteopetrosis
Chronic, severe anemia
Hydrocephalus (enlargement of the ventricles; see Chapter 184)
Masses
Cysts
Arteriovenous malformations
Subdural fluid collections/hematoma
Neoplasm
Megalencephaly (enlargement of the brain)
Embryological disorder causing abnormal proliferation of brain tissue
• Neurofibromatosis
• Tuberous sclerosis
• Sturge-Weber syndrome
• Sotos syndrome
• Riley-Smith syndrome
• Hemi-megalencephaly
Accumulation of abnormal metabolic substances
• Alexander disease
• Canavan disease
• Gangliosidoses
• Mucopolysaccharidoses
Benign causes
Benign extracerebral collections of infancy
Familial macrocephaly

Schizencephaly is characterized by clefts within the cerebral hemispheres that extend from the cortical surface to the ventricular cavity. Unilateral clefts can cause isolated congenital hemiparesis, whereas bilateral schizencephaly causes spastic quadriparesis and associated intellectual disability. Affected individuals are at high risk for focal epilepsy.

A severe defect in cortical migration, **lissencephaly** results in a smooth brain without sulcation (agyria). The normal six-layered cortex does not develop. Affected children have difficult-to-control seizures and profound developmental retardation. This anomaly most commonly is part of a genetic disorder, which may be x-linked (*DCX* mutations) or caused by de novo autosomal-dominant gene mutations (*Lis-1* mutations). In **pachygyria**, the gyri are few in number and too broad. In **polymicrogyria**, the gyri are too many and too small. Sometimes pachygyria and polymicrogyria affect an entire hemisphere, producing enlargement of that hemisphere and a clinical syndrome of severe, medically intractable seizures that begin in early infancy. **Gray matter heterotopias** are abnormal islands within the central white matter of neurons that have never completed the migratory process.

TABLE 187.2 Causes of Microcephaly

PRIMARY MICROCEPHALY	SECONDARY (ACQUIRED) MICROCEPHALY
Microcephaly vera	Infections (congenital)
Chromosomal disorders	Rubella
Trisomy 21	Cytomegalovirus
Trisomy 13	Toxoplasmosis
Trisomy 18	Syphilis
5p microdeletion	Human immunodeficiency virus (HIV)
Angelman syndrome	Zika virus
Prader-Willi syndrome	Infections (noncongenital)
Central nervous system (CNS) malformation	Meningitis
Holoprosencephaly	Encephalitis
Encephalocele	Stroke
Hydranencephaly	Toxic
CNS migrational disorder	Radiation exposure—fetal
Lissencephaly	Fetal alcohol syndrome
Schizencephaly	Maternal phenylketonuria
Pachygyria	Hypoxic-ischemic or other severe brain injury
Micropolygyria	Periventricular leukomalacia
Agenesis of the corpus callosum	Systemic disease
Sex-linked microcephaly syndromes	Chronic cardiac or pulmonary disease
Smith-Lemli-Opitz syndrome	Chronic renal disease
Cornelia de Lange syndrome	Malnutrition
Seckel dwarfism syndrome	Craniosynostosis totalis
Cockayne syndrome	
Rubinstein-Taybi syndrome	
Hallermann-Streiff syndrome	

Suggested Readings

Blume HK. Pediatric headache: a review. *Pediatr Rev*. 2012;33:562–576.

Fenichel GM. *Fenichel's Clinical Pediatric Neurology: A Signs and Symptoms Approach*. 7th ed. Philadelphia: Saunders; 2013.

Gillam-Krakauer M, Carter BS. Neonatal hypoxia and seizures. *Pediatr Rev*. 2012;33:387–397.

Glauser T, Shinnar S, Gloss D, et al. Evidence-based guideline: treatment of convulsive status epilepticus in children and adults: report of the guideline committee of the American Epilepsy Society. *Epilepsy Curr*. 2016;16:48–61.

Jacobs H, Gladstein J. Pediatric headache: a clinical review. *Headache*. 2012;52:333–339.

Kliegman RM, Stanton BMD, St. Geme J, et al. *Nelson Textbook of Pediatrics*. 20th ed. Philadelphia: Saunders; 2015.

Kruer MC. Pediatric movement disorders. *Pediatr Rev*. 2015;36:104–116.

Peredo DE, Hannibal MC. The floppy infant: evaluation of hypotonia. *Pediatr Rev*. 2009;30:e66–e76.

Richer L, Billinghurst L, Linsdell MA, et al. Drugs for the acute treatment of migraine in children and adolescents. *Cochrane Database Syst Rev*. 2016;(4):CD005220.

Schunk JE, Schutzman SA. Pediatric head injury. *Pediatr Rev*. 2012;33:398–411.

Tsao CY. Muscle disease. *Pediatr Rev*. 2014;35:49–59.

www.epilepsydiagnosis.org.

PEARLS FOR PRACTITIONERS

CHAPTER 179

Neurology Assessment

- The pediatric neurological examination varies with age; the newborn is unique, with many transient and primitive reflexes, which provide assessment of the functional integrity of the brainstem and basal ganglia.
- Careful evaluations of social, cognitive, language, fine motor and gross motor skills, and their age appropriateness are key in the neurological assessment of children.
- Watching a child creep, crawl, cruise, or walk is the best global assessment for the motor and coordination systems.

CHAPTER 180

Headache and Migraine

- There are four temporal patterns of childhood headache: acute; acute recurrent; chronic progressive; and chronic nonprogressive or chronic daily.
- Additional investigation is warranted for headaches in the presence of an abnormal neurological exam (especially papilledema), symptoms of increased intracranial pressure, atypical headache, progressive chronic headache, signs of increased intracranial pressure, or "worst headache of my life."
- Symptoms of increased intracranial pressure include early morning vomiting or headache that wakens the child from sleep.

CHAPTER 181

Seizures

- Focal seizures with retained awareness (previously termed simple partial seizures) arise from a specific anatomical focus.
  - Clinical symptoms include motor (tonic, clonic, myoclonic), sensory, psychic, or autonomic abnormalities, but consciousness is preserved.
- Focal seizures with altered awareness (previously termed complex partial seizures) can have similar sensorimotor signs but also have associated alteration of consciousness.
- The clinical hallmark of absence seizures is a brief (less than 15 seconds) loss of awareness accompanied by eyelid fluttering or simple automatisms, such as fumbling with the fingers and lip smacking. Absence seizures usually begin between 4 and 6 years of age.
- Children with febrile seizures have an excellent prognosis, and daily antiseizure medication to prevent febrile seizures is not recommended.
- Infantile spasms are clusters of brief contractions of the neck, trunk, and arm muscles, followed by a phase of sustained muscle contraction lasting less than 2 seconds. Rapid initiation of effective therapy offers the best chance for favorable neurodevelopmental outcomes.
- Initial management of status epilepticus is with a benzodiazepine and should begin if the seizure persists longer than 5 minutes.
  - If the seizure does not resolve after two doses of benzodiazepine, a second-line agent must be administered, typically phenobarbital for newborns and infants and intravenous fosphenytoin, valproic acid, or levetiracetam for older children.
- Psychogenic nonepileptic seizures (PNES) may be the manifestation of conversion disorders or malingering.
  - Children with epilepsy may, consciously or subconsciously, exhibit concurrent PNES.
  - Careful assessment and intervention for abuse, as well as other social stressors, is a key component of the care of children with PNES.

CHAPTER 182

Weakness and Hypotonia

- Weakness is a decreased ability to voluntarily and actively move muscles; hypotonia is a state of low muscle resistance to movement.
- An upper motor neuron pattern of weakness with increased deep tendon reflexes, spasticity, and extensor plantar responses may be caused by tumors, traumatic brain injury, infections, stroke, demyelinating syndromes, spinal cord trauma or mass, metabolic diseases, or neurodegenerative diseases.
- Acute spinal cord lesions, such as infarction or compression, may produce a flaccid, areflexic paralysis that mimics lower motor neuron disease. Lesions of the spinal cord are best delineated with magnetic resonance imaging.
- Spinal muscular atrophy is a genetic disease characterized by progressive degeneration of anterior horn cells, which results in weakness.
- Guillain-Barré syndrome (acute inflammatory demyelinating polyradiculoneuropathy) is a postinfectious autoimmune peripheral neuropathy that can occur after an infection and is the most common cause of acute flaccid paralysis in children. It presents with areflexia, flaccidity, and symmetrical ascending weakness.
- Muscular dystrophies are characterized by progressive myofiber degeneration and the gradual replacement of muscle by fibrotic tissue. Duchenne muscular dystrophy is the most common muscular dystrophy.
- The acute onset of focal neurological deficits in a child is stroke until proven otherwise.
  - The most common causes of pediatric stroke are autoimmune vasculitis, infection, cardioembolic infarcts due to congenital heart disease, sickle cell anemia, or coagulation disorders, dehydration, vascular malformations, and head trauma.

CHAPTER 183

Ataxia and Movement Disorders

- The most common causes of acute ataxia in childhood are postinfectious acute cerebellar ataxia and drug intoxications.
- Movement disorders in children are typically hyperkinetic.
- Tics are rapid, purposeless, involuntary, stereotyped movements and typically involve the face, eyes, shoulder, and arm. Approximately 25% of children have transient tics.
- A child who is unsteady and has erratic eye movements may have opsoclonus myoclonus and should be evaluated for occult neuroblastoma.

CHAPTER 184

Altered Mental Status

- In childhood, the most common causes of coma are toxins, infections, head trauma, hypoxia-ischemia (cardiac arrest, near-drowning), and seizures.
- Computed tomography is the preferred head imaging technique in emergency situations because it can be performed rapidly without sedation and accurately identifies acute hemorrhages and mass lesions.
- Cerebral herniation is a medical emergency. Signs include altered mental status, signs of increased intracranial pressure (ICP) with dilated pupil or miosis, hemiparesis, decorticate or decerebrate posturing, and irregular respirations.
- Lumbar puncture is contraindicated in the setting of an intracranial mass lesion or clear hydrocephalus, because withdrawal of cerebrospinal fluid (CSF) can change pressures between the intracranial compartments and promote brainstem shifts and herniation.
- Head trauma may result in concussion, posttraumatic intracranial hemorrhage, skull fractures, or cranial nerve or cervical spine injuries.
  - Concussion is the rapid onset of short-lived neurological impairment that typically resolves spontaneously.
    - Symptoms may include headache, slowed reaction times, emotional lability, drowsiness, loss of consciousness, or amnesia.
  - Epidural, subdural, parenchymal, and subarachnoid intracranial hemorrhages can occur following head trauma.
    - Intracranial bleeding accompanied by neurological deterioration requires prompt assessment for likely evacuation of the blood.
  - Linear, diastatic, and minimally depressed fractures necessitate no specific treatment; fractures with more than 0.5-1.0 cm depression usually require surgical elevation.

CHAPTER 185

Neurodegenerative Disorders

- Neurodegenerative disorders encompass a large heterogeneous group of diseases that result from specific genetic and biochemical defects and varied unknown causes.
  - Neuronal degenerative disorders affect gray matter.
    - Early signs are seizures and intellectual impairment
  - Leukodystrophies affect white matter.
    - Early signs include upper motor neuron signs and progressive spasticity
- Mitochondrial diseases represent a clinically heterogeneous group of disorders in oxidative phosphorylation.
  - Abrupt symptoms often manifest during physiological stress (febrile illness, fasting).

CHAPTER 186

Neurocutaneous Disorders

- Abnormalities of skin, teeth, hair, and nails may indicate abnormal brain development, as all are derived from ectoderm.

CHAPTER 187

Congenital Malformations of the Central Nervous System

- CNS malformations include disorders of the spinal cord, neural tube formation, structure specification (neuronal migration), brain growth, and skull growth and shape.
  - Spina bifida is the defective closure of the caudal neural tube and ranges in severity from insignificant defects of vertebral arches to myelomeningocele.
    - An elevated alpha-fetoprotein in mother's blood suggests myelomeningocele in the fetus.
    - Children with myelomeningocele often have an associated Chiari type II malformation.
- Defective closure of the rostral neural tube produces anencephaly or encephaloceles.
  - Holoprosencephaly represents varying degrees of failure of the forebrain to divide into two distinct cerebral hemispheres.
- Hydranencephaly is a condition in which the brain presumably develops normally, but is destroyed by an intrauterine, probably vascular, accident.
- Schizencephaly and lissencephaly are disorders or neuronal migration that result in abnormal neurological development and often are associated with treatment-resistant epilepsy.

DERMATOLOGY

Mary Kim | Yvonne E. Chiu

CHAPTER 188

Dermatology Assessment

Approximately one in three Americans of any age has at least one recognizable skin disorder at any time. The most common cutaneous diseases encountered in community settings are dermatophytosis, acne vulgaris, seborrheic dermatitis, atopic dermatitis (eczema), verrucae (warts), tumors, psoriasis, vitiligo, and infections such as herpes simplex and impetigo. The most common diagnoses in children attending pediatric dermatology clinics include atopic dermatitis, impetigo, tinea capitis, acne vulgaris, verrucae vulgaris, and seborrheic dermatitis.

HISTORY

The age of the patient, onset, duration, progression, associated cutaneous symptoms (pain, pruritus), previous treatments, and associated systemic signs or symptoms (fever, malaise, weight loss) are important clues. Obtaining an accurate description of the original lesion improves diagnostic accuracy. Patients often do not consider a topical antibiotic or antiitch medication as treatment. As over-the-counter remedies may alter the appearance of a rash, it is important to probe deeply with related questions in the history. Other important information includes a history of allergies, environmental exposure, travel history, previous treatment, affected contacts, and family history.

PHYSICAL EXAMINATION

A careful examination of the skin requires a visual and a tactile assessment. Examination of the skin over the entire body must be performed systematically. Mucous membranes, hair, nails, and teeth, all of ectodermal origin, also may be involved in cutaneous disorders and should be assessed.

COMMON MANIFESTATIONS

Decision-Making Algorithms
Available @ StudentConsult.com

Alopecia
Vesicles and Bullae
Fever and Rash

A descriptive nomenclature of skin lesions helps with generating a differential diagnosis and with communication between health care providers. Determination of the primary lesion and secondary change is the cornerstone of dermatological diagnosis. A **primary lesion** is defined as the basic lesion that arises de novo and is most characteristic of the disease process (Table 188.1

TABLE 188.1 Primary Skin Lesions

LESION	DESCRIPTION
Macule	Flat, nonpalpable lesion <1 cm in diameter
Patch	Similar to macule, but >1 cm in diameter
Papule	Elevated, solid lesion <1 cm in diameter
Plaque	Similar to papule, but >1 cm in diameter; has a flat and broad surface in contrast to a nodule
Nodule	Similar to papule, but >1 cm in diameter; has a rounded surface in contrast to a plaque
Tumor	Similar to nodule, but implies a neoplastic growth rather than an inflammatory process
Vesicle	Fluid-filled (usually clear or straw-colored) epidermal lesion <1 cm in diameter
Bulla	Similar to vesicle, but >1 cm in diameter
Pustule	Pus-filled epidermal lesion, which often is surrounded by erythema
Purpura	Red-purple macule or papule resulting from extravasated blood into the skin; does not blanch with pressure
Petechia	Similar to purpura, but less than a few millimeters in diameter
Ecchymosis	Larger, hemorrhagic patch or plaque resulting from extravasated blood
Wheal (hive)	Pink, edematous papules and plaques that vary greatly in size and configuration; characterized by transient nature with individual lesions resolving within 24 hr
Telangiectasia	Collection of small superficial red blood vessels
Milia	Superficial, white, small epidermal keratin cysts
Comedo	Plug of keratin and sebum within the orifice of a hair follicle, which can be open (blackhead) or closed (whitehead); characteristic lesion of acne vulgaris
Cyst	Papule or nodule with an epidermal lining and filled with solid material

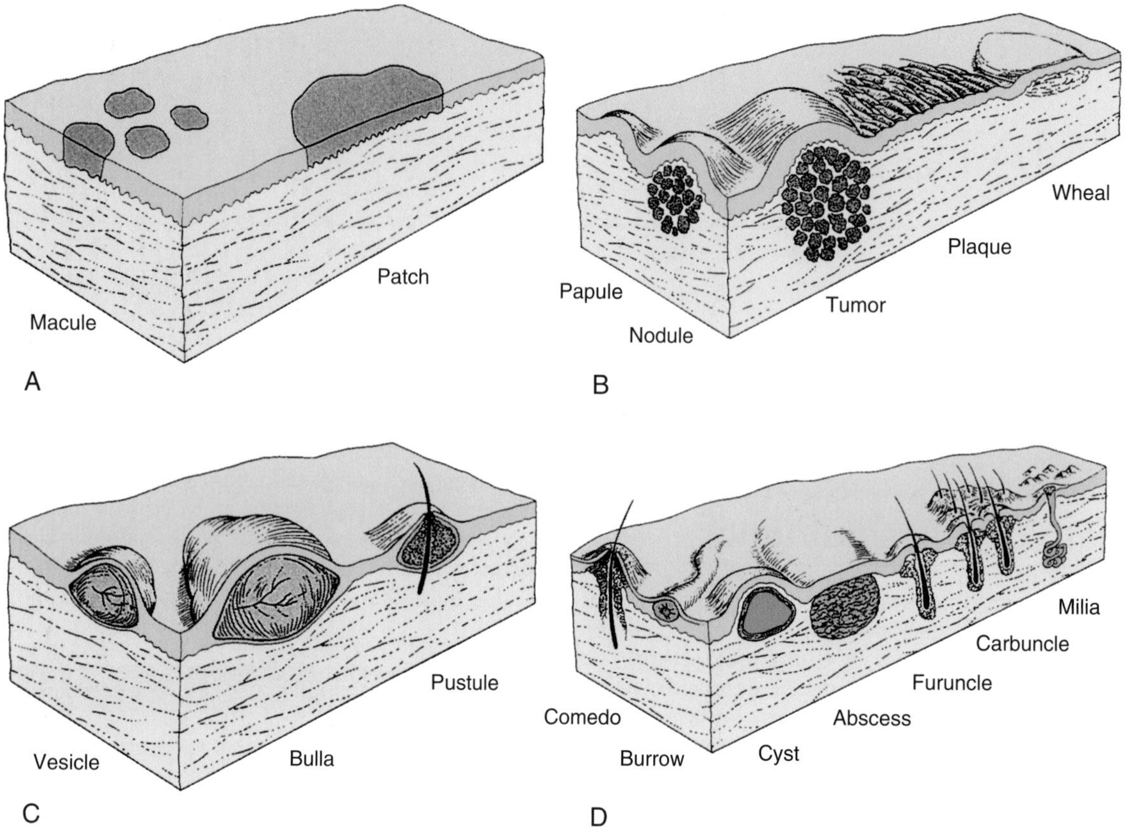

FIGURE 188.1 Morphology of Primary Skin Lesions. **(A)** Flat lesions. **(B)** Palpable lesions. **(C)** Fluid-filled lesions. **(D)** Special primary lesions. (From Swartz MH. *Textbook of Physical Diagnosis: History and Examination.* Philadelphia: WB Saunders; 1989.)

and Fig. 188.1). Primary lesions are often not seen on a patient at the time of presentation, as most lesions are altered by time or external factors such as medication applied, secondary infection, or physical manipulation (e.g., scratching). A search for the primary lesion often proves worthwhile and focuses the differential diagnosis to a category of lesion that is specific for the underlying diagnosis. On occasion, two different types of primary lesions may be present. In most cases, **secondary lesions** are the result of the effects of the primary lesion (Table 188.2). They may be created by scratching or secondary infection and may be seen in the absence of a primary lesion.

The color, texture (e.g., rough, smooth), configuration (e.g., annular, serpiginous, linear), location, and distribution (e.g., localized, widespread, symmetrical, dermatomal) of the lesion should be recorded. Lesions on mucous membranes are usually short-lived and harder to definitively diagnose. Lesions in thick-skinned areas, such as the palms and soles, may be particularly difficult to characterize.

INITIAL DIAGNOSTIC EVALUATION AND TESTS

A thorough history and physical examination are usually sufficient for diagnosis because of the visibility of the skin. Adjunctive tests at the time of examination include potassium hydroxide (KOH) examination for fungi and dermatophytes, skin scrapings for scabies, cytological examination (Tzanck test) for herpesvirus and varicella-zoster virus infection, and Wood

TABLE 188.2 Secondary Skin Lesions

LESION	DESCRIPTION
Scale	Results from abnormal keratinization; may be fine or sheet-like
Crust	Dried collection of serum and cellular debris
Erosion	Shallow depression with loss of the superficial epidermis
Ulcer	Deeper depression with loss of the entire epidermis into dermis; heals with scarring
Atrophy	Thinning of epidermis (surface appears shiny and translucent) or dermis (skin is depressed with epidermis intact)
Scar	Thickened, firm, and discolored collection of connective tissue that results from dermal damage; initially pink, but lightens with time
Sclerosis	Circumscribed or diffuse hardening of skin
Lichenification	Accentuated skin lines/markings that result from thickening of the epidermis due to rubbing
Excoriation	Superficial linear erosion that is caused by scratching
Fissure	Linear break within the skin surface that usually is painful

light examination for the yellowish-gold fluorescence of tinea versicolor, depigmentation (e.g., vitiligo), or hypopigmentation (e.g., ash leaf macules of tuberous sclerosis). A skin biopsy may be performed to help with the diagnosis. The biopsy specimen can be accomplished by either shave or punch biopsy. Both are simple in-office procedures. Occasionally, laboratory or imaging studies are necessary.

CHAPTER 189

Acne

ETIOLOGY

Acne vulgaris (or acne) is a chronic inflammatory disorder that affects areas with the greatest concentration of sebaceous glands, such as the face, chest, and back. The pathogenesis of acne is multifactorial. Gender, age, genetic factors, and environment are all major contributing factors. Stress may trigger acne, possibly by affecting hormone levels. A high glycemic diet and milk intake may be associated with acne, although remain controversial as potential causes.

Acne is caused by chronic inflammation of the pilosebaceous unit (hair follicle with an associated sebaceous gland). The primary event in all acne lesions is the development of the **microcomedo**, which results from the obstruction of the hair follicle with keratin, increased sebum production from sebaceous glands, and overgrowth of normal skin flora, leading to pilosebaceous occlusion and enlargement. Androgens are a potent stimulus of the sebaceous gland. The subsequent inflammatory component and pustule formation results from proliferation of *Propionibacterium acnes (P. acnes)*, a commensal organism of the skin. The pathogenesis of acne thus involves three components: increased sebum production, hyperkeratosis, and bacterial proliferation. Effective treatment focuses on minimizing these factors.

EPIDEMIOLOGY

Acne is the most common skin disorder in adolescents, occurring in 85% of teenagers. The incidence is similar in both sexes, although boys often are more severely affected. Acne may begin as early as 8 years of age and may continue into adulthood.

CLINICAL MANIFESTATIONS

Acne primarily affects areas with increased sebaceous gland density, such as the face, upper chest, and back. Superficial plugging of the pilosebaceous unit results in noninflammatory small (1- to 2-mm) **open (blackhead)** and **closed (whitehead) comedones.** An open comedo is less likely to become inflammatory than a closed comedo. Rupture of a comedo into adjacent dermis and proliferation of *P. acnes* induce an inflammatory response and development of inflammatory **papules** and **pustules**. Larger, skin-colored or red cysts and nodules represent deeper plugging and **cystic acne**. Increased and persistent inflammation, especially with rupture of a deep cyst, increases the risk of scarring.

The diagnosis of acne is usually not difficult because of the characteristic and chronic lesions. Laboratory studies and imaging studies are usually not necessary to diagnose acne. Screening tests may be necessary if there are signs of hyperandrogenism due to polycystic ovarian syndrome (irregular menses, hirsutism, insulin resistance) or an underlying androgen-secreting tumor (irregular menses, hirsutism, deepening voice, clitoromegaly).

TREATMENT

The mainstays of treatment of acne are topical comedolytic agents and topical antibiotics. Creams, lotions, gels, foams, and solutions are available. Gels and solutions are commonly used because acne skin is generally greasier and these agents tend to be drying. They also have the tendency to be irritating and may not be as well tolerated. Creams and lotions are better tolerated but may not be as effective.

The comedolytic agents (salicylic acid, azelaic acid, tretinoin, adapalene, tazarotene) produce superficial desquamation and, subsequently, relieve follicular obstruction. They are a mainstay of first-line therapy. The topical retinoids (tretinoin, adapalene, tazarotene) are based on the vitamin A molecule. They decrease keratin and sebum production and have some antiinflammatory and antibacterial activity; thus they can be the most effective when used as monotherapy.

Topical antimicrobials (benzoyl peroxide, dapsone) and topical antibiotics (erythromycin, clindamycin) are anti-inflammatory and inhibit *P. acnes* proliferation. Erythromycin efficacy has decreased as *P. acnes* has become increasingly resistant to this antibiotic and should no longer be used. Topical antibiotics should be combined with an antimicrobial, such as benzoyl peroxide, to prevent the development of resistance. Combination therapy of a topical comedolytic agent and a topical antimicrobial is more effective than either agent alone for inflammatory acne.

Oral antibiotics (tetracycline, doxycycline, minocycline) are typically used for deeper cystic lesions but should always be used in combination with a topical regimen. Tetracyclines are the most effective antibiotics because of their significant antiinflammatory activity. Tetracyclines should not be used in children 8 years of age and younger. As with topical erythromycin, oral erythromycin is no longer used because of bacterial resistance. Given their increased risk of bacterial resistance and reported associations with inflammatory bowel disease, Candida, and *Clostridium difficile* infections, judicious use of systemic antibiotics in the treatment of acne vulgaris is emphasized for those who treat acne.

For recalcitrant or severe nodulocystic acne, oral isotretinoin may be instituted. Isotretinoin, an oral analog of vitamin A, normalizes follicular keratinization, reduces sebum production, and decreases 5α-dihydrotestosterone formation and androgen receptor-binding capacity. A course of isotretinoin (0.5-1 mg/kg/day to reach a cumulative dose of 120-150 mg/kg) is the only medication that can permanently alter the course of acne and induce a durable remission. Because of the high incidence of adverse effects, it should be used only by physicians familiar with this medication. Isotretinoin therapy requires careful patient selection, pretreatment counseling, and laboratory monitoring. It is teratogenic and must not be used immediately before or during pregnancy.

For females, hormonal agents can also be considered for anti-acne therapy. These include the estrogen-containing combined oral contraceptives (although use should be limited to those without contraindications) and spironolactone.

COMPLICATIONS

Acne has significant and frequently devastating effects on an adolescent's body image and self-esteem. There may be little correlation between severity and psychosocial impact. Scarring may result in permanent morbidity.

PROGNOSIS

Classically, acne lasts 3-5 years, although some individuals may have disease for 15-20 years. Only early treatment with isotretinoin may alter the natural course of acne. Acne lesions often heal with temporary postinflammatory erythema and hyperpigmentation. Depending on the severity, chronicity, and depth of involvement, pitted, atrophic, or hypertrophic scars may develop. **Cystic acne** has the highest incidence of scarring because rupture of a deep cyst induces the greatest inflammation, although scarring may be caused by milder pustular or even comedonal acne.

PREVENTION

Greasy hair and cosmetic preparations should be avoided because they exacerbate preexisting acne. There are no effective means for preventing acne, although a low milk or low glycemic diet may improve acne. Repetitive cleansing with soap and water or use of astringents or abrasives removes only surface lipids; their use makes the skin appear less oily but does not prevent formation of microcomedones and may paradoxically worsen acne.

CHAPTER 190

Atopic Dermatitis

ETIOLOGY

Atopic dermatitis is a chronic inflammatory disease with no known cure. It is associated with significant psychosocial morbidity and decreased health-related quality of life. For many affected individuals, atopic dermatitis is the skin manifestation of atopy accompanied by asthma and allergic rhinitis.

Atopic dermatitis manifests with a defective skin barrier, reduced innate immune responses, and exaggerated immune responses to allergens and microbes. Both genetic predisposition and environmental factors play a role in the development of atopic dermatitis. Genes associated with skin barrier dysfunction and inflammation have been linked with atopic dermatitis. Inflammatory mediators involved include predominantly T helper (T_H) cells, with the T_H2 pathway implicated early in acute lesions and a T_H1 predominance found in chronic lesions. Langerhans cells, immunoglobulin (Ig)E, and eosinophils play a prominent role, as well as many other inflammatory mediators. Environmental and contact allergens, infections, irritants, extremes of temperature, sweat, and lack of humidity can exacerbate the condition, as can scratching or rubbing. Triggers are somewhat variable from individual to individual.

EPIDEMIOLOGY

Atopic dermatitis is the most common skin disease in children, with an estimated prevalence of up to 20% of children. Only 1-2% of adults manifest disease. In addition to genetic factors, an environmental influence contributes. Atopic dermatitis occurs more frequently in urban areas and in higher socioeconomic classes. Prevalence is lower in areas where industrial pollution is less and where eosinophil-mediated infections such as helminthic infections are endemic.

Patients generally have a family history of atopy. Children with atopic dermatitis are predisposed to the development of allergy and allergic rhinitis, referred to as the *atopic march.* Asthma develops in up to half of children with atopic dermatitis, and allergic rhinitis develops even more frequently. Food allergies are commonly present in children with atopic dermatitis but are a rare cause of atopic dermatitis itself.

CLINICAL MANIFESTATIONS

Atopic dermatitis is a chronic, relapsing skin disease characterized by xerosis, pruritus, and characteristic skin findings. The condition generally improves with age and remits in adulthood, although some childhood cases will continue into adulthood.

Characteristic lesions of atopic dermatitis are erythematous papules or plaques with ill-defined borders and overlying scale or hyperkeratosis. Weeping may be present in acute stages, which then develops into yellow crust. Lesions can be secondarily excoriated and result in hemorrhagic crusting and lichenification in older lesions. Formation of fissures is common in both acute and chronic lesions. Temporary hypo- and hyperpigmentation can be seen after lesions resolve, but atopic dermatitis is not usually scarring unless secondary features become severe (e.g., infection or scratching).

Characteristic locations vary with the age of the patient. Infantile atopic dermatitis typically affects the face and extensor surfaces of the extremities and is often generalized. Childhood lesions predominate in flexural surfaces (antecubital and popliteal fossae), wrists, ankles, hands, and feet (Fig. 190.1). The adult phase occurs after puberty and manifests in the flexural areas, including the neck, as well as predominant involvement on the face, hands, fingers, toes, and the upper arms and back.

Secondary bacterial infection, most commonly with *Staphylococcus aureus* or less commonly with *Streptococcus pyogenes*, is frequently present. Patients are at increased risk for infections with cutaneous viruses and can develop disseminated skin infections with viruses such as herpes simplex virus (HSV; eczema herpeticum), varicella-zoster virus, coxsackievirus (eczema coxsackium), smallpox virus (eczema vaccinatum), and molluscum contagiosum. Atopic skin is more susceptible to fungal infections as well. Signs of concomitant infection include acute worsening of disease in an otherwise well-controlled patient, resistance to standard therapy, fever, and presence of pustules, fissures, punched out erosions, or exudative or crusted lesions (Fig. 190.2). Eczema herpeticum and eczema vaccinatum can be life threatening if not treated.

LABORATORY AND IMAGING STUDIES

Diagnosis of atopic dermatitis is based on clinical signs and symptoms. Skin biopsy findings are generally characteristic but not exclusively diagnostic and can overlap with other skin

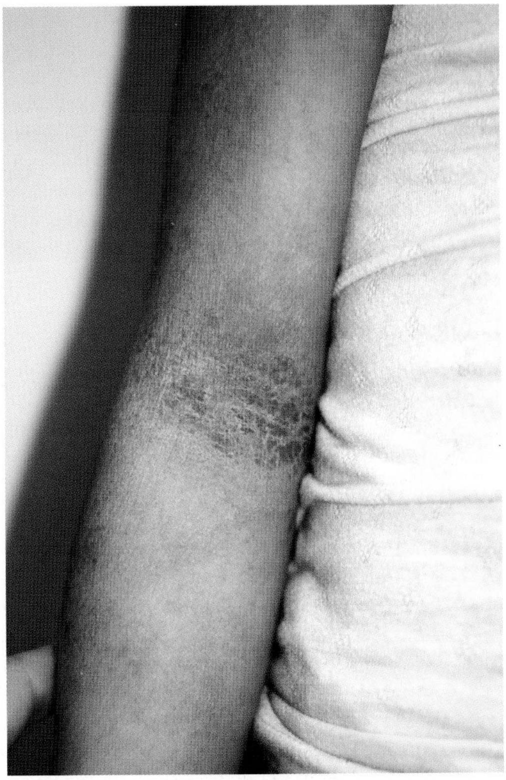

FIGURE 190.1 Atopic dermatitis (arm).

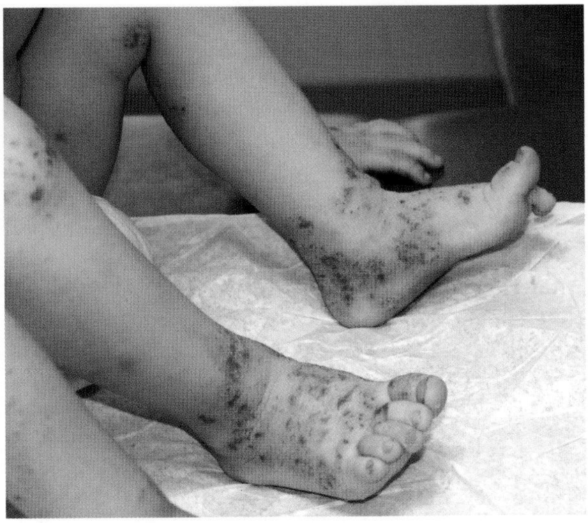

FIGURE 190.2 Atopic dermatitis with *Staphylococcus* superinfection.

conditions. Peripheral blood eosinophilia and elevated IgE levels can be found but are not specific and not routinely obtained. Skin prick testing or measurement of specific IgE antibody levels can detect sensitization to food and environmental allergens, although false-positive findings occur.

DIFFERENTIAL DIAGNOSIS

The differential diagnosis of atopic dermatitis is extensive, but the history of a relapsing pruritic condition in the setting of atopy and skin lesions in a characteristic distribution is typical.

The lesions of **seborrheic dermatitis** have circumscribed and well-defined borders. The scale or hyperkeratosis is thicker, greasy, and yellowish. The distribution of seborrheic dermatitis is different from that of atopic dermatitis, typically involving the scalp, eyebrows, perinasal region, upper chest, and back. The two conditions occasionally coexist.

Psoriasis tends to localize on the elbows, knees, lower back, and scalp. The lesions of psoriasis on exposed surfaces are salmon color at the base with an overlying hyperkeratosis that is much thicker with silver coloration. They are generally very well demarcated, oval or round, thick plaques.

Allergic contact dermatitis has a distribution limited to one area of the body corresponding to contact with the allergen. The lesions generally make well-demarcated, bizarre, linear, square, or angulated shapes corresponding to the source. **Nickel dermatitis** is common and results from contact sensitization to nickel in metals. It occurs in characteristic locations, such as the periumbilical area (where metal from pant buttons rub against skin); on the ear lobule or neck (where earrings contact skin); circumferentially around the neck (necklaces); and under rings or wristbands. Patients with atopic dermatitis can have concomitant contact dermatitis as well.

TREATMENT

Ideal therapy for atopic dermatitis includes three main components: frequent liberal use of bland moisturizers to restore the skin barrier, avoidance of triggers of inflammation, and use of topical antiinflammatory medication to affected areas of skin when needed. Control of pruritus and infection should be considered on an individual basis. If topical therapy and these measures are inadequate, systemic therapy with immunosuppressive agents or ultraviolet light therapy may be indicated.

A daily short bath with warm but not hot water is generally recommended, although this is controversial and there are some who advocate less frequent bathing. A moisturizing cream or ointment should be applied to the entire body immediately afterward to trap moisture. Application of topical medications is also most effective immediately after bathing. Additional information for patients and families can be found at the website of the National Eczema Association for Science and Education (http://www.nationaleczema.org).

Common triggers of inflammation in atopic dermatitis include rubbing or scratching, contact with saliva or acidic foods, soaps and detergents, wool or other harsh materials, fragranced products, sweat, highly chlorinated pools, low humidity, tobacco smoke, dust mites, animal dander, environmental pollens, and molds. Exposure to these triggers should be limited whenever possible. Infections that are unrelated to skin disease, such as an upper respiratory infection, can also exacerbate atopic dermatitis. Food allergy is commonly seen in patients with atopic dermatitis but typically presents with urticaria or anaphylaxis rather than exacerbation of the atopic dermatitis.

Topical corticosteroids are the mainstay of antiinflammatory therapy for atopic dermatitis. Hundreds of topical corticosteroids are available and are classified according to strength from I to VII. Class I is the highest potency and class VII is the lowest potency. Potency varies according to the steroid molecule (active ingredient), and, for a given ingredient, strength can vary according to relative concentration and vehicle base. Enhanced penetration occurs in areas of natural occlusion (flexures such as axillae and groin), with external occlusion (diapers or bandages), in areas of open skin (excoriations), and with heat or hydration. Use of wet wraps with topical corticosteroid application takes advantage of this principle of heat and hydration for enhanced penetration for recalcitrant lesions. Class I and II steroids are typically avoided in young children or in areas of thinner skin or enhanced penetration.

Corticosteroids are available in different vehicles. In general, ointments are preferred because of their increased efficacy, occlusive nature, and tolerability. Creams may be slightly less effective for a given steroid ingredient, but may be more cosmetically acceptable for older patients or in warmer climates. Lotions may cause more irritation and are generally less potent. Sprays, foams, solutions, and gels can be especially useful for hair-bearing areas. Creams, lotions, sprays, solutions, and gels can be particularly irritating when applied to atopic skin and should generally be avoided on areas of open skin.

Topical corticosteroids should be used in conjunction with adequate skin care, such as avoiding triggers of inflammation and frequent application of moisturizers. Twice-daily application of corticosteroids is recommended. The goal is to limit the need for antiinflammatory medications and thereby avoid potential for adverse effects. Local side effects such as skin atrophy, striae, acne, and hypopigmentation are related to corticosteroid potency, site of application, and duration of application. Systemic side effects of adrenal suppression or Cushing syndrome can result with application of a potent topical corticosteroid to large surface areas or occluded areas at risk of enhanced penetration.

Topical **calcineurin inhibitors** (also referred to as topical immune modulators) such as topical tacrolimus and pimecrolimus may be part of the treatment regimen for atopic dermatitis. These agents selectively inhibit T-cell proliferation by inhibiting calcineurin and subsequent interleukin 2 production. There is no potential for skin atrophy; thus these agents are particularly useful for face or genital lesions. They are currently approved for intermittent therapy as second-line treatments for mild to moderate atopic dermatitis. Long-term studies, combined with other modalities for treatment, are underway.

Sedating antihistamines (e.g., diphenhydramine, hydroxyzine) have only mild effect on pruritus but can improve the sleeplessness due to scratching during the night. A dose before bedtime is most effective. Additional daytime doses can be added on an individual basis when needed. Nonsedating antihistamines are of little benefit in controlling the pruritus of atopic dermatitis.

Short-term administration of systemic corticosteroids is rarely indicated for cases of severe disease and may be considered when adequate topical therapy failed or is being instituted. Systemic corticosteroid courses should be adequately tapered and used in conjunction with an appropriate atopic skin care regimen. Rebound flare of atopic dermatitis is common following withdrawal of corticosteroids and should be anticipated to avoid misinterpretation of the natural disease severity. Long-term and frequent repeated courses should be avoided to prevent adverse effects.

Ultraviolet light therapy (UVB, narrow band UVB, UVA, or UVA1) can be an option for moderate to severe cases in older children. Typically light therapy is administered two to three times weekly until improvement is seen and then is tapered or discontinued once the acute flare has resolved. More frequent use of light therapy in children is hindered by requirements for frequent office visits, ability to cooperate with standing in a light box while wearing protective goggles, and risk of long-term skin damage, including the potential for skin cancer development with excessive UV light exposure. Systemic immunosuppressants such as cyclosporine methotrexate, azathioprine, or mycophenolate mofetil can be effective therapies for atopic dermatitis in severe cases.

COMPLICATIONS

Decision-Making Algorithm
Available @ StudentConsult.com

Fever and Rash

An increased tendency toward bacterial, viral, and fungal skin infections is due to an impaired skin barrier and decrease in innate immune proteins in the skin as well as maladaptive secondary immune responses.

Secondary impetigo with *S. aureus* is the most common secondary skin infection found in atopic dermatitis. Group A streptococcus infection is also common. Infection manifests with pustules, erythema, crusting, flare of disease, or lack of response to adequate antiinflammatory therapy. Localized lesions can be treated with topical mupirocin. Widespread and generalized lesions require oral antibiotic therapy, most commonly with a first-generation cephalosporin such as cephalexin. Methicillin-resistant *S. aureus* infection is increasingly common, and antibiotic therapy should be tailored based on local resistance rates and patient factors. Diagnosis of superinfection may be made clinically, but a superficial bacterial culture can confirm the diagnosis and provide antimicrobial susceptibilities. Treatment should include a concomitant atopic skin care routine including the continued use of topical corticosteroids. Although secondary skin infection with *S. aureus* is common, progression to cellulitis or septicemia is unusual. Rarely, intravenous antibiotics may be required. Children with colonization and frequent infections may benefit from dilute bleach baths two to three times weekly; one-fourth to one-half cup of household bleach is added to a half-full or full bathtub.

Eczema herpeticum (Kaposi varicelliform eruption) is one of the potentially serious infectious complications in atopic dermatitis. After HSV infection, an eruption of multiple, pruritic, vesiculopustular lesions occurs in a disseminated pattern, both within plaques of atopic dermatitis and on normal-appearing skin. These characteristically rupture and form crusted umbilicated papules and punched-out hemorrhagic erosions (Fig. 190.3). Irritability, anorexia, and fever can also be seen. Systemic and central nervous system disease have been reported. Bacterial superinfection of eroded areas of the skin often occurs. Diagnosis can be made rapidly from a scraping of the skin lesion stained with Giemsa or Wright's stain **(Tzanck test),** although these are not highly sensitive. These stains allow microscopic visualization of the presence of multinucleated giant cells indicative of HSV or varicella-zoster virus infection. Vesicle fluid can also be sent for polymerase chain reaction (PCR) detection of HSV DNA, rapid direct fluorescent antibody testing, or viral culture. Laboratory confirmation of infection is important because similar clinical manifestations can occur with bacterial infections.

The psychosocial impact of atopic dermatitis can be significant. There is often disfigurement, lack of sleep from pruritus resulting in irritability and fatigue, and limitations

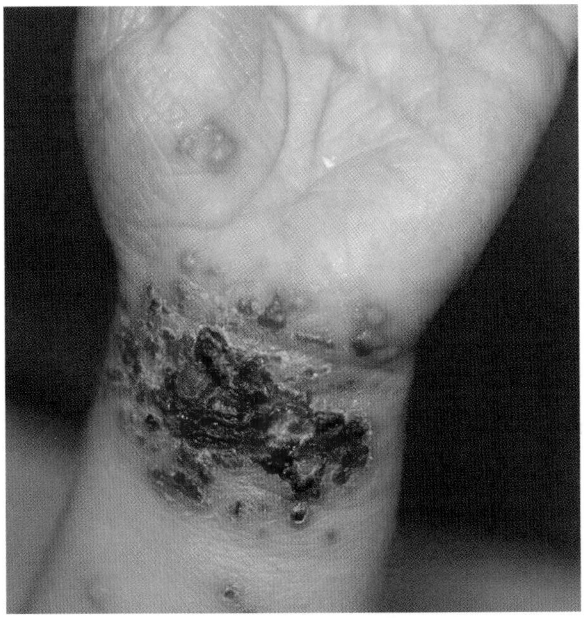

FIGURE 190.3 Eczema herpeticum (hand).

on participation in sports. Significant time, as well as financial strain, is involved in caring for a child with atopic dermatitis. Thus management should address these potential issues and provide adequate anticipatory guidance.

PROGNOSIS

Atopic dermatitis frequently remits during childhood and is much less common after puberty. The condition is generally most severe and widespread in infancy and early childhood. Relapse of disease in adults can occur and commonly manifests as face or hand dermatitis. Frequently, adults have generalized dry skin and are aware that their skin is sensitive to many over-the-counter preparations. Patients with atopic dermatitis can also develop asthma and allergic rhinitis. Asthma is more commonly associated with more severe skin disease.

PREVENTION

Individual flares of atopic dermatitis can be prevented by avoiding triggers of inflammation and can be lessened with frequent moisturizer application. Evidence suggests that breast feeding for at least 4 months, with or without formula supplementation, decreases the incidence and severity of atopic dermatitis in individuals at high risk (i.e., those who have a first-degree relative with atopic dermatitis). For infants at high risk who are not exclusively breast fed, there is modest evidence that the onset of atopic dermatitis may be delayed or prevented by the use of extensively hydrolyzed casein-based formulas. There is no convincing evidence that an antigen avoidance diet in pregnant or lactating mothers prevents the development of atopic disease. Early introduction of peanuts among children at high risk for this allergy (i.e., infants with severe eczema, egg allergy, or both) significantly decreased the frequency of the development of peanut allergy in these infants in one large randomized study.

CHAPTER 191

Contact Dermatitis

ETIOLOGY AND EPIDEMIOLOGY

Inflammation in the top layers of the skin, caused by direct contact with a substance, is divided into two subtypes: irritant contact dermatitis and allergic contact dermatitis. **Irritant contact dermatitis** is observed after the skin surface is exposed to an irritating chemical or substance. Contact dermatitis may occur in any age, and girls are more frequently affected than boys. **Allergic contact dermatitis** is a cell-mediated immune reaction, also called type IV or delayed-type hypersensitivity. The antigens, or haptens, involved in allergic contact dermatitis readily penetrate the epidermis and are bound by Langerhans cells, the antigen-presenting cells of the skin. The hapten is presented to T lymphocytes and an immune cascade follows.

CLINICAL MANIFESTATIONS

Irritant contact dermatitis is characterized by ill-defined, scaly, pink or red patches and plaques (Fig. 191.1). The eruption is localized to skin surfaces that are exposed to the irritant. Irritant contact dermatitis is observed frequently on the dorsal surfaces of the hands in patients, often from repeated handwashing or exposure to irritating chemicals.

Diaper dermatitis is a common problem in infants and most commonly is a form of irritant contact dermatitis. The dermatitis is caused by irritation from urine and feces, typically affecting the perianal region and the buttocks while sparing the protected groin folds and other occluded areas. Secondary infection by *Candida albicans* or bacterial pathogens may complicate diaper dermatitis as well.

Allergic contact dermatitis may be acute (such as *Rhus* dermatitis) or chronic (such as nickel dermatitis). Acute lesions are bright pink, pruritic patches, often in linear or sharply marginated bizarre configurations. Within the patches are clear vesicles and bullae (Fig. 191.2). Signs and symptoms of the disease may be delayed for 7-14 days after exposure if the patient has not been sensitized previously. On re-exposure, symptoms begin within hours and are usually more severe. The eruption may persist for weeks. Chronic lesions are pink, scaly, pruritic

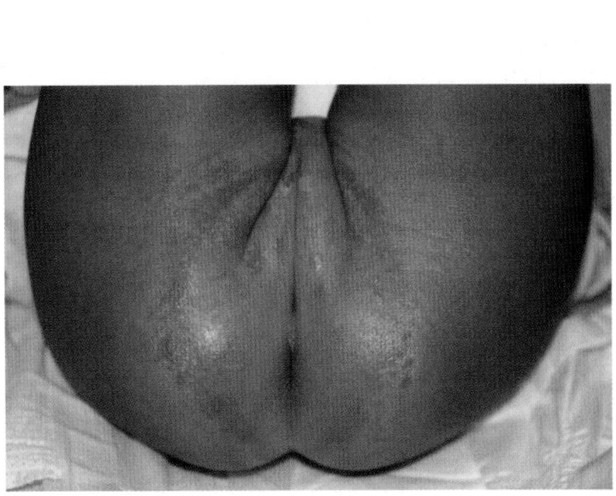

FIGURE 191.1 Irritant diaper dermatitis.

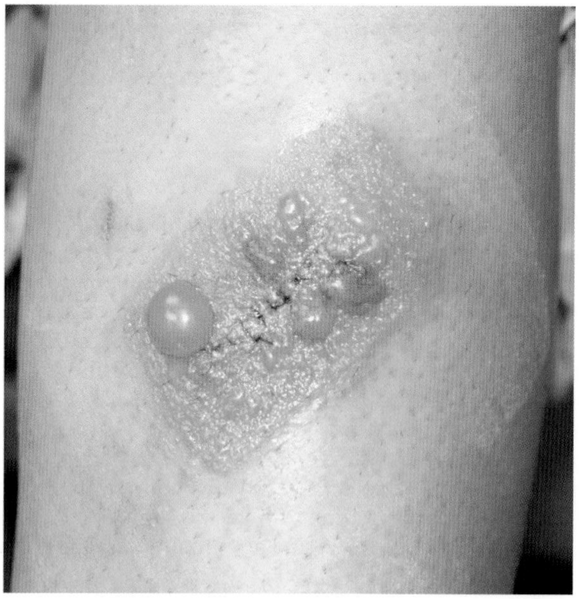

FIGURE 191.2 Allergic contact dermatitis to tincture of benzoin.

plaques, often mimicking atopic dermatitis. Even intermittent exposure can result in a persistent dermatitis.

LABORATORY AND IMAGING STUDIES

The diagnosis is established by clinical presentation and history of exposure to a recognized irritant or allergen. Skin-prick testing and serum IgE levels are not helpful in determining the cause of allergic contact dermatitis. Patch testing may be used to determine the allergen causing the reaction in difficult cases.

DIFFERENTIAL DIAGNOSIS

The distribution and appearance of the dermatitis and a detailed exposure history are the most useful diagnostic tools. Involvement of the lower legs and distal arms suggests exposure to plants of the *Rhus* species (poison ivy or poison oak), especially when linear configurations of lesions are present. Dermatitis of the ears (earrings), wrist (bracelet or watch), or periumbilical region (belt buckle or pant buttons) suggests a metal allergy to nickel. Distribution on the dorsal surfaces of the feet indicates a shoe allergy, usually to dyes, rubber, or leather. Topical antibiotics (neomycin) and fragrances (soaps, perfumes, cosmetics) are frequent causes of allergic contact dermatitis.

Diaper rashes caused by *Candida* are quite common. Irritant contact dermatitis primarily affects the prominent, exposed surfaces, whereas *Candida* primarily affects intertriginous areas. The two are frequently present simultaneously, as secondary *Candida* infection may complicate irritant dermatitis.

Psoriasis, seborrheic dermatitis, and Langerhans cell histiocytosis can present with an erythematous rash in the diaper area. Referral to a dermatologist should be considered for any child with a severe rash or with a diaper rash that does not respond to conventional therapy.

TREATMENT

Topical corticosteroids are effective in treatment of allergic and irritant contact dermatitis. High-potency corticosteroids, and even short courses of oral corticosteroids, may be necessary for severe reactions of allergic contact dermatitis. Oral antihistamines may be required to control itching.

Treatment of candidal diaper dermatitis consists of topical nystatin or topical azole antifungals. Low-potency topical corticosteroids are frequently used in addition to topical antifungal therapy to treat the irritant component of the diaper dermatitis when present concomitantly.

COMPLICATIONS

In addition to superinfection of diaper dermatitis by *C. albicans*, bacterial superinfection may complicate any form of contact dermatitis. This is especially common if the skin barrier is no longer intact because of blistering or scratching.

PREVENTION

Every effort should be made to identify the trigger of allergic or irritant contact dermatitis. With allergic contact dermatitis, re-exposure often leads to increasingly severe reactions.

CHAPTER 192

Seborrheic Dermatitis

ETIOLOGY

Seborrheic dermatitis is a common, chronic inflammatory disease that has different clinical presentations at different ages. Seborrheic dermatitis classically presents in infants as cradle cap or dermatitis in the intertriginous areas of the axillae, groin, antecubital and popliteal fossae, and umbilicus. It is seen in adolescents as dandruff. The pathogenesis of seborrheic dermatitis is unclear, but it is theorized that there is an abnormal inflammatory response to commensal *Malassezia* species in sebum-rich areas. Areas prone to seborrheic dermatitis include the scalp, eyebrows, eyelids, nasolabial folds, external auditory canals, and posterior auricular folds.

CLINICAL MANIFESTATIONS

Seborrheic dermatitis in infants begins during the first month and persists during the first year of life. It is also called **cradle cap** because of the thick, greasy and waxy, yellow-white scaling and crusting of the scalp (Fig. 192.1). It is usually prominent on the vertex of the scalp, but it may be diffuse. Greasy, scaly, erythematous, nonpruritic patches and plaques may extend to the face and posterior auricular folds, sometimes involving the entire body. Diaper and intertriginous areas can have sharply demarcated, shiny, erythematous patches with minimal scale. Hypopigmentation may persist after the inflammation has faded. The eruption is usually asymptomatic, which helps differentiate it from infantile atopic dermatitis, which is pruritic.

Classic seborrheic dermatitis during adolescence is typically localized to the scalp. The mild form is commonly known as **dandruff,** a fine, white, dry scaling of the scalp with minor itching. Additional findings of seborrheic dermatitis vary from

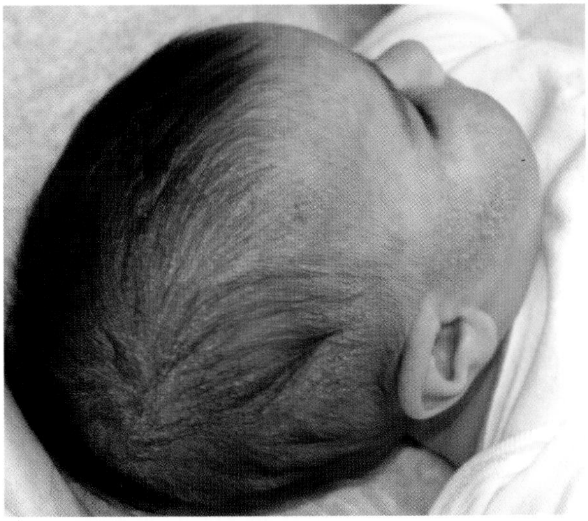

FIGURE 192.1 Seborrheic dermatitis (cradle cap).

diffuse, brawny scaling to focal areas of thick, oily, yellow crusts with underlying erythema. The external auditory canals, eyebrows, eyelids, and intertriginous areas may be involved as well. Pruritus may be minimal or severe.

LABORATORY AND IMAGING STUDIES

Laboratory studies and imaging studies are not necessary to diagnose seborrheic dermatitis. Fungal cultures and potassium hydroxide studies may be necessary to help differentiate seborrheic dermatitis of the scalp from tinea capitis (see Chapter 98).

DIFFERENTIAL DIAGNOSIS

Seborrheic dermatitis in an infant may be difficult to differentiate from atopic dermatitis, and in fact, some cases may represent an overlap. In a teenager, seborrheic dermatitis of the scalp and psoriasis of the scalp may have very similar clinical findings; it may be very difficult to differentiate the two disorders, especially if there are no other cutaneous findings to provide additional clues. Intractable, severe, generalized seborrheic dermatitis suggests Langerhans cell histiocytosis. Intractable seborrheic dermatitis, accompanied by chronic diarrhea and failure to thrive, suggests erythroderma desquamativum (Leiner disease) or acquired immunodeficiency syndrome (AIDS).

TREATMENT

Seborrheic dermatitis of the scalp is usually asymptomatic and generally does not require treatment. Minor amounts of scale can be removed easily by frequent shampooing. For infants with cradle cap, oil (such as mineral oil or olive oil) may be gently massaged into the scalp and left on for a few minutes before gently brushing out the scale and shampooing. Daily shampooing with ketoconazole, zinc pyrithione, selenium sulfide, or salicylic acid shampoos can treat scalp scale. Seborrheic dermatitis with inflamed lesions responds rapidly to treatment with low-potency steroids two times daily.

The response to treatment is usually rapid. Secondary bacterial infection can occur but is uncommon. Intractable disease and other complications warrant further evaluation for other etiologies.

PROGNOSIS

Cradle cap is self-limited and resolves during the first year of life. Seborrheic dermatitis does not cause permanent hair loss. For teenagers, continued use of an antiseborrheic shampoo is often required for control of dandruff.

PREVENTION

Frequent shampooing, especially with early signs of seborrheic dermatitis, may help prevent progression.

OTHER PAPULOSQUAMOUS DERMATOSES

Pityriasis Rosea

Pityriasis rosea is a benign, self-limited eruption that may occur at any age, with peak incidence during adolescence. A solitary 2- to 5-cm, pink, oval patch with central clearing, the so-called **herald patch**, is the first manifestation of the eruption. The herald patch typically is found on the trunk or proximal thigh and is often misdiagnosed as fungal or eczematous in origin. One to 2 weeks later, a generalized eruption occurs on the torso and proximal extremities. Multiple 0.5- to 2-cm, oval to oblong, red or tan macules with a fine, bran-like scale are characteristically arranged parallel to skin tension lines (**Christmas-tree pattern**). Rarely the eruption may have an inverse distribution involving the axillae and groin or a papular or papulovesicular appearance. Mild prodromal symptoms may be present with the appearance of the herald patch, and pruritus is present in 25% of cases. The eruption lasts 4-14 weeks, with gradual resolution. Residual hyperpigmentation or hypopigmentation can take additional months to clear. Treatment is unnecessary, though pruritus can be managed with oral antihistamines, phototherapy, and low-potency topical corticosteroids.

Psoriasis

Psoriasis is a common papulosquamous condition characterized by well-demarcated, erythematous, scaling papules and plaques. Psoriasis occurs at all ages, including infancy, with onset of 30% of cases during childhood. The disease is characterized by a chronic and relapsing course, although spontaneous remissions can occur. Infections (especially *Streptococcus pyogenes*), stress, trauma, and medications may cause disease exacerbations. Various subtypes of psoriasis exist. The most common variety is **plaque-type psoriasis (psoriasis vulgaris)**, which can be localized or generalized. The lesions consist of round, well-demarcated, red plaques measuring 1- to 7-cm with micaceous scale, which is distinctive in its thick, silvery appearance with pinpoint bleeding points revealed on removal of the scales **(Auspitz sign)**. The lesions of psoriasis have a distinctive distribution involving the extensor aspect of the elbows and knees, posterior occipital scalp, periumbilical region, lumbosacral region, and intergluteal cleft. Children often have facial lesions involving the superomedial aspect of the eyelids. Nail plate involvement is common and includes pitting, onycholysis, subungual hyperkeratosis, and oil staining (reddish brown subungual macular discoloration). **Guttate** (numerous small papules and plaques diffusely distributed on the torso), **erythrodermic** (covering large body surface areas), **inverse** (moist red patches affecting body folds), and **pustular** forms may occur.

The foundation of therapy is topical corticosteroids. Treatment of psoriasis with oral corticosteroids can induce pustular psoriasis and should be avoided. Because of the risk of atrophy, striae, and telangiectases, especially when potent fluorinated corticosteroid preparations are administered long term, the goal is to use the least potent corticosteroid necessary. Topical vitamin D analogs, salicylic acid, and tar preparations are useful adjuvants to topical corticosteroids. Phototherapy with ultraviolet B (UVB) light can be useful as secondary therapy in older children. Extensive plaque or guttate, erythrodermic, and pustular psoriasis may necessitate systemic treatments with immune suppressive medication (methotrexate, cyclosporine, tumor necrosis factor-α antagonists). Disease triggers such as infection or medications should be identified and removed.

CHAPTER 193

Pigmented Lesions

Birthmark is a term that describes congenital anomalies of the skin. It should not be used as a definitive diagnosis because congenital skin lesions vary greatly in their appearance and prognosis. The differential diagnosis of various birthmarks is listed in Table 193.1.

DERMAL MELANOSIS

The most frequently encountered pigmented lesion is **dermal melanosis**, which occurs in 70-90% of African-American, Hispanic, Asian, and Native American infants and in approximately 5% of white infants. This is a congenital lesion caused by entrapment of melanocytes in the dermis during their migration from the neural crest into the epidermis. Although most of these lesions are found in the lumbosacral area (Mongolian spot), they also occur at other sites, such as the buttocks, flank, extremities, or rarely, the face (Fig. 193.1). Single or multiple, poorly demarcated, gray-blue patches up to 10 cm in size may be present. Most lesions gradually disappear during the first few years of life; aberrant lesions in unusual sites are more likely to persist.

TABLE 193.1 Common Birthmarks

COLOR/LESION	BIRTHMARK	LOCATION	OTHER FEATURES
Brown/macule or patch	Café-au-lait macule	Variable	May be associated with genetic syndromes
Brown (<20 cm)/patch or plaque	Congenital melanocytic nevus	Variable	Low risk of melanoma
Brown (>20 cm)/patch or plaque	Giant congenital melanocytic nevus	Trunk most common	Risk of melanoma and neuromelanosis
Brown or skin-colored/plaque	Epidermal nevus	Variable, trunk and neck	May enlarge with time
Red/patch	Port-wine stain (nevus flammeus)	Variable, face most common	May be associated with Sturge-Weber syndrome
Red/patch	Salmon patch (nevus simplex)	Glabella, eyelids, nape of neck	Improves or resolves with time
Red/papule or plaque	Hemangioma	Variable	May be associated with liver hemangiomas, airway hemangiomas, and PHACE syndrome
Gray-blue/patch	Dermal melanosis	Lower trunk (Mongolian spot); face (nevus of Ota); posterior shoulder (nevus of Ito)	Nevus of Ota may be associated with ocular pigmentation
Blue-purple/plaque	Venous, lymphatic, or mixed malformation	Variable	Intermittent swelling and pain
Yellow-orange/plaque	Nevus sebaceus	Head and neck	Malignant and benign tumors may arise within
Yellow-orange/papule	Juvenile xanthogranuloma	Head and neck most common	Spontaneously involutes
Yellow-brown/papule or plaque	Mastocytoma	Variable	Spontaneously involutes
Hypertrichosis/plaque	Smooth muscle hamartoma	Trunk	
Hypertrichosis/tumor	Plexiform neurofibroma	Trunk most common	Associated with neurofibromatosis type 1
White/patch	Nevus anemicus	Variable	Surrounding redness and telangiectasia
White/patch	Nevus depigmentosus	Variable	

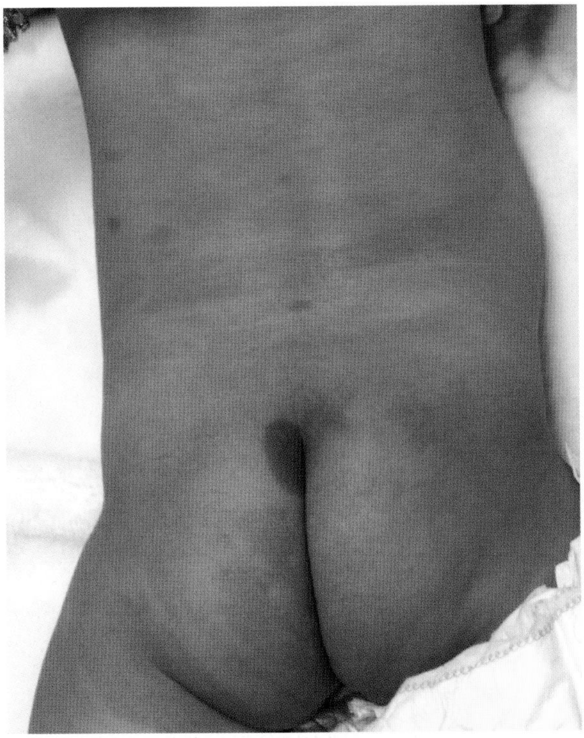

FIGURE 193.1 Dermal hypermelanosis (back).

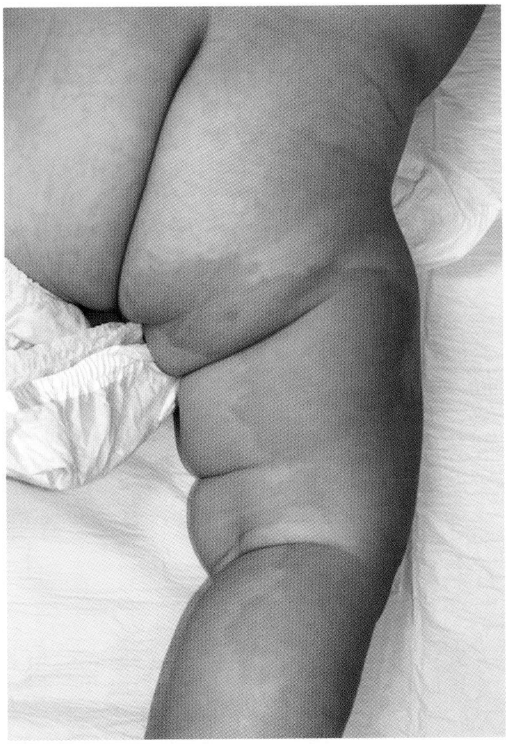

FIGURE 193.2 Café-au-lait spots (leg).

CAFÉ-AU-LAIT MACULES

Café-au-lait macules are pigmented macules or patches, which may be present in a newborn but tend to develop during childhood (Fig. 193.2). They range in color from very light brown to a chocolate brown. Up to five café-au-lait macules

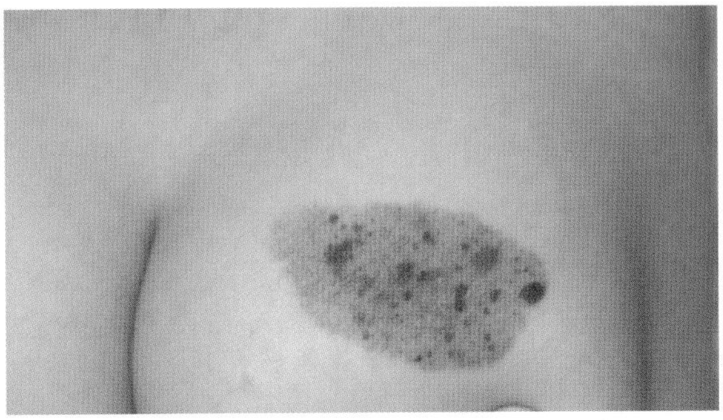

FIGURE 193.3 Congenital melanocytic nevus (buttock).

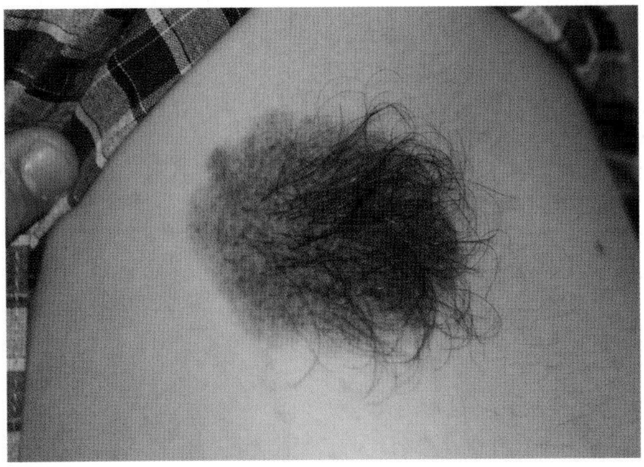

FIGURE 193.4 Hairy congenital nevus.

are found in 1.8% of newborns and 25-40% of normal children, and have no significance. Children with six or more café-au-lait macules (0.5 cm in diameter before puberty or greater than 1.5 cm in diameter after puberty), especially when accompanied by **axillary or inguinal freckling,** should be evaluated carefully for additional stigmata of neurofibromatosis type 1. Other disorders also associated with café-au-lait macules include the other forms of neurofibromatosis, Legius syndrome, tuberous sclerosis, McCune-Albright syndrome, Noonan syndrome, and Russell-Silver syndrome.

CONGENITAL MELANOCYTIC NEVI

Approximately 1-2% of newborns have **congenital melanocytic nevi.** Smaller lesions (as opposed to giant pigmented nevi) are brown patches or plaques, often with an oval or lancet configuration. Lesions may resemble café-au-lait macules initially, but darker pigmentation, variegated speckles, textural changes, and elevation develop with time and help to differentiate these lesions (Fig. 193.3). Thick, dark, coarse hair frequently is associated with congenital melanocytic nevi (Fig. 193.4). These lesions vary in site and size but are most often solitary. Congenital melanocytic nevi pose a very slightly increased risk for the development of malignant melanoma, usually during adulthood. Surgical removal may be considered to improve the cosmetic appearance of the patient or to reduce the likelihood of malignant transformation, although some patients and physicians elect for observation. Excisional biopsy is indicated when malignant change is suspected.

GIANT CONGENITAL MELANOCYTIC NEVI

Giant congenital melanocytic nevi are defined as nevi that would be approximately 20 cm in length in adulthood; in a neonate, this translates to 9 cm on the head and neck and 6 cm on the rest of the body. These lesions appear as color variegated, light brown to black patches or plaques, sometimes with smaller macules and papules **(satellite nevi)** in addition. The affected skin may be smooth, nodular, or leathery. Prominent, dark hypertrichosis is often present. **Neuromelanosis**, the presence of melanocytes in the central nervous system, may be associated with giant congenital melanocytic nevi. Affected patients may be asymptomatic or have hydrocephalus and seizures; in symptomatic patients, death often results during early childhood. **Malignant melanoma** develops in approximately 2-10% of patients with giant congenital melanocytic nevi, in either the cutaneous lesion or the neural melanocytes. In contrast to small and medium congenital melanocytic nevi, melanoma is more likely to develop during childhood. Because of the incidence of malignant degeneration and extensive deformity, surgical excision should be considered for resectable lesions. The use of tissue expansion techniques has greatly improved the capability for surgical removal of large lesions.

ACQUIRED MELANOCYTIC NEVI

Acquired melanocytic nevi are common skin lesions. Melanocytic nevi may occur at any age; however, the lesions develop most rapidly in prepubertal children and teenagers. Melanocytic nevi are well-delineated, round to oval, brown macules and papules. Lesions are most common on the face, upper torso, and arms. Family history, fair skin, and sun exposure are considered major risk factors. Irregular pigmentation, rapid growth, bleeding, and a change in configuration or borders suggest signs of malignant degeneration and biopsy should be performed. Malignant melanoma is rare in childhood; however, there is an alarming increase in incidence in adolescence, especially in those who use indoor tanning. Education of parents and children regarding the risks of sun exposure, appropriate sun protection, and recognition of worrisome lesions is important.

CHAPTER 194

Vascular Anomalies

Vascular anomalies can be divided into two major categories: tumors and malformations. Vascular tumors are characterized by hypercellularity, proliferation, and growth. Vascular malformations, however, are developmental defects derived from the capillary, venous, arterial, or lymphatic vessels. In contrast to hemangiomas, vascular malformations remain relatively static and grow very slowly over time. Differentiating between these entities is important because they have different prognoses and clinical implications.

VASCULAR TUMORS

Infantile Hemangiomas

Decision-Making Algorithms
Available @ StudentConsult.com

Neck Masses
Stridor

Infantile hemangiomas are the most common soft tissue tumors of infancy, occurring in approximately 5-10% of 1-year-old infants. In newborns, hemangiomas may originate as a pale white macule with threadlike telangiectasia. When the tumor proliferates, it assumes its most recognizable form as a bright red, lobulated plaque or nodule (superficial type, Fig. 194.1). Hemangiomas that lie deeper in the skin are soft, warm masses with a blue discoloration (deeper type). Frequently, hemangiomas have both a superficial and a deep component (mixed type). They range from a few millimeters to several centimeters in diameter and are usually solitary; 20% of affected children have multiple lesions. Hemangiomas occur predominantly in females (3:1) and have an increased incidence in low birth weight infants. Approximately 55% are present at birth; the rest develop in the first weeks of life. Superficial hemangiomas reach their maximal size by 6-8 months, but deep hemangiomas may grow for 12-14 months. They then undergo slow, spontaneous resolution, which takes 3-10 years.

Despite the benign nature of most cutaneous hemangiomas, there may be the risk of functional compromise or permanent disfigurement, depending on the location and extent. Ulceration, the most frequent complication, can be painful and increases the risk of infection, hemorrhage, and scarring. Areas frequently associated with complications include the periocular region, lip, nasal tip, beard, face (large lesions), groin, and buttocks.

Periorbital hemangiomas pose considerable risk to vision and should be monitored carefully. Amblyopia can result from the hemangioma, causing obstruction of the visual axis or pressure on the globe, resulting in astigmatism. If there is any concern, the patient should have urgent evaluation by an ophthalmologist. Treatment may be indicated to prevent blindness. **Subglottic hemangiomas** manifest as hoarseness and stridor; progression to respiratory failure may be rapid. Symptomatic airway hemangiomas develop in more than 50% of infants with extensive facial hemangiomas on the chin and

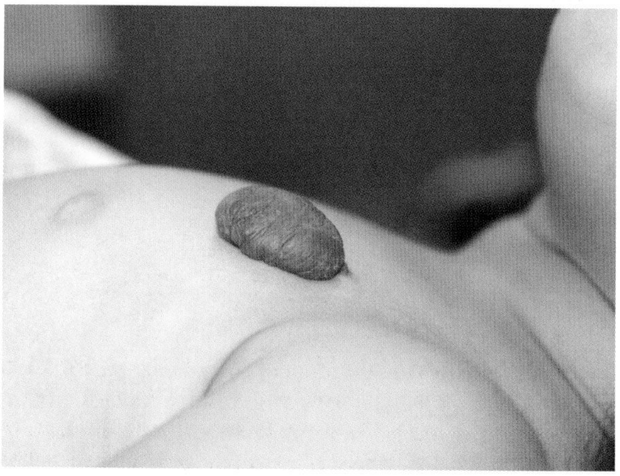

FIGURE 194.1 Hemangioma (chest).

jaw (beard distribution); any infant with a beard hemangioma should be urgently referred for laryngoscopy. Multiple cutaneous (diffuse hemangiomatosis) and large facial hemangiomas may be associated with visceral hemangiomas. Extensive cervicofacial hemangiomas may be associated with multiple anomalies, including posterior fossa malformations, hemangiomas, arterial anomalies of the cerebrovasculature, coarctation of aorta and cardiac defects, and eye abnormalities **(PHACE syndrome).** **Lumbosacral hemangiomas** suggest an occult spinal dysraphism with or without anorectal and urogenital anomalies. Magnetic resonance imaging of the spine is indicated in all patients with large midline cutaneous hemangiomas in the lumbosacral area.

Most hemangiomas do not necessitate medical intervention and involute spontaneously; however, if complications arise and treatment is warranted, oral propranolol or topical timolol are the mainstays of therapy.

Pyogenic Granuloma

A pyogenic granuloma is an acquired, benign vascular tumor commonly seen in children. Initially, the lesions appear as pink-red papules that often arise after minor trauma, growing rapidly over a period of weeks into a bright red, vascular, often pedunculated papule measuring 2-10 mm. The lesions often have the appearance of granulation tissue and are very friable. They may occur anywhere on the body, but the head, neck, and upper extremities are most commonly affected. When traumatized, these lesions may bleed profusely, often requiring emergent medical attention. Surgical excision is the most definitive treatment option, although pulsed dye laser can be useful for very small lesions.

VASCULAR MALFORMATIONS

Port-Wine Stain

Port-wine stains (nevus flammeus, capillary malformation) are malformations of the superficial capillaries of the skin. These lesions are present at birth and should be considered permanent developmental defects. They do not enlarge after birth; any apparent increase in size is caused by growth of the child. A port-wine stain may be localized to any body surface, but facial lesions are the most common. They are pink-red, sharply demarcated macules and patches in infancy (Fig. 194.2). With time, they darken to a purple or *port-wine* color and may develop a pebbly or slightly thickened surface. Vascular blebs may form within the lesions and become symptomatic or bleed. The most successful treatment modality in use is the pulsed dye laser, which can result in 80-90% improvement in these lesions after a series of treatment sessions and can avoid future complications associated with vascular dilation. Treatment is more effective if undertaken in infancy. Overgrowth of underlying bone can occur and is frequently seen with facial lesions. Affected patients often need maxillofacial intervention from malalignment that develops.

Most port-wine stains occur as isolated defects and do not indicate systemic malformations. Rarely, they may suggest ocular defects or specific neurocutaneous syndromes. **Sturge-Weber syndrome** (encephalotrigeminal angiomatosis) may occur with a facial port-wine stain, usually in the cutaneous distribution of the first branch of the trigeminal nerve. Other features include leptomeningeal angiomatosis, mental retardation, seizures, hemiparesis contralateral to the facial lesions, ipsilateral intracortical calcification, and frequent ocular manifestations

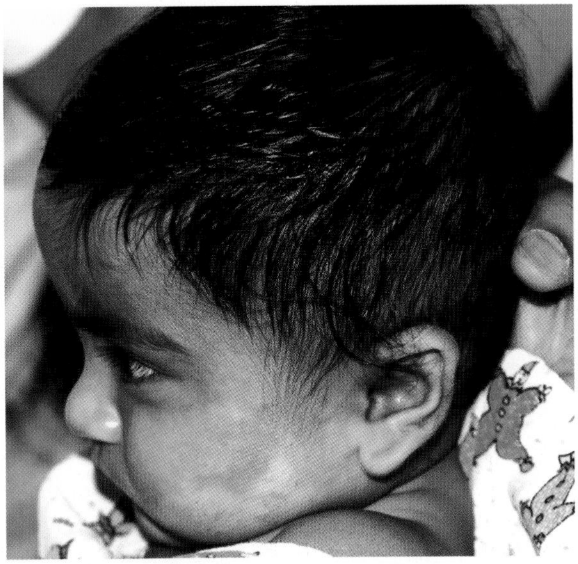

FIGURE 194.2 Port-wine stain (face).

such as buphthalmos, glaucoma, angioma of the choroid, hemianoptic defects, and optic atrophy. Anticonvulsant therapy and neurosurgical procedures have been of value in some patients. Glaucoma can occur in association with port-wine stains located on the eyelid, even in the absence of Sturge-Weber syndrome, and these patients need lifelong monitoring of ocular pressures. **Klippel-Trénaunay-Weber** syndrome is characterized by the triad of capillary and venous malformations, venous varicosities, and hyperplasia of the soft tissues—and often bone—of the involved area. The lower limb is most commonly affected. A port-wine stain overlying the spine may rarely be a marker of spinal dysraphism or an intraspinal vascular malformation.

Nevus Simplex

A nevus simplex (salmon patch, stork bite, angel's kiss) is a vascular birthmark that is present in 70% of normal newborns. They are red, irregular, macular patches resulting from dilation of dermal capillaries and are usually found on the nape of the neck, the eyelids, and the glabella. Most of the facial lesions fade by 1 year of age, but lesions on the neck may persist for life. Surveys of adult populations confirm the persistence of the nuchal lesions in approximately 25% of the population.

CHAPTER 195

Erythema Multiforme, Stevens-Johnson Syndrome, and Toxic Epidermal Necrolysis

Erythema multiforme (EM), Stevens-Johnson syndrome (SJS), and toxic epidermal necrolysis (TEN) are acute hypersensitivity reactions characterized by cutaneous and mucosal necrosis. These syndromes represent a hypersensitivity reaction to a precipitating cause, usually infectious organisms or drugs. These disorders were historically thought to represent a spectrum of the same disease process, and inconsistent use of these disease names led to further confusion. A consensus definition was published in 1993, and current literature favors that EM is distinct from the SJS/TEN spectrum of disease. The differential diagnosis of vesiculobullous eruptions is listed in Table 195.1.

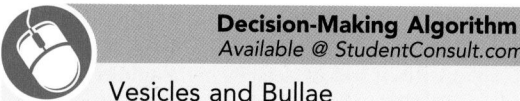

Decision-Making Algorithm
Available @ StudentConsult.com
Vesicles and Bullae

TABLE 195.1 Vesiculobullous Eruptions

ENTITY	CLINICAL CLUES
INFECTIOUS	
Bacterial	
Staphylococcal scalded skin syndrome	Generalized, tender erythema Nikolsky sign Occasionally associated with underlying infection such as osteomyelitis, septic arthritis, pneumonia Desquamation and moist erosions observed, especially in intertriginous areas More common in children younger than 5 yr of age
Bullous impetigo	Localized blisters from staphylococcal infection
Viral	
Herpes simplex	Grouped vesicles on erythematous base May be recurrent at same site—lips, eyes, cheeks, hands Reactivated by fever, sunlight, trauma, stress
Varicella	Crops of vesicles on erythematous base ("dewdrops on rose petal") Highly contagious May see multiple stages of lesions simultaneously Associated with fever
Herpes zoster	Grouped vesicles on erythematous base limited to one or several adjacent dermatomes Thoracic dermatomes most commonly involved in children Usually unilateral Burning, pruritus
Hand-foot-mouth syndrome (coxsackievirus infection)	Prodrome of fever, anorexia, sore throat Oval blisters in acral distribution, usually few in number Shallow, oral erosions on erythematous base in oral mucosa Highly infectious Peak incidence in late summer and in fall
HYPERSENSITIVITY	
Erythema multiforme	Target lesions on acral sites May have involvement of mucosal surfaces Associated with herpes simplex virus infection
Stevens-Johnson syndrome and toxic epidermal necrolysis	Prodrome of fever, headache, malaise, sore throat, cough, vomiting, diarrhea Extensive epidermal necrosis with mucosal involvement Frequently related to drugs (e.g., sulfonamides, anticonvulsants) Nikolsky sign
EXTRINSIC	
Contact dermatitis	Irritant or allergic Distribution dependent on the irritant or allergen Distribution helpful in identifying cause
Insect bites	Occur occasionally following flea or mosquito bites May be hemorrhagic bullae Often in linear or irregular clusters Very pruritic
Burns	Irregular shapes and configurations May be suggestive of abuse Bullae with second- and third-degree injuries
Friction	Usually on acral surfaces May be related to footwear Often activity-related
MISCELLANEOUS	
Urticaria pigmentosa	Red-brown macules and papules; bullous lesions are rare Darier sign Lesions appear in infancy and spontaneously resolve in childhood
Miliaria crystallina	Clean, 1- to 2-mm superficial vesicles occurring in crops Rupture spontaneously Intertriginous areas, especially neck and axillae
Hereditary: epidermolysis bullosa, incontinentia pigmenti, epidermolytic hyperkeratosis	
Autoimmune: linear immunoglobulin A disease, bullous pemphigoid, dermatitis herpetiformis	

Modified from Nopper AJ, Rabinowotz RG. Rashes and skin lesions. In: Kliegman RM, ed. Practical Strategies in Pediatric Diagnosis and Therapy. *Philadelphia: WB Saunders; 1996.*

ERYTHEMA MULTIFORME

EM is a common, self-limiting, acute hypersensitivity syndrome characterized by the abrupt onset of round, deep red, well-demarcated macules and papules with a dusky gray or bullous center. The size may range from a few millimeters to a few centimeters, but most lesions are approximately 1 cm in diameter. The classic **target lesion** consists of three concentric rings; the outermost is red, the intermediate is white, and the center is a dusky red or purple. These can progress to edematous plaques or bullae. If blistering occurs, it is circumscribed and involves less than 10% of the body surface area. Cutaneous lesions are symmetrically distributed and commonly involve acral areas such as the hands, feet, elbows, and knees. Involvement of the ocular, oral, and genital mucosa can be seen in some cases.

Most EM cases in children are precipitated by herpes simplex virus infection, although the infection may no longer be apparent by the time EM develops. Other infectious organisms may also trigger EM. Symptomatic treatment is usually sufficient. Oral antihistamines help suppress pruritus, stinging, and burning. The use of systemic corticosteroids is controversial but may be considered for severe mucosal disease. Antiviral medications targeting herpes simplex virus do not alter the course of the EM, although children with recurrent EM may be candidates for prophylactic antivirals. The prognosis is excellent, with most lesions lasting no more than 2 weeks. Healing occurs without scarring.

STEVENS-JOHNSON SYNDROME AND TOXIC EPIDERMAL NECROLYSIS

SJS, TEN, and SJS/TEN overlap are severe, life-threatening disorders thought to represent the same disease continuum. They are usually preceded by a prodrome of fever, malaise, and upper respiratory symptoms 1-14 days before the onset of cutaneous lesions. Red macules appear suddenly and tend to coalesce into large patches, with a predominant distribution over the face and trunk. Atypical targets may be present, causing diagnostic confusion initially with EM, although the atypical targets lack the characteristic three zones. Skin lesions evolve rapidly into bullae and areas of necrosis. SJS is defined as epidermal detachment of less than 10% of the body surface area, whereas SJS/TEN overlap has 10-30% and TEN has greater than 30% body surface area involvement. Any mucosal surface may be involved. The upper and lower lips are generally swollen and bright red with erosions and hemorrhagic crusts. The remainder of the oral mucosa may also be involved. Early in the disease process, there is bilateral conjunctival injection; this usually progresses to conjunctival erosions. There may be erosions of the penile, vaginal, or perianal mucosa. Urogenital, esophageal, and tracheal surfaces may be involved in the most severe cases.

Drugs are the most common causes of SJS/TEN in children. The most common drugs implicated are nonsteroidal antiinflammatory drugs, sulfonamides, anticonvulsants, and antibiotics. Other precipitating factors are viral infections, bacterial infections, syphilis, and deep fungal infections.

SJS/TEN can occur at any age. The diagnosis of SJS/TEN is clinical; there are no diagnostic tests. Confusion with EM, Kawasaki disease, and bacterial toxin-mediated diseases (scarlet fever, toxic shock syndrome, and staphylococcal scalded skin syndrome) may occur. Patients with Kawasaki disease have conjunctival injection and hyperemia of the mucous membranes. Necrosis of the mucosal surfaces does not occur; blistering, erosions, and severe crusting are not observed. The mucosal changes of staphylococcal scalded skin syndrome are minor, and frank erosions are not present. The blistering of the skin is more superficial and favors intertriginous regions. *Mycoplasma pneumoniae* may induce a SJS/TEN-like disorder that is newly recognized as a distinct disease called mycoplasma pneumonia-associated mucocutaneous disease.

SJS/TEN is a serious illness with a mortality rate as high as 35% for severe cases of TEN. Prompt discontinuation of the offending agent is key. No controlled clinical trials regarding medical therapy exist, although early initiation of intravenous immunoglobulin has been proposed. Supportive care is another essential component of therapy. A multidisciplinary care team is often necessary. Sepsis is the major cause of morbidity and mortality, so meticulous wound care is crucial, with stringent surveillance for cutaneous infections and use of antibiotics as warranted. Parenteral or nasogastric feeding should be instituted early to accelerate the healing process. Careful fluid management and monitoring of electrolytes are critical. Ocular complications are a major cause of long-term morbidity, making early involvement of an ophthalmologist important.

CHAPTER 196

Cutaneous Infestations

Arthropods are common in the environment. Although many can bite or sting humans, only a few infest humans. Arachnids (mites) are the most common, parasitizing humans and animals by burrowing into the skin and depositing eggs within the skin.

SCABIES

Decision-Making Algorithm
Available @ StudentConsult.com
Vesicles and Bullae

Scabies is caused by the mite *Sarcoptes scabiei*. The female mite burrows into the epidermis and deposits her eggs, which mature in 10-14 days. The disease is highly contagious, as infested humans do not manifest the typical signs or symptoms for 3-4 weeks, facilitating transmission. An immunocompetent person with scabies typically harbors only 10-20 mites.

The clinical presentation varies depending on the age of the patient, duration of infestation, and immune status of the patient. Severe and paroxysmal itching is the hallmark, with complaints of itching that is frequently worse than the eruption would suggest. Most children exhibit an eczematous eruption composed of red, excoriated papules and nodules. The classic linear papule or burrow is often difficult to find. Distribution is the most diagnostic finding; the papules are found in the axillae, umbilicus, groin, penis, instep of the foot, and web spaces of the fingers and toes (Fig. 196.1). Infants infested with

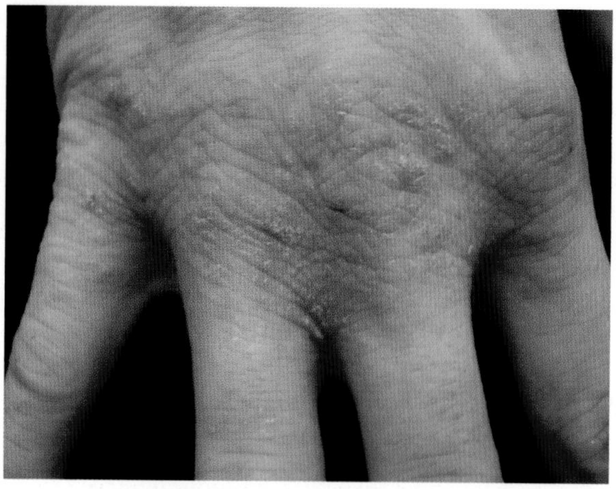

FIGURE 196.1 Scabies (hand).

scabies have diffuse erythema, scaling, and pinpoint papules. Pustules, vesicles, and nodules are much more common in infants and may be more diffusely distributed. The face and scalp usually are spared in adults and older children, but these areas are usually involved in infants. Nodular lesions may represent active infection or prolonged hypersensitivity lesions following resolution of infestation. Immunocompromised or neurologically impaired persons may develop a severe form of the disease known as **Norwegian** or **crusted scabies**, with infestation of 2 million live mites at one time.

The diagnosis of scabies can be confirmed by microscopic visualization of the mite, eggs, larvae, or feces in scrapings of papules or burrows examined under oil immersion. Skin biopsy is rarely necessary but may be useful if lesions have become nodular.

Curative treatment is achieved by a 12-hour (overnight) application of permethrin 5% cream applied to the entire body. Because permethrin is not effective against the eggs, the treatment should be repeated 1 week later to kill any subsequently hatched larvae. All household members and close contacts should be treated simultaneously, even if asymptomatic. Bed linens, towels, and clothes worn for the previous 2 days before treatment should be machine-washed in hot water and machine-dried using high heat; heat is the most effective scabicide. Items that are not washable may be dry-cleaned or placed in a sealed plastic bag for 7 days.

Secondary bacterial infection may occur but is uncommon. In contrast to the pediculoses, scabies is not a vector for infections. Pruritus may persist for 7-14 days after successful therapy because of a prolonged hypersensitivity reaction, which does not indicate treatment failure. Inadequate treatment or reinfestation should be suspected if new lesions develop after treatment.

PEDICULOSES

Three species of lice infest humans: *Pediculus humanus capitis,* the **head louse**; *Pthirus pubis,* the **pubic louse** or **crab louse**; and *Pediculus humanus humanus* (also known as *Pediculus humanus corporis*), the **body louse**. Lice are wingless insects 2-4 mm in length that cannot fly or jump. Transmission usually occurs by direct contact with another infested individual. Indirect spread through contact with fomites or personal belongings, such as hairbrushes, combs, or caps, is much less frequent.

Pediculosis differs from scabies infestation in that the louse resides on the hair or clothing and intermittently feeds on the host by piercing the skin. The *bite* causes small urticarial papules and itching. Head lice live close to the skin and may live for 30 days, depositing 100-400 eggs as **nits** on hair shafts, usually within 6 mm of the scalp.

Head lice are seen most frequently in early school-age children. Head lice infestations are unrelated to hygiene and are not more common among children with long hair or with dirty hair. It is estimated that 6-12 million persons in the United States and 1-3% of persons in developed countries are infested with head lice each year. In the United States, head lice infestation is rare among African Americans and may be more common in girls, which is attributed to their tendency to play more closely with one another than boys do.

Pubic lice are transmitted by sexual contact. Their presence in children may be a sign of child abuse. Body lice are firm evidence of poor hygiene, such as infrequent washing and clothing changes.

Itching, if present, is the primary symptom. Pediculosis capitis usually causes pruritus behind the ears or on the nape of the neck, or a crawling sensation in the scalp. Pediculosis pubis usually causes pruritus in the groin. Eyelash involvement in children may cause crusting and blepharitis. Pediculosis corporis causes pruritus that, because of repeated scratching, may result in lichenification or secondary bacterial infection. Excoriations and crusting, with or without associated regional lymphadenopathy, may be present.

Infestation with the head louse may be asymptomatic and has little morbidity. The diagnosis can be confirmed by visualizing a live louse. A fine-toothed comb to trap lice is more effective than simply looking at the hair. Wet combing is more time-consuming, but dry combing produces static that may propel the lice away from the comb.

Nits represent the outer casing of the louse ova. Viable nits have an intact operculum (cap) on the nonattached end and a developing louse within the egg. **Brown nits** located on the proximal hair shaft suggest active infestation. **White nits** located on the hair shaft 4 cm or farther from the scalp indicate previous infestation. Because nonviable nits can remain stuck in the hair for weeks to months after an infestation has resolved, many children with nits do not have active lice infestation.

The treatment of head lice is controversial because of resistance to many established options. Permethrin (1%) and pyrethrin-based products (0.17-0.33%) (pyrethroids) are over-the-counter options. Because 20-30% of eggs may survive one treatment, a second treatment should be applied in 9-10 days. Drug resistance to pyrethroids is on the rise. Malathion (0.5%) lotion, benzyl alcohol (5%) lotion, spinosad (0.9%) topical suspension, and ivermectin (0.5%) lotion may be used as alternatives for resistant cases.

Everyone in the family should be checked for head lice and treated if live lice are found to reduce the risk of reinfestation. Bed linens, towels, and clothes worn for the previous 2 days before treatment should be machine-washed in hot water and machine-dried using high heat. Items that are not washable may be dry-cleaned or placed in a sealed plastic bag for 2 weeks. Brushes and combs should be soaked in dish detergent or rubbing alcohol for 1 hour. Rugs, furniture, mattresses, and car seats should be vacuumed thoroughly.

Manual removal of nits after treatment is not necessary to prevent spread. Children treated for head lice should return to school immediately after completion of the first effective treatment or first wet combing, regardless of the presence of remaining nits. There is no evidence that *no nit* or *nit-free* policies reduce transmission of head lice. If required for return to school, nit removal is best achieved by wetting the hair and combing with a fine-toothed metal comb.

Excoriations can become secondarily infected with skin bacteria, usually *Staphylococcus* and *Streptococcus.* The body louse functions as a vector for potentially serious infectious diseases, including **epidemic typhus,** caused by *Rickettsia prowazekii*; **louse-borne relapsing fever,** caused by *Borrelia recurrentis*; and **trench fever,** caused by *Bartonella quintana.* These louse-borne infections are rare in the United States. In contrast to body lice, head lice and pubic lice are not associated with transmission of other infections.

Suggested Readings

Eichenfield LF, Frieden IJ. *Neonatal and Infant Dermatology.* 3rd ed. London: Saunders; 2015.
Eichenfield LF, Krakowski AC, Piggott C. Evidence-based recommendations for the diagnosis and treatment of pediatric acne. *Pediatrics.* 2013;131:S163–S186.
Eichenfield LF, Tom WL, Berger TG. Guidelines of care for the management of atopic dermatitis: Section 2. Management and treatment of atopic dermatitis with topical therapies. *J Am Acad Dermatol.* 2014;71:116–132.
Eichenfield LF, Tom WL, Chamlin SL. Guidelines of care for the management of atopic dermatitis: Section 1. Diagnosis and assessment of atopic dermatitis. *J Am Acad Dermatol.* 2014;70:338–351.
Holland KE, Drolet BA. Infantile hemangioma. *Pediatr Clin North Am.* 2010;57:1069–1083.
Paller AS, Mancini AJ. *Hurwitz Clinical Pediatric Dermatology.* 5th ed. Philadelphia: Elsevier; 2015.
Schachner LA, Hansen RC. *Pediatric Dermatology.* 4th ed. Philadelphia: Saunders; 2014.
Zaenglein AL, Pathy AL, Schlosser BJ. Guidelines of care for the management of acne vulgaris. *J Am Acad Dermatol.* 2016;74:945–973.

PEARLS FOR PRACTITIONERS

CHAPTER 188

Dermatology Assessment

- Common cutaneous conditions in pediatrics include atopic dermatitis, impetigo, tinea capitis, acne vulgaris, verrucae vulgaris, and seborrheic dermatitis.
- Obtaining a thorough history with regard to the age of the patient, onset, duration, progression, associated cutaneous symptoms (pain, pruritus), previous treatments, and associated systemic signs or symptoms (fever, malaise, weight loss) is important.
- Characterizing and describing the primary and secondary skin lesions is important for diagnosis and communication with other health care providers.

CHAPTER 189

Acne

- Acne vulgaris is the most common skin condition in adolescents.
- The pathogenesis of acne involves increased sebum production, hyperkeratosis, and bacterial proliferation. Treatment is aimed at decreasing these factors.

CHAPTER 190

Atopic Dermatitis

- Atopic dermatitis is the most common skin disease in children and is associated with allergic rhinitis, asthma, and food allergies. Both genetic and environmental factors play a role in the development of atopic dermatitis.
- Treatment of atopic dermatitis is aimed at decreasing inflammation.
- Complications of atopic dermatitis include secondary impetigo and eczema herpeticum.

CHAPTER 191

Contact Dermatitis

- Contact dermatitis is a delayed type IV hypersensitivity reaction that occurs when the skin is directly exposed to irritating chemicals or substances (irritant contact dermatitis) or allergens in predisposed individuals.
- Diaper dermatitis is commonly due to irritant contact dermatitis from urine and feces, frequently complicated by secondary candida and bacterial infections.
  - Differential diagnosis for diaper dermatitis includes psoriasis, seborrheic dermatitis, and Langerhans cell histiocytosis. Referral to a pediatric dermatologist should be made in recalcitrant, difficult-to-treat cases.
- Treatment of contact dermatitis is generally avoidance of irritating substances, allergens, barriers, and topical corticosteroids.

CHAPTER 192

Seborrheic Dermatitis

- Seborrheic dermatitis is a common, chronic inflammatory disease that presents as cradle cap or dermatitis in intertriginous areas in infants and dandruff in adolescents.
- The pathogenesis of seborrheic dermatitis is unclear, but it is theorized that there is an abnormal inflammatory response to commensal *Malassezia* species in sebum-rich areas.

- Treatment for seborrheic dermatitis is generally not needed, but oils, shampoos, and topical steroids can be used if needed.
- Pityriasis rosea is a benign, self-limited eruption that starts with a herald patch, which precedes a generalized eruption on the torso and extremities in a Christmas-tree pattern.
- Psoriasis is a common papulosquamous disorder with various subtypes, including plaque-type psoriasis (psoriasis vulgaris), guttate, erythrodermic, and pustular.
  - Treatments for psoriasis include topical corticosteroids, topical vitamin D analog, salicyclic acid, tar preparations, phototherapy, and systemic immunosuppressants.

CHAPTER 193

Pigmented Lesions

- Dermal melanosis is the most frequently encountered pigmented lesion. The gray-blue lesions are typically found in the lumbosacral area, buttocks, flank, extremities, or rarely, the face.
- Café-au-lait macules are light- to chocolate-brown pigmented macules or patches that can be found in normal newborns and children.
  - Children with six or more café-au-lait macules (0.5 cm in diameter before puberty or greater than 1.5 cm in diameter after puberty), especially when accompanied by axillary or inguinal freckling, should be evaluated carefully for additional stigmata of neurofibromatosis type 1.
  - Other disorders also associated with café-au-lait macules include the other forms of neurofibromatosis, Legius syndrome, tuberous sclerosis, McCune-Albright syndrome, Noonan syndrome, and Russell-Silver syndrome.
- There is an increased risk of neuromelanosis and malignant melanoma when congenital melanocytic nevi are giant (>20 cm in length in adulthood, or 9 cm on the head and neck and 6 cm on the rest of the body in a neonate).

CHAPTER 194

Vascular Anomalies

- Infantile hemangiomas are the most common soft tissue tumors of infancy and present as superficial, deep, or mixed types.
  - They undergo spontaneous involution after a rapid growth phase.
  - They do not need to be treated unless they are symptomatic and/or pose risks that can lead to functional compromise or permanent disfigurement, in which case oral propranolol is the mainstay of therapy.
- Infantile hemangiomas can have visceral involvement and be associated with other underlying anomalies.
  - Evaluation for airway hemangiomas should be undertaken in infants with a beard hemangioma.
  - Large lumbosacral hemangiomas should be investigated with a magnetic resonance imaging (MRI) of the spine.

CHAPTER 195

Erythema Multiforme, Stevens-Johnson Syndrome, and Toxic Epidermal Necrolysis

- Erythema multiforme (EM) is a common, self-limiting, acute hypersensitivity syndrome characterized by the abrupt onset of round, deep red, well-demarcated macules and papules with a dusky gray or bullous center (targetoid).
  - EM can be precipitated by infections (most commonly herpes simplex virus) or medications.
- Stevens-Johnson syndrome (SJS), toxic epidermal necrolysis (TEN), and SJS/TEN overlap are severe, life-threatening disorders thought to represent the same disease continuum. They are precipitated by medications.
  - SJS is defined as epidermal detachment of less than 10% of the body surface area, whereas SJS/TEN overlap has 10-30% and TEN has greater than 30% body surface area involvement.

CHAPTER 196

Cutaneous Infestations

- Scabies is caused by the mite *Sarcoptes scabiei.*
  - Curative treatment for scabies is achieved by a 12-hour (overnight) application of permethrin 5% cream applied to the entire body and repeated in 1 week. All household members and close contacts should be treated for scabies simultaneously, even if asymptomatic.
- Household treatment for scabies and pediculosis includes machine washing (in hot water) and machine drying (using high heat) all bed linens, towels, and clothes worn in the previous 2 days. Items that are not washable may be dry-cleaned or placed in a sealed plastic bag for 7 days (scabies) and 14 days (pediculosis).

SECTION 26

ORTHOPEDICS

Kevin D. Walter | J. Channing Tassone

CHAPTER 197

Orthopedics Assessment

To care for the pediatric patient, one must understand the growth and development of the musculoskeletal system as well as common orthopedic terms (Table 197.1). Providers should recognize common mechanisms for congenital and acquired orthopedic disorders (Table 197.2).

TABLE 197.1 Common Orthopedic Terminology

Abduction	Movement away from midline
Adduction	Movement toward or across midline
Apophysis	Bone growth center that has a muscular insertion but is not considered a growth plate (e.g., tibial tubercle)
Arthroscopy	Surgical exploration of a joint using an arthroscope
Arthroplasty	Surgical reconstruction of a joint
Arthrotomy	Surgical incision into a joint; an "open" procedure
Deformation	Changes in limb, trunk, or head due to mechanical force
Dislocation	Displacement of bones at a joint
Equinus	Plantar flexion of the forefoot, hindfoot, or entire foot
Femoral anteversion	Increased angulation of the femoral head and neck with respect to the frontal plane
Malformation	Defect in development that occurs during fetal life (e.g., syndactyly)
Osteotomy	Surgical division of a bone
Pes cavus	High medial arch of the foot
Pes planus	Flat foot
Rotation, internal	Inward rotation (toward midline)
Rotation, external	Outward rotation (away from midline)
Subluxation	Incomplete loss of contact between two joint surfaces
Tibial torsion	Rotation of the tibia in an internal or external fashion
Valgus/valgum	Angulation of a bone or joint in which the apex is toward the midline (e.g., knock-knee)
Varus/varum	Angulation of a bone or joint in which the apex is away from the midline (e.g., bowlegs)

GROWTH AND DEVELOPMENT

The ends of the long bones contain a much higher proportion of cartilage in the skeletally immature child than in an adult (Figs. 197.1 and 197.2). The high cartilage content allows for a unique vulnerability to trauma and infection (particularly in the metaphysis).

The physis is responsible for the longitudinal growth of the long bones. Articular cartilage allows the ends of the bone to enlarge and accounts for growth of smaller bones, such as the tarsals. The periosteum provides for circumferential growth. Trauma, infection, nutritional deficiency (rickets), inborn errors of metabolism (mucopolysaccharidoses), and

TABLE 197.2 Mechanisms of Common Pediatric Orthopedic Problems

CATEGORY	MECHANISM	EXAMPLE(S)
CONGENITAL		
Malformation	Teratogenesis before 12 wk of gestation	Spina bifida
Disruption	Amniotic band constriction	Extremity amputation
	Fetal varicella infection	Limb scar/atrophy
Deformation	Neck compression	Torticollis
Dysplasia	Abnormal cell growth or metabolism	Osteogenesis imperfecta Skeletal dysplasias
ACQUIRED		
Infection	Pyogenic-hematogenous spread	Septic arthritis, osteomyelitis
Inflammation	Antigen-antibody reaction	Systemic lupus erythematosus
	Immune mediated	Juvenile idiopathic arthritis
Trauma	Mechanical forces, overuse	Child abuse, sports injuries, unintentional injury, fractures, dislocations, tendinitis
Tumor	Primary bone tumor	Osteosarcoma
	Metastasis to bone from other site	Neuroblastoma
	Bone marrow tumor	Leukemia, lymphoma

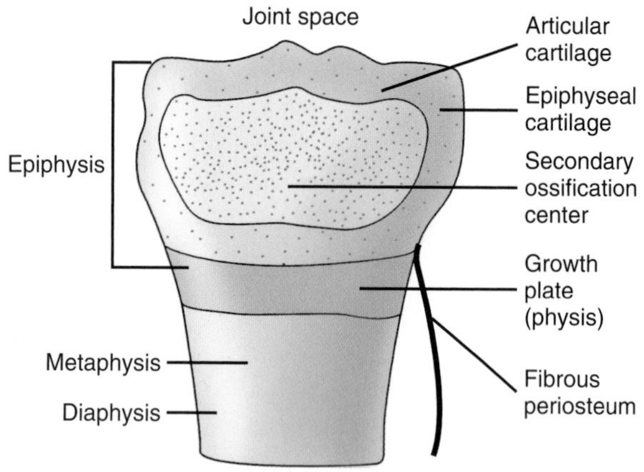

FIGURE 197.1 Schematic of long bone structure.

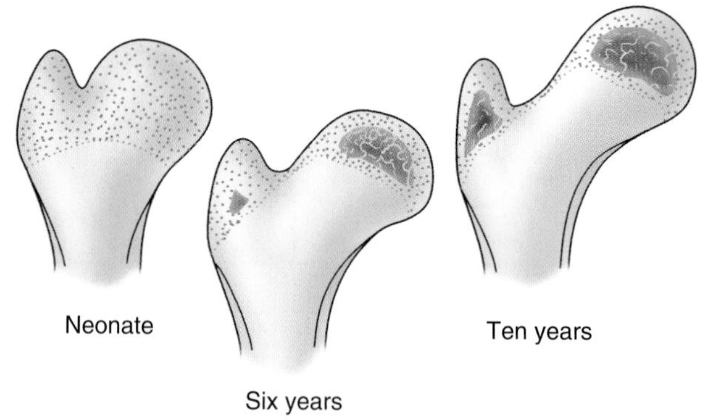

FIGURE 197.2 The ends of long bones at various ages. Lightly stippled areas represent cartilage composition, whereas heavily darkened areas are zones of ossification. (From Tachjidan MO. *Congenital Dislocation of the Hip*. New York: Churchill Livingstone; 1982:105.)

other disorders (renal tubular acidosis, hypothyroid) may affect each of the growth processes and produce distinct aberrations.

DEVELOPMENTAL MILESTONES

Neurological maturation, marked by achievement of developmental motor milestones, is important for normal musculoskeletal development (see Section 2). A neurological disorder may cause a secondary musculoskeletal abnormality (e.g., extremity contractures in Duchenne muscular dystrophy). Thus normal motor development must be included in the definition of a normal musculoskeletal system.

Infants

Decision-Making Algorithms
Available @ StudentConsult.com

In-Toeing, Out-Toeing, and Toe-Walking
Bowlegs and Knock-Knees

In utero positioning of the fetus may affect the angular and torsional alignment (temporary or permanent) of the skeletal system, especially of the lower extremity (Fig. 197.3). The newborn's hips are externally rotated. Pes planus and genu varum are common. Infants are usually born with a flexed posture, which usually decreases to neutral within the first 4-6 months. The foot is often flat and *tucked under* at birth; the ankle will be inverted, and the forefoot is adducted when compared with the hindfoot. The lateral border of the foot must straighten out, even with dorsiflexion, to be considered secondary to in utero positioning.

The head and neck may also be distorted by in utero positioning. The spine and upper extremities are less likely to be affected. By the age of 3-4 years, the effects of in utero positioning have usually resolved.

Gait

Normal gait has a stance phase and swing phase; each leg should have symmetrical timing with each phase. The stance phase represents 60% of the gait and begins with foot contact (usually the heel strike) and ends with the toe-off. During the swing phase (40%), the foot is off the ground. The gait cycle is the interval between stance phases on the same limb.

Toddlers will generally walk independently by 18 months of age. Their externally rotated gait is usually inconsistent, is characterized by short, rapid steps, and does not have the reciprocal arm swing. Gait coordination improves over time, with a normal gait usually achieved by the time a child enters elementary school.

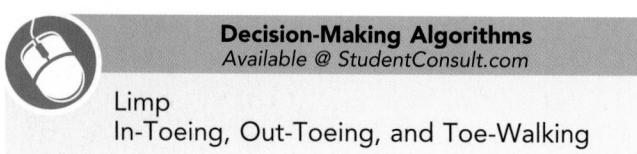

Decision-Making Algorithms
Available @ StudentConsult.com

Limp
In-Toeing, Out-Toeing, and Toe-Walking

Limping Child

The differential diagnosis for a limping child is often categorized by age and presence or absence of a painful limp (Table 197.3). The gluteus medius muscle stabilizes the pelvis during the stance phase, preventing the pelvis from dropping toward the leg in swing phase. An **antalgic gait** is a painful limp; the stance phase and stride of the affected limb are shortened to decrease the discomfort of weight bearing on the affected limb. The **Trendelenburg gait** has a normal stance phase but excessive swaying of the trunk. **Waddling gait** refers to a bilateral decrease in function of the gluteus muscles.

Toe walking is a common complaint in early walkers. A physician should evaluate any child older than 3 years of age who still toe walks. Although this is most likely habit, a neuromuscular disorder (cerebral palsy, tethered cord), Achilles tendon contracture (heel cord tightness), or a leg-length discrepancy should be considered.

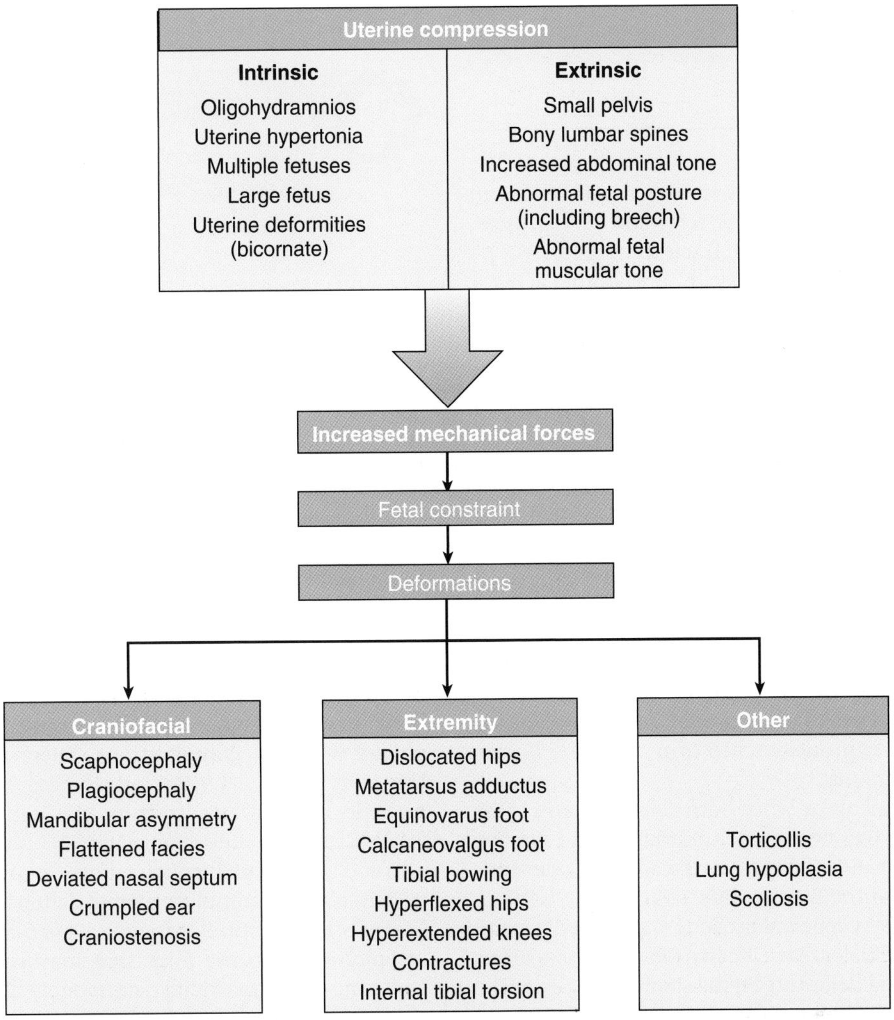

FIGURE 197.3 Deformation abnormalities resulting from uterine compression.

TABLE 197.3 Differential Diagnosis of Limping in Children

AGE GROUP	DIAGNOSTIC CONSIDERATIONS
Early walker: 1-3 yr of age	*Painful limp* Septic arthritis and osteomyelitis Transient monarticular synovitis Occult trauma ("toddler's fracture") Intervertebral diskitis Malignancy *Painless limp* Developmental dysplasia of the hip Neuromuscular disorder Cerebral palsy Lower extremity length inequality
Child: 3-10 yr of age	*Painful limp* Septic arthritis, osteomyelitis, myositis Transient monarticular synovitis Trauma Rheumatological disorders Juvenile idiopathic arthritis Intervertebral diskitis Malignancy *Painless limp* Developmental dysplasia of the hip Legg-Calve-Perthes disease Lower extremity length inequality Neuromuscular disorder Cerebral palsy Muscular dystrophy (Duchenne)
Adolescent: 11 yr of age to maturity	*Painful limp* Septic arthritis, osteomyelitis, myositis Trauma Rheumatological disorder Slipped capital femoral epiphysis: acute; unstable Malignancy *Painless limp* Slipped capital femoral epiphysis: chronic; stable Developmental dysplasia of the hip: acetabular dysplasia Lower extremity length inequality Neuromuscular disorder

CHAPTER 198

Fractures

Fractures account for 10-15% of all childhood injuries. The anatomical, biomechanical, and physiological differences in children account for unique fracture patterns and management. Fracture terminology helps describe fractures (Table 198.1).

The pediatric skeleton has a higher proportion of cartilage and a thicker, stronger, and more active periosteum capable of producing a larger callus more rapidly than in an adult. The thick periosteum may decrease the rate of displaced fractures and stabilize fractures after reduction. Because of the higher proportion of cartilage, the skeletally immature patient can withstand more force before deformation or fracture than adult bone. As children mature into adolescence, the rate of healing slows and approaches that of adults.

PEDIATRIC FRACTURE PATTERNS

Buckle or **torus fractures** occur after compression of the bone; the bony cortex does not truly break. These fractures will typically occur in the metaphysis and are stable fractures that heal in approximately 4 weeks with immobilization. A common example is a fall onto an outstretched arm causing a buckle fracture in the distal radius.

Complete fractures occur when both sides of bony cortex are fractured. This is the most common fracture and may be classified as comminuted, oblique, transverse, or spiral, depending on the direction of the fracture line.

Greenstick fractures occur when a bone is angulated beyond the limits of plastic deformation. The bone fails on the tension side and sustains a bend deformity on the compression side. The force is insufficient to cause a complete fracture (Fig. 198.1).

Bowing fractures demonstrate no fracture line evident on radiographs, but the bone is bent beyond its limit of plastic deformation. This is not a true fracture but will heal with periosteal reaction.

TABLE 198.1	Useful Fracture Terminology
Complete	The bone fragments separate completely
Incomplete	The bone fragments are still partially joined
Linear	Referring to a fracture line that is parallel to the bone's long axis
Transverse	Referring to a fracture line that is at a right angle to the bone's long axis
Oblique	Referring to a fracture line that is diagonal to the bone's long axis
Spiral	Referring to a twisting fracture
Comminution	A fracture that results in several fragments
Compaction	The bone fragments are driven into each other
Angulation	The fragments have angular malalignment
Rotation	The fragments have rotational malalignment
Shortening	The fractured ends of the bones overlap
Open	A fracture in which the bone has pierced the skin

Physeal Fractures

Decision-Making Algorithms
Available @ StudentConsult.com

Limp
Extremity Pain

Fractures involving the growth plate constitute about 20% of all fractures in the skeletally immature patient. These fractures are more common in males (2:1 male-female ratio). The peak incidence is 13-14 years in boys and 11-12 years in girls. The distal radius, distal tibia, and distal fibula are the most common locations.

Ligaments frequently insert onto epiphyses. Thus traumatic forces to an extremity may be transmitted to the physis, which is not as biomechanically strong as the metaphysis; it may fracture with mechanisms of injury that may cause sprains in the adult. The growth plate is most susceptible to torsional and angular forces.

Physeal fractures are described using **Salter-Harris classification,** which allows for prognostic information regarding premature closure of the growth plate and poor functional outcomes. The higher the type number, the more likely the patient will have complications. There are five main groups (Fig. 198.2):

- Type I: transverse fracture through the physis; growth disturbance is unusual
- Type II: fracture through a portion of the physis and metaphysis; most common type of Salter-Harris fracture (75%)
- Type III: fracture through a portion of the physis and epiphysis into the joint that may result in complication because of intraarticular component and because of disruption of the growing or hypertrophic zone of the physis
- Type IV: fracture through the metaphysis, physis, and epiphysis with a high risk of complication
- Type V: a crush injury to the physis with a poor functional prognosis

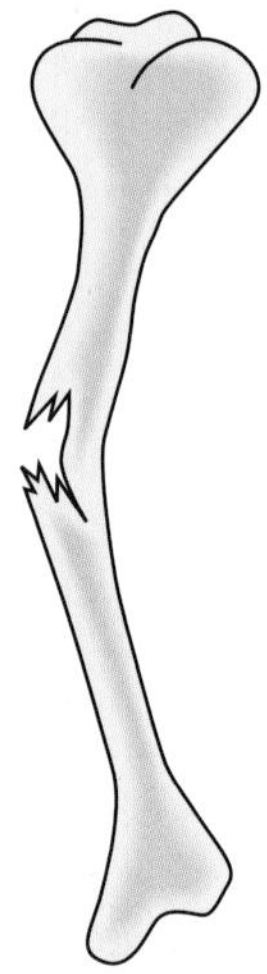

FIGURE 198.1 The greenstick fracture is an incomplete fracture. (Modified from White N, Sty R. Radiological evaluation and classification of pediatric fractures. *Clin Pediatr Emerg Med.* 2002;3:94–105.)

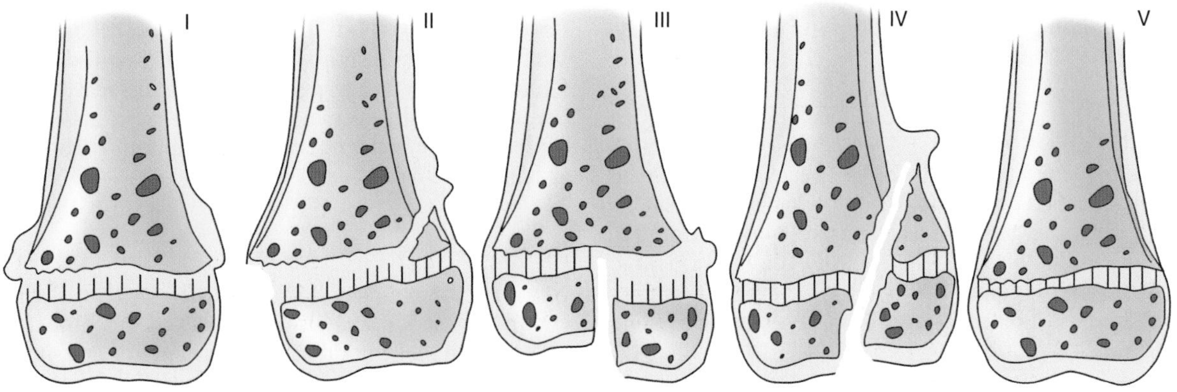

FIGURE 198.2 The types of growth plate injury as classified by Salter and Harris. See text for descriptions of types I to V. (From Salter RB, Harris WR. Injuries involving the epiphyseal plate. *J Bone Joint Surg Am*. 1963;45:587–622.)

Types I and II fractures can often be managed by closed reduction and do not require perfect alignment. A major exception is the type II fracture of the distal femur, which is associated with a poor outcome unless proper anatomical alignment is obtained. Types III and IV fractures require anatomical alignment for successful treatment. Type V fractures are rare and often result in premature closure of the physis.

MANAGEMENT OF PEDIATRIC FRACTURES

The majority of pediatric fractures can be managed with closed methods. Some fractures need closed reduction to improve alignment. Approximately 4% of pediatric fractures require internal fixation. Patients with open physes are more likely to require internal fixation if they have one of the following fractures:

- Displaced epiphyseal fractures
- Displaced intraarticular fractures
- Fractures in a child with multiple injuries
- Open fractures
- Unstable fractures

The goal of internal fixation is to improve and maintain anatomical alignment. This is usually done with Kirschner wires, Steinmann pins, and cortical screws with subsequent external immobilization in a cast until healing is satisfactory. After healing, the hardware is frequently removed to prevent incorporation into the callus and prevent physeal damage.

External fixation without casting may be necessary for pelvic fractures causing hemodynamic instability. Fractures associated with soft tissue loss, burns, and neurovascular damage may benefit from external fixation.

SPECIAL CONCERNS

Remodeling

Fracture remodeling occurs because of a combination of periosteal resorption and new bone formation. Many pediatric fractures do not need perfect anatomical alignment for proper healing. Younger patients have greater potential for fracture remodeling. Fractures that occur in the metaphysis, near the growth plate, may undergo more remodeling. Fractures angulated in the plane of motion also remodel very well. Intraarticular fractures, angulated or displaced diaphyseal fractures, rotated fractures, and fracture deformity not in the plane of motion tend not to remodel as well.

Overgrowth

Overgrowth occurs in long bones as the result of increased blood flow associated with fracture healing. Femoral fractures in children younger than 10 years of age will frequently overgrow 1-3 cm. This is the reason end-to-end alignment for femur and long-bone fractures may not be indicated. After 10 years of age, overgrowth is less of a problem, so end-to-end alignment is recommended.

Progressive Deformity

Fractures and injuries to the physis can result in premature closure. If it is a partial closure, the consequence may be an angular deformity. If it is a complete closure, limb shortening may occur. The most commonly affected locations are the distal femur and the distal and proximal tibia.

Neurovascular Injury

Fractures and dislocations may damage adjacent blood vessels and nerves. The most common location is the distal humerus **(supracondylar fracture)** and the knee (dislocation and physeal fracture). It is necessary to perform and document a careful neurovascular examination distal to the fracture (pulse, sensory, and motor function).

Compartment Syndrome

Compartment syndrome is an **orthopedic emergency** that results from hemorrhage and soft tissue swelling within the tight fascial compartments of an extremity. This can result in muscle ischemia and neurovascular compromise unless it is surgically decompressed. The most common sites are the lower leg (tibial fracture) and arm (supracondylar fracture).

Affected patients have severe pain and will eventually have decreased sensation in the dermatomes supplied by the nerves located in the compartment. Swollen and tight compartments and pain with passive stretching are present. This can happen underneath a cast and may actually occur when a cast is applied too tightly. It is important to educate all patients with fractures on the signs of compartment syndrome and ensure that they realize it is an emergency.

Toddler's Fracture

This is an oblique fracture of the distal tibia without a fibula fracture. There is often no significant trauma. Patients are usually 1-3 years old but can be as old as 6 and present with limping and pain with weight bearing. There may be minimal swelling and pain. Initial radiographs do not always show the fracture; if symptoms persist, a repeat x-ray in 7-10 days may be helpful.

Child Abuse

Decision-Making Algorithm
Available @ StudentConsult.com

Extremity Pain

Child abuse must always be considered in the differential diagnosis of a child with fractures, especially in those younger than 3 years (see Chapter 22). Common fracture patterns that should increase the index of suspicion include multiple fractures in different stages of radiographic healing, metaphyseal corner fractures (twisting and shaking), fractures too severe for the history, or fractures in nonambulatory infants. Although spiral fractures of long bones were historically considered pathognomonic for abuse, they can be seen in nonabuse situations.

When there is concern for child abuse, the child should have a full evaluation, which may include admission to the hospital. A thorough and well-documented physical examination should focus on soft tissue injuries, the cranium, and a funduscopic examination for retinal hemorrhages or detachment. A skeletal survey or a bone scan may be helpful in identifying other fractures.

CHAPTER 199

Hip

The hip is a ball (femoral head) and socket (acetabulum) joint that is important for skeletal stability. The femoral head and acetabulum are interdependent for normal growth and development. The femoral neck and head, which contain the capital femoral epiphysis, are intraarticular. The blood supply to this region is unique because the blood vessels are extraosseous and lie on the surface of the femoral neck, entering the epiphysis peripherally. Thus the blood supply to the femoral head is vulnerable to trauma, infection, and other causes that may increase intraarticular pressure. Damage to the blood supply can lead to **avascular necrosis**.

DEVELOPMENTAL DYSPLASIA OF THE HIP

In developmental dysplasia of the hip (DDH), the hips may be dislocated or dislocatable at birth. The femoral head and acetabulum develop from the same mesenchymal cells; by 11 weeks' gestation, the hip joint is formed. There are two types of DDH: teratological and typical. **Teratological dislocations** occur early in utero and are usually associated with neuromuscular disorders (spina bifida, arthrogryposis). **Typical dislocations** occur in the neurologically normal infant and can occur before or after birth. The true incidence of DDH is unknown, but it may be as high as 1.5 cases per 1,000 infants.

Etiology

Newborn infants have ligamentous laxity that, if significant enough in the hip, may lead to spontaneous dislocation and reduction of the femoral head. Persistence of this spontaneous pattern can lead to pathological changes, such as flattening of the acetabulum, muscle contractures that limit motion, and joint capsule tightening. The left hip is affected three times as often as the right hip, possibly because of in utero positioning.

Physiological risk factors for DDH include a generalized ligamentous laxity, perhaps from maternal hormones that are associated with pelvic ligament relaxation (estrogen and relaxin). Female infants are at higher risk (9 : 1); family history is positive in 20% of all patients with DDH.

Other risk factors include breech presentation, firstborn child (60%), oligohydramnios, and postnatal infant positioning. In breech presentations, the fetal pelvis is situated in the maternal pelvis. This can increase hip flexion and limit overall fetal hip motion, causing further stretching of the already lax joint capsule and exposing the posterior aspect of the femoral head. The altered relationship between the acetabulum and femoral head causes abnormal acetabular development. Postnatal positioning of the hips in a tight swaddle with the hips adducted and extended can displace the hip joint.

Congenital muscular torticollis, metatarsus adductus, and clubfoot are associated with DDH. An infant with any of these three conditions should receive a careful examination of the hips.

Clinical Manifestations

Every newborn requires a screening physical examination for DDH; further evaluation through at least the first 18 months of life is part of the physical examination for toddlers. DDH evolves over time, so the examination may change as the patient ages. The examination starts with inspection for asymmetrical thigh and gluteal folds with the hips and knees flexed. A relative shortening of the femur with asymmetrical skin folds is a positive **Galeazzi sign** and indicates DDH. Range of motion should be assessed with the pelvis stabilized and the child supine on the examining table, not in the parent's lap (Fig. 199.1). Hip abduction should easily reach or exceed 75 degrees, and hip adduction should reach 30 degrees. Limitations may indicate contractures associated with DDH, especially decreased abduction.

The **Barlow test** attempts to dislocate an unstable hip (Fig. 199.2). The examiner should stabilize the infant's pelvis with one hand and grasp the abducted and flexed thigh in the other hand. The hip should be flexed to 90 degrees. Next, begin to adduct the hip while applying a posterior force to the anterior hip. A hip that can be dislocated in this method is readily felt (clunk feeling) and is a positive test. It may reduce spontaneously once the posterior force is removed, or the examiner may need to perform the Ortolani test.

The **Ortolani test** may reduce a dislocated hip (Fig. 199.3). The examiner should stabilize the pelvis and hold the leg in the

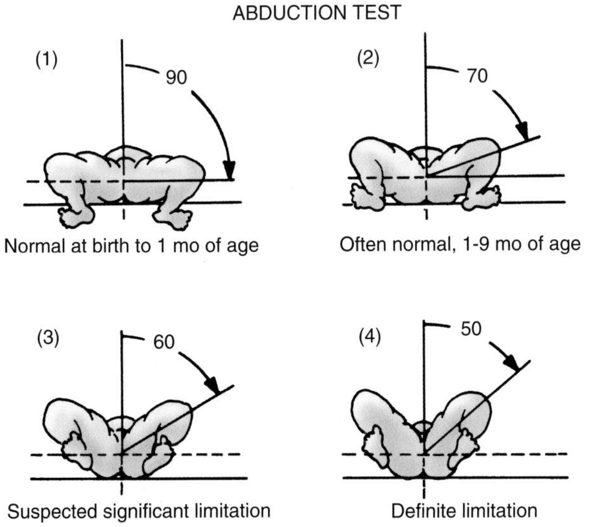

FIGURE 199.1 Hip abduction test. Place the infant supine, flex the hips 90 degrees, and fully abduct the hips. Although the normal abduction range is broad, hip disease should be suspected in any patient who lacks more than 30-45 degrees of abduction. (From Chung SMK. *Hip Disorders in Infants and Children*. Philadelphia: Lea & Febiger; 1981:69.)

same method as for the Barlow test. The infant's hip should be in 90 degrees of flexion. Abduct the hip while applying anterior pressure to the posterior thigh. A positive test is the palpable reduction of the dislocation, which may be felt (clunk). After 2 months of age, the hip may develop muscular contractures, preventing positive Ortolani tests.

These tests should be performed with only gentle force and done one hip at a time. The test may need to be repeated multiple times, as they can be difficult to interpret. A click, which is not pathological, may occur from breaking the surface tension of the hip joint or snapping gluteal tendons.

Bilateral fixed dislocations present a diagnostic dilemma because of the symmetry on exam. The **Klisic test** is useful in this situation; it is done by placing the third finger over the greater trochanter and the index finger over the anterior superior iliac spine, then drawing an imaginary line between the two. The line should point to the umbilicus in a normal child. However, in a dislocated hip, the greater trochanter is elevated, which causes the line to project lower (between the umbilicus and pubis). This test is helpful in identifying bilateral DDH, which can otherwise be difficult to diagnose because of the symmetry found on examination.

Older children with unrecognized DDH may present with limping. A patient with increased lumbar lordosis and a waddling gait may have an unrecognized bilateral DDH.

Radiographic Evaluation

Ultrasound is used for initial evaluation of infants with DDH. Ultrasonography is necessary for girls with a positive family history or breech presentation in both sexes. This should be obtained after 6 weeks of age to avoid confusion with physiological laxity. Because the femoral head begins to ossify at 4-6 months of age, plain radiographs can be misleading until patients are older.

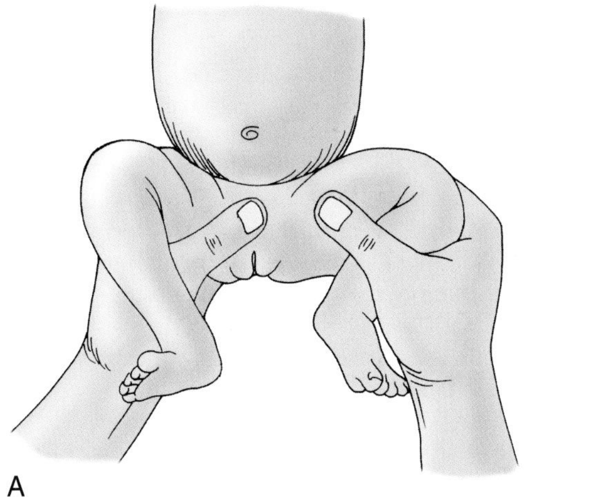

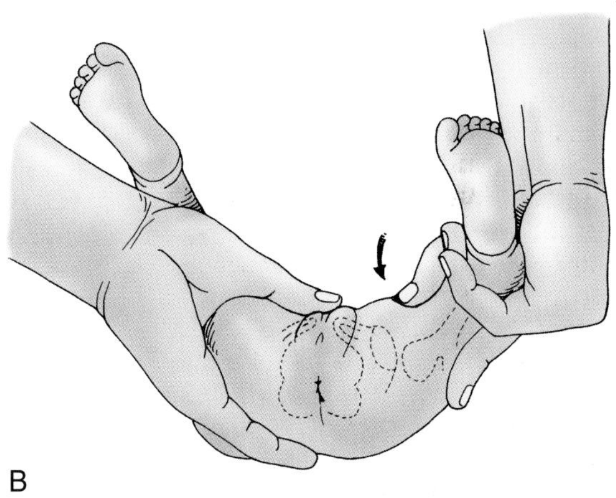

FIGURE 199.2 Barlow (dislocation) test. Reverse of Ortolani test. If the femoral head is in the acetabulum at the time of examination, the Barlow test is performed to discover any hip instability. **(A)** The infant's thigh is grasped as shown and adducted with gentle downward pressure. **(B)** Dislocation is palpable as the femoral head slips out of the acetabulum. Diagnosis is confirmed with the Ortolani test.

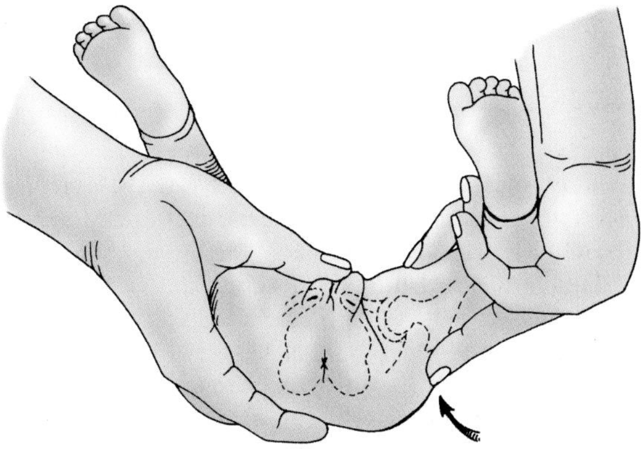

FIGURE 199.3 Ortolani (reduction) test. With the infant relaxed and content on a firm surface, the hips and knees are flexed to 90 degrees. The hips are examined one at a time. The examiner grasps the infant's thigh with the middle finger over the greater trochanter and lifts the thigh to bring the femoral head from its dislocated posterior position to opposite the acetabulum. Simultaneously the thigh is gently abducted, reducing the femoral head in the acetabulum. In a positive finding, the examiner senses reduction by a palpable, nearly audible *clunk*.

Treatment

The treatment of DDH is individualized and depends on the child's age at diagnosis. The goal of treatment is a stable reduction that results in normal growth and development of the hip. If DDH is suspected, the child should be sent to a pediatric orthopedic specialist.

The **Pavlik harness** is an effective treatment up to 6 months of age. It provides hip flexion to just over 90 degrees and limits adduction to no more than neutral. This positioning redirects the femoral head toward the acetabulum. The hip must be reduced within 1-2 weeks of beginning the Pavlik harness, although the infant will need more time in the device. The Pavlik harness is successful in treating approximately 95% of dysplastic or subluxated hips, and 80% successful for treatment of true dislocations. Persistently dislocated hips should not remain in a Pavlik harness for more than 2 weeks for fear of iatrogenic acetabular damage. Patients failing the Pavlik harness warrant treatment with an abduction orthosis.

Children over 6 months or those who have failed nonoperative treatment should undergo closed reduction using a hip spica cast. This is done under general anesthesia; reduction is evaluated with an intraoperative arthrogram then confirmed by postoperative computed tomography (CT) or magnetic resonance imaging (MRI). If closed reduction fails, open reduction is indicated. Patients over 18 months of age may require a pelvic and femoral osteotomy.

Complications

The most important and severe complication of DDH is iatrogenic avascular necrosis of the femoral head. This can occur from excessive flexion or abduction during positioning of the Pavlik harness or hip spica cast. Infants under 6 months of age are at highest risk. Pressure ulcers can occur with prolonged casting. Redislocation or subluxation of the femoral head and residual acetabular dysplasia can occur.

TRANSIENT MONOARTICULAR SYNOVITIS

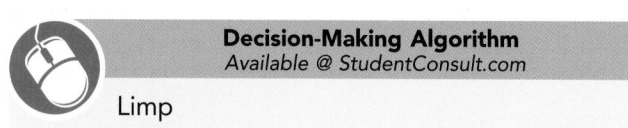

Decision-Making Algorithm
Available @ StudentConsult.com

Limp

Transient synovitis, also known as **toxic synovitis**, is a common cause of limping in children. It is a diagnosis of exclusion because **septic arthritis** and **osteomyelitis** of the hip must be excluded (see Chapters 117 and 118).

Etiology and Epidemiology

The etiology of transient synovitis is uncertain, but possible causes are viral illness and hypersensitivity. Approximately 70% of children diagnosed with transient synovitis have an upper respiratory tract viral infection in the preceding 7-14 days. Biopsies have revealed nonspecific synovial hypertrophy. Hip joint aspirations, when necessary, are negative for bacterial culture or signs of bacterial infection.

The mean age at onset is 6 years, with a range of 3-8 years. It is twice as common in male children.

Clinical Manifestations and Evaluation

The patient or family will describe an acute onset of pain in the groin/hip, anterior thigh, or knee. Irritation of the obturator nerve can cause referred pain in the thigh and knee when the pathology is at the hip. Patients with transient synovitis are often afebrile, walk with a painful limp, and have normal to minimally elevated white blood cell count, C-reactive protein, and erythrocyte sedimentation rate compared with bacterial diseases of the hip (Table 199.1). Table 197.3 lists the differential diagnosis of a limping child.

Anteroposterior and frog-leg radiographs of the hip are usually normal. Ultrasonography may reveal a joint effusion. It is mandatory to rule out septic arthritis in the presence of effusion with a joint aspiration and cell count.

Treatment

The mainstay of treatment is bed rest and minimal weight bearing until the pain resolves. Nonsteroidal antiinflammatory medication is usually sufficient to decrease pain. Limiting strenuous activity and exercise for 1-2 weeks following recovery is helpful. Follow-up will help ensure that there is no deterioration. Lack of improvement necessitates further evaluation for more serious disorders.

LEGG-CALVE-PERTHES DISEASE

Etiology and Epidemiology

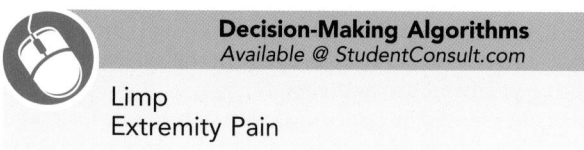

Decision-Making Algorithms
Available @ StudentConsult.com

Limp
Extremity Pain

Legg-Calve-Perthes disease (LCPD) is idiopathic **avascular necrosis (osteonecrosis)** of the capital epiphysis of the femoral head. The etiology is unclear, but it is likely caused by an interruption of the blood supply to the capital femoral epiphysis. There may be an associated hypercoagulability state (factor V Leiden).

TABLE 199.1 Differences Between Bacterial Infection and Transient Synovitis

BACTERIAL INFECTION*	TRANSIENT SYNOVITIS
Elevated joint fluid cell count	Afebrile
Fever—temperature >38.5°C	
Leukocytosis	Normal WBC count
ESR >20 mm/hr	Normal ESR and CRP
Refusal to walk	Painful limp
Hip held in external rotation, abduction, and flexion	Hip held normally
Severe pain and tenderness	Moderate pain and mild tenderness

*Examples: Septic arthritis, osteomyelitis of hip.
CRP, C-reactive protein; *ESR*, erythrocyte sedimentation rate; *WBC*, white blood cell.

LCPD commonly presents in patients 3-12 years of age, with a mean age of 7 years. It is four to five times more common in boys.

Clinical Manifestations

Patients may not present for several weeks because of minimal discomfort; the classic presentation is a child with an atraumatic, painless limp. There may be mild or intermittent hip/groin, anterior thigh, or knee pain. Decreased internal rotation and abduction with some discomfort, thigh muscle spasm, and anterior thigh muscular atrophy may be present. Patients have delayed bone age.

Radiological Evaluation

Anteroposterior and frog-leg radiographs of both hips are usually adequate for diagnosis and management. It is necessary to document the extent of the disease and follow its progression. MRI and bone scan are helpful to diagnose early LCPD.

Treatment and Prognosis

LCPD is usually a self-limited disorder that should be followed by a pediatric orthopedist. Initial treatment focuses on pain control and restoration of hip range of motion. The goal of treatment is prevention of complications, such as femoral head deformity and secondary osteoarthritis (OA).

Containment is important in treating LCPD; the femoral head is contained inside the acetabulum, which acts like a mold for the capital femoral epiphysis as it reossifies. Nonsurgical containment uses abduction casts and orthoses, whereas surgical containment is accomplished with osteotomies of the proximal femur and pelvis.

The short-term prognosis is determined by the magnitude of the femoral head deformity after healing has completed. It is improved by early diagnosis, good follow-up, and compliance with the treatment plan. Older children and children with a residual femoral head deformity are more likely to develop OA. The incidence of OA in patients who developed LCPD after 10 years of age is close to 100%; it is negligible in children with onset before 5 years of age. Patients between 6 and 9 years of age have a risk of OA of less than 40%.

SLIPPED CAPITAL FEMORAL EPIPHYSIS

Decision-Making Algorithms
Available @ StudentConsult.com

Limp
Extremity Pain

Etiology and Epidemiology

Slipped capital femoral epiphysis (SCFE) is an adolescent hip disorder that is an orthopedic emergency. The incidence is 10.8 per 100,000, and it is slightly higher in males. African-American and Hispanic populations are at higher risk. Approximately 20% of patients with SCFE will have bilateral involvement at presentation, and another 20-40% may progress to bilateral involvement. The average age is 10-16 years, with a mean of 12 years in boys and 11 years in girls. Additional risk factors for SCFE include obesity, trisomy 21, and endocrine disorders (hypothyroid, pituitary tumor, growth hormone deficiency).

Classification

SCFE is classified as stable or unstable. Unstable patients refuse to ambulate even with crutches. Stable patients have an antalgic gait. SCFE can also be characterized as acute (symptoms <3 weeks) or chronic (symptoms >3 weeks). Acute-on-chronic SCFE is seen when more than 3 weeks of symptoms are accompanied by an acute exacerbation of pain and difficulty/inability to bear weight.

Clinical Manifestation

The presentation is variable, based on severity and type of slip. Patients will often report hip or knee pain, limp or inability to ambulate, and decreased hip range of motion. There may or may not be a traumatic event. *Any knee pain mandates an examination of the hip, as hip pathology can cause referred pain to the anterior thigh and knee along the obturator nerve.* The patient usually holds the affected extremity in external rotation. As the hip is flexed, it will progressively externally rotate. There is usually a limitation of internal rotation, but there may also be a loss of flexion and abduction. If the patient can bear weight, it is typically an antalgic gait with the affected leg in external rotation. It is important to examine both hips to determine bilateral involvement.

Radiological Evaluation

Anteroposterior and frog-leg radiographs are indicated. Patients with known SCFE or with a high index of suspicion should not undergo frog-leg lateral radiographs. Instead, a cross table lateral radiograph reduces the risk of iatrogenic progression. The earliest sign of SCFE is widening of the physis without slippage **(preslip condition).** Klein's line (Fig. 199.4) is helpful in assessing the anteroposterior radiograph for SCFE. The slippage can be classified radiographically as type I (0-33% displacement), type II (34-50%), or type III (>50%). The likelihood of complications increases with degree of displacement.

Treatment

Patients with SCFE should be immediately made non–weight bearing and referred to a pediatric orthopedist. The goal is to prevent further slippage, enhance physeal closure, and minimize complications, which is usually accomplished with internal fixation in situ with a single cannulated screw. More severe cases may require surgical hip dislocation and reduction to realign the epiphysis. There is controversy surrounding the prophylactic fixation of the nonaffected side. Assessment for endocrine disorders is important, particularly in children outside the range of 10-16 years of age.

Complications

The two most serious complications of SCFE are **chondrolysis** and **avascular necrosis.** Chondrolysis is destruction of the articular cartilage. It is associated with more severe slips and with intraarticular penetration of operative hardware. This can

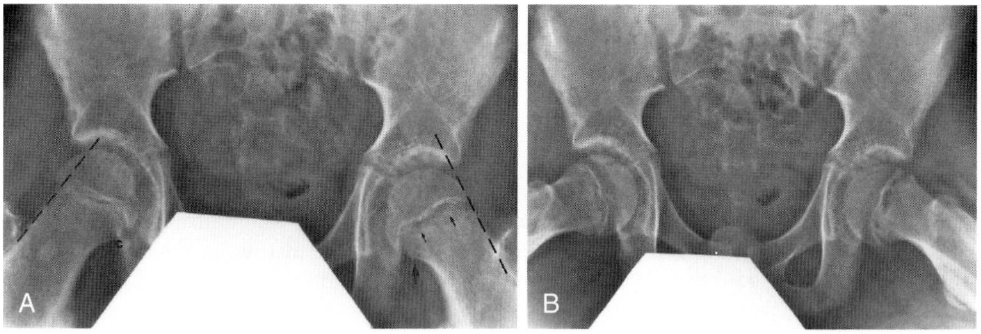

FIGURE 199.4 Slipped capital femoral epiphysis. **(A)** Anteroposterior radiograph reveals a widened physis *(small arrows)* and decreased height of the epiphysis on the left. In addition, there is loss *(large arrow)* of the Capener triangle *(c)* (normal double density of the medial metaphysis superimposed on the posterior acetabular rim on *right*) and an abnormal lateral femoral neck line (normal on *right*). **(B)** Frog, lateral view confirms the inferomedial position of the slipped capital femoral epiphysis. (From Blickman H. *Pediatric Radiology, the Requisites.* 2nd ed. St Louis: Mosby; 1998:244.)

lead to severe OA and disability. Avascular necrosis occurs when there is a disruption of the blood supply to the capital femoral epiphysis. This usually happens at the time of injury but may occur during forced manipulation of an unstable slip. Avascular necrosis may occur in up to 50% of unstable SCFEs and may lead to OA.

CHAPTER 200

Lower Extremity and Knee

Torsional (in-toeing and out-toeing) and angular (physiological bowlegs and knock knees) variations in the legs are common reasons that parents seek medical attention for their child. Most of these concerns are physiological and resolve with normal growth. Understanding the natural history allows physicians to reassure the family and to identify nonphysiological disorders that necessitate further intervention. Physiological disturbances are referred to as variations; pathological disturbances are called deformities.

TORSIONAL VARIATIONS

The femur is internally rotated (anteversion) about 30 degrees at birth, decreasing to about 10 degrees at maturity. The tibia begins with up to 30 degrees of internal rotation at birth and can decrease to a mean of 15 degrees at maturity.

Torsional variations should not cause a limp or pain. Unilateral torsion raises the index of suspicion for a neurological (hemiplegia) or neuromuscular disorder.

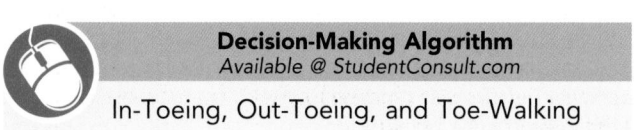

In-Toeing

Decision-Making Algorithm
Available @ StudentConsult.com
In-Toeing, Out-Toeing, and Toe-Walking

TABLE **200.1** Common Causes of In-Toeing and Out-Toeing

IN-TOEING	OUT-TOEING
Internal femoral torsion or anteversion	External femoral torsion or retroversion
Internal tibial torsion	External tibial torsion
Metatarsus adductus	Calcaneovalgus feet
Talipes equinovarus (clubfoot)	Hypermobile pes planus (flatfoot)
Developmental dysplasia	Slipped capital femoral epiphysis

Femoral Anteversion

Internal femoral torsion or femoral anteversion is the most common cause of in-toeing in children 2 years or older (Table 200.1). It is at its worst between 4 and 6 years of age, and then resolves. It occurs twice as often in girls. Many cases are associated with generalized ligamentous laxity. The etiology of femoral anteversion is likely congenital and is common in individuals with abnormal sitting habits such as *W-sitting.*

Clinical Manifestations. The family may give a history of W-sitting, and there may be a family history of similar concerns when the parents were younger. The child may have *kissing kneecaps* due to increased internal rotation of the femur. While walking, the entire leg will appear internally rotated, and with running, the child may appear to have an *egg-beater* gait where the legs flip laterally. The flexed hip will have internal rotation increased to 80-90 degrees (normal 60-70 degrees) and external rotation limited to about 10 degrees. Radiographic evaluation is usually not indicated.

Internal Tibial Torsion

Decision-Making Algorithm
Available @ StudentConsult.com
In-Toeing, Out-Toeing, and Toe-Walking

This is the most common cause of in-toeing in a child *younger* than 2 years old. When it is the result of in utero positioning, it may be associated with metatarsus adductus.

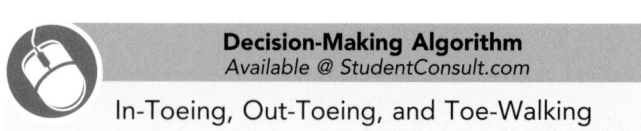

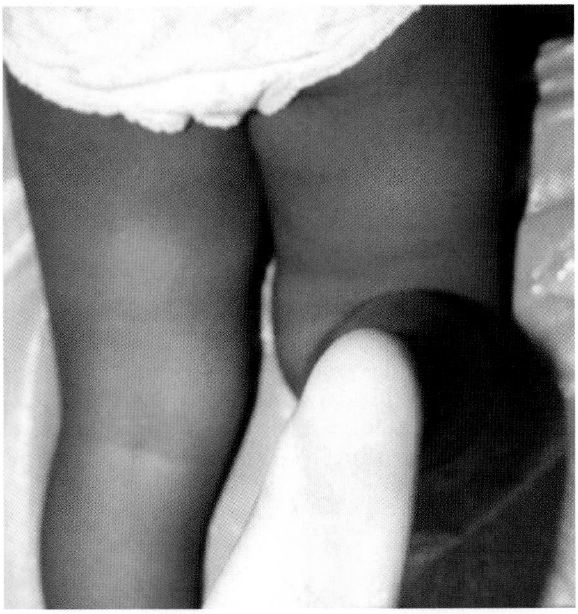

FIGURE 200.1 Thigh-foot angle measurement. The thigh-foot angle is useful for assessment of tibial torsion. The patient lies prone, with knees flexed to 90 degrees. The long axis of the thigh is compared to the long axis of the foot to determine the thigh-foot angle. Negative angles are associated with internal tibial torsion, and positive angles are associated with external tibial torsion.

Clinical Manifestations. The child will present with a history of in-toeing. The degree of tibial torsion may be measured using the **thigh-foot angle** (Fig. 200.1). The patient lies prone on a table with the knee flexed to 90 degrees. The long axis of the foot is compared with the long axis of the thigh. An inwardly rotated foot represents a negative angle and internal tibial torsion. If follow-up is warranted, measurements should be done at each visit to document improvement.

Treatment of In-Toeing

The mainstay of management is to identify patients who have pathological reasons for in-toeing and reassurance and follow-up to document improvement for patients with femoral anteversion and internal tibial torsion. It can take until 7-8 years of age for correction, so it is important to inform families of the appropriate timeline. Braces (Denis Browne splint) do not improve these conditions. Fewer than 1% of all patients with in-toeing will need surgical intervention because of functional disability or cosmetic appearance.

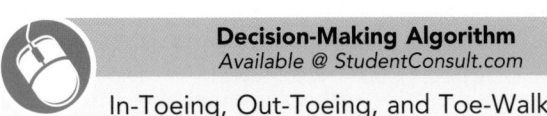

Out-Toeing

Decision-Making Algorithm
Available @ StudentConsult.com
In-Toeing, Out-Toeing, and Toe-Walking

External Tibial Torsion

External tibial torsion is the most common cause of out-toeing and may be associated with a calcaneovalgus foot (see Chapter 201). This is often related to in utero positioning. It may improve over time, but because the tibia rotates externally with age, external tibial torsion can worsen. It may be an etiological factor for patellofemoral syndrome, especially when combined with femoral anteversion. Treatment is usually observation and reassurance, but patients with dysfunction and cosmetic concerns may benefit from surgical intervention.

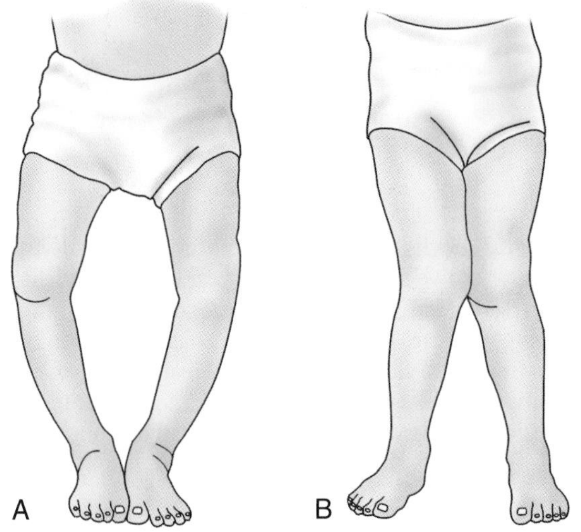

FIGURE 200.2 Bowleg and knock-knee deformities. **(A)** Bowleg deformity. Bowlegs are referred to as varus angulation (genu varum) because the knees are tilted away from the midline of the body. **(B)** Knock-knee or valgus deformity of the knees. The knee is tilted toward the midline. (From Scoles P. *Pediatric Orthopedics in Clinical Practice.* Chicago: Year Book Medical Publishers; 1982:84.)

ANGULAR VARIATIONS

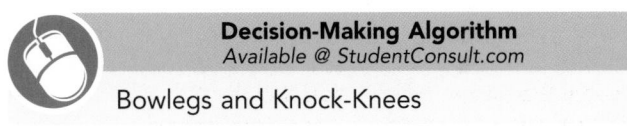

Decision-Making Algorithm
Available @ StudentConsult.com
Bowlegs and Knock-Knees

The majority of patients who present with knock-knees **(genu valgum)** or bowlegs **(genu varum)** are normal (Fig. 200.2). Infants are born with maximum genu varum. The lower extremity straightens out around 18 months of age. Children typically progress to maximal genu valgum around 4 years. The legs are usually straight to a slight genu valgum in adulthood.

It is important to inquire about family history and assess overall height. A child who is two standard deviations below normal with angular deformities may have skeletal dysplasia. Dietary history should be obtained, as rickets (see Chapter 31) may cause angular deformities. For genu valgum, following the intermalleolar distance (distance between the two tibial medial malleoli with the knees touching) is used. Measurement of the intercondylar distance (the distance between the medial femoral condyles with the medial malleoli touching) is used for genu varum. These measurements track improvement or progression. When obtaining radiographs, it is important to have the patella, not the feet, facing forward. In the child with external tibial torsion, having the feet facing forward gives the false appearance of bowlegs.

Genu Valgum

Decision-Making Algorithm
Available @ StudentConsult.com

Bowlegs and Knock-Knees

Physiological knock-knees are most common in 3- to 4-year-olds and usually resolve between 5 and 8 years of age. Patients with asymmetrical genu valgum or severe deformity may have underlying disease causing their knock-knees (e.g., renal osteodystrophy, skeletal dysplasia). Treatment is based on reassurance of the family and patient. Surgical intervention may be indicated for severe deformities, gait dysfunction, pain, and cosmesis.

Genu Varum

Decision-Making Algorithm
Available @ StudentConsult.com

Bowlegs and Knock-Knees

Physiological bowlegs are most common in children older than 18 months with symmetrical genu varum. This will generally improve as the child approaches 2 years of age. The most important consideration for genu varum is differentiating between physiological genu varum and Blount disease (tibia vara).

Tibia Vara (Blount Disease)

Decision-Making Algorithms
Available @ StudentConsult.com

Extremity Pain
Bowlegs and Knock-Knees

Tibia vara is the most common pathological disorder associated with genu varum. It is characterized by abnormal growth of the medial aspect of the proximal tibial epiphysis, resulting in a progressive varus deformity. Blount disease is classified according to age of onset:

- Infantile (1-3 years)
- Juvenile (4-10 years)
- Adolescent (>11 years)

Late-onset Blount disease is less common than infantile disease. The cause is unknown, but it is felt to be secondary to growth suppression from increased compressive forces across the medial knee.

Clinical Manifestations

Infantile tibia vara is more common in African Americans, females, and obese patients. Many patients were early walkers. Nearly 80% of patients with infantile Blount disease have bilateral involvement. It is usually painless. The patients will often have significant internal tibial torsion and lower extremity leg-length discrepancy (LLD). There may also be a palpable medial tibial metaphyseal beak.

Late-onset Blount disease is more common in African Americans, males, and markedly obese patients. Only 50% have bilateral involvement. The initial presentation is usually painful bowlegs. Late-onset Blount disease is usually not associated with palpable metaphyseal beaking, significant internal tibial torsion, or significant LLD.

Radiological Evaluation

Weight-bearing anteroposterior and lateral radiographs of both legs are necessary for the diagnosis of tibia vara. Fragmentation, wedging, and beak deformities of the proximal medial tibia are the major radiological features of infantile Blount disease. In late-onset Blount disease, the medial deformity may not be as readily noticeable. It can be very difficult to tell the difference between physiological genu varum and infantile Blount disease on radiographs in patients younger than 2 years of age.

Treatment

Once the diagnosis of Blount disease is confirmed, treatment should begin immediately. Orthotics to unload the medial compressive forces can be used in children younger than 3 years of age with a mild deformity. Compliance with this regimen can be difficult. Nonoperative management of more severe Blount disease is contraindicated. Any patient older than 4 years should undergo surgical intervention. Patients with moderate to severe deformity and patients who fail orthotic treatment also require surgical intervention. Proximal tibial valgus osteotomy with fibular diaphyseal osteotomy is the usual procedure performed.

LEG-LENGTH DISCREPANCY

Decision-Making Algorithm
Available @ StudentConsult.com

In-Toeing, Out-Toeing, and Toe-Walking

LLD is common and may be due to differences in the femur, tibia, or both bones. The differential diagnosis is extensive, but common causes are listed in Table 200.2. The majority of the lower extremity growth comes from the distal femur (38%) and the proximal tibia (27%).

Measuring Leg-Length Discrepancy

Clinical measurements using bony landmarks (anterior superior iliac spine to medial malleolus) are inaccurate. The **teloradiograph** is a single radiograph of both legs that can be done in very young children. The **orthoradiograph** consists of three slightly overlapping exposures of the hips, knees, and ankles. The **scanogram** consists of three standard radiographs of the hips, knees, and ankles with a ruler next to the extremities. A **computed tomography (CT) scanogram** is the most accurate measure of LLD but also has the highest radiation exposure. Technology such as EOS/slot scanning is an extremely accurate, reduced-radiation alternative to CT scan. The measured discrepancy is followed using Moseley and Green-Anderson graphs.

TABLE 200.2	Common Causes of Leg-Length Discrepancy
Congenital	Coxa vara Clubfoot Hypoplasia
Developmental	Developmental dysplasia of the hip (DDH) Legg-Calve-Perthes disease (LCPD)
Neuromuscular	Hemiplegia Disuse secondary to developmental delay
Infectious	Physeal injury secondary to osteomyelitis
Tumors	Fibrous dysplasia Physeal injury secondary to irradiation or neoplastic infiltration Overgrowth
Trauma	Physeal injury with premature closure Malunion (shortening of extremity) Overgrowth of healing fracture
Syndrome	Neurofibromatosis Beckwith-Wiedemann syndrome Klippel-Trenaunay syndrome

Treatment

Treating LLD is complex. The physician must take into account the estimated adult height, discrepancy measurements, skeletal maturity, and the psychological aspects of the patient and family. LLD greater than 2 cm usually requires treatment. Shoe lifts can be used, but they will often cause psychosocial problems for the child and may make the shoes heavier and less stable. Surgical options include shortening of the longer extremity, lengthening of the shorter extremity, or a combination of the two procedures. Discrepancies less than 5 cm are treated by epiphysiodesis (surgical physeal closure) of the affected side, whereas discrepancies greater than 5 cm are treated by lengthening. Current use of removable implants, which permit growth modulation without permanent impact on growth plates, has allowed for early and more accurate treatment.

KNEE

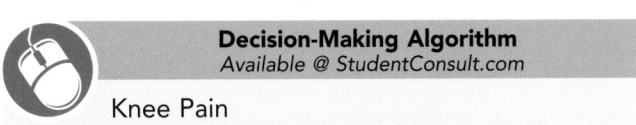

Decision-Making Algorithm
Available @ StudentConsult.com

Knee Pain

The knee joint is constrained by soft tissues rather than the usual geometric fit of articulating bones. The medial and lateral collateral ligaments as well as the anterior and posterior cruciate ligaments maintain knee stability. Weight and force transmission can cross articular cartilage and the meniscus. The patellofemoral joint is the extensor mechanism of the knee and a common site of injury in the adolescent (Fig. 200.3).

Knee effusion or swelling is a common sign of injury. When the fluid accumulates rapidly after an injury, it is usually a hemarthrosis (blood in the joint) and may indicate a fracture, ligamentous disruption (often of the anterior cruciate ligament [ACL]), or meniscus tear. Unexplained knee effusion may occur with arthritis (septic, Lyme disease, viral, postinfectious, juvenile idiopathic arthritis, systemic lupus erythematosus). It may also occur as a result of overactivity and hypermobile joint syndrome (ligamentous laxity). An aspiration and laboratory evaluation of unexplained effusion can help expedite a diagnosis.

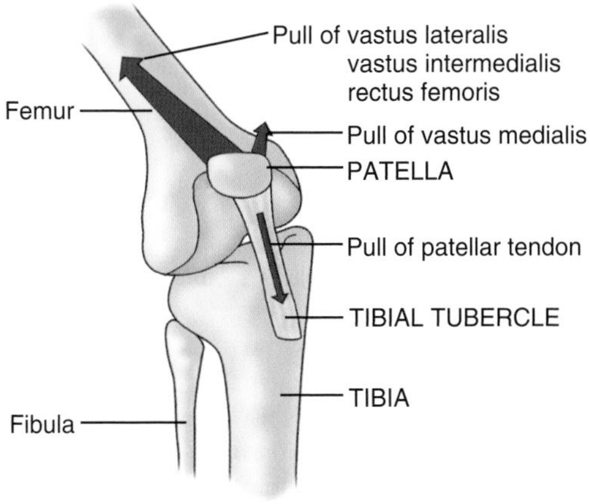

FIGURE 200.3 Diagram of the knee extensor mechanism. The major force exerted by the quadriceps muscle tends to pull the patella laterally out of the intercondylar sulcus. The vastus medialis muscle pulls medially to keep the patella centralized. (Modified from Smith JB. Knee problems in children. *Pediatr Clin North Am.* 1986;33:1439.)

Discoid Lateral Meniscus

Each meniscus is normally semilunar in shape; rarely the lateral meniscus will be disk shaped. A normal meniscus is attached at the periphery and glides anteriorly and posteriorly with knee motion. The discoid meniscus is less mobile and may tear more easily. When there is inadequate posterolateral attachment, the discoid meniscus can displace anteriorly with knee flexion, causing an audible click. Most commonly, patients will present in late childhood or early adolescence after an injury with knee pain and swelling. The anteroposterior radiographs can show increased joint space and a squared-off appearance of the lateral femoral condyle; magnetic resonance imaging (MRI) can confirm the diagnosis. Treatment is usually arthroscopic excision of tears and reshaping of the meniscus.

Popliteal Cyst

A popliteal cyst **(Baker cyst)** is commonly seen in the middle childhood years. The cause is the distension of the gastrocnemius and semimembranous bursa along the posteromedial aspect of the knee by synovial fluid. In adults, Baker cysts are associated with meniscus tears. In childhood, the cysts are usually painless and benign. They often spontaneously resolve, but it may take several years. Knee radiographs are normal. The diagnosis can be confirmed by ultrasound. Treatment is reassurance because surgical excision is indicated only for progressive cysts or cysts that cause disability.

Osteochondritis Dissecans

Decision-Making Algorithms
Available @ StudentConsult.com

Knee Pain
Extremity Pain

Osteochondritis dissecans (OCD) occurs when an area of bone adjacent to the articular cartilage suffers a vascular insult and separates from the adjacent bone. It most commonly affects the lateral aspect of the medial femoral condyle. Patients may complain of knee pain or swelling. The lesions can be seen on anteroposterior, lateral, and tunnel view radiographs. MRI can be helpful in determining the extent of the injury. In young patients with intact articular cartilage, the lesion will often revascularize and heal with rest from activities. The healing process may take several months and requires radiographic follow-up to document healing. With increasing age, the risk for articular cartilage damage and separation of the bony fragment increases. Older patients are more likely to need surgical intervention. Any patient with a fracture of the articular cartilage is unlikely to improve without surgical intervention. Patients with OCD should be referred to a specialist.

Osgood-Schlatter Disease

Decision-Making Algorithm
Available @ StudentConsult.com

Knee Pain

Osgood-Schlatter disease is a common cause of knee pain at the insertion of the patellar tendon on the tibial tubercle. The stress from a contracting quadriceps muscle is transmitted through the developing tibial tubercle, which can cause microfractures and apophysitis. It usually occurs after a growth spurt and is more common in boys. The age at onset is typically 11 years for girls and 13-14 years for boys.

Patients will present with pain during and after activity as well as have tenderness and local swelling over the tibial tubercle. Radiographs may be necessary to rule out infection, tumor, or avulsion fracture.

Rest and activity modification are paramount for treatment. Pain control medications and icing may be helpful. Lower extremity flexibility and strengthening exercise programs are important. The course is usually benign, but symptoms frequently last 1-2 years. Complications can include bony enlargement of the tibial tubercle and avulsion fracture of the tibial tubercle.

Patellofemoral Disorders

Decision-Making Algorithm
Available @ StudentConsult.com

Knee Pain

The patellofemoral joint is a complex joint that depends on a balance between restraining ligaments of the patella, muscular forces around the knee, and alignment for normal function. The interior surface of the patella has a V-shaped bottom that moves through a matching groove in the femur called the trochlea. When the knee is flexed, the patellar ligaments and the majority of the muscular forces pulling through the quadriceps tendon move the patella in a lateral direction. The vastus medialis muscle counteracts the lateral motion, pulling the patella toward the midline. Problems with function of this joint usually result in anterior knee pain.

Idiopathic anterior knee pain is a common complaint in adolescents. It is particularly prevalent in adolescent female athletes. Previously, this was referred to as chondromalacia of the patella, but this term is incorrect as the joint surfaces of the patella are normal. It is now known as **patellofemoral pain syndrome** (PFPS). The patient will present with anterior knee pain that worsens with activity, going up and down stairs, and soreness after sitting in one position for an extended time. There is usually no associated swelling. The patient may complain of a grinding sensation under the kneecap. Palpating and compressing the patellofemoral joint with the knee extended elicits pain. Patients often have weak hip musculature or poor flexibility in the lower extremities. Radiographs are rarely helpful but may be indicated to rule out other diagnoses such as OCD.

Treatment is focused on correcting the biomechanical problems that are causing the pain. This is usually done using an exercise program emphasizing hip girdle and vastus medialis strengthening with lower extremity flexibility. Antiinflammatory medication, ice, and activity modifications may also be helpful. Persistent cases should be referred to an orthopedic or sports medicine specialist.

One must exclude **recurrent patellar subluxation** and **dislocation** when evaluating a patient with PFPS. Acute traumatic dislocation will usually cause significant disability, swelling, and pain. Patients with recurrent dislocations often have associated ligamentous laxity, genu valgum, and femoral anteversion. The initial treatment is nonoperative and may involve a brief period of immobilization, followed by an aggressive physical therapy program designed to strengthen the quadriceps and improve function of the patellofemoral joint. Continued subluxation or recurrent dislocation is failure of this treatment plan, and surgical repair is usually necessary.

CHAPTER 201

Foot

In newborns and non–weight-bearing infants, the difference between posturing and deformity is important. Posturing is the habitual position in which the infant holds the foot; passive range of motion is normal. Deformity produces an appearance similar to posturing, but passive motion is restricted. Most pediatric foot disorders are painless. Foot pain is more common in older children (Table 201.1).

TABLE 201.1 Differential Diagnosis of Foot Pain by Age	
AGE GROUP	**DIAGNOSTIC CONSIDERATIONS**
0-6 years	Poorly fitting shoes Fracture Puncture wound Foreign body Osteomyelitis Cellulitis Juvenile idiopathic arthritis Hair tourniquet Leukemia
6-12 years	Poorly fitting shoes Trauma (fracture, sprain) Juvenile idiopathic arthritis Puncture wound Sever disease Accessory tarsal navicular Hypermobile flatfoot Oncological (Ewing sarcoma, leukemia)
12-18 years	Poorly fitting shoes Stress fracture Trauma (fracture, sprain) Foreign body Ingrown toenail Metatarsalgia Plantar fasciitis Achilles tendinopathy Accessory ossicles (navicular, os trigonum) Tarsal coalition Avascular necrosis of metatarsal (Freiberg infarction) or navicular (Kohler disease) Plantar warts

CLUBFOOT (TALIPES EQUINOVARUS)

Decision-Making Algorithm
Available @ StudentConsult.com

In-Toeing, Out-Toeing, and Toe-Walking

A clubfoot deformity involves the entire leg, not just the foot. It affects 1 in 1,000 newborns and is bilateral in one half of cases. The tarsals in the affected foot are hypoplastic; the talus is most affected. The muscles of the limb are hypoplastic because of the abnormal tarsal interactions, which leads to a generalized limb hypoplasia, mainly affecting and shortening the foot. There is usually atrophy of the calf musculature.

Etiology

Family history is important. Clubfoot can be congenital, teratological, or positional. Although congenital clubfoot (75% of all cases) is usually an isolated abnormality, every infant should be assessed for developmental dysplasia of the hip. Teratological clubfoot is associated with a neuromuscular disorder, such as myelomeningocele, arthrogryposis, or other syndromes. Positional clubfoot is a normal foot that was held in the deformed position in utero.

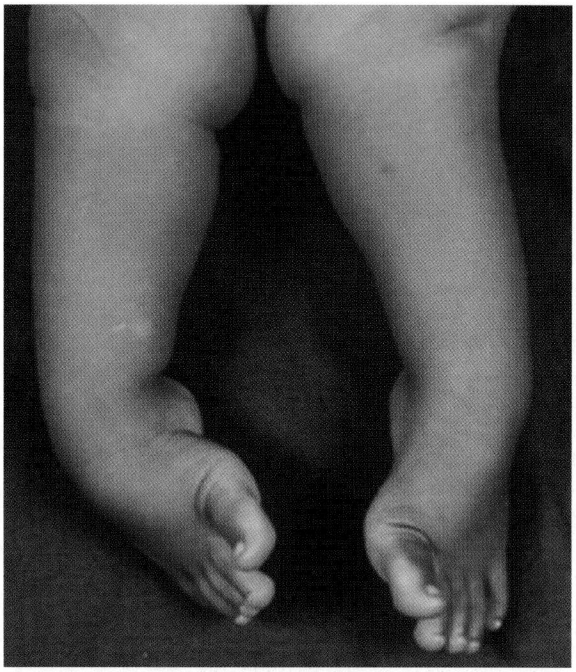

FIGURE 201.1 Clinical picture demonstrating clubfoot deformity. (From Kliegman RM, Behrman RE, Jenson HB, et al. *Nelson's Textbook of Pediatrics*. 18th ed. Philadelphia: Saunders; 2007:2778.)

Clinical Manifestations

The diagnosis is seldom confused with other disorders (Fig. 201.1). The presence of clubfoot should prompt a careful search for other abnormalities. The infant will have hindfoot equinus and varus, forefoot adduction, and varying degrees of rigidity. All are secondary to the abnormalities of the talonavicular joint. Calf atrophy and foot shortening are more noticeable in older children.

Radiological Evaluation

In infants, radiographs and advanced imaging are rarely necessary for assessment because their tarsals have incomplete ossification. The navicular ossifies at about 3 years of age for girls and 4 years for boys. As children age, radiographs can be used to follow the tibial calcaneal and lateral talocalcaneal angles and to assess navicular positioning.

Treatment

The goal of treatment is to correct the deformity and preserve mobility. Nonoperative treatment involves the Ponseti method of serial casting. The Ponseti method also relies on a percutaneous tenotomy of the Achilles tendon to help correct the equinus deformity.

About 20% of patients will require an anterior tibialis tendon transfer in early childhood. Rarely, more aggressive surgical procedures may need to be done. Complications of untreated clubfoot include severe disability. Complications of treated clubfoot include recurrence and stiffness.

METATARSUS ADDUCTUS

Decision-Making Algorithm
Available @ StudentConsult.com
In-Toeing, Out-Toeing, and Toe-Walking

Metatarsus adductus is the most common foot disorder in infants. It is characterized by a convexity of the lateral foot (Fig. 201.2) and is caused by in utero positioning. It is bilateral in half of cases. Occurring equally in boys and girls, it is more common in first-born children because of the smaller primigravid uterus. Two percent of infants with metatarsus adductus have **developmental dysplasia of the hip**.

Clinical Manifestations

The forefoot is adducted and sometimes supinated, but the midfoot and hindfoot are normal. The lateral border of the foot is convex, while the medial border is concave. Ankle dorsiflexion and plantar flexion are normal. With the midfoot and hindfoot stabilized, the deformity can be pushed beyond a neutral position (into abduction). Older children may present with an in-toeing gait.

Treatment

True metatarsus adductus resolves spontaneously over 90% of the time without treatment, so reassurance is all that is needed. Metatarsus adductus that does not improve within 2 years needs evaluation by a pediatric orthopedist. Persistent cases may benefit from serial casting or bracing, and potentially surgery. The deformity is not associated with a disability.

It is important to differentiate among metatarsus adductus, **metatarsus varus,** and **skewfoot.** Metatarsus varus looks like metatarsus adductus, but it is an uncommon rigid deformity that will need serial casting. Skewfoot is an uncommon deformity that is characterized by hindfoot plantar flexion, midfoot abduction, and forefoot adduction, giving the foot a Z or serpentine appearance. This needs to be managed very carefully with serial casting and surgery to help reduce the risk of disability in adulthood.

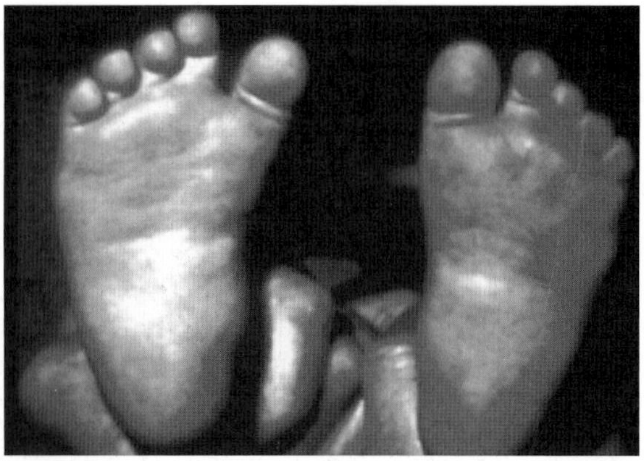

FIGURE 201.2 Clinical picture of metatarsus adductus with a normal foot on opposite side. (From Kliegman RM, Behrman RE, Jenson HB, et al. *Nelson's Textbook of Pediatrics*. 18th ed. Philadelphia: Saunders; 2007:2777.)

CALCANEOVALGUS FOOT

The calcaneovalgus foot is another common foot disorder in newborns that is secondary to in utero positioning. It is characterized by a hyperdorsiflexed foot with forefoot abduction and heel valgus. It is usually unilateral. The appearance may be quite severe dorsiflexion, but it is not a rigid deformity like congenital vertical talus. Simulated weight-bearing radiographs may be necessary for questionable diagnoses. The calcaneovalgus foot will appear normal or have minimal hindfoot valgus.

This disorder requires no treatment beyond reassurance. Parents can be taught passive stretching exercises for their infant's foot. Most affected infants realign by 2 years. A calcaneovalgus foot can be associated with bowing of the tibia, which resolves spontaneously, but a leg length discrepancy may exist.

HYPERMOBILE PES PLANUS (FLEXIBLE FLATFOOT)

Hypermobile or pronated feet are seen in 15% of adults. The child with flatfeet is usually asymptomatic and has no activity limitations. Newborn and toddler flatfoot is the result of ligamentous laxity and fat in the medial longitudinal arch. This is called **developmental flatfoot** and usually improves by 6 years of age. In older children, flatfoot is typically the result of generalized ligamentous laxity, and there is often a positive family history. Hypermobile flatfoot can be thought of as a normal variant.

Clinical Manifestations

In the non–weight-bearing position, the older child with a flexible flatfoot will have a medial longitudinal arch. When weight bearing, the foot pronates (arch collapse) with varying degrees of hindfoot valgus. Subtalar motion (essentially all ankle motion except plantar and dorsiflexion) is normal. Any loss of subtalar motion may indicate a rigid flatfoot, which can be related to tarsal coalition, neuromuscular disorders (cerebral palsy), and heel cord contractures. Radiographs of hypermobile flatfeet are usually not indicated.

Treatment

Hypermobile pes planus cannot be diagnosed until after 6 years of age; before that, it is developmental pes planus. Reassurance that this is a normal variant is very important. Patients who are symptomatic with activity may require education on proper, supportive footwear, orthotics/arch supports, and heel cord stretching.

TARSAL COALITION

Patients with tarsal coalition will usually present with a **rigid flatfoot** (loss of inversion and eversion at the subtalar joint). Coalition is produced by a congenital fusion or failure of segmentation of two or more tarsal bones. The attachment may be fibrous, cartilaginous, or osseous. Tarsal coalition can be unilateral or bilateral and will often become symptomatic in early adolescence. The most common forms of tarsal coalition are **calcaneonavicular** and **talocalcaneal.**

Clinical Manifestations

Decision-Making Algorithms
Available @ StudentConsult.com
Limp
Extremity Pain

The patient will usually present with hindfoot pain, which may radiate laterally because of peroneal muscle spasm. Symptoms are exacerbated by sports, and young athletes can present with frequent *ankle sprains.* There is a familial component. Pes planus is usually present in both weight-bearing and non–weight-bearing positions. There is usually a loss of subtalar motion, and passive attempts at joint motion may produce pain.

Radiological Evaluation

Anteroposterior, lateral, and oblique radiographs should be obtained, but they may not always clearly identify the disorder. The oblique view often identifies the calcaneonavicular coalition. Computed tomography (CT) is the gold standard for diagnosis of tarsal coalition. Even patients with obvious calcaneonavicular coalition on plain radiographs should have a CT scan to rule out a second coalition.

Treatment

Coalitions that are asymptomatic (the majority) do not need treatment. Nonoperative treatment for patients with pain consists of cast immobilization for a few weeks and foot orthotics. The symptoms will often return, necessitating surgery. Surgical excision of the coalition and soft tissue interposition to prevent reossification can be very effective.

CAVUS FOOT

Cavus foot is characterized by increased height of the medial longitudinal arch **(high arch)** and frequently hindfoot varus. It can be classified as physiological or neuromuscular. Most patients with physiological cavus foot are asymptomatic. A thorough neurological examination on all patients with a cavus foot is important. Patients with painful high arches have a high risk of neurological (tethered cord) and neuromuscular disease, and there is a strong association with **Charcot-Marie-Tooth disease,** a familial neuropathy. The underlying disorder should be treated first. Nonoperative treatment using orthotics is usually not helpful. Progressive, symptomatic cavus foot will likely need surgical reconstruction.

IDIOPATHIC AVASCULAR NECROSIS

Decision-Making Algorithms
Available @ StudentConsult.com
Limp
Extremity Pain

Kohler disease (tarsal navicular) and **Freiberg disease** (head of the second metatarsal) are uncommon and due to avascular necrosis. Patients will present with pain at the affected site with activity and weight bearing. Infection, fracture, and neoplasm should be excluded. Treatment consists of immobilization and activity restriction. The majority of the patients will improve upon subsequent revascularization and re-formation of bone.

SEVER DISEASE (CALCANEAL APOPHYSITIS)

Decision-Making Algorithm
Available @ StudentConsult.com
Extremity Pain

Sever disease is a common cause of heel pain among active young people. The mean age of presentation for girls is about 9 years of age and for boys about 11-12 years. Approximately 60% of cases are bilateral. Sever disease is caused by the forces of the calf musculature through the Achilles tendon at the calcaneal apophysis, causing microfracture. As the child ages and the apophysis begins to close, the pain disappears.

Clinical Manifestations

The common presentation is a young athlete who develops heel pain with activity that decreases with rest. Swelling is rare, but limping may be associated with Sever disease. The child will have pain to palpation of the posterior calcaneus and often tight heel cords. Radiographs are rarely indicated, but with persistent pain they should be done to exclude infection or tumor.

Treatment

Activity modification, icing, and antiinflammatory medications can be helpful. A program designed to improve heel cord flexibility and overall ankle strength may decrease symptoms. Heel elevation using heel wedges or heel cups can be helpful.

TOE DEFORMITIES

Curly toes are the most common deformity of the lesser toes. The fourth and fifth toes are most commonly affected. Curly toes are characterized by flexion at the proximal interphalangeal joint with lateral rotation of the toe. It is caused by contractures of the flexor digitorum brevis and longus tendons. Some curly toes will spontaneously resolve by 3-4 years of age. Persistent deformity may be treated by surgical tenotomy.

Polydactyly (extra toes) is usually found on the initial newborn physical examination. When the extra toe is adjacent to the fifth toe and attached by only a stalk of soft tissue or skin, simple ligation or amputation is effective. When the deformity involves the great toe or middle toes, or when the extra digit has cartilage or bone, delayed surgical intervention is indicated. **Syndactyly** (fusion of toes) is more common than polydactyly. It is usually a benign cosmetic problem. Both syndactyly and polydactyly may be associated with malformation syndromes (Table 201.2).

TABLE 201.2 Disorders Associated With Syndactyly and Polydactyly

POLYDACTYLY	SYNDACTYLY
Ellis-van Creveld syndrome	Apert syndrome
Rubinstein-Taybi syndrome	Carpenter syndrome
Carpenter syndrome	de Lange syndrome
Meckel-Gruber syndrome	Holt-Oram syndrome
Polysyndactyly	Orofaciodigital syndrome
Trisomy 13	Polysyndactyly
Orofaciodigital syndrome	Fetal hydantoin syndrome
	Laurence-Moon-Biedl syndrome
	Fanconi pancytopenia
	Trisomy 21
	Trisomy 13
	Trisomy 18

CHAPTER 202

Spine

SPINAL DEFORMITIES

A simplified classification of the common spinal abnormalities, scoliosis and kyphosis, is presented in Table 202.1.

TABLE 202.1 Classification of Spinal Deformities

SCOLIOSIS
Idiopathic
Infantile
Juvenile
Adolescent
Congenital
Failure of formation
Wedge vertebrae
Hemivertebrae
Failure of segmentation
Unilateral bar
Bilateral bar
Mixed
Neuromuscular
Neuropathic diseases
Upper motor neuron disease
Cerebral palsy
Spinocerebellar degeneration
Friedreich ataxia
Syringomyelia
Spinal cord tumor
Spinal cord trauma
Lower motor neuron disease
Myelodysplasia
Poliomyelitis
Spinal muscular atrophy
Charcot-Marie-Tooth disease
Myopathic diseases
Duchenne muscular dystrophy
Arthrogryposis
Other muscular dystrophies
Syndromes
Neurofibromatosis
Marfan syndrome
Compensatory
Leg-length inequality
KYPHOSIS
Postural roundback
Scheuermann disease
Congenital kyphosis

Modified from the Terminology Committee of the Scoliosis Research Society, 1975.

Clinical Manifestations

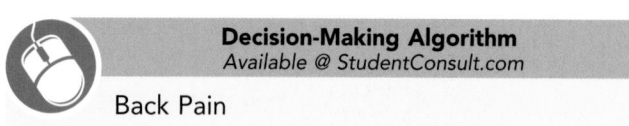

Decision-Making Algorithm
Available @ StudentConsult.com

Back Pain

Most patients will present for evaluation of an asymmetrical spine, which is usually pain free. A complete physical examination is necessary for any patient with a spinal deformity because the deformity can indicate an underlying disease. The back is examined from behind (Fig. 202.1). First, the levelness of the pelvis is assessed. Leg-length discrepancy produces pelvic obliquity, which often results in **compensatory scoliosis.** When the pelvis is level, the spine is examined for symmetry and spinal curvature with the patient upright. Cutaneous lesions (hemangioma, skin dimple, or hair tuft) should be noted. The spine should be palpated for areas of tenderness.

The patient is then asked to bend forward with the hands directed between the feet **(Adams forward bend test).** The examiner should inspect for asymmetry in the spine. The presence of the hump in this position is the hallmark for scoliosis. The area opposite the hump is usually depressed because of spinal rotation. Scoliosis is a rotational malalignment of one vertebra on another, resulting in rib elevation in the thoracic spine and paravertebral muscle elevation in the lumbar spine. With the patient still in the forward flexed position, inspection from the side can reveal the degree of roundback. A sharp forward angulation in the thoracolumbar region indicates a **kyphotic deformity**. It is important to examine the skin for café-au-lait spots **(neurofibromatosis),** hairy patches, and nevi **(spinal dysraphism).** Abnormal extremities may indicate skeletal dysplasia, whereas heart murmurs can be associated with Marfan syndrome. It is essential to do a full neurological examination to determine whether the scoliosis is idiopathic or secondary

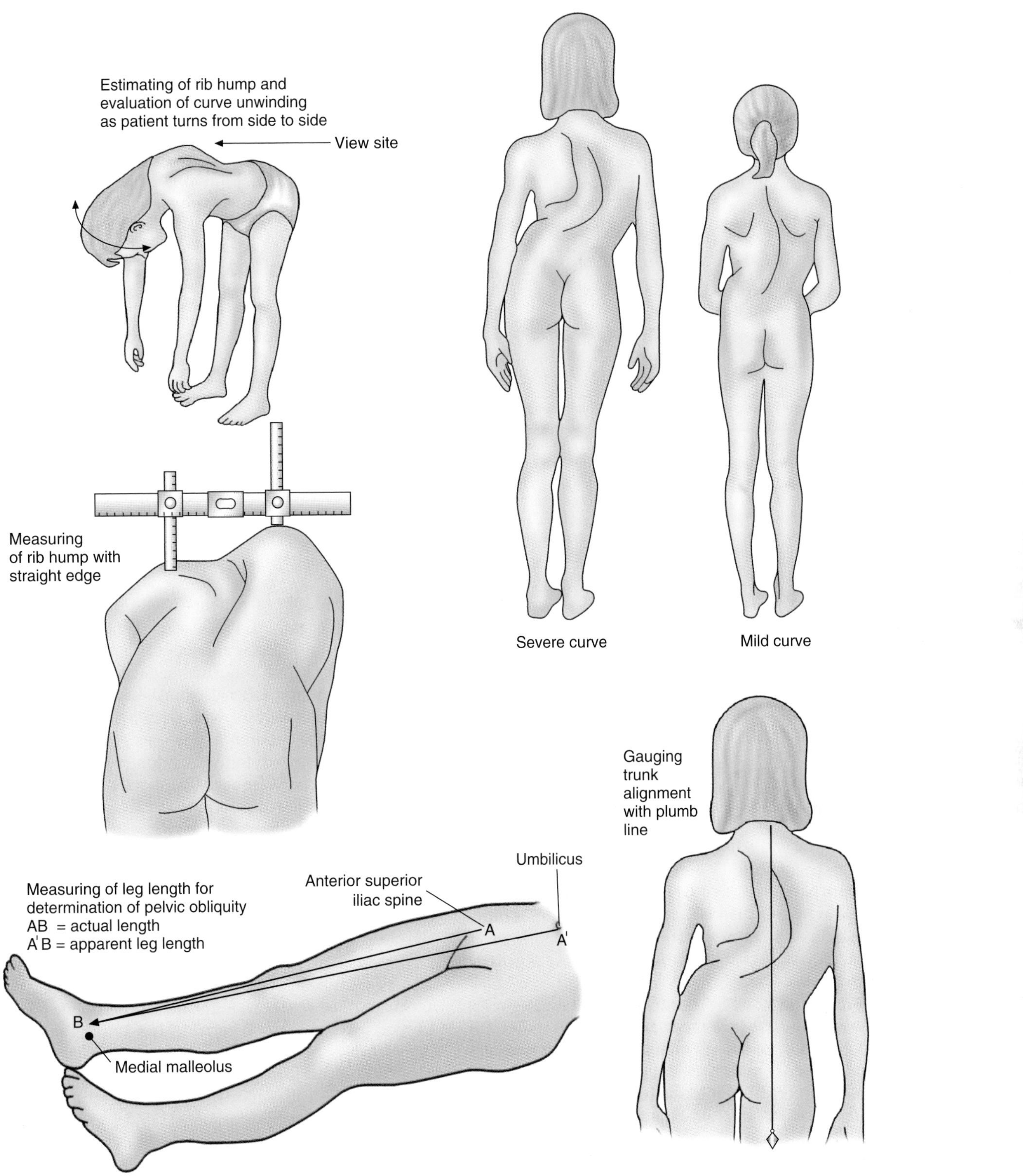

FIGURE 202.1 Clinical evaluation of a patient with scoliosis.

to an underlying neuromuscular disease, and to assess whether the scoliosis is producing any neurological sequelae.

Radiological Evaluation

Initial radiographs should include a posteroanterior and lateral standing film of the entire spine. The iliac crests should be visible to help determine skeletal maturity. The degree of curvature is measured from the most tilted or end vertebra of the curve superiorly and inferiorly to determine the Cobb angle (Fig. 202.2). Newer imaging modalities such as slot scanning or EOS provide the ability to obtain accurate measurements with much lower radiation than radiographs.

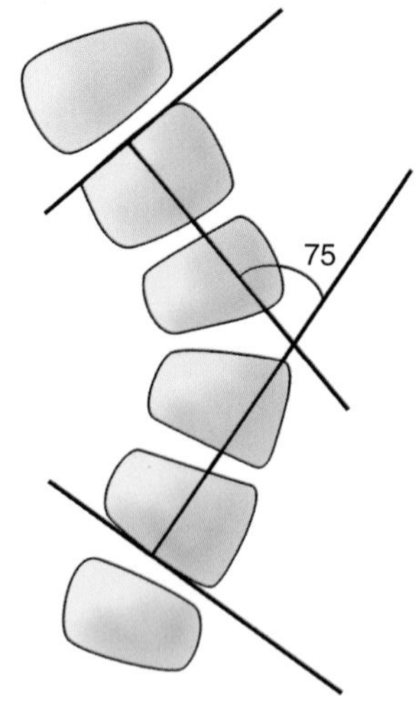

FIGURE 202.2 Cobb method of scoliotic curve measurement. Determine the end vertebrae of the curve: they are at the upper and lower limits of the curve and tilt most severely toward the concavity of the curve. Draw two perpendicular lines, one from the bottom of the lower body and one from the top of the upper body. Measure the angle formed. This is the accepted method of curve measurement according to the Scoliosis Research Society. Curves of 0-20 degrees are mild; 20-40 degrees, moderate; and greater than 40 degrees, severe.

SCOLIOSIS

Alterations in normal spinal alignment that occur in the anteroposterior plane are termed scoliosis. Most scoliotic deformities are idiopathic. Scoliosis may also be congenital, neuromuscular, or compensatory from a leg-length discrepancy.

Idiopathic Scoliosis

Etiology and Epidemiology

Idiopathic scoliosis is the most common form of scoliosis. It occurs in healthy, neurologically normal children. Approximately 20% of patients have a positive family history. The incidence is slightly higher in girls than boys, and the condition is more likely to progress and require treatment in females. There is some evidence that progressive scoliosis may have a genetic component as well.

Idiopathic scoliosis can be classified in three categories: **infantile** (birth to 3 years), **juvenile** (4-10 years), and **adolescent** (>11 years). Idiopathic adolescent scoliosis is the most common cause (80%) of spinal deformity. The right thoracic curve is the most common pattern. Juvenile scoliosis is uncommon but may be underrepresented because many patients do not seek treatment until they are adolescents. In any patient younger than 11 years of age, there is a greater likelihood that scoliosis is not idiopathic. The prevalence of an intraspinal abnormality in a child with congenital scoliosis is approximately 40%.

Clinical Manifestations

Idiopathic scoliosis is a painless disorder 70% of the time. A patient with pain requires a careful evaluation. Any patient presenting with a left-sided curve has a high incidence of intraspinal pathology (syrinx or tumor). Evaluation of the spine with magnetic resonance imaging (MRI) is indicated in these cases.

Treatment

Treatment of idiopathic scoliosis is based on the skeletal maturity of the patient, the size of the curve, and whether the spinal curvature is progressive or nonprogressive. Initial treatment for scoliosis is likely observation and repeat radiographs to assess for progression. No treatment is indicated for nonprogressive deformities. The risk factors for curve progression include gender, curve location, and curve magnitude. Girls are five times more likely to progress than boys. Younger patients are more likely to progress than older patients.

Typically, curves under 25 degrees are observed. Progressive curves between 20 degrees and 50 degrees in a skeletally immature patient are treated with bracing. A radiograph in the orthotic is important to evaluate correction. Curves greater than 50 degrees usually require surgical intervention.

Congenital Scoliosis

Abnormalities of the vertebral formation during the first trimester may lead to structural deformities of the spine that are evident at birth or early childhood. Congenital scoliosis can be classified as follows (Fig. 202.3):

Partial or complete failure of vertebral formation (wedge vertebra or hemivertebra)

Partial or complete failure of segmentation (unsegmented bars)

Mixed

More than 60% of patients have other associated abnormalities, such as VACTERL association (vertebral defects, imperforate anus, cardiac anomalies, tracheoesophageal fistula, renal anomalies, limb abnormalities such as radial agenesis) or Klippel-Feil syndrome. Renal anomalies occur in 20% of children with congenital scoliosis, with renal agenesis being the most common; 6% of children have a silent, obstructive uropathy suggesting the need for evaluation with ultrasonography. Congenital heart disease occurs in about 12% of patients. **Spinal dysraphism** (tethered cord, intradural lipoma, syringomyelia, diplomyelia, and diastematomyelia) occurs in approximately 20% of children with congenital scoliosis. These disorders are frequently associated with cutaneous lesions on the back and abnormalities of the legs and feet (e.g., cavus foot, neurological changes, calf atrophy). MRI is indicated in evaluation of spinal dysraphism.

The risk of spinal deformity progression in congenital scoliosis is variable and depends on the growth potential of the malformed vertebrae. A unilateral unsegmented bar typically progresses, but a block vertebra has little growth potential. About 75% of patients with congenital scoliosis will show some progression that continues until skeletal growth is complete, and about 50% will require some type of treatment. Progression can be expected during periods of rapid growth (before 2 years and after 10 years).

Treatment of congenital scoliosis hinges on early diagnosis and identification of progressive curves. Orthotic treatment is not helpful in congenital scoliosis. Early spinal surgery should be performed once progression has been documented. This can help prevent major deformities. Patients with large curves that cause thoracic insufficiency should undergo surgery immediately.

Neuromuscular Scoliosis

Progressive spinal deformity is a common and potentially serious problem associated with many neuromuscular disorders, such

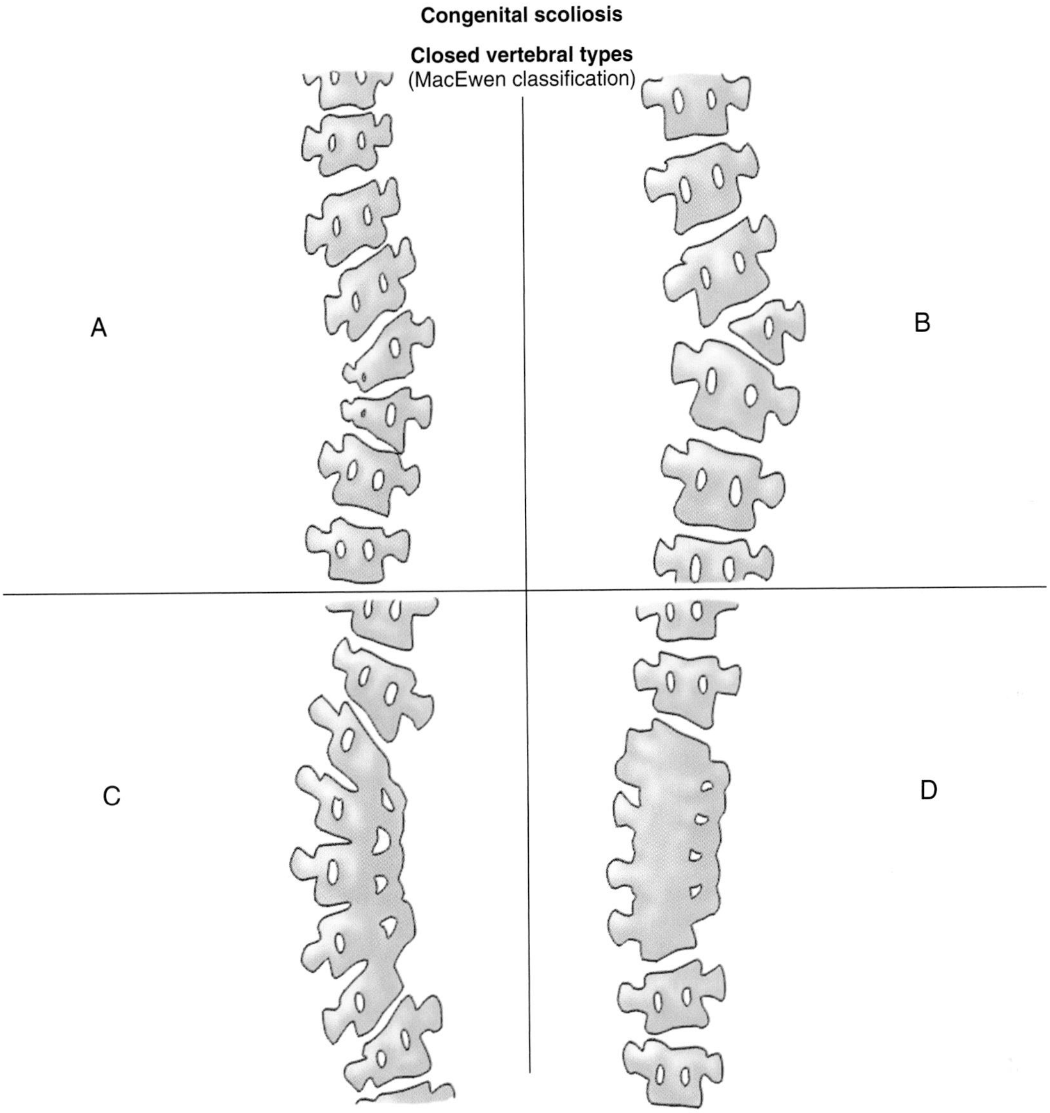

FIGURE 202.3 Types of closed vertebral and extravertebral spinal anomalies that result in congenital scoliosis. **(A)** Partial unilateral failure of formation (wedge vertebra). **(B)** Complete unilateral failure of formation (hemivertebra). **(C)** Unilateral failure of segmentation (congenital bar). **(D)** Bilateral failure of segmentation (block vertebra).

as cerebral palsy, Duchenne muscular dystrophy, spinal muscular atrophy, and spina bifida. Spinal alignment must be part of the routine examination for a patient with neuromuscular disease. Once scoliosis begins, progression is usually continuous. The magnitude of the deformity depends on the severity and pattern of weakness, whether the underlying disease process is progressive, and the amount of remaining musculoskeletal growth. Nonambulatory patients have a higher incidence of spinal deformity than ambulatory patients. In nonambulatory patients, the curves tend to be long and sweeping, produce pelvic obliquity, involve the cervical spine, and also produce restrictive lung disease. If the child cannot stand, then a supine or seated anteroposterior radiograph of the entire spine, rather than a standing posteroanterior view, is indicated.

The goal of **treatment** is to prevent progression and loss of function. Nonambulatory patients are more comfortable and independent when they can sit in a wheelchair without external support. Progressive curves can impair sitting balance, which affects quality of life. Orthotic treatment is usually ineffective in neuromuscular scoliosis. Surgical intervention may be necessary with frequent fusion to the pelvis.

Compensatory Scoliosis

Adolescents with a leg-length discrepancy (Chapter 200) may have a positive screening examination for scoliosis. Before correction of the pelvic obliquity, the spine curves in the same direction as the obliquity. However, with identification and correction of any pelvic obliquity, the curvature should resolve, and treatment should be directed at the leg-length discrepancy. Thus it is important to distinguish between a structural and compensatory spinal deformity.

KYPHOSIS

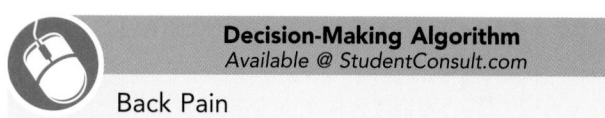

Decision-Making Algorithm
Available @ StudentConsult.com
Back Pain

Kyphosis refers to a roundback deformity or to increased angulation of the thoracic or thoracolumbar spine in the sagittal plane. Kyphosis can be postural, structural (Scheuermann kyphosis), or congenital.

Postural Roundback

Postural kyphosis is secondary to poor posture. It is voluntarily corrected in the standing and prone positions. The patient may also have increased lumbar lordosis. Radiographs are usually unnecessary if the kyphosis fully corrects. If not, radiographs will reveal no vertebral abnormalities. Treatment, if needed, is aimed at improving the child's posture.

Scheuermann Kyphosis

Scheuermann disease is the second most common cause of pediatric spinal deformity. It occurs equally in males and females. The etiology is unknown, but there may be hereditary factors. Scheuermann kyphosis is differentiated from postural roundback on physical examination and by radiographs.

A patient with Scheuermann disease cannot correct the kyphosis with standing or lying prone. When viewed from the side in the forward flexed position, patients with Scheuermann disease will have an abrupt angulation in the mid to lower thoracic region (Fig. 202.4), and patients with postural roundback show a smooth, symmetrical contour. In both conditions, lumbar lordosis is increased. However, half of patients with Scheuermann disease will have atypical back pain, especially with thoracolumbar kyphosis. The **classic radiological findings** of Scheuermann kyphosis include the following:

Narrowing of disk space
Loss of anterior height of the involved vertebrae producing wedging of 5 degrees or more in at least three consecutive vertebrae
Irregularities of the vertebral endplates
Schmorl nodes

Treatment of Scheuermann kyphosis is similar to idiopathic scoliosis. It is dependent on the degree of deformity, skeletal maturity, and the presence or absence of pain. Nonoperative treatment begins with bracing. Surgical fusion is done for patients who have completed growth, have a severe deformity, or have intractable pain.

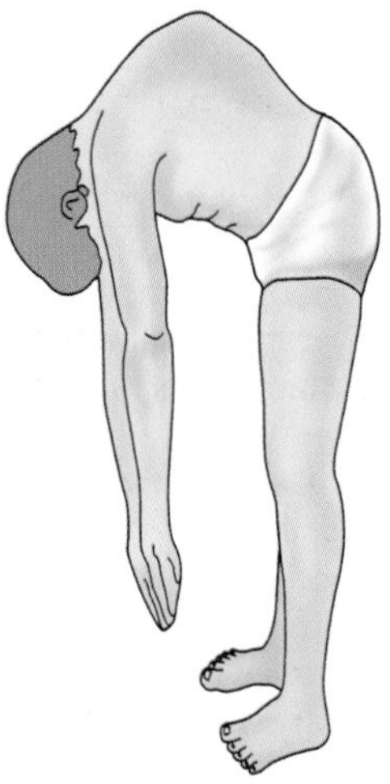

FIGURE 202.4 Note the sharp break in the contour of a child with kyphosis. (From Behrman RE. *Nelson Textbook of Pediatrics*. 14th ed. Philadelphia: WB Saunders; 1992.)

Congenital Kyphosis

Congenital kyphosis is a failure of the formation of all or part of the vertebral body (with preservation of posterior elements) or failure of anterior segmentation of the spine, or both. Severe deformities are found at birth and tend to rapidly progress. Progression will not cease until the end of skeletal growth. A progressive spine deformity may result in neurological deficit. Treatment of congenital kyphosis is often surgical.

TORTICOLLIS

Etiology and Epidemiology

Torticollis is usually first identified in newborns because of a head tilt. Torticollis is usually secondary to a shortened sternocleidomastoid muscle (muscular torticollis). This may result from in utero positioning or birth trauma. Acquired torticollis may be related to upper cervical spine abnormalities or central nervous system pathology (mass lesion). It can also occur in older children during a respiratory infection (potentially secondary to lymphadenitis) or local head or neck infection, and it may herald psychiatric diagnoses.

Clinical Manifestations and Evaluation

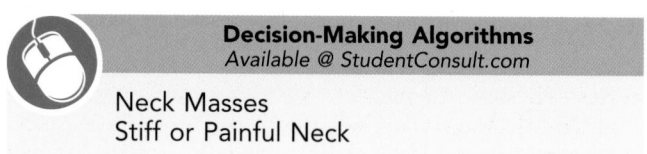

Decision-Making Algorithms
Available @ StudentConsult.com
Neck Masses
Stiff or Painful Neck

Infants with muscular torticollis have the ear tilted toward the clavicle on the ipsilateral side. The face will look upward toward the contralateral side. There may be a palpable swelling or fibrosis in the body of the sternocleidomastoid shortly after birth, which is often the precursor of a contracture. Congenital muscular torticollis is associated with skull and facial asymmetry **(plagiocephaly)** and developmental dysplasia of the hip.

After a thorough neurological examination, anteroposterior and lateral radiographs should be obtained. The goal is to rule out a nonmuscular etiology. A computed tomography (CT) scan or MRI of the head and neck is necessary for persistent neck pain, neurological symptoms, and persistent deformity.

Treatment

Treatment of muscular torticollis is aimed at increasing the range of motion of the neck and correcting the cosmetic deformity. Stretching exercises of the neck can be very beneficial for infants. Surgical management is indicated if patients do not improve with adequate stretching exercises in physical therapy. Postoperative physical therapy is needed to decrease the risk of recurrence. Treatment in patients with underlying disorders should target the disorder.

BACK PAIN IN CHILDREN

Etiology and Epidemiology

Back pain in the pediatric population should always be approached with concern. In contrast to adults, in whom back pain is frequently mechanical or psychological, back pain in children may be the result of organic causes, especially in preadolescents. Back pain lasting longer than a week requires a detailed investigation. In the pediatric population, approximately 85% of children with back pain for greater than 2 months have a specific lesion: 33% are post-traumatic (spondylolysis, occult fracture), 33% are developmental (kyphosis, scoliosis), and 18% have an infection or tumor. In the remaining 15%, the diagnosis is undetermined.

Clinical Manifestations and Management

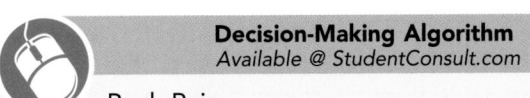

Decision-Making Algorithm
Available @ StudentConsult.com

Back Pain

The history must include the onset and duration of symptoms. The location, character, and radiation of pain are important. Neurological symptoms (muscle weakness, sensory changes, and bowel or bladder dysfunction) must be reviewed. Medical history and family history should be obtained, with a focus on back pain, rheumatological disorders, and neoplastic processes. The review of systems should include detailed questions on overall health, fever, chills, recent weight loss, and recent illnesses. Physical examination should include a complete musculoskeletal and neurological evaluation. Spinal alignment, range of motion, areas of tenderness, and muscle spasm should be noted. **Red flags** for childhood back pain include persistent or increasing pain, systemic findings (e.g., fever, weight loss), neurological deficits, bowel or bladder dysfunction, young age (under 4 is strongly associated with tumor), night waking, pain that restricts activity, and a painful left thoracic spinal curvature.

Anteroposterior and lateral standing films of the entire spine with bilateral oblique views of the affected area should be obtained. Secondary imaging with bone scan, CT scan, or MRI may be necessary for diagnosis. MRI is very useful for suspected intraspinal pathology. Laboratory studies, such as a complete blood count, erythrocyte sedimentation rate (ESR), C-reactive protein (CRP), and specialized testing for juvenile idiopathic arthritis and ankylosing spondylitis, may be indicated.

The differential diagnosis of pediatric back pain is extensive (Table 202.2). Treatment depends on the specific diagnosis. If serious pathology has been ruled out and no definite diagnosis has been established, an initial trial of physical therapy with close follow-up for reevaluation is recommended.

TABLE 202.2 Differential Diagnosis of Back Pain
INFECTIOUS DISEASES
Diskitis (most common before the age of 6 years)
Vertebral osteomyelitis (pyogenic or tuberculous)
Spinal epidural abscess
Pyelonephritis
Pancreatitis
RHEUMATOLOGICAL DISEASES
Juvenile idiopathic arthritis
Reactive arthritis
Ankylosing spondylitis
Psoriatic arthritis
Inflammatory bowel disease
DEVELOPMENTAL DISEASES
Scheuermann kyphosis
Scoliosis (left thoracic)
Spondylolysis
Spondylolisthesis
TRAUMATIC AND MECHANICAL ABNORMALITIES
Hip and pelvic abnormalities (sacroiliac joint dysfunction)
Herniated nucleus pulposus (intervertebral disk)
Overuse injuries (facet syndrome)
Vertebral stress fractures (spondylolysis, spondylolisthesis)
Vertebral compression fracture (steroid, sickle cell anemia)
Upper cervical spine instability (atlantoaxial instability)
NEOPLASTIC DISEASES
Primary vertebral tumors (osteogenic sarcoma)
Metastatic tumor (neuroblastoma)
Primary spinal tumor (astrocytoma)
Bone marrow malignancy (leukemia, lymphoma)
Benign tumors (eosinophilic granuloma, osteoid osteoma)
OTHER
Conversion disorder
Juvenile osteoporosis

SPONDYLOLYSIS AND SPONDYLOLISTHESIS

Etiology and Epidemiology

Spondylolysis is a defect in the pars interarticularis. Spondylolisthesis refers to bilateral defects with anterior slippage of the superior vertebra on the inferior vertebra. The lesions are not present at birth, but about 5% of children will have the lesion by 6 years of age. It is most common in adolescent athletes, especially those involved in sports that involve repetitive back extension. Classically, this was an injury seen in gymnasts and divers. However, with increased intensity and year-round sports, the incidence is increasing. Football interior linemen (extension while blocking), soccer players (extension while shooting), and basketball players (extension while rebounding) are examples of athletes at higher risk. The most common location of spondylolysis is L5, followed by L4.

Spondylolisthesis is classified according to the degree of slippage:

- Grade 1: less than 25%
- Grade 2: 25-50%
- Grade 3: 50-75%
- Grade 4: 75-99%
- Grade 5: complete displacement or spondyloptosis

The most common location of spondylolisthesis is L5 on S1.

Clinical Manifestations

Decision-Making Algorithm
Available @ StudentConsult.com

Back Pain

Patients will often complain of an insidious onset of low back pain persisting over 2 weeks. The pain tends to worsen with activity and with extension of the back and improves with rest. There may be some radiation of pain to the buttocks. A loss of lumbar lordosis may occur due to muscular spasm. Pain is present with extension of lumbar spine and with palpation over the lesion. Patients with spondylolisthesis may have a palpable *step off* at the lumbosacral area. A detailed neurological examination should be done, especially because spondylolisthesis can have nerve root involvement.

Radiological Evaluation

Anteroposterior, lateral, and oblique radiographs of the spine should be obtained. The oblique views may show the classic *Scotty dog* findings associated with spondylolysis. The lateral view will allow measurement of spondylolisthesis. Unfortunately, plain radiographs do not regularly reveal spondylolysis, so advanced imaging may be needed. The most helpful form of advanced imaging among CT, bone scan, single photon emission CT (SPECT), or MRI continues to be debated. MRI should be considered in patients with neurological deficits.

Treatment

Spondylolysis

Painful spondylolysis requires activity restriction. Bracing is controversial but may help with pain relief. Patients benefit from an aggressive physical therapy plan to improve lower extremity flexibility and increase core strength and spinal stability. There is evidence that some patients with an acute spondylolysis can achieve bony union and that these patients have a decreased incidence of low back pain and degenerative change in the low back as they age when compared with spondylolysis patients with nonunion. Rarely, surgery is indicated for intractable pain and disability.

Spondylolisthesis

Decision-Making Algorithm
Available @ StudentConsult.com

Back Pain

Patients with spondylolisthesis require periodic evaluation for progression of their slippage. Treatment of spondylolisthesis is based on grading:

- Grade 1: Same treatment as spondylolysis. Failure of nonoperative management may lead to surgical fusion.
- Grade 2: Reasonable to try nonoperative management, but if the slippage is progressing, surgical intervention may be needed. Any patient with neurological symptoms requires surgical intervention.
- Grades 3-5: Spinal fusion is usually required to prevent further slippage or damage.

DISKITIS

Decision-Making Algorithms
Available @ StudentConsult.com

Back Pain
Stiff or Painful Neck

Diskitis is an intervertebral disk space infection that does not cause associated vertebral osteomyelitis (see Chapter 117). The most common organism is *Staphylococcus aureus.* The infection can occur at any age but is more common in patients under 6 years of age.

Clinical Manifestations

Children may present with back pain, abdominal pain, pelvic pain, irritability, and refusal to walk or sit. Fever is an inconsistent symptom. The child typically holds the spine in a straight or stiff position, generally has a loss of lumbar lordosis due to paravertebral muscular spasm, and refuses to flex the lumbar spine. The white blood cell count is normal or elevated, but the ESR and CRP are usually high.

Radiological Evaluation

Radiographic findings vary according to the duration of symptoms before diagnosis. Anteroposterior, lateral, and oblique radiographs of the lumbar or thoracic spine will typically show a narrow disk space with irregularity of the adjacent vertebral body end plates. In early cases, bone scan or MRI may be helpful because they will be positive before findings are noticeable on plain radiographs. MRI can also be used to differentiate between diskitis and the more serious condition of vertebral osteomyelitis.

Treatment

Intravenous antibiotic therapy is the mainstay of treatment. Blood cultures may occasionally be positive and identify the infectious agent. Aspiration and needle biopsy are reserved for children who are not responding to empirical antibiotic treatment. Symptoms should resolve rapidly with antibiotics, but intravenous antibiotics should be continued for 1-2 weeks and be followed by 4 weeks of oral antibiotics. Pain control can be obtained with medications and temporary orthotic immobilization of the back.

CHAPTER 203

Upper Extremity

SHOULDER

The shoulder actually comprises four joints:

- Glenohumeral joint (commonly referred to as the shoulder joint)
- Acromioclavicular joint
- Sternoclavicular joint
- Scapulothoracic joint

The glenohumeral joint has minimal geometric stability because the relatively small glenoid fossa articulates with the proportionately larger head of the humerus. The low level of intrinsic stability allows for a large range of motion. The rotator cuff muscles help give the glenohumeral joint more stability, but they need normal contact of the glenohumeral joint to be successful. The scapulothoracic movement also expands the range of motion of the shoulder, but like the glenohumeral joint, it requires strong, coordinated musculature to function efficiently.

Sprengel Deformity

Sprengel deformity is the congenital elevation of the scapula. There are varying degrees of severity; it is usually unilateral. There is restricted scapulothoracic motion (especially with abduction), so most of the shoulder motion is through the glenohumeral joint. There is usually associated hypoplasia of the periscapular muscles. Webbing of the neck and low posterior hairline can be associated problems. There is an association with congenital syndromes, such as Klippel-Feil anomaly, so a thorough history and examination are necessary. Mild forms with a cosmetic deformity and mild loss of shoulder motion do not need surgical correction. Severe forms may have a bony connection (omovertebral) between the scapula and lower cervical spine. Moderate and severe forms may need surgical repositioning of the scapula in early childhood to improve cosmesis and function.

Brachial Plexus Injuries

Obstetric brachial plexus palsy is discussed in Section 11. **Brachial plexopathy** is an athletic injury, commonly referred to as a **stinger** or **burner.** The symptoms are often likened to a *dead arm.* There is pain (often burning), weakness, and numbness in a single upper extremity. There are three mechanisms of injury:

1. Traction caused by lateral flexion of the neck away from the involved upper extremity
2. Direct impact to the brachial plexus at Erb's point
3. Compression caused by neck extension and rotation toward the involved extremity

Symptoms are always unilateral and should resolve within 15 minutes. It is paramount to assess the *cervical spine* for serious injury. Bilateral symptoms, lower extremity symptoms, persistent symptoms, or recurrent injury are all signs of more serious disease and may need a more extensive work-up and cervical spine stabilization. Athletes may return to activity if there are no red flags on history or physical examination and the athlete has full pain-free range of motion and strength in the neck and affected extremity.

Glenohumeral Dislocation

Shoulder dislocation is uncommon in childhood but becomes more frequent in adolescence. The younger the patient is at presentation, the more likely it is that the patient will have recurrent dislocation. Anterior dislocation is the most common. If assessment of the neurovascular status of the affected extremity reveals any compromise, urgent reduction is needed to prevent further complications. Patients will need radiographs to assess for fractures of the glenoid (Bankhart lesion) and humeral head (Hill-Sachs lesion). Most patients will require a brief period of protection in a sling or shoulder immobilizer, as well as pain control. As symptoms resolve, a gentle range-of-motion program, followed by an aggressive strengthening program, should be done. Recurrence rate may be nearly 90% for contact sport athletes, so there is controversy surrounding early surgical intervention at the first dislocation.

Overuse Injuries

The incidence of overuse injuries is increasing because of increased opportunities for athletic participation as well as higher levels of intensity during sports. Overuse injuries are inflammatory responses in tendons and bursae that are subjected to repetitive motions and trauma (e.g., rotator cuff tendinitis in swimmers). These injuries are uncommon in children but may be seen in adolescents. Bony injury, such as physeal fractures and apophysitis, must be ruled out before making the diagnosis of a soft tissue overuse injury. Overuse injuries in the shoulder can be provoked by joint laxity.

The patient will often present with discomfort over the affected area that worsens with activity. Physical examination usually reveals tenderness to palpation and often weakness of the associated muscles due to pain. It is important to assess for glenohumeral stability. Radiographs may be indicated for acute trauma or when symptoms are not improving. Treatment consists of activity modification, icing, antiinflammatory medication, and a physical therapy program aimed at strengthening, increasing flexibility, and improving posture.

Proximal Humeral Epiphysiolysis

Proximal humeral epiphysiolysis is commonly referred to as **Little Leaguer's shoulder.** It most commonly occurs in 9–14 year olds who participate in overhead (tennis, volleyball) and throwing sports, particularly baseball pitchers. It is a stress injury that potentially can be a fracture (epiphysiolysis) of the proximal humeral physis. Most patients present with pain during or after throwing. There may be tenderness to palpation over the proximal humerus; if the athlete has been resting for a few days, examination may be normal. Radiographs should include comparison views to assess the physis. There may be widening of the proximal humeral physis in the affected arm, but the films may be normal. Treatment is rest from the offending activity, followed by a rehabilitation program designed to improve strength in the shoulder muscles. Pitchers should also be encouraged to follow youth pitching guidelines published by Little League baseball.

ELBOW

The elbow consists of three articulations:
1. Ulnar-humeral joint
2. Radial-humeral joint
3. Proximal radioulnar joint

Collectively, these joints produce a hinge-type joint that allows for supination (palm up) and pronation (palm down) positioning of the hand. The elbow has excellent geometric stability, and the musculature around the elbow primarily produces flexion and extension.

Radial Head Subluxation

Decision-Making Algorithm
Available @ StudentConsult.com
Extremity Pain

Radial head subluxation is more commonly known as **nursemaid's elbow.** Because the radial head is not as bulbous in infants and young children, the annular ligament that passes around it can partially slip off the radial head with traction across the elbow (Fig. 203.1). The subluxation is usually caused by a quick pull on the extended elbow when a child is forcefully lifted by the hand or when the child falls while holding hands with an adult. After a subluxation, the child usually holds the hand in a pronated position and will refuse to use the hand or move the elbow. Moving the hand into the supinated position while applying pressure to the radial head will usually reduce the injury. Usually radiographs are not necessary unless reduction cannot be obtained or there is concern for fracture (swelling and bruising). Once the injury is reduced, the child will begin using the arm again without complaint. Parents should be educated about the mechanism of injury and encouraged to avoid that position. There is a high rate of recurrence for this injury. The problem generally resolves with maturation, but some children with high recurrence rates may benefit from casting or, rarely, surgical intervention.

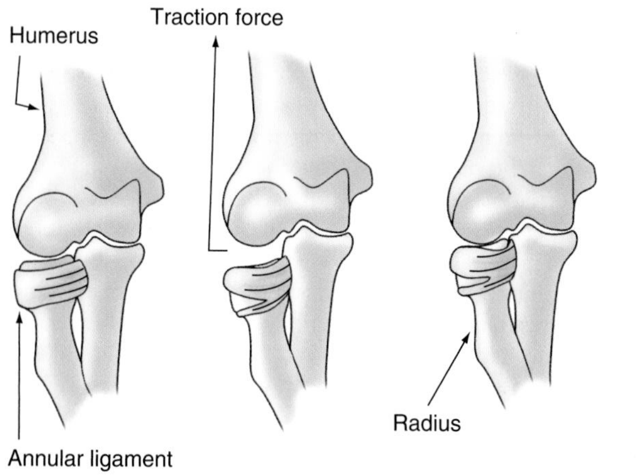

FIGURE 203.1 Nursemaid's elbow. The annular ligament is torn when the arm is pulled. The radial head moves distally, and when traction is discontinued, the ligament is carried into the joint. (From Rang M. *Children's Fractures*. Philadelphia: JB Lippincott; 1974:121.)

Panner Disease

Decision-Making Algorithm
Available @ StudentConsult.com
Extremity Pain

Panner disease is an osteochondritis of the capitellum (lateral portion of distal humeral epiphysis) that occurs spontaneously in late childhood. Clinical features include elbow pain, decreased range of motion, and tenderness to palpation over the capitellum. Radiographs reveal fragmentation of the capitellum. Treatment is activity restriction and follow-up radiographs to demonstrate spontaneous reossification of the capitellum over several months. There is usually no need for further treatment or imaging studies. This is not to be confused with osteochondritis dissecans of the capitellum, which usually will occur in adolescents involved with throwing sports.

Throwing Injuries

The elbow is especially vulnerable to throwing injuries in the skeletally immature athlete. These occur from excessive and repetitive tension forces across the radial aspect of the elbow and compression forces across the lateral aspect of the elbow. These injuries are commonly known as Little Leaguer's elbow.

Decision-Making Algorithm
Available @ StudentConsult.com
Extremity Pain

Although this injury is most common in baseball players who throw frequently (pitcher, catcher, third base, and shortstop), it also occurs in football quarterbacks and tennis players. Patients will usually complain of pain over the medial elbow with throwing that may last for a few days afterward. There may be associated swelling and lateral or posterior elbow pain. Radiation of pain may be secondary to ulnar neuropathy. There is often a flexion contracture of the elbow when compared to the opposite side. Palpation of the medial epicondyle, radial head, capitellum, lateral epicondyle, and olecranon process often reveals tenderness. Ulnar (medial) collateral ligament stability should be assessed. Radiographs should include the contralateral elbow for comparison. Radiographic findings in Little Leaguer's elbow can vary and may include normal anatomy, medial humeral epicondyle apophyseal avulsion fracture, osteochondritis dissecans of the capitellum, radial head abnormalities, and foreign bodies in the elbow. MRI may be helpful.

Treatment depends on the underlying diagnosis but always includes pain control and rest from activity. *Classic Little Leaguer's elbow* refers to medial humeral epicondyle apophysitis. These athletes benefit from rest, ice, antiinflammatory medication, and a physical therapy program aimed at upper body strengthening. Throwing mechanics and the pitching guidelines published by Little League Baseball/Softball should be reviewed with these players. Switching players to a lower throwing position (e.g., first base) after rehabilitation, to avoid pitching for the remainder of the season, is often recommended.

WRIST AND HAND

Multiple small joints, a delicately balanced intrinsic muscle system, a powerful extrinsic muscle system, dense sensory innervation, and specialized skin combine to make the hand a highly mobile and sensitive yet powerful anatomical part. The extrinsic muscles originate in the forearm and the intrinsic muscles are located in the hand and coordinate small, delicate movements. The movements of opening the hand, extending and spreading the fingers, and then clenching the hand into a fist requires coordinated function of the intrinsic and extrinsic muscles. Tenderness of direct palpation of the bones raises the concern for fracture. **Scaphoid fracture** is the most common carpal bone fracture in the pediatric population. It requires immobilization in a thumb spica cast, whereas displaced fractures require surgical intervention. **Salter-Harris fractures of the distal radius** are also very common. In young gymnasts, there is increased risk for injury at the distal radial physis from repetitive impact and upper extremity weight bearing. This is commonly called **gymnast's wrist** and requires absolute rest from impact and weight bearing to prevent premature closure of the growth plate.

Ganglion cysts are synovial fluid-filled cysts about the wrist. The most common location is the dorsum of the wrist near the radiocarpal joint, followed by the volar radial aspect of the wrist. The defect is in the joint capsule, which allows synovial fluid into the soft tissues with wrist use, where it can become walled off with fibrous tissue. Often, in skeletally immature patients, the process is benign and disappears over time. Large ganglion cysts or cysts that are painful and interfere with function may require more aggressive therapy. Aspiration and steroid injection into the cyst may be helpful, but many will recur. Surgical excision will remove the tract that attaches to the wrist joint, so it is usually curative.

Finger Abnormalities

Polydactyly (extra digits) occurs in simple and complex varieties (see Table 201.2). Skin tags and digit remnants that occur near the metacarpophalangeal joint of the fifth digit and thumb that do not have palpable bones or possess voluntary motion are simple varieties. These may be excised or ligated in the nursery. Complex deformities should be referred to a pediatric orthopedist for amputation. **Syndactyly** (fused digits) are concerning because of the possibility of shared structures and the tethering effects on bone growth (see Table 201.2). All patients with syndactyly should be referred for treatment options.

Trigger thumb and **trigger finger** are secondary to isolated thickening of the flexor tendons. As the thickened nodule enlarges, it may catch in a bent position, then snap or *trigger* straight as it passes through the first pulley that anchors the tendon. Ultimately, as it enlarges, it cannot pass through at all and produces a flexion deformity at the interphalangeal joints. The nodule may be palpable near the metacarpophalangeal joint. These children should be referred for surgical correction.

CHAPTER 204

Benign Bone Tumors and Cystic Lesions

Benign bone tumors and cystic lesions are common in childhood. Some represent fibrous dysplasia. Others are benign bone cysts (unicameral) or benign bone tumors (osteoid osteoma). Subacute osteomyelitis **(Brodie abscess)** and eosinophilic granulomas are lesions not associated with abnormal bone or cartilage growth. Some of these lesions can produce pain, limp, and pathological fractures. Others can be incidental findings on radiographs. The prognosis is usually excellent. A brief differential diagnosis of bone tumors and their management is listed in Table 204.1. Malignant bone tumors are discussed in Section 21.

TABLE 204.1 Benign Bone Tumors and Cysts

DISEASE	CHARACTERISTICS	RADIOGRAPHIC FINDINGS	TREATMENT	PROGNOSIS
Osteochondroma (osteocartilaginous exostosis)	Common; distal metaphysis of femur, proximal humerus, proximal tibia; painless, hard, nontender mass	Bony outgrowth, sessile or pedunculated	Excision, if symptomatic	Excellent; malignant transformation rare
Multiple hereditary exostoses	Osteochondroma of long bones; bone growth disturbances	As above	As above	Recurrences
Osteoid osteoma	Pain relieved by aspirin; femur and tibia; found predominantly in boys	Dense sclerosis surrounds small radiolucent nidus, <1 cm	As above	Excellent
Osteoblastoma (giant osteoid osteoma)	As above, but more destructive	Osteolytic component; size >1 cm	As above	Excellent
Enchondroma	Tubular bones of hands and feet; pathological fractures, swollen bone; Ollier disease if multiple lesions are present	Radiolucent diaphyseal or metaphyseal lesion; may calcify	Excision or curettage	Excellent; malignant transformation rare

Continued

TABLE 204.1 Benign Bone Tumors and Cysts—cont'd

DISEASE	CHARACTERISTICS	RADIOGRAPHIC FINDINGS	TREATMENT	PROGNOSIS
Nonossifying fibroma	Silent; rare pathological fracture; late childhood, adolescence	Incidental radiographic finding; thin sclerotic border, radiolucent lesion	None or curettage with fractures	Excellent; heals spontaneously
Eosinophilic granuloma	Age 5-10 years; skull, jaw, long bones; pathological fracture; pain	Small, radiolucent without reactive bone; punched-out lytic lesion	Biopsy, excision rare; irradiation	Excellent; may heal spontaneously
Brodie abscess	Insidious local pain; limp; suspected as malignancy	Circumscribed metaphyseal osteomyelitis; lytic lesions with sclerotic rim	Biopsy; antibiotics	Excellent
Unicameral bone cyst (simple bone cyst)	Metaphysis of long bone (femur, humerus); pain, pathological fracture	Cyst in medullary canal, expands cortex; fluid-filled unilocular or multilocular cavity	Curettage; steroid injection into lesion	Excellent; some heal spontaneously
Aneurysmal bone cyst	As above; contains blood, fibrous tissue	Expands beyond metaphyseal cartilage	Curettage, bone graft	Excellent

Suggested Reading

DiFiori JP, Benjamin HJ, Brenner JS, et al. Overuse injuries and burnout in youth sports: a position statement from the American Medical Society for Sports Medicine. *Br J Sports Med.* 2014;48:287–288.

Herman MJ, Martinek M. The limping child. *Pediatr Rev.* 2015;36(5):184–197.

Herring JA. *Tachdjian's Pediatric Orthopedics.* 5th ed. Philadelphia: Saunders; 2013.

Kliegman RM, Stanton BF, St. Geme JW, et al, eds. *Nelson Textbook of Pediatrics.* 20th ed. Philadelphia: Saunders; 2015.

Miller MD, Thompson SR. *DeLee & Drez's Orthopaedic Sports Medicine: Principles and Practices.* 4th ed. Philadelphia: Saunders; 2015.

Shipman SA, Helfand M, Moyer VA, et al. Screening for developmental dysplasia of the hip: a systemic literature review for the U.S. Preventive Services Task Force. *Pediatrics.* 2006;117:e557–e576.

Stein CJ, Micheli LJ. Overuse injuries in youth sports. *Phys Sports Med.* 2010;38:102–108.

Wenger DR, Pring ME, Rang M. *Rang's Children's Fractures.* 3rd ed. Philadelphia: Lippincott Williams & Wilkins; 2005.

Wilson JC, Rodenberg RE. Apophysitis of the lower extremities. *Contemp Pediatr.* 2011;28:38–46.

PEARLS FOR PRACTITIONERS

CHAPTER 197

Orthopedics Assessment

- Orthopedic rough guide to developmental milestones
  - Sit independently at 6 months
  - Pull to stand at 10 months
  - Cruising at 12 months
  - Walk at 18 months
- Lower extremity angular profile
  - Genu varum (bowlegs)—birth and begin to straighten out by 18 months
  - Genu valgum (knock knees)—maximum at 4 years old and resolve by 5-8 years of age
  - Pathological genu verum: Blount disease (Tibia Vara) and Rickets
- The limping child differential diagnosis
  - Painful
    - Septic arthritis, osteomyelitis, diskitis
    - Transient monoarticular synovitis
    - Toddler's fracture or trauma
    - Malignancy
    - Rheumatological disorders in older children
    - Acute slipped capital femoral epiphysis (SCFE) in adolescents
  - Painless
    - Development dysplasia of the hip
    - Neuromuscular disorder
    - Leg length inequality
    - Legg-Calve-Perthes disease in older children
    - Muscular dystrophy in older children
    - Chronic, stable SCFE in adolescents

CHAPTER 198

Fractures

- Salter-Harris Fracture Types
  - I—transverse through physis
  - II—through physis into metaphysis
  - III—through physis into epiphysis (joint)
  - IV—through both metaphysis and epiphysis
  - V—crush to the physis
- Signs/symptoms of acute compartment syndrome producing neurovascular injury

- Pain out of proportion, exacerbated by passive stretch or muscle contraction
- Later findings: pallor, pulselessness, paresthesia, poikliothermia (cold)
- Common sites at risk include supracondylar and tibial fractures

CHAPTER 199

Hip

- Development dysplasia of the hip
  - Risk factors: first born, female, breech, family history, oligohydramnios
  - Associated lesions include congenital torticollis, metatarsus adductus, and clubfoot
  - Ortolani test reduces dislocated hip
  - Barlow test dislocates unstable hip
  - Galeazzi sign indicates dislocated hip
  - Klisic test is helpful to diagnose bilateral dislocations
  - Treatment is Pavlik harness through 6 months of age
- Legg-Calve-Perthes disease
  - Avascular necrosis of the femoral head
  - Classic presentation is painless limp in elementary school-aged boy
  - Mean age is 7 years
  - Delayed treatment increases risk of arthritis
- Transient monoarticular synovitis often follows a recent viral illness, with no fever and normal to minimally elevated white blood cell (WBC), erythrocyte sedimentation rate (ESR), and C-reactive protein (CRP)
- Septic arthritis has elevated WBC, ESR, CRP, and elevated joint fluid cell count. Patients are usually febrile and hold hip in flexion and external rotation.
- Slipped capital femoral epiphysis
  - Mean age is 12 years in males and 11 years in females
  - Risk factors: adolescent, obese, trisomy 21, endocrine disorder
  - May present as isolated hip or knee pain
  - Hip held externally rotated, especially when moved into hip flexion
  - Treat as orthopedic emergency—non-weight bearing and immediate referral

CHAPTER 200

Lower Extremity and Knee

- Tarsal coalition
  - Rigid flatfoot with decreased subtalar motion
  - Imaging is diagnostic (x-rays and computed tomography)
  - Treat with rest and immobilization or surgical excision
- Apophysitis
  - Osgood Schlatter disease at tibial tubercle
  - Sever disease at posterior calcaneus
  - Sinding Larsen Johansson syndrome at inferior pole of patella
  - Treat with rest, stretching, and ice
  - Internal tibial torsion is the most common cause of in-toeing in children <2 years of age
  - Internal femoral torsion (anteversion) may be seen in children with W-sitting positions
  - Acute swelling of the knee joint after injury may indicate a hemarthrosis
  - Chondromalacia of the patella is an incorrect term; the proper term is patellofemoral pain syndrome

CHAPTER 201

Foot

- Clubfoot (talipes equinovarus) may be congenital, teratological, or positional
- Clubfoot is often seen with developmental hip dysplasia
- Metatarsus adductus is a common foot disorder in infants; it resolves spontaneously in >90% of infants
- Hypermobile pes planus (flatfoot) are pronated feet associated with generalized ligamentous laxity, in children over 6 years of age
- A cavus foot (high arch) is associated with Charcot-Marie-Tooth disease (genetic neuropathy)

CHAPTER 202

Spine

- Scoliosis
  - Coronal curvature greater than 10 degrees
  - Adam's forward bend test shows trunk asymmetry
  - Congenital scoliosis has abnormal bony morphology
  - Neuromuscular scoliosis is associated with underlying disorder
  - Idiopathic scoliosis—no clear etiology
  - Treat
    - <25 degrees—observation
    - 20-50 degree curve or if progressing—bracing
    - 50+ degree curve—spinal fusion
- Kyphosis
  - Postural—normal bony structure
  - Scheuermann kyphosis
    - >5 degree anterior wedging on 3 consecutive vertebral bodies
    - Treat with bracing if skeletally immature; observation or surgical correction if skeletally mature
  - Congenital—abnormal bony structure that often requires bracing or surgery to treat

CHAPTER 203

Upper Extremity

- Brachial plexus birth injury
  - Moro reflex will give true neurological function
  - Differential diagnosis: clavicle or humerus fracture
- Radial head subluxation (nursemaid's elbow)
  - Mechanism—pulling the outstretched arm of a child
  - Treatment is reduction, usually with supination of forearm and flexion of elbow

INDEX

A

AAFP (American Academy of Family Physicians), on immunization, 364–365
AAP (American Academy of Pediatrics), 99
  on immunization, 364–365
ABC (airway, breathing, and circulation), for acute illness or injury, 145, 146*t*
Abdomen
  anemia and, 569*t*
  of newborn, 231
Abdominal muscles, during exhalation, 507
Abdominal pain, 467–472
  acute, 468
    diagnostic approach to, 468, 469*t*
    differential diagnosis of, 468, 469*t*–470*t*
    distinguishing features of, 468, 470*t*
    onset of, 468
  functional (recurrent), 468–471
    differential diagnosis of, 470, 471*t*
    distinguishing features of, 470–471
    suggested evaluation of, 470–471, 472*t*
    treatment of, 471–472
    warning signs in, 470–471, 472*t*
  general considerations with, 468
  due to irritable bowel syndrome, 468–471, 471*t*
  referred, 468
  somatic, 468
  somatoparietal, 468
  visceral, 468
Abdominal trauma, due to child abuse, 81
Abdominal tuberculosis, 454
Abdominal x-ray, in functional constipation, 50
Abducens nerve, assessment of, 683
Abduction, 739*t*
Abnormal temper tantrums, 44*t*
Abnormal uterine bleeding (AUB), 276–277, 276*t*
ABO blood group incompatibility, 247
Abortions, adolescent, 2
ABPA (allergic bronchopulmonary aspergillosis)
  asthma *vs.*, 314
  in cystic fibrosis, 527
Abscess, 722*f*
  breast, 100
  Brodie, 426, 765, 765*t*–766*t*
  of lung, 405–407
  peritonsillar, upper airway obstruction due to, 517*t*
  renal, 416
  retropharyngeal, upper airway obstruction due to, 517*t*
Absence seizures, 688–689
  atypical, 689
Absolute neutrophil count (ANC), in immunocompromised person, 434–435
Abuse. *see* Child abuse; Physical abuse
Acanthosis nigricans, 646
  Crouzon syndrome with, 170*t*
Access to care, 1, 3
Accessory muscles of exhalation, 507
Accessory muscles of inspiration, 507
Acebutolol, maternal use of, 238*t*
Acetaminophen
  as analgesia, 166*t*
  toxicity, 162*t*
Acetazolamide, maternal use of, 238*t*
Achondroplasia (ACH), genetic basis for, 170*t*
Acid-base balance, 139
Acid-base disorders, 138–142
  clinical assessment of, 139
  metabolic acidosis as, 139–141, 139*t*
  metabolic alkalosis as, 141–142, 141*t*
  mixed, 139
  respiratory acidosis as, 142*t*
  respiratory alkalosis as, 142*t*
  simple, 139, 139*t*
Acid-labile subunit, 650–651
Acid lipase deficiency, 210*t*–212*t*
Acidemia, 139
Acidosis, 139
  due to diabetic ketoacidosis, 642
  fetal, 220
  lactic, 140
    due to mitochondrial disorders, 214
  metabolic, 139–141, 139*t*
  respiratory, 142*t*
ACIP (Advisory Committee on Immunization Practices), on immunization, 364–365
Acne, 723–724
  cystic, 723
  vulgaris, 723
Acoustic reflectometry, for otitis media, 396
Acquired antiphospholipid antibodies, 589
Acquired epileptic aphasia, 690
Acquired immunodeficiency syndrome (AIDS), 457–461
  clinical manifestations of, 458–460, 459*t*
  complications of, 461
  differential diagnosis of, 460
  epidemiology of, 458
  etiology of, 457–458
  laboratory and imaging studies for, 460
  prevention of, 461
  prognosis for, 461
  treatment of, 460–461, 460*t*
Acquired thrombocytopenia, 584
Acrocyanosis, in newborn, 232
Acrodermatitis enteropathica, 121
Activated charcoal, for poisoning, 164
Activated partial thromboplastin time (aPTT), 584*t*
  prolonged, in hemophilia, 587
Activated platelets, 580
Acute bacterial meningitis, 387*t*
Acute bronchospasm, 335*t*–336*t*
Acute chest syndrome, in sickle cell disease, 576–577, 577*t*
Acute conjunctivitis, 430, 431*t*
Acute disseminated encephalomyelitis (ADEM), 389
Acute dystonic reactions, 703
Acute gastroenteritis, 410–413
  clinical manifestations of, 412
  complications and prognosis of, 413
  differential diagnosis of, 412
  etiology and epidemiology of, 410–412, 410*t*
  laboratory and imaging studies in, 412
  prevention of, 413
  treatment of, 412–413
Acute gastrointestinal hypersensitivity, 335*t*–336*t*
Acute hemolytic transfusion reaction, 590*t*
Acute illness or injury, 145–166
  cardiopulmonary arrest as, 147–149, 147*t*
    airway in, 147
    breathing in, 147–148
    circulation in, 147
    drugs in, 148–149, 148*t*
    pediatric advanced life support and cardiopulmonary resuscitation in, 147
  common manifestations of, 145, 146*t*
  diagnostic tests and imaging of, 146
  history of, 145
  initial assessment of, 145
  initial diagnostic evaluation for, 145–146
  physical examination of, 145, 146*t*
  resuscitation for, 146–147
  screening tests for, 145–146
Acute kidney injury (AKI)
  causes of, 625*t*
  clinical manifestations of, 625
  diagnostic studies of, 625–626
  etiology of, 625
  laboratory and clinical evaluation of, 625*t*
  nonoliguric, 625
  oliguric, 625
  prognosis for, 626
  treatment of, 626
Acute labyrinthitis, ataxia due to, 702
Acute lymphoid/lymphoblastic leukemia (ALL), 603
  classification of, 603
  clinical manifestations of, 603
  differential diagnosis of, 604
  epidemiology of, 603
  laboratory and imaging studies of, 603–604
  prognosis for, 604–605, 605*t*
  risk factors for, 597*t*
  T-cell, 603
  treatment of, 604
Acute mastoiditis, otitis media and, 397
Acute myeloid leukemia (AML)
  clinical manifestations of, 603
  epidemiology of, 603
  risk factors for, 597*t*
Acute neuritis, in varicella zoster virus, 378
Acute otitis media (AOM), 395
  defined, 396*t*
Acute painful events, in sickle cell disease, 577
Acute phase reactants, in infectious diseases, 361–362
Acute phase response, in infectious diseases, 361–362
Acute renal failure (ARF), 625–627
  classification of, 626*t*
  clinical manifestations of, 625
  diagnostic studies of, 625–626
  etiology of, 625
Acute respiratory distress syndrome (ARDS), 149, 149*t*, 524
Acute retroviral syndrome, 384, 458
Acute rheumatic fever, 393
Acute salicylate intoxication, 140
Acute water intoxication, 133

Page numbers followed by "*f*" indicate figures, and "*t*" indicate tables.

Acyclovir
for encephalitis, 390
for varicella zoster virus, 379
Acylcarnitine profile, plasma, 199*t*
Acylglycine profile, urine, 199*t*
Adalimumab, for juvenile idiopathic arthritis, 352
Adams forward bend test, 756–757
Adapalene, for acne, 723
Adaptive immune system, 289
Addison disease, 676–678
Adduction, 739*t*
Adenoidal hypertrophy, 519
Adenoma sebaceum, 681, 715
with developmental disabilities, 30*t*
Adenopathy, with anemia, 568
Adenosine
for cardiopulmonary resuscitation, 148*t*
for dysrhythmias, 543–544
Adenotonsillar hypertrophy, 515
Adenoviruses, conjunctivitis from, 430
ADH. *see* Antidiuretic hormone
ADHD. *see* Attention-deficit/hyperactivity disorder
Adjunctive therapy, for meningitis, 388
Adjuvant therapy, 601
Adolescent(s)
abortions, 2
birthrate in, 2
constitutional delay in, 656
defined, 15
developmental age of, 267, 270*t*
eating disorders in, 281–283
anorexia nervosa as, 281–283, 282*f*
clinical features of, 283
treatment and prognosis for, 283, 283*t*
bulimia nervosa as, 282–283, 283*t*
issues that can trigger, 282*t*
risk factors for, 282*f*
slippery slope to, 282*f*
treatment and prognosis for, 283*t*
ethical principles related to, 4–5
genetic assessment of, 178
interviewing of, 267–270, 270*t*
confidentiality in, 267, 270*t*
developmental age and, 267, 270*t*
on risk-taking behavior, 267, 270*t*
SCAG tool for, 268*f*–269*f*
STEP guide for, 270*f*
leading causes of death in, 267, 267*t*
legal rights of, 267, 270*t*
obesity and, 107–108
overview and assessment of, 267–273
as parent, 88
physical growth and development of, 14, 270–273
for boys, 271–273, 272*f*
changes associated with, 273
for girls, 270–271, 271*f*–272*f*
normal variations in, 274–275
breast asymmetry and masses as, 274, 274*t*
gynecomastia as, 274–275, 274*t*
irregular menses as, 274
physiological leukorrhea as, 274
physician-patient relationship with, 19
psychological development of, 267, 270*t*, 273
psychosocial assessment of, 15–16
early, 15
late, 16
middle, 15–16
reaction to divorce by, 94
sexual maturity rating for, 14
sleep, 53
substance use and abuse by, 2
well care of, 273–275
Adolescent(s) *(Continued)*
early, 273
late, 273
middle, 273
pelvic examination in, 273–274
physical examination in, 273, 273*t*
Adolescent gynecology, 275–281
contraception in, 278–281
barrier methods for, 280–281
condoms as, 280
sponge, caps, and diaphragm as, 280
coitus interruptus for, 281
emergency postcoital, 280–281, 281*t*
intrauterine devices for, 279
oral and anal for, 281
rhythm method (periodic coital abstinence) for, 281
steroidal, 278–281
combined hormonal contraceptives for, 279–280, 279*t*–280*t*
contraceptive patch for, 279–280
contraceptive vaginal ring for, 279–280
hormonal injections and implants for, 278–279
long-acting reversible contraceptives for, 278–279
progesterone-only pill or minipill for, 280
menstrual disorders in, 275–277
abnormal uterine bleeding as, 276–277
amenorrhea as, 275–276
dysmenorrhea as, 277
irregular menses as, 274–275
pregnancy in, 277–278
continuation of, 278
diagnosis of, 278
termination of, 278
rape in, 281
Adoption, 89
Adrenal adenomas, 660
Adrenal carcinomas, 660
Adrenal cortex, 674
Adrenal corticosteroids, maternal use of, 238*t*
Adrenal gland, physiology of, 674
Adrenal gland dysfunction, 674–678, 680
Addison disease, 676–678
adrenal insufficiency, 674–675
Cushing syndrome, 678
11-hydroxylase deficiency, 676
21-hydroxylase deficiency, 675–676
Adrenal hemorrhage, 675
Adrenal hyperplasia
congenital. *see* Congenital adrenal hyperplasia
lipoid, 675*f*
mild (late-onset) or nonclassic, 675
Adrenal insufficiency, 674–675
clinical and biochemical features of, 677*t*
clinical manifestations of, 676*t*
Adrenarche
in boys, 271–273, 272*f*
in girls, 270–271, 271*f*–272*f*
Adrenoleukodystrophy (ALD), 713
genetic basis for, 174*t*
X-linked, 711*t*–712*t*, 713
Adult health challenges, 2
Adult tapeworm infections, 452*t*
Advanced care, 6
Adventitious breath sounds, 510*t*
Adverse drug reactions, 338–339
accelerated, 338
classification of, 338
clinical manifestations of, 338
complications of, 339
defined, 338
differential diagnosis of, 339
epidemiology of, 338
etiology of, 338, 338*t*
Adverse drug reactions *(Continued)*
immediate (anaphylactic), 338
immunological, 338, 338*t*
laboratory and imaging studies for, 338–339
late, 338
nonimmunological, 338, 338*t*
prevention of, 339
prognosis for, 339
treatment of, 339
Advisory Committee on Immunization Practices (ACIP), on immunization, 364–365
Advocacy, 4
Aeroallergens, in asthma, 314
Aerosol therapy, 512, 512*f*
Afebrile pneumonia, 403
Afferent pupillary defect, 683
African tick-bite fever, 439*t*–442*t*
African trypanosomiasis, 439*t*–442*t*
Afterload, in heart failure, 553, 554*t*
Afterload reduction
for cardiomyopathies, 557*t*, 558
for heart failure, 554, 555*t*
for ventricular septal defect, 545–546
Agammaglobulinemia, 294, 295*t*
autosomal recessive, 294
X-linked, 294
Age, tantrums and, 43–44, 44*f*
Age-related macular degeneration, 306
Ages and Stages Questionnaires, 17
Agonal respiration, 509*t*
β_2-Agonists, for asthma
long-acting, 315
short-acting, 315–316
Agoraphobia, 62
AH_{50} test, 306
AIRE (autoimmune regulator) gene, in chronic mucocutaneous candidiasis, 298
Airway(s), endoscopic evaluation of, 511
Airway hemorrhage, 525
Airway hyperresponsiveness, in asthma, 313
Airway management, for burns, 159
Airway patency, in rapid cardiopulmonary assessment, 146*t*
Airway remodeling, in asthma, 313
Airway resistance, 508
AIS (arterial ischemic stroke), 699
Alagille syndrome, 494
Albright hereditary osteodystrophy, 669
Albuterol, for asthma, 315
Alcohol
acute effects of, 284*t*–285*t*
as teratogen, 237*t*
use, during pregnancy, 90
ALD (adrenoleukodystrophy), genetic basis for, 174*t*
Alertness, assessment of, 682
Alfentanil, as analgesia, 166*t*
Algid malaria, 449
Alkalemia, 139
Alkali agents, ingestion of, 160–162
Alkalosis
metabolic, 141–142, 141*t*
respiratory, 142*t*
Alkylating agents, for cancer, 601*t*–602*t*
ALL. *see* Acute lymphoid/lymphoblastic leukemia
Allergen, 311
Allergen immunotherapy, for allergic rhinitis, 325
Allergic bronchopulmonary aspergillosis (ABPA)
asthma *vs.*, 314
in cystic fibrosis, 527
Allergic conjunctivitis, 433*t*
Allergic contact dermatitis, 727, 728*f*
Allergic eosinophilic esophagitis, 335*t*–336*t*

Allergic eosinophilic gastroenteritis, 335t–336t
Allergic proctocolitis, 335t–336t
Allergic rhinitis, 323–325
clinical manifestations of, 323
complications of, 325
differential diagnosis of, 323–324
epidemiology of, 323
episodic, 323
etiology of, 323
laboratory and imaging studies of, 323
perennial, 323
prognosis and prevention of, 325
seasonal, 323
treatment of, 324–325
immunotherapy for, 325
pharmacotherapy for, 324–325
Allergic rhinoconjunctivitis, 335t–336t
Allergic salute, 312, 323
Allergic shiners, 312, 323
Allergic transfusion reaction, 590t
Allergy, 311–339, 724, 727
allergen in, 311
assessment of, 311–313
diagnostic imaging in, 313
history in, 312
initial diagnostic evaluation in, 312–313
physical examination in, 312
screening tests in, 312–313
atopy in, 311
contact, 311–312, 727–728, 728f
drug, 338–339
accelerated, 338
classification of, 338
clinical manifestations of, 338
complications of, 339
defined, 338
differential diagnosis of, 339
epidemiology of, 338
etiology of, 338, 338t
immediate (anaphylactic), 338
immunological, 338, 338t
laboratory and imaging studies for, 338–339
late, 338
nonimmunological, 338, 338t
prevention of, 339
prognosis for, 339
treatment of, 339
food, 334–338
with atopic dermatitis, 725
clinical manifestations of, 335, 335t–336t
complications of, 337
diagnosis of, 335–337
etiology and epidemiology of, 334–335
laboratory and imaging studies for, 335
prognosis and prevention of, 337–338
treatment of, 337
vomiting due to, 473t
hypersensitivity reactions in, 311, 311t
type I (anaphylactic), 311, 311t
immediate, 311t
late-phase, 311
type II (antibody cytotoxicity), 311, 311t
type III (immune complex), 311, 311t
arthus reaction in, 311
serum sickness in, 311
type IV (cellular immune-mediated, delayed type), 311–312, 311t
insect, 333–334
clinical manifestations of, 333, 333t
complications of, 334
differential diagnosis of, 334
epidemiology of, 333
etiology of, 333
laboratory and imaging studies for, 334
prevention of, 334
Allergy *(Continued)*
prognosis for, 334
treatment of, 334
Allergy skin testing, for asthma, 314
Alopecia, in systemic lupus erythematosus, 353
Alper disease, 213–214
Alpha-chain hemoglobinopathies, 575
Alpha-fetoprotein (AFP) maternal serum screening for, 179
Alport syndrome, hematuria due to, 622–623
Alstrom syndrome, obesity in, 106t
Alternative pathway, of complement activation, 304–305, 305f
Alternative splicing, 169
Altruism, 4
Alveolar bleeding, 525
Alveolar-capillary membrane, gas diffusion across, 508
Alveolar cyst disease, 452
Alveolar macrophages, as lung defense mechanisms, 508
Alveolar ventilation, 508
Alveoli, 507
Amblyomma cajennense, 444
Amblyopia, 33
Amebiasis, 411–412
Amebic dysentery, 412
Amegakaryocytic thrombocytopenia, 584
Amenorrhea, 275–276
athletic, 658
in congenital adrenal hyperplasia, 275
endocrine evaluation for, 275
history and physical examination for, 275
in polycystic ovary syndrome, 275
primary, 659
defined, 275
progesterone withdrawal test for, 275
secondary, defined, 275
therapy for, 275–276
in Turner syndrome, 275
American Academy of Family Physicians (AAFP), on immunization, 364–365
American Academy of Pediatrics (AAP), 99
on immunization, 364–365
American dog tick, 444
American trypanosomiasis (Chagas disease), 439t–442t
Amino acid(s), in parenteral nutrition, 131
Amino acid analysis
neonatal screening for, 197, 198t
specialized testing for, 197
Amino acid disorder(s), 201–205
of ammonia disposal, 204–205, 204f
argininosuccinate lyase deficiency as, 204
ornithine carbamoyltransferase deficiency as, 204
of metabolism, 201
homocystinuria as, 203, 203f
maple syrup urine disease as, 203–204, 203f
phenylketonuria as, 200f, 201–202
tyrosinemias as, 202–203, 202f
that affect specific transport mechanisms in kidney and intestine, 205
cystinuria as, 205
Hartnup syndrome as, 205
Amino acid profile
plasma, 199t
urine, 199t
Amino acid substitution, in sickle cell disease, 576
Aminopterin, as teratogen, 237t
5-Aminosalicylic acid (5-ASA), for ulcerative colitis, 491
Amiodarone
for cardiopulmonary resuscitation, 148t
maternal use of, 238t
Ammonia
disposal, disorders of, 204–205, 204f
in renal function, 617
Amniocentesis, 177
Amniotic fluid, meconium-stained, 226, 245
Amoxicillin
for Lyme disease, 444
for sinusitis, 395
for streptococcal pharyngitis, 393–394
Amoxicillin-clavulanate, for sinusitis, 395
Amphetamines
acute effects of, 284t–285t
toxicity, 162t
Anabolic steroids, acute effects of, 284t–285t
Anakinra, for juvenile idiopathic arthritis, 352
Anal stenosis, constipation due to, 476t
Analgesia, 165–166, 166t
Anaphylactic hypersensitivity reactions, 311, 311t
Anaphylactoid reaction, 328–330
Anaphylatoxins, 328, 330
Anaphylaxis, 328–332
biphasic, 331
clinical manifestations of, 330
common causes of, 329t
differential diagnosis of, 331
epidemiology of, 330
etiology of, 328
due to insect bites, 333
laboratory and imaging studies for, 330–331
prevention of, 331–332
protracted, 331
treatment of, 331, 332f
Anaplasma phagocytophilum, 439t–442t, 445–446, 446f
Anaplasmosis, 439t–442t, 445–446
clinical manifestations of, 445
complications and prognosis of, 446
differential diagnosis of, 446
epidemiology of, 445
etiology of, 445
human, 445
laboratory and imaging studies, 446
prevention of, 446
treatment for, 446
Anaplastic large cell lymphoma (ALCL), 605
Anatomic dead space, 508
Anatomic evaluation, for chronic liver disease, 500t
Ancylostoma braziliense, 450t
Ancylostoma duodenale, 450, 450t
Androgen insensitivity syndrome, 672–673
complete, 659
Anemia, 566–580, 567f, 591–592
aplastic, 574
etiology and epidemiology of, 574
laboratory studies of, 574
treatment of, 574
classification of, 566, 567f
clinical manifestations of, 567–568, 568t–569t
differential diagnosis of, 568–580
etiology of, 566
Fanconi, 574–575
clinical manifestations of, 574
etiology and epidemiology of, 574
marrow replacement in, 575
pancytopenia resulting from destruction of cells, 575
treatment of, 575
hemolytic, 566, 567f, 575–580
autoimmune, 580
caused by disorders extrinsic to the red blood cell, 579–580
clinical manifestations of, 579–580, 579f
etiology of, 579–580, 579f
laboratory diagnosis of, 580

Anemia *(Continued)*
prognosis for, 580
treatment of, 580
due to enzymopathies, 578
clinical manifestations of, 578
epidemiology of, 578
etiology of, 578
glucose-6-phosphate dehydrogenase (G6PD) deficiency as, 566
laboratory studies of, 578
prevention of, 578
pyruvate kinase deficiency as, 566
treatment of, 578
due to major hemoglobinopathies, 575
alpha-chain hemoglobinopathies, 575
beta-chain hemoglobinopathies, 575
due to membrane disorders, 578–579
clinical manifestations of, 579
etiology of, 578–579
laboratory diagnosis of, 579
treatment of, 579
due to sickle cell disease, 576–578
clinical manifestations of, 576–577, 577*t*
etiology and epidemiology of, 576, 576*t*
laboratory diagnosis of, 577
treatment of, 577–578
due to β-thalassemia major, 575–576
clinical manifestations of, 575
etiology and epidemiology of, 575
treatment of, 575–576
hypochromic, microcytic, 566, 567*f*, 568–574
due to iron deficiency, 568–571
clinical manifestations of, 570
epidemiology of, 570, 570*t*
etiology of, 570
prevention of, 571
treatment of, 571, 571*t*
due to lead poisoning, 571
thalassemia minor as, 571
etiology and epidemiology of, 571, 572*f*, 572*t*
laboratory testing for, 571
treatment of, 571
of inflammation, 571–573
iron deficiency, 568–571
clinical manifestations of, 570
diagnosis of, 120
epidemiology of, 570, 570*t*
etiology of, 570
prevention of, 571
treatment of, 120, 571, 571*t*
laboratory studies in, 568, 570*f*
macrocytic, 566, 567*f*, 574–575
due to marrow failure/pancytopenia, 574
differential diagnosis of, 574
etiology of, 574
microangiopathic hemolytic, 624
in newborn, 247–249
due to blood group incompatibility, 247
blood loss, 249
due to decreased red blood cell production, 247
diagnosis and management of, 249
differential diagnosis of, 248*f*
due to erythroblastosis fetalis, 247
etiology of, 247
due to hemolytic disease, 249
due to increased red blood cell destruction, 247–249
normocytic, 566, 567*f*, 571–574
etiology and treatment of, 571–574, 573*t*
oncological emergencies, 600*t*
pernicious, 117
physiological, 247
presentation of, 564*t*
Anergy, in tuberculosis, 453
Anesthetic agents, maternal use of, 238*t*
Aneuploidy, 179–182
monosomies as, 181–182
Turner syndrome as, 181–182
trisomies as, 180–181
Down syndrome as, 180
Klinefelter syndrome as, 181
trisomy 13 as, 180–181
trisomy 18 as, 180, 181*t*
Aneurysm(s)
cerebral, in autosomal dominant polycystic kidney disease, 630
coronary artery, in Kawasaki disease, 347
Aneurysmal bone cyst, 765*t*–766*t*
Angel dust, acute effects of, 284*t*–285*t*
Angelman syndrome (AS), genetic basis for, 176
Angel's kiss, 733
Angina
Ludwig, 393
Vincent, 393
Angioedema, 328–332
acute, 328, 335*t*–336*t*
chronic, 328–329
clinical manifestations of, 330
differential diagnosis of, 331
epidemiology of, 330
etiology of, 328
hereditary, 329, 329*t*, 331*t*
idiopathic, 331*t*
laboratory and imaging studies for, 330–331
physical, 328–329
prevention of, 331–332
recurrent, 330, 331*t*
treatment of, 331
upper airway obstruction due to, 517*t*
Angiography, of pulmonary embolism
CT, 526
pulmonary, 526
Angiomas, in Sturge-Weber syndrome, 715, 733
Angiomatosis, encephalotrigeminal, port-wine stain in, 733
Angioneurotic edema, hereditary, genetic basis for, 170*t*
Angiostrongyliasis, abdominal, 450*t*
Angiostrongylus cantonensis, 450*t*
Angiostrongylus costaricensis, 450*t*
Animal dander, asthma and, 315*t*
Anion gap, 140
in metabolic acidosis, 162*t*
Anions, in body fluids, 125
Aniridia Wilms tumor association, 182
Ankylosing spondylitis, juvenile, 351*t*
Anomalous innominate artery, 521
Anorectal malformations, 489
constipation due to, 476*t*
Anorectal manometry, for Hirschsprung disease, 489–490
Anorexia nervosa, 281–283, 282*f*
clinical features of, 283
delayed puberty due to, 658
treatment and prognosis for, 283, 283*t*
Anovulation, 276
Antagonism, of antimicrobial drugs, 367–368
Antalgic gait, 740
Anterior pituitary gland, 637–638
Anterior pituitary hormone function testing, 639*t*
Anterior uveitis, 433*t*
Anthrax, 439*t*–442*t*
Anthropometric data, for obesity, 107
Antiarrhythmics, for cardiomyopathies, 557*t*
Antibiotic-lock therapy, 438
Antibiotics, 726
for acne, 723
oral, 723
topical, 723
Antibiotics *(Continued)*
for cystic fibrosis, 529
for infectious diseases, 362
for infective endocarditis, 409
for pneumonia, 408
prophylaxis, for severe combined immunodeficiency, 299
topical, for acne, 723
Antibody cytotoxicity hypersensitivity reactions, 311, 311*t*
Antibody deficiency disease, 294–295, 294*f*, 295*t*
agammaglobulinemia as, 294, 295*t*
autosomal recessive, 294
X-linked, 294
antibody deficiency syndrome as, 295, 295*t*
common variable immunodeficiency as, 294–295, 295*t*
IgA deficiency as, 295, 295*t*
IgG subclass deficiency as, 295, 295*t*
transient hypogammaglobulinemia of infancy as, 295, 295*t*
Anti-CCP antibody, in juvenile idiopathic arthritis, 350–351
Anticholinergics, toxicity, 162*t*
Anticoagulant, for cardiomyopathies, 557*t*
Anticongestive medications, in truncus arteriosus, 552
Anticonvulsants
for anxiety disorders, 64
for autism spectrum disorder (ASD), 71
for bipolar disorders, 68
Antidepressants
for depressive disorders, 66
for somatic symptom and related disorders (SSRDs), 61
Antidiuretic hormone (ADH)
in regulation of intravascular volume, 125
in renal function, 617, 619*f*
in sodium balance, 131
Antidysrhythmic drugs, 544*t*
Antiemetic medications, for vomiting, 473
Antihistamines
for allergic rhinitis, 325
first-generation, 325
second-generation, 325
for atopic dermatitis, 726
for urticaria and angioedema, 331
Antiinfective therapy, 367–368
antagonism in, 367–368
definitive, 367
drug-drug interactions and, 367–368
drug susceptibilities in, 367
empirical or presumptive, 367
site and nature of the infection and, 367
synergism, 367–368
Antiinflammatory doses, for Kawasaki disease, 348
Antiinflammatory medications, for pericarditis, 558
Antimetabolites, for cancer, 601*t*–602*t*
Antimicrobial therapy, for pneumonia, 404*t*
Antinuclear antibody
in juvenile idiopathic arthritis, 350
in systemic lupus erythematosus, 354
Antioxidant, 117
Antiphospholipid syndrome, maternal, 235
Antipsychotics
for autism spectrum disorder (ASD), 71
for schizophrenia spectrum disorders, 72–73
Anti-Rh-positive immune globulin (RhoGAM), 248–249
Antithrombin, 589
Antithrombin III, in hemostasis, 581
Antithrombotic doses, for Kawasaki disease, 348
α1-Antitrypsin deficiency, 494
Anuria, fluid therapy for, 127, 127*t*

Anus
  anteriorly displaced, constipation due to, 476*t*
  imperforate, 489
    constipation due to, 476*t*
Anxiety disorders, 61–64
  agoraphobia, 62
  attention-deficit/hyperactivity disorder (ADHD) and, 64
  bipolar and related disorders and, 67–68
  characteristics of, 62*t*
  defined, 61
  generalized anxiety disorder (GAD), 62
  management of, 63
  panic disorder, 61–62
  selective mutism, 63
  separation anxiety disorder (SAD), 63, 63*t*
  social anxiety disorder, 63, 64*t*
  specific phobias, 63
  unspecified, 62
AOM (acute otitis media), 395
  defined, 396*t*
Aorta
  fetal, Doppler examination of, 220
  overriding, in tetralogy of Fallot, 549
Aortic stenosis, 548
Apgar examination, 225, 225*t*
Aphasia, 682
  acquired epileptic, 690
Apid stings, allergic reactions to, 333
Aplasia cutis congenita, in trisomy 13, 180–181
Aplastic anemia, 574. *see also* Anemia, aplastic
Aplastic crisis(es)
  in chronic hemolytic anemia, 574
  in sickle cell disease, 576, 577*t*
  transient, erythema infectiosum and, 377
Apnea, 514–515
  categories of, 514*t*
  central, 246, 514, 514*t*
  defined, 246
  etiology of, 514–515
  mixed, 246
  obstructive, 246
    sleep, 514–515, 514*t*
  of prematurity, 246, 514, 514*t*
Apnea-hypopnea index (AHI), 515
Apneustic respiration, 509*t*
Apophysis, 739*t*
Apophysitis, calcaneal, 755
  clinical manifestations of, 755
  treatment of, 755
Apparent life-threatening event (ALTE), 515
Appearance, of newborn, 227
Appendicitis, 493–494
  abdominal pain due to, 470*t*
  clinical manifestations of, 493
  etiology and epidemiology of, 493
  laboratory and imaging studies for, 493, 493*t*
  treatment of, 494
  vomiting due to, 473*t*
Appendicular ataxia, 700
Appetite suppression, in attention-deficit/hyperactivity disorder (ADHD), 47
Arboviruses, encephalitis from, 389
Arch, high, 755
ARF. *see* Acute renal failure
Argininosuccinate lyase (ASL) deficiency, 205
Ariboflavinosis, 113
Arm recoil, in newborn, 229*f*
Arm span, 651
Arousal, 703
Arrhythmias. *see* Dysrhythmia(s)
Arsenic, for cancer, 601*t*–602*t*
Arterial blood gas, in respiratory failure, 150
Arterial blood gas analysis, 511
Arterial clots, in hemostatic disorders, 583
Arterial ischemic stroke (AIS), 699
Arterial switch, in transposition of great arteries, 551
Artery-to-pulmonary shunt, for tricuspid atresia, 551
Arthralgias, in systemic lupus erythematosus, 353
Arthritis
  in Henoch-Schönlein purpura, 345
  infectious, 428–430
    clinical manifestations of, 428–429
    complications and prognosis of, 430
    differential diagnosis of, 429, 433*t*
    epidemiology of, 428
    etiology of, 428
    juvenile idiopathic arthritis *vs.*, 352*t*
    laboratory and imaging studies for, 429
    pathogenic organisms causing, 428*t*
    prevention of, 430
    treatment of, 429–430, 430*t*
  juvenile idiopathic. *see* Juvenile idiopathic arthritis
  Lyme, 429*t*
  poststreptococcal, 352*t*
  reactive, 428
    juvenile idiopathic arthritis *vs.*, 352*t*
    synovial fluid findings in, 429*t*
  in rheumatic diseases, 343
  due to rheumatic fever, 556
  in systemic lupus erythematosus, 353
Arthritis-dermatitis syndrome, 428
Arthrocentesis, for juvenile idiopathic arthritis, 351
Arthrogryposis multiplex congenita, 185
Arthroplasty, 739*t*
Arthroscopy, 739*t*
Arthrotomy, 739*t*
Arthus reaction, 311
Articular cartilage, 740*f*
Artificial airway, 513
Arylsulfatase A deficiency, 210*t*–212*t*
Arytenoid cartilages, 507
AS (Angelman syndrome), genetic basis for, 176
Ascariasis, 450
  intestinal, 450*t*
  pulmonary, 450
Ascaris lumbricoides, 450, 450*t*
Ascites, with chronic liver disease, 497, 500*t*
Ascorbic acid deficiency, 112, 114*t*
ASD. *see* Atrial septal defect
ASD (autism spectrum disorder), 70–73, 70*t*
Ash leaf spots, 715
Asparaginase, for cancer, 601*t*–602*t*
Aspartylglucosaminidase deficiency, 210*t*–212*t*
Aspergillosis, allergic bronchopulmonary
  asthma *vs.*, 314
  in cystic fibrosis, 527
Asphyxia
  birth, etiology of, 225*t*
  effects of, 224*t*
  intrauterine, 225
  metabolic acidosis during, 222
  pallida, 233
Aspiration, foreign body, 521–522
  bronchiolitis and, 402
Aspirin
  for Kawasaki disease, 348
  maternal use of, 238*t*
Aspirin exacerbated respiratory disease, 324
Assault, 92
Association, in dysmorphology, 184
Asthma, 313–321, 335*t*–336*t*, 520
  cardiogenic, 402
  clinical manifestations of, 313
  complications of, 316, 320*f*
  differential diagnosis of, 314, 314*t*
  epidemiology of, 313
Asthma *(Continued)*
  etiology of, 313
  factors contributing to severity of, 314, 315*t*
  laboratory and imaging studies of, 313–314
  persistent, 316–321, 321*t*
  prevention of, 321
  prognosis for, 316–321, 318*t*
  respiratory failure due to, 149
  status asthmatic in, 316
  treatment of, 314–316, 315*t*
    approach to, 316
      stepwise, 316, 317*f*–318*f*
    for exacerbations, 320*f*
    long-term control medications in, 314–315
      biologics as, 315
      inhaled corticosteroids as, 314–315, 319*f*
      leukotriene modifiers as, 315
      long-acting β_2-agonists as, 315
      mepolizumab as, 315
      omalizumab as, 315
      theophylline as, 315
    quick-relief medications in, 315–316
      anticholinergic agents as, 316
      oral corticosteroids as, 316
      short-acting β_2-agonists as, 315–316
    rules of two for, 316
    self-management guidelines in, 321, 322*f*
      adherence in, 321
      peak flow monitoring in, 321
  triad, 321*t*
Astroviruses, diarrhea from, 410*t*
Asymmetric tonic neck reflex, 14, 682*t*
Ataxia, 684, 700–703
  due to acute labyrinthitis, 702
  appendicular, 700
  due to brain tumors, 701
  clinical manifestations of, 700
  defined, 700–702
  due to drug intoxication, 700
  etiologies of, 700–702, 701*t*
  Friedreich, 702
    genetic basis for, 173*t*
  due to inborn errors of metabolism, 702
  due to neuroblastoma, 701–702
  postinfectious acute cerebellar, 700–701
  truncal, 700
Ataxia-telangiectasia, 298, 299*t*, 702
Atelectasis, 510*t*
  in respiratory distress syndrome, 242
Atenolol, maternal use of, 238*t*
Athetosis, 702–703
Athlete's foot, 381*t*. *see also* Tinea pedis
Athletic amenorrhea, 658
ATM gene, in ataxia-telangiectasia, 298
Atomoxetine, for attention-deficit/hyperactivity disorder (ADHD), 47
Atonic seizures, 689
Atopic dermatitis, 325–328, 335*t*–336*t*, 724–727
  with bacterial superinfection, 726, 727*f*
  clinical manifestations of, 326, 326*f*, 724, 725*f*
  complications of, 328, 726–727, 727*f*
  differential diagnosis of, 326, 327*t*, 725
  epidemiology of, 326, 724
  etiology of, 325–326, 724
  laboratory and imaging studies for, 326, 327*t*, 724–725
  lichenified plaques in, 326, 326*f*
  prevention of, 328, 727
  prognosis for, 328, 727
  treatment of, 326–328, 725–726
Atopic march, 724
Atopy, 311
Atrial contractions, premature, 543
Atrial dysrhythmias, 542–543
Atrial fibrillation, 543
Atrial flutter, 543, 544*t*

Atrial natriuretic peptide, in regulation of intravascular volume, 125
Atrial pacemaker, wandering, 542
Atrial septal defect (ASD), 546, 546*f*
Atrophy, 722*t*
Atropine
for cardiopulmonary resuscitation, 148*t*
for organophosphate poisoning, 164*t*–165*t*
Attachment, 91
in infancy, 15
Attention-deficit/hyperactivity disorder (ADHD), 45–47
anticipatory guidance for, 47
anxiety disorders and, 64
clinical symptoms of, 46, 46*t*
co-morbidities in, 46
complications of, 47
diagnosis of, 46
differential diagnosis of, 46–47
etiology of, 45
evaluation of, 46
laboratory and imaging studies in, 46
physical examination for, 46
treatment of, 47
Atypical hemolytic uremic syndrome, 306
Atypical lymphocytes
in infectious diseases, 362
in lymphadenitis, 384
Atypical pneumonia, 402–403
Auditory brainstem response (ABR), 35
Aura, migraine, 686
Auscultation, in cardiovascular system assessment, 536
Auspitz sign, in psoriasis, 729–730
Autism, screening for, 17–18
Autism spectrum disorder (ASD), 70–73, 70*t*
Autoantibodies
manifestations of, 345*t*
in systemic lupus erythematosus, 353
Autocrine action, of hormones, 637, 637*f*
Autoimmune encephalitis, 389
Autoimmune hemolytic anemia, 580
Autoimmune hepatitis, 500, 500*t*
Autoimmune polyglandular syndrome type I, 667
Autoimmune polyglandular syndrome type II, 667
Autoimmune regulator *(AIRE)* gene, in chronic mucocutaneous candidiasis, 298
Autoimmune thrombocytopenic purpura of childhood (childhood ITP), 584–585
Autonomic nerves, dysfunction of, in Guillain-Barré syndrome, 695
Autonomy, 4
in early childhood, 15
in end-of-life decision making, 8
Autosomal dominant disorders, 170–171
achondroplasia due to, 170*t*
Crouzon syndrome with acanthosis nigricans due to, 170*t*
hereditary angioneurotic edema due to, 170*t*
Marfan syndrome due to, 170*t*
myotonic dystrophy due to, 170*t*
neurofibromatosis 1 due to, 170*t*
neurofibromatosis 2 due to, 170*t*
nonsyndromic craniosynostosis due to, 170*t*
pedigree drawing of, 170*f*
penetrance in, 170, 170*f*
thanatophoric dysplasia due to, 170*t*
variable expressivity of, 171
Autosomal dominant (AD) inheritance
pedigree of, 173*f*
rules of, 171*t*
Autosomal recessive agammaglobulinemia, 294
Autosomal recessive disorders, 171
consanguinity and, 177
cystic fibrosis due to, 173*t*
Friedreich ataxia due to, 173*t*
Gaucher disease due to, 173*t*
phenylketonuria due to, 173*t*
sickle cell disease due to, 173*t*
Autosomal recessive (AR) inheritance, rules of, 173*t*
Autosomes, 169
Avascular necrosis, 747–748
idiopathic, 755
Avian influenza (bird flu), 403
Azathioprine, for ulcerative colitis, 491
Azelaic acid, for acne, 723
Azithromycin
for *Chlamydia* infection, 423
for pertussis, 401
for streptococcal pharyngitis, 393–394

B

B cells, 289–290
Babesia, 439, 439*t*–442*t*
Babesiosis, 439*t*–442*t*
Babinski reflex, 682*t*
Babinski response, 684
Babinski sign, 231–232
Baby bottle caries, 479
Baby-cereals, as complementary food, 101
Bacille Calmette-Guérin (BCG) vaccine, 454, 457
Bacillus anthracis, 439*t*–442*t*
Back pain, 761, 761*t*
Back to Sleep initiative, 22
Back-to-sleep program, 515–516
Bacteremia, 417
catheter-associated, 437–438
fever and, 368
in nephrotic syndrome, 621
occult, 369
Bacterial colonization, of newborn, 222
Bacterial conjunctivitis, 433*t*
Bacterial diarrhea, fever due to, 368
Bacterial diseases, zoonotic, 439*t*–442*t*
Bacterial enteritis, gastrointestinal bleeding due to, 477*t*
Bacterial gastroenteritis, vomiting due to, 473*t*
Bacterial infections
in immunocompromised person, 434–435
superficial, 379–380
cellulitis as, 380
folliculitis as, 380
impetigo as, 379–380
perianal dermatitis as, 380
viral infections *vs.*, 363*t*, 368–369
Bacterial meningitis, 707
causes of, 386*t*
Bacterial tracheitis, 399
upper airway obstruction due to, 517*t*
Bacterial vaginosis, 417–418, 418*t*, 422*t*
Bag/mask ventilation, for respiratory failure, 150
Baker cyst, 751
Balloon angioplasty, for coarctation of aorta, 548
Balloon atrial septostomy, for transposition of great arteries, 551
Balloon valvuloplasty
for aortic stenosis, 548
for pulmonary stenosis, 548
Barbiturates, maternal use of, 238*t*
Bardet-Biedl syndrome, obesity in, 106*t*
Bare lymphocyte syndrome, 297*t*, 298
Barium enema, for Hirschsprung disease, 489–490
Barium esophagram, 511
Barium upper gastrointestinal (GI) series, for gastroesophageal reflux, 481
Barlow test, 231, 745*f*
Bart hemoglobin, 575
Bartonella henselae, 383, 439*t*–442*t*
conjunctivitis from, 430
Bartter syndrome, 135–136, 136*t*
Basophilic stippling, 571
Batten disease, 210*t*–212*t*
Batteries, ingestion of, 162
Battle sign, 710
Baylisascaris procyonis, 450–451, 450*t*
Becker muscular dystrophy, 696
Beckwith-Wiedemann syndrome, 184, 648
Beclomethasone HFA, for asthma, 319*f*
Bed bug bites, allergic reactions to, 333
Bed rest, for rheumatic fever, 556
Bee stings, allergic reactions to, 333
Behavioral assessment, issues in, 18–19, 18*t*
Behavioral disorders, 41–58
attention-deficit/hyperactivity disorder (ADHD), 45–47
crying, 41–43
colic and, 41–43
normal development, 41, 41*f*
elimination, control of, 47–51
pediatric sleep disorders, 52–56
temper tantrums, 43–45
Behavioral insomnia of childhood, pediatric sleep disorders and, 55
Behavioral issues, screening for, 18*t*, 19
Behavioral management, in attention-deficit/hyperactivity disorder (ADHD), 47
Behavioral sleep disorders, 54*t*–55*t*
Behavioral training, for functional constipation, 50
Bell palsy, 683
Belt-positioning booster seat, 22
Beneficence, 4
in end-of-life decision making, 8
Benign fibroadenomas, 274
Benzathine penicillin
for rheumatic fever, 556
for streptococcal pharyngitis, 394*t*
Benzodiazepines
for anxiety disorders, 64
maternal use of, 238*t*
for status epilepticus, 691, 691*t*
Benzoyl peroxide, for acne, 723
Bereavement, 95–96
Bernard-Soulier syndrome, 586
Beta cells, in insulin-dependent diabetes mellitus, 640
Beta-chain hemoglobinopathies, 575
Beta-chain synthesis, in β-thalassemia major, 575
Bi-level positive airway pressure (BiPAP), 515
Bicarbonate, for cardiopulmonary resuscitation, 148*t*
Bidirectional cavopulmonary shunt, for tricuspid atresia, 551
Bidirectional Glenn procedure, for tricuspid atresia, 551
Biemond syndrome, obesity in, 106*t*
Bilateral renal agenesis, 629
Bilateral Wilms tumor, 611
Bilharziasis, 451
Biliary atresia, extrahepatic, 494
Bilirubin
in breast-fed infants, 100
in fetus, 251
Bilirubin diglucuronide, 250
Bilirubin encephalopathy, 251
Biliverdin, 249–250
Biophysical profile, of fetus, 220
Biopsy
lung, 512
rectal, for Hirschsprung disease, 489–490
small bowel, for celiac disease, 489–490

Biopsychosocial influences, on health and illness, 3
Biopterin metabolism, disorders, 201–202
Biot respiration, 509*t*
Biotinidase deficiency, 206
  neonatal screening for, 197
Bipolar and related disorders, 66–68
  anxiety disorders and, 67–68
  bipolar I disorder, 66, 67*t*
  bipolar II disorder, 66
  cyclothymic disorder, 66–67
  specifiers for, 67
  treatment of, 68
  unspecified, 66
Bipolar I disorder (BD), 66, 67*t*
Bipolar II disorder, 66
Bird flu, 403
Birth(s)
  history of, in genetic assessment, 178
  preterm, 1, 218
Birth injury, 233–234
Birth weight
  low, 218–219
  very low, 219
Birthmarks, 730, 730*t*
Birthrate, in adolescent, 2
Bisacodyl, for functional constipation, 52*t*
Bisacodyl suppository, for functional constipation, 51*t*
Bisacodyl tablet, for functional constipation, 51*t*
Black-legged tick, 443. *see also* Deer tick
  Western, 443
Blackfly bites, allergic reactions to, 333
Blackhead, 723
Blackwater fever, 449
Bladder outlet obstruction, 630
Blalock-Taussig procedure, for tricuspid atresia, 551
Bleeding
  causes of, 583*f*
  gastrointestinal, 476–478
  in hematological disorders, 563
  rectal, evaluation of, 478*t*
  spontaneous, 587
Bleeding disorders. *see* Hemostatic disorders
Bleeding time, 583, 584*t*
Blepharitis, 431, 433*t*
Blinatumomab, for cancer, 601*t*–602*t*
β-blockers
  for cardiomyopathies, 557*t*
  for heart failure, 554
Blood-brain barrier, in chemotherapy, 601
Blood component therapy, 589–590, 593
Blood cultures, 362
Blood gas analysis, for respiratory distress in newborns, 241
Blood glucose testing, for type 1 diabetes, 645
Blood group sensitization, maternal, 236*t*
Blood loss, anemia and, 567–568
  in newborn, 249
Blood pressure
  in cardiovascular system assessment, 535
  classification of, 627*t*
Blood smear, 584*t*
Blood urea nitrogen (BUN)
  in acute renal failure, 619
  in dehydration, 128
Blood volume, 125
  of newborn, 247
Bloodstream infection, catheter-related, 437
Blount disease, 750
Blue cohosh herbal tea, maternal use of, 238*t*
BMI. *see* Body mass index
Body composition, fluid in, 125, 126*f*
Body lice, 736
Body mass index (BMI)
  defined, 11
  growth charts of, 12*f*
  obesity and, 105–107, 107*t*
Body plethysmography, 511
Body temperature
  instability of, in infants younger than 3 months of age, 368
  normal, 368
  regulatory system for, 368
Boils, 380
Bonding, in infancy, 15
Bone(s)
  growth and development of, 739, 740*f*
  structure of, 740*f*
Bone and mineral diseases, important physiological changes in, 670*t*
Bone cyst
  aneurysmal, 765*t*–766*t*
  unicameral, 765*t*–766*t*
Bone destruction, in osteomyelitis, 426
Bone marrow
  biopsy, in aplastic anemia, 574
  infiltration, by malignant cells, 573
Bone marrow abnormalities, due to lysosomal storage diseases, 210*t*–212*t*
Bone marrow aspiration (BMA), for cancer, 599*t*
Bone marrow examination, in hematological disorders, 563
Bone marrow failure, 574
  pancytopenia resulting from, 584
Bone marrow replacement, in aplastic anemia, 575
Bone mineral accretion, 119
Bone morphogenetic receptor-2 (*BMPR2*) gene, 524
Bone scan, for cancer, 599*t*
Bone tumors, 765, 765*t*–766*t*
Bordetella holmesii, 401
Bordetella parapertussis, 401
Bordetella pertussis, 400
Borrelia, 439*t*–442*t*
Borrelia burgdorferi, 439*t*–442*t*
  infection from, 443–444
Bottle mouth, 479
Botulism, infant, 696
Boutonneuse fever, 439*t*–442*t*
Bowing fractures, 742
Bowleg, 749, 749*f*
Boys, growth and development of, 271–273
BPD (bronchopulmonary dysplasia), 244–245
Brachial plexopathy, 763
Brachial plexus injuries, 763
  in newborn, 233
Brachycephaly, 183*t*, 185
Brachydactyly, 183*t*
Bradycardia, fetal, 220
Bradypnea, 509*t*
Brain, congenital anomalies of, 716–717
Brain cancers, risk factors for, 597*t*
Brain cell swelling, in hyponatremia, 133
Brain hemorrhage, due to hypernatremia, 134
Brain herniations, 705–706, 705*t*
  foremen magnum, 705*t*
  subfalcian, 705*t*
  transtentorial (central), 705–706, 705*t*
  uncal, 705–706, 705*t*
Brain tumors
  ataxia due to, 701
  vomiting due to, 473*t*
Branched chain amino acids, metabolism of, 203*f*
Branched chain ketoaciduria, 203
Branching enzyme, 200*t*
Break bone fever, 446
Breast, of newborn, 228*f*
Breast abscess, 100
Breast-feeding, 99–100, 100*f*
  adequacy of, 99–100
  common problems with, 100
  maternal contraindications and recommendations for, 101*t*
  maternal drug use and, 100
Breast-feeding jaundice, 100
Breast milk, composition of, 102*t*
Breast milk jaundice, 100
Breast tenderness, 100
Breastfeeding, initiation and maintenance of, 2
Breath holding spells, 514, 514*t*
Breath sounds, 510*t*
Breathing
  control of, 513–516, 514*f*
    disorders of
      apnea as, 514–515, 514*t*
      brief resolved unexplained event as, 515
      sudden infant death syndrome as, 515–516, 516*t*
  in newborn resuscitation, 225–226
  in rapid cardiopulmonary assessment, 146*t*
  work of, 509–510
Breathing patterns, abnormal, 509*t*
Brentuximab, for cancer, 601*t*–602*t*
Bridging therapy, in juvenile idiopathic arthritis, 352
Brief psychotic disorder, 72, 72*t*
Brief resolved unexplained event (BRUE), 515
Broca aphasia, 682
Brodie abscess, 426, 765, 765*t*–766*t*
Bromides, maternal use of, 238*t*
Bronchi, mainstem, 507
Bronchiectasis, 405–407, 520
Bronchiolitis, 401–402, 522
  clinical manifestations of, 401–402
  complications and prognosis of, 402
  differential diagnosis of, 402
  epidemiology of, 401
  etiology of, 401
  laboratory and imaging studies for, 402
  prevention of, 402
  treatment of, 402
  viral, 401
Bronchiolitis obliterans, 407
Bronchoalveolar lavage, 511
Bronchopneumonia, 402–403
Bronchopulmonary dysplasia (BPD), 244–245, 522
Bronchoscopy, rigid, 511
Bronchospasm, 510*t*
Broviac catheters, 437
Brown dog tick, 444
Brucella, 439*t*–442*t*
Brucellosis, 439*t*–442*t*
BRUE. *see* Brief resolved unexplained event
Bruises, due to child abuse, 80–81, 81*f*
Buckle fracture, 742
Budesonide DPI, for asthma, 319*f*
Budesonide inhaled, for asthma, 319*f*
Bulbar weakness, 694*t*
Bulimia nervosa, 282–283, 283*t*
Bulla, 721*t*, 722*f*
Bullous impetigo, 379, 734*t*
Bullous rash, infections with fever and, 373*t*–374*t*
Bullying, 92
Bumblebee stings, allergic reactions to, 333
Burkitt lymphoma
  clinical manifestations of, 605
  endemic (African) form of, 605
  etiology of, 605, 606*t*
  sporadic (North American) form of, 605
Burner, 763

Burns, 158–160
  due to child abuse, 81, 81*f*
  clinical manifestations of, 158–159, 159*f*
  complications of, 159, 160*t*
  deep partial-thickness, 158
  epidemiology of, 158
  etiology of, 158
  first-degree, 158
  full-thickness, 158
  inhalation injuries, 158
  laboratory and imaging studies of, 159
  prevention of, 160
  prognosis for, 160
  second-degree, 158
  superficial, 158
  superficial partial-thickness, 158
  third-degree, 158
  treatment of, 159
  vesiculobullous eruptions due to, 734*t*
Burrow, 722*f*
Bursitis, suppurative, 429
Button batteries, ingestion of, 162

C

C1-esterase inhibitor deficiency, acquired, 331*t*
C1-inhibitor, laboratory studies of, 306
C1-inhibitor deficiency, 306
  treatment of, 306
C3 deficiency, 306
Café au lait macules, 681, 731, 731*f*
  differential diagnosis pf, 730*t*
Café-au-lait spots, 714, 714*f*
  with developmental disabilities, 30*t*
CAH. *see* Congenital adrenal hyperplasia
Calcaneal apophysitis, 755
  clinical manifestations of, 755
  treatment of, 755
Calcaneovalgus foot, 754
Calcidiol, 118
Calcineurin inhibitors, topical, for atopic dermatitis, 726
Calcinosis, in juvenile dermatomyositis, 356
Calcinosis universalis, in juvenile dermatomyositis, 356
Calcitriol, 118
  in renal function, 617
Calcium, 669
Calcium chloride, for cardiopulmonary resuscitation, 148*t*
Calcium deficiency, 119–120
Caliciviruses (noroviruses), diarrhea from, 410*t*
Caloric intake, growth and, 11
Calories, in parenteral nutrition, 131
CAM (complementary and alternative medicine), 3
Camptodactyly, 183*t*
Campylobacter jejuni, 439*t*–442*t*
  diarrhea from, 410*t*, 411
  and Guillain-Barré syndrome, 695
Campylobacteriosis, 439*t*–442*t*
Cancer
  assessment of, 595–596, 596*f*
    common manifestations in, 595, 598*t*
    differential diagnosis in, 596
    history in, 595, 597*t*
    initial diagnostic evaluation in, 596
      diagnostic imaging in, 596, 599*t*
      screening tests in, 596
    physical examination in, 595
  childhood
    incidence of, 595, 596*f*
    risk factors for, 597*t*
  common manifestations of, 595, 598*t*
  differential diagnosis of, 596
  emergencies with, 599, 600*t*
  prevention of, 599
Cancer treatment, 599–601, 613–614
  adverse effects of, 601, 603*t*
  chemotherapy as, 601, 601*t*–602*t*
  for oncological emergencies, 599, 600*t*
  other therapies for, 601
  radiation therapy as, 601
  surgery for, 599
Candida albicans infection, oropharyngeal, 480
Candidal diaper dermatitis, 728
Candidiasis, 381*t*
  chronic mucocutaneous, 298, 299*t*
  vulvovaginal, 423*t*
Canthus, 183*t*
Capillary hemangiomas, 228–229
Capillary leak, systemic, due to burns, 159
Capnocytophaga canimorsus, 439*t*–442*t*
Captopril
  for heart failure, 555*t*
  maternal use of, 238*t*
Caput succedaneum, 233
Carbohydrate disorder, 199–201
  fructosuria as, 201
  galactokinase deficiency as, 201
  galactosemia as, 201
  glycogen storage diseases as, 199–201, 200*f*, 200*t*
  hereditary fructose intolerance as, 201
Carbon dioxide
  end-tidal, 511
  in pulmonary physiology, 507
Carbon monoxide
  in bilirubin production, 249–250
  toxicity, 162*t*
Carboplatin, for cancer, 601*t*–602*t*
Carboxyhemoglobin assessment, for burns, 159
Carbuncle, 380, 722*f*
Carcinoma, of thyroid, 668
Cardiac arrhythmias. *see* Dysrhythmia(s)
Cardiac catheterization, in cardiovascular system assessment, 540, 540*f*
Cardiac murmurs. *see* Heart murmurs
Cardiac output
  cardiopulmonary arrest and, 147
  oxygen delivery and, 149
Cardiac silhouette, 539, 539*f*
Cardiac syncope, 541*t*
Cardiac transplantation, for cardiomyopathies, 557*t*, 558
Cardiogenic asthma, 402
Cardiomegaly
  in coarctation of aorta, 548
  in hypoplastic left heart syndrome, 553
  in truncus arteriosus, 552
Cardiomyopathies, 213–214, 556–558
  clinical manifestations of, 558
  etiology of, 556, 557*t*
  imaging studies for, 558
  in sickle cell disease, 577*t*
  treatment of, 558
Cardiopulmonary assessment, rapid, 146*t*
Cardiovascular support, for shock, 153, 153*t*
Cardiovascular system, 535–560
  assessment of, 535–540
    history in, 535, 536*t*
    laboratory and imaging tests in, 538–540
      cardiac catheterization as, 540, 540*f*
      chest radiography as, 539, 539*f*
      echocardiography as, 539–540, 540*f*
      electrocardiography as, 538–539, 538*f*
      pulse oximetry as, 538
    physical examination in, 535–538
      auscultation in, 536
      clicks in, 536
      heart murmurs in, 536–538
      heart sounds in, 536, 537*t*
      inspection in, 535
      palpation in, 535
Cardioversion
  in cardiopulmonary resuscitation, 148–149, 148*t*
  synchronized, for dysrhythmias, 543–544
Carditis, due to heart failure, 556, 556*t*
Care coordination, for anxiety disorders, 64
Caries, dental, 479–480
Carmustine, for cancer, 601*t*–602*t*
Carnitine(s), plasma, 199*t*
Carotid bruit, 538*t*
Carotid sinus syncope, 541*t*
Carpenter syndrome, obesity in, 106*t*
Carriers, for genetic disorders, 170
Carvedilol, for heart failure, 555*t*
Caseous lymph node, skeletal tuberculosis and, 454
Cat eye syndrome, 183
Cat-scratch disease, 384, 439*t*–442*t*
Cataract, in galactosemia, 201
Catarrhal stage, of pertussis, 400
CATCH 22 syndrome, 298
Catch-down growth, 13
Catch-up growth, 11–13, 112
Catecholamines, in neuroblastoma, 609
Cathartic, for poisoning, 164
Catheter-related infections, 437*t*
  bloodstream, 437
Catheter-related sepsis, due to parenteral nutrition, 131
Catheter-related thrombosis, 437
Cations, in body fluids, 125
Caustic ingestions, 160–162
Caustic injuries, 484
Cavernous hemangiomas, 228–229
Cavopulmonary shunt, bidirectional, for tricuspid atresia, 551
Cavus foot, 755
CD. *see* Crohn disease
Cefdinir, for otitis media, 396–397
Cefixime, after rape, 281
Cefotaxime, for meningitis, 388
Ceftriaxone
  after rape, 281
  for gonorrhea, 422
  for Lyme disease, 444
  for meningitis, 388
  for otitis media, 396–397
Celiac disease, 335*t*–336*t*, 492
  clinical manifestations of, 492
  constipation due to, 476*t*
  etiology and epidemiology of, 492
  laboratory and imaging studies for, 492
  treatment of, 492
Cellular compartment disorders, due to inborn errors of metabolism, 193*t*
Cellular immune-mediated hypersensitivity, 311–312, 311*t*
Cellulitis, 380
  orbital, 395, 433*t*
  periorbital, 433*t*
  preseptal (periorbital), 395
Central apnea, 514, 514*t*
Central catheter, peripherally inserted, for parenteral nutrition, 131
Central chemoreceptors, in control of ventilation, 513, 514*f*
Central diabetes insipidus, 133–134
Central line associated bloodstream infection (CLABSI), 437
Central nervous system (CNS)
  congenital malformations of, 716–717
    of brain, 716–717
    of spinal cord, 716
  due to lysosomal storage diseases, 210*t*–212*t*
  of newborn, 14

Central nervous system abnormalities, delayed puberty due to, 657
Central nervous system depression, in newborn, 227
Central nervous system perfusion, in rapid cardiopulmonary assessment, 146*t*
Central nervous system reflexes
  of child, 684
  of infancy, 682*t*
Central nervous system shunts, infections associated with, 438–439
Central nervous system tumors, 607–608, 614
  clinical manifestations of, 607
  complications of, 608
  differential diagnosis of, 608
  epidemiology of, 607
  etiology of, 607
  laboratory/imaging studies in, 607, 608*f*
  prognosis for, 608, 608*t*
  treatment of, 608
Central pontine myelinolysis
  hyponatremia and, 133
  rehydration and, 129
Central venous catheters, infections associated with, 437
Central wheal, in allergen-specific IgE in vivo skin testing, 312–313
Cephalexin, for streptococcal pharyngitis, 394*t*
Cephalhematoma, 730*t*
  in newborn, 233
Cephalosporins
  allergic reaction to, 338
  for streptococcal pharyngitis, 393–394
Cephalothin, maternal use of, 238*t*
Cerebellar ataxia, postinfectious acute, 700–701
Cerebellar mutism, central nervous system and, 608
Cerebral aneurysms, in autosomal dominant polycystic kidney disease, 630
Cerebral edema, 129
  due to diabetic ketoacidosis, 641
Cerebral palsy (CP), 37–38, 37*t*–38*t*
Cerebrohepatorenal syndrome, 208–209
Cerebrosidase, nephropathic, 210*t*–212*t*
Cerebrospinal fluid (CSF) analysis, 684–685, 685*t*
  for cancer, 599*t*
  for neonatal meningitis, 256
Cerebrospinal fluid rhinorrhea, 324*t*
Cerebrospinal leak, 710
Cerebrovascular accidents, in sickle cell disease, 577*t*
Cervical cancer, 382
Cervical lymphadenitis
  etiology of, 383
  suppurative, 384
Cervical lymphadenopathy, in Kawasaki disease, 347
Cervical spine injuries, 710
Cervicitis, nongonococcal, 423
Cestodes, parasitic, pediatric syndrome caused by, 452*t*
Cetirizine, for allergic rhinitis, 325
CFTR gene, pancreatic insufficiency and, 501
CH_{50} test, 306
Chagas disease, congenital infection with, 260*t*
Chalasia, vomiting *vs.*, 472
Chalazion, 431
Chancre, 423
Chancroid, 419, 421*t*
Charcoal, activated, for poisoning, 164
Charcot-Marie-Tooth disease, 695
  cavus foot in, 755
CHARGE association, choanal atresia in, 324
CHCs. *see* Combined hormonal contraceptives
Chédiak-Higashi syndrome (CHS), 301*t*
Chelation therapy, for β-thalassemia major, 575–576
Chemical(s), as teratogens, 176
Chemoprophylaxis
  for malaria, 449
  for meningitis, 388–389
Chemoreceptors, in control of ventilation
  central, 513, 514*f*
  peripheral, 513, 514*f*
Chemotherapy, 601, 601*t*–602*t*
  adjuvant, 601
  adverse effects of, 601, 603*t*
  in blood-brain barrier, 601
  high-dose, 609
  for leukemia, 604
  neoadjuvant, 601
  resistance to, 601
  vomiting due to, 473*t*
Cherub appearance, in GH deficiency, 655
Chest
  anemia and, 569*t*
  of newborn, 230
Chest compressions, 147
Chest motion, 510*t*
Chest pain, 541–542, 542*t*
Chest percussion, 513
Chest physiotherapy, 513
  for cystic fibrosis, 529
Chest radiography, 510–511
Chest tubes, for pleural effusion, 532
Chest wall disorders, 529–532
  pectus carinatum as, 530
  pectus excavatum as, 529
Chest x-ray (CXR)
  for asthma, 314
  for cancer, 596, 599*t*
  in cardiovascular system assessment, 539, 539*f*
Cheyne-Stokes respiration, 509*t*
Chiari type II malformation, 716
Chickenpox, 378–379
  clinical manifestations of, 378
  complications and prognosis of, 379
  differential diagnosis of, 378–379
  epidemiology of, 378
  etiology of, 378
  laboratory and imaging studies for, 378
  prevention of, 379
  treatment of, 379
Chikungunya virus, 446–447
Child abuse, 80–84
  fracture due to, 744
  management of, 84, 85*f*
  physical, 80–82, 80*t*
    abdominal trauma due to, 81
    bruises due to, 80–81, 81*f*
    burns due to, 81, 81*f*
    differential diagnosis of, 81–82, 83*t*
    fractures due to, 81, 82*f*
    head trauma due to, 81, 82*f*
    subdural hemorrhage due to, 256–257
  sexual, 82–84
Child-centered approach, in elimination, 47–48
Child neglect, 80
Child Protective Services (CPS), 83
Child with special needs, 28–38
  cerebral palsy, 37–38, 37*t*–38*t*
  hearing impairment, 34–36, 35*t*
  management of, 31–32
    counseling principles for, 32
    interdisciplinary team intervention for, 32
    intervention in primary care setting for, 31–32, 32*t*
  mental retardation, 33, 33*t*–34*t*
  multifaceted team assessment of, 28–31
    educational, 29–31
    medical, 28, 29*t*–30*t*
Child with special needs *(Continued)*
    motor, 28
    psychological, 28–29, 31*t*
    of social environment, 31
  speech-language impairment, 36–37, 36*t*
  vision impairment, 33–34
Childhood antecedents, of adult health conditions, 1
Childhood extreme obesity, 104–105
Childhood-onset schizophrenia, 72
Childhood thrombocytopenic syndromes, differential diagnosis of, 585*f*
Children
  ethical principles related to, 4–5
  laboratory results in various types of thyroid function in, 665*t*
Children with special health care needs (SHCN), 28
Children's Somatization Inventory, for somatic symptom and related disorders (SSRDs), 61
Chinese liver fluke, 451*t*
Chlamydia trachomatis, 422–423
  clinical features of infections caused by, 420*t*
  congenital infection with, 260*t*, 263
  pelvic inflammatory disease due to, 420–421
  pneumonia from, 403, 407*t*
Chlamydial conjunctivitis, 431
Chlamydophila pneumoniae, pneumonia from, 403, 407*t*
Chlamydophila psittaci, 439*t*–442*t*
Chloral hydrate, for sedation, 166*t*
Chloroquine, for malaria, 449
Choanal atresia (stenosis), 227*t*, 324, 324*t*
  upper airway obstruction due to, 518
Cholangiopancreatography, endoscopic retrograde, 503
Cholecalciferol, 118
Cholecystitis, abdominal pain due to, 470*t*
Cholelithiasis, abdominal pain due to, 470*t*
Cholera-like enterotoxin, 411
Cholestasis, 494
  chronic, 498
  clinical manifestations of, 494
  etiology and epidemiology, 494
  laboratory and imaging studies for, 494, 497*t*, 498*f*
  treatment of, 494
Cholestatic liver disease, due to parenteral nutrition, 131
Cholinergics, toxicity, 162*t*
Chondritis, *Pseudomonas*, 425–426
Chondrolysis, 747–748
"ChooseMyPlate," 103–104, 103*f*, 103*t*
Chordee, 632
Chorea, 702
  due to heart failure, 556, 556*t*
Choriomeningitis, lymphocytic, 439*t*–442*t*
Chorionic villus sampling (CVS), 179
Choroiditis, 433*t*
Chromatin, 169
Chromium deficiency, 119*t*
Chromosomal deletion syndrome, 182–183
  of chromosome 22q11.2 deletion syndromes, 182–183
  cri du chat syndrome as, 182
  Williams syndrome as, 182
Chromosomal disorder, 179–183
  due to abnormalities in number (aneuploidy), 179–182
    monosomies as, 179–182
      monosomies as, 181–182
      Turner syndrome as, 181–182
    trisomies as, 180–181
      Down syndrome as, 180
      Klinefelter syndrome as, 181

Chromosomal disorder *(Continued)*
trisomy 13 as, 180–181
trisomy 18 as, 180, 181*t*
due to chromosomal deletions, 182–183
aniridia Wilms tumor association as, 182
of chromosome 22q11.2 deletion syndromes, 182–183
cri du chat syndrome as, 182
Williams syndrome as, 182
due to chromosome duplication, 183
cat eye syndrome as, 183
inverted duplication chromosome 15 as, 183
Chromosome(s), sex, 169
Chromosome 15, inverted duplication, 183
Chromosome 22q11.2 deletion syndromes, 182–183
Chromosome analysis, in genetic assessment, 179
Chromosome duplication syndromes, 183
cat eye syndrome as, 183
inverted duplication chromosome 15 as, 183
Chronic autoimmune lymphocytic thyroiditis, 645
Chronic blood loss, in iron deficiency anemia, 570
Chronic granulomatous disease (CGD), 301*t*, 303
Chronic idiopathic thrombocytopenic purpura, 585
Chronic illnesses
in children and adolescents, 267, 267*t*
in hospital admission, 1
Chronic kidney disease (CKD), 626–627
complications and treatments of, 627*t*
etiology and epidemiology of, 626
prognosis for, 627
treatment of, 627
Chronic kidney disease-mineral bone disorder (CKD-MBD), 626–627
Chronic lung disease, 244–245
in sickle cell disease, 577*t*
Chronic major depressive disorder. *see* Persistent depressive disorder
Chronic mucocutaneous candidiasis, 298, 299*t*
Chronic myeloid leukemia (CML), 603
Chronic respiratory failure, 149
Chvostek sign, 235
Cigarette smoke, around children, 91
Ciliary dyskinesia, primary, 523
Ciliary elevator system, in pneumonia, 403
Ciliated epithelium, as lung defense mechanism, 508
Circadian rhythm disorders, 54*t*–55*t*
pediatric sleep disorders and, 55
treatment of, 56
Circulating toxins, 580
Circulation
in cardiopulmonary resuscitation, 147
in rapid cardiopulmonary assessment, 146*t*
transition from fetal to neonatal, 222
Cis-retinoic acid, for neuroblastoma, 609
Cisgender, 84*t*
Cisplatin, for cancer, 601*t*–602*t*
CKD. *see* Chronic kidney disease
Classical pathway, of complement activation, 304–305, 305*f*
Cleft lip and palate, 480
Clicks, 536
Clindamycin
for acne, 723
for streptococcal pharyngitis, 394*t*
Clinodactyly, 183*t*
Clitoral enlargement, in newborn, 231
Clonidine, for attention-deficit/hyperactivity disorder (ADHD), 47
Clonorchiasis, 451*t*
Clonorchis sinensis, 451*t*
C-loop, in midgut malrotation, 488
Clostridium difficile, diarrhea from, 410*t*, 411
Clot retraction, 580
Clotting factors, disorders of, 586, 592
disseminated intravascular coagulation in, 588, 588*t*–589*t*
etiology of, 586
hemophilia in, 586–587, 586*t*
thrombosis in, 589, 589*f*
vitamin K deficiency in, 588
von Willebrand disease in, 587–588
Club drugs, 283
Clubbing, digital, 510, 510*f*
in cystic fibrosis, 527
Clubfoot, 753–754, 753*f*
Clue cells, in vulvovaginitis, 419*f*
CMV (cytomegalovirus)
congenital infection with, 260*t*, 261–262
in immunocompromised person, 435
pneumonia and, 403
Coagulation
hemostasis and, 580
simplified pathways of, 582*f*
Coagulation disorder(s)
disseminated intravascular coagulation as, 580, 588
with fulminant liver failure, 500*t*
gastrointestinal bleeding due to, 477*t*
in newborn, clinical manifestations and differential diagnoses of, 253–254
thrombosis as, 589
von Willebrand disease as, 587–588
Coagulation factors, 252–253
Coagulopathy. *see also* Coagulation disorder(s)
presentation of, 564*t*
Coarctation of aorta, 548
Cobb angle, 757, 758*f*
Cocaine
acute effects of, 284*t*–285*t*
neonatal addiction to and withdrawal from, 235
toxicity, 162*t*
use, during pregnancy, 90
Cochlear implants, 36
Cockroach allergens, asthma and, 315*t*
Codeine, as analgesia, 166*t*
Codon, 169
Cognitive-behavioral methods, in somatic symptom and related disorders (SSRDs), 61
Cognitive-behavioral therapy (CBT)
for bipolar disorders, 68
for depressive disorders, 66
for OCD, 69
Cognitive deficits, in iron deficiency anemia, 570
Cognitive development, milestones of, 17*t*
Cohen syndrome, obesity in, 106*t*
Cold, common, 323–324, 391
Cold caloric stimulation, 703–704
Cold injury, of infant, 234
Cold sores, 382
Colic, 41–43
anticipatory guidance and management of, 43
clinical manifestations of, 42, 42*f*
differential diagnosis of, 43
epidemiology of, 41–42
etiology of, 41
medications for, 43
physical examination of, 42
prognosis for, 43
Colicky crying, 41
Colitis
allergic, gastrointestinal bleeding due to, 477*t*
pseudomembranous, gastrointestinal bleeding due to, 477*t*
Colitis *(Continued)*
Trichuris, 450*t*
ulcerative, 490*t*, 491
Collaboration, 4
Collagen vascular diseases
assessment of, 343, 344*t*
common manifestations in, 343–345, 345*t*
diagnostic imaging in, 345
history in, 343
initial diagnostic evaluation in, 345
laboratory testing in, 345
physical examination in, 343
differential diagnosis of, 344*t*
Collecting ducts, 617
Colonic malformations, constipation due to, 476*t*
Colonic stricture, constipation due to, 476*t*
Colonopathy, fibrosing, due to lipase, 529
Colony-stimulating factors, 564*f*, 566
Color blindness, genetic basis for, 174*t*
Colorado tick fever, 439*t*–442*t*
Columella, 183*t*
Coma, 703
due to inborn errors of metabolism, 192, 195*t*
due to poisoning, 160
Combined hormonal contraceptives (CHCs), 279–280, 279*t*–280*t*
Combined immunodeficiency diseases, 296–299, 297*t*
autosomal recessive, 297–298
bare lymphocyte syndrome as, 297*t*, 298
clinical manifestations of, 297
DiGeorge syndrome as, 297*t*, 298
hyper-IgM syndrome as, 297*t*
autosomal recessive, 296
due to defects in NEMO, 296
X-linked, 296, 296*f*
Omenn syndrome as, 297–298, 297*t*
reticular dysgenesis as, 297*t*
severe, 297, 297*t*
autosomal recessive, 297–298
clinical manifestations of, 297–298
due to deficiencies in adenosine deaminase and purine nucleoside phosphorylase, 298
X-linked, 297–298
Combined ventricular hypertrophy, in truncus arteriosus, 552
Comedo(nes), 721*t*, 722*f*, 723
Common cold, 323–324, 391
Common variable immunodeficiency (CVID), 294–295, 295*t*
Common warts (verruca vulgaris), 382
Communication, 4
Comparative genomic hybridization, microarray, 179
Compartment syndrome, 743–744
Compassion, 4
Compensatory scoliosis, 756, 759
Complement assays, 293
Complement component cascade, 305*f*
Complement evaluation, in angioedema, 331*t*
Complement proteins, disorder of, 304
Complement system
disorders of, 304–306, 304*t*, 305*f*
etiology of, 304–306
laboratory studies of, 306
treatment for, 306
Complementary and alternative medicine (CAM), 3
Complete blood count
for anemia, 568
for gastrointestinal symptoms, 467
for infectious diseases, 362
Complete heart block, 544*t*
Compulsions, in OCD, 68

Computed tomography (CT)
angiography, of pulmonary embolism, 526
of brain and spinal cord, 685
for cancer, 596, 599t
of chest, 511
contrast-enhanced, for infectious diseases, 362–363
for increased intracranial pressure, 708
for infectious diseases, 362–363
for kidney structure, 620
scanogram, of leg-length discrepancy, 750
for seizures, 691
for trauma patient, 155
Concussion, 709, 709t
Conditioning therapy, for enuresis, 49
Condoms, 280
Conduction, heat loss via, 234
Condylomata acuminata, 382, 419, 424
Condylomata lata, 423
Confidentiality, 4
of adolescent interview, 267, 270t
ethical issues in, 5
Health Insurance Portability and Accountability Act (HIPAA) on, 5
limited, 4
Confusional arousals, 54t–55t
Confusional migraine, 706
Congenital adrenal hyperplasia (CAH), 662
amenorrhea due to, 275
Congenital adrenal mineralocorticoid deficiency, 674–675
Congenital anomalies, life-threatening, 227t
Congenital anomalies of the kidney and urinary tract (CAKUT), 626
Congenital central hypoventilation syndrome (CCHS), 514
Congenital complete heart block, 543
Congenital diaphragmatic hernia, 246, 522
Congenital heart disease, 180
acyanotic, 545–548
aortic stenosis as, 548
atrial septal defect as, 546, 546f
coarctation of aorta as, 548
endocardial cushion defect as, 547, 547f
etiology and epidemiology of, 545, 545t
patent ductus arteriosus as, 546–547, 546f
pulmonary stenosis as, 547–548
ventricular septal defect as, 545–546, 545f
congenital malformation syndromes associated with, 536t
cyanotic, 549–553
extracardiac complications of, 553t
hypoplastic left heart syndrome as, 552–553, 552f
with polycythemia, 584
presenting symptoms in, 549t
tetralogy of Fallot as, 549–550, 550f
total anomalous pulmonary venous return as, 552, 552f
transposition of great arteries as, 550–551, 550f
tricuspid atresia as, 551, 551f
truncus arteriosus as, 551–552, 551f
ductal-dependent, 227t
Congenital hemolytic disorders, 567–568
Congenital hypopituitarism, 639
Congenital hypoplastic anemia, 573, 573t
Congenital hypotonia, benign, 699
Congenital infections, 259–264, 260t
Congenital lobar emphysema, 522
Congenital malformation syndromes, with congenital heart disease, 536t
Congenital malformations, 169
association in, 184
defined, 184
diagnosis of, 186
Congenital malformations (Continued)
due to disruptions of development, 184
due to extrinsic factors, 184
history for
family, 184
pregnancy, 184
due to inborn errors of metabolism, 195–196
due to intrinsic factors, 184
laboratory evaluation of, 186
minor, 184
multiple, 184
physical examination of, 184–186
craniofacial, 185
of extremities, 185
of genitalia, 185–186
growth in, 184–185
of neck, 185
of trunk, 185
sequence in, 184
Congenital melanocytic nevi, 228–229, 731–732, 731f
differential diagnosis of, 730t
giant, 730t, 732
hairy, 731–732, 731f
Congenital myasthenic syndromes, 696
Congenital myopathies, 697–698
Congenital pulmonary airway malformations (CPAMs), 522, 523f
Congenital rubella syndrome, 375
Congenital scoliosis, 758
Congenital thyroxine-binding globulin deficiency, 665–666
Congenital tuberculosis, 454
Congestive heart failure. see Heart failure
Conjunctival erythema, in Kawasaki disease, 347
Conjunctivitis
acute, 430
allergic, 433t
bacterial, 431, 433t
chlamydial, 431
epidemiology of, 431
gonococcal, 431
hyperpurulent, 431
inclusion, 431
neonatal, 430, 432t–433t
viral, 430, 433t
Connective tissue disease
assessment of, 343, 344t
common manifestations in, 343–345, 345t
diagnostic imaging in, 345
history in, 343
initial diagnostic evaluation in, 345
laboratory testing in, 345
physical examination in, 343
juvenile idiopathic arthritis vs., 352t
Conotruncal anomaly face syndrome, 182–183
Consanguinity, and autosomal recessive inheritance, 177
Consciousness
depression of, transient, recurrent, 706
disorders of, 703–706
acute, 703–706
assessment of, 703–705
clinical manifestations of, 705–706, 705t
etiology of, 705
laboratory and diagnostic imaging of, 706
prognosis for, 706
treatment of, 706
Consolidation, of lung, 510t
Constipation, 475–476
defined, 49
differential diagnosis of, 475, 476t
distinguishing features of, 475–476
functional, 49–51
clinical manifestations of, 49–50
complications of, 51
Constipation (Continued)
defined, 475
differential diagnosis of, 50, 475, 476t
epidemiology of, 49
etiology of, 49
evaluation of, 476
prevention of, 51
treatment of, 50–51, 50t–52t, 476
Constitutional delay, short stature due to, 653
Constitutional short stature, 13
Contact allergies, 311–312, 728f
Contact dermatitis, 335t–336t, 725, 727–728
allergic, 727, 728f
atopic vs., 725
clinical manifestations of, 727–728, 727f–728f
complications of, 728
differential diagnosis of, 728
etiology and epidemiology of, 727
irritant, 727–728
laboratory and imaging studies for, 728
prevention of, 728
treatment of, 728
vesiculobullous eruptions due to, 734t
Containment, 747
Continuous, machine-like murmur, with patent ductus arteriosus, 546–547
Continuous murmurs, 538
Continuous positive airway pressure (CPAP), 515, 521
Contraception, 278–281
barrier methods for, 280–281
condoms as, 280
sponge, caps, and diaphragm as, 280
coitus interruptus for, 281
emergency postcoital, 280–281, 281t
intrauterine devices for, 279
oral and anal for, 281
rhythm method (periodic coital abstinence) for, 281
steroidal, 278–281
combined hormonal contraceptives for, 279–280, 279t–280t
contraceptive patch for, 279–280
contraceptive vaginal ring for, 279–280
hormonal injections and implants for, 278–279
long-acting reversible contraceptives for, 278–279
progesterone-only pill or minipill for, 280
Contraceptive patch, 279–280
Contraceptive vaginal ring, 279–280
Contrast-enhanced CT, for infectious diseases, 362–363
Convalescent stage, of pertussis, 400
Convection, heat loss via, 234
Conversion disorder, 59, 60t
Convulsion(s). see also Seizure(s)
benign neonatal, 690
simple febrile, 689
Cooley anemia, 575–576
Coombs test, 579f
Coordination, of movement, 684
Copper deficiency, 119t
Cor pulmonale, 524–525
Cordocentesis, 220
Corn syrup, for functional constipation, 52t
Corneal reflex, 683
Coronary artery aneurysms, in Kawasaki disease, 347
Coronary artery disease, syncope due to, 541t
Corpus callosum, agenesis of, 716–717
Corrin ring, 117
Corticospinal tract, 693

Corticosteroids, 725–726
for asthma
inhaled, 314–315, 319*f*
oral, 316
for atopic dermatitis
systemic, 726
topical, 327, 725–726
for autoimmune hemolysis, 580
intranasal, for allergic rhinitis, 324–325
for juvenile dermatomyositis, 356
for juvenile idiopathic arthritis, 352
for systemic lupus erythematosus, 355
topical, 726
for atopic dermatitis, 725–726
complications of, 726
for urticaria and angioedema, 331
Cortisol deficiency, hypoglycemia due to, 649
Cough
evaluation of, 509
as lung defense mechanism, 509
whooping, 400
Cough syncope, 541*t*
Coumarin, as teratogen, 237*t*
Counter-regulatory hormones, defects in, 649
Cow's milk-based formulas, 100–101
Coxiella burnetii, 439*t*–442*t*
Coxsackievirus infection, vesiculobullous eruptions due to, 734*t*
Coxsackieviruses, conjunctivitis from, 430
CP. *see* Cerebral palsy
CPAP. *see* Continuous positive airway pressure
CPS (Child Protective Services), 83
Crab louse, 425
Cracked lips, in Kawasaki disease, 347
Crackles, 510
Cradle cap, 728, 729*f*
Cranial nerve evaluation, 682–683
of cranial nerve I, 683
of cranial nerve II, 683
of cranial nerves III, IV, and VI, 683
of cranial nerve V, 683
of cranial nerve VII, 683
of cranial nerve VIII, 683
of cranial nerves IX and X, 683
of cranial nerve XII, 683
Cranial nerve palsies, 708
Craniopharyngioma, 639
delayed puberty due to, 657
Craniosynostosis, 681
Craniotabes, 118, 229
Creatine biosynthesis, disorders of, 199*t*
Creatinine clearance, 619
Creatinine concentration, in dehydration, 128
Cri du chat syndrome, 182
Cricoid ring, 507
Crigler-Najjar syndrome, hyperbilirubinemia due to, 250
Crohn disease (CD), 490*t*, 491
Croup (laryngotracheobronchitis), 398–400, 518
clinical manifestations of, 399
complications and prognosis of, 400
differential diagnosis of, 399
etiology and epidemiology of, 398–399
laboratory and imaging studies for, 399, 399*f*
spasmodic, 399
upper airway obstruction due to, 517*t*
treatment of, 399–400
upper airway obstruction due to, 517*t*
Crouzon syndrome, with acanthosis nigricans, genetic basis for, 170*t*
Crust, 722*t*
Crusted impetigo, 379
Crying, 41–43
colic and, 41–43
anticipatory guidance and management of, 43
Crying *(Continued)*
clinical manifestations of, 42, 42*f*
differential diagnosis of, 43
epidemiology of, 41–42
etiology of, 41
medications for, 43
physical examination of, 42
prognosis for, 43
duration of, 41
frequency of, 41
intensity of, 41
normal development, 41, 41*f*
Cryoprecipitate, 590*t*
Cryptosporidium parvum, diarrhea from, 410*t*, 411–412
CT. *see* Computed tomography
Cullen sign, 502
Cultures, 3, 8–9
for infectious diseases, 362
Cushing syndrome, 678
obesity in, 106*t*
Cushing triad, 708
Custody, 94
Cutaneous infections, 379–383
Cutaneous infestation(s), 735–737
pediculoses as, 736–737
scabies as, 735–736
Cutaneous larva migrans, 450*t*
CVID (common variable immunodeficiency), 294–295, 295*t*
CVS (chorionic villus sampling), 179
CXR. *see* Chest x-ray
Cyanide, toxicity, 162*t*
Cyanosis
central, 232
in newborn, 232, 232*t*, 241
perioral, 535
peripheral, 535
with respiratory distress, 549*t*
due to respiratory failure, 149
without respiratory distress, 549*t*
Cyanotic congenital heart disease, with polycythemia, 584
Cyanotic heart disease, maternal, 236*t*
Cyclic antidepressants, toxicity, 162*t*
Cyclic vomiting syndrome, 472, 473*t*, 486–487
clinical manifestations of, 487
epidemiology of, 486–487
etiology of, 486–487
laboratory and imaging studies for, 487
treatment of, 487
Cyclophosphamide
for cancer, 601*t*–602*t*
for juvenile dermatomyositis, 356
for systemic lupus erythematosus, 355
Cyclospora cayetanensis, diarrhea from, 410*t*
Cyclosporine
for atopic dermatitis, 726
for juvenile dermatomyositis, 356
Cyclothymic disorder, 66–67
Cyst(s), 722*f*
bone
aneurysmal, 765*t*–766*t*
unicameral, 765*t*–766*t*
duplication
gastrointestinal bleeding due to, 477*t*
vomiting due to, 473*t*
ganglion, 765
laryngeal, 519
leptomeningeal, 710
ovarian, 662
pancreatic pseudocyst, 502
popliteal (Baker), 751
Cystathionine β-synthase deficiency, 203
Cysteinyl leukotriene receptor antagonists, for asthma, 315
Cystic acne, 723
Cystic fibrosis (CF), 526–529
clinical manifestations of, 526–528, 527*t*
complications of, 527*t*
constipation due to, 476*t*
diagnostic studies for, 528–529, 528*t*
etiology and epidemiology of, 526
genetic basis for, 173*t*
intestinal atresia in, 488
pancreatic insufficiency due to, 501
treatment of, 529
Cystic fibrosis transmembrane conductance regulator (CFTR), 526
Cystinosis, in Fanconi syndrome, 140
Cystinuria, 205
Cystitis, 416
Cystourethrogram, voiding, for urinary tract infection, 417
Cytogenetic analysis, for leukemia, 603–604
Cytokine, in hematopoiesis, 564*f*
Cytokine synthesis, test for, 293
Cytomegalovirus (CMV)
congenital infection with, 260*t*, 261–262
in immunocompromised person, 435
pneumonia and, 403
Cytosine arabinoside (Ara-C), for cancer, 601*t*–602*t*

D

Dacryoadenitis, 433*t*
Dacryocystitis, 431, 433*t*
Dactinomycin, for cancer, 601*t*–602*t*
Dactylitis, in sickle cell disease, 577*t*
Danazol, for C1-inhibitor deficiency, 306
Dander, asthma and, 315*t*
Dandruff, 728
Dandy-Walker malformation, 716–717
Danon disease, 210*t*–212*t*
Darier sign, 331
Dasatinib, for cancer, 601*t*–602*t*
Date rape, 92
Date-rape drugs, 283
Dating violence, 92
Daunorubicin, for cancer, 601*t*–602*t*
DDH. *see* Developmental dysplasia of the hip
Death and dying
cause of, 2, 2*t*
explaining to child of, 95–96
of parent or family member, 95–96
understanding, 7
unexpected, 6
Debranching enzyme, 200*f*, 200*t*
Decerebrate posturing, 705
Deciduous teeth, 479
Decongestants, for allergic rhinitis, 325
Decorticate posturing, 705
Deep tendon reflexes, 682, 684
Deep venous thrombi, in hemostatic disorders, 583
Deer tick, 443
DEET (*N,N*-diethyl-*m*-toluamide), for prevention of zoonoses, 439
Deferoxamine, for iron poisoning, 164*t*–165*t*
Defibrillation, in cardiopulmonary resuscitation, 148–149, 148*t*
Definitive antiinfective therapy, 367
Deformation, 184
defined, 739*t*
mechanism of, 739*t*
due to uterine compression, 741*f*
Degenerative disorders, 711–714, 711*t*–712*t*
acquired illnesses mimicking, 714
with focal manifestations, 713
gray matter (neuronal), 711
hereditary and metabolic, 711–713
white matter (leukodystrophies), 711

Deglutition syncope, 541t
Degree of effort, 509–510
Dehydration, 127–128
approach to, 128
assessment of degree of, 128t
calculation of fluid deficit in, 128
from diarrhea, 412
fluid management of, 129t
hypernatremic, 129, 130f
hyponatremic, 129
laboratory evaluation of, 128
mild, 127–128
moderate, 127–128
monitoring and adjusting therapy for, 129, 129t
oral rehydration for, 129
severe, 127–128
Dehydroepiandrosterone (DHEA), 656
Delayed hemolytic transfusion reaction, 590t
Delayed sleep phase disorder, 54t–55t
Delayed-type hypersensitivity, 293, 311–312, 311t
Deletion 9q34, obesity in, 106t
Delivery, history of, in genetic assessment, 178
Delivery room care
resuscitation in, 225, 226f
algorithm for, 226f
breathing in, 225–226
specific conditions requiring, 232–234
cyanosis as, 232, 232t
shock as, 233
routine, 222–227
vitamin K prophylaxis in, 222
Delta agent, 413
Dementia
acquired illnesses mimicking, 714
with focal manifestations, 713
gray matter (neuronal), 711
hereditary and metabolic, 711–713
white matter (leukodystrophies), 711
Dengue fever, 446
Dennie lines, 312
in atopic dermatitis, 326
Dennie-Morgan folds, 312
in atopic dermatitis, 326
Dental caries, 479–480
Denver Developmental Screening Test II, 17
Depression, somatic symptom and related disorders (SSRDs) and, 59
Depressive disorders, 64–68
disruptive mood dysregulation disorder (DMDD), 65
major depressive disorder (MDD), 64, 65t
persistent depressive disorder, 65
premenstrual dysphoric disorder (PDD), 65
specifiers for, 65
treatment of, 66
unspecified, 65
Deprivation dwarfism, 653
Dermacentor andersoni, 444
Dermacentor variabilis, 444
Dermal melanosis, 730, 731f
Dermatitis
atopic, 325–328, 335t–336t, 724–727
contact, 335t–336t, 725, 727–728
diaper, 727
candidal, 728
irritant contact, 727–728, 727f
nickel, 725, 727–728
papulosquamous, 729–730
perianal, 380
Rhus, 727–728
seborrheic, 728–730
Dermatitis herpetiformis, 335t–336t
Dermatoglyphics, 185
Dermatographism, 329
Dermatology assessment, 721–723
common manifestations in, 721–722
of primary skin lesions, 721, 721t, 722f
of secondary skin lesions, 721, 722t
history in, 721
initial diagnostic evaluation and screening tests in, 722–723
physical examination in, 721
Dermatomyositis, juvenile, 355–356
Dermatophytosis, 380
Desensitization, for penicillin allergy, 339
Desloratadine, for allergic rhinitis, 325
Desmopressin
for enuresis, 49
for hemophilia, 587
for von Willebrand disease, 588
Desquamation, in Kawasaki disease, 347
Development
of adolescents
changes associated with, 273
for girls, 270–271, 271f–272f
normal variations in, 274–275
breast asymmetry and masses as, 274, 274t
gynecomastia as, 274–275, 274t
irregular menses as, 274
physiological leukorrhea as, 274
physical
for boys, 271–273, 272f
for girls, 270–271, 271f–272f
of bones, 739, 740f
defined, 11
disorders of, 16–19
disruptions of, 184
history of, in genetic assessment, 178
normal, 14–16
physical, 14
in adolescent, 14
in later infancy, 14
in newborn period, 14
in school age/preadolescent, 14
psychosocial, 15–16
in adolescence, 15–16
in early childhood, 15
in infancy, 15
of school readiness, 15, 15t
Developmental delay, constipation due to, 476t
Developmental dysplasia of the hip (DDH), 744–746
Barlow (dislocation) test for, 744, 745f
clinical manifestations of, 744–745
complications of, 746
etiology of, 744
Galeazzi sign in, 744
hip abduction test for, 745f
Klisic test for, 745
Ortolani (reduction) test for, 744–745, 745f
radiographic evaluation of, 745
teratological dislocation of, 744
treatment of, 746
typical dislocation in, 744
Developmental hematology, 563–566, 564f
Developmental hemostasis, 581, 592
Developmental milestones, 14, 17t, 740
for infants, 740, 741f
Developmental screening, 16–18
Developmental surveillance, 16–18
Deviated septum, 324t
Dexamethasone
for cancer, 601t–602t
for central nervous system tumors, 608
for croup, 399–400
for meningitis, 388
Dexmedetomidine, for sedation, 166t
Dextrose
for cardiopulmonary resuscitation, 148t
in parenteral nutrition, 131
Diabetes Control and Complications Trial, 643–644
Diabetes mellitus (DM), 639–646, 678–679
autoimmune evolution of, 640f
classification of, 640t
constipation due to, 476t
cystic fibrosis-related, 527
definition of, 639–640
honeymoon period in, 643
maternal, 236t
maturity-onset, of youth, 646
type 1, 640–641
chronic autoimmune lymphocytic thyroiditis, 645
clinical manifestations of, 641
complications of, 645
diabetic ketoacidosis due to, 641–645
clinical presentation of, 641
complications of, 643
pathophysiology of, 641, 642f
transition to outpatient management of, 643
treatment of, 642–643
epidemiology of, 640–641
etiology of, 640
hypoglycemia in, 645
outpatient management of, 643
blood glucose testing in, 645
goals of, 643–644
insulin regimens in, 644
long-term glycemic control, 645
nutrition in, 644
prognosis for, 645
type 2, 645–646
clinical manifestations of, 646
differential diagnosis of, 646
epidemiology of, 645–646
pathophysiology of, 645
therapy for, 646
Diabetic ketoacidosis (DKA), 641–645
clinical presentation of, 641
complications of, 643
pathophysiology of, 641, 642f
transition to outpatient management of, 643
treatment of, 642–643
Dialysis, for poisoning, 164
Diamond-Blackfan syndrome, 573, 573t
Diaper dermatitis, 727–728
candidal, 728
irritant contact, 727–728, 727f
Diaphoresis, due to heart failure, 535
Diaphragm
contraceptive, 280
during inspiration, 507
Diaphragmatic hernia, 227t
congenital, 246
Diaphysis, 740f
Diarrhea, 120–121, 412, 473–475
acute, 474
adjusting fluid therapy for, 127t
bacterial, fever due to, 368
bloody, evaluation of, 478t
causes of, 410t
chronic, 474
complications and prognosis of, 413
dehydration from, 412
differential diagnosis of, 412, 474–475, 474t
distinguishing features of, 475
etiology and epidemiology of, 410–412, 410t
functional, 474–475
infective, 410
mechanisms of, 411t
laboratory and imaging studies in, 412
malabsorption, 450t
osmotic, 474–475
prevention of, 413

Diarrhea *(Continued)*
secretory, 474
toddler's, 474–475
traveler's, 413
treatment of, 412–413
Diastematomyelia, 716
Diastolic murmurs, 536–538
Diazepam
for neonatal seizures, 256
for status epilepticus, 691, 691*t*
DIC. *see* Disseminated intravascular coagulation
Diet
for celiac disease, 492
of normal child and adolescent, 102–104
of normal infant, 99–102
breast-feeding in, 99–100, 100*f*
complementary foods for, 101–102
formula feeding in, 100–101
recommendations, 103–104, 103*t*
of toddlers and older children, 103
Dietary history
in anemia, 567–568
in obesity, 107, 107*t*
Dietary iron deficiency anemia, 570
Dietary protein-induced enteropathy, 335*t*–336*t*
Difficult child, 16
Diffusion, of gases across alveolar-capillary membrane, 508
Diffusion defect, hypoxemia due to, 508*t*
DiGeorge syndrome, 182–183, 297*t*, 298
Digestive system, 467–505
assessment of, 467–478
diagnostic imaging in, 467
history in, 467
physical examination in, 467
screening tests in, 467
Digital clubbing, 510, 510*f*
in cystic fibrosis, 527
Digitalis, for heart failure, 555*t*
Digoxin, for ventricular septal defect, 545–546
Dihydrobiopterin reductase, 201–202
1,25-Dihydroxyvitamin D (1,25- [OH]2-D), 118
Dilated cardiomyopathies, 557*t*
clinical manifestations of, 558
etiology of, 556
imaging studies for, 558
treatment of, 558
Dilated nail-fold capillaries, in juvenile dermatomyositis, 355–356
Dinutuximab
for cancer, 601*t*–602*t*
for neuroblastoma, 609
Diphenhydramine, for allergic rhinitis, 325
Diphtheria and tetanus toxoids and acellular pertussis (DTaP) vaccine, 364*f*–365*f*
Diphtheria vaccine, 363–364
Diplegia, due to cerebral palsy, 37*t*
Diplopia, 683
Direct antiglobulin test (DAT), 579*f*
Direct DNA analysis, 186
Directly observed therapy (DOT), for tuberculosis, 456
Discipline, 22–25
Discoid lateral meniscus, 751
Discoid lupus, 353
Diskitis, 762
Dislocation, 739*t*
Disorders of sexual development (DSD)
ovotesticular, 673
sex chromosome, 673
Disruptions
of development, 184
orthopedic problems due to, 739*t*
Disruptive mood dysregulation disorder (DMDD), 65
Disseminated gonococcal infections, 421–422
arthritis of, 428
Disseminated intravascular coagulation (DIC), 580, 588
clinical manifestations of, 588, 589*t*
etiology of, 588, 588*t*
in newborn, 252
oncological emergencies, 600*t*
due to thrombotic microangiopathy, 585–586
treatment of, 588
Distal convoluted tubule (DCT), 617
Distal intestinal obstruction syndrome (DIOS), 527
Distal tubule, 617, 619*f*
Distraction, in temper tantrum, 45
Distributive justice, 6
Diuretics
for cardiomyopathies, 557*t*, 558
for heart failure, 555*t*
for patent ductus arteriosus, 547
Diverticulum, Meckel, 490
abdominal pain due to, 470*t*
gastrointestinal bleeding due to, 477*t*
Divorce, 93–95
outcome of, 94–95
reaction of different ages, 94
role of pediatrician in, 95, 95*t*
Dizziness, etiology of, 541*t*
DKA. *see* Diabetic ketoacidosis
DM. *see* Diabetes mellitus
DMD. *see* Duchenne muscular dystrophy
DNA (deoxyribonucleic acid), 169
DNA analysis, direct, in genetic assessment, 179
Dobutamine
for heart failure, 555*t*
for shock, 153*t*
Dolichocephalic, defined, 185
Doll's eye maneuver, 683, 703–704
Donovanosis, 419, 421*t*
Dopamine
for heart failure, 555*t*
for shock, 153*t*
Doppler examination, of fetal aorta or umbilical arteries, 220
Double-stranded DNA, antibodies to, in systemic lupus erythematosus, 354
Down syndrome (DS), 180
newborn assessment for, 227*t*
obesity in, 106*t*
Doxorubicin, for cancer, 601*t*–602*t*
Doxycycline, 530
for *Chlamydia* infection, 423
for Lyme disease, 444
Drowning, 157–158
Drowsiness, after traumatic brain injury, 710
Drug(s)
anemia and, 567–568
associated with neutropenia, 302*t*
constipation due to, 476*t*
maternal
small for gestational age due to, 239*t*
as teratogens, 237*t*
vomiting due to, 473*t*
Drug abuse, during pregnancy, 100, 236*t*
Drug addiction, neonatal, 235
to cocaine, 235
to opiates, 235
Drug-drug interactions, 367–368
Drug intoxication, ataxia due to, 700
Drug reactions, adverse, 338–339
Drug susceptibilities, 367
Drug toxicity, therapeutic monitoring for, 164*t*
Drug withdrawal, neonatal, 235
from cocaine, 235
from opiates, 235
Dry powder inhaler (DPI), 512
DS (Down syndrome), 180
newborn assessment for, 227*t*
obesity in, 106*t*
DTaP (diphtheria and tetanus toxoids and acellular pertussis) vaccine, 364*f*–365*f*
Duchenne muscular dystrophy (DMD), 696–697
clinical manifestations of, 696–697
etiology of, 696
genetic basis for, 174*t*
laboratory and diagnostic studies of, 697
treatment of, 697
Ductal-dependent congenital heart disease, 227*t*
Ductus arteriosus
closure of, 222
patent, 221–222, 546–547, 546*f*
clinical manifestations of, 244–245, 546
etiology and epidemiology of, 546
imaging studies for, 547
respiratory distress syndrome and, 241–244
treatment of, 547
Ductus venosus, 221–222
Duke clinical criteria, Modified, for infective endocarditis, 409, 409*t*
Duodenal atresia, 227*t*, 488
Duodenal hematoma, 157
Duodenal ulcer, abdominal pain due to, 470*t*
Duplication cysts
gastrointestinal bleeding due to, 477*t*
vomiting due to, 473*t*
Dust mites, asthma and, 315*t*
Dwarfism
Laron, 651
psychosocial or deprivation, 653
zinc deficiency, 120–121
Dysentery, 412
amebic, 412
diarrhea due to, 474
Trichuris, 450*t*
Dysgerminomas, 674
Dyshormonogenesis, 665
Dyskeratosis congenita, 573*t*
Dyskinesias, 702
Dysmenorrhea
primary, 277
secondary, 277
treatment of, 277, 277*t*
Dysmetria, 684
Dysmorphic features, due to inborn errors of metabolism, 195–196
Dysmorphology, 169
association in, 184
defined, 183–184
diagnosis of, 186
due to disruptions of development, 184
due to extrinsic factors, 184
history for
family, 184
pregnancy, 184
due to intrinsic factors, 184
laboratory evaluation of, 186
malformation sequence in, 184
minor, 184
multiple, 184
physical examination of, 184–186
craniofacial, 185
of extremities, 185
of genitalia, 185–186
growth in, 184–185
of neck, 185
of trunk, 185
sequence in, 184
Dysostosis multiplex, due to lysosomal storage diseases, 210*t*–212*t*
Dyspepsia, nonulcer, 485–486, 486*t*
Dysphagia, 511
Dysplasias, 739*t*

Dyspnea
exertional, due to pulmonary stenosis, 547
due to pulmonary edema, 524
Dysrhythmia(s), 542–544
atrial, 542–543
in children, 544*t*
etiology and differential diagnosis of, 542–543, 543*t*
heart block as, 543
poisoning and, 162, 163*t*
syncope due to, 541*t*
treatment of, 543–544, 544*t*
ventricular, 543
Dysthymia. *see* Persistent depressive disorder
Dystonia, 703
in glutaric acidemia, 206
Dystrophin, 696
Dystrophy, 693*t*
Becker, 696
Duchenne, 696–697
clinical manifestations of, 696–697
etiology of, 696
genetic basis for, 174*t*
laboratory and diagnostic studies of, 697
treatment of, 697
facioscapulohumeral, 697
limb-girdle, 697
myotonic, 697

E

EAEC (enteroaggregative *E. coli*), 410*t*, 411
Ear(s)
anemia and, 569*t*
with developmental disabilities, 30*t*
of newborn, 228*f*
swimmer's. *see* Otitis externa
Early childhood, developing autonomy in, 15
Early childhood caries (ECCs), 101
East African sleeping sickness, 439*t*–442*t*
Easy child, 16
Eating disorders, 281–283
anorexia nervosa as, 281–283, 282*f*
clinical features of, 283
treatment and prognosis for, 283, 283*t*
bulimia nervosa as, 282–283, 283*t*
issues that can trigger, 282*t*
risk factors for, 282*f*
slippery slope to, 282*f*
treatment and prognosis for, 283*t*
Ebola virus, 446
EBV (Epstein-Barr virus), infectious mononucleosis due to, 384, 385*f*
Ecchymosis(es), 583, 721*t*
ECF. *see* Extracellular fluid
Echinococcosis, 452, 452*t*
alveolar, 452*t*
unilocular, 452*t*
Echinococcus granulosus, 452
Echinococcus multilocularis, 452
Echinococcus vogeli, 452
Echocardiography, in cardiovascular system assessment, 539–540, 540*f*
Eclampsia, 218
ECMO (extracorporeal membrane oxygenation)
for heart failure, 555*t*
for meconium aspiration syndrome, 245
for primary pulmonary hypertension of the newborn, 245
Ecstasy, acute effects of, 284*t*–285*t*
Ecthyma, 380
Ecthyma gangrenosum, 380
Eczema, 724. *see also* Atopic dermatitis
with developmental disabilities, 30*t*
herpeticum
in atopic dermatitis, 328, 724
herpes zoster virus and, 382
varicella zoster virus and, 378–379
vaccinatum, in atopic dermatitis, 328, 724
Edema
hereditary angioneurotic, genetic basis for, 170*t*
in nephrotic syndrome, 620
in newborn, 228–229
due to renal disease, 617
Edetate calcium disodium (EDTA), for lead poisoning, 164*t*–165*t*
Edrophonium, maternal use of, 238*t*
Educational intervention, for child with special needs, 32
EEG (electroencephalography), 685
for seizures, 691
Egg cases, of pubic lice, 425
EHEC (enterohemorrhagic *E. coli*), 410*t*, 411
Ehlers-Danlos syndrome
hypermobility in, 357
hypotonia in, 699
Ehrlichia chaffeensis, 439*t*–442*t*, 445–446, 446*f*
Ehrlichia ewingii, 439*t*–442*t*, 445
Ehrlichiosis, 439, 439*t*–442*t*, 445–446
clinical manifestations of, 445
complications and prognosis of, 446
differential diagnosis of, 446
epidemiology of, 445
etiology of, 445
human monocytic, 439*t*–442*t*, 445
laboratory and imaging studies, 446
prevention of, 446
sennetsu, 439*t*–442*t*
treatment for, 446
EIEC (enteroinvasive *E. coli*), 410*t*, 411
Ejection clicks, 536
in aortic stenosis, 548
Ejection murmurs, 536
adolescent, 538*t*
due to atrial septal defect, 546
systolic, 536
due to aortic stenosis, 548
in total anomalous pulmonary venous return, 552
Elbow, 764
Little Leaguer's, 764
nursemaid's, 764, 764*f*
Panner disease of, 764
radial head subluxation of, 764, 764*f*
throwing injuries of, 764
Electrocardiographic (ECG) changes
in hyperkalemia, 138
in hypokalemia, 136
Electrocardiography, in cardiovascular system assessment, 538–539, 538*f*
Electroconvulsive therapy (ECT), for depressive disorders, 66
Electroencephalography (EEG), 685
for seizures, 691
Electrolyte, in parenteral nutrition, 131
Electrolyte imbalances, in diabetic ketoacidosis, 642–643
Electromyography, 685
Elimination, control of, 47–51
enuresis, 48–49
functional constipation and soiling, 49–51
normal development of, 47–48
Elliptocytosis, hereditary, etiology of, 566, 578–579
EM (erythema multiforme), 331, 733–735, 734*t*
Emancipated minors, 5
Emboli, septic, 410
Embolism, pulmonary, 526
Embryonic hemoglobins, 566
Emergencies, oncological, 599, 600*t*
Emergency postcoital contraception, 280–281
Emotional aspects, of pediatric practice, 3
Empathy, 4
Empirical antiinfective therapy, 367
Empyema, 405, 530–531
Enalapril
for heart failure, 555*t*
maternal use of, 238*t*
Encephalitis, 389–391
autoimmune, 389
causes of, 389*t*
clinical manifestations of, 389–390
complications and prognosis of, 390–391
differential diagnosis of, 390
epidemiology of, 389
etiology of, 389
laboratory and imaging studies for, 390
prevention of, 391
treatment for, 390
Encephalomyelitis
acute disseminated, 389
due to measles, 375
Encephalomyelopathy, subacute necrotizing, 711*t*–712*t*
Encephalopathy
bilirubin, 251
hepatic, 497–498
stages of, 499*t*
treatment of, 500*t*
hypoxic-ischemic, in newborn, 257–258
clinical manifestations of, 257–258, 257*t*
prognosis for, 257
seizures due to, 255–256
due to inborn errors of metabolism, 192, 193*t*
Encephalotrigeminal angiomatosis, port-wine stain in, 733
Enchondroma, 765*t*–766*t*
Encopresis, 49, 475–476
End-of-life care, 6–7
End-of-life issues, 6–9
access to comprehensive and compassionate palliative care, 6–7
acknowledgment and support provisions for caregivers, 7
bereavement in, 7
cognitive issues in, 7
commitment to quality improvement in, 7
cultural, religious, and spiritual concerns about, 7–8
in dignity of patients and families, 6
interdisciplinary resources in, 7
End-tidal carbon dioxide, 511
Endocardial cushion defect, 547, 547*f*
Endocardial cushion tissue, 545
Endocarditis, infective, 408–410
causes of, 408*t*
clinical manifestations of, 408
complications and prognosis of, 410
culture-negative, 409
differential diagnosis of, 409
etiology of, 408
laboratory studies and imaging of, 409
modified Duke clinical criteria for, 409, 409*t*
prevention of, 410
subacute, 408
treatment of, 409
Endocervicitis, 419
Endocrine disorders, manifestations of, 637
Endocrine evaluation, of growth hormone secretion, 651
Endocrine system, 637
Endocrinology assessment, 637–639, 678
Endometriosis, dysmenorrhea due to, 277

Endophthalmitis, 431–432, 433*t*
Endoscopic evaluation, of airways, 511
Endoscopic retrograde cholangiopancreatography (ERCP), 503
Endoscopy
for gastroesophageal reflux, 481
for gastrointestinal symptoms, 467, 468*f*
Endotracheal tubes, 513
Endovascular infections, 408
Enema, for functional constipation, 51*t*
Energy deficiency, due to inborn errors of metabolism, 193
Engorgement, 100
ENPP1 gene mutations, obesity in, 106*t*
Entamoeba histolytica, diarrhea from, 410*t*
Enteric adenoviruses, diarrhea from, 410*t*
Enteritis. *see* Gastroenteritis
Enteroaggregative *E. coli* (EAEC), 410*t*, 411
Enterobiasis, 451
Enterobius vermicularis, 450*t*, 451
Enterocolitis
food protein-induced, 335*t*–336*t*
due to Hirschsprung disease, 489–490
necrotizing, 254–255
gastrointestinal bleeding due to, 477*t*
Enterohemorrhagic *E. coli* (EHEC), 410*t*, 411
Enteroinvasive *E. coli* (EIEC), 410*t*, 411
Enteropathogenic *E. coli* (EPEC), 410*t*, 411
Enteropathy, dietary protein-induced, 335*t*–336*t*
Enterotoxigenic *E. coli* (ETEC), 410*t*, 411
Enteroviruses
conjunctivitis from, 431*t*
meningitis from, 387
Enthesitis, in rheumatic diseases, 343
Enuresis, 48–49
clinical manifestations of, 48
complications of, 49
differential diagnosis of, 48
epidemiology of, 48
etiology of, 48
prevention of, 49
treatment of, 49
Enuresis alarm, 49
Environmental control, for asthma, 314, 315*t*
Environmental sleep disorders, 54*t*–55*t*
Enzootic cycle, 439
Enzyme defects, 676
Enzymes, for cancer, 601*t*–602*t*
Enzymopathies, in hemolytic anemia, 567*f*, 578, 592
clinical manifestations of, 578
epidemiology of, 578
etiology of, 578
glucose-6-phosphate dehydrogenase (G6PD) deficiency as, 566, 578
laboratory studies of, 578
prevention of, 578
pyruvate kinase deficiency as, 566, 578
treatment of, 578
Eosinophil(s), values of, 565*t*
Eosinophilia
disorders associated with, 312, 312*t*
in infectious diseases, 362
nonallergic rhinitis with, 323, 324*t*
Eosinophilic esophagitis, 482–483
clinical manifestations of, 482
complications with, 483
etiology and epidemiology of, 482
laboratory and imaging studies for, 482, 482*f*
treatment and prognosis for, 482
vomiting due to, 473*t*
Eosinophilic granuloma, 765*t*–766*t*
Eosinophilic meningitis, 450*t*
Eotaxins, functions of, 290*t*
EPEC (enteropathogenic *E. coli*), 410*t*, 411
Epidemic keratoconjunctivitis, 430
Epidemic typhus, 737
Epidermal nevus, 730*t*
Epidural analgesia, 166
Epidural hemorrhages, 709–710
Epiglottis, 507
Epiglottitis
croup and, 399
upper airway obstruction due to, 517*t*, 518
Epilepsy. *see also* Seizure(s)
benign childhood, with centrotemporal spikes, 690
defined, 687
myoclonic, 689
juvenile, 690
rolandic, 690
status epilepticus in, 690–691
management of, 691*t*
Epilepsy syndrome, 688*t*, 690
Epinephrine
for anaphylaxis, 331
for cardiopulmonary resuscitation, 148, 148*t*
for croup, 399–400
deficiencies in, 649
for food allergies, 337
in newborn resuscitation, 227
for shock, 153*t*
Epiphyseal cartilage, 740*f*
Epiphyseal growth plate, 425
Epiphysiolysis, proximal humeral, 763
Epiphysis, 740*f*
Episcleritis, 433*t*
Episodic disorders, 681
Episodic rhinitis, 323
Epstein-Barr virus (EBV) infection, 573*t*
infectious mononucleosis due to, 384, 385*f*
in X-linked lymphoproliferative disease, 298–299
Equinus, 739*t*
Erb-Duchenne paralysis, in newborn, 233
Ergocalciferol, 118
Erosion, 722*t*
Erysipelas, 380
Erysipeloid, 439*t*–442*t*
Erysipelothrix rhusiopathiae, 439*t*–442*t*
Erythema infectiosum (fifth disease), 377–378
clinical manifestations of, 377
complications and prognosis of, 378
differential diagnosis of, 377
epidemiology of, 377
etiology of, 377
laboratory and imaging studies in, 377
prevention of, 378
treatment of, 377
Erythema marginatum, due to heart failure, 556, 556*t*
Erythema migrans, 443
Erythema multiforme (EM), 331, 733–735, 734*t*
vesiculobullous eruptions due to, 734*t*
Erythema nodosum, infections with fever and, 373*t*–374*t*
Erythema toxicum, 228–229
Erythematous flare, in allergen-specific IgE in vivo skin testing, 312–313
Erythroblastosis fetalis
newborn anemia due to, 247
predicting severity of, 247–248
Erythrocyte P antigen, erythema infectiosum and, 377
Erythrocytic phase, of *Plasmodium* life cycle, 447
Erythroderma, diffuse, infections with fever and, 373*t*–374*t*
Erythroid cells, in hematopoiesis, 563
Erythroid colony-forming unit, 563–566
Erythromycin, for acne, 723
Erythropoiesis, 563–566
embryonic, 247
ineffective, 575
Erythropoietin, 563–566, 617–618
Escherichia coli
diarrhea from, 410*t*, 411
urinary tract infections due to, 416
Esophageal atresia, 483
Esophageal disorders, 480–487
caustic injuries as, 484
eosinophilic esophagitis as, 482–483, 482*f*
esophageal atresia as, 483
due to foreign bodies, 483–484
gastroesophageal reflux as, 480–482, 481*t*
pill ulcers as, 484
tracheoesophageal fistula as, 483, 483*f*
Esophageal foreign bodies, 483–484
Esophageal impedance monitoring, for gastroesophageal reflux, 481
Esophageal pH probe monitoring, 24-hour, for gastroesophageal reflux, 481
Esophageal reflux, abdominal pain due to, 470*t*
Esophageal varices, 497
gastrointestinal bleeding due to, 477*t*
Esophagitis, 485–486, 486*t*
allergic eosinophilic, 335*t*–336*t*
Esophagram, barium, 511
Etanercept, for juvenile idiopathic arthritis, 352
ETEC (enterotoxigenic *E. coli*), 410*t*, 411
Ethical decision making, 4
Ethical issues
in end-of-life decision making, 8
in genetic testing and screening, 5–6
in practice, 5–6
Ethical principles, related to infants, children, and adolescents, 4–5
Ethics, 4–6, 9
in health care, 4
religious issues and, 6
Ethylene glycol, 140
toxicity, 162*t*
Etonogestrel implant, 278–279
Etoposide, for cancer, 601*t*–602*t*
Eunuchoid proportions, 656
Euphoria, in bipolar I disorder (BD), 66
Euvolemic hyponatremia, 132
Evaporation, heat loss via, 234
Ewing sarcoma, 611
clinical manifestations of, 612
diagnosis of, 612
differential diagnosis of, 612
epidemiology of, 611
laboratory/imaging studies in, 612
prognosis for, 613
risk factors for, 597*t*
treatment of, 612
Exchange transfusion, for indirect hyperbilirubinemia, 252
Excoriation, 722*t*
Exercise intolerance, due to heart failure, 535
Exertional dyspnea, due to pulmonary stenosis, 547
Exhalation, 507
Exit site infection, 437
Exocrine pancreatic insufficiency, in cystic fibrosis, 527, 529
Exons, 169
Exostoses
multiple hereditary, 765*t*–766*t*
osteocartilaginous, 765*t*–766*t*
Expiratory reserve volume, 508*f*
Extensor plantar reflex, 684
External cardiac massage, in newborn resuscitation, 226–227
External genitalia, differentiation of male and female, 671*f*

External intercostal muscles, during inspiration, 507
External tibial torsion, 749
Extinction, 16, 25
Extracellular fluid (ECF), 125
Extracorporeal membrane oxygenation (ECMO)
  for heart failure, 555*t*
  for meconium aspiration syndrome, 245
  for primary pulmonary hypertension of the newborn, 245
Extrahepatic biliary atresia, 494
Extramedullary hematopoiesis, in hematological disorders, 563
Extrapulmonary shunt, hypoxemia due to, 508*t*
Extrapulmonary tuberculosis, 455
Extremities
  anemia and, 569*t*
  congenital malformations of, 185
  of newborn, 231
Extremity fractures, in newborn, 234
Extrinsic pathways, in coagulation, 580
Extrinsic tracheal compression, 521, 521*f*
Exudates, 530–531
Eye(s)
  anemia and, 569*t*
  with developmental disabilities, 30*t*
  dysmorphology of, 185
  of newborn, 228*f*
Eye movements, assessment of, 683
Eyelid scrub, for blepharitis, 431

F

FA (Friedreich ataxia), 702
  genetic basis for, 173*t*
Fabry disease, 210*t*–212*t*
Face
  congenital malformations of, 183*t*
  with developmental disabilities, 30*t*
  of newborn, 230
Facial nerve, assessment of, 683
Facial nerve injury, in newborn, 233
Facial weakness, 694*t*
Facioscapulohumeral dystrophy, 697
Factitious disorder, 60–61, 61*t*
Factitious hyperinsulinemia, 649
Factor 5 Leiden, 589
Factor VIII deficiency, 586–587
  genetic basis for, 174*t*
Factor 9 deficiency, 586–587
Failure to thrive, 77–79, 109
  clinical manifestations of, 77–79
  complications of, 79
  diagnosis of, 77–79
  etiology of, 77, 78*t*
  malnutrition and, 109
  treatment of, 79, 79*t*
Famciclovir
  for herpes simplex virus infection, 424
  for varicella zoster virus, 379
Familial hemophagocytic lymphohistiocytosis, 573*t*
Familial hypophosphatemic rickets, 670, 670*t*
Familial male-limited precocious puberty, 662
Familial short stature, 13
Family
  defined, 87
  functions of, 87–88, 88*t*
  single-parent, 88
  traditional, 88
Family dysfunction
  defined, 87
  for emotional support, education, and socialization, 91
  for physical needs, 90–91
Family history
  for dysmorphology, 184
  in genetic assessment, 178
Family structure, 88–90
  adoption as, 89
  foster care as, 89–90
  with sexual minority parents, 88–89
  single-parent families as, 88
Fanconi anemia, 573*t*, 574–575
  clinical manifestations of, 574
  etiology and epidemiology of, 574
  marrow replacement in, 575
  treatment of, 575
Fanconi syndrome, 621
  proximal renal tubular acidosis and, 140
Farber lipogranulomatosis, 210*t*–212*t*
Fasciculations, 684
  spinal muscular atrophy, 694
Fasciitis, necrotizing, 380
Fascioliasis, 451*t*
Fasciolopsiasis, 451*t*
Fasciolopsis buski, 451*t*
Fat metabolic disorder(s), 207–208
Fat-soluble vitamins, 114*t*, 117–119
Fatal injuries, 154
Fatigability, due to pulmonary stenosis, 547
Fatigue, due to heart failure, 535
Fatty acid(s), catabolism of, 207, 207*f*
Fatty acid disorder(s)
  carnitine deficiency as, 208
  of fatty acid oxidation, 207–208
  glutaric aciduria type II, 208
Fatty acid oxidation disorders, 207–208
  of ketogenesis, 649–650
Fatty liver disease, nonalcoholic, 501
FBN1 gene, in Marfan syndrome, 171
Febrile nonhemolytic transfusion reaction, 590*t*
Febrile paroxysms, 447
Febrile seizures, 689
  complex, 689
  simple, 689
Fecalith, in appendicitis, 493
Feeding jejunostomy, for gastroesophageal reflux, 481*t*
Femoral anteversion, 739*t*, 748
  clinical manifestations of, 748
Femoral pulses, in coarctation of aorta, 548
Femur, 751*f*
Fentanyl, as analgesia, 166*t*
Ferrous sulfate, for iron deficiency anemia, 120
Fetal acidosis, 220
Fetal alcohol spectrum disorder (FASD), 90, 176–177
Fetal alcohol syndrome (FAS), 90
Fetal aorta, Doppler examination of, 220
Fetal growth, 219, 220*t*
Fetal heart rate monitoring, 220
Fetal hemoglobin, 220–221, 247, 566
Fetal hydrops, 240
  respiratory distress in newborn due to, 240
Fetal-maternal hemorrhage, 249
Fetal maturity, 219
Fetal size, 219
Fetal well-being, 220
Fetus
  assessment of, 219–220, 220*t*
  diseases of, 239–240
    hydrops fetalis as, 240
    intrauterine growth restriction and small for gestational age as, 239–240, 239*t*
Fever
  blackwater, 449
  dengue, 446
  factitious, 371
  in immunocompromised person, 434–435, 435*f*, 436*t*
Fever *(Continued)*
  infections with rash and, 373–379
    differential diagnosis of, 373*t*–374*t*
    erythema infectiosum (fifth disease) as, 377–378
    measles (rubeola) as, 373–375
    roseola infantum (exanthem subitum), 376–377
    rubella (German or 3-day measles), 375–376
    varicella-zoster virus infection (chickenpox and zoster), 378–379
  in infectious diseases, 361
  in Kawasaki disease, 347
  normal body temperature and, 368
  Q, 439*t*–442*t*
  rat-bite, 439*t*–442*t*
  relapsing, 439*t*–442*t*
    louse-borne, 737
  rheumatic, 556, 556*t*
  in rheumatic diseases, 343
  scarlet, 393
  of short duration, 368
  trench, 737
  of unknown origin, 368, 370*f*
    causes of, in children, 371*t*–372*t*
    screening tests for, 371
  without a focus, 368–371
    bacteremia and, 368
    in children 3 months to 3 years of age, 369–370, 369*f*
    in infants younger than 3 months of age, 368–369
    pattern of, 368
    sepsis and, 368
Fever blisters, 382
Fexofenadine, for allergic rhinitis, 325
FGFR3 gene, in achondroplasia, 171
Fiber supplements, for irritable bowel syndrome, 471–472
Fibrillation(s), 685
  atrial, 543
  ventricular, 544*t*
Fibrinogen, 583
Fibrinolysis, in hemostasis, 581
Fibrinolytic agents, for thrombosis, 589
Fibroma, nonossifying, 765*t*–766*t*
Fibromyalgia, 358
Fibrosing colonopathy, due to lipase, 529
Fibrous periosteum, 740*f*
Fibula, 751*f*
Filiform warts, 382
Fine motor-adaptive development, milestones of, 17*t*
Finger
  abnormalities of, 765
  trigger, 765
Fire ant bites, allergic reactions to, 333
First-degree heart block, 543, 544*t*
First heart sound (S_1), 536
FISH (fluorescent in situ hybridization), 179
Fissure, 722*t*
Fitz-Hugh-Curtis syndrome, 420–421
Flat warts (verruca plana), 382
Flatfoot
  developmental, 754
  flexible, 754
  rigid, 754–755
Flavoprotein metabolism, 207*f*
Flea bites, allergic reactions to, 333
Flexible bronchoscopy, 511
Flexible flatfoot, 754
Floppy infant, 698
Fluid
  in body composition, 125, 126*f*
  in cardiopulmonary resuscitation, 148*t*

Fluid deficit, calculation of, 128
Fluid management, for burns, 159
Fluid restriction, for heart failure, 555*t*
Fluid resuscitation
  for dehydration, 128
  for intussusception, 493
Fluid therapy, maintenance, 125–126, 126*t*
Flumazenil, for benzodiazepine poisoning, 164*t*–165*t*
Flunisolide, for asthma, 319*f*
Flunitrazepam, acute effects of, 284*t*–285*t*
Fluorescent in situ hybridization (FISH), 179
Fluorescent treponemal antibody-absorption (FTA-ABS) test, 424
Fluoride deficiency, 119*t*, 121
Fluoride supplementation, 479
Fluorosis, 121, 479
Fluoxetine
  maternal use of, 238*t*
  as teratogens, 237*t*
Fluticasone HFA/MDI/DPI, for asthma, 319*f*
Flutter, atrial, 543, 544*t*
Fly bites, allergic reactions to, 333
FMR-1 gene, in fragile X syndrome, 176
FMRP (fragile X mental retardation protein), 176
Focal segmental glomerulosclerosis (FSGS), 620
Folate deficiency, 114–116, 114*t*
  in anemia, 567*f*
Folic acid antagonists, as teratogens, 237*t*
Folliculitis, 380
  hot tub, 380
Fontan procedure, for tricuspid atresia, 551
Fontanelles, 229
Food(s), adverse reactions to, 334–338
  clinical manifestations of, 335, 335*t*–336*t*
  complications of, 337
  diagnosis of, 335–337
  etiology and epidemiology of, 334–335
  laboratory and imaging studies for, 335
  prognosis and prevention of, 337–338
  treatment of, 337
Food-borne causes, of diarrhea, 410–411
Food protein-induced enterocolitis syndrome, 335*t*–336*t*
Foot, 752–755
  calcaneovalgus, 754
  cavus, 755
  club, 753–754, 753*f*
  deformity, posturing *vs.*, 752
  hypermobile pes planus (flexible flatfoot), 754
  idiopathic avascular necrosis of, 755
  metatarsus adductus, 754, 754*f*
  Sever disease (calcaneal apophysitis) of, 755
  skew, 754
  tarsal coalition of, 754–755
  toe deformities of, 755, 756*t*
Foot pain, differential diagnosis of, 752, 753*t*
Forced expiratory flow (FEF), 511
Forced expired volume in first second (FEV_1), 511
Forced vital capacity (FVC), 511
Forchheimer spots, in rubella, 375
Forehead, dysmorphology of, 185
Foreign bodies
  esophageal, 483–484
  in nose, 324
  upper airway obstruction due to, 517*t*
Foreign body aspiration, 521–522
  bronchiolitis and, 402
Formicid stings, allergic reactions to, 333
Formoterol, for asthma, 315
Formula feeding, 100–101
  cow's milk-based, 100–101
  soy-based, 100–101, 102*t*
  standard, 100–101, 102*t*
Forward-facing car seat, 22
Fosphenytoin, for status epilepticus, 691, 691*t*
Foster care, 2, 89–90
Fostering optimal development, 23*t*–24*t*
Founder effect, with inborn errors of metabolism, 196–197
Fourth heart sound (S_4), 536
Fraction of inspired oxygen (FiO_2), low, hypoxemia due to, 508*t*
Fracture(s), 742–744
  angulation, 742*t*
  bowing, 742
  buckle or torus, 742
  due to child abuse, 81, 82*f*, 744
  comminution, 742*t*
  compaction, 742*t*
  complete, 742, 742*t*
  greenstick, 742, 742*f*
  incomplete, 742*t*
  linear, 742*t*
  management of pediatric, 743
  oblique, 742*t*
  open, 742*t*
  patterns, pediatric, 742–743
  physeal, 742–743
  rotation, 742*t*
  Salter-Harris classification of, 742, 743*f*
  shortening, 742*t*
  skull, 710
  special concerns with, 743–744
    compartment syndrome as, 743–744
    neurovascular injury as, 743
    overgrowth as, 743
    progressive deformity as, 743
    remodeling as, 743
  spiral, 742*t*
  terminology for, 742*t*
  toddler's, 744
  transverse, 742*t*
Fracture remodeling, 743
Fragile X mental retardation protein (FMRP), 176
Fragile X syndrome (FRAX), genetic basis for, 174*t*, 176
Frameshift mutation, 169
Francisella tularensis, 439*t*–442*t*
Free fatty acids, in serum glucose regulation, 647
Freiberg disease, 755
Fremitus, vocal, 510*t*
Fresh frozen plasma, 590*t*
Friction, vesiculobullous eruptions due to, 734*t*
Friedreich ataxia (FA), 702
  genetic basis for, 173*t*
Fröhlich syndrome, obesity in, 106*t*
Fructose intolerance, hereditary, 201
Fructosuria, 201
FTO gene polymorphism, obesity in, 106*t*
α-Fucosidase L deficiency, 210*t*–212*t*
Fucosidosis, 210*t*–212*t*
Fulminant liver failure, 494–497
  clinical manifestations of, 497
  etiology and epidemiology of, 494, 499*t*
  laboratory and imaging studies for, 497
  treatment of, 497, 500*t*
Fumarylacetoacetate hydrolase deficiency, 202
Functional abdominal pain (FAP). *see* Abdominal pain, functional (recurrent)
Functional constipation, 49–51
  clinical manifestations of, 49–50
  complications of, 51
  differential diagnosis of, 50
  epidemiology of, 49
  etiology of, 49
  prevention of, 51
  treatment of, 50–51, 50*t*–52*t*
Functional residual capacity (FRC), 507–508, 508*f*
Fundoplication procedure, for gastroesophageal reflux, 481*t*
Funeral, children at, 96
Fungal infections
  in immunocompromised person, 434–435
  superficial, 380–381, 381*t*
Fungal meningitis, 387*t*
Fungemia, catheter-associated, 437–438
Furosemide, for heart failure, 555*t*
Furuncles (boils), 380, 722*f*
Fusobacterium necrophorum, 393

G

GAD. *see* Generalized anxiety disorder
Gadolinium-enhanced magnetic resonance imaging, in infectious diseases, 362–363
Gag reflex, 683
Gait
  antalgic, 740
  assessment of, 684
  Trendelenburg, 740
  waddling, 740
Galactocerebroside β-galactosidase deficiency, 210*t*–212*t*
Galactokinase deficiency, 201
Galactose-1-phosphate uridyltransferase deficiency, 201, 201*f*
Galactose-6-sulfatase deficiency, 210*t*–212*t*
Galactosemia, 201
  clinical manifestations of, 201
  genetic basis for, 196*t*
  hypoglycemia due to, 650
  laboratory manifestations of, 201
  treatment of, 201
Galactosialidosis, 210*t*–212*t*
α-Galactosidase deficiency, 210*t*–212*t*
β-Galactosidase deficiency, 210*t*–212*t*
Galactosyl ceramide lipidosis, 210*t*–212*t*
Galeazzi sign, 744
Gallbladder disease, in sickle cell disease, 577*t*
Gallstones, in anemia, 567–568
Ganglion cysts, 765
Gangliosidosis
  GM_1 (generalized, infantile), 210*t*–212*t*
  GM_2, 210*t*–212*t*
Gardnerella vaginalis, 417–418
Gastric lavage, for poisoning, 164
Gastritis, vomiting due to, 473*t*
Gastroenteritis
  acute, 410–413
    clinical manifestations of, 412
    complications and prognosis of, 413
    differential diagnosis of, 412
    etiology and epidemiology of, 410–412, 410*t*
    laboratory and imaging studies in, 412
    prevention of, 413
    treatment of, 412–413
  allergic eosinophilic, 335*t*–336*t*
  bacterial, vomiting due to, 473*t*
  viral, vomiting due to, 473*t*
Gastroesophageal reflux (GER), 480–482
  clinical manifestations of, 481
  epidemiology of, 480–481
  etiology of, 480–481
  infantile, 472
  laboratory and imaging studies for, 481
  physiological, 480
  treatment of, 481–482, 481*t*
  vomiting *vs.*, 472, 473*t*
Gastroesophageal reflux disease (GERD), 481
Gastrointestinal bleeding, 476–478
  differential diagnosis of, 477
  distinguishing features of, 477, 477*t*
  evaluation of, 477, 478*t*
  treatment of, 477–478, 478*f*

Gastrointestinal decontamination, for poisoning, 164
Gastrointestinal disorders, manifestations of, 467–478
  abdominal pain as, 467–472
  constipation and encopresis as, 475–476
  diarrhea as, 473–475
  gastrointestinal bleeding as, 476–478
  vomiting as, 472–473
Gastrointestinal involvement, in Henoch-Schönlein purpura, 346
Gastrointestinal losses, adjusting fluid therapy for, 127*t*
Gastrointestinal symptoms, poisoning and, 163
Gastroschisis, 227*t*, 231, 489
Gaucher disease, 712
  genetic basis for, 173*t*
Gender dysphoria, 87
Gender expression, 84*t*
Gender identity, 87
Gender roles, 84*t*, 87
Gene(s), 169
Generalized anxiety disorder (GAD), 62
Genetic assessment, 177–179
  history in
    delivery and birth, 178
    of development, 178
    family, 178
    laboratory evaluation, 179
      chromosome analysis in, 179
      direct DNA analysis in, 179
      fluorescent in situ hybridization in, 179
      microarray comparative genomic hybridization in, 179
      whole exome sequencing, 179
    physical examination, 179
    of pregnancy, 178
  preconception and prenatal counseling of, 177–178
    adolescent and adult, 178
    familial factors, 177
    maternal factors in, 177–178
    postnatal, 178
    screening in, 177
Genetic disorder(s)
  autosomal dominant, 170–171
  autosomal recessive, 171
  due to expansion of trinucleotide repeat, 176
  due to genomic imprinting, 176
  mitochondrial inheritance, 175
    heteroplasmy in, 175
    hypertrophic pyloric stenosis as, 174–175
    MELAS as, 175
    neural tube defects as, 175
  types of, 169
  due to uniparental disomy, 175
    Angelman syndrome due to, 176
    Prader-Willi syndrome as, 175–176
  X-linked recessive, 172
Genetic testing and screening
  ethical issues in, 5–6
  for primary immunodeficiency, 293
Genetics, 169–173
Genital herpes, 421*t*, 424
  primary, 424
  secondary, recurrent or reactivation eruptions of, 424
Genital ulcers, 419, 421*t*
Genital warts (condylomata acuminata), 382, 419, 423*t*, 425
Genitalia
  congenital malformations of, 185–186
  of newborn, 228*f*, 231
Genomic imprinting, 176
Genomics, 169–173
Genu valgum, 749*f*, 750
Genu varum, 749*f*, 750
Germ cell tumors, malignant, risk factors for, 597*t*
Germinomas, 662
Gestation. *see also* Pregnancy
  multiple, 217
Gestational age
  fetus, 219
  large for, 228, 228*f*
  of newborn, 227–228, 229*f*–230*f*
    and abnormal fetal growth patterns, 228
    cumulative score in, 227–228
    neurological criteria in, 227–228
    physical criteria in, 227–228, 228*f*
  small for, 228, 230*f*, 239–240
    complications of, 220*t*
    management of, 239–240
    and mortality rate, 230*f*
Gestational diabetes, 237
GH. *see* Growth hormone
Ghent nosology, 172*t*
Ghon complex, 453
Gianotti-Crosti syndrome, 413
Giant cell (Hecht) pneumonia, due to measles, 375
Giant congenital melanocytic nevi, 732
Giant coronary artery aneurysms, in Kawasaki disease, 347
Giant pigmented nevi, 228–229, 731–732
Giardia lamblia, diarrhea from, 410*t*, 411–412
Gingivostomatitis, 393
Girls, growth and development of, 270–271
Gitelman syndrome, 135–136, 136*t*
Glabella, 183*t*
Glands, 637
Glanzmann thrombasthenia, 586
Glasgow Coma Scale, 155, 155*t*, 703, 704*t*, 710
Glenn procedure, bidirectional, for tricuspid atresia, 551
Glenohumeral dislocation, 763
Glenohumeral joint, 763
Globin chains, in erythropoiesis, 563–566
Glomerular filtration, 617
Glomerulonephritis (GN), 622–624
  acute postinfectious, 622
  clinical manifestations of, 622–623
  diagnostic studies of, 623
  etiology and epidemiology of, 622
  prognosis and prevention of, 623–624
  therapy for, 623
Glomerulosclerosis, focal segmental, nephrotic syndrome due to, 620
Glottis, 507
Glucagon
  for β-blocking agents, 164*t*–165*t*
  deficiencies in, 649
Glucocerebrosidase deficiency, 210*t*–212*t*
  genetic basis for, 173*t*
Gluconeogenesis
  and hypoglycemia, 649
  in serum glucose regulation, 647
Glucose, serum, regulation, 647, 648*f*
Glucose-6-phosphate dehydrogenase (G6PD) deficiency
  African variant of, 578
  in anemia, 566
  clinical manifestations of, 578
  epidemiology of, 578
  etiology of, 578
  genetic basis for, 174*t*
  laboratory studies of, 578
  Mediterranean variant of, 578
  phagocytic disorders in, 301*t*
  type B, 578
Glucose tolerance, impaired, 639–640
Glucosylceramide lipidosis, 210*t*–212*t*
Glucuronosyltransferase deficiency, 250
Glutaric acidemia I, 206, 207*f*
Glutaric acidemia type II, 208
Glutaryl-CoA dehydrogenase deficiency, 207*f*
Glycerin suppositories, for functional constipation, 51*t*–52*t*
Glycogen, 199
  synthesis and degradation, 200*f*
Glycogen storage diseases (GSDs), 199–201, 200*f*, 200*t*, 649
Glycogen synthetase, 200*f*
Glycogenolysis, in serum glucose regulation, 649
Glycohemoglobin (HgbA1c), 645
Glycolytic enzymes, in erythropoiesis, 563–566
Glycosaminoglycans, 209
GM_1 gangliosidosis, 210*t*–212*t*
GM_2 gangliosidosis, 210*t*–212*t*
GN. *see* Glomerulonephritis
Goiter, endemic, maternal, 236*t*
GoLYTELY (polyethylene glycol), for poisoning, 164
Gonadarche, 656
Gonadoblastomas, 674
Gonococcal conjunctivitis, 431
Gonococcal infections, disseminated, 421–422
Gonococcemia, differential diagnosis of, 344*t*
Gonorrhea *(Neisseria gonorrhoeae)*, 421–422
  clinical features of, 420*t*
  congenital infection with, 259–261
  disseminated gonococcal infections due to, 421–422
Gordon syndrome, 138
Gottron papules, in juvenile dermatomyositis, 355–356
Gower sign, 684, 696
  in juvenile dermatomyositis, 355
Graduated extinction, for pediatric sleep disorders, 56
Graft-*versus*-host disease (GVHD)
  acute, 307–308
  chronic, 307–308
  with hematopoietic stem cell transplantation, 307
  oncological emergencies, 600*t*
  in severe combined immunodeficiency, 299
Gram-negative anaerobic bacilli, pneumonia due to, 407*t*
Granulocyte colony-stimulating factor (G-CSF), in hematopoiesis, 564*f*, 566
Granulocyte-macrophage colony-stimulating factor (GM-CSF), in hematopoiesis, 564*f*, 566
Granuloma
  eosinophilic, 765*t*–766*t*
  pyogenic, 733
Granuloma inguinale, 419, 421*t*
Graphesthesia, 684
Grasp reflex, 682*t*
Graves disease, 667–668
  clinical manifestations of, 667
  drugs for, 667–668
  maternal, 236, 236*t*
  radioiodine for, 668
  surgery, 668
  thyroid storm for, 668
  treatment of, 667
Gray matter heterotopias, 717
Great arteries, transposition of, 550–551, 550*f*
Greenstick fractures, 742, 742*f*
Grey Turner sign, 502
Gross motor development, milestones of, 17*t*
Group A *Streptococcus*, 392
  osteomyelitis due to, 425
  pharyngitis due to, 392–394
    causes of, 392*t*
    clinical manifestations of, 392–393

Group A *Streptococcus (Continued)*
complications and prognosis of, 394
differential diagnosis of, 393
epidemiology of, 392
etiology of, 392
laboratory evaluation of, 393
treatment of, 393–394, 394*t*
pneumonia due to, 407*t*
Group B *Streptococcus*
osteomyelitis due to, 425
pneumonia due to, 407*t*
Growing pain, 356–357
diagnosis of, 356–357
Growth abnormalities, 651–656
short stature. *see* Short stature
Growth and development, 11–40
of adolescents, 270–273
for boys, 271–273, 272*f*
changes associated with, 273
for girls, 270–271, 271*f*–272*f*
normal variations in, 274–275
breast asymmetry and masses as, 274, 274*t*
gynecomastia as, 274–275, 274*t*
irregular menses as, 274
physiological leukorrhea as, 274
benchmarks for, 11, 11*t*
of bones, 739, 740*f*
catch-down, 13
catch-up, 11–13
defined, 11
disorders of, 11, 13
hormonal effects on, 650*t*
linear, patterns of, 653*f*
measurement of, 651
normal, 11–13, 650–651
Growth chart
of body mass index, 12*f*
of head circumference, 12*f*
of length, 12*f*
of stature, 12*f*
Growth factors, mechanisms of action of, 637*f*
Growth failure
in anemia, 568
defined, 651
screening tests, 655*t*
in sickle cell disease, 577*t*
Growth hormone (GH)
physiology of, 650–651
resistance, 651
secretion, endocrine evaluation of, 651
Growth hormone-binding protein, 650–651
Growth hormone deficiency, 653–656
classic congenital or idiopathic, 653
clinical manifestations of, 655
diagnosis of, 655
etiology and epidemiology of, 653
hypoglycemia due to, 649
obesity in, 106*t*
treatment of, 655–656
tumor and, 653
Growth hormone-releasing factor, 650–651
Growth patterns, evaluation of, 11, 13*t*
Growth plate, 740*f*
Grunting, 509–510
Guanfacine, for attention-deficit/hyperactivity disorder (ADHD), 47
Guillain-Barré syndrome, 695
Gustatory rhinitis, 324
Guttate psoriasis, 729–730
Gymnast's wrist, 765
Gynecological issue
contraception in, 278–281
barrier methods for, 280–281
condoms as, 280
sponge, caps, and diaphragm as, 280
Gynecological issue *(Continued)*
coitus interruptus for, 281
emergency postcoital, 280–281, 281*t*
intrauterine devices for, 279
oral and anal for, 281
rhythm method (periodic coital abstinence) for, 281
steroidal, 278–281
combined hormonal contraceptives for, 279–280, 279*t*–280*t*
contraceptive patch for, 279–280
contraceptive vaginal ring for, 279–280
hormonal injections and implants for, 278–279
long-acting reversible contraceptives for, 278–279
progesterone-only pill or minipill for, 280
menstrual disorders as, 275–277
abnormal uterine bleeding as, 276–277
amenorrhea as, 275–276
dysmenorrhea as, 277
irregular menses as, 274–275
pregnancy as, 277–278
continuation of, 278
diagnosis of, 278
termination of, 278
rape as, 281
Gynecomastia, 663
in adolescent boy, 274

H

H_1 antihistamines, for anaphylaxis, 331
H_2 receptor antagonist, for gastroesophageal reflux, 481*t*
Haddon matrix, 154
Haemophilus ducreyi, 419
Haemophilus influenzae, conjunctivitis from, 430
Haemophilus influenzae type b (Hib)
osteomyelitis from, 425
pneumonia from, 403, 407*t*
Haemophilus influenzae type b (Hib) conjugate vaccine, 363–364, 364*f*–365*f*
Hair grooming, syncope due to, 541*t*
Hair tufts, over lumbosacral spine, 228
Hairy congenital nevus, 731–732, 731*f*
Hallucinogens, acute effects of, 284*t*–285*t*
Haloperidol, maternal use of, 238*t*
Hamartomas, 660
smooth muscle, 730*t*
Hand-foot-mouth syndrome, vesiculobullous eruptions due to, 734*t*
HANE (hereditary angioneurotic edema), genetic basis for, 170*t*
Hantavirus, 439*t*–442*t*
Haptenation, in adverse drug reactions, 338
Hartnup syndrome, 205
Harvester ant bites, allergic reactions to, 333
Hashimoto thyroiditis, 666–667
Haverhill fever, 439*t*–442*t*
Hay fever, 323
HBIG (hepatitis B immunoglobulin), 416
HBsAg (hepatitis B surface antigen), 413–414
HBV. *see* Hepatitis B virus
HCV. *see* Hepatitis C virus
HD (Huntington disease), genetic basis for, 170*t*
HDV (hepatitis D virus), 413, 414*t*
Head
anemia and, 569*t*
congenital malformations of, 183*t*, 185
with developmental disabilities, 30*t*
Head circumference
benchmarks for, 11, 11*t*
growth chart of, 12*f*
in neurology assessment, 681
Head louse, 736
Head tilt, 683
Head trauma. *see also* Traumatic brain injury
due to child abuse, 81, 82*f*
Headache, 685–687
acute, 686*t*
recurrent, 686*t*
after traumatic brain injury, 710
chronic
daily, 686*t*
nonprogressive, 686*t*
progressive, 686*t*
clinical manifestations of, 686, 686*f*, 686*t*
diagnostic studies for, 686–687
etiology and epidemiology of, 685–686
temporal patterns of, 686, 686*t*
treatment for, 687
Health care, pediatric
changing morbidity and, 3
culture and, 3
current challenges in, 1
health disparities in, 3
landscape of, 1–2, 2*t*
other health issues affecting, 2–3
in society, 1
Health care-associated infections, 437
Health care team, 1
Health insurance coverage, 1
Health Insurance Portability and Accountability Act (HIPAA), 5
Health maintenance or supervision visits, 11–14, 19
anticipatory guidance in, 22–25, 23*t*–24*t*
dental care in, 22
fostering optimal development in, 22–25
immunizations in, 22
nutritional assessment in, 22
safety issues in, 22
screening tests in, 17, 20–22
for anemia, 20–21
for cholesterol, 21, 21*t*
for depression, 22
hearing and vision, 20
for lead, 21, 21*t*
newborn, 20
for sexually transmitted infection, 21–22
for tuberculosis, 21, 21*t*
topics for, 19, 19*t*
Hearing, with developmental disabilities, 30*t*
Hearing assessment, 683
Hearing deficit, 18, 18*t*
Hearing impairment, in child, with special needs, 34–36, 35*t*
Hearing loss, otitis media and, 397
Hearing screening, 20
of children 3 years of age and older, 20
of infants and toddlers, 20
Heart
boot-shaped, 550
congenital diaphragmatic, 246
with developmental disabilities, 30*t*
of newborn, 231
normal, 540*f*
Heart block, 543
Heart disease, congenital
acyanotic, 545–548
aortic stenosis as, 548
atrial septal defect as, 546, 546*f*
coarctation of aorta as, 548
endocardial cushion defect as, 547, 547*f*
etiology and epidemiology of, 545, 545*t*
patent ductus arteriosus as, 546–547, 546*f*
pulmonary stenosis as, 547–548
ventricular septal defect as, 545–546, 545*f*
congenital malformation syndromes associated with, 536*t*
cyanotic, 549–553
extracardiac complications of, 553*t*

Heart disease, congenital *(Continued)*
hypoplastic left heart syndrome as, 552–553, 552*f*
presenting symptoms in, 549*t*
tetralogy of Fallot as, 549–550, 550*f*
total anomalous pulmonary venous return as, 552, 552*f*
transposition of great arteries as, 550–551, 550*f*
tricuspid atresia as, 551, 551*f*
truncus arteriosus as, 551–552, 551*f*
ductal-dependent, 227*t*
Heart failure, 553–554
clinical manifestations of, 554
etiology and epidemiology of, 553, 554*f*, 554*t*
by age group, 555*t*
imaging studies for, 554
treatment of, 554, 555*t*
ventricular function curve in, 553, 554*f*
Heart murmurs, 535–538
continuous, 538
diastolic, 536–538
ejection, 536
frequency or pitch of, 537
holosystolic, 536
intensity of, 537*t*
in newborn, 231
normal or innocent, 538, 538*t*
Still's, 538*t*
systolic, 536
timing of, 537*f*
vibratory, 538*t*
Heart rate
in cardiovascular system assessment, 535
in heart failure, 554*t*
Heart sounds, 536, 537*t*
Heat-labile (cholera-like) enterotoxin, 411
Heat loss, mechanisms of, 234
Heat-stable enterotoxin, 411
Heat stress, in newborn, 234
Hecht pneumonia, due to measles, 375
Heel to ear, in newborn, 229*f*
Height, growth chart of, 12*f*
Heinz bodies, in G6PD deficiency, 578
Helicobacter pylori, in peptic ulcer disease, 485–486
Heliotrope discoloration, in juvenile dermatomyositis, 355–356
Helium dilution, 511
HELLP syndrome, 218
Helminthiases, 449–452
ascariasis, 450
enterobiasis as, 451
hookworm infections of, 450
neurocysticercosis, 452
schistosomiasis as, 451–452
visceral larva migrans as, 450–451
Helper T cells (CD4 cells), HIV infected by, 458
Hemangioma(s), 732–733, 732*f*
capillary, 228–229
cavernous, 228–229
complications of, 732
defined, 732
with developmental disabilities, 30*t*
differential diagnosis of, 730*t*
lumbosacral, 732–733
periorbital, 732–733
in PHACE syndrome, 732–733
subglottic, 732–733
treatment of, 732–733
Hemarthroses, 587
Hematemesis, evaluation of, 478*t*
Hematocrit, values of, 565*t*
Hematological abnormalities, in systemic lupus erythematosus, 354–355
Hematological disorders
juvenile idiopathic arthritis *vs.*, 352*t*
presentation of, 563, 564*t*
Hematological values, during infancy and childhood, 563, 565*t*
Hematology, 563–593
developmental, 563–566, 564*f*
Hematology assessment, 563–566, 591
developmental hematology and, 563–566, 564*f*
history in, 563
initial diagnostic evaluation in, 563, 565*t*
physical examination and common manifestations in, 563, 564*t*
Hematomas
duodenal, 157
in hemostatic disorders, 583
subdural, in newborn, 256–257
Hematopoiesis, 564*f*
embryonic, 247
extramedullary, 563
Hematopoietic stem cell transplantation (HSCT), 306–308
in aplastic anemia, 574
complications of, 307–308
immunodeficiency diseases curable by, 306, 307*t*
major histocompatibility complex compatibility in, 307
for sickle cell disease, 577–578
Hematuria, 622–624
benign familial, 622–623
clinical manifestations of, 622–623
diagnostic studies of, 623, 623*f*
differential diagnosis of, 622*t*
etiology and epidemiology of, 622
gross, 622
microscopic, 622
therapy for, 623
Heme, in erythropoiesis, 563–566
Heme iron, 120
Hemiparesis (hemiplegia), due to cerebral palsy, 37*t*
Hemochromatosis, in β-thalassemia major, 575–576
Hemodynamics, for cardiomyopathies, 557*t*
Hemoglobin
fetal, 220–221, 247, 566
production of, 566
values of, 565*t*
Hemoglobin A, 566
Hemoglobin C, 575
Hemoglobin D, 575
Hemoglobin E, 575
Hemoglobin electrophoresis, for hemoglobinopathies, 577
Hemoglobin F, 247, 566
Hemoglobin level(s)
after birth, 247
in anemia, 566
Hemoglobin-oxygen dissociation curve, fetal, 220–221, 222*f*
Hemoglobin S, 575
Hemoglobin SS disease. *see also* Sickle cell disease
anemia of, 576
Hemoglobinopathies, 592
alpha-chain, 575
beta-chain, 575
in hemolytic anemia, 567*f*
major, 575
Hemolysis
acute episode of, 578
isoimmune, 579
in newborn
diagnosis and management of, 249
nonimmune causes of, 249
Hemolytic anemia, 566, 567*f*, 575–580
autoimmune, 580
caused by disorders extrinsic to the red blood cell, 579–580, 592
clinical manifestations of, 579–580, 579*f*
etiology of, 579–580, 579*f*
laboratory diagnosis of, 580
prognosis for, 580
treatment of, 580
due to enzymopathies, 578
clinical manifestations of, 578
epidemiology of, 578
etiology of, 578
glucose-6-phosphate dehydrogenase (G6PD) deficiency as, 566
laboratory studies of, 578
prevention of, 578
pyruvate kinase deficiency as, 566
treatment of, 578
due to major hemoglobinopathies, 575
alpha-chain hemoglobinopathies, 575
beta-chain hemoglobinopathies, 575
due to membrane disorders, 578–579
clinical manifestations of, 579
etiology of, 578–579
laboratory diagnosis of, 579
treatment of, 579
due to sickle cell disease, 576–578
clinical manifestations of, 576–577, 577*t*
etiology and epidemiology of, 576, 576*t*
laboratory diagnosis of, 577
treatment of, 577–578
due to β-thalassemia major, 575–576
clinical manifestations of, 575
etiology and epidemiology of, 575
treatment of, 575–576
Hemolytic crisis, in sickle cell disease, 577*t*
Hemolytic disease, of the newborn, 249
Hemolytic uremic syndrome (HUS), 411, 585–586, 624
clinical manifestations of, 624
diagnostic studies of, 624
etiology and epidemiology of, 624
gastrointestinal bleeding due to, 477*t*
laboratory findings with, 624*t*
in thrombotic microangiopathy, 580
treatment and prognosis for, 624
Hemophagocytic activity, in juvenile idiopathic arthritis, 352
Hemophagocytosis syndrome, from roseola infantum, 377
Hemophilia, 581–582, 586–587, 586*t*
Hemophilia A, 586–587, 586*t*
genetic basis for, 174*t*
Hemophilia B, 586–587, 586*t*
Hemoptysis, due to pulmonary hemorrhage, 525
Hemorrhage
airway, 525
alveolar, 525
brain, due to hypernatremia, 134
fetal-maternal, 249
intracranial
in NATP, 584
in newborn, 256–257
in newborn
intraventricular. *see* Intraventricular hemorrhage (IVH), in newborn
periventricular, 257
retinal, 233
subarachnoid, 257
subconjunctival, 233
subdural, 256–257
pulmonary, 525–526, 525*t*
subarachnoid, 709–710
aneurysmal, 686*t*
in newborn, 255

Hemorrhage *(Continued)*
subdural, 709–710
due to child abuse, 81, 82*f*
in newborn, 256–257
Hemorrhagic disease of newborn, 118–119
due to vitamin K deficiency, 253
Hemorrhagic disorders. *see* Hemostatic disorders
Hemorrhagic stroke, 699
Hemorrhoids, gastrointestinal bleeding due to, 477*t*
Hemosiderosis, idiopathic pulmonary, 525
Hemostasis
developmental, 581, 592
normal, 580–581, 581*f*, 592
Hemostatic disorders, 580–589, 592–593
clinical manifestations of, 582–583
differential diagnosis of, 583–589
disorders of clotting factors, 586
disorders of platelets in, 583, 585*f*
function, 586
disseminated intravascular coagulation, 588, 588*t*–589*t*
hemolytic uremic syndrome in, 585–586
idiopathic thrombocytopenic purpura in, 584–585
other disorders in, 585–586
thrombocytopenia
resulting from decreased platelet production, 584
resulting from peripheral destruction, 584
thrombosis, 589
thrombotic microangiopathy in, 585–586
thrombotic thrombocytopenic purpura in, 585–586
vitamin K deficiency, 588
von Willebrand disease, 587–588
Wiskott-Aldrich syndrome in, 585
etiology and epidemiology of, 581–582, 582*t*, 583*f*
laboratory testing in, 583, 584*t*
Hemotympanum, 710
Henoch-Schönlein purpura (HSP), 345–347
clinical manifestations of, 345–346, 346*f*
complications of, 347
differential diagnosis of, 346, 346*t*
epidemiology of, 345
etiology of, 345
laboratory and imaging studies of, 346
prognosis for, 347
treatment of, 347
Heparin
for disseminated intravascular coagulation, 588
for thrombosis, 589
Hepatic encephalopathy, 497
stages of, 499*t*
treatment of, 500*t*
Hepatic failure, due to inborn errors of metabolism, 195*t*
Hepatic fibrosis, 630
Hepatic synthetic function, for gastrointestinal symptoms, 467
Hepatitis
autoimmune, 500, 500*t*
neonatal, 494
viral, 413–416
clinical manifestations of, 413–414, 415*f*
complications of, 415
differential diagnosis of, 415
epidemiology of, 413
etiology of, 413
laboratory and imaging studies and, 414
laboratory and imaging studies for, 500*t*
prevention of, 415–416
treatment of, 415
vomiting due to, 473*t*
Hepatitis A (HepA) vaccine, 363–364, 364*f*–365*f*, 415–416
Hepatitis A virus (HAV), 413, 414*t*
clinical manifestations of, 415*f*
laboratory studies for, 414
Hepatitis B surface antigen (HBsAg), 413
Hepatitis B (HepB) vaccine, 363–364, 364*f*–365*f*, 416
Hepatitis B virus (HBV), 413, 414*t*
clinical manifestations of, 415*f*
complications and prognosis of, 415
congenital infection with, 260*t*
laboratory studies for, 414
in transfusion, 590
treatment of, 415
Hepatitis C virus (HCV), 413, 414*t*
clinical manifestations of, 415*f*
complications and prognosis for, 415
laboratory studies for, 414
in transfusion, 590
treatment of, 415
Hepatitis D virus (HDV), 413, 414*t*
Hepatitis E virus (HEV), 413, 414*t*
Hepatoblastoma, risk factors for, 597*t*
Hepatocellular carcinoma, risk factors for, 597*t*
Hepatocellular function, impaired, 498
Hepatomegaly, 649
in glycogen storage diseases, 199
due to inborn errors of metabolism, 195*t*
Hepatorenal syndrome, 497
Hepatosplenomegaly
in anemia, 568
in hematological disorders, 563
Herald patch, in pityriasis rosea, 729
Hereditary angioedema (HAE), 306, 329, 329*t*, 331*t*
with normal C1 inhibitor, 329
Hereditary angioneurotic edema (HANE), genetic basis for, 170*t*
Hereditary cancer syndrome, genetic assessment of, 178
Hereditary elliptocytosis, etiology of, 566, 578–579
Hereditary fructose intolerance, 201
hypoglycemia due to, 650
Hereditary motor sensory neuropathy (HMSN), 695
Hereditary pyropoikilocytosis, 578–579
Hereditary spherocytosis
clinical manifestations of, 579
etiology of, 566, 578–579
laboratory diagnosis of, 579
treatment of, 579
Hering-Breuer reflex, 513
Hernia
congenital diaphragmatic, 246
umbilical, 231
Heroin, acute effects of, 284*t*–285*t*
Herpangina, 393
Herpes gingivostomatitis, 382
Herpes gladiatorum, 382
Herpes labialis, 382
Herpes simplex virus (HSV), 424
congenital infection with, 260*t*, 262
conjunctivitis from, 430
encephalitis from, 389
pneumonia from, 407*t*
superficial infections due to, 381–382
superinfection with, in atopic dermatitis, 328, 724, 727*f*
varicella zoster virus and, 378–379
vesiculobullous eruptions due to, 734*t*
Herpesvirus B, 439*t*–442*t*
Herpetic whitlow, 382
Hers disease, 200*t*
Heterophyes heterophyes, 451*t*
Heterophyiasis, 451*t*
Heteroplasmy, 175
Heterozygous, 170
Hexamethonium bromide, maternal use of, 238*t*
Hexosaminidase A deficiency, 210*t*–212*t*
Hexose monophosphate shunt pathway, 578
HGV (hepatitis G virus), 413, 414*t*
HHV-6 (human herpesvirus type 6), roseola infantum due to, 376
HHV-7 (human herpesvirus type 7), roseola infantum due to, 376
Hib (*Haemophilus influenzae* type b)
osteomyelitis from, 425
pneumonia from, 403, 407*t*
Hib (*Haemophilus influenzae* type b) conjugate vaccine, 363–364, 364*f*–365*f*
Hickman catheters, 437
High-altitude pulmonary edema, 524
High-dose chemotherapy, for neuroblastoma, 609
High-performance liquid chromatography, for hemoglobinopathies, 577
Hip, 744–748
developmental dysplasia of, 744–746
Legg-Calvé-Perthes disease of, 746–747
slipped capital femoral epiphysis of, 747–748
transient monoarticular synovitis, 746, 746*t*
Hip abduction test, 744, 745*f*
HIPAA (Health Insurance Portability and Accountability Act), 5
Hirschsprung disease, 489–490
constipation due to, 475, 476*t*
History
for cancer, 595, 597*t*
for dysmorphology
family, 184
pregnancy, 184
family, 178
in genetic assessment
of delivery and birth, 178
of development, 178
laboratory evaluation, 179
physical examination, 179
in hematology assessment, 563
in neurology assessment, 681
perinatal, 221*t*
of skin disorders, 721
HIV. *see* Human immunodeficiency virus
Hives, 328, 721*t*
HMSN. *see* Hereditary motor sensory neuropathy
Hodgkin lymphoma (HL)
clinical manifestations of, 605
epidemiology of, 605
etiology of, 605
laboratory/imaging studies in, 606
prognosis for, 607
risk factors for, 597*t*
treatment of, 606
Holocarboxylase deficiency, 206
clinical manifestations of, 206
treatment of, 206
Holoprosencephaly, 639, 717
Holosystolic murmurs, 536
Homocysteine
metabolism of, 203*f*
plasma total, 199*t*
Homocysteinemia, 589
Homocystinuria, 203
Homosexuality, 86, 86*t*
Homovanillic acid, in neuroblastoma, 609
Homozygous, 170
Honesty, 4
Honeybee stings, allergic reactions to, 333
Hookworm iron deficiency, 450*t*
Hordeola, 431

Horizontal transmission, of HIV, 458
Hormones, 637, 637*f*
for cancer, 601*t*–602*t*
deficiency, 637
Horner syndrome, 683
in newborn, 233
Hornet stings, allergic reactions to, 333
Hospital admissions, 2
Hot spot mutational, 171
Hot tub folliculitis, 380
HPS (hypertrophic pyloric stenosis), genetic basis for, 174–175
HPV. *see* Human papillomavirus
HSCT. *see* Hematopoietic stem cell transplantation
HSP. *see* Henoch-Schönlein purpura
HSV. *see* Herpes simplex virus
Human chorionic gonadotropin (HCG), maternal serum screening for, 177
Human herpesvirus type 6 (HHV-6), roseola infantum due to, 376
Human herpesvirus type 7 (HHV-7), roseola infantum due to, 376
Human immunodeficiency virus (HIV), 457–461
clinical manifestations of, 458–460, 459*t*
complications of, 461
congenital infection with, 260*t*
differential diagnosis of, 460
epidemiology of, 458
horizontal transmission of, 458
laboratory and imaging studies for, 460
prevention of, 461
prognosis for, 461
in transfusion, 590
treatment of, 460–461, 460*t*
vertical transmission of, 458
Human papillomavirus (HPV), 382
genital warts due to, 419, 423*t*
Human papillomavirus (HPV) vaccines, 363–364, 364*f*–365*f*
Human parvovirus B19, erythema infectiosum and, 377
Humidified high flow nasal cannula (HFNC), 512
Hunter syndrome, 713
Huntington disease (HD), genetic basis for, 170*t*
Hurler syndrome, 713
HUS. *see* Hemolytic uremic syndrome
Hyaline membrane disease. *see* Respiratory distress syndrome
Hydralazine, for heart failure, 555*t*
Hydranencephaly, 717
Hydrocarbon ingestion, 160
Hydrocephalus, 707
obstructive, 707
treatment of, 708
vomiting due to, 473*t*
Hydronephrosis, 227*t*
Hydrops fetalis, 218, 240
Hydroxychloroquine
for juvenile dermatomyositis, 356
for systemic lupus erythematosus, 355
11-hydroxylase deficiency, 676
21-hydroxylase deficiency, 138, 675–676
genetic basis for, 173*t*
Hydroxymethylglutaryl-CoA lyase deficiency, 208
Hydroxyurea, in sickle cell disease, 577–578
25-Hydroxyvitamin D (25-[OH]-D), 118
Hydroxyzine, for allergic rhinitis, 325
Hymenolepis diminuta, 452*t*
Hymenolepis nana, 452*t*
Hymenoptera stings, allergic reactions to, 333
Hyper-IgE syndrome, 299, 299*t*
disorders of neutrophil migration in, 303
Hyper-IgM syndrome, 297*t*
autosomal recessive, 296
due to defects in NEMO, 296
X-linked, 296, 296*f*
Hyperacute renal graft rejection, in thrombotic microangiopathy, 580
Hyperammonemia
etiology of, 195*t*
in later infancy and childhood, 192, 194*f*
neonatal
moderate, 192
severe, 192
treatment of, 205
Hyperbilirubinemia
conjugated
differential diagnosis of, 496*t*
direct, 251
in newborn, 251, 251*t*
in newborn, 249–254
kernicterus (bilirubin encephalopathy) due to, 251
unconjugated, indirect, 250–251, 251*t*
Hypercalcemia, oncological emergencies, 600*t*
Hypercalciuria, hematuria due to, 623
Hypercholesterolemia, in nephrotic syndrome, 620
Hypercoagulable states, 582*t*
Hyperdynamic precordium, with patent ductus arteriosus, 546–547
Hyperemia, in otitis media, 396
Hyperextension, 357*f*
Hyperglycemia
due to diabetic ketoacidosis, 642
due to poisoning, 162*t*
Hypergonadotropic hypogonadism, 658–659
Hyperinflation, 520
Hyperinsulinemia
factitious, 649
hypoglycemia due to, 648
Hyperinsulinism
congenital, 648
obesity in, 106*t*
Hyperirritable skin, in atopic dermatitis, 325–326
Hyperkalemia, 137–138
causes of, 137*t*
clinical manifestations of, 138
diagnosis of, 138
etiology of, 137–138
factitious, 137
oncological emergencies, 600*t*
treatment of, 138, 138*t*
Hyperkeratosis, 202–203
Hyperkinetic movement, 702
Hyperleukocytosis, oncological emergencies, 600*t*
Hyperlucent lung, unilateral, 407
Hypermetabolic response, to burns, 159
Hypermobile pes planus, 754
Hypermobility, benign, 357, 357*f*, 357*t*
Hypermobility syndromes, 357
Hypernatremia, 133–134, 133*f*
Hypernatremic dehydration, 129, 130*f*
Hyperosmolality, 131–132
Hyperparathyroidism, 670*t*
maternal, 236*t*
Hyperphenylalaninemia, maternal, 202
Hyperphosphatemia
in infant, 235
oncological emergencies, 600*t*
Hyperpnea, 509*t*
Hyperpurulent conjunctivitis, 431
Hypersensitivity reactions, 311, 311*t*
of food, 334–338
clinical manifestations of, 335, 335*t*–336*t*
complications of, 337
Hypersensitivity reactions *(Continued)*
diagnosis of, 335–337
etiology and epidemiology of, 334–335
laboratory and imaging studies for, 335
prognosis and prevention of, 337–338
treatment of, 337
type I (anaphylactic), 311, 311*t*
immediate, 311*t*
late-phase, 311
type II (antibody cytotoxicity), 311, 311*t*
type III (immune complex), 311, 311*t*
Arthus reaction in, 311
serum sickness in, 311
type IV (cellular immune-mediated, delayed type), 311–312, 311*t*
Hypersplenism, in pancytopenia, 575
Hypertelorism, 185
Hypertension
causes of, 628*t*
clinical manifestations of, 628
in coarctation of aorta, 548
definition of, 627
diagnostic studies of, 628
essential, 627
etiology of, 627
intracranial. *see also* Intracranial pressure (ICP), increased
idiopathic, 707–708
maternal, 236*t*
portal, 497
prognosis for, 628
pulmonary
arterial, 524–525
persistent (primary), of newborn, 222, 246
syncope due to, 541*t*
due to renal disease, 627
treatment of, 628
Hyperthermia, malignant, 698
Hyperthyroidism, 667–668
clinical manifestation of, 667*t*
congenital, 668
neonatal, 236
Hypertonic phosphate, for functional constipation, 51*t*
Hypertransfusion program, for β-thalassemia major, 575–576
Hypertrophic cardiomyopathies, 557*t*
clinical manifestations of, 558
etiology of, 556
imaging studies for, 558
treatment of, 558
Hypertrophic pyloric stenosis (HPS), genetic basis for, 174–175
Hyperuricemia, oncological emergencies, 600*t*
Hyperventilation, in seizures, 688–689
Hyperviscosity syndrome, in newborn, 252
Hypervitaminosis A, 117
Hypervolemic hyponatremia, 132
Hypocalcemia, 669–670
neonatal seizures due to, 255
in newborn, 228–229
due to poisoning, 162*t*
Hypochromic, microcytic anemia, 566, 567*f*, 568–574
due to iron deficiency, 568–571
clinical manifestations of, 570
epidemiology of, 570, 570*t*
etiology of, 570
prevention of, 571
treatment of, 571, 571*t*
due to lead poisoning, 571
thalassemia minor as, 571
etiology and epidemiology of, 571, 572*f*, 572*t*
laboratory testing for, 571
treatment of, 571

Hypoglycemia, 646–650, 679
classification of, 647*t*
clinical manifestations of, 646–647
definition of, 646
diagnosis of, 650
emergency management of, 650
with fulminant liver failure, 500*t*
in glycogen storage diseases, 199
ketotic, due to inborn errors of metabolism, 195
due to medications and intoxications, 650
metabolic disorders of, 650
neonatal seizures due to, 255
pathophysiology of, 647–649
disrupted metabolic response pathways, 649–650
energy stores, 649
hormonal signal in, 647–649
counter-regulatory hormone defects, 649
factitious hyperinsulinemia, 649
and hyperinsulinemia, 648
idiopathic ketotic hypoglycemia, 649
due to poisoning, 162*t*
symptoms and signs of, 648*t*
with type 1 diabetes mellitus, 645
Hypoglycemic disorders, due to inborn errors of metabolism, 193*t*
Hypogonadotropic hypogonadism, 656
Hypoketotic hypoglycemia, 208
Hypomagnesemia, 669
neonatal seizures due to, 255
in newborn, 234–235
Hypomania, in bipolar I disorder (BD), 66
Hyponatremia, 131–133, 132*f*
Hyponatremic dehydration, 129
Hypoparathyroidism
primary, 669, 670*t*
pseudo-, 653, 669, 670*t*
transient, 669
Hypoperfusion, 549*t*
Hypophosphatemic rickets, 173
Hypopituitarism
acquired, 639
diagnostic evaluation of, 638*t*
idiopathic, 657
Hypoplastic left heart syndrome, 552–553, 552*f*
Hypoplastic nail, 183*t*
Hypoplastic right ventricle, 551
Hypoproteinemia, in nephrotic syndrome, 620
Hypospadias, 185, 632
Hypothalamic corticotropin-releasing hormone (CRH), 674
Hypothalamic deficiency, 639
Hypothalamic dysfunction, obesity with, 106*t*
Hypothalamic gliomas, 662
Hypothalamic gonadotropin-releasing hormone (GnRH), 656
Hypothalamic-pituitary axis, 637–638, 638*f*
disorders of, 638–639
interrelationships of, 664*f*
Hypothalamus, 637–638, 638*f*
Hypothyroidism, 658, 665–667
acquired, 666–667
causes of, 665*t*
congenital, 665–666
clinical manifestations of, 666
symptoms and signs of, 666*t*
Hypothyroidism, obesity in, 106*t*
Hypotonia, 684, 692–700. *see also* Weakness
benign congenital, 699
central (without significant weakness), 698–699
neonatal and infantile, 698–699, 698*f*
Hypoventilation
congenital central, 514
hypoxemia due to, 508*t*
Hypovolemic hyponatremia, 132
Hypoxemia
causes of, 508*t*
during drowning, 157
in newborn, treatment of, 241
Hypoxia, disorders of consciousness with, 703
Hypoxic-ischemic encephalopathy, in newborn, 257–258
clinical manifestations of, 257–258, 257*t*
prognosis, 257
seizures due to, 255–256
Hypoxic-ischemic injury, due to drowning, 158
Hypoxic pulmonary vasoconstriction, 508
Hypoxic spells, in tetralogy of Fallot, 550
Hypsarrhythmia, 690

I

I-cell disease, 210*t*–212*t*
Ibuprofen, maternal use of, 238*t*
ICP. *see* Intracranial pressure
Icteric phase, of viral hepatitis, 413
Idiogenic osmoles, 129
Idiopathic aplastic anemia, 573*t*
Idiopathic hypopituitarism, 657
Idiopathic intracranial hypertension, 707–708
Idiopathic ketotic hypoglycemia, 649
Idiopathic nephrotic syndrome, 620
Idiopathic pulmonary hemosiderosis, 525
Idiopathic scoliosis, 758
Idiopathic thrombocytopenic purpura (ITP), 584–585
bleeding disorder in newborn due to, 254
clinical manifestations of, 585
diagnosis of, 585
etiology of, 584–585
maternal, 235–236, 236*t*, 584
neonatal thrombocytopenia due to, 254
prognosis for, 585
treatment of, 585
Iduronate 2-sulfatase deficiency, 210*t*–212*t*
α-L-Iduronidase deficiency, 210*t*–212*t*
Ifosfamide, for cancer, 601*t*–602*t*
Ig replacement therapy, for severe combined immunodeficiency, 299–300
IgA nephropathy, 622
Ileal atresia, 227*t*
Illness, 54*t*–55*t*
Illness anxiety disorder, 59, 60*t*
Illness Attitude Scales and Soma Assessment Interview, for somatic symptom and related disorders (SSRDs), 61
Imatinib, for cancer, 601*t*–602*t*
Imipramine
for enuresis, 49
maternal use of, 238*t*
Immobilization, physiological changes due to, 670*t*
Immotile cilia syndrome, 523
Immune-mediated mechanisms, in thrombocytopenia resulting from peripheral destruction, 584
Immunization, 363–366
active, 363
administration of, 365
adverse events after, 366
catch-up, 364–365
schedules for, 365*f*
contraindications to, 365–366
informed consent for, 365
passive, 363
and prophylaxis, 363–366
recommended schedules for, 364*f*
Immunocompromised person, infection in, 434–437
clinical manifestations of, 436
differential diagnosis of, 436
Immunocompromised person, infection in *(Continued)*
epidemiology of, 435, 435*f*
etiology of, 434–435, 434*t*
laboratory tests and imaging for, 436
prevention of, 436–437
treatment of, 436
Immunodeficiency, 117
common variable, 294–295, 295*t*
fever due to, 371
general management of, 299, 300*t*
severe combined, 297, 297*t*
autosomal recessive, 297–298
clinical manifestations of, 297–298
due to deficiencies in adenosine deaminase and purine nucleoside phosphorylase, 298
X-linked, 297–298
Immunodeficiency diseases
antibody deficiency disease, 294–295, 294*f*, 295*t*
agammaglobulinemia as, 294, 295*t*
autosomal recessive, 294
X-linked, 294
antibody deficiency syndrome as, 295, 295*t*
common variable immunodeficiency as, 294–295, 295*t*
IgA deficiency as, 295, 295*t*
IgG subclass deficiency as, 295, 295*t*
transient hypogammaglobulinemia of infancy as, 295, 295*t*
assessment, 289–293
adaptive immune system and, 289
clinical characteristics of, 291*t*
due to defects in anatomic-mucociliary barrier, 289, 289*t*
diagnostic evaluation of, 292–293, 292*f*
imaging in, 293
laboratory tests in, 292–293, 293*t*
differential diagnosis of, 291–292, 291*t*
history of, 290–291
innate immune system and, 289, 290*t*
physical examination for, 291
combined, 296–299, 297*t*
autosomal recessive, 297–298
bare lymphocyte syndrome as, 297*t*, 298
clinical manifestations of, 297
DiGeorge syndrome as, 297*t*, 298
hyper-IgM syndrome as, 297*t*
autosomal recessive, 296
due to defects in NEMO, 296
X-linked, 296, 296*f*
Omenn syndrome as, 297–298, 297*t*
reticular dysgenesis as, 297*t*
severe, 297, 297*t*
autosomal recessive, 297–298
clinical manifestations of, 297–298
due to deficiencies in adenosine deaminase and purine nucleoside phosphorylase, 298
X-linked, 297–298
due to lymphocyte disorders. *see* Lymphocyte disorders
secondary, 291*t*
Immunoglobulin, intravenous, for autoimmune hemolysis, 580
Immunoglobulin A (IgA) deficiency, 295, 295*t*
Immunoglobulin E (IgE)
disorders associated with elevated, 312, 312*t*
in food allergies, 337*t*
Immunoglobulin G (IgG) subclass deficiency, 295, 295*t*
Immunomodulating drugs, topical, for atopic dermatitis, 327–328
Immunophenotype, of leukemia, 603–604
Immunosuppression, immunization and, 366

Immunotherapy, for allergic rhinitis, 325
Impact seizures, 710
Imperforate anus, 489
  constipation due to, 476*t*
Impetigo, 379–380
  bullous, 379
  nonbullous, 379
Impetigo, bullous, 734*t*
Implanted venous access systems (Port-a-Cath), 437
In-toeing, 748–749
  common causes of, 748*t*
  due to femoral anteversion, 748
  due to internal tibial torsion, 748–749
  treatment of, 749
In vitro serum testing, for antigen-specific IgE, 312–313, 313*t*
In vivo skin testing, for allergen-specific IgE, 313, 313*t*
Inactivated poliovirus (IPV) vaccine, 364*f*–365*f*
Inborn errors of metabolism
  assessment of, 191
    clinical, and laboratory findings, 196, 196*t*
  ataxia due to, 702
  clinical presentation of, 191–196
    congenital malformations or dysmorphic features in, 195–196
    energy deficiency in, 193
    ketosis and ketotic hypoglycemia in, 193–195
    specific organ, 192–193, 195*t*
    storage disorders, 196
    toxic, 191–192
  genetic aspects of, 196–197
    identification of molecular pathology as, 197
    mechanisms of inheritance as, 196–197
  hyperammonemia in
    etiology of, 195*t*
    in later infancy and childhood, 192, 194*f*
    metabolic acidosis in, 192, 196*t*
    neonatal
      moderate, 192
      severe, 192
  incidence of, 192*t*
  metabolic acidosis due to, 140
  neonatal screening for, 197–199
    confirmatory testing principles of, 197
    disorders identified by, 197
    specialized laboratory and clinical testing after, 197–199, 199*t*
    strategy of, 197
  overview of treatment for, 199
  signs and symptoms of, 191
Inclusion conjunctivitis, 431
Incontinentia pigmenti, 173
Individualized educational plan (IEP), 28
Indomethacin, maternal use of, 238*t*
Induction chemotherapy, for leukemia, 604
Infancy
  bonding and attachment in, 15
  obesity and, 107–108
  physical development in later, 14
Infant(s)
  crying, 41. *see also* Crying
  ethical principles related to, 4–5
  genetic assessment of, 178
  hearing and vision screening of, 20
  low birth weight of, 218–219
  mortality, 2, 218
  very low birth weight of, 219
Infant botulism, 696
Infantile beriberi, 113
Infantile hypotonia, 698–699, 698*f*
Infantile spasms, 690
Infantometer, 651
Infection(s)
  assessment, 289–293
    adaptive immune system and, 289
    clinical characteristics of, 291*t*
    due to defects in anatomic-mucociliary barrier, 289, 289*t*
    diagnostic evaluation of, 292–293, 292*f*
      imaging in, 293
      laboratory tests in, 292–293, 293*t*
    differential diagnosis of, 291–292, 291*t*
    history of, 290–291
    innate immune system and, 289, 290*t*
    physical examination for, 291
  congenital (TORCH), 259–264, 260*t*
    with chlamydia, 263–264
    with *Chlamydia trachomatis*, 260*t*
    with cytomegalovirus, 261–262
    with herpes simplex virus, 260*t*, 262
    with HIV, 260*t*
    with *Mycobacterium tuberculosis*, 260*t*
    with *Neisseria gonorrhoeae*, 260*t*, 263
    with parvovirus, 260*t*
    with rubella, 260*t*, 261
    with toxoplasmosis, 261
    with *Trypanosoma cruzi*, 260*t*
    with varicella-zoster virus, 260*t*
    with Zika virus, 264
  cutaneous (superficial)
    bacterial, 379–380
      cellulitis as, 380
      folliculitis as, 380
      impetigo as, 379–380
      perianal dermatitis as, 380
    fungal, 380–381, 381*t*
    viral, 381–383
      from herpes simplex virus, 381–382
      from human papillomaviruses (warts), 382
      molluscum contagiosum as, 383
  with fever and rash, 373–379
    differential diagnosis of, 373*t*–374*t*
    erythema infectiosum (fifth disease) as, 377–378
    measles (rubeola) as, 373–375
    roseola infantum (exanthem subitum), 376–377
    rubella (German or 3-day measles), 375–376
    varicella-zoster virus infection (chickenpox and zoster), 378–379
  in immunocompromised person, 434–437
    clinical manifestations of, 436
    differential diagnosis of, 436
    epidemiology of, 435, 435*f*
    etiology of, 434–435, 434*t*
    laboratory tests and imaging for, 436
    prevention of, 436–437
    treatment of, 436
  maternal
    effect on fetus or newborn, 236*t*
    as teratogens, 176
  medical devices-associated, 437–439
    from central nervous system shunts, 438–439
    peritoneal dialysis-associated infections as, 438
    from urinary catheters, 438
    from vascular devices, 437–438
    ventilator-associated pneumonia as, 438
  with neutropenia, 302*t*
  orthopedic problems due to, 739*t*
  in sickle cell disease, 577*t*
Infectious arthritis, juvenile idiopathic arthritis *vs.*, 352*t*
Infectious diseases, 361–461
  assessment of, 361–363
    diagnostic imaging in, 362–363
    differential diagnosis in, 361
    history in, 362*t*
    initial diagnostic evaluation in, 361
    physical examination in, 361
    screening tests in, 361–362
  localizing manifestations of, 363*t*
  in transfusion reactions, 590
  viral *vs.* bacterial, 363*t*, 368–369
Infectious mononucleosis, 384
Infectious pyogenic infection, synovial fluid findings in, 429*t*
Infectious rhinitis, 323–324
Infective endocarditis, 408–410
  causes of, 408*t*
  clinical manifestations of, 408
  complications and prognosis of, 410
  culture-negative, 409
  differential diagnosis of, 409
  etiology of, 408
  laboratory studies and imaging of, 409
  modified Duke clinical criteria for, 409
  prevention of, 410
  subacute, 408
  treatment of, 409
Inflammation, orthopedic problems due to, 739*t*
Inflammatory bowel disease (IBD), 490–491
  abdominal pain due to, 470*t*
  clinical manifestations of, 490, 490*t*
  epidemiology and etiology of, 490–491
  gastrointestinal bleeding due to, 477*t*
  juvenile idiopathic arthritis *vs.*, 351*t*
  laboratory and imaging studies for, 491, 491*t*
  synovial fluid findings in, 429*t*
  treatment of, 491
Inflammatory diseases, fever due to, 371
Infliximab, for juvenile idiopathic arthritis, 352
Influenza, avian, 403
Influenza A (H5N1), 403
Influenza vaccines, 364*f*
  for prevention of pneumonia, 407–408
Infuse-a-Port (implanted venous access systems), infections associated with, 437
Inhalants, acute effects of, 284*t*–285*t*
Inhalation challenge tests, 511
Inheritance patterns
  autosomal dominant disorders, 170–171, 170*t*
  autosomal recessive disorders, 171
  mitochondrial, 175
    MELAS due to, 175
  multifactorial disorders (polygenic inheritance), 173–175
    hypertrophic pyloric stenosis as, 174–175
    neural tube defects as, 175
    uniparental disomy as, 175
  pedigree drawing of, 169–170, 170*f*
Inhibin, in puberty, 656
Inhibitors, for hemophilia, 587
Inhibitory factors, in hemostasis, 581
Injury(ies), 2
  birth, 233–234
  prevention of, 23*t*–24*t*, 154–155
    educations for, 154–155
    epidemiology of, 154
    etiology of, 154
Innate immune system, 289, 290*t*
Innocent bystander, 580
Innocent murmurs, 538, 538*t*
Innominate artery, anomalous, extrinsic tracheal compression due to, 521
Inotropic agents
  for cardiomyopathies, 557*t*, 558
  for heart failure, 555*t*
Insect allergies, 333–334

Insect bites, vesiculobullous eruptions due to, 734*t*
Insensible losses, 126
Insomnia of childhood, 54*t*–55*t*
Inspiration, 507
Inspiratory reserve volume, 508*f*
Inspiratory stridor, due to laryngomalacia, 518
Insulin
carbohydrate ratio, 644
long-acting, 644
multiple daily injections of, 643
representative profiles of, 644*t*
sensitivity, 644
short-acting, 644
subcutaneous, 643
Insulin deficiency, in cystic fibrosis, 527
Insulin-like growth factor-1, 650–651
Insulin-like growth factor-binding protein, 650–651
Insulin pumps, 643
Insulin therapy, hypokalemia due to, 135
Integrity, 4
Intercostal retractions, 509–510
Interferon-γ (IFN-γ), functions of, 290*t*
Interleukin-1 (IL-1), functions of, 290*t*
Interleukin-2 (IL-2), functions of, 290*t*
Interleukin-3 (IL-3), functions of, 290*t*
Interleukin-4 (IL-4), functions of, 290*t*
Interleukin-5 (IL-5), functions of, 290*t*
Interleukin-6 (IL-6), functions of, 290*t*
Interleukin-7 (IL-7), functions of, 290*t*
Interleukin-8 (IL-8), functions of, 290*t*
Interleukin-9 (IL-9), functions of, 290*t*
Interleukin-10 (IL-10), functions of, 290*t*
Interleukin-12 (IL-12), functions of, 290*t*
Interleukin-13 (IL-13), functions of, 290*t*
Interleukin-17 (IL-17), functions of, 290*t*
Interleukin-18 (IL-18), functions of, 290*t*
Internal intercostal muscles, during exhalation, 507
Internal tibial torsion, 748–749, 749*f*
Interstitial edema, 523–524
Interstitial fluid, 125
Interstitial pneumonitis, 402–403
Interstitial process, 510*t*
Intertriginous areas, dermatitis in, 728
Intestinal atresia, 488–489
clinical manifestations of, 488
etiology and epidemiology of, 488–489
laboratory and imaging studies for, 488
treatment of, 489
types of, 489*f*
vomiting due to, 473*t*
Intestinal injury, 157
Intestinal obstruction
abdominal pain due to, 470*t*
due to congenital anomaly, 227*t*
Intestinal tract disorders, 487–494
anorectal malformations as, 489
appendicitis as, 493–494, 493*t*
celiac disease as, 492
gastroschisis as, 489
Hirschsprung disease as, 489–490
inflammatory bowel disease as, 490–491, 491*t*
intestinal atresia as, 488–489, 489*f*
intussusception as, 492–493
Meckel diverticulum as, 490
midgut malrotation as, 487–488, 487*f*–488*f*
omphalocele as, 489
Intimate partner violence, 91, 92*t*
Intracellular fluid (ICF), 125
Intracranial hemorrhage
in NATP, 584
in newborn, 256–257
Intracranial pressure (ICP), increased, 706–708
due to bacterial meningitis, 707
causes of, 707*t*
in central nervous system, 607
clinical manifestations of, 708
etiology of, 706–708, 707*t*
due to hydrocephalus, 707, 707*t*
due to idiopathic intracranial hypertension, 707–708
laboratory and diagnostic studies for, 708
oncological emergencies, 600*t*
treatment of, 708
Intramedullary destruction, in pancytopenia, 575
Intramuscular influenza vaccine, 363–364
Intrapulmonary shunting, 523–524
hypoxemia due to, 508*t*
Intrauterine growth restriction (IUGR), 239–240
complications of, 219
management of, 239–240
Intravascular volume, regulation of, 125
Intravenous (IV) fluids, during labor, 238*t*
Intravenous immunoglobulin (IVIG)
for autoimmune hemolysis, 580
complications of, 299–300
for Guillain-Barré syndrome, 695
Intraventricular hemorrhage (IVH), in newborn
diagnosis of, 257
seizures due to, 255
Intrinsic factor, 117
Intrinsic pathways, in coagulation, 580
Introns, 169
Intubation, 513
Intussusception, 492–493
abdominal pain due to, 470*t*
clinical manifestations of, 492
etiology and epidemiology of, 492
gastrointestinal bleeding due to, 477*t*
ileocolonic, 492
laboratory and imaging studies for, 492–493
treatment of, 493
vomiting due to, 473*t*
Inverse psoriasis, 729–730
Inverted duplication chromosome 15, 183
Involucrum, 426
Iodides, maternal use of, 238*t*
radioactive, 238*t*
Iodine, radioactive
maternal use of, 238*t*
as teratogens, 237*t*
Iodine deficiency, 119*t*
IP-10, functions of, 290*t*
Ipecac syrup, for poisoning, 164
Ipratropium bromide
for allergic rhinitis, 325
for asthma, 316
IPV (inactivated poliovirus) vaccine, 364*f*–365*f*
Iridocyclitis, 433*t*
in juvenile idiopathic arthritis, 350
Iris coloboma, in cat eye syndrome, 183
Iron, toxicity of, 162*t*
Iron deficiency, 119*t*, 120
hookworm, 450*t*
Iron deficiency anemia, 568–571, 591
clinical manifestations of, 570
diagnosis of, 120
epidemiology of, 570, 570*t*
etiology of, 570
prevention of, 571
treatment of, 120, 571, 571*t*
Iron-fortified cereals, as complementary food, 101
Iron intake, for toddlers and older children, 104
Irregular sleep-wake pattern, 54*t*–55*t*
Irritable bowel syndrome, abdominal pain due to, 468–471, 470*t*
Irritant contact dermatitis, 727
Irritant diaper dermatitis, 727*f*
Isoelectric focusing, for hemoglobinopathies, 577
Isoimmune hemolysis, 579
Isolation effect, with inborn errors of metabolism, 196–197
Isoleucine, metabolism of, 203*f*
Isoniazid (INH), for tuberculosis, 455–456, 457*t*
Isospora belli, diarrhea from, 410*t*
Isotonic crystalloids, 146
Isotonic fluid, for third space losses, 127
Isotretinoin
for acne, 723
for cancer, 601*t*–602*t*
as teratogens, 237*t*
Isovaleric acidemia, 206, 206*f*
neonatal screening for, 198*t*
ITP. *see* Idiopathic thrombocytopenic purpura
IUGR. *see* Intrauterine growth restriction
IV (intravenous) fluids, during labor, 238*t*
IVIG (intravenous immunoglobulin)
for autoimmune hemolysis, 580
complications of, 299–300
for Guillain-Barré syndrome, 695
Ixodes pacificus, 443
Ixodes scapularis, 443, 445

J

Jarisch-Herxheimer reaction, 424
JAS (juvenile ankylosing spondylitis), 351*t*
Jaundice, 649
due to anemia, 567–568
breast-feeding, 100
breast milk, 100, 250
differential diagnosis of, 494, 495*f*
on first day of life, 250
in hematological disorders, 563
due to inborn errors of metabolism, 195*t*
physiological, 250
in pyloric stenosis, 485
JDM. *see* Juvenile dermatomyositis
Jejunostomy, feeding, for gastroesophageal reflux, 481*t*
JIA. *see* Juvenile idiopathic arthritis
Jock itch, 381*t*
Joint custody, 94
Joint hypermobility, 357
Joint space, 740*f*
Jones criteria, for rheumatic fever, 556, 556*t*
Juice intake, for toddlers and older children, 103
Justice, 4
distributive, 6
Juvenile ankylosing spondylitis (JAS), 351*t*
Juvenile dermatomyositis (JDM), 355–356
clinical manifestations of, 355–356
complications of, 356
diagnostic criteria for, 356*t*
differential diagnosis of, 356
epidemiology of, 355
etiology of, 355
laboratory and imaging studies of, 356
prognosis for, 356
treatment of, 356
Juvenile idiopathic arthritis (JIA), 349–353
clinical presentation of, 349–351, 350*f*, 350*t*
complications of, 352
differential diagnosis of, 344*t*, 351–352, 352*t*
epidemiology of, 349
etiology of, 349
laboratory and imaging studies for, 351
oligoarticular, 350
polyarticular, 350–351
prognosis for, 352–353
spondyloarthropathies and, 351, 351*t*
systemic, 351
treatment of, 352

Juvenile laryngeal papillomatosis, 519
Juvenile pernicious anemia, 117
Juvenile polyp, gastrointestinal bleeding due to, 477*t*
Juvenile rheumatoid arthritis. *see* Juvenile idiopathic arthritis

K

Kallmann syndrome, 657
Kaposi varicelliform eruption
  in atopic dermatitis, 328, 726, 727*f*
  herpes zoster virus and, 382
  varicella zoster virus and, 378–379
Karyotype, 180
Kasabach-Merritt syndrome, 253, 580
Kasai procedure, 494
Katayama fever, 452
Kawasaki disease (KD), 347–349, 735
  clinical manifestations of, 347–348
    in acute phase, 347, 348*f*
    in convalescent phase, 347–348
    incomplete (atypical), 348
    in subacute phase, 347
  complications of, 348, 349*t*
  differential diagnosis of, 344*t*, 348, 348*t*–349*t*
  epidemiology of, 347
  etiology of, 347
  laboratory and imaging studies for, 348
  prognosis for, 349
  Stevens-Johnson syndrome *vs.*, 735
  treatment of, 348
Kehr sign, 156
Keratitis, 202–203, 430, 433*t*
Keratoconjunctivitis, epidemic, 430
Keratolytic agents, for acne, 723
Keratosis pilaris, 312
  in atopic dermatitis, 326
Kerion, 381*t*
Kerley B lines, in pulmonary edema, 524
Kernicterus, 251
Ketamine, for sedation, 166*t*
Ketoacidosis, diabetic, 641–645
Ketoaciduria, branched chain, 203
Ketogenesis
  fatty acid oxidation disorders of, 649–650
  in insulin-dependent diabetes mellitus, 640–641
Ketone bodies
  in diabetic ketoacidosis, 641
  formation of, 207*f*
Ketosis
  due to defects in propionate pathway, 205
  due to inborn errors of metabolism, 195
Ketotic hypoglycemia, due to inborn errors of metabolism, 195
Kidney disease(s)
  chronic, 626–627
    complications and treatments of, 627*t*
    etiology and epidemiology of, 626
    prognosis for, 627
    treatment of, 627
  polycystic, 629–630
    autosomal dominant, 630
    autosomal recessive, 630
Kindergarten readiness, 15
Kingella kingae, osteomyelitis from, 425
Kissing kneecaps, 748
Klinefelter syndrome (KS), 181, 659, 673
  gynecomastia and, 663
Klippel-Trénaunay-Weber syndrome, port-wine stain in, 733
Klisic test, 745
Klumpke paralysis, 233
Knee(s), 751–752
  discoid lateral meniscus, 751
  effusion or swelling, 751
Knee(s) *(Continued)*
  extensor mechanism of, 751, 751*f*
  knock-, 749, 749*f*
  Osgood-Schlatter disease of, 752
  osteochondritis dissecans of, 752
  patellofemoral disorders of, 752
  popliteal cyst of, 751
Knee pain, idiopathic anterior, 752
Kneecaps, kissing, 748
Knock-knee deformities, 749, 749*f*
Knowledge of limits, 4
Kohler disease, 755
Koplik spots, 373–374
Kostmann syndrome, neutropenia in, 301
Krabbe disease, 210*t*–212*t*, 712
KS. *see* Klinefelter syndrome
Kugelberg-Welander syndrome, 694
Kussmaul respirations, 509*t*
  in diabetic ketoacidosis, 641
Kwashiorkor, 110–111
Kyphosis, 760
  classification of, 756*t*
  congenital, 760
  postural roundback, 760
  Scheuermann, 760, 760*f*

L

L/S (lecithin to sphingomyelin) ratio, 248
La belle indifference, 59
La Crosse encephalitis, 389
Laboratory studies, for obesity, 107
Labyrinthitis
  acute, ataxia due to, 702
  vomiting due to, 473*t*
Lactate, metabolism of, 214*f*
Lactic acidosis, 140
  due to mitochondrial disorders, 214
Lactose intolerance, abdominal pain due to, 470*t*
Lactulose, for functional constipation, 52*t*
Lacy, reticulated rash, in erythema infectiosum, 377
LAD-I (leukocyte adhesion deficiency type I), 302–303
LAD-II (leukocyte adhesion deficiency type II), 303
Ladd bands, in midgut malrotation, 487–488, 487*f*
Lamina papyracea, 395
Lamp-2 deficiency, 210*t*–212*t*
Landau-Kleffner syndrome, 690
Landau posture, 698
Langerhans cell histiocytosis, 326, 729
Language development, milestones of, 17*t*
Language function, assessment of, 682
Lanugo, 228*f*
Lap and shoulder seat belts, 22
Large for gestational age, 228
Laron dwarfism, 651
Laron syndrome, 655
Laryngeal cysts, 519
Laryngeal hemangioma, upper airway obstruction due to, 519
Laryngeal mask airway (LMA), 513
Laryngeal webs, 519
Laryngomalacia, 518
  clinical manifestations of, 518
  diagnostic studies for, 518
  etiology of, 517*t*, 518
  treatment of, 518
Laryngotracheobronchitis, 398–400
  clinical manifestations of, 399
  complications and prognosis of, 400
  differential diagnosis of, 399
  etiology and epidemiology of, 398–399
  laboratory and imaging studies for, 399, 399*f*
  spasmodic, 399
Laryngotracheobronchitis *(Continued)*
  treatment of, 399–400
  upper airway obstruction due to, 517*t*, 518
Lateral meniscus, discoid, 751
Laurence-Moon-Bardet-Biedl syndrome, 653
LBW (low birth weight) infants, 218–219
LCHAD (long-chain hydroxyacyl-CoA dehydrogenase) deficiency, 207, 207*f*
  neonatal screening for, 198*t*
Lead, maternal ingestion of, 238*t*
Lead poisoning, in hypochromic, microcytic anemia, 571, 591
Lecithin to sphingomyelin (L/S) ratio, 248
Lectin pathway, of complement activation, 304–305, 305*f*
Leflunomide, for juvenile idiopathic arthritis, 352
Left-shift, in infectious diseases, 362
Left-to-right shunts, 545
Left ventricular diastolic volume, in heart failure, 554*t*
Left ventricular hypertrophy
  due to aortic stenosis, 548
  due to tricuspid atresia, 551
Left ventricular outflow tract (LVOT) obstruction, syncope due to, 541*t*
Leg discomfort, in coarctation of aorta, 548
Leg-length discrepancy (LLD), 750–751
  common causes of, 751*t*
  measuring, 750
  treatment of, 751
Leg ulceration, in sickle cell disease, 577*t*
Legal blindness, 33
Legal issues, 5, 9
Legg-Calvé-Perthes disease (LCPD), 746–747
  clinical manifestations of, 747
  etiology and epidemiology of, 746–747
  radiological evaluation for, 747
  treatment and prognosis for, 747
Legionella pneumophila, 405
Legionnaires disease, 405
Leigh disease, 213–214
Leishmania, 439*t*–442*t*
Leishmania donovani complex, 439*t*–442*t*
Leishmaniasis, 439*t*–442*t*
  visceral, 439*t*–442*t*
Lemierre syndrome, 393
Length, growth chart of, 12*f*
Lennox-Gastaut syndrome, 690
Leptin receptor gene deficiency, obesity in, 106*t*
Leptomeningeal cyst, 710
Leptospira spp., 439*t*–442*t*
Leptospirosis, 439*t*–442*t*
Lethargy, 703
  due to intussusception, 492
Leucine, metabolism of, 203*f*
Leukemia, 180, 603–605, 614
  acute lymphoid/lymphoblastic. *see* Acute lymphoid/lymphoblastic leukemia
  acute myeloid. *see* Acute myeloid leukemia
  chronic myeloid, 603
  clinical manifestations of, 603
  complications of, 604
  differential diagnosis of, 344*t*, 604
  epidemiology of, 603
  etiology of, 603
  laboratory and imaging studies for, 603–604
  prognosis for, 604–605, 605*t*
  treatment of, 604
Leukocyte adhesion deficiency, 301*t*
  type I (LAD-I), 302–303
  type II (LAD-II), 303
Leukocyte esterase, in urine, 619–620
Leukocytes, values of, 565*t*
Leukocytosis, 362

Leukodystrophy
adreno-, genetic basis for, 174*t*
metachromatic, 210*t*–212*t*
Leukokoria, in newborn, 230
Leukomalacia, periventricular, in newborn, 257
Leukorrhea, physiological, *vs.* sexually transmitted infections, 422*t*
Leukotriene modifiers, for asthma, 315
Levalbuterol, for, for asthma, 315–316
Levocetirizine, for allergic rhinitis, 325
Lichenification, 722*t*
Liddle syndrome, 136
Lidocaine, for cardiopulmonary resuscitation, 148*t*
Lifestyle modifications, for migraines, 687
Ligament of Treitz, in midgut malrotation, 487–488
Limb-girdle muscular dystrophy, 697
Limb weakness
distal, 694*t*
ophthalmoplegia and, 694*t*
Limit-setting subtype, behavioral insomnia of childhood, 55
Limits, knowledge of, 4
Limping child, 740, 741*t*
Lipase, fibrosing colonopathy due to, 529
Lipid emulsion, in parenteral nutrition, 131
Lipidoses, 210*t*–212*t*
Lipoma, sacral, constipation due to, 476*t*
Lisch nodules, 714
Lissencephaly, 717
Listeria monocytogenes, 439*t*–442*t*
Listeriosis, 439*t*–442*t*
Lithium
for bipolar disorders, 68
as teratogens, 237*t*
Little Leaguer's elbow, 764
Little Leaguer's shoulder, 763
Liver disease, 494–501
cholestasis as, 494, 497*t*, 498*f*
chronic, 497–498
clinical manifestations of, 497–498
etiology and epidemiology of, 497
laboratory and imaging studies for, 498, 500*t*
treatment of, 498, 501*t*
fulminant liver failure as, 494–497, 499*t*–500*t*
Liver failure
fulminant, 494–497
clinical manifestations of, 497
etiology and epidemiology of, 494, 499*t*
laboratory and imaging studies for, 497
treatment of, 497, 500*t*
in galactosemia, 201
Liver function tests
for chronic liver disease, 500*t*
for gastrointestinal symptoms, 467
Liver phosphorylase deficiency, 200*t*
LLD. *see* Leg-length discrepancy
Lobar pneumonia, 402–403
Local anesthetics, 166
Lomustine, for cancer, 601*t*–602*t*
Long-chain hydroxyl-CoA dehydrogenase (LCHAD) deficiency, 207, 207*f*
neonatal screening for, 198*t*
Long-term penicillin prophylaxis, for rheumatic fever, 556
Loop of Henle, 617, 619*f*
Loratadine, for allergic rhinitis, 325
Lorazepam
for sedation, 166*t*
for status epilepticus, 691, 691*t*
Loss-of-function mutation, 176
Louse-borne infections, 737
Louse-borne relapsing fever, 737
Low birth weight (LBW) infants, 218–219
Lower airway disease, 519–526
acute respiratory distress syndrome, 524
asthma as. *see* Asthma
bronchiolitis as. *see* Bronchiolitis
bronchopulmonary dysplasia as, 522
clinical manifestations of, 520
congenital lung anomalies, 522
cor pulmonale as, 524–525
diagnostic studies for, 520
differential diagnosis of, 520–526
etiology of, 519–520, 520*t*
due to extrinsic tracheal compression, 521, 521*f*
due to foreign body aspiration, 521–522
pneumonia as. *see* Pneumonia
primary ciliary dyskinesia as, 523
pulmonary arterial hypertension as, 524–525
pulmonary edema as, 523–524
pulmonary embolism as, 526
pulmonary hemorrhage as, 525–526, 525*t*
tracheoesophageal fistula as. *see* Tracheoesophageal fistula
tracheomalacia as, 520–521
Lower extremity, 748–752
angular variations in, 749–750
genu valgum as, 749*f*, 750
genu varum as, 749*f*, 750
tibia vara (Blount disease) as, 750
leg-length discrepancy in, 750–751, 751*t*
torsional variations in, 748–749
common causes of, 748*t*
due to external tibial torsion, 749
in-toeing as, 748–749
common causes of, 748*t*
due to femoral anteversion, 748
due to internal tibial torsion, 748–749, 749*f*
treatment of, 749
out-toeing as, 749
common causes of, 748*t*
due to external tibial torsion, 749
Lower motor neuron disease, 694–698, 694*t*
of anterior horn cells, 693*t*, 694
Duchenne muscular dystrophy as, 696–697
infant botulism as, 696
laboratory and diagnostic studies for, 698
malignant hyperthermia with, 698
muscle diseases as, 697–698. *see also* Muscular disease(s)
myasthenia gravis as, 696
myotonic dystrophy as, 697
peripheral neuropathy as, 695–696
spinal muscular atrophy as, 694–695
topography of, 694*t*
upper motor neuron lesions and, 693*t*
Lower motor neurons, 692–693
Lower motor unit, 693
Lower respiratory tract infection, 402–403
LP. *see* Lumbar puncture
LSD (lysergic acid diethylamide), acute effects of, 284*t*–285*t*
Lubricant, for functional constipation, 52*t*
Ludwig angina, 393
Lumbar puncture (LP)
for increased intracranial pressure, 708
for infectious diseases, 362
for leukemia, 603–604
traumatic, 684–685
Lumbosacral hemangioma, 732–733
Lumbosacral spine, hair tufts over, 228
Lung(s)
anatomy of, 507
of newborn, 230
physiology, 507–509
defense mechanisms in, 508–509
pulmonary mechanics in, 507–508, 508*f*
respiratory gas exchange in, 508, 508*t*
unilateral hyperlucent, 407
Lung abscess, 405–407
Lung biopsy, 512
Lung capacities, 508*f*
Lung compliance, 508
Lung defense mechanisms, 508–509
Lung development, 241
Lung disease
chronic, 244–245
restrictive, 508
Lung volumes, 508*f*
Lupus, discoid, 353
Lupus nephritis, 355
Luteinizing hormone, in puberty, 656
LVOT (left ventricular outflow tract) obstruction, syncope due to, 541*t*
Lyme disease, 429, 439*t*–442*t*, 443–444
clinical manifestations of, 443, 443*f*
complications and prognosis, 444
differential diagnosis of, 344*t*, 444
early disseminated, 443
epidemiology of, 443, 443*f*
etiology of, 443
laboratory and imaging studies for, 443–444
late, 443
prevention of, 444
synovial fluid findings in, 429*t*
treatment of, 444
Lymphadenitis, 383
cervical
etiology of, 383
suppurative, 384
Lymphadenopathy, 383–386
clinical manifestations of, 383–384
complications and prognosis for, 385–386
differential diagnosis for, 385
epidemiology of, 383
etiology of, 383
generalized, 383, 383*t*
in hematological disorders, 563
inguinal, 384*t*
in Kawasaki disease, 347
laboratory and imaging studies for, 384–385
prevention of, 386
regional, 384*t*
treatment for, 385
Lymphangitis, 383
Lymphatic malformation, differential diagnosis of, 730*t*
Lymphocutaneous syndromes, 383, 384*t*
Lymphocyte disorders, 293–300
antibody deficiency diseases due to, 294–295, 294*f*, 295*t*
agammaglobulinemia as, 294, 295*t*
autosomal recessive, 294
X-linked, 294
antibody deficiency syndrome as, 295, 295*t*
common variable immunodeficiency as, 294–295, 295*t*
IgA deficiency as, 295, 295*t*
IgG subclass deficiency as, 295, 295*t*
transient hypogammaglobulinemia of infancy as, 295, 295*t*
combined immunodeficiency diseases due to, 296–299
etiology and clinical manifestation of, 294–299
other
ataxia-telangiectasia as, 298, 299*t*
chronic mucocutaneous candidiasis as, 298, 299*t*
hyper-IgE syndrome as, 299, 299*t*
Nijmegen breakage syndrome as, 299*t*
Wiskott-Aldrich syndrome as, 298, 299*t*
X-linked lymphoproliferative syndrome as, 298–299, 299*t*
prevention and newborn screening of, 300
treatment of, 299–300

Lymphocyte phenotyping, 293
Lymphocytes, 566
atypical
in infectious diseases, 362
in lymphadenitis, 384
values of, 565*t*
Lymphocytic choriomeningitis, 439*t*–442*t*
Lymphocytosis, pertussis and, 400–401
Lymphoma, 605–607, 614
anaplastic large cell, 605
Burkitt
clinical manifestations of, 605
etiology of, 605, 606*t*
clinical manifestations of, 605
complications of, 607
defined, 605
diagnosis of, 605
differential diagnosis of, 606
epidemiology of, 605
etiology of, 605, 606*t*
Hodgkin. *see* Hodgkin lymphoma
laboratory/imaging studies in, 606, 606*f*
large cell, 606*t*
lymphoblastic, 606*t*
non-Hodgkin. *see* Non-Hodgkin lymphoma
prognosis for, 607
treatment of, 606–607
Lymphoproliferative disease
B-cell, with hematopoietic stem cell transplantation, 307
X-linked, 386
Lymphoproliferative syndrome, 303
Lysosomal α-glucosidase deficiency, 200*t*
Lysosomal enzyme activity, 209
Lysosomal membrane, storage diseases caused by defective synthesis of, 210*t*–212*t*
Lysosomal proteolysis, storage diseases caused by, 210*t*–212*t*
Lysosomal storage disorders, 209
diagnostic testing for, 209
treatment strategies for, 209
Lysosomes, 209

M

M-CHAT-R (Modified Checklist for Autism in Toddlers-Revised), 17–18
M-CSF (macrophage colony-stimulating factor), 564*f*
MAC (membrane attack complex), 304–305, 305*f*
Macro-orchidism, with developmental disabilities, 30*t*
Macrocephaly, 681, 717, 717*t*
in glutaric acidemia I, 206
Macrocytic anemia, 574–575, 591
Macrolides, for pertussis, 401
Macrophage activation syndrome (MAS), 352
Macrophage colony-stimulating factor (M-CSF), 564*f*
Macroscopic analysis, 619–620
Macular rash, infections with fever and, 373*t*–374*t*
Macule, 721*t*, 722*f*
Maculopapular rash, infections with fever and, 373*t*–374*t*
Magnesium citrate
for functional constipation, 51*t*
for poisoning, 164
Magnesium hydroxide (milk of magnesia), for functional constipation, 52*t*
Magnesium sulfate, maternal use of, 238*t*
Magnetic resonance imaging (MRI), 186
of brain and spinal cord, 685
for cancer, 596, 599*t*
in central nervous system, 607, 608*f*
of chest, 511
Magnetic resonance imaging (MRI) *(Continued)*
with gadolinium enhancement, for infectious diseases, 362–363
for increased intracranial pressure, 708
for infectious diseases, 362
for kidney structure, 620
for seizures, 691
Mainstem bronchi, 507
Maintenance water
adjustments in, 127*t*
components of, 126*t*
Major depressive disorder (MDD), 64, 65*t*
Major determinant, in skin testing for penicillin allergy, 339
Major hemoglobinopathies, 575
Major histocompatibility complex (MHC) compatibility, in hematopoietic stem cell transplantation, 307
Malar butterfly rash, in systemic lupus erythematosus, 353, 354*f*
Malar region, dysmorphology of, 185
Malaria, 447–449
algid, 449
clinical manifestations of, 447
complications and prognosis of, 449
differential diagnosis of, 449
epidemiology of, 447
etiology of, 447
laboratory and imaging studies for, 447–449
prevention of, 449
treatment of, 449
Male sex determination, 672*f*
Malformations, 169, 183–184
association in, 184
congenital, 169
defined, 183–184, 739*t*
diagnosis of, 186
due to disruptions of development, 184
due to extrinsic factors, 184
history for
family, 184
pregnancy, 184
due to inborn errors of metabolism, 195–196
due to intrinsic factors, 184
laboratory evaluation of, 186
life-threatening, 232–233
mechanisms of, 739*t*
minor, 184
multiple, 184
physical examination of, 184–186
craniofacial, 185
of extremities, 185
of genitalia, 185–186
growth in, 184–185
of neck, 185
of trunk, 185
sequence of, 184
Malignancies, fever due to, 371
Malignant germ cell tumors, risk factors for, 597*t*
Malignant hypertension, in thrombotic microangiopathy, 580
malignant hyperthermia, 698
Malignant melanoma, 732
giant congenital nevi and, 732
Malignant melanoma, maternal, 236*t*
Malingering, in somatic symptom and related disorders (SSRDs), 61
Mallory-Weiss syndrome, gastrointestinal bleeding due to, 477*t*
Malnutrition
definitions of, 110*t*
in failure to thrive, 78*t*, 109. *see also* Failure to thrive
kwashiorkor as, 110–111
marasmus as, 110
maternal, effect on infants, 1
Malnutrition-infection cycle, 79
Maltreatment, 2
Mandibular region, dysmorphology of, 185
α-Mannosidase deficiency, 210*t*–212*t*
Mannosyl phosphotransferase deficiency, 210*t*–212*t*
Mantoux test, 454
Maple syrup urine disease (MSUD), 203–204
clinical manifestations of, 203
definitive diagnosis of, 204
laboratory manifestations of, 204
neonatal screening for, 198*t*
Marasmus, 110
Marcus Gunn pupil, 683
Marfan syndrome (MS), 171
diagnostic criteria for, 171
genetic basis for, 170*t*
hypermobility in, 357
hypotonia in, 699
Marijuana, acute effects of, 284*t*–285*t*
Markers, for cancer, 599*t*
Maroteaux-Lamy syndrome, 210*t*–212*t*
Marrow failure, in macrocytic anemia, 574
Masculinization, in male, 673*t*
Mass lesions, 706–707
upper airway obstruction due to, 519
Mastocytoma, 730*t*
Mastoiditis, acute, otitis media and, 397
Maternal assessment, 217–218
Maternal blood, ingested, gastrointestinal bleeding due to, 477*t*
Maternal deprivation, growth failure due to, 653
Maternal disease, affecting newborn, 235–237, 236*t*
antiphospholipid syndrome as, 235
diabetes mellitus as, 236*t*–237*t*, 237
hyperthyroidism as, 236, 236*t*
idiopathic thrombocytopenia as, 235–236, 236*t*
other, 237
systemic lupus erythematosus as, 236, 236*t*
teratogens, 176
Maternal history, in cardiovascular system assessment, 535
Maternal hyperphenylalaninemia, 202
Maternal infections, as teratogens, 176
Maternal medications
small for gestational age due to, 239*t*
that may adversely affect newborn, 238*t*
Mature minors, 5
Maturity
fetal, 219
pulmonary, 219–220
of newborn
neurological criteria in, 227–228
physical criteria for, 227–228
Maturity-onset diabetes of youth, 646
MCAD (medium-chain acyl-CoA dehydrogenase) deficiency, 207–208
McArdle disease, 200*t*
McCune-Albright syndrome, 660
MCD (multicystic renal dysplasia), 629
MDI (metered dose inhaler), 512
Mean mid-expiratory flow rate ($FEF_{25-75\%}$), 511
Measles, mumps, and rubella (MMR) vaccine, 363–364, 364*f*–365*f*, 375
Measles (rubeola), 373–375
black, 373–374
clinical manifestations of, 373–374
complications and prognosis of, 375
differential diagnosis of, 374
epidemiology of, 373
etiology of, 373
laboratory and imaging studies in, 374

Measles (rubeola) *(Continued)*
modified, 374
mumps, and rubella (MMR) vaccine, 363–364, 364*f*–365*f*, 375
prevention of, 375
treatment of, 374–375
Mechanical counterpulsation, for heart failure, 555*t*
Mechanical ventilation, 513
for bronchopulmonary dysplasia, 245
pulmonary air leaks due to, 244
for respiratory failure, 150
Meckel diverticulum, 490
abdominal pain due to, 470*t*
gastrointestinal bleeding due to, 477*t*
Meconium aspiration pneumonia, 245
Meconium aspiration syndrome, 245–246
Meconium ileus
in cystic fibrosis, 527, 529
intestinal atresia in, 488
Meconium-stained amniotic fluid, 226
Mediastinal deviation, 510*t*
Mediastinal lymphadenopathy, 605
Medical conditions
psychological factors in, 59–60, 60*t*
psychotic disorder due to, 72
Medical decision making, 4
Medical devices, infections associated with, 437–439
Medical history, in genetic assessment, 178
Medications. *see* Drug(s)
Mediterranean spotted fever, 439*t*–442*t*
Medium-chain acyl-CoA dehydrogenase (MCAD) deficiency, 207–208
neonatal screening for, 198*t*
Mefloquine, for malaria, 449
Megacolon, toxic, 490
Megakaryocytes, 566
Megakaryocytic cells, in hematopoiesis, 563
Melanocortin 4 receptor gene mutation, obesity in, 106*t*
Melanocytic nevi, 730*t*
acquired, 732
congenital, 228–229, 731–732, 731*f*
differential diagnosis of, 730*t*
giant, 730*t*, 732
hairy, 731–732, 731*f*
Melanoma, malignant, 732
giant congenital nevi and, 732
maternal, 236*t*
Melanosis
dermal, 730, 730*t*, 731*f*
pustular, 228–229
MELAS (mitochondrial encephalomyopathy with lactic acidosis and strokelike episodes), 175
Melia, 183*t*
Membrane attack complex (MAC), 304–305, 305*f*
Membrane disorders, in hemolytic anemia, 578–579, 592
clinical manifestations of, 579
etiology of, 578–579
laboratory diagnosis of, 579
treatment of, 579
Membrane rupture
premature, 218
prolonged, 218
Membranoproliferative glomerulonephritis (MPGN), 620
type II, 306
Membranous nephropathy, 620
Membranous septum, 545
Menaquinone, 118
Menarche, 270–271, 656
Meningitis, 386–389
aseptic, 386
bacterial, 707
causes of, 386*t*
clinical manifestations of, 387
complications and prognosis for, 388
differential diagnosis of, 388
epidemiology of, 386–387
etiology of, 386
fever due to, 368
laboratory and imaging studies for, 387–388, 387*t*
in newborn, 258–259
partially treated, 386, 387*t*
prevention of, 388–389
recurrence of, 388
relapse of, 388
treatment of, 388, 388*t*
tuberculous, 453–454
viral, 387*t*
vomiting due to, 473*t*
Meningocele, 716
Meningococcal vaccines, 364*f*–365*f*
Meningococcus prophylaxis, 366
Meningoencephalitis, 387*t*, 389
Meningomyelocele, 227*t*
constipation due to, 476*t*
Menstrual disorders, 275–277
abnormal uterine bleeding as, 276–277
amenorrhea as, 275–276
definition of, 276*t*
dysmenorrhea as, 277
irregular menses as, 274–275
Mental health condition, 3
Mental motor milestones, 740
Mental retardation, in child, with special needs, 33, 33*t*–34*t*
Mental status
altered, 703–711
due to respiratory failure, 149
evaluation, 682
Mepivacaine, maternal use of, 238*t*
Mepolizumab, for asthma, 315
6-Mercaptopurine
for cancer, 601*t*–602*t*
for ulcerative colitis, 491
Mescaline, acute effects of, 284*t*–285*t*
Metabolic acidosis, 139–141, 139*t*
due to inborn errors of metabolism, 192, 196*t*
in newborn, 222
due to poisoning and, 162, 162*t*
Metabolic alkalosis, 141–142, 141*t*
causes of, 141*t*
chloride-resistant, 141
chloride responsive, 141
clinical manifestations of, 141
diagnosis of, 141
etiology of, 141
hypokalemic, in pyloric stenosis, 485
treatment of, 141–142
Metabolic compensation, appropriate, 139
Metabolic disorder(s), 191–215
assessment of, 191–199, 192*f*
clinical presentation of, 191–196
congenital malformations or dysmorphic features in, 195–196
energy deficiency in, 193
hyperammonemia
etiology of, 195*t*
in later infancy and childhood, 192, 194*f*
moderate neonatal, 192
severe neonatal, 192
ketosis and ketotic hypoglycemia in, 193–195
metabolic acidosis in, 192, 196*t*
Metabolic disorder(s) *(Continued)*
specific organ, 192–193, 195*t*
toxic, 191–192
genetic aspects of, 196–197
identification of molecular pathology as, 197
mechanisms of inheritance as, 196–197
neonatal screening for. *see* Neonatal screening, for inborn errors of metabolism
overview of treatment for, 199
storage as, 196
vomiting due to, 473*t*
Metabolic syndrome, 646
Metabolic testing, for chronic liver disease, 500*t*
Metachromatic leukodystrophy, 210*t*–212*t*, 712
Metagonimiasis, 451*t*
Metagonimus yokogawai, 451*t*
Metaphase analysis, in genetic assessment, 179
Metaphysis, 740*f*
Metatarsal, head of the second, idiopathic avascular necrosis of, 755
Metatarsus adductus, 754, 754*f*
Metatarsus varus, 754
Metered dose inhaler (MDI), 512
Methadone, as analgesia, 166*t*
Methanol ingestion, metabolic acidosis due to, 140
Methicillin-resistant *Staphylococcus aureus*, pneumonia from, 407*t*
Methicillin-susceptible *Staphylococcus aureus*, pneumonia from, 407*t*
Methimazole, maternal use of, 238*t*
Methionine, metabolism of, 203*f*
Methotrexate
for cancer, 601*t*–602*t*
for juvenile dermatomyositis, 356
for juvenile idiopathic arthritis, 352
Methyl mercury, as teratogen, 237*t*
Methylene blue, for nitrite poisoning, 164*t*–165*t*
Methylmalonic acidemia, 205
clinical manifestations of, 205
neonatal screening for, 198*t*
treatment of, 205
Methylprednisolone, for systemic lupus erythematosus, 355
Methylxanthines, for apnea of prematurity, 246
Metoclopramide, for gastroesophageal reflux, 481*t*
Metorchiasis, 451*t*
Metorchis conjunctus, 451*t*
Metronidazole, for trichomoniasis, 424
MHC (major histocompatibility complex) compatibility, in hematopoietic stem cell transplantation, 307
Micaceous scale, in psoriasis, 729–730
Microangiopathy, thrombotic, 580, 585–586
Microarray comparative genomic hybridization, 186
Microcephaly, 681, 717, 718*t*
Microcomedo, 723
Microcytic anemia, hypochromic, 566, 567*f*, 568–574
due to iron deficiency, 568–571
clinical manifestations of, 570
epidemiology of, 570, 570*t*
etiology of, 570
prevention of, 571
treatment of, 571, 571*t*
due to lead poisoning, 571
thalassemia minor as, 571
etiology and epidemiology of, 571, 572*f*, 572*t*
laboratory testing for, 571
treatment of, 571
Microhemagglutination assay-*T. pallidum* (MHA-TP), 424

Micronutrient deficiencies, 112–121, 113*t*
of fat-soluble vitamins, 114*t*, 117–119
malnutrition with, 112
of minerals, 119–121, 119*t*
of water-soluble vitamins, 112–117, 114*t*
Micronutrients, 112
Microphallus, 673
Microscopic analysis, 619–620
Microsporidia, diarrhea from, 410*t*
Micturition syncope, 541*t*
Mid-diastolic murmur, due to ventricular septal defect, 545
Midazolam
for sedation, 166*t*
for status epilepticus, 691, 691*t*
Middle ear effusion, persistent, otitis media and, 397
Midface, dysmorphology of, 185
Midgut malrotation, 487–488
clinical manifestations of, 488
etiology and epidemiology of, 487–488, 487*f*
laboratory and imaging studies for, 488
treatment of, 488
with volvulus, 487–488, 488*f*
vomiting due to, 473*t*
Midparental height determination, growth chart and, 13
Migraine, 685–687
clinical manifestations of, 686, 686*f*, 686*t*
confusional, 706
diagnostic studies for, 686–687
etiology and epidemiology of, 685–686
treatment of, 687
vomiting due to, 473*t*
Mild to moderate visual impairment, 34
Milia, 228–229, 721*t*, 722*f*
Miliaria, 228–229
crystallina, vesiculobullous eruptions due to, 734*t*
Miliary tuberculosis, 453
Military deployment, 3
Milk intake
adequacy of, 99–100
for toddlers and older children, 103
Milk intolerance, vomiting due to, 473*t*
Milk of molasses, for functional constipation, 51*t*
Miller Fisher variant, of Guillain-Barré syndrome, 695
Milrinone
for heart failure, 555*t*
for shock, 153*t*
Mineral, in parenteral nutrition, 131
Mineral bone disorder, chronic kidney disease, 626–627
Mineral deficiencies, 119–121, 119*t*
Mineral endocrinology, 669–670, 680
Mineral oil, for functional constipation, 51*t*–52*t*
Minimal change nephrotic syndrome, 620
Minor determinant, in skin testing for penicillin allergy, 339
Minors
emancipated, 5
mature, 5
Minute dog tapeworm, 452
Minute ventilation, 513
MIP-1α, functions of, 290*t*
MiraLAX (polyethylene glycol powder), for functional constipation, 52*t*
Misoprostol, as teratogen, 237*t*
Missense mutation, 169
Mitochondrial disorders, 213–214, 713
genetics of, 214
inborn errors of metabolism due to, 196*t*
MELAS as, 175
signs and symptoms of, 213–214
treatment of, 214
Mitochondrial DNA (mtDNA), 175
Mitochondrial encephalomyopathy with lactic acidosis and strokelike episodes (MELAS), 175
Mitochondrial function, biochemical abnormalities in, 214
Mitochondrial genome, 213*f*
Mitochondrial inheritance, 175
heteroplasmy in, 175
MELAS as, 175
Mitochondrion(ia), function of, 214
Mixed malformation, differential diagnosis of, 730*t*
Mixed marasmus-kwashiorkor, 111
Mixed venous oxygen saturation, in shock, 152–153
ML (mucolipidosis[es]), 210*t*–212*t*
Mobitz type I heart block, 544*t*
Mobitz type II heart block, 544*t*
Möbius syndrome, in newborn, 233
Modified Checklist for Autism in Toddlers-Revised (M-CHAT-R), 17–18
Mold, asthma and, 315*t*
Molecular tests, 362
Molluscum contagiosum, 383
Mometasone DPI, for asthma, 319*f*
Mongolian spots, 228, 730, 730*t*, 731*f*
Monkeypox, 439*t*–442*t*
Monoclonal antibodies, for cancer, 601*t*–602*t*
Monocytes, values of, 565*t*
Monosomy(ies), 181–182
Turner syndrome as, 181–182
Montelukast, for asthma, 315
Morbidity, changing, 3
Morbilliform rash, in juvenile idiopathic arthritis, 351
Moro reflex, 14, 233, 682*t*
Morphine
as analgesia, 166*t*
maternal use of, 238*t*
Mortality, infant, 2
Mosaicism, 180
Motion sickness, vomiting due to, 473*t*
Motor examination, 682, 684
of bulk, 684
of coordination, 684
of gait, 684
in neonate, 682
of reflexes, 684
of strength, 684
of tone, 684
Motor intervention, for child with special needs, 32
Motor sensory neuropathy, hereditary, 695
Motor vehicle accidents, 2
Motor vehicle crashes, 22
Mouth. *see also* Oral cavity
anemia and, 569*t*
bottle, 479
of newborn, 230
Mouth sores, in systemic lupus erythematosus, 353
Movement disorders, 702–703
causes of, 702*t*
MPS (mucopolysaccharidoses), 210*t*–212*t*
MRI. *see* Magnetic resonance imaging
MS. *see* Marfan syndrome
MSUD. *see* Maple syrup urine disease
mtDNA (mitochondrial DNA), 175
MTTL1 gene, in MELAS, 175
Muckle-Wells syndrome, 331
Mucolipidosis(es) (ML), 210*t*–212*t*
Mucopolysaccharidoses (MPS), 210*t*–212*t*, 713
Mucopurulent cervicitis, 420*t*
Multicystic renal dysplasia (MCD), 629
Multifactorial disorders
hypertrophic pyloric stenosis due to, 174–175
neural tube defects due to, 175
Multiple acyl-CoA dehydrogenase deficiency, 208
Multiple gestation, 217
Multiple hereditary exostoses, 765*t*–766*t*
Multiple malformation syndrome, 184
Multiple organ dysfunction, in respiratory failure, 150
Multiple sulfatase deficiency, 210*t*–212*t*
Multisystem disease, constipation due to, 476*t*
Munchausen syndrome, 649
fever due to, 371
Munchausen syndrome by proxy, fever due to, 371
Murine typhus-like illness, 439*t*–442*t*
Murmurs. *see* Heart murmurs
Muscle bulk, in motor examination, 684
Muscle fasciculations, 684–685
in spinal muscular atrophy, 694
Muscle fibrillations, 685
Muscle phosphofructokinase deficiency, 200*t*
Muscle phosphorylase deficiency, 200*t*
Muscle tone
in motor examination, 684
in neonate, 682
Muscular disease(s)
congenital myopathies as, 697–698
Duchenne muscular dystrophy as, 696–697
Emery-Dreifuss muscular dystrophy as, 697
facioscapulohumeral dystrophy as, 697
limb-girdle muscular dystrophy as, 697
metabolic myopathies as, 698
myotonic dystrophy as, 697
Muscular dystrophy, 693*t*
Becker, 696
congenital, 697
constipation due to, 476*t*
Duchenne, 696–697
clinical manifestations of, 696–697
etiology of, 696
laboratory and diagnostic studies of, 697
treatment of, 697
facioscapulohumeral, 697
limb-girdle, 697
myotonic, 697
Muscular septum, 545
Musculoskeletal pain syndromes, 356–358
benign hypermobility as, 357, 357*f*, 357*t*
defined, 343
growing pain as, 356–357
juvenile idiopathic arthritis *vs.*, 352*t*
myofascial pain syndrome and fibromyalgia as, 358
Mutation, 169
frameshift, 169
hot spot, 171
loss-of-function, 176
missense, 169
nonsense, 169
point, 169
single-gene, 169
spontaneous, 171
Mutism, selective, 63
Myasthenia gravis, 696
congenital, 696
diagnostic studies of, 696
juvenile, 696
maternal, 236*t*
transient neonatal, 696
Myasthenic syndrome, congenital, 696
Mycobacteria, nontuberculous, lymphadenitis and, 384
Mycobacterial diseases, zoonotic, 439*t*–442*t*
Mycobacteriosis, 439*t*–442*t*

Mycobacterium fortuitum, 439*t*–442*t*
Mycobacterium kansasii, 439*t*–442*t*
Mycobacterium marinum, 439*t*–442*t*
Mycobacterium tuberculosis, 452
Mycoplasma pneumoniae
pneumonia due to, 407*t*
Stevens-Johnson syndrome due to, 735
Myelitis, transverse, 694
Myeloid cells, in hematopoiesis, 563
Myelomeningocele, 716
Myeloperoxidase deficiency, 301*t*
Myeloproliferative disorder, transient, 604
Myocardial contractility, in heart failure, 553
Myocarditis, syncope due to, 541*t*
Myoclonic epilepsy, 689
juvenile, 690
Myoclonus, 703
Myofascial pain syndrome, 358
Myonecrosis, 380
Myopathies
congenital, 697–698
endocrine, 698
metabolic, 698
mitochondrial, 698
Myositis, in rheumatic diseases, 343
Myotonia, 697
Myotonic dystrophy, 697
clinical manifestations of, 697
etiology and epidemiology of, 697
genetic basis for, 170*t*
maternal, 236*t*

N

N-acetylcysteine, for acetaminophen poisoning, 164*t*–165*t*
N-acetylgalactosamine-4-sulfatase deficiency, 210*t*–212*t*
Nail, hypoplastic, 183*t*
Nail-fold capillaries, dilated, in juvenile dermatomyositis, 355–356
Naloxone
in newborn resuscitation, 227
for opiate poisoning, 164*t*–165*t*
Naltrexone, for autism spectrum disorder (ASD), 71
Nanophyetiasis, 451*t*
Nanophyetus salmincola, 451*t*
Naphthalene, maternal use of, 238*t*
Narcotics
constipation due to, 476*t*
maternal use of, 238*t*
toxicity, 162*t*
Nasal alae, 183*t*
Nasal cannula, 512
Nasal flaring, 509–510
Nasal influenza vaccine, 363–364
Nasal polyposis, in cystic fibrosis, 527
Nasal polyps, 324
Nasal smear, for upper respiratory tract infection, 391
Nasal sores, in systemic lupus erythematosus, 353
Nasal turbinates, 507
Nasolabial fold, 183*t*
Nasopharyngoscopy, 511
National Childhood Vaccine Injury Act, 366
National Practitioner Data Bank, 3–4
National Vaccine Injury Compensation Program, 366
NBS (New Ballard Score), 229*f*
NCL (neuronal ceroid lipofuscinosis), 210*t*–212*t*
NCVs (nerve conduction velocities), 685
Nebulizer, 512
Necator americanus, 450, 450*t*
Neck
congenital malformations of, 185
of newborn, 230
Necrotic eschar, infections with fever and, 373*t*–374*t*
Necrotizing enterocolitis (NEC), 254–255
gastrointestinal bleeding due to, 477*t*
Necrotizing fasciitis, 380
Needle biopsy, 512
Negative-pressure ventilation, for tuberculosis, 457
Negative reinforcement, 16
Neglect, 80
Neisseria gonorrhoeae
clinical features of infections caused by, 420*t*
congenital infection with, 260*t*, 263
conjunctivitis from, 430
disseminated gonococcal infections from, 421–422
pelvic inflammatory disease from, 420–421
Neisseria meningitidis, prophylaxis for, 366
Neisseria meningitidis vaccine, 363–364
NEMO (nuclear factor κB essential modulator), in hyper-IgM syndrome, 296
Neoadjuvant chemotherapy, 601
Neonatal alloimmune thrombocytopenic purpura (NATP), 584
Neonatal conjunctivitis, 432*t*–433*t*
Neonatal drug addiction and withdrawal, 235
from cocaine, 235
from opiates, 235
Neonatal hepatitis, 494
Neonatal hypotonia, 698–699
Neonatal mortality, 218, 219*t*
Neonatal physiology, transition from fetal to, 218, 221*t*
Neonatal screening, for inborn errors of metabolism, 198*t*
confirmatory testing principles of, 197
disorders identified by, 197, 198*t*
specialized laboratory and clinical testing after, 197–199, 199*t*
strategy of, 197
Nephritis, lupus, 355
Nephrogenic diabetes insipidus, 133–134
Nephrolithiasis, 631
Nephrology assessment, 617–620
common manifestations in, 618*t*
history in, 617
physical examination in, 617
Nephropathic cystinosis, 210*t*–212*t*
Nephrotic syndrome (NS), 620–622
clinical manifestations of, 621
complications of, 621
congenital, 620–621
diagnostic studies of, 621
differential diagnosis of, 621
edema in, 620
etiology and epidemiology of, 620–621
hypercholesterolemia in, 620
hypoproteinemia in, 620
idiopathic, 620
minimal change, 620
primary, 620, 620*t*
prognosis for, 622
proteinuria in, 620–622
secondary, 620, 620*t*
treatment of, 621
Nerve conduction velocities (NCVs), 685
Nerves, anemia and, 569*t*
Neural crest cells, 608–609
Neural tube defects (NTDs)
genetic basis for, 175
maternal screening for, 179
newborn assessment for, 227*t*
Neuralgia, postherpetic, 379
Neuraminidase deficiency, 210*t*–212*t*
Neuroblastoma, 608–609, 614
ataxia due to, 701–702
clinical manifestations of, 609
complications of, 609
differential diagnosis of, 609
epidemiology of, 609
etiology of, 608–609
laboratory/imaging studies in, 609
prognosis for, 609
risk factors for, 597*t*
treatment of, 609, 610*t*
Neuroborreliosis, 443
Neurocardiogenic syncope, 541*t*
Neurocutaneous disorders, 714–716
neurofibromatosis type 1, 714–715, 714*f*
Sturge-Weber syndrome as, 715–716, 733
tuberous sclerosis complex as, 715
Neurocysticercosis, 452, 452*t*
Neurodegenerative disorders, 711–714, 711*t*–712*t*
acquired illnesses mimicking, 714
with focal manifestations, 713
gray matter (neuronal), 711
hereditary and metabolic, 711–713
white matter (leukodystrophies), 711
Neurodevelopmental therapy, 32
Neurofibromas, 714–715
plexiform, 730*t*
Neurofibromatosis, with spinal deformities, 756–757
Neurofibromatosis 1, 171, 714–715
genetic basis for, 170*t*
Neurofibromatosis 2, 715
genetic basis for, 170*t*
Neurogenic bladder, 628–629
Neurogenic pulmonary edema, 524
Neuroimaging, 685
Neurological criteria, for newborn maturity and gestational age, 227–228
Neurology assessment, 681–685
of child, 682
cranial nerve evaluation in, 682–683
of cranial nerve I, 683
of cranial nerve II, 683
of cranial nerves III, IV, and VI, 683
of cranial nerve V, 683
of cranial nerve VII, 683
of cranial nerve VIII, 683
of cranial nerves IX and X, 683
of cranial nerve XII, 683
mental status and developmental evaluation in, 682
motor examination in, 682, 684
of bulk, 684
of coordination, 684
of gait, 684
of reflexes, 684
of strength, 684
of tone, 684
sensory examination in, 682, 684
special diagnostic procedures in, 684–685
cerebrospinal fluid analysis as, 684–685, 685*t*
electroencephalography, 685
electromyography and nerve conduction studies as, 685
neuroimaging as, 685
history in, 681
of neonate, 681–682
mental status in, 682
motor examination and tone in, 682
of posture, 682
reflexes in, 682, 682*t*
physical examination in, 681
Neuromuscular criteria, for newborn maturity and gestational age, 229*f*

Neuromuscular disease
of anterior horn cells, 693t–694t, 694
clinical sign of, 693t
Duchenne muscular dystrophy as, 696–697
infant botulism as, 696
laboratory and diagnostic studies for, 698
malignant hyperthermia with, 698
metabolic myopathies as, 698
muscle diseases as, 697–698
myasthenia gravis as, 696
myotonic dystrophy as, 697
neonatal and infantile hypotonia as, 698–699, 698f
peripheral neuropathy as, 695–696
spinal muscular atrophy as, 694–695
topography of, 694t
upper motor neuron lesions and, 693t
Neuromuscular scoliosis, 758–759
Neuronal ceroid lipofuscinosis (NCL), 210t–212t, 711t–712t, 712–713
Neuronal migration, disorders of, 717
Neuropathy, peripheral, 695–696
Neurosyphilis, 424
Neutropenia, 301
autoimmune, 302
benign congenital, 301
congenital, 301t
cyclic, 301, 301t
drug-associated, 302t
in immunocompromised person, 434–435, 435f, 436t
infection-associated, 302t
isoimmune, 301–302
maternal, 236t
in Kostmann syndrome, 301
mechanisms of, 302t
oncological emergencies, 600t
presentation of, 564t
in reticular dysgenesis, 301
in Schwachman-Diamond syndrome, 301
severe congenital, 301
Neutrophil chemotactic defects, 303–304
Neutrophil disorders, 300–304
etiology and clinical manifestations of, 300–303
of function, 303
laboratory diagnosis of, 303–304
of migration, 302–303, 303f
leukocyte adhesion deficiency
type I, 302–303
type II, 303
of numbers, 300–302
prognosis and prevention of, 304
treatment for, 304
Neutrophil function
disorders of, 303
in Chediak-Higashi syndrome, 303
in chronic granulomatous disease, 303
test for, 293
Neutrophil migration, disorders of, 302–303, 303f
in leukocyte adhesion deficiency
type I, 302–303
type II, 303
Neutrophil number, disorders of, 300–302
autoimmune neutropenia as, 302
benign congenital neutropenia as, 301
cyclic neutropenia as, 301, 301t
drug-associated, 302t
infection-associated, 302t
in Kostmann syndrome, 301
mechanisms of, 302t
in reticular dysgenesis, 301
in Schwachman-Diamond syndrome, 301
severe congenital neutropenia as, 301
Neutrophils
precursors, production of, 566
values of, 565t
Nevus(i)
acquired, 732
anemicus, 730t
depigmentosus, 730t
epidermal, 730t
flammeus, 228, 733
differential diagnosis, 730t
in Klippel-Trénaunay-Weber syndrome, 733
in Sturge-Weber syndrome, 733
of Ito, 730t
melanocytic, 730t
acquired, 732
congenital, 228–229, 731–732, 731f
giant, 732
hairy, 731–732, 731f
differential diagnosis of, 730t
of Ota, 730t
satellite, 732
sebaceous, 730t
simplex, 228
New Ballard Score (NBS), 229f
Newborn(s)
anemia in, 247–249. *see also* Anemia, in newborn
bacterial colonization of, 222
birth injury, 233–234
coagulation disorders in, 252–253
clinical manifestations and differential diagnoses of, 253–254
congenital infections in, 259–264, 260t
cyanosis in, 232, 232t
hemolytic disease of, 249
hyperbilirubinemia in, 249–254
direct conjugated, etiology of, 251
indirect unconjugated
etiology of, 250–251
kernicterus (bilirubin encephalopathy) due to, 251
hypocalcemia in, 234–235
hypoxic-ischemic encephalopathy in, 257–258
intracranial hemorrhage in, 256–257
life-threatening congenital anomalies for, 227t
maternal diseases affecting, 235–237, 236t
meningitis in, 258–259
necrotizing enterocolitis in, 254–255
neurology assessment of, 681–682
mental status in, 682
motor examination and tone in, 682
reflexes in, 682, 682t
persistent pulmonary hypertension of, 222
polycythemia (hyperviscosity syndrome) in, 252
respiratory disease of, 240–246
due to apnea of prematurity, 246
etiology of, 240t, 247
due to hydrops fetalis, 240
due to infection, 240
initial laboratory evaluation of, 241t
due to meconium aspiration syndrome, 240, 245–246
due to primary pulmonary hypertension, 246
due to pulmonary hypoplasia, 240
due to respiratory distress syndrome, 241–243
bronchopulmonary dysplasia due to, 244–245
clinical manifestations of, 242, 243f
complications of, 243–245
lung development and, 241, 242f
patent ductus arteriosus due to, 243–244
potential causes of, 243t
prevention and treatment of, 242–243
Newborn(s) *(Continued)*
pulmonary air leaks due to, 244
and retinopathy of prematurity, 245
due to transient tachypnea, 245
treatment of
for hypoxemia, 241
for metabolic acidosis, 241
for respiratory acidosis, 241
supportive care for, 246
resuscitation of, 222–227
routine delivery room care for, 222–227
vitamin K prophylaxis in, 222
screening, 223t–224t
seizures in, 255–258
benign familial, 255
clinical characteristics of, 256t
diagnostic evaluation of, 256
differential diagnosis of, 255
focal clonic, 256t
focal tonic, 256t
generalized tonic, 256t
myoclonic, 256t
treatment of, 256
sepsis in, 258–259
acquired in utero, 258
bacterial, 258
early-onset, 258–259
incidence of, 258
late-onset, 259
preterm, 258
shock, 233
temperature regulation in, 234
transient myeloproliferative disorder of, 604
transient tachypnea of, 222, 245
Newborn assessment, 220–231
Apgar examination in, 225
genetic, 178
of gestational age, 227–231
and abnormal fetal growth patterns, 228
neurological criteria in, 227–228
physical criteria for, 227–228, 228f
neurological, 231–234
perinatal history in, 221t
physical examination in, 227–231
of abdomen, 231
of appearance, 227
of extremities, 231
of face, eyes, and mouth, 230
of genitalia, 231
of heart, 231
of hips, 231
of lungs, 230
of neck and chest, 230
of skin, 228–229
of spine, 231
of vital signs, 227
Newborn period, physical development in, 14
NF-κB (nuclear factor κB) essential modulator (NEMO), in hyper-IgM syndrome, 296
NF1 gene, 171
Niacin deficiency, 113, 114t
Nickel dermatitis, 725, 727–728
Nicotinamide, 113
Nicotine, acute effects of, 284t–285t
Niemann-Pick disease, 711t–712t, 712
Night blindness, 117
Nighttime anxiety/ fears, 54t–55t
Nikolsky sign, 734t
Nipples, supernumerary, 230
Nissen procedure, for gastroesophageal reflux, 481t
Nitric oxide analysis, exhaled, for asthma, 314
Nitrite test, in urinalysis, 619–620
Nitroblue tetrazolium test, for chronic granulomatous disease, 303–304
Nitroprusside, for heart failure, 555t

Nits, 736
of pubic lice, 425
N,N-Diethyl-*m*-toluamide (DEET), for prevention of zoonoses, 439
Nodular lymphoid hyperplasia, gastrointestinal bleeding due to, 477*t*
Nodule, 721*t*, 722*f*
Non-Hodgkin lymphoma (NHL)
epidemiology of, 605
etiology of, 605
prognosis for, 607
risk factors for, 597*t*
subtypes of, 606*t*
treatment of, 606–607
Non-nucleoside reverse transcriptase inhibitor (NNRTI), for HIV, 460
Non-REM (NREM) sleep, 52
Nonadherence, in tuberculosis, 456
Nonalcoholic fatty liver disease, 501
Nonallergic, noninfectious rhinitis, 324, 324*t*
Nonallergic rhinitis with eosinophilia syndrome, 323, 324*t*
Nonbullous impetigo, 379
Noncompliance, in tuberculosis, 456
Nongonococcal urethritis and cervicitis, 423
Nonheme iron, 120
Noninvasive ventilation, 150, 513
Nonmaleficence, 4
in end-of-life decision making, 8
Nonossifying fibroma, 765*t*–766*t*
Nonsense mutation, 169
Nonsteroidal antiinflammatory drugs (NSAIDs)
as analgesia, 166*t*
gastrointestinal bleeding due to, 477*t*
for juvenile idiopathic arthritis, 352
Nonstress test, of fetal well-being, 220
Nonsyndromic craniosynostosis, genetic basis for, 170*t*
Nontreponemal antibody tests, 424
Nontuberculous mycobacteria, lymphadenitis and, 384
Nonulcer dyspepsia, 485–486, 486*t*
Norepinephrine, for shock, 153*t*
Normal saline, for functional constipation, 51*t*
Normal temper tantrums, 44*t*
Normocytic anemia, 571–574, 591
North American liver fluke, 451*t*
Nose, 507
as filter, 508
foreign bodies in, 324
skier's, 324
Nosocomial infections, 437
NSAIDs. *see* Nonsteroidal antiinflammatory drugs
NTDs. *see* Neural tube defects
Nucleated red cells, values of, 565*t*
Nucleic and amplification test (NAAT), 412
Nucleotide reverse transcriptase inhibitor (NRTI) , for HIV, 460
Nucleotides, 169
Nursemaid's elbow, 764, 764*f*
Nutrition
of adolescent, 102–104
and growth, 653
of normal infant, 99–102
breast-feeding in, 99–100, 100*f*
complementary foods for, 101–102
formula feeding in, 100–101
parenteral. *see* Parenteral nutrition
recommendations to, 103–104, 103*t*
of toddlers and older children, 103
for type 1 diabetes mellitus, 644
Nutritional counseling, 23*t*–24*t*
Nutritional evaluation, for chronic liver disease, 500*t*
Nutritional management, for failure to thrive, 79
Nutritional rehabilitation, 112
Nutritional support, for burns, 159
Nystagmus, 683

O

Obesity, 2–3, 104–109
assessment of, 107
clinical manifestations of, 105–107, 106*t*
complications of, 105*t*
definitions of, 104–105
epidemiology of, 105
prevention of, 107–109, 108*t*
treatment of, 109
Obsessions, in OCD, 68
Obsessive-compulsive disorder (OCD), 68–70, 69*t*
Obstructive hydrocephalus, 707
Obstructive sleep apnea (OSA), 54*t*–55*t*
pediatric sleep disorders and, 56
syndrome, 514–515, 514*t*
Obstructive stenotic lesions, congenital heart disease due to, 545
Obtunded patients, 703
Occult blood, 568
OCD (osteochondritis dissecans), 752
Ocular examination, in neurology assessment, 681
Ocular hypertelorism, 183*t*
Ocular infections, 430–432
clinical manifestations of, 431
complications and prognosis of, 432
differential diagnosis of, 431–432
epidemiology of, 431
etiology of, 430
laboratory and imaging studies for, 431
prevention of, 432
treatment of, 432, 432*t*
Ocular larva migrans, 450–451, 450*t*
Oculocephalic vestibular reflexes, 683, 703–704
Oculomotor nerve, assessment of, 683
Oculovestibular response, 703–704
OI (oxygenation index), for primary pulmonary hypertension of the newborn, 246
Oligodactyly, 185
Oligohydramnios, 217–218
Oligosaccharide chromatography, urine, 199*t*
Oliguria, fluid therapy for, 127, 127*t*
Omalizumab, for asthma, 315
Omenn syndrome, 297–298, 297*t*
Omphalitis, 231
Omphalocele, 227*t*, 231, 489
Oncological disorders, juvenile idiopathic arthritis *vs.*, 352*t*
Oncology assessment, 595–596, 596*f*, 613
common manifestations in, 595, 598*t*
differential diagnosis in, 596
history in, 595, 597*t*
initial diagnostic evaluation in, 596
diagnostic imaging in, 596, 599*t*
screening tests in, 596
physical examination in, 595
Oncospheres, in echinococcosis, 452
Onychomycosis, 380, 381*t*
Open adoptions, 89
Ophthalmia neonatorum, 430
treatment of, 432
Ophthalmoplegia
and limb weakness, 694*t*
progressive external, 213–214
Opiate
acute effects of, 284*t*–285*t*
neonatal addiction to and withdrawal from, 235
use, during pregnancy, 90
Opioids, as analgesia, 166*t*
Opisthorchiasis, 451*t*
Opisthorchis viverrini, 451*t*
Opsoclonus-myoclonus, neuroblastoma and, 701–702
Opsomyoclonus, neuroblastoma and, 609
Optic gliomas, 662
Optic nerve, assessment of, 683
Optic nerve hypoplasia, 639
Optimal educational settings, in attention-deficit/hyperactivity disorder (ADHD), 47
Oral allergy syndrome, 335*t*–336*t*
Oral cavity, 479–480
cleft lip and palate of, 480
deciduous and primary teeth in, 479, 479*t*
dental caries in, 479–480
effects of systemic disease on, 479
thrush of, 480
Oral glucose tolerance test (OGTT), 639
Oral iron, therapeutic trial of, for iron deficiency anemia, 571
Oral rehydration solution (ORS), 129, 413
Oral tolerance, 334
Orbital cellulitis, 395, 433*t*
Orchidopexy, 633
Orf, 439*t*–442*t*
Organ-directed therapeutics, for shock, 153–154
Organ donation, 8
Organic acid disorders, 205–206
biotinidase deficiency as, 206
glutaric acidemia I as, 206, 207*f*, 208
holocarboxylase deficiency as, 206
isovaleric acidemia as, 206, 206*f*
methylmalonic acidemia as, 205, 206*f*
neonatal screening for, 197–198, 198*t*
propionic acidemia as, 205, 206*f*
treatment of, 206
Organic acid metabolism, disorders of, hypoglycemia due to, 650
Organic acid profile, urine, 199*t*
Organic sleep disorders, 54*t*–55*t*
Orientia tsutsugamushi, 439*t*–442*t*
Ornithine carbamoyltransferase (OTC) deficiency, 204
ORS. *see* Oral rehydration solution
Orthopedic disorders
juvenile idiopathic arthritis *vs.*, 352*t*
mechanisms of, 739*t*
Orthopedics, common terminology in, 739*t*
Orthopedics assessment, 739–740
developmental milestones in, 740
for infants, 740, 741*f*
of gait, 740
growth and development in, 739–740, 740*f*
of limping child, 740, 741*t*
of toe walking, 740
Orthoradiograph, of leg-length discrepancy, 750
Ortolani (reduction) test, 744–745, 745*f*
OSA. *see* Obstructive sleep apnea
Osgood-Schlatter disease, 752
Osmolality, regulation of, 125
Osmotic fragility test, 579
Osmotic gap, in diarrhea, 475
Osmotics, for functional constipation, 52*t*
Ossification center, secondary, 740*f*
Osteoblastoma, 765*t*–766*t*
Osteochondritis dissecans, 752
Osteochondroma, 765*t*–766*t*
Osteoid osteoma, 765*t*–766*t*
Osteomalacia, 118, 670
Osteomyelitis, 425–428
acute hematogenous, 425
chronic, 425
clinical manifestations of, 426
complications and prognosis of, 427–428
culture-negative, 425
differential diagnosis for, 427
epidemiology of, 426
etiology of, 425–426, 426*f*

Osteomyelitis *(Continued)*
fever due to, 368
hematogenous, complications and prognosis of, 427–428
laboratory and imaging studies in, 426–427, 427*f*
multifocal, recurrent, 425–426
prevention of, 428
subacute, 425
focal, 425–426
treatment for, 427, 427*t*
vertebral, 426
Osteoporosis, 119
Osteosarcoma, 611
clinical manifestations of, 612
epidemiology of, 611
etiology of, 611
laboratory/imaging studies in, 612
prognosis for, 613
risk factors for, 597*t*
treatment of, 612
Osteotomy, 739*t*
Ostiomeatal complex, 394
Otalgia, in otitis media, 396
Otitis externa, 397–398
clinical manifestations of, 398
complications and prognosis of, 398
differential diagnosis of, 398
epidemiology of, 398
etiology of, 397–398
laboratory and imaging studies of, 398
malignant, 397–398
Otitis media, 395–397
clinical manifestations of, 395–396, 397*f*
due to common cold, 391–392
complications and prognosis of, 397
definition of, 396*t*
differential diagnosis of, 396
with effusion, 396
epidemiology of, 395
etiology of, 395
laboratory and imaging studies, 396
prevention of, 397
recurrent, 395
treatment of, 396–397, 396*t*
with tympanic perforation, 398
vomiting due to, 473*t*
Otitis prone, 395
Otoacoustic emission, 35
Otorrhea
in otitis media, 396
tympanostomy tube, 398
Out-toeing, 749
common causes of, 748*t*
due to external tibial torsion, 749
Ovarian cysts, 662
Ovarian failure, 659
Overgrowth syndrome, 184–185
Overuse injuries, of shoulder, 763
Oxycodone, acute effects of, 284*t*–285*t*
Oxygen
administration of, 512
for carbon monoxide poisoning, 164*t*–165*t*
delivery, 145
for heart failure, 555*t*
in pulmonary physiology, 507
supplemental, 512
supplementation, 146
Oxygenation index (OI), for primary pulmonary hypertension of the newborn, 246
Oxytocin, maternal use of, 238*t*
Oxytocin challenge test, 220

P

P wave, 539
Pachygyria, 717
Packed RBCs, 589–590, 590*t*
PAH. *see* Pulmonary arterial hypertension
PAH (phenylalanine hydroxylase) deficiency, 173*t*
Pain
analgesia for, 166
back, 761
clinical manifestations and management of, 761
differential diagnosis of, 761, 761*t*
etiology and epidemiology of, 761
red flags in, 761
chest, 541–542, 542*t*
in sickle cell disease, 577*t*
Palivizumab, for bronchiolitis, 402
Palliative care, 6–9
access to comprehensive and compassionate palliative care, 6–7
acknowledgment and support provisions for caregivers, 7
bereavement in, 7
cognitive issues in, 7
commitment to quality improvement of, 7
cultural, religious, and spiritual concerns about, 7–8
in dignity of patients and families, 6
interdisciplinary resources in, 7
Palliative shunt surgery, 550
Pallor
in anemia, 567–568
in hematological disorders, 563
Palpation, in cardiovascular system assessment, 535
Palpebral fissure, 183*t*
Pancreatic disease, 501–503
pancreatic insufficiency as, 501–502
pancreatitis as
acute, 502–503, 502*t*
chronic, 503
Pancreatic enzymes, for pancreatic insufficiency, 502
Pancreatic injury, 157
Pancreatic insufficiency, 501–502
exocrine, in cystic fibrosis, 527, 529
Pancreatic pseudocyst, 502
Pancreatitis
abdominal pain due to, 470*t*
acute, 502–503
clinical manifestations of, 502–503
etiology and epidemiology of, 502, 502*t*
laboratory and imaging studies for, 503
treatment of, 503
chronic, 503
clinical manifestations of, 503
etiology and epidemiology of, 503
laboratory and imaging studies for, 503
treatment of, 503
vomiting due to, 473*t*
Pancytopenia, 573*t*, 574, 591
differential diagnosis of, 574
etiology of, 574
resulting from bone marrow failure, 584
resulting from destruction of cells, 575
Panencephalitis, subacute sclerosing, due to measles, 375
Panic attack, 61–62
Panic disorder, 61–62
Panner disease, 764
Pansystolic murmur, due to ventricular septal defect, 545
Pantothenic acid deficiency, 114*t*
Papilledema, 686, 686*f*
Papules, 721*t*, 722*f*
in acne, 723
Papulosquamous dermatoses, 729–730
Paracentesis, for peritonitis, 504
Parachute reflex, 682*t*
Paracrine action, of hormones, 637, 637*f*
Paragonimiasis, 451*t*
Paragonimus africanus, 451*t*
Paragonimus heterotremus, 451*t*
Paragonimus kellicotti, 451*t*
Paragonimus skjabini, 451*t*
Paragonimus uterobilateralis, 451*t*
Paragonimus westermani, 451*t*
Parainfluenza virus, croup from, 398–399
Paralysis
flaccid, areflexic, 694
due to hypokalemia, 136
periodic, 698
tick, 695–696
Parameningeal infection, 387*t*
Paraneoplastic syndromes, 609
Paraphimosis, 632
Parapneumonic effusion, 407, 530–531
Parasitic diseases, 447–452
ascariasis, 450
helminthiases as, 449–452
enterobiasis as, 451
hookworm infections of, 450
neurocysticercosis, 452
schistosomiasis as, 451–452
visceral larva migrans, 450–451
protozoal, 447–449
malaria as, 447–449
toxoplasmosis, 449
Parasomnias, 54*t*–55*t*
pediatric sleep disorders and, 55
Parathyroid bone, 669–670, 680
Parathyroid hormone, 669
Parechoviruses, meningitis from, 387
Parenteral nutrition, 130–131
access for, 131
for burn patients, 159
complications of, 131
composition of, 131
indications for, 130–131, 130*t*
Parenteral penicillin, 263
Parenting, 25
Parents' Evaluation of Developmental Status (PEDS), 17
Parinaud oculoglandular syndrome, 430
Parinaud syndrome, 384
Paronychia, viral, 382
Paroxysmal disorders, 687–692, 687*t*. *see also* Seizure(s)
Paroxysmal nocturnal hemoglobinuria, 573*t*
Paroxysmal stage, of pertussis, 400
Partial thromboplastin time (PTT), 583
activated, 584*t*
prolonged, in hemophilia, 587
in newborn, 253
Partial vision, 33
Parvovirus infection, 573*t*
congenital, 260*t*
Pasteurella multocida, 439*t*–442*t*
osteomyelitis from, 425
Patch, 721*t*, 722*f*
Patella, 751*f*
Patellar dislocation, recurrent, 752
Patellar subluxation, recurrent, 752
Patellofemoral disorders, 752
Patellofemoral joint, 752
Patellofemoral pain syndrome (PFPS), 752
Patent airway, 147
Patent ductus arteriosus (PDA), 221–222, 546–547, 546*f*
clinical manifestations of, 244, 546
etiology and epidemiology of, 546
imaging studies for, 547
respiratory distress syndrome and, 243–244
treatment of, 244, 547

Paternalism, 4
Pathogen-associated molecular patterns, 289
Patient-controlled analgesia, 166
Pavlik harness, for developmental dysplasia of the hip, 746
PCD. *see* Primary ciliary dyskinesia
PDA. *see* Patent ductus arteriosus
Peak expiratory flow rate (PEFR), 511
  in asthma, 316
Peak flow monitoring, for asthma, 321
Pectus carinatum, 530
Pectus excavatum, 529
Pediatric acute-onset neuropsychiatric syndrome (PANS), 68
Pediatric advanced life support and cardiopulmonary resuscitation, 147
Pediatric autoimmune neuropsychiatric disorders associated with streptococcal (PANDAS) infection, 68
Pediatric sleep disorders, 52–56, 54*t*–55*t*
  clinical manifestations and evaluation of, 53–55
  differential diagnosis of, 55–56
  epidemiology of, 53
  prevention and treatment of, 56, 56*t*
Pediculoses, 736–737
  capitis, 736
  corporis, 736
  pubis, 736
  treatment of, 736
Pediculosis pubis (crabs), 423*t*
Pediculus humanus capitis, 736
Pediculus humanus corporis, 736
Pediculus humanus humanus, 736
Pedigree
  drawing, 169–170, 170*f*
  for dysmorphology, 184
  in genetic assessment, 178
  in hematology assessment, 563
PEFR (peak expiratory flow rate), 511
  in asthma, 316
Pellagra, 113
Pelvic inflammatory disease, 420–421, 420*t*
  dysmenorrhea due to, 277
PEM. *see* Protein-energy malnutrition
Penicillamine, as teratogen, 237*t*
Penicillin
  allergic reaction to, 338
    desensitization for, 339
    skin testing for, 339
  for streptococcal pharyngitis, 393–394
Penicillin G
  for Lyme disease, 444
  for syphilis, 424
Penicillin V, for pharyngitis, 394
Penicilloyl polylysine, in skin testing for penicillin allergy, 339
Penis, disorders of, 632
Peptic ulcer disease, 485–486
  clinical manifestations of, 486, 486*t*
  etiology and epidemiology of, 485–486
  gastrointestinal bleeding due to, 477*t*
  laboratory and imaging studies for, 486
  risk factors for, 485–486, 486*t*
  treatment of, 486
  vomiting due to, 473*t*
Peptide hormones, 637
Percussion, 510*t*
Perennial allergic rhinitis, 323
Perianal dermatitis, 380
Pericardiocentesis, for pericarditis, 558
Pericarditis, 558, 559*t*
Perinatal care, 1
Perinatal history, 221*t*
  present, 221*t*
  prior, 221*t*
Perinatal mortality, 218, 219*t*
Perinatal period, obesity and, 107–108
Periodic breathing, 509*t*
Periodic fever, aphthous stomatitis, pharyngitis, and cervical adenitis (PFAPA) syndrome, 393
Periodic paralysis, 698
Periorbital cellulitis, 395, 433*t*
Periorbital hemangioma, 732–733
Periosteal elevation, in osteomyelitis, 426
Periosteal fat line, loss of, in osteomyelitis, 426
Peripheral chemoreceptors, in control of ventilation, 513, 514*f*
Peripheral destruction
  in pancytopenia, 575
  thrombocytopenia resulting from, 584
Peripheral neuropathy, 695–696
  in chronic inflammatory demyelinating polyneuropathy, 695
  in Guillain-Barré syndrome, 695
  in hereditary motor sensory neuropathy (Charcot-Marie-Tooth disease), 695
  in tick paralysis, 695–696
Peripheral pulmonary stenosis murmur, 538*t*
Peripherally inserted central catheter (PICC), 437
  for parenteral nutrition, 131
Peristaltic waves, in pyloric stenosis, 485
Peritoneal dialysis-associated infections, 438
Peritonitis, 504–505
  in nephrotic syndrome, 621
  tuberculous, 454
Peritonsillar abscess, upper airway obstruction due to, 517*t*
Periventricular hemorrhage, in newborn, 257
Periventricular leukomalacia, in newborn, 257
Permanent teeth, 479*t*
Permethrin, for prevention of zoonoses, 439
Pernicious anemia, 117
Peroxisomal disorders, 208–209
Peroxisomes, 208–209
Persistent depressive disorder, 65
Persistent middle ear effusion, otitis media and, 397
Persistent pulmonary hypertension of the newborn (PPHN), 222, 246
Personal-social development, milestones of, 17*t*
Pertussis, 400–401
  complications and prognosis of, 401
  differential diagnosis of, 401
  epidemiology of, 400
  etiology of, 400
  laboratory and imaging studies for, 400–401
  prevention of, 401
  treatment of, 401
Pertussis vaccine, 363–364
Pes cavus, 739*t*
  in hereditary motor sensory neuropathy, 695
Pes planus, 739*t*
  hypermobile, 754
Petechiae, 721*t*
  in anemia, 568
  in hematological disorders, 563
  in hemostatic disorders, 583
Petechial-purpuric rash, infections with fever and, 373*t*–374*t*
PFPS (patellofemoral pain syndrome), 752
PHACE syndrome, 732–733
Phagocytic disorders, 301*t*
Phagocytosis, 301*t*
Pharmacodynamics, 367
Pharmacokinetics, 367
Pharmacotherapy
  for anxiety disorders, 63–64
  for enuresis, 49
Pharyngitis, 392–394
  causes of, 392*t*
  clinical manifestations of, 392–393
  complications and prognosis of, 394
  differential diagnosis of, 393
  epidemiology of, 392
  etiology of, 392
  laboratory evaluation of, 393
  treatment of, 393–394, 394*t*
Pharynx, 507
Phencyclidine, acute effects of, 284*t*–285*t*
Phenobarbital
  maternal use of, 238*t*
  for status epilepticus, 691, 691*t*
Phenylalanine, metabolism of, 202*f*
Phenylalanine hydroxylase (PAH) deficiency, 173*t*
Phenylephrine, for allergic rhinitis, 325
Phenylketonuria (PKU), 201–202, 202*f*
  genetic basis for, 173*t*, 198*t*, 201–202
  maternal, 236*t*
  outcome of, 202
  as teratogens, 176
  treatment of, 202
Phenytoin
  for status epilepticus, 691, 691*t*
  as teratogen, 237*t*
Philtrum, 183*t*
Phimosis, 632
Phlebitis, due to parenteral nutrition, 131
Phobias, 63
Phosphate, 669
Phosphorylase kinase deficiency, 200*t*
Photosensitivity, in systemic lupus erythematosus, 353
Phototherapy, for indirect hyperbilirubinemia, 252
PHOX2B gene, in congenital central hypoventilation syndrome, 514
Phrenic nerve palsy, 233
Phthirus pubis, 425
Phylloquinone, 118
Physeal fractures, 742–743
Physical abuse, 80–82, 80*t*
  abdominal trauma due to, 81
  bruises due to, 80–81, 81*f*
  burns due to, 81, 81*f*
  differential diagnosis of, 81–82, 83*t*
  fractures due to, 81, 82*f*
  head trauma due to, 81, 82*f*
Physical activity history, for obesity, 107
Physical criteria, for newborn maturity and gestational age, 227–228, 228*f*
Physical examination
  for cancer, 595
  in cardiovascular system assessment, 535–538
  in hematology assessment, 563, 564*t*
  in hemostatic disorders, 583
  in neurology assessment, 681
  of newborn, 227–231
  for obesity, 107
  for skin disorders, 721
Physical maturation, changes associated with, 273
Physiological nadir, 566
Physiological stability, in anemia, 568
Physis, 740*f*
Pica, 571
Pierre Robin sequence, 184
Pierre Robin syndrome, 227*t*
Pigmented lesions, 730–732
  acquired nevi as, 732
  café au lait macules as, 731, 731*f*
  congenital melanocytic nevi as, 731–732, 731*f*
    giant, 732
    hairy, 731–732, 731*f*
  dermal melanosis as, 730, 731*f*
  differential diagnosis of, 730, 730*t*

Pigmented nevi, giant, 731–732
Pill ulcers, 484
Pimecrolimus, for atopic dermatitis, 327–328
Pinworm, 450*t*, 451
Pituitary function, assessment of, 638
Pituitary hormone, 637–638, 638*f*
Pituitary thyroid-stimulating hormone (TSH), 663
Pityriasis rosea, 729
PKU. *see* Phenylketonuria
Placenta previa, 217
Placental abruption, 217
Placing reflex, 682*t*
Plagiocephaly, 183*t*, 185
  and torticollis, 760
Plague, 439*t*–442*t*
Plain x-rays, for infectious diseases, 362–363
Plantar surface, of newborn, 228*f*
Plantar warts, 382
Plaque, 721*t*, 722*f*
Plasma, fresh frozen, 590*t*
Plasma creatinine, 619
Plasma lipids, alterations in, 580
Plasma osmolality, 125
Plasma water, 125
Plasminogen, 589
Plasmodium, 447, 448*t*
  life cycle of, 447, 448*f*
Plasmodium falciparum, 448*t*
Plasmodium knowlesi, 448*t*
Plasmodium malariae, 448*t*
Plasmodium ovale, 448*t*
Plasmodium vivax, 448*t*
Platelet concentrate, 590*t*
Platelet count, 583, 584*t*
Platelet function, disorders of, 586
Platelet function analyzer (PFA), 584*t*
Platelet plug, in hemostasis, 580
Platelets
  activated, 580
  disorders of, 583, 592
  production, decreased, thrombocytopenia resulting from, 584
Pleiotropy, 171
Pleura disorders, 529–532
  pleural effusion as, 530–532
  pneumomediastinum as, 530
  pneumothorax as, 530
Pleural effusion, 405, 510*t*, 530–532
  clinical manifestations of, 531
  diagnostic studies for, 531–532, 531*t*
  etiology of, 530–531, 531*f*
  treatment of, 532
Plexiform neurofibroma, 730*t*
Pluripotential progenitor stem cells, 563
Pneumatic otoscopic examination, 36
Pneumatic otoscopy, in otitis media, 396
Pneumatic vests, 513
Pneumatocele, 407
Pneumatosis intestinalis, due to necrotizing enterocolitis, 254–255
Pneumococcal polysaccharide vaccines, 364*f*–365*f*
Pneumocystis jiroveci, in immunocompromised person, 434–435
Pneumomediastinum, 530
Pneumonia, 120–121, 402–408, 523
  afebrile, 403, 404*t*
  atypical, 402–403
  broncho-, 402–403
  clinical manifestations of, 403–405
  complications and prognosis for, 407
  differential diagnosis of, 406, 406*t*
  epidemiology of, 403
  etiology of, 402–403, 404*t*
  fever due to, 368
Pneumonia *(Continued)*
  giant cell (Hecht), due to measles, 375
  in immunocompromised persons, 403
  laboratory and imaging studies for, 405–406, 405*f*–406*f*
  lobar, 402–403
  meconium aspiration, 245
  in neonates, 403, 404*t*
  prevention of, 407–408
  treatment of, 406, 407*t*
  ventilator-associated, 438
  viral, 403
  vomiting due to, 473*t*
Pneumonitis, 402–403
  interstitial, 402–403
Pneumothorax, 244*f*, 510*t*, 530
  due to assisted ventilation in newborn, 244
  clinical manifestations of, 530
  diagnostic studies for, 530
  etiology of, 530
  in newborn, 227
  secondary, 530
  spontaneous primary, 530
  tension, 530
  treatment of, 530
Point mutation, 169
Poisoning, 160–165
  clinical manifestations of, 160, 161*t*
  complications of, 160–163
    coma as, 160
    direct toxicity as, 160–162
    dysrhythmias as, 162, 163*t*
    gastrointestinal symptoms as, 163
    metabolic acidosis as, 162, 162*t*
    seizures as, 163
  epidemiology of, 160
  etiology of, 160
  laboratory and imaging studies of, 163, 164*t*
  prevention of, 165
  prognosis for, 165
  treatment of, 163–164
    enhanced elimination for, 164
    gastrointestinal decontamination for, 164
    specific antidotes for, 164, 164*t*–165*t*
    supportive care for, 163–164
Polio vaccine, 363–364
Pollen-food allergy syndrome, 335*t*–336*t*
Polyarthritis, due to heart failure, 556*t*
Polycystic kidney disease (PKD), 629–630
  autosomal dominant, 630
  autosomal recessive, 630
Polycystic ovary syndrome, amenorrhea due to, 275
Polycythemia
  cyanotic congenital heart disease with, 584
  in newborn, 252
  presentation of, 564*t*
Polydactyly, 183*t*, 185
  of digits, 765
  of toes, 755, 756*t*
Polydipsia, in insulin-dependent diabetes mellitus, 641
Polyethylene glycol (GoLYTELY), for poisoning, 164
Polyethylene glycol electrolyte solution, for functional constipation, 51*t*
Polygenic inheritance, 173–174
  hypertrophic pyloric stenosis due to, 174–175
  neural tube defects due to, 175
Polyhydramnios, 218
Polymerase chain reaction (PCR), 362
  for HIV, 460
Polymicrogyria, 717
Polymorphonuclear cells, as lung defense mechanisms, 508
Polyp, juvenile, gastrointestinal bleeding due to, 477*t*
Polysomnography, 55, 515
Polyuria, fluid therapy for, 127, 127*t*
Pompe disease, 200*t*, 698
Popliteal angle, in newborn, 229*f*
Popliteal cyst, 751
Population, 1–3, 8–9
  changing morbidity and, 3
  culture and, 3
  current challenges in, 1
  health disparities in, 3
  landscape of, 1–2, 2*t*
  other health issues affecting, 2–3
  in society, 1
Pork tapeworm, 452
Port-a-Cath (implanted venous access systems), infections associated with, 437
Port-wine stain, 228, 733, 733*f*
  differential diagnosis of, 730*t*
  in Klippel-Trénaunay-Weber syndrome, 733
  in Sturge-Weber syndrome, 715, 733
Portal hypertension, 497
Portion sizes, age-appropriate, 108–109
Portosystemic shunts, 498
Positive reinforcement, 16
Positron emission tomography (PET), for cancer, 596, 599*t*
Post-traumatic stress disorder, due to domestic violence, 91
Posterior fossa, tumors in, ataxia due to, 701
Posterior fossa syndrome, central nervous system and, 608
Posterior urethral valves, 630
Posterior uveitis, 433*t*
Postexposure prophylaxis, for measles, 375
Postherpetic neuralgia, 379
  varicella zoster virus and, 378
Postmenopausal osteoporosis, 119
Postmitotic maturing cells, 563
Postnatal genetic assessment, 178
Postobstructive pulmonary edema, 524
Postpericardiotomy syndrome, 558
Postseptal cellulitis, 395, 433*t*
Poststreptococcal arthritis (PsA), 352*t*
Poststreptococcal glomerulonephritis (PSGN)
  clinical manifestations of, 622–623
  etiology and epidemiology of, 622
  therapy for, 623
Posttransplant lymphoproliferative disorder (PTLD), 435
Posttraumatic seizures, 710
Postural roundback, 760
Posture
  assessment of, 683
  of newborn, 229*f*, 682
  vs. foot deformity, 752
Potassium, for diabetic ketoacidosis, 642–643
Potassium disorders, 134–138
  hyperkalemia as, 137–138
  hypokalemia as, 134–137, 135*t*
Pott disease, 454
Pott puffy tumor, 395
Potter syndrome, 217–218, 227*t*, 629
Poverty, health disparities and, 3
PPD-S (purified protein derivative standard), 454
PPHN (persistent pulmonary hypertension of the newborn), 222
PR interval, 539
Prader-Willi syndrome (PWS), 653
  genetic basis for, 175–176, 183–184
  hypotonia in, 698–699
  obesity in, 106*t*
Pralidoxime, for organophosphate poisoning, 164*t*–165*t*

Preadoption visit, 89
Precocious puberty, 659–663
  central, 660
  classification of, 659–660
  differential diagnosis of, 661*t*
  familial male-limited, 662
  GnRH-dependent, 660
  GnRH-independent, 660–662
Preconception genetic assessment, 177–178
  adolescent and adult, 178
  familial factors in, 177
  maternal factors in, 177–178
  postnatal, 178
  screening in, 177
Precordium, hyperdynamic, with patent ductus arteriosus, 546–547
Prednisolone, for croup, 399–400
Prednisone, 527
  for asthma, 316
  for cancer, 601*t*–602*t*
  for Henoch-Schönlein purpura, 347
  for idiopathic thrombocytopenic purpura, 585
  for nephrotic syndrome, 621
  for serum sickness, 333
Preeclampsia, 218
Pregnancy
  adolescent, 277–278
    continuation of, 278
    diagnosis of, 278
    termination of, 278
  assessment during, 217
  complications of, 217
    hydrops fetalis as, 218
    maternal medical, 217
    with multiple gestations, 218
    obstetric, 217
    oligohydramnios as, 217–218
    placenta previa as, 217
    placental abruption as, 217
    polyhydramnios as, 218
    preeclampsia/eclampsia as, 218
    premature rupture of membranes as, 218
    prolonged rupture of membranes as, 218
    vaginal bleeding as, 217
  genetic assessment during, 177–179
    familial factors in, 177
    maternal factors, 177–178
    postnatal, 178
    screening in, 177
  high-risk, 217
  maternal diseases during, 235
    antiphospholipid syndrome as, 235
    diabetes mellitus as, 236*t*–237*t*, 237
    hyperthyroidism as, 236
    idiopathic thrombocytopenic purpura as, 235–236, 236*t*
    other, 237
    systemic lupus erythematosus as, 236, 236*t*
  toxemia of, 218
  vomiting due to, 473*t*
Pregnancy history
  for dysmorphology, 184
  in genetic assessment, 184
Prehospital trauma care, 155
Preicteric phase, of viral hepatitis, 413
Preload, in heart failure, 553, 554*t*
Premature atrial contractions, 543
Premature pubarche, 663
Premature rupture of membranes, 218
Premature ventricular contractions (PVCs), 543, 544*t*
Prematurity
  apnea of, 246, 514, 514*t*
  retinopathy of, 245
Premenstrual dysphoric disorder (PDD), 65
Premutation carriers, in fragile X syndrome, 176
Prenatal care, 1
Prenatal genetic assessment, 177–178
  adolescent and adult, 178
  familial factors in, 177
  maternal factors in, 177–178
  postnatal, 178
  screening in, 177
Prenatal history, in cardiovascular system assessment, 535
Prerenal azotemia, 625
  due to shock, 154
Preschool children
  obesity in, 107–108
  reaction to divorce by, 94
Preschool readiness, 15
Preseptal (periorbital) cellulitis, 395
Preslip condition, 747
Presumptive antiinfective therapy, 367
Preterm births, 1, 218
Preterm infants, sepsis in, 258
Priapism, in sickle cell disease, 577, 577*t*
Primaquine, maternal use of, 238*t*
Primary ciliary dyskinesia (PCD), 523
Primary enuresis, 48
Primary hypoparathyroidism, 669, 670*t*
Primary survey, of trauma patient, 155
Primary teeth, 479, 479*t*
Primitive neonatal reflexes, 14
Procedural sedation, 165
Proctocolitis, allergic, 335*t*–336*t*
Professionalism, 3–4
Progesterone withdrawal test, for amenorrhea, 275
Progressive primary disease, 453
Progressive symptoms, in neurology assessment, 681
Prolonged QT syndrome, 539
Prolonged rupture of membranes, 218
Promoter sequence, 169
Pronator drift, 684
Proopiomelanocortin deficiency, obesity in, 106*t*
Properdin, 304–305
  deficiency of, 306
Prophase analysis, in genetic assessment, 179
Prophylaxis, 366
  immunization and, 363–366
  for meningococcus, 366
  postexposure, for measles, 375
  primary, 366
  for rabies, 366
  secondary, 366
  for tetanus, 366, 367*t*
Propionate pathway, 206*f*
Propionibacterium acnes, 723
Propionic acidemia, 205, 206*f*
  clinical manifestations of, 206
  neonatal screening for, 198*t*, 205
  treatment of, 206
Propofol, for sedation, 166*t*
Propranolol, maternal use of, 238*t*
Propylthiouracil, maternal use of, 238*t*
Prostaglandin E_1
  for coarctation of aorta, 548
  for hypoplastic left heart syndrome, 553
  for transposition of great arteries, 551
Protein C, 581, 589
Protein carrier, 363–364
Protein-energy malnutrition (PEM), 109
Protein S, 581, 589
Proteinuria, 620–622
  asymptomatic, 620
  clinical manifestations of, 621
  complications of, 621
  diagnostic studies of, 621
  differential diagnosis of, 621
  etiology and epidemiology of, 620–621
Proteinuria *(Continued)*
  fixed, 620
  glomerular, 620
  persistent, 620
  postural, 621
  prognosis for, 622
  symptomatic, 620
  transient, 620
  treatment of, 621
  tubular, 620
Prothrombin time (PT), 583, 584*t*
  in newborn, 253
Proton-pump inhibitor, for gastroesophageal reflux, 481*t*
Protozoal disease, 447–449
  malaria as, 447–449
  toxoplasmosis, 449
  zoonotic, 439*t*–442*t*
Proximal humeral epiphysiolysis, 763
Proximal tubule, 617, 619*f*
Pruritus ani, 451
PsA (poststreptococcal arthritis), 352*t*
Pseudo-Hurler polydystrophy, 210*t*–212*t*
Pseudocyst, pancreatic, 502
Pseudoephedrine, for allergic rhinitis, 325
Pseudohypertrophy, 684
Pseudohypoaldosteronism (PHA) type 1, 138
Pseudohyponatremia, 131–132
Pseudohypoparathyroidism, 653, 669, 670*t*
  obesity in, 106*t*
Pseudomembranous colitis, gastrointestinal bleeding due to, 477*t*
Pseudomonas aeruginosa
  conjunctivitis from, 430
  in cystic fibrosis, 527
  folliculitis due to, 380
  osteomyelitis from, 425–426
  otitis externa from, 397–398
  pneumonia from, 407*t*
Pseudomonas chondritis, 425–426
Pseudoparalysis, from osteomyelitis, 426
Pseudoseizures, 689–690
Pseudotumor cerebri, 707–708
PSGN. *see* Poststreptococcal glomerulonephritis
Psilocybin, acute effects of, 284*t*–285*t*
Psittacosis, 439*t*–442*t*
Psoriasis, 729–730
  plaque-type, 729–730
  treatment of, 730
  vs. atopic dermatitis, 725
  vulgaris, 729–730
Psychiatric disorders, 59–73
  anxiety disorders, 61–64
  autism spectrum disorder and schizophrenia spectrum disorders, 70–73
  depressive disorders and bipolar disorders, 64–68
  in medical conditions, 59–60, 60*t*
  obsessive-compulsive disorder (OCD), 68–70, 69*t*
  somatic symptom and related disorders (SSRDs), 59–61, 60*t*
Psychogenic nonepileptic seizures, 689–690
Psychological development, of adolescent, 270*t*
Psychological intervention, for child with special needs, 32
Psychological problems, in sickle cell disease, 577*t*
Psychosocial assessment, 15–16
  of adolescence, 15–16
  of bonding and attachment in infancy, 15
  of developing autonomy in early childhood, 15
  of early childhood, 15
  of infancy, 15
  of school readiness, 15, 15*t*

Psychosocial behaviors, modification of, 16
Psychosocial dwarfism, 653
Psychosocial issues, 77–96
bereavement as, 93–96
child abuse and neglect as, 80–84
divorce as, 93–96
failure to thrive as, 77–79
family structure and function as, 87–91
homosexuality and gender identity as, 84–87
separation as, 93–96
violence as, 91–93
Psychosocial problems, 3
Psychosocial short stature, 79
Psychosocial treatments, for schizophrenia spectrum disorders, 73
Psychotherapy, for depressive disorders, 66
Psychotropics, constipation due to, 476*t*
PT (prothrombin time), 583, 584*t*
in newborn, 253
PTT (partial thromboplastin time), 583
activated, 584*t*
prolonged, in hemophilia, 587
in newborn, 253
Pubarche, 656
in boys, 271–273, 272*f*
in girls, 270–271, 271*f*–272*f*
isolated premature, 663
Pubertal development
for boys, 271–273, 272*f*
for girls, 270–271, 271*f*–272*f*
variations in, 274–275, 663
breast asymmetry and masses as, 274, 274*t*
gynecomastia as, 274–275, 274*t*
irregular menses as, 274
physiological leukorrhea as, 274
Puberty, 656–663, 679–680
delayed, 656–659
classification of, 657*t*
due to CNS abnormalities, 657
due to constitutional delay, 656
differential diagnostic feature of, 658*t*
evaluation of, 659
due to hypergonadotropic hypogonadism, 658–659
due to hypogonadotropic hypogonadism, 656, 658
due to idiopathic hypopituitarism, 657
due to isolated gonadotropin deficiency, 657
due to Kallmann syndrome, 657
primary amenorrhea as, 659
treatment of, 659
physiology of, 656
precocious, 659–663
central, 660
classification of, 659–660
differential diagnosis of, 661*t*
familial male-limited, 662
GnRH-dependent, 660
GnRH-independent, 660–662
Pubic hair growth
in boys, 271–273, 272*f*
in girls, 270–271, 271*f*–272*f*
Pubic lice, 736
Public health, legal issues in, 5
Pulmonary air leaks, due to assisted ventilation in newborn, 244
Pulmonary angiography, of pulmonary embolism, 526
Pulmonary arterial hypertension (PAH), 524–525
Pulmonary blood flow, in cardiovascular system assessment, 539
Pulmonary capillaritis, 525
Pulmonary capillary blood flow, 508
Pulmonary disease, physical signs of, 510*t*
Pulmonary edema, 523–524
in coarctation of aorta, 548
Pulmonary embolism, 526
Pulmonary function testing, 511
Pulmonary hemorrhage, 525–526, 525*t*
Pulmonary hemosiderosis, 335*t*–336*t*
idiopathic, 525
Pulmonary hypoplasia, 240, 246, 522
Pulmonary maturity, of fetus, 219–220
Pulmonary mechanics, 507–508, 508*f*
Pulmonary physiology, 507–509
lung defense mechanisms in, 508–509
pulmonary mechanics in, 507–508, 508*f*
respiratory gas exchange in, 508, 508*t*
Pulmonary sequestration, 522
Pulmonary stenosis, 547–548
murmur, in tetralogy of Fallot, 549
in tetralogy of Fallot, 549
Pulmonary surfactant, 219–220
in lung development, 242
Pulmonary toxicity, due to poisoning, 160
Pulse oximetry, 511
for bronchiolitis, 402
in cardiovascular system assessment, 538
for respiratory failure, 150
Pulse pressure
in cardiovascular system assessment, 535
in dilated cardiomyopathy, 558
with patent ductus arteriosus, 546–547
Pulsed Doppler studies, 620
Puncture wounds, osteomyelitis from, 425–426
Punishment, 16
physical (corporal), 25
Pupil, Marcus Gunn, 683
Pupillary defect, afferent, 683
Pupillary light reactions, 683
Purified protein derivative standard (PPD-S), 454
Purine nucleotides, 169
Purpura, 721*t*
in anemia, 568
in hematological disorders, 563
in hemostatic disorders, 583
idiopathic thrombocytopenic, 584–585
bleeding disorder in newborn due to, 254
clinical manifestations of, 585
diagnosis of, 585
etiology of, 584–585
maternal, 235–236, 236*t*
neonatal thrombocytopenia due to, 254
prognosis for, 585
treatment of, 585
neonatal alloimmune thrombocytopenic, 584
palpable, 345
thrombotic thrombocytopenic, 585–586, 624
in thrombotic microangiopathy, 580
Pustular melanosis, 228–229
Pustular rash, infections with fever and, 373*t*–374*t*
Pustules, 721*t*, 722*f*
in acne, 723
PVCs (premature ventricular contractions), 543, 544*t*
PWS. *see* Prader-Willi syndrome
Pyelogram, intravenous, 620
Pyelonephritis, 416
abdominal pain due to, 470*t*
Pyloric stenosis, 472, 484–485
clinical manifestations of, 485
etiology and epidemiology of, 484–485
laboratory and imaging studies for, 485, 485*f*
treatment of, 485
vomiting due to, 473*t*, 485
Pyogenic granuloma, 733
Pyrazinamide, for tuberculosis, 455–456, 457*t*
Pyridostigmine, maternal use of, 238*t*
Pyridoxal phosphate, 113–114
Pyrimethamine, for toxoplasmosis, 449
Pyrogens, 368
Pyropoikilocytosis, hereditary, 578–579
Pyruvate, metabolism of, 214*f*
Pyruvate kinase deficiency
in anemia, 566
in enzymopathies, 578
Pyuria, 417

Q

Q fever, 439*t*–442*t*
QRS complex, 539
QT interval, 539
Quad screen, 177
Quadriplegia, due to cerebral palsy, 37*t*
Quartan periodicity, of *P. malariae*, 447

R

Rabies, 439*t*–442*t*
prophylaxis for, 366
Rabies immune globulin (RIG), 366
Raccoon eyes, 710
Rachitic rosary, 118
Radial head subluxation, 764, 764*f*
Radiation
heat loss via, 234
as teratogen, 177, 237*t*
Radiation therapy, 601
adverse effects of, 601, 603*t*
Radioactive iodine
maternal use of, 238*t*
as teratogens, 237*t*
Radiofrequency ablation, 543–544
Radiographs, for cancer, 596
Radioiodine, 668
Radiology, for gastrointestinal symptoms, 467
Radionuclide scans, 362
Radioulnar synostosis, 185
Radius, distal, Salter-Harris fractures of, 765
RAG1 (recombinase activating gene 1), in severe combined immunodeficiency, 297–298
RAG2 (recombinase activating gene 2), in severe combined immunodeficiency, 297–298
Rales, 510
Ramsay Hunt syndrome, varicella zoster virus and, 378
RANTES, functions of, 290*t*
Rape, 281
date, 92
defined, 281
forensic material from, 281
therapy after, 281
Rapid eye movement (REM) sleep, 52
Rapid plasma reagin (RPR) test, 424
Rapid tests, 362
Rapidly progressive glomerulonephritis, 622
Rash
infections with fever and, 373–379
differential diagnosis of, 373*t*–374*t*
erythema infectiosum (fifth disease) as, 377–378
measles (rubeola) as, 373–375
roseola infantum (exanthem subitum), 376–377
rubella (German or 3-day measles), 375–376
varicella-zoster virus infection (chickenpox and zoster), 378–379
in juvenile dermatomyositis, 355–356
in juvenile idiopathic arthritis, 351
in systemic lupus erythematosus, 353
Rat-bite fever, 439*t*–442*t*
Raynaud phenomenon, in systemic lupus erythematosus, 353
Re-feeding syndrome, 79

Reactivation pulmonary tuberculosis, 453
Reactive arthritis, 428
  juvenile idiopathic arthritis *vs.*, 352*t*
  synovial fluid findings in, 429*t*
Rear-facing safety seat, 22
Rebuck skin window, 303–304
Recoil, 682
Recombinant factor concentrates, 590*t*
Recombinant factor VIIa, 590*t*
Recombinase activating gene 1 *(RAG1)*, in severe combined immunodeficiency, 297–298
Recombinase activating gene 2 *(RAG2)*, in severe combined immunodeficiency, 297–298
Rectal biopsy, for Hirschsprung disease, 489–490
Rectal structure, anemia and, 569*t*
Red blood cell (RBC)
  decreased production of, newborn anemia due, 247
  disorders extrinsic to, hemolytic anemia caused by, 579–580
  production, 563–566
  transfusion of, 589–590
Red blood cell aplasias, 573*t*
Red reflex, in newborn, 230
Red strawberry tongue, 393
5α-Reductase deficiency, 673
Reed-Sternberg cells, 606
Refeeding syndrome, 112
Reflex rhinitis, 324
Reflexes
  of child, 684
  of neonates, 682, 682*t*
  primitive, 682
    neonatal, 14
Reflux, vesicoureteral. *see* Vesicoureteral reflux
Reflux nephropathy, 628–629
Regurgitation, vomiting *vs.*, 472
Rehydration, oral, 129
Reinforcement
  negative, 16
  positive, 16
Relapsing fever, 439*t*–442*t*
  louse-borne, 737
Reliability, 4
Religious issues, ethics and, 6
Renal abscess, 416
Renal agenesis, 227*t*
Renal disease
  common manifestations of, 618, 618*t*
  imaging studies of, 620
  primary, 618, 618*t*
  risk factors for, 617
  secondary, 618
Renal failure
  acute kidney injury, 625–626
  chronic kidney disease, 626–627
    complications and treatments of, 627*t*
    etiology and epidemiology of, 626
    prognosis for, 627
    treatment of, 627
  with fulminant liver failure, 500*t*
  indications for renal replacement therapy, 626*t*
  treatment of, 626
Renal hypoplasia/dysplasia, 629
Renal injury, 156–157
  in hemolytic uremic syndrome, 624
Renal involvement
  in Henoch-Schönlein purpura, 346
  in systemic lupus erythematosus, 353
Renal medullary carcinoma, risk factors for, 597*t*
Renal output, altered, fluid therapy for, 127*t*
Renal physiology, 617–618, 619*f*
Renal salvage, for shock, 154
Renal tubular acidosis
  distal, 140
  hyperkalemic, 140
  proximal, 140
Renal tubular function, disordered, in galactosemia, 201
Renal ultrasound, 625–626
Renin, in renal function, 617
Renin-angiotensin system, 125
Replacement solution, for gastrointestinal losses, 126–127, 127*t*
Replacement therapy, 126–127
  for hemophilia, 587
Research, children as human subject in, 6
Reserpine, maternal use of, 238*t*
Residual volume (RV), 507–508, 508*f*
Respect for others
  autonomy and, 4
  in professionalism, 4
Respiration
  agonal, 509*t*
  apneustic, 509*t*
  Biot, 509*t*
  Cheyne-Stokes, 509*t*, 705–706
  Kussmaul, 509*t*
Respiratory acidosis, 142*t*
  in newborn, 241
Respiratory alkalosis, 142*t*
Respiratory compensation, appropriate, 139, 139*t*
Respiratory disease
  assessment of
    breathing patterns in, 509*t*
    endoscopic evaluation of airways in, 511
    examination of sputum in, 511–512
    history in, 509
    imaging techniques in, 510–511
    lung biopsy in, 512
    measures of respiratory gas exchange in, 511
    physical examination in, 509–510, 509*t*–510*t*, 510*f*
    pulmonary function testing in, 511
  of newborn, 240–246
  therapeutic measures for, 512–513
    aerosol therapy as, 512, 512*f*
    chest physiotherapy and clearance techniques as, 513
    intubation as, 513
    mechanical ventilation as, 513
    oxygen administration as, 512
    tracheostomy as, 513
Respiratory distress
  cyanosis with/without, 549*t*
  with desaturation, 549*t*
  with normal saturation, 549*t*
Respiratory distress syndrome (RDS), 241–243
  acute, 149
  bronchopulmonary dysplasia due to, 244–245
  clinical manifestations of, 242, 243*f*
  lung development and, 241, 242*f*
  patent ductus arteriosus due to, 221–222
  potential causes of, 243*t*
  prevention and treatment of, 242–243
  pulmonary air leaks due to, 244
  and retinopathy of prematurity, 245
Respiratory failure, 145, 149–151
  acute, due to shock, 154
  chronic, 149
  clinical manifestations of, 149
  complications of, 150
  differential diagnosis of, 150
  epidemiology of, 149
  etiology of, 149
  hypercarbic, 149–150
  hypoxemic, 149
Respiratory failure *(Continued)*
  hypoxic, 150
  laboratory and imaging studies of, 149–150
  mixed forms of, 150
  prevention of, 150–151
  prognosis for, 150
  treatment of, 150
Respiratory gas exchange, 508, 508*t*
  measures of, 511
Respiratory rate
  assessment of, 509, 509*t*
  in cardiovascular system assessment, 535
  of newborn, 227
Respiratory support, for shock, 153–154
Respiratory syncytial virus (RSV)
  bronchiolitis and, 401
  croup from, 398–399
Respiratory system, 507–532
  anatomy of, 507
  assessment of, 507–513
    breathing patterns in, 509*t*
    history in, 509
    physical examination in, 509–510, 509*t*–510*t*, 510*f*
  physiology of, 507–509
    lung defense mechanisms in, 508–509
    pulmonary mechanics in, 507–508, 508*f*
    respiratory gas exchange in, 508, 508*t*
Responsibility, 4
Rest, for heart failure, 555*t*
Restless legs syndrome, 54*t*–55*t*
Restrictive cardiomyopathies, 557*t*
  clinical manifestations of, 558
  etiology of, 556
  imaging studies for, 558
  treatment of, 558
Restrictive lung disease, 508
Resuscitation, 146–147
  for drowning, 157
  fluid, for shock, 153
  of newborn, 225, 226*f*
    breathing in, 225–226
    cyanosis as, 232, 232*t*
    specific conditions requiring, 232–234
      life-threatening congenital malformations as, 232–233
      shock as, 233
Reticular dysgenesis, neutropenia in, 301
Reticulate bodies, in *Chlamydia* infection, 423
Reticulocytes
  count of, 568
  in erythropoiesis, 563–566
  values of, 565*t*
Retinoblastoma, risk factors for, 597*t*
Retinoids, topical, for acne, 723
Retinol, 117
Retinopathy of prematurity, 245
Retrolental fibroplasia, 245
Retropharyngeal abscess, upper airway obstruction due to, 517*t*
Retroviral syndrome, acute, 384
Rett syndrome, 173, 711*t*–712*t*, 713
  genetic basis for, 183–184
Reye syndrome, hyperammonemia *vs.*, 192
Rh antigen system, 247–248
Rh blood group incompatibility, erythroblastosis fetalis due to, 247–248
Rh sensitization
  management of, 248
  maternal, 236*t*
Rhabdomyolysis, 213–214
  due to hypokalemia, 136
Rhabdomyosarcoma (RMS), 611
  alveolar, 612
  clinical manifestations of, 612
  differential diagnosis of, 612

Rhabdomyosarcoma (RMS) *(Continued)*
  embryonal, 612
  epidemiology of, 611
  laboratory/imaging studies in, 612
  prognosis for, 613
  risk factors for, 597*t*
  treatment of, 612
Rheumatic diseases
  assessment of, 343–345, 344*t*
    common manifestations in, 343–345, 345*t*
    diagnostic imaging in, 345
    differential diagnosis of, 344*t*
    history in, 343
    initial diagnostic evaluation in, 345
    laboratory testing in, 345
    physical examination in, 343
  of childhood, 343–358
Rheumatic fever, 556, 556*t*
  differential diagnosis of, 344*t*
Rheumatoid arthritis, synovial fluid findings in, 429*t*
Rhinitis
  allergic, 323–325, 391
  defined, 323
  differential diagnosis of, 323–324, 324*t*
  episodic, 323
  gustatory, 324
  infectious, 323–324
  medicamentosa, 324
  nonallergic, 324
    noninfectious, 324, 324*t*
  reflex, 324
  vasomotor, 324
Rhinosinusitis, chronic infectious, 323–324
Rhipicephalus sanguineus, 444
Rhodopsin, 117
RhoGAM, (anti-Rh-positive immune globulin), 248–249
Rhonchi, 510
Rib notching, in coarctation of aorta, 548
Riboflavin deficiency, 113, 114*t*
Rickets, 118, 670
  clinical manifestations of, 118
  diagnosis of, 118
  familial hypophosphatemic, 670*t*
  vitamin D-resistant, 173
Rickettsia africae, 439*t*–442*t*
Rickettsia akari, 439*t*–442*t*
Rickettsia conorii, 439*t*–442*t*
Rickettsia felis, 439*t*–442*t*
Rickettsia prowazekii, 439*t*–442*t*
Rickettsia rickettsii, 439, 439*t*–442*t*, 444–445
Rickettsia typhi, 439*t*–442*t*
Rickettsial diseases, 439*t*–442*t*
Rickettsialpox, 439*t*–442*t*
Rifampin, for tuberculosis, 455–456, 457*t*
Right axis deviation, in tetralogy of Fallot, 550
Right-to-left shunts, 549
Right ventricular hypertrophy
  in hypoplastic left heart syndrome, 553
  in tetralogy of Fallot, 549–550
Right ventricular impulse
  in tetralogy of Fallot, 549
  in total anomalous pulmonary venous return, 552
Rigid bronchoscopy, 511
Rigidity, 684
Ring form, in *Plasmodium* life cycle, 447
Ringworm, 381*t*
Ristocetin cofactor assay, in von Willebrand disease, 587
Rituximab, for cancer, 601*t*–602*t*
RNA polymerase chain reaction, for HIV, 460
Rocky Mountain spotted fever, 439*t*–442*t*
  clinical manifestations of, 444–445, 445*f*
  complications and prognosis of, 445
  differential diagnosis of, 445
  epidemiology of, 444
  etiology of, 444
  laboratory and imaging studies for, 445
  prevention of, 445
  treatment of, 445
Rolandic epilepsy, 690
Rome III criteria, for pediatric functional gastrointestinal syndromes, 471*t*
Rooting reflex, 14, 231–232, 682*t*, 683
ROP (retinopathy of prematurity), 245
Roseola infantum (exanthem subitum), 376–377
  clinical manifestations of, 376
  complications and prognosis for, 377
  differential diagnosis for, 376–377
  epidemiology of, 376
  etiology of, 376
  laboratory and imaging studies for, 376
  treatment for, 377
Rotation
  external, 739*t*
  internal, 739*t*
Rotavirus (RV), diarrhea from, 410*t*
Rotavirus (RV) vaccines, 363–364, 364*f*–365*f*
RPR (rapid plasma reagin) test, 424
RSV (respiratory syncytial virus)
  bronchiolitis and, 401
  croup from, 398–399
Rubella (German or 3-day measles), 375–376
  clinical manifestations, 375
  complications and prognosis for, 376
  congenital, 260*t*, 261
  differential diagnosis for, 376
  epidemiology of, 375
  etiology of, 375
  laboratory and imaging studies for, 375–376
  prevention of, 376
  as teratogen, 176
  treatment for, 376
Rubella vaccine, 376
  contraindications to, 376
Rules of two, for asthma, 316
Rupture of the membranes
  premature, 218
  prolonged, 218
RV (rotavirus), diarrhea from, 410*t*
RV (rotavirus) vaccines, 363–364, 364*f*–365*f*

S

Sacral lipoma, constipation due to, 476*t*
Sacral teratoma, constipation due to, 476*t*
SAD. *see* Separation anxiety disorder
Salicylates
  intoxication, metabolic acidosis due to, 140
  for rheumatic fever, 556
  toxicity, 162*t*
Salicylic acid, for acne, 723
Salla disease, 210*t*–212*t*
Salmeterol, for asthma, 315
Salmon-colored rash, in juvenile idiopathic arthritis, 351
Salmon fluke, 451*t*
Salmon patch, 228, 730*t*, 733
Salmonella
  diarrhea from, 410*t*
  nontyphoidal, 411, 439*t*–442*t*
  osteomyelitis due to, 426
Salmonellosis, 439*t*–442*t*
Salt intake, for toddlers and older children, 104
Salter-Harris classification, 742, 743*f*
Sandhoff disease, 711*t*–712*t*
Sanfilippo syndrome, 210*t*–212*t*, 711*t*–712*t*, 713
Sarcoma(s), 611–613, 615
  clinical manifestations of, 611–612
  complications of, 613
  differential diagnosis of, 612
  epidemiology of, 611
  etiology of, 611
  Ewing. *see* Ewing sarcoma
  laboratory/imaging studies of, 612
  prognosis for, 613
  treatment of, 612
Sarcoptes scabiei, 735
SARS (severe acute respiratory syndrome), 403
Satellite nevi, 732
Scabies, 735–736
  atopic dermatitis *vs.*, 326
  clinical presentation of, 735–736, 736*f*
  diagnosis of, 736
  Norwegian or crusted, 735–736
  treatment of, 736
SCAD (short-chain acyl-CoA dehydrogenase) deficiency, 207, 207*f*
SCAG (Structured Communication Adolescent Guide), 268*f*–269*f*
Scalding injuries, due to child abuse, 81, 81*f*
Scale, 722*t*
Scalene muscles, during inspiration, 507
Scanogram, of leg-length discrepancy, 750
Scaphocephaly, 183*t*
Scaphoid fracture, 765
Scar, 722*t*
Scarf sign, in newborn, 229*f*
Scarlet fever, 393
Scheuermann kyphosis, 760
  radiological findings of, 760, 760*f*
  treatment of, 760
Schistosoma haematobium, 451, 451*t*
Schistosoma japonicum, 451, 451*t*
Schistosoma mansoni, 451, 451*t*
Schistosoma mekongi, 451, 451*t*
Schistosomiasis, 451–452, 451*t*
  intestinal or hepatic, 451*t*
  urinary, 451*t*
Schistosomiasis intercalatum, 451
Schizencephaly, 717
Schizoaffective disorder, 72
Schizogony, of *Plasmodium* life cycle, 447
Schizophrenia spectrum disorders, 71–73, 72*t*
Schizophreniform disorder, 72
Schnitzler syndrome, 331
School-age children
  obesity and, 107–108
  physical development in, 14
  reaction to divorce by, 94
School readiness, 15, 15*t*
Schwachman-Diamond syndrome, neutropenia in, 301
SCID. *see* Severe combined immunodeficiency
Scleritis, 433*t*
Sclerosis, 722*t*
Scoliosis
  adolescent, 758
  classification of, 756*t*
  clinical evaluation of, 757*f*
  compensatory, 756, 759
  congenital, 758, 759*f*
    treatment of, 758
  idiopathic, 758
    clinical manifestations of, 758
    etiology and epidemiology of, 758
    treatment of, 758
  infantile, 758
  juvenile, 758
  neuromuscular, 758–759
    treatment of, 759
  thoracic, 529

Screening
anemia, 20–21
autism, 17–18
cholesterol, 21, 21*t*
depression, 22
developmental, 16–18
hearing, 20
of children 3 years of age and older, 20
of infants and toddlers, 20
language, 18, 18*t*
lead, 21, 21*t*
newborn, 20
critical congenital heart disease (CCHD), 20
hearing, 20
hemoglobin electrophoresis, 20
metabolic, 20
sexually transmitted infection, 21–22
tuberculosis, 21, 21*t*
vision, 20
of children 3 years of age and older, 20
of infants and toddlers, 20
Screening tests
for cancer, 596
in well child, 17, 20–22
for anemia, 20–21
for cholesterol, 21, 21*t*
for depression, 22
hearing and vision, 20
for lead, 21, 21*t*
newborn, 20
for sexually transmitted infection, 21–22
for tuberculosis, 21, 21*t*
Screening tools, for somatic symptom and related disorders (SSRDs), 61
Scrofula, 454
Scrotum, abnormalities of, 632–633
Scrub typhus, 439*t*–442*t*
Scurvy, 112
Seasonal allergic rhinitis, 323
Seborrheic dermatitis, 728–730
atopic *vs*., 725, 729
clinical manifestations of, 728–729, 729*f*
differential diagnosis of, 729
etiology of, 728
laboratory and imaging studies of, 729
prevention of, 729
prognosis for, 729
treatment of, 729
Second-degree heart block, 543, 544*t*
Second hand cigarette smoke, 91
Second heart sound (S_2), 536
abnormal, 537*t*
in tetralogy of Fallot, 549
in total anomalous pulmonary venous return, 552
in tricuspid atresia, 551
in truncus arteriosus, 551
Second impact syndrome, 709
Secondary enuresis, 48
Secondary ossification center, 740*f*
Secondary pneumothorax, 530
Secondary survey, of trauma patient, 155
Sedation, 165–166, 166*t*
Sedatives, acute effects of, 284*t*–285*t*
Sedentary behavior, obesity and, 109
Sedentary lifestyle, 2
Seizure(s), 687–692, 733
absence, 688–689
atonic, 689
atypical, 689
due to inborn errors of metabolism, 195*t*
myoclonic, 689
causes of, 688*t*
classification of, 687, 688*t*
clonic, 688
Seizure(s) *(Continued)*
differential diagnosis of, 687, 687*t*
in epilepsy syndrome, 688*t*, 690
etiology and epidemiology of, 687, 687*t*–688*t*
febrile, 689
complex, 689
simple, 689
focal, 687–688, 689*t*
with altered awareness, 687–688
with retained awareness, 687
generalized, 688–690
impact, 710
laboratory and diagnostic evaluation of, 691
long-term therapy for, 691–692, 692*f*, 692*t*
neonatal, 255–256
benign familial, 255
clinical characteristics of, 256*t*
diagnostic evaluation of, 256
focal clonic, 256*t*
focal tonic, 256*t*
generalized tonic, 256*t*
myoclonic, 256*t*
poisoning and, 163
posttraumatic, 710
pseudo-, 689–690
psychogenic nonepileptic, 689–690
status epilepticus with, 690–691
management of, 691*t*
in Sturge-Weber syndrome, 733
tonic, 688
tonic-clonic, 688
Selective mutism, 63
Selective serotonin reuptake inhibitors (SSRIs)
for anxiety disorders, 64
for autism spectrum disorder (ASD), 71
for depressive disorders, 66
for OCD, 69
Selenium deficiency, 119*t*
Self-awareness, 4
Self-improvement, 4
Self-management strategies, for somatic symptom and related disorders (SSRDs), 61
Senna, for functional constipation, 52*t*
Sennetsu ehrlichiosis, 439*t*–442*t*
Sensory and motor neuropathy, 117
Sensory examination, 682, 684
Separation anxiety disorder (SAD), 63, 63*t*
Separations, 95
Sepsis
bacterial, 258
catheter-related, 131
clinical manifestations of, 259
early-onset
clinical manifestations of, 259
treatment for, 259
fever and, 368
incidence of, 258
in newborn, 258–259
acquired in utero, 258
Septic arthritis, fever due to, 368
Septic emboli, 410
Septic thrombophlebitis, 437
Septooptic dysplasia, 639
Sequence, of malformations, 184
Sequestration crisis, in sickle cell disease, 577*t*
Sequestrum, in osteomyelitis, 425–426
Serological tests, 362
Serositis, in rheumatic diseases, 343
Serum immunoglobulin levels, for immunodeficiency disorders, 292
Serum sickness, 311, 332–333
clinical manifestations of, 332–333
epidemiology of, 332
etiology of, 332
laboratory and imaging studies for, 333
treatment and prevention of, 333
Sever disease, 755
clinical manifestations of, 755
treatment of, 755
Severe acute respiratory syndrome (SARS), 403
Severe combined immunodeficiency (SCID), 297, 297*t*
autosomal recessive, 297–298
clinical manifestations of, 297–298
due to deficiencies in adenosine deaminase and purine nucleoside phosphorylase, 298
hematopoietic stem cell transplantation for, 307
X-linked, 297–298
Severe visual impairment, 33
Sex chromosomes, 169
Sex steroids, in puberty, 656
Sexual abuse, 82–84
Sexual development
abnormal, 672–673
classification of, 671
diagnosis of, 673–674
disorders of, 670–674, 680
ovotesticular, 673
sex chromosome, 673
normal, 670–671
treatment of, 674
Sexual infantilism, 657*t*
differential diagnostic features of, 658*t*
Sexual maturity rating, 14
Sexual phase, of *Plasmodium* life cycle, 447
Sexual precocity, 659–663
classification of, 659–660, 660*t*
differential diagnosis of, 661*t*
evaluation of, 662
laboratory evaluation of, 662
pharmacological therapy of, 662*t*
treatment of, 662–663
Sexuality, development of, 84–86
Sexually transmitted infections (STIs), 274, 419–425
abnormal uterine bleeding due to, 276
chlamydia *(Chlamydia trachomatis)* as, 422–423
clinical features of, 420*t*
pelvic inflammatory disease due to, 420–421
genital ulcers from, 419, 421*t*
genital warts (condylomata acuminata) as, 382, 419, 423*t*, 425
gonorrhea *(Neisseria gonorrhoeae)* as, 421–422
clinical features of, 420*t*
disseminated gonococcal infections due to, 421–422
granuloma inguinale as, 419, 421*t*
herpes simplex virus infection (genital herpes) as, 419, 424
lymphadenopathy due to, 384*t*
mucopurulent cervicitis as, 420*t*
pediculosis pubis (crabs) as, 423*t*
pelvic inflammatory disease, 420–421, 420*t*
syphilis *(Treponema pallidum)* as, 419, 421*t*, 423–424
trichomoniasis *(Trichomonas vaginalis)* as, 419, 422*t*, 424–425
urethritis as, 419
vaginal discharge from, 419
vulvovaginal candidiasis as, 423*t*
SGA. *see* Small for gestational age
Shagreen patches, 715
Shawl sign, in juvenile dermatomyositis, 355–356
Shiga-like toxin, 411
Shiga toxin, 411
Shigella, diarrhea from, 410*t*
Shigella dysenteriae, 411

Shock, 145, 151–154
cardiogenic, 152
clinical manifestations of, 152
classification of, 151*t*
clinical manifestations of, 152
complications of, 154
differential diagnosis of, 153
dissociative, 152
clinical manifestations of, 152
distributive, 151–152
clinical manifestations of, 152
epidemiology of, 151
etiology of, 151
hypovolemic, 151
clinical manifestations of, 152
laboratory and imaging studies of, 152–153
in newborn, 233
obstructive, 152
clinical manifestations of, 152
prevention of, 154
prognosis for, 154
Short bowel syndrome, parenteral nutrition for, 130–131
Short-chain acyl-CoA dehydrogenase (SCAD) deficiency, 207, 207*f*
Short stature, 650–656, 679
caused by growth hormone deficiency, 653–656
causes of, 652*t*
constitutional, 13
due to constitutional delay, 653
differential diagnosis and therapy of, 654*t*
familial, 13
genetic or familial, 653
of nonendocrine causes, 651–653
psychosocial, 79
Shortness of breath, due to heart failure, 535
Shoulder, 763
brachial plexus injuries of, 763
glenohumeral dislocation of, 763
Little Leaguer's, 763
overuse injuries of, 763
proximal humeral epiphysiolysis of, 763
Sprengel deformity of, 763
Shoulder, drooping of, 683
Shprintzen syndrome, 182–183
Shunts, central nervous system, infections associated with, 438–439
Shwachman-Diamond syndrome, 301*t*
Sialidosis type I, 210*t*–212*t*
Sialidosis type II, 210*t*–212*t*
Sickle cell disease, 576–578, 592
clinical manifestations of, 576–577, 577*t*
etiology and epidemiology of, 576, 576*t*
genetic basis for, 173*t*
laboratory diagnosis of, 577
treatment of, 577–578
SIDS. *see* Sudden infant death syndrome
Silent stroke, in sickle cell disease, 577
Silver nitrate instillation, in newborn, 222
Single gene mutations, 169
Single-parent families, 88
Sinus arrhythmia, 542
Sinus rhythm, 542
Sinus tachycardia, 544*t*
Sinus venosus defect, 546
Sinusitis, 394–395
chronic, 394
clinical manifestations of, 394
complications and prognosis for, 395
epidemiology of, 394
etiology of, 394
laboratory and imaging studies for, 395
prevention of, 395
treatment for, 395
Skeletal radiographs, 186
Skeletal tuberculosis, 454
Skewfoot, 754
Skier's nose, 324
Skin
anemia and, 569*t*
of newborn, 228–229
Skin color, in cardiovascular system assessment, 535
Skin disorder, 721
assessment of, 721
history in, 721
initial diagnostic evaluation and screening tests in, 722–723
physical examination in, 721
common manifestations of, 721–722
with primary lesions, 721, 721*t*, 722*f*
with secondary lesions, 721, 722*t*
Skin lesions
primary, 721, 721*t*, 722*f*
secondary, 721, 722*t*
Skull, of newborn, 229
Skull fractures, 710
in newborn, 233–234
Slapped cheek rash, 377
SLE. *see* Systemic lupus erythematosus
Sleep, normal, 52–56
Sleep disturbances, in attention-deficit/hyperactivity disorder (ADHD), 47
Sleep-onset association subtype, behavioral insomnia of childhood, 55
Sleep position, 23*t*–24*t*
Sleep terrors, 54*t*–55*t*
Sleepwalking, 54*t*–55*t*
Slipped capital femoral epiphysis, 747–748
classification of, 747
clinical manifestation of, 747
complications of, 747–748
etiology and epidemiology of, 747
radiological evaluation for, 747, 748*f*
treatment of, 747
Slow to warm up child, 16
Sly syndrome, 210*t*–212*t*, 711*t*–712*t*, 713
Small bowel biopsy, for celiac disease, 489–490
Small for gestational age (SGA), 239–240
complications of, 220*t*, 228
management of, 239–240
Small molecule pathway inhibitors, for cancer, 601*t*–602*t*
SMART goals, 109
Smell, assessment of, 683
Smooth muscle hamartoma, 730*t*
Sniffing position, in epiglottitis, 399
Social anxiety disorder, 63, 64*t*
Social aspects, of pediatric practice, 3
Social (pragmatic) communication disorder (SCD), 71
Social disruptions, 54*t*–55*t*
Social phobia. *see* Social anxiety disorder
Social stress, 3
Sodium balance, regulation of, 125
Sodium benzoate, for hyperammonemia, 205
Sodium bicarbonate, 148
for cyclic antidepressants poisoning, 164*t*–165*t*
Sodium disorders, 131–134
hypernatremia as, 133–134, 133*f*
hyponatremia as, 131–133, 132*f*
Sodium excretion, 131
Sodium intoxication, 133
Sodium phenylacetate, for hyperammonemia, 205
Sodium restriction, for heart failure, 555*t*
Sodoku, 439*t*–442*t*
Soiling, 49–51. *see also* Encopresis
Solid cereals, as complementary food, 101
Somatic pain, in appendicitis, 493
Somatic symptom and related disorders (SSRDs), 59–61, 60*t*
prevalence of, 59
screening tools for, 61
treatment of, 61
Somatostatin, for chronic pancreatitis, 503
Somatostatin release inhibitory factor, 650–651
Somnolence syndrome, central nervous system and, 608
Sorbitol
for functional constipation, 52*t*
for poisoning, 164
Sotos syndrome, 184–185
Southeast Asian liver fluke, 451*t*
Southern tick-associated rash illness (STARI), 439*t*–442*t*, 444
Soy-based formulas, 100–101, 102*t*
Soy protein intolerance, vomiting due to, 473*t*
Spasmodic croup, 399
Spasms, infantile, 690
Spasticity, 684
Specifiers
for bipolar and related disorders, 67
for depressive disorders, 65
Speculum examination, for adolescents, 274
Speech-language impairment, in child, with special needs, 36–37, 36*t*
Spherocytosis, hereditary
clinical manifestations of, 579
etiology of, 566, 578–579
laboratory diagnosis of, 579
treatment of, 579
Sphingolipidoses, 712
Sphingomyelin lipidosis A, 210*t*–212*t*
Sphingomyelin lipidosis B, 210*t*–212*t*
Sphingomyelinase deficiency, 210*t*–212*t*
Spina bifida, 716
occulta, 716
Spinal cord, congenital anomalies of, 716
Spinal cord abnormalities, constipation due to, 476*t*
Spinal cord compression, oncological emergencies, 600*t*
Spinal cord injuries, in newborn, 233
Spinal cord injury without radiological abnormality (SCIWORA), 156
Spinal cord lesions, weakness due to, 694
Spinal deformities, 756–757
classification of, 756*t*
clinical manifestations of, 756–757
kyphosis as, 760
classification of, 756*t*
congenital, 760
postural roundback, 760
Scheuermann, 760, 760*f*
radiological evaluation of, 757, 758*f*
scoliosis as. *see* Scoliosis
Spinal dysraphism, 756–758
Spinal muscular atrophy, 683, 694–695
clinical manifestations of, 694
etiology of, 694
laboratory and diagnostic studies for, 694–695
treatment for, 695
Spine, 756–762
back pain of, 761, 761*t*
deformities of, 756–757
classification of, 756*t*
clinical manifestations of, 756–757
kyphosis as, 760
classification of, 756*t*
congenital, 760
postural roundback, 760
Scheuermann, 760, 760*f*
radiological evaluation of, 757, 758*f*
scoliosis as. *see* Scoliosis
diskitis as, 762

Spine *(Continued)*
of newborn, 231
spondylolysis and spondylolisthesis of, 761–762
torticollis of, 760–761
Spirillum minus, 439*t*–442*t*
Spirochetal diseases, zoonotic, 439*t*–442*t*
Spirometry, 511
for asthma, 313–314, 316
Spitting up, 480
vomiting *vs.*, 472
Spleen, injury to, 156
Splenectomy, for hereditary spherocytosis, 579
Splenic dysfunction, in sickle cell disease, 576
Splenic infarction, in sickle cell disease, 576
Splenic sequestration crisis, in sickle cell disease, 576
Splenomegaly, in anemia, 567–568
Spondylitis, juvenile ankylosing, 351*t*
Spondyloarthropathies, 351, 351*t*
Spondylolisthesis, 761–762
classification of, 762
clinical manifestations of, 762
etiology and epidemiology of, 761–762
radiological evaluation of, 762
treatment of, 762
Spondylolysis, 761–762
clinical manifestations of, 762
etiology and epidemiology of, 761–762
radiological evaluation of, 762
treatment of, 762
Spontaneous bacterial peritonitis, 504
Spontaneous bleeding, 587
Spontaneous mutation, 171
Spontaneous primary pneumothorax, 530
Spore-forming intestinal protozoa, diarrhea from, 410*t*
Sporogony, of *Plasmodium* life cycle, 447
Spot urine protein/creatinine, 620
Sprengel deformity, 763
Spur cells, 580
Sputum, examination of, 511–512
Square window wrist, in newborn, 229*f*
SSPE (subacute sclerosing panencephalitis), 375
St. Vitus dance, due to rheumatic fever, 556
Stage MS, neuroblastoma, 609
Stanozolol, for C1-inhibitor deficiency, 306
Staphylococcal scalded skin syndrome, 734*t*, 735
Staphylococcus aureus
in cystic fibrosis, 527
osteomyelitis from, 425
subacute focal, 425–426
treatment of, 427
pneumonia from, 407*t*
Starvation, 79
Static neurological abnormalities, 681
Stature
with developmental disabilities, 30*t*
growth chart of, 12*f*
Status asthmaticus, 316
Status epilepticus, 690–691
management of, 691*t*
Steatorrhea, in cystic fibrosis, 527
Steeple sign, in croup, 399
Steinert disease, genetic basis for, 170*t*
STEP guide, for adolescent interviewing, 267, 270*f*
Stepped down therapy, for asthma, 316, 317*f*–318*f*
Stepped up therapy, for asthma, 316, 317*f*–318*f*
Stepwise approach, to asthma management, 316, 317*f*–318*f*
Stereognosis, 684
Sternocleidomastoid muscles, during inspiration, 507
Steroid hormones, 637
Steroidal contraception, 278–281
combined hormonal contraceptives for, 279–280, 279*t*–280*t*
contraceptive patch for, 279–280
contraceptive vaginal ring for, 279–280
hormonal injections and implants for, 278–279
long-acting reversible contraceptives for, 278–279
progesterone-only pill or minipill for, 280
Stertor, 516
Stevens-Johnson syndrome (SJS), 733–735, 734*t*
Stilbestrol, as teratogen, 237*t*
Still's murmur, 538*t*
Stimson line, in measles, 373–374
Stimulants
for attention-deficit/hyperactivity disorder (ADHD), 47
for autism spectrum disorder (ASD), 71
for bipolar disorders, 68
for functional constipation, 52*t*
Stimulation, appropriate, 91
Stinger, 763
STIs. *see* Sexually transmitted infections
Stomach disorders, 480–487
peptic disease as, 485–486, 486*t*
pyloric stenosis as, 484–485, 485*f*
Stool, of breast-fed infant, 99–100
Stool impaction, in functional constipation, 49
Stool softener, for functional constipation, 476
Stop codons, 169
Storage disorders, 196
caused by defective synthesis of lysosomal membrane, 210*t*–212*t*
caused by defects in lysosomal proteolysis, 210*t*–212*t*
caused by dysfunction of lysosomal transport proteins, 210*t*–212*t*
Stork bite, 733
Stranger anxiety, 15
Strawberry tongue
in Kawasaki disease, 347
red, 393
white, 393
Strength, in motor examination, 684
Streptobacillus moniliformis, 439*t*–442*t*
Streptococcal carriage, 393
Streptococcal infection
in OCD, 68
in rheumatic fever, 556
Streptococcal pharyngitis, 392–394
causes of, 392*t*
clinical manifestations of, 392–393
complications and prognosis of, 394
differential diagnosis of, 393
epidemiology of, 392
etiology of, 392
laboratory evaluation of, 393
treatment of, 393–394, 394*t*
Streptococcus
group A, 392
osteomyelitis due to, 425
pharyngitis due to, 392–394
causes of, 392*t*
clinical manifestations of, 392–393
complications and prognosis of, 394
differential diagnosis of, 393
epidemiology of, 392
etiology of, 392
laboratory evaluation of, 393
treatment of, 393–394, 394*t*
pneumonia due to, 407*t*
group B
osteomyelitis due to, 425
pneumonia due to, 407*t*
Streptococcus pneumoniae
conjunctivitis from, 430
immunization against, 388–389
osteomyelitis due to, 425
pneumonia from, 403
Streptococcus pneumoniae vaccine, 363–364
Streptococcus pyogenes, pharyngitis from, 392
Streptomycin, as teratogen, 237*t*
Stridor, 510
croup and, 398–399
inspiratory, due to laryngomalacia, 518
due to subglottic stenosis, 518–519
due to upper airway obstruction, 516
String sign, in pyloric stenosis, 485
Stroke, 699–700
clinical manifestations of, 699–700
diagnostic tests and imaging for, 700
differential diagnosis of, 700
etiology of, 699, 699*t*
hemorrhagic, 699
in sickle cell disease, 577
treatment of, 700
Stroke volume, oxygen delivery and, 151
Strongyloides stercoralis, 450*t*
Structured Communication Adolescent Guide (SCAG), 268*f*–269*f*
Stunting
failure to thrive and, 77
marasmus and, 110
zinc deficiency and, 120–121
Stupor, 703, 705
Sturge-Weber syndrome, 715, 733
Styes, 431
Subacute bacterial endocarditis prophylaxis, 550
Subacute necrotizing encephalomyelopathy, 711*t*–712*t*, 713
Subacute sclerosing panencephalitis (SSPE), 375
Subarachnoid hemorrhages, 709–710
aneurysmal, 686*t*
in newborn, 255
Subconjunctival hemorrhage, in newborn, 233
Subcutaneous nodules, due to heart failure, 556, 556*t*
Subdural hematoma, in newborn, 256–257
Subdural hemorrhages, 709–710
due to child abuse, 81, 82*f*
in newborn, 256–257
Subependymal giant cell astrocytomas, 715
Subependymal nodules, 715
Subgaleal bleed, in newborn, 233
Subglottic hemangioma, 732–733
Subglottic space, 507
Subglottic stenosis, 518–519
Subluxation, 739*t*
Substance abuse
by adolescents, 2, 283–284, 284*t*
acute and chronic effects of, 284
acute overdose due to, 284, 284*t*–285*t*
treatment for, 284
maternal, during pregnancy, 90
Substance/medication-induced psychotic disorders, 72
Substernal retractions, 509–510
Succimer acid, for lead poisoning, 164*t*–165*t*
Succinylacetone, urine or blood, 199*t*
Sucking reflex, 14
Sudden infant death syndrome (SIDS), 515–516
differential diagnosis of, 516*t*
etiology and epidemiology of, 515
with medium-chain acyl-CoA dehydrogenase deficiency, 207–208
prevention of, 515–516
Sufentanil, as analgesia, 166*t*
Suffocation, fatal injury due to, 154
Suicide, in bipolar disorders, 68
Sulfadiazine, 449

Sulfasalazine, for ulcerative colitis, 491
Sulfatases deficiency, 210*t*–212*t*
Sulfonamides, maternal use of, 238*t*
Sulfonylurea, maternal use of, 238*t*
Superficial infections
bacterial, 379–380
cellulitis as, 380
folliculitis as, 380
impetigo as, 379–380
perianal dermatitis as, 380
fungal, 380–381, 381*t*
viral, 381–383
from herpes simplex virus as, 381–382
from human papillomaviruses (warts), 382
molluscum contagiosum as, 383
Superior vena cava syndrome, oncological emergencies, 600*t*
Supplemental oxygen, 512
Supportive care
for cancer, 601
for poisoning, 163–164
for Stevens-Johnson syndrome and toxic epidermal necrolysis, 735
Suppurative bursitis, 429
Supraclavicular retractions, 509–510
Supracondylar fracture, 743
Supracristal septum, 545
Supraventricular tachycardia (SVT), 543, 544*t*
Surfactant, 219–220
Susceptibilities, to antiinfective drugs, 367
Sutures, of newborn, 229
Swallowing study, videofluoroscopic, 520
Sweat test, for cystic fibrosis, 528, 528*t*
Swimmer's ear, 397–398. *see also* Otitis externa
Swinging flashlight test, 683
Swyer-James syndrome, 407
Sydenham chorea, due to rheumatic fever, 556, 556*t*
Sympathomimetics
maternal use of, 238*t*
toxicity, 162*t*
Symptomatic hyponatremia, 133
Synchronized cardioversion, for dysrhythmias, 543–544
Syncope, 540–541, 706
cardiac, 541*t*
carotid sinus, 541*t*
clinical manifestations of, 540–541
cough (deglutition), 541*t*
diagnostic studies for, 541
etiology of, 540, 541*t*
micturition, 541*t*
neurocardiogenic (vasopressor), 541*t*
Syndactyly, 183*t*, 185
of finger, 765
of toes, 755, 756*t*
Syndrome of inappropriate antidiuretic hormone (SIADH), 132
Synergism, of antimicrobial drugs, 367–368
Synophrys, 183*t*
Synovial fluid findings, in various joint diseases, 429*t*
Synovitis
in juvenile idiopathic arthritis, 349
in rheumatic diseases, 343
toxic or transient, 428
transient monoarticular, 746
clinical manifestations and evaluation of, 746, 746*t*
etiology and epidemiology of, 746
treatment for, 746
Syphilis *(Treponema pallidum)*, 419, 423–424
clinical features of, 421*t*
congenital, 262–263, 423
latent, 423
neuro-, 424
Syphilis *(Treponema pallidum) (Continued)*
primary, 423
secondary, 423
tertiary, 423
Syrup of ipecac, for poisoning, 164
Systematic ignoring, for pediatric sleep disorders, 56
Systemic capillary leak, due to burns, 159
Systemic diseases, cardiac manifestations of, 536*t*
Systemic inflammatory response syndrome (SIRS), 151–152
Systemic lupus erythematosus (SLE), 353–355
clinical manifestations of, 353, 353*t*–354*t*
complications of, 355
differential diagnosis of, 344*t*, 355
epidemiology of, 353
etiology of, 353
laboratory and imaging studies for, 354–355
maternal, 236, 236*t*
prognosis for, 355
synovial fluid findings in, 429*t*
treatment of, 355
Systolic murmurs, 536
ejection, 536
due to aortic stenosis, 548
in total anomalous pulmonary venous return, 552
in truncus arteriosus, 551

T

T-cell proliferation, 293
T cells, 289–290
Tachycardia
due to respiratory failure, 149
sinus, 544*t*
supraventricular, 543, 544*t*
ventricular, 543, 544*t*
Tachypnea, 509*t*
due to heart failure, 535
due to respiratory failure, 149
transient, of newborn, 222
Tacrolimus, for atopic dermatitis, 327–328
Taenia solium, 452, 452*t*
Talipes equinovarus, 753–754, 753*f*
Tanner stages
in boys, 271–273, 272*f*
in girls, 270–271, 271*f*–272*f*
Tantrums, 43–45. *see also* Temper tantrums
anticipatory guidance and management of, 45
clinical manifestations of, 43–44, 44*f*, 44*t*
differential diagnosis of, 44–45
epidemiology of, 43
etiology of, 43
physical examination for, 44
Tapeworm
echinococcosis from, 452
neurocysticercosis from, 452
Tardive dyskinesia, 703
Target lesions, in erythema multiforme, 735
Targeted therapies, for cancer, 601
Tarsal coalition, 754–755
calcaneonavicular, 754–755
clinical manifestations of, 755
radiological evaluation of, 755
talocalcaneal, 754–755
treatment of, 755
Tarsal navicular, idiopathic avascular necrosis of, 755
Tarui disease, 200*t*
Tay-Sachs disease, 210*t*–212*t*, 711*t*–712*t*, 712
Tazarotene, for acne, 723
Teeth
deciduous (primary), 479, 479*t*
eruption of, 479, 479*t*
delayed, 479
Teeth *(Continued)*
natal, 479
permanent, 479*t*
TEF. *see* Tracheoesophageal fistula
Telangiectasia, 721*t*
with developmental disabilities, 30*t*
Telecanthus, 183*t*
Teloradiograph, of leg-length discrepancy, 750
Temper tantrums, 43–45
anticipatory guidance and management of, 45
clinical manifestations of, 43–44, 44*f*, 44*t*
differential diagnosis of, 44–45
epidemiology of, 43
etiology of, 43
physical examination for, 44
Temperament, 16
Temperature instability, in infants younger than 3 months of age, 368
Temperature regulation, in newborn, 234
Tender points, in myofascial pain syndromes, 358
Tension pneumothorax, 530
Tension-type headaches, 686
Teratogenic agents, 176–177
Teratoma, sacral, constipation due to, 476*t*
Tertian periodicity, of *P. vivax* and *P. ovale*, 447
Tertiary survey, of trauma patient, 155
Testes
detorsion and fixation of, 633
undescended, 632
Testosterone-like drugs, as teratogens, 237*t*
Tet spells, 550
Tetanus, prophylaxis for, 366, 367*t*
Tetanus and diphtheria toxoids and acellular pertussis (Tdap) vaccine, 364*f*–365*f*
Tetanus vaccine, 363–364
Tetany, neonatal, 235
Tethered cord, constipation due to, 476*t*
Tetracycline
for acne, 723
as teratogen, 237*t*
Tetralogy of Fallot, 549–550, 550*f*
TGF-β (transforming growth factor-β), functions of, 290*t*
Thalassemia(s), 591
α-Thalassemia minor, 571, 575
β-Thalassemia major, 575–576
β-Thalassemia minor, 571
Thalassemia minor, in hypochromic, microcytic anemia, 571
etiology and epidemiology of, 571, 572*f*, 572*t*
laboratory testing for, 571
treatment of, 571
Thalidomide, as teratogen, 237*t*
Thanatophoric dysplasia, 170*t*
Thelarche, 270–271, 656
isolated premature, 663
Theophylline, for asthma, 315
Thermal environment, neutral, of newborn, 234
Thiamine deficiency, 113, 114*t*
Thiazides, maternal use of, 238*t*
Thigh-foot angle, 749, 749*f*
Thin basement membrane disease, 622–623
Third-degree heart block, 543
Third heart sound (S_3), 536
Third space losses, 127
Thoracic scoliosis, 529
Thoracoscopic procedure, 512
Thoracotomy, 512
Threats, by parents, 25
Threshold, in hypertrophic pyloric stenosis, 174–175
Throat culture, for streptococcal pharyngitis, 393
Thrombin, in hemostasis, 580
Thrombin time, 584*t*

Thrombocytopenia, 583
bleeding disorder in newborn due to, 254
due to decreased platelet production, 584
in hemolytic uremic syndrome, 624
isoimmune
maternal, 236*t*
in newborn, 254
maternal
idiopathic purpura, 235–236, 236*t*
isoimmune, 236*t*
oncological emergencies, 600*t*
due to peripheral destruction, 584
presentation of, 564*t*
Thrombocytopenia with absent radii syndrome, 584
Thrombocytopenic purpura
idiopathic. *see* Idiopathic thrombocytopenic purpura
neonatal alloimmune, 584
thrombotic, 585–586, 624
in thrombotic microangiopathy, 580
Thromboembolism, in nephrotic syndrome, 621
Thrombophlebitis, 437
septic, 437
Thrombopoietin, 566
Thrombosis, 589, 593
catheter-related, 437
clinical manifestations of, 589
diagnostic and imaging studies in, 589
etiology of, 589, 589*f*
presentation of, 564*t*
treatment of, 589
Thrombotic microangiopathy, 580, 585–586
Thrombotic thrombocytopenic purpura, 585–586, 624
in thrombotic microangiopathy, 580
Thrush, 480
Thumb, trigger, 765
Thumb sign, in epiglottitis, 399
Thyroid disease, 665–668, 680
hypothyroidism, 665–667
laboratory results of, 665*t*
physiology and development of, 663–665
Thyroid hormone, and GH secretion, 651
Thyroid tumors, 668
Thyrotropin-releasing hormone (TRH), 663
Thyroxine (T_4), 663
Thyroxine-binding globulin, 664
Tibia, 751*f*
Tibia vara (Blount disease), 750
Tibial torsion, 739*t*
external, 749
internal, 748–749, 749*f*
Tibial tubercle, 751*f*
Tic(s), 703
Tick paralysis, 695–696
Tidal volume (TV), 507–508, 508*f*
Timeout, 25
Tinea capitis, 380, 381*t*, 729
Tinea corporis, 380, 381*t*
Tinea cruris, 380, 381*t*
Tinea pedis, 380, 381*t*
Tinea unguium, 381*t*
Tinea versicolor, 381*t*
Tissue factor pathway inhibitor, in hemostasis, 581
Tobacco smoke, asthma and, 315*t*
Tocolytic-β agonist agents , maternal use of, 238*t*
α-Tocopherol, 117
Toddlers
hearing and vision screening of, 20
nutritional issues for, 103
Toddler's fracture, 744
Toe(s)
curly, 755
extra, 755, 756*t*
fusion, 755, 756*t*
Toe deformities, 755, 756*t*
Toe walking, 740
Tolerance, oral, 334
Toluene, as teratogen, 237*t*
Tone, in motor examination, 684
Tongue, strawberry
in Kawasaki disease, 347
red, 393
white, 393
Tonic neck reflex, 682
Tonsillar hypertrophy, 519
Tonsillitis, 393
Tonsillopharyngitis, 393
Toothbrush, introduction of, 102
Topoisomerase inhibitors, for cancer, 601*t*–602*t*
Topotecan, for cancer, 601*t*–602*t*
TORCH infection(s), 259–264, 260*t*
Torticollis, 760–761
Torus fracture, 742
Total anomalous pulmonary venous return, 552, 552*f*
Total body surface area, 159
Total body water (TBW), 125, 126*f*
Total lung capacity (TLC), 507–508, 508*f*
Tourette syndrome, 703
Toxemia
of pregnancy, 218
in thrombotic microangiopathy, 580
Toxic epidermal necrolysis (TEN), 733–735, 734*t*
Toxic ingestions, metabolic acidosis due to, 140
Toxic megacolon, 490
Toxic stress, 2
Toxic syndromes, 162*t*
Toxic synovitis, 428, 746, 746*t*
Toxocara canis, 450–451, 450*t*
Toxocara cati, 450–451, 450*t*
Toxoids, for immunization, 363–364
Toxoplasma gondii, 439*t*–442*t*, 449
congenital infection with, 259–261
in immunocompromised person, 434–435
Toxoplasmosis, 439*t*–442*t*, 449
congenital infection with, 260*t*, 261
Trachea, 507
Tracheal compression
extrinsic, 521, 521*f*
oncological emergencies, 600*t*
Tracheitis, bacterial, 399
upper airway obstruction due to, 517*t*
Tracheoesophageal fistula (TEF), 227*t*, 483, 521
clinical manifestations of, 483, 483*f*
complications with, 483
etiology and epidemiology of, 483
laboratory and imaging studies for, 483
treatment and prognosis for, 483
Tracheomalacia, 520–521
Tracheostomy, 513
Traffic light diet, 107–108
Tranquilizers, acute effects of, 284*t*–285*t*
Transcellular shift, of potassium, 135
Transcription, 169
Transcutaneous electrodes, for respiratory gas exchange measurements, 511
Transesophageal echocardiography (TEE), in cardiovascular system assessment, 540
Transforming growth factor-β (TGF-β)
functions of, 290*t*
in Marfan syndrome, 171
Transfusion, 589–590
for autoimmune hemolysis, 580
commonly used, 590*t*
reactions of, evaluation of, 590*t*
Transgender, 84*t*, 87
Transient aplastic crisis, erythema infectiosum and, 377
Transient erythroblastopenia, 573*t*
of childhood, 573–574
Transient hypogammaglobulinemia of infancy as, 295, 295*t*
Transient hypoparathyroidism, 669
Transient monoarticular synovitis, 746, 746*t*
Transient myeloproliferative disorder, 604
Transient neonatal hypocalcemia, 669
Transient synovitis, 428
Transient tachypnea of the newborn, 222, 245
Transplantation, for heart failure, 555*t*
Transposition, of great arteries, 550–551, 550*f*
Transtentorial (central) herniation, 705–706
Transudates, 530–531
Transverse myelitis, 694
Trauma, 155–157. *see also* Injury(ies)
abdominal, 156
assessment and resuscitation for, 155
clinical manifestations of, 156–157
complications of, 157
epidemiology of, 155
etiology of, 155
head, 156
informed care, 93
intestinal, 157
laboratory and imaging studies of, 155, 156*t*
liver, 156
orthopedic problem due to, 739*t*
pancreatic, 157
prevention of, 157
prognosis for, 157
renal, 156–157
spleen, 156
thoracic, 156
treatment of, 156–157
Traumatic brain injury
due to cervical spine injuries, 710
concussion in, 709, 709*t*
due to CSF leak, 710
disorders of consciousness due to, 703, 709–711
drowsiness, headache, and vomiting after, 710
evaluation and treatment for, 710
Glasgow Coma Scale for, 710
intracranial hemorrhage in, 709–711, 709*t*
due to posttraumatic seizures, 710
prognosis for, 710–711
due to skull fractures, 710
Traumatic intracranial hemorrhage, 709–711, 709*t*
Traveler's diarrhea, 411, 413
Trematodes, parasitic, pediatric syndromes caused by, 451*t*
Tremor, 703
Trench fever, 737
Trench mouth, 393
Trendelenburg gait, 740
Treponema pallidum, 419, 423–424
congenital infection with, 260*t*
Treponemal antibody tests, 424
Tretinoin (vitamin A analog)
for acne, 723
for cancer, 601*t*–602*t*
Triad asthma, 321*t*
Triamcinolone acetonide, for asthma, 319*f*
Triatoma bites, anaphylaxis due to, 333
Trichinella spiralis, 450*t*
Trichinellosis, 450*t*
Trichomonas vaginalis, 419, 424–425
Trichuris dysentery, 450*t*
Tricuspid atresia, 551, 551*f*
Trifunctional protein, in fatty acid catabolism, 207, 207*f*
Trigeminal nerve, assessment of, 683
Triiodothyronine (T_3), 663
Trimethadione, as teratogen, 237*t*
Trimethoprim-sulfamethoxazole (TMP-SMX)
for HIV, 461
for pertussis, 401

Trinucleotide repeat, expansion of, 176
Triptans, for migraine, 687
Trisomic rescue, 180
Trisomy(ies), 180–181
  Down syndrome as, 180
  Klinefelter syndrome as, 181
  trisomy 13 as, 180–181
  trisomy 18 as, 180, 181*t*
Trisomy 13, 180–181
Trisomy 18, 180, 181*t*
Trisomy 21, newborn assessment for, 227*t*
Trochlear nerve, assessment of, 683
Trophozoite, of *Plasmodium* life cycle, 447
Trousseau sign, 235, 669
Truncal ataxia, 700
Truncus arteriosus, 551–552, 551*f*
Trunk, congenital malformations of, 185
Trunk incurvation reflex, 682*t*
Trypanosoma brucei gambiense, 439*t*–442*t*
Trypanosoma brucei rhodesiense, 439*t*–442*t*
Trypanosoma cruzi, 439*t*–442*t*
  congenital infection with, 260*t*
Trypanosomiasis
  African, 439*t*–442*t*
  American, 439*t*–442*t*
Trypsin, 502
Tryptophan, 113
Tubercle bacilli, 453–454
Tuberculin skin test, 454*t*–455*t*
Tuberculosis, 452–457
  abdominal, 454
  clinical manifestations of, 453–454
  complications and prognosis of, 457
  diagnosis of
    culture for, 454–455
    imaging in, 455, 456*f*
    tuberculin skin test for, 454*t*–455*t*
  differential diagnosis of, 455
  epidemiology of, 453
  etiology of, 452
  extrapulmonary, 455
  laboratory and imaging studies for, 454–455
  latent, 453
  miliary, 453
  prevention of, 457
  primary progressive, 453
  pulmonary
    primary, 453
    reactivation, 453
  skeletal, 454
  synovial fluid findings in, 429*t*
  transmission of, 453
  treatment for, 455–456, 457*t*
  urogenital, 454
Tuberculous meningitis, 387*t*, 453–454
Tuberculous peritonitis, 454
Tuberculous pleural effusion, 453
Tuberous sclerosis
  complex, 715
  infantile spasms due to, 690
Tubers, 715
Tubular function, 617
Tubulin inhibitors, for cancer, 601*t*–602*t*
Tularemia, 439*t*–442*t*
Tumor(s), 721
  orthopedic problem due to, 739*t*
  of skin, 721*t*, 722*f*
  syncope due to, 541*t*
  of thyroid, 668
Tumor lysis syndrome, 599, 600*t*
Tunnel infection, 437
Turner syndrome, 181–182, 653, 673
  amenorrhea due to, 275
  obesity in, 106*t*
Twin-to-twin transfusion syndrome, 218
Twinning, 218
Two-point discrimination, 684
TYK2 gene, in hyper-IgE syndrome, 299
Tympanic membranes, of newborn, 230
Tympanic perforation, otitis media with, 398
Tympanocentesis, for otitis media, 396–397
Tympanogram, for otitis media, 396
Tympanometry, 36
  for otitis media, 396
Tympanostomy tube otorrhea, 398
Tympanostomy tubes, otitis externa and, 397–398
Typhus
  endemic
    flea-borne, 439*t*–442*t*
    louse-borne, 439*t*–442*t*
  epidemic, 737
Typical syncopal events, 540–541
Tyrosinemia(s)
  neonatal screening for, 198*t*
  type I, 202
  type II, 202–203
  type III, 202–203
Tzanck test, 726

U

UBE3A gene, in Angelman syndrome, 176
UC. *see* Ulcerative colitis
Ulcer(s), 722*t*
  duodenal, abdominal pain due to, 470*t*
  genital, 419, 421*t*
  peptic, 485–486
  pill, 484
Ulcerative colitis (UC), 490*t*, 491
Ultrasonography
  of chest, 511
  for infectious diseases, 362–363
  for infective arthritis, 429
  of kidney, 620
  for urinary tract infection, 417
Ultraviolet light therapy, for atopic dermatitis, 726
Umbilical arteries, Doppler examination of, 220
Umbilical cord, clamping or milking (stripping) of, 247
Umbilical hernia, 231
Uncal herniation, 705–706
Undernutrition, pediatric, 109–112, 110*f*
  complications of, 112
  in failure to thrive, 109
  kwashiorkor as, 110–111
  marasmus as, 110
  mixed marasmus-kwashiorkor as, 111
  physical signs of, 111*t*
  treatment of, 111–112
Undescended testes, 632
Unicameral bone cyst, 765*t*–766*t*
Unilateral hyperlucent lung, 407
Unilateral renal agenesis, 629
Unilocular cyst disease, 452
Unintentional injury, 154
Uniparental disomy, 175
  Angelman syndrome due to, 176
  Prader-Willi syndrome as, 175–176
Unmodified extinction, for pediatric sleep disorders, 56
Unspecified anxiety disorder, 62
Unspecified bipolar and related disorder, 66
Unspecified depressive disorder, 65
Upper airway obstruction, 516–519
  acute, causes of, 517*t*
  adenoidal and tonsillar hypertrophy, 519
  due to angioedema, 517*t*
  due to bacterial tracheitis, 517*t*
  due to choanal stenosis (atresia), 518
  clinical manifestations of, 516
  due to croup (laryngotracheobronchitis), 517*t*
Upper airway obstruction *(Continued)*
  diagnostic studies for, 517–518
  differential diagnosis of, 518–519
    age-related, 516*t*
  due to epiglottitis, 517*t*
  etiology of, 516
  due to foreign body, 517*t*
  due to laryngomalacia, 518
  due to mass lesions, 519
  due to peritonsillar abscess, 517*t*
  due to retropharyngeal abscess, 517*t*
  due to spasmodic croup, 517*t*
  due to subglottic stenosis, 518–519
  supraglottic *vs.* subglottic, 517*t*
  due to vocal cord paralysis, 519
Upper extremity, 763–765
  elbow in, 764
    Panner disease of, 764
    radial head subluxation of, 764, 764*f*
    throwing injuries of, 764
  shoulder in, 763
    brachial plexus injuries of, 763
    glenohumeral dislocation of, 763
    overuse injuries of, 763
    proximal humeral epiphysiolysis of, 763
    Sprengel deformity of, 763
  wrist and hand in, 765
    finger abnormalities of, 765
    fracture of, 765
    ganglion cysts of, 765
Upper respiratory tract infection, 391–392
  clinical manifestations of, 391
  complications and prognosis for, 391–392
  differential diagnosis for, 391
  epidemiology of, 391
  etiology of, 391
  laboratory and imaging studies for, 391
  prevention of, 392
  treatment for, 391
Upper-to-lower segment ratio, 651
Urea cycle, 204*f*
Ureaplasma urealyticum, pneumonia from, 403
Urethritis, 419
  nongonococcal, 423
Urinalysis, 619–620
  for urinary tract infection, 417
Urinary anion gap, 617
Urinary ascites, 630
Urinary catheters, infections associated with, 438
Urinary concentrating capacity, 617–618
Urinary schistosomiasis, 451*t*
Urinary tract
  congenital and developmental abnormalities of, 629–630
    etiology and epidemiology of, 629–630
  and genital disorders, 631–633
Urinary tract infection (UTI), 416–417
  clinical manifestations of, 416
  common manifestations of, 618
  complications and prognosis of, 417
  differential diagnosis, 417
  epidemiology of, 416
  etiology of, 416
  fever due to, 368
  laboratory and imaging studies in, 416–417
  prevention of, 417
  treatment of, 417
  urinary catheters and, 438
  vomiting due to, 473*t*
Urinary tract obstruction, 630
  clinical manifestations of, 630
  diagnostic imaging of, 630
  site and etiology of, 630*t*
  treatment of, 630
Urinary tract stones, 631

Urine amino acid profile, 199*t*
Urine culture, for urinary tract infection, 417
Urine output, water loss and, 127
Urine specific gravity, in dehydration, 128
Urogenital tuberculosis, 454
Urolithiasis, 623, 631
abdominal pain due to, 470*t*
Urology assessment, 617–620
common manifestations in, 618, 618*t*
history in, 617
laboratory studies in, 619–620
physical examination in, 617
Urticaria, 328–332
acute, 328, 329*t*, 335*t*–336*t*
cholinergic, 329
chronic, 328–329, 329*t*
clinical manifestations of, 330, 330*f*
cold, 329
differential diagnosis of, 331
epidemiology of, 330
etiology of, 328, 329*t*
laboratory and imaging studies for, 330–331, 331*t*
physical, 328–329
pigmentosa, vesiculobullous eruptions due to, 734*t*
prevention of, 331–332
treatment of, 331
Urticarial rash, infections with fever and, 373*t*–374*t*
Urticarial vasculitis, 331
Uterine abnormalities, intrauterine growth restriction and small for gestational age due to, 239*t*
Uterine compression, deformation abnormalities resulting from, 741*f*
UTI. *see* Urinary tract infection
Uveitis
anterior, 433*t*
in juvenile idiopathic arthritis, 350
posterior, 433*t*

V

V/Q (ventilation-perfusion) matching, 508
V/Q (ventilation-perfusion) mismatching, 508, 508*t*
Vaccine Adverse Event Reporting System (VAERS), 366
Vaccines and vaccinations, 363–364
catch-up schedules for, 365*f*
contraindications to, 365–366
informed consent for, 365
recommended schedules for, 364*f*
VACTERL association, 184
tracheoesophageal fistula and, 483
VAERS (Vaccine Adverse Event Reporting System), 366
Vagal maneuvers, 543–544
Vaginal bleeding, during pregnancy, 217
Vaginal discharge, physiological, 419, 422*t*
Vaginal sponge, 280
Vaginitis
due to *Gardnerella vaginalis*, 417–418
nonspecific, 417–418
vulvo-. *see* Vulvovaginitis
Vaginosis, bacterial, 417–418, 418*t*, 422*t*
Valacyclovir
for herpes simplex virus infection, 424
for varicella zoster virus, 379
Valgum, 739*t*
Valgus, 739*t*
Valine, metabolism of, 203*f*
Valproate, as teratogen, 237*t*
Valproic acid, for status epilepticus, 691, 691*t*
Value differences, ethical problems due to, 4
Vanillylmandelic acid, in neuroblastoma, 609
Variable expressivity, 171
Varicella, vesiculobullous eruptions due to, 734*t*
Varicella vaccine, 363–364, 364*f*–365*f*
Varicella-zoster immunoglobulin (VZIG), 379
in immunocompromised person, 437
Varicella-zoster virus infection (chickenpox and zoster), 378–379
clinical manifestations of, 378
complications and prognosis of, 379
congenital infection with, 260*t*
differential diagnosis of, 378–379
epidemiology of, 378
etiology of, 378
in immunocompromised person, 435
laboratory and imaging studies for, 378
prevention of, 379
treatment of, 379
Varices, esophageal, 497
gastrointestinal bleeding due to, 477*t*
Varum, 739*t*
Varus, 739*t*
Vascular anomalies, 732–733
Vascular catheters, infections associated with, 437
Vascular device infections, 437–438
Vascular malformation(s), 733
defined, 732
port-wine stain (nevus flammeus) as, 733, 733*f*
pyogenic granuloma as, 733
salmon patch stain (nevus simplex) as, 733
Vascular ring, extrinsic tracheal compression due to, 521
Vasculitis
angioedema *vs.*, 331*t*
in rheumatic diseases, 343
urticarial, 331
Vasoactive substances, 146–147
Vasoconstriction, hypoxic pulmonary, 508
Vasomotor rhinitis, 324
Vasoocclusive painful events, in sickle cell disease, 576
Vasopressin, in renal function, 617
Vasopressor syncope, 541*t*
VCUG (voiding cystourethrogram), for urinary tract infection, 417
Vector borne infection, 439–447
Vegetation, in infective endocarditis, 408
Velocardiofacial syndrome, 182–183, 298
Venereal Disease Research Laboratory (VDRL) test, 424
Venom immunotherapy, for insect allergies, 334
Venous hum, 538, 538*t*
Venous malformation, differential diagnosis of, 730*t*
Ventilation, 147
Ventilation-perfusion (V/Q) matching, 508
Ventilation-perfusion (V/Q) mismatching, 508, 508*t*
Ventilator-associated pneumonia, 438
Ventricular contractions, premature, 543, 544*t*
Ventricular dysrhythmias, 543
Ventricular fibrillation, 544*t*
Ventricular function curve, 553, 554*f*
Ventricular septal defect, 545–546, 545*f*
clinical manifestations of, 545
etiology and epidemiology of, 545
imaging studies for, 545
perimembranous, 545
in tetralogy of Fallot, 549
treatment of, 545–546
tricuspid atresia with, 551*f*
Ventricular tachycardia, 543, 544*t*
Ventriculoperitoneal shunt, for hydrocephalus, 708
Vernix caseosa, 228
Verruca
plana, 382
vulgaris, 382
Vertebral osteomyelitis, 426
Vertical transmission, of HIV, 458
Very long chain acyl-CoA dehydrogenase (VLCAD) deficiency, 207, 207*f*
neonatal screening for, 198*t*
Very low birth weight (VLBW) infants, 219
Vesicle, 721*t*, 722*f*
Vesicoureteral reflux (VUR), 628–629
classification of, 629*f*
clinical manifestations of, 629
complications of, 629
diagnostic studies of, 629
etiology and epidemiology of, 628–629
treatment of, 629
Vesicular rash, infections with fever and, 373*t*–374*t*
Vesicular stomatitis, 439*t*–442*t*
Vesiculobullous eruptions, 734*t*
Vespid stings, allergic reactions to, 333
Vibratory murmur, 538*t*
Vibrio cholerae, diarrhea from, 410*t*
Vibrio parahaemolyticus, diarrhea from, 410*t*
Video-assisted thoracoscopic surgery (VATS), for pleural effusion, 532
Video endoscopy, for gastrointestinal symptoms, 467
Videofluoroscopic swallowing study, 520
Vinblastine, for cancer, 601*t*–602*t*
Vincent angina, 393
Vincristine, for cancer, 601*t*–602*t*
Violence, 3, 91–93
dating, 92
intimate partner, 91, 92*t*
prevention of, 23*t*–24*t*
technology and, 93
youth, 92
Viral conjunctivitis, 433*t*
Viral disease, zoonotic, 439*t*–442*t*
Viral gastroenteritis, vomiting due to, 473*t*
Viral hepatitis, 413–416
laboratory and imaging studies for, 500*t*
Viral infections
asthma and, 315*t*
bacterial infections *vs.*, 363*t*, 368–369
superficial, 381–383
from herpes simplex virus as, 381–382
from human papillomaviruses (warts), 382
molluscum contagiosum as, 383
Viral meningitis, 387*t*
Viral opportunistic infections, in immunocompromised person, 435
Viral paronychia, 382
Virilization, in the female, 672*t*
Virus-associated hemophagocytic syndrome, 573*t*
Visceral larva migrans, 450–451, 450*t*
Visceral pain, in appendicitis, 493
Visceral trauma, in newborn, 234
Vision impairment, in child, with special needs, 33–34
Vision screening, 20
of children 3 years of age and older, 20
of infants and toddlers, 20
Visual acuity, 683
Visual evoked response, 34
Vital capacity (VC), 507–508, 508*f*
Vital signs, of newborn, 227
Vitamin A, as teratogen, 237*t*
Vitamin A analog (tretinoin)
for acne, 723
for cancer, 601*t*–602*t*
Vitamin A deficiency, 114*t*, 117
Vitamin B_6 deficiency, 113–114, 114*t*

Vitamin B_{12} deficiency, 114*t*, 116–117
in anemia, 567*f*
Vitamin D, 669
as teratogen, 237*t*
Vitamin D deficiency, 114*t*, 118, 670*t*
nutritional, 670
Vitamin D_2, 118
Vitamin D_3, 118
Vitamin deficiencies, 113*t*
fat-soluble, 114*t*, 117–119
treatment of, 115*t*–116*t*
water-soluble, 112–117, 114*t*
Vitamin E deficiency, 114*t*, 117, 580
Vitamin K deficiency, 114*t*, 118–119, 588
coagulation disorders due to, 253
Vitamin K prophylaxis, for newborn, 222
Vitamin K_1, 118
Vitamin K_2, 118
VLBW (very low birth weight) infants, 219
VLCAD (very long chain acyl-CoA dehydrogenase) deficiency, 207, 207*f*
neonatal screening for, 198*t*
Vocal cord paralysis, 519
Vocal fremitus, 510*t*
Voice signs, 510*t*
Voiding cystourethrogram (VCUG), 620, 629
for urinary tract infection, 417
Voiding dysfunction, 631–632
Volume depletion, 129
Volume expansion, 125
Volume overload, 125
Volume status, regulation of, 125
Volvulus, 227*t*
gastrointestinal bleeding due to, 477*t*
midgut malrotation with, 487–488, 488*f*
Vomiting, 472–473
after traumatic brain injury, 710
cyclic, 472
differential diagnosis of, 472, 473*t*
distinguishing features of, 472–473
treatment of, 473
von Willebrand disease, 581–582, 586*t*, 587–588
clinical manifestations of, 587
etiology of, 587
laboratory testing in, 587
treatment of, 588
von Willebrand factor (VWF)
antigen, 587
containing concentrate, 588
in hemostasis, 580
VP-16, for cancer, 601*t*–602*t*
Vulnerable child syndrome, 91
Vulvovaginal candidiasis, 423*t*
Vulvovaginitis, 417–419
characteristics of, 418*t*
clinical manifestations of, 419
complications and prognosis of, 419
differential diagnosis for, 419
epidemiology of, 418
etiology of, 417–418
laboratory and imaging studies for, 419
prevention of, 419
treatment for, 419
VUR. *see* Vesicoureteral reflux
VWF. *see* von Willebrand factor
VZIG (Varicella-zoster immunoglobulin), 379
in immunocompromised person, 437

W

Waddling gait, 740
WAGR (Wilms tumor, aniridia, genitourinary anomalies, and mental retardation) syndrome, 182
Wandering atrial pacemaker, 542
Warfarin, for thrombosis, 589
Warts
common, 382
filiform, 382
genital, 382, 419, 425
clinical features of, 423*t*
plantar, 382
Wasp stings, allergic reactions to, 333
Water
in body composition, 125, 126*f*
plasma, 125
total body, 125, 126*f*
Water balance, sodium excretion and, 131
Water losses
hypernatremia from, 133
insensible, 126
Water-soluble vitamins, 112–117, 114*t*
Weakness, 692–700
clinical manifestations of, 693*t*
disorders causing, 693*t*
etiology of, 692–693
facial and bulbar, 694*t*
hypotonia without significant, 698–699
limb
distal, 694*t*
ophthalmoplegia and, 694*t*
due to lower motor neuron diseases, 694–698, 694*t*
Duchenne muscular dystrophy as, 696–697
infant botulism as, 696
muscle diseases as, 697–698
myasthenia gravis as, 696
myotonic dystrophy as, 697
peripheral neuropathy as, 695–696
spinal muscular atrophy as, 694–695
malignant hyperthermia, 698
in neonatal and infantile hypotonia, 698–699, 698*f*
proximal, 694*t*
due to spinal cord lesions, 694
due to stroke, 699–700, 699*t*
due to upper motor neuron diseases, 693–694
etiology and epidemiology of, 693–694
Weight
benchmarks for, 11, 11*t*
growth charts for, 12*f*
Well child, evaluation of, 19–25
anticipatory guidance in, 22–25, 23*t*–24*t*
dental care in, 22
fostering optimal development in, 22–25
immunizations in, 22
nutritional assessment in, 22
safety issues in, 22
screening tests in, 17, 20–22
for anemia, 20–21
for cholesterol, 21, 21*t*
for depression, 22
hearing and vision, 20
for lead, 21, 21*t*
newborn, 20
for sexually transmitted infection, 21–22
for tuberculosis, 21, 21*t*
topics for, 19, 19*t*
Wenckebach heart block, 543, 544*t*
Werdnig-Hoffmann disease, 694
Wernicke aphasia, 682
Wessel's rule of threes, in colic, 41
West African sleeping sickness, 439*t*–442*t*
West Nile virus, encephalitis from, 389
West syndrome, 690
Western black-legged tick, 443
Wet beriberi, 113
Wheal, 721*t*, 722*f*
Wheezing, 510
causes of, 520*t*
differential diagnosis of, 402
White reflex, in newborn, 230
White strawberry tongue, 393
Whitehead, 723
Whitlow, herpetic, 382
Whole blood, in transfusion, 589–590
Whole-bowel irrigation, for drug toxicity, 164
Whole exome sequencing, in genetic assessment, 179
Whooping cough, 400
Williams syndrome, 182
Wilms tumor, aniridia, genitourinary anomalies, and mental retardation (WAGR) syndrome, 182
Wilms tumors, 610–611, 614
bilateral, 611
clinical manifestations of, 610
differential diagnosis of, 611
etiology and epidemiology of, 610
laboratory/imaging studies in, 611
prognosis and complications of, 611
risk factors for, 597*t*
treatment of, 611
Wilson disease, 499–500, 711*t*–712*t*, 713
Window period, for hepatitis B virus, 414
Wireless capsule endoscopy, for gastrointestinal symptoms, 467, 468*f*
Wiskott-Aldrich syndrome, 298, 299*t*, 585
Wolman disease, 210*t*–212*t*
Wood smoke, asthma and, 315*t*
Wood tick, 444
Wound care, for burns, 159
Wrist, square window, in newborn, 229*f*

X

X chromosome, 171
X-linked adrenoleukodystrophy, 711*t*–712*t*, 713
X-linked agammaglobulinemia, 294
X-linked dominant inheritance, 173
G6PD deficiency due to, 174*t*
hemophilia A due to, 174*t*
incontinentia pigmenti due to, 173
Rett syndrome due to, 173
vitamin D-resistant rickets due to, 173
X-linked hyper-IgM syndrome, 296, 296*f*
X-linked lymphoproliferative disease, 386
X-linked lymphoproliferative syndrome, 298–299, 299*t*
X-linked recessive inheritance, 172
pedigree of, 174*f*
rules of, 174*t*
X-linked thrombocytopenia, isolated, 298
X-Prep (senna), for functional constipation, 51*t*
Xanthogranuloma, juvenile, 730*t*
Xerophthalmia, 117
Xerosis, 117

Y

Y chromosome, 171
Yale-Brown Obsessive-Compulsive Scale (Y-BOCS), 69
Yeast infections, superficial, 381*t*
Yellow jacket stings, allergic reactions to, 333
Yersinia enterocolitica, 439*t*–442*t*
diarrhea from, 410*t*, 411
Yersinia pestis, 439*t*–442*t*
Yersinia pseudotuberculosis, 439*t*–442*t*
Yersiniosis, 439*t*–442*t*
Youth violence, 92

Z

Zafirlukast, for asthma, 315
Zellweger syndrome, 208–209
Zidovudine, for HIV, 461
Zika virus, 447
congenital infection with, 264
Zileuton, for asthma, 315
Zinc deficiency, 119*t*, 120–121

Zinc deficiency dwarfism, 120–121
Zoonoses, 439–447
  anaplasmosis as, 445–446
  defined, 439
  ehrlichiosis as, 445–446
  Lyme disease as, 443–444
  Rocky Mountain spotted fever as, 444–445
Zoonoses *(Continued)*
  spread of, 439
  West Nile virus as, 446
Zoster, 378–379
  clinical manifestations of, 378
  complications and prognosis of, 379
  differential diagnosis of, 378–379
Zoster *(Continued)*
  epidemiology of, 378
  etiology of, 378
  laboratory and imaging studies for, 378
  prevention of, 379
  treatment of, 379
  vesiculobullous eruptions due to, 734*t*